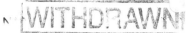

NORMAL CLINICAL PATHOLOGY DATA

Normal values of laboratory data vary widely, depending on the patient's sex, breed, and age, and on the laboratory. The values in these tables are approximations for use as guidelines only.

Routine Chemistry Results

Test	Units	Canine	Feline
Albumin	g/dL	3.0–4.2	2.3–3.5
ALP	U/L	1–145	1–80
ALT	U/L	5–65	19–91
Amylase	U/L	235–870	170–1250
Anion Gap		6–16	8–20
AST	U/L	10–56	9–53
Bilirubin, total	mg/dl	0.0–0.4	0.0–0.6
BUN	mg/dL	6–24	14–33
BUN/creatinine		5.1–34.1	6.1–31.7
Calcium	mg/dL	9.5–11.5	8.9–11.3
Chloride	mEq/L	108–121	117–128
Cholesterol	mg/dL	115–300	50–150
CK	U/L	55–309	55–382
CO_2	mEq/L	15–26	12–21
Creatinine	mg/dL	0.5–1.5	0.6–1.4
GGT	U/L	–	0.0–4.0
Glucose	mg/dL	80–125	50–150
Lipase	U/L	60–500	10–220
Mg^+	mg/dL	1.4–2.2	1.8–2.6
Osmol		282–303	299–319
Phosphorus	mg/dL	2.2–6.6	3.8–8.2
Potassium	mEq/L	3.6–5.6	3.9–6.3
SDH	U/L	–	–
Sodium	mEq/L	141–151	149–158
Total protein	g/dL	4.7–7.3	5.5–7.6
TG	mg/dL	20–85	0–105
Uric acid	mg/dL	0.0–0.9	0.2–0.8
Bile acid pre	μmol/L	0–5	0–3
Bile acid pos	μmol/L	<15	<10
Ammonia	μg/dL	19–120	100–300
D-Xylose	mg/dL	70–90	
Methemalb	mg/dL	0–5	
Free plasma hemoglobin	mg/dL	<10	<10
Protein/creatinine ratio			
Normal		<0.5	
Borderline		0.5–1.0	
Abnormal		>1.0	

Arterial Blood Gas Reference Range

pH		7.35–7.48	7.23–7.43
pCO_2	mm Hg	24–38	29–42
pO_2	mm Hg	85–100	78–100
HCO_3	mmol/L	17–25	15–22
Ionized calcium	mg/dL	4.93–5.65	4.93–5.65

Hematology

Test	Units	Canine	Feline
WBC	×10–3/μL	4.1–13.3	3.4–15.7
RBC	×10–6/μL	5.71–8.29	5.74–10.5
HGB	g/dL	13.5–19.9	8.8–16.0
HCT	%	38.5–56.7	26.1–46.7
MCV	fl	64–73	39.2–50.6
MCH	pg	21.8–26.0	12.9–17.7
MCHC	g/dL	33.6–36.6	31.5–36.5
RDW	%	12.5–16.5	15.6–21.2
TPP	g/dL	5.8–7.2	5.7–7.5
FIB	g/dL	0.2–0.4	0.15–0.3
PLT	/μL	160–425	160–489
MPV	fl	6.0–11.0	9.3–19.7
PCT	%	0.11–0.35	0.15–0.89
PDW	10 (GSD)	15.3–18.1	15.3–19.7
Reticulocytes	/μL	0–1.5	0–0.4
(punctate)	/μL	0	1.4–10.4

Differential	Percent		
Bands	%	0–1	0–1
Segments	%	51–84	34–84
Lymphocytes	%	8–38	7–60
Monocytes	%	1–9	0–5
Eosinophils	%	0–9	0–12
Basophils	%	0–1	0–2

Differential	Absolute		
Bands	×10–3	0–0.13	0–0.16
Segments	×10–3	2.1–11.2	1.2–13.2
Lymphocytes	×10–3	0.3–5.1	0.2–9.4
Monocytes	×10–3	0–1.2	0–0.8
Eosinophils	×10–3	0–1.2	0–1.9
Basophils	×10–3	0–0.13	0–0.3

Normal Values, Urinalysis

	DOG	CAT
Color	Light yellow	Light yellow
Turbidity	Clear	Clear
Specific gravity	1.015–1.045	1.015–1.060
Volume	24–40 ml /kg. / day	22–30 ml /kg. / day
Protein, ketones, glucose, hemoglobin, urobilinogen	Negative	Negative
Bilirubin	Negative–trace	Negative
pH	5.0–7.0	5.0–7.0

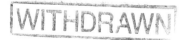

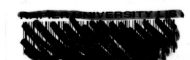

Kirk and Bistner's

••

Handbook of
**Veterinary Procedures
and Emergency Treatment**

Kirk and Bistner's

Handbook of
Veterinary Procedures
and Emergency Treatment

Seventh Edition

Stephen I. Bistner, B.S., D.V.M.

Diplomate, American College of Veterinary
  Ophthalmologists
Professor of Veterinary Medicine
School of Veterinary Medicine
University of Minnesota
St. Paul, Minnesota

Richard B. Ford, D.V.M., M.S.

Diplomate, American College of Veterinary
  Internal Medicine
Professor of Medicine
College of Veterinary Medicine
North Carolina State University
Raleigh, North Carolina

Mark R. Raffe, D.V.M., M.S.

Diplomate, American College of Veterinary
  Anesthesiologists and American College
  of Veterinary Emergency and Critical Care
Formerly Associate Professor, Division
  of Comparative Anesthesiology and
  Emergency Medicine
School of Veterinary Medicine
University of Minnesota
St. Paul, Minnesota

W.B. SAUNDERS COMPANY
A Harcourt Health Sciences Company
Philadelphia   London   Toronto   Montreal   Sydney   Tokyo

W.B. SAUNDERS COMPANY
A Harcourt Health Sciences Company

The Curtis Center
Independence Square West
Philadelphia, Pennsylvania 19106

Library of Congress Cataloging-in-Publication Data

Bistner, Stephen I.
Kirk and Bistner's handbook of veterinary procedures and emergency treatment / Stephen I. Bistner, Richard B. Ford, Mark R. Raffe.—7th ed.

p.   cm.

Rev. ed. of: Kirk and Bistner's handbook of veterinary procedures & emergency treatment. © 1995.

Includes bibliographical references and index.

ISBN 0–7216–7166–7

1. Veterinary medicine Handbooks, manuals, etc.   2. First aid for animals Handbooks, Manuals, etc.   I. Ford, Richard B., D.V.M.   II. Raffe, Mark R. III. Title.   IV. Title: Handbook of veterinary procedures and emergency treatment.

SF748.B57 2000   636.089—dc21

99–41999

Kirk and Bistner's Handbook of Veterinary Procedures and
Emergency Treatment   ISBN 0–7216–7166–7

Printed in the United States of America.

Last digit is the print number: 9   8   7   6   5   4   3   2   1

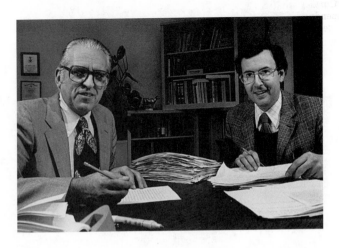

Dedication

The seventh edition of the *Handbook of Veterinary Procedures and Emergency Treatment* is dedicated to Dr. Robert Kirk. This edition of the *Handbook* marks the fourth decade in which we the authors, editors, and numerous contributors have attempted to serve veterinary medicine.

Bob Kirk is my (SIB) mentor and friend. When I was an intern and Dr. Kirk a faculty member at Cornell University in the 1960s, we conceived the concept of developing a practical, utility-centered handbook that could be used as a reference in companion animal medicine. The hallmark of a distinguished teacher is the ability to condense and edit material to make it understandable. Bob Kirk has a gift for doing this, as evidenced by his years as a Professor of Veterinary Medicine and as editor of *Current Veterinary Therapy* and *Small Animal Dermatology*, as well as by his years of continuing education lectures. When we first published the *Handbook* in 1969, we had great difficulty in deciding what was critical to the practicing veterinarian and entry-level student. With ensuing editions, this task became much more difficult and the critical core of information dramatically increased. Bob Kirk was able to help us maintain the structure of the *Handbook* through five editions. We are most appreciative of his friendship and ability as a teacher and author.

CONTRIBUTORS

Dennis Aron, D.V.M.
Department of Small Animal Medicine, College of Veterinary Medicine, University of Georgia, Athens, Georgia
Fractures and Musculoskeletal Trauma and Orthopedic Examination

Susan Bunch, D.V.M., Ph.D., Dipl. A.C.V.I.M.
North Carolina State University, College of Veterinary Medicine, Raleigh, North Carolina
Examination of the Gastrointestinal System

Teresa C. DeFrancesco, D.V.M., Dipl. A.C.V.I.M. (Cardiology)
North Carolina State University, College of Veterinary Medicine, Raleigh, North Carolina
Cardiac Emergencies, Hypertension, Electrocution, Examination of the Cardiovascular System

Stephen DiBartola, D.V.M., Dipl. A.C.V.I.M.
The Ohio State University, College of Veterinary Medicine, Columbus, Ohio
Urinary Emergencies and Fluid Therapy

Ava Firth, D.V.M., M.V.S., M.A.C.V.Sc., Dipl. A.C.V.E.C.C.
University of Minnesota, School of Veterinary Medicine, St. Paul, Minnesota
Poisonings

Elizabeth Hardie, D.V.M., Ph.D., Dipl. A.C.V.S.
North Carolina State University, College of Veterinary Medicine, Raleigh, North Carolina
Gastrointestinal Emergencies

Eleanor Hawkins, D.V.M., Dipl. A.C.V.I.M.
North Carolina State University, College of Veterinary Medicine, Raleigh, North Carolina
Respiratory Emergencies and Examination Respiratory System

Mike Henson, D.V.M.
Clinical Instructor, University of Minnesota School of Veterinary Medicine, St. Paul, Minnesota
Bleeding and Coagulation Emergencies

Mark Jackson, D.V.M., Ph.D.
Assistant Professor of Medicine, North Carolina State University, College of Veterinary Medicine, Raleigh, North Carolina
Basic Clinical Nutrition

Lynne Johnson, L.V.T.
Idexx Laboratories, Inc., Westbrook, Maine
*In Hospital Laboratory Clinical Pathology and Emergency
Monitoring Techniques*

Margaret V. Root Kustritz, D.V.M., Ph.D., Dipl. A.C.T.
Assistant Professor, University of Minnesota, School of
Veterinary Medicine, St. Paul, Minnesota
Emergencies of the Genital System

Jody Lulich, D.V.M., Ph.D., Dipl. A.C.V.I.M.
Associate Professor, University of Minnesota School of
Veterinary Medicine, St. Paul, Minnesota
Urinalysis

Carl A. Osborne, D.V.M., Ph.D., Dipl. A.C.V.I.M.
Professor, University of Minnesota School of Veterinary
Medicine, St. Paul, Minnesota
Urinalysis

Michael E. Peterson, D.V.M.
Clarkston, Washington
Envenomation–Snake Bites

Robert Rosenthal, D.V.M., Ph.D., Dipl. A.C.V.I.M., Dipl. A.C.V.R.
Veterinary Specialists of Rochester, Rochester, New York
Oncology–Basic Management Techniques

Steven F. Swaim, D.V.M., Ph.D.
Department of Small Animal Medicine and Surgery, School of
Veterinary Medicine, Auburn University, Auburn, Alabama
Burns and Soft Tissue Injury, Bandaging Techniques

Carrie Wood, D.V.M., Dipl. A.C.V.I.M. (Oncology)
Assistant Clinical Specialist, University of Minnesota, School of
Veterinary Medicine, St. Paul, Minnesota
Oncologic Emergency

PREFACE

It was just over 30 years ago that Drs. Kirk and Bistner edited the first edition of the *Handbook of Veterinary Procedures and Emergency Treatment*. Looking back at the original 1969 edition offers some striking insights into the many changes introduced into the profession over this relatively short period. It was a time when only four vaccines existed for dogs (distemper, hepatitis, leptospirosis, and rabies), when ether and phencyclidine [sic], a.k.a. "Angel Dust," were listed in the chart of "Common Drug Doses," and when a discussion of electrocardiography could be published, in its entirety, on page 143. Indeed, things have changed. Yet, in many respects, the first edition was remarkably advanced for its time. Topics ranging from the use of diagnostic radioisotopes and bronchoscopy to procedural techniques still applicable today highlight the fact that the *Handbook* has played a fundamental role in defining the standards of care in companion animal practice as we know it today.

Thirty years later, as the seventh edition of the *Handbook* goes to press, that philosophy remains unchanged. The objective of this edition remains very much the same as that outlined by the original edition: *to provide an efficient, highly practical resource fundamental in today's practice environment*. To that end, we are indebted to the nineteen contributing authors of this edition, whose experience and expertise in their respective specialties have so richly enhanced this text. The extensive revisions and updates incorporated into this edition are part of an ongoing effort to augment the continuing education demands facing our profession today.

In recognition of their resilience, tenacity, insight, and, most importantly, patience, we wish to extend our special thanks to the staff at the W.B. Saunders Company, who have again led us through the interminable maze of publishing a book . . . and we remain good friends.

It is also important to note that this edition marks a significant milestone in the history of the *Handbook*, with Dr. Stephen Bistner's retirement as the principal contributing editor. An author and editor for this and each of the previous six editions, Steve's contributions are deeply ingrained in the quality of this text and the value it brings to veterinary medicine. For your vision, your tireless efforts, and organizational skills . . . we thank you!

THE EDITORS

Prehospital Management
of the Injured Animal

Survey the Scene

1. CALL FOR HELP! It usually requires more than one person to assist at the accident scene.
2. If an injury has occurred in a traffic zone, alert oncoming traffic of the injured animal in the road. Do not become injured because traffic cannot identify you. Wave a piece of clothing or other object to alert oncoming traffic.
3. If the animal is conscious, prevent being injured while moving to a safe location. Use a belt or rope to make a muzzle to prevent injury. If this is not possible, cover the head and forelimb area with a coat, blanket, or drop cloth before moving.
4. If the animal is unconscious, or conscious but immobile, move to a safe location with a back support device that may be made from a board, box, door, blanket, or sheet.

Initial Examination

1. Is there a patent airway? If airway noises are present or the animal is stuporous, gently and carefully extend the head and neck. Extend the tongue if possible. Wipe mucus, blood, or vomitus from mouth. In unconscious animal maintain head and neck stability.
2. Look for signs of breathing. If no evidence of breathing or gum color is blue, begin mouth-to-mouth breathing. Encircle muzzle area with hands to pinch down on gums and blow into nose at 15 to 20 times per minute.
3. Cardiac function? Check pulse on inside of hindlimbs or over chest. If none is noted, begin steps for external cardiac massage.
4. Bleeding? Use a clean cloth (white preferred), towel, paper towel, or disposable diaper to cover the wound. Apply firm pressure to begin slowing blood loss. Place "counter pressure" over the femoral or brachial arteries to decrease blood flow. Use a rope or belt to make and apply a tourniquet. Use a tool or stick to turn the tourniquet tight enough. If abdominal swelling is noted, tightly bind the abdomen with a towel or elastic bandage.
5. Cover wounds. Keep wounds moist with a homemade saline solution of 1 teaspoon salt per quart of water. Use clean bandaging material as noted above. Penetrating wounds of the thorax and abdomen should be covered with wet pressure dressings as soon as possible.
6. Fractures? Immobilize fractures with a splint made from broom handles, sticks, or rolled up newspapers. Muzzle the awake animal prior to splintage. Use a single splint and tie limb above and below fracture site with bandages, belts, cord, or other tie material. If no splints are available, bind leg to other side (mountaineer's splint).
7. Skin protection. Apply cool compresses to burn areas including skin loss associated with pavement injuries. Remove and replace as the compress warms to body temperature.
8. Wrap to conserve heat. If the animal is shivering or in shock, wrap in a blanket, towel, or plastic garbage bag.

Preparation for Transport to an Emergency Facility

1. Call ahead! Let the facility know you are coming.
2. Line upholstery with plastic or sheeting to prevent spoilage.
3. Move injured animal carefully. Use the same approach as moving from the pavement.
4. DRIVE SAFELY! Don't turn one accident into two.

NOTICE

Veterinary Medicine is an ever-changing field. Standard safety precautions must be followed, but as new research and clinical experience broaden our knowledge, changes in treatment and drug therapy become necessary or appropriate. Readers are advised to check the product information currently provided by the manufacturer of each drug to be administered to verify the recommended dose, the method and duration of administration, and contraindications. It is the responsibility of the treating veterinarian, relying on experience and the knowledge of the animal, to determine dosages and the best treatment for the animal. Neither the publisher nor the editor assumes any responsibility for any injury and/or damage to animals or property.

THE PUBLISHER

CONTENTS

Section I

EMERGENCY CARE

INITIAL EMERGENCY EXAMINATION AND MANAGEMENT

Examination of the acutely injured animal that is unconscious, in shock, or suffering from acute hemorrhage or respiratory distress must proceed simultaneously with lifesaving treatment. Because there is no time for a detailed history taking, diagnosis is based on physical examination and simple diagnostic aids. The process of examination and the rapid classification of emergency cases by the urgency with which treatment is required is known as *triage*. For the following conditions, immediate recognition and prompt treatment are lifesaving.

............PRIMARY SURVEY OF THE EMERGENCY PATIENT

1. General examination.
    a. Visually inspect the animal. Note level of consciousness and behavior.
    b. Note body conformation and limb posture.
    c. Note respiratory rate, pattern, and effort.
    d. Note for presence of bleeding.
    e. Note external wounds and condition of wounds.
2. Examine the head and neck.
    a. Note bleeding from nose, ears, or oral cavity.
    b. Evaluate airway patency by listening for wheezing, stridor, or exaggerated breath sounds on auscultation. Check mucous membrane color.
    c. Palpate neck for integrity of airway. Check for tracheal location or displacement, subcutaneous emphysema, and other indications of cervical wounds.
3. Examine breathing status.
    a. Look for wounds over thorax and abdomen.
    b. Check symmetry and integrity of chest wall.
    c. Auscultate thorax to check for lung and heart sounds.
4. Examine the cardiovascular system.
    a. Palpate peripheral pulse for strength, rate, and regularity. Assess heart sounds, mucous membrane color, and capillary refill time.
5. Examine the musculoskeletal system.
    a. Note symmetry of spine.
    b. Palpate limbs and pelvis.
    c. Palpate abdomen and flank regions.

............EMERGENCY RESUSCITATION MEASURES

1. *Is the animal breathing?*
    a. Clear the air passage by rolling the patient's tongue forward, and remove any debris obstructing the passageway; suction may be necessary.
    b. Perform tracheal intubation or a tracheotomy as indicated to ensure airway patency.
    c. Cover any open wounds of the throat or chest, and perform thoracentesis or tube thoracostomy, if needed. Use a cover dressing with antibiotic or povidone-iodine ointment.
    d. Institute artificial respiration, if necessary.
    e. Administer oxygen, if necessary.
2. *If the animal is breathing, are respiratory patterns normal?*
    a. Is inspiratory distress present? It is characterized by extension of the head and neck; the commissures of the mouth are pulled back; the ribs

are extended and pulled out; the thoracic inlet and intercostal muscles are accentuated. Are there any obstructions in the posterior pharynx or larynx? Is there any evidence of laryngeal paralysis?

    b. Is there any evidence of expiratory distress? This is characterized by prolonged and forced expiration with accentuated abdominal lift, expiratory wheeze, and protrusion of the anus on expiration. Is the "bellows" (lung, pleural space, and diaphragm) working normally? If the bellows is not working properly, does the problem involve the upper airway or the lower airway, including the thoracic cavity and lungs? (see Respiratory Emergencies, p. 235).

3. *Is there a heartbeat?* If not, institute cardiopulmonary resuscitation (CPR) (see pp. 4–5).

4. *Is the heartbeat normal?* What is the heart rhythm and is it normal? Are there underlying cardiac arrhythmias? (see p. 61).

5. *Is the femoral pulse palpable?* (If it is, blood pressure must be at least 75 mm Hg.) Is the pulse full and bounding or weak and thready? If the pulse is weak and thready, consider shock therapy (see p. 32).

6. *What is the core body temperature?*

7. *Is there any evidence of external hemorrhage?*

    a. Control external hemorrhage with local counterpressure or regional compression using external wrapping with elastic bandage material over a sterile dressing pack. Pressure point occlusion of superficial arteries is used for wounds of wide area. If abdominal hemorrhage is suspected, place a cotton roll on the ventral abdomen prior to external wrapping.

    b. Establish a large-bore intravenous (IV) line (see p. 542). If this cannot be done owing to cardiovascular collapse, place an intraosseous needle (bone marrow needle) in the humeral tubercle, intratrochanteric fossa of the femur, or the tibial crest, and use for fluid and drug infusion.

    c. Administer resuscitation fluids. Use 4 mL/kg of a 7% sodium chloride and 10 mL/kg dextran 70 or hetastarch solution. Expand fluid compartment with 40 to 90 mL/kg of fluids such as lactated Ringer's solution. Infusion time is doubled for intraosseous needles. Administer whole blood, plasma, plasma expanders such as hetastarch and dextrans, or fluids in conjunction with other forms of treatment for shock (see p. 32).

    d. Acute body cavity bleeding into the thorax or abdomen will require emergency surgery to stop hemorrhage.

8. *Temporarily immobilize fractures.* Attempt to keep the animal in lateral recumbency. Place animals suspected of having spinal cord injuries on boards to be moved. Cover open wounds using pressure to control bleeding where necessary.

9. *Relieve pain by the use of analgesics.* In unstable patients, opioid-class analgesics are preferred.

10. *Perform an initial physical examination to assess the degree of injury.* Use the mnemonic, A CRASH PLAN, below to evaluate all areas of the animal.

⋯⋯⋯⋯⋯SECONDARY SURVEY OF THE INJURED PATIENT

Perform a physical examination using the mnemonic A CRASH PLAN.

    A—Airway. Perform careful visualization, palpation, and auscultation of the oral cavity, pharynx, and neck.

    C and *R*—Cardiovascular and Respiratory. Perform careful visualization, palpation, auscultation, and percussion of the chest *bilaterally*. Begin monitoring and recording of respiratory rate and depth.

    A—Abdomen. Examine the inguinal, caudal thoracic, and paralumbar re-

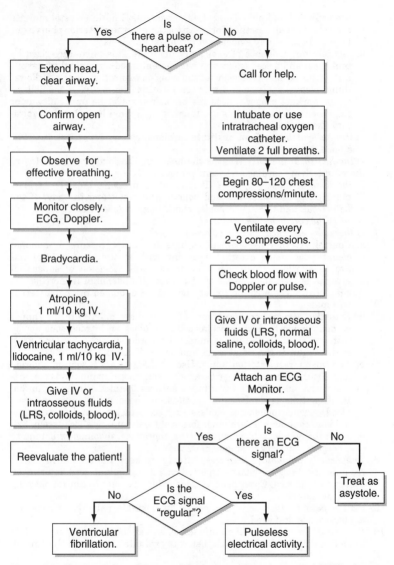

Figure 1–1. Basic cardiopulmonary life support. (See also p. 55.) ECG, electrocardiogram; IV, intravenous; LRS, lactated Ringer's solution.

gions. This examination includes visualization; clipping of hair for the detection of bruises and punctures; palpation; percussion; and auscultation for bowel sounds.

S—Spine. Perform neurologic examination from C1 to the last caudal vertebra.

H—Head. Examine eyes, ears, nose, mouth, teeth, and all cranial nerves.

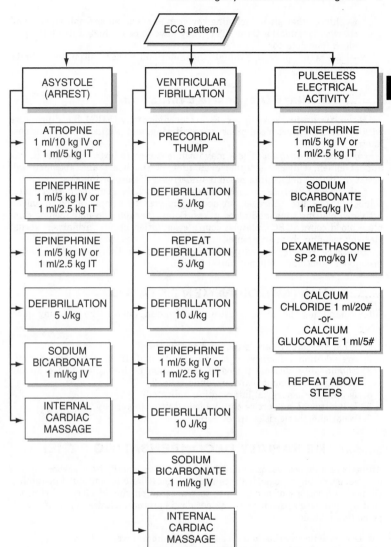

Figure 1–2. Advanced cardiopulmonary life support. (See also p. 60.) ECG, electrocardiogram; IV, intravenous; IT, intratracheal; SP, sodium phosphate.

P—Pelvis. Examine the perineum, perianal, and rectal areas. The external genitalia of the male and female are also included.
L—Limbs. Examine pectoral and pelvic extremities, evaluating muscles, skin, and tendons.
A—Arteries (peripheral). Palpate brachial and femoral pulses bilaterally.

Evaluate other sites, including the cranial tibial, superficial palmar, and coccygeal (caudal) arteries. They may have to be evaluated using Doppler blood flow detector.

N—Nerves (peripheral). Evaluate the motor and sensory output to the limbs and tail.

...........Ancillary Diagnostic Evaluation

Hemodynamic Techniques Electrocardiography (ECG), blood pressure with direct or indirect blood pressure monitoring, and perfusion with pulse oximetry.

Imaging Techniques These may include survey radiography of the thorax and abdomen. Ultrasonographic evaluation of the heart and abdomen will assist in further delineating possible underlying disease or injuries.

Laboratory Testing Immediate tests will include hematocrit (Hct), total solids, glucose, urea nitrogen, urine specific gravity, peripheral blood smear, activated clotting time, and blood gases. Delayed evaluation may include complete blood count (CBC), platelet count, coagulation profile, urinalysis, serum electrolytes, and chemistry panel.

Invasive Testing Invasive testing may include thoracentesis, abdominocentesis, and diagnostic peritoneal lavage.

...........SUMMARY OF PATIENT STATUS

After completing the initial physical examination, answer the following questions:

1. What supportive care is required at this time?
2. Are additional diagnostic procedures indicated? If so, which procedures?
3. Should an additional period of observation be instituted before further definitive treatment plans are undertaken?
4. Is immediate surgical intervention indicated?
5. Is additional supportive care indicated prior to surgery?
6. What anesthetic risks are evident?

...........THE RAPIDLY DECOMPENSATING PATIENT

Animals that do not respond to initial resuscitation usually have severe ongoing or preexisting physiologic disturbances that contribute to continued instability. Clinical indications of nonresponse to resuscitation should alert the clinician that a rapid decompensation of the patient is present. Clinical signs of decompensation include:

1. Decreased or markedly increased body temperature.
2. Poor peripheral vascular perfusion.
3. Poor renal output.
4. Confusion.
5. Depression.
6. Tachycardia.
7. Changing Hct values.
8. Distended and painful abdomen.
9. Cardiac arrhythmias.
10. Abnormal ventilatory patterns with signs of respiratory difficulty.
11. Indications of gastrointestinal blood loss via emesis or defecation.

The most frequently seen clinical problems associated with the decompensating patient are:

1. Internal hemorrhage (see p. 181).
2. Pneumothorax (see p. 242).
3. Coagulopathies—disseminated intravascular coagulation (DIC) (see pp. 44 and 46).
4. Bowel and gastric rupture (see p. 115).
5. Central nervous system (CNS) edema and hemorrhage (see p. 155).
6. Sepsis or septic shock—fever, pain, hypovolemia, abnormal patterns of ventilation, abnormal levels of consciousness, tachycardia, tachypnea, and lowered blood glucose levels (see p. 62).
7. Rupture of the urinary bladder (see p. 19).
8. Oliguria (see p. 122).
9. Acute renal failure (see p. 122).

REFERENCES

Betts CW, Crane SW: Manual of Small Animal Surgical Therapeutics. New York, Churchill Livingstone, 1986.
Crowe DT: Triage and trauma management. *In* Murtaugh RM, Kaplan P, eds: Veterinary Emergency and Critical Care Medicine. St Louis, Mosby–Year Book, 1992.
DeCamp M, Deming R: Post-traumatic multisystem organ failure. JAMA 260:530–534, 1988.
Haskins SC: Overview of emergencies in intensive care. *In* Sherding RG, ed: Medical Emergencies. New York, Churchill Livingstone, 1985.
Kirby R: Critical care: The overview. Vet Clin North Am Small Anim Pract 19:1007, 1989.
Kirby R: The critical trauma patient. *In* Proceedings of the American Animal Hospital Association, 1986, 106–115.
Matthews KA: Veterinary Emergency and Critical Care Manual. Guelph, Ont, Canada, Lifelearn, 1996.
Short CE, Irvin K, Gleed RD, et al: Trauma Management in Cats. Santaa Barbara, Calif, Veterinary Practice, 1985.
Wingfield WE: Veterinary Emergency Medicine Secrets. Philadelphia, Hanley & Belfus, 1997.
Wingfeld WE, Van Pelt D: Respiratory and cardiopulmonary arrest in dogs and cats: 265 cases (1986–1991). J Am Vet Med Assoc 200, 1992.

....

EMERGENCY TREATMENT OF SPECIFIC CONDITIONS

Management of Pain in the Trauma Patient

Rational management of pain requires an understanding of underlying mechanisms involved in pain and an appreciation of how analgesic agents interact to disrupt pain mechanisms. It is important to appreciate that pain is not a uniform syndrome; many aspects associated with pain origin, transmission, perception, and response must be understood.

...........DEFINITION OF PAIN

The definition of pain has been philosophically debated over the ages, and has changed as knowledge has increased. In its simplest form, *pain is a perception*. Until recognition of a noxious stimulus occurs in the cerebral cortex, no response or adaptation results.

...........EPIDEMIOLOGY OF PAIN

Multiple factors and causes produce pain in humans and domestic animal species. Generally, two major pain subclasses are acute and chronic pain, the terms being relative to the duration and intensity of clinical signs. Specific categories and causes of pain are listed below:

Acute Pain	Chronic Pain
Trauma	Arthritis
Thermal	Cancer
Postoperative	Neurologic–diabetes mellitus
Musculoskeletal	Musculoskeletal
Visceral/pleural	Sympathetic dystrophies

Understanding the origin and duration of pain symptoms is important so that appropriate therapy can be instituted on a rational basis.

............CLINICAL SIGNS OF PAIN

1. Inappetence or decreased activity.
2. Guarding or splinting of the affected area.
3. Licking, chewing, or scratching at a specific body site.
4. Restlessness; will not sleep or lie down, constantly pacing.
5. Vocalization.
6. Mydriasis; wide-eyed appearance.
7. Tachypnea.
8. Tachycardia.
9. Dysrhythmias—premature ventricular complexes (PVCs), premature atrial contractions (PACs).
10. Hyperglycemia.

............PHYSIOLOGIC IMPACT OF PAIN

Pain produces a physiologic response that is similar to other "stress" states. Pain response has been shown to be similar to stress triggers, including emotional, noxious impulses, temperature changes, shock, starvation, sepsis, and wound hormones. The pattern of neuroendocrine response to pain includes the following features:

Catabolism—characterized by increased adrenocorticotropic hormone (ACTH), cortisol, antidiuretic hormone (ADH), growth hormone (GH), cyclic adenosine monophosphate (cAMP), catecholamine, renin, angiotensin, aldosterone, and glucagon levels.
Metabolic—increased carbohydrate metabolism, protein catabolism, lipolysis.
Water and electrolyte flux—retention of water and sodium, decreased functional extracellular fluid (ECF).
Cardiorespiratory—increased cardiac output, vasoconstriction, hypoxemia, hyperventilation.
Psychologic—fear, anxiety, sleeplessness.

Pain relief will attenuate most of the changes noted above. Variable reduction in plasma cortisol, GH, ADH, β-endorphin, aldosterone, epinephrine, norepinephrine, renin, and aldosterone is noted based on anesthetic technique and drugs selected. Epidural anesthesia blunts the adrenal response to sympathetic efferents; the magnitude of neuroendocrine response is greatest with this technique. General anesthesia variably maintains the response to pain. Opiates variably inhibit these responses. It appears that the relationship between administration of analgesics and systemic response to pain is a central issue. Prophylactic administration of analgesics blunts response; analgesics administered following pain perception are not as effective; higher doses are generally necessary to achieve an equivalent level of analgesia.

..........METHODS TO REDUCE PAIN

> A spectrum of techniques have been reported to provide pain relief in acute pain states. The important issue is to differentiate *pathologic*, or *injury-associated pain*, from *physiologic*, or *normal protective pain*. Pathologic pain should be treated with techniques and agents to reduce ongoing pain stimuli; physiologic pain is protective and should be minimally inhibited.

..........NURSING CARE AND PHYSICAL SUPPORT

Providing clean, dry, warm housing and good basic nursing care will reduce pain levels. Adequate bedding and housing of appropriate type, attention to the physical and psychological needs of the animal, and minimizing disturbances to allow for rest are of great importance. Stabilization and support of injured areas by appropriate bandaging and splintage are important in reducing pain. Local application of cold (ice) or heat as indicated will also reduce pain.

..........Analgesic Drugs

..........When Are Analgesic Drugs Indicated?

The "art" of pain management is decision making regarding analgesic drug use. The simplest answer is treat if you believe that pain is a real possibility. New studies indicate better patient response and lower drug requirements if analgesics are administered *prior to pain recognition* (preemptive analgesia). Surgical procedures, including orthopedic, ocular, thoracic, and major abdominal surgeries, often require postoperative analgesics. Trauma or other insults that induce pain will also require therapy. Behavioral or species differences may dictate treatment. For example, certain breeds such as huskies, collies, or Afghan hounds appear more painful.

..........Peripheral-Acting Agents

Local anesthetic agents are the major class used as peripheral-acting analgesics. Their mechanism of action is to block transmission of pain impulses at nociceptors or peripheral nerves. They may be used to block specific nerves or to inhibit nerve "zones" by regional techniques. Although all local anesthetic agents are capable of providing pain relief, agents with long duration of action are preferred for management reasons. Bupivacaine and etidocaine are examples of long-acting local anesthetic drugs that are used for pain relief. A single dose of bupivicaine or etidocaine injected at the site of pain will provide analgesia for 6 to 10 hours. Addition of 1:200,000 epinephrine immediately prior to injection of the local anesthetic agent will increase the duration of action by 15% to 30%. Despite this additional duration, we do not routinely admix epinephrine with local anesthetic drugs unless it is felt that readministration is impractical for management reasons.

..........Systemic Analgesia

Opioids The opioids affect impulse processing and transmission at multiple levels of the spinal cord. Opioids interact with specific receptors to inhibit

Table 1–1. Analgesics Used in the Intensive Care Unit

Drug	Dose (mg/kg)	Route	Dose Interval (hr)*	Comments
Opioid agonist†				
Morphine	0.05–0.4 (dog)	IV	1–4	
	00.2–1.0 (dog)	IM, SC	2–6	
	0.05–0.2 (cat)	IM, SC	2–6	Observe cats for excitement
Oxymorphone	0.02–0.1 (dog)	IV		
	0.02–0.05 (cat)	IM, SC	2–4	
	0.05–0.02 (dog)	IM	2–6	
Meperidine	0.05–0.1 (cat)	IM		Do not administer bolus IV
	1.0–4.0 (dog)	IM	0.5–1.0	
Opioid agonist–antagonists				
Butorphanol	0.2–1.0 (dog)	IM, IV, SC	1–4	
	0.1–0.4 (cat)	IM, IV, SC	1–4	
Pentazocine	1.0–3.0 (dog)	IM, IV	0.5–3.0	Inconsistent effectiveness
Nalbuphine	0.5–1.5 (dog)	IM, IV	1–6	
Opioid partial agonist				
Buprenorphine	0.005–0.02 (dog)	IM, IV	4–12	Effects may be difficult to reverse
	0.005–0.01 (cat)			
Nonsteroidal anti-inflammatory agents				
Aspirin	10 (dog)	PO	12	GI hemorrhage
	10 (cat)	PO	48	
Phenylbutazone	20 (dog)	PO	24	Do not exceed 80 mg/day
Flunixin meglumine	0.5–1.0 (dog)	IV	24	GI hemorrhage and renal ischemia; avoid methoxyflurane

*For continuous IV infusion, administer the first dose as a bolus and immediately begin infusion administration of the same dose over the anticipated dose interval. The infusion rate should be increased or decreased to achieve and maintain the desired effect.

†For the first IV dose, start with a low dose and then repeat it every 5 to 10 minutes to effect. Once effective analgesia is achieved, plan on repeating the total dose at regular intervals.

From Hansen B: Analgesics in cardiac, surgical, and intensive care patients. In Kirk RW, ed: Current Veterinary Therapy XI. Small Animal Practice. Philadelphia, WB Saunders, 1992, p 84.

pain signal transmission from the dorsal root zone to higher centers. They may also act at neuronal transmission sites in the hind- and forebrain. The thalamus and cerebral cortex appear to have a high density of opioid receptors. In addition to modulating effects at the spinal cord level, activation of central receptors inhibits pain signal transmission to higher centers, thus blocking perception of the painful stimulus.

Traditional opioids represented by morphine, oxymorphone, meperidine, and fentanyl activate multiple receptor subclasses. Expected patient responses (species variable) may include one or more of the following characteristics: analgesia, bradycardia, respiratory depression, urine retention, reduced gastrointestinal (GI) motility, and histamine release (morphine, meperidine). The change in level of consciousness is variable by species. Depression may occur in dogs, primates, rats, and rabbits. Excitation may occur in cats. This behavior response is related to the receptor density and distribution in the brain areas associated with behavior. Specific members of this class and their actions are as follows:

Morphine The "gold standard" of analgesia, morphine is commonly used in dogs; use in other species produces variable response.

Advantages—Inexpensive, provides sedation and restraint plus analgesia, long-lasting (3 to 6 hours), can be given by many routes including intramuscular (IM), subcutaneous (SC), intravenous (IV), intra-articular, and epidural.

Disadvantages—A scheduled substance with record requirements due to potential human abuse potential, dose-related respiratory depression, vomiting, and histamine release following IV injection.

Oxymorphone A semisynthetic morphine analogue. Is used in dogs and cats for analgesia and preanesthesia. It can provide immediate pain relief if administered IV. It produces sedation, restraint, and analgesia in dogs; other species require tranquilizer coadministration.

Advantages—Provides sedation and restraint plus analgesia, medium duration of effect (2 to 4 hours), can be given by many routes including IV, IM, SC, intra-articular, and epidural. Does not produce significant cardiovascular effects.

Disadvantages—Relatively expensive. A scheduled substance with record requirements due to potential human abuse potential, dose-related respiratory depression following IV injection.

Meperidine A semisynthetic morphine analogue that has less potency than morphine.

Advantages—Inexpensive, provides sedation and restraint plus analgesia, short-acting (1 to 2 hours), can be given by many routes including IM, SC, intra-articular, and epidural.

Disadvantages—A scheduled substance with record requirements due to potential human abuse potential, dose-related cardiovascular and respiratory depression, hypotension, vomiting, histamine release following IV injection.

Fentanyl Synthetic morphine analogue.

Advantages—Rapid onset following IV administration, provides sedation and analgesia, short-lasting (0.5 to 1.0 hour), can be given by many routes including IM, SC, intra-articular, transdermal, and epidural.

Disadvantages—A scheduled substance with record requirements due to potential human abuse potential, dose-related respiratory depression, bradycardia following parenteral administration, short duration of activity, auditory sensitization.

Newer opioid agents represented by partial agonist and agonist-antagonist drugs selectively activate receptor subtypes. The response produced is based on the receptors activated. Opioid antagonists "antagonize" opioid effects at the receptor sites.

Butorphanol

Advantages—Can be used in many species. Can be given by all routes of administration. Provides mild sedation and restraint plus analgesia, short- to medium-acting (1 to 4 hours), can be given by many routes including IM, SC, intra-articular, and epidural. Some respiratory depression, but limited by receptor profile.

Disadvantages—Short duration of action; intermediate expense.

Buprenorphine A synthetic morphine analogue.

Advantages—Inexpensive, provides sedation and restraint plus analgesia, long-lasting (6 to 12 hours), can be given by many routes, including IV, IM, and SC.

Disadvantages—A scheduled substance with record requirements due to potential human abuse potential, dose-related respiratory depression, slow onset (30 to 60 minutes); some effects may not be reversed by naloxone.

Pentazocine Similar actions to butorphanol.

Advantages—Inexpensive, provides slight sedation and restraint plus analgesia, short-acting (1 to 3 hours), can be given by many routes, including IM, SC, IV, and oral (PO).

Disadvantages—A scheduled substance with record requirements due to potential human abuse potential, dose-related respiratory depression, inconsistent patient response.

Tranquilizer Agents These are useful in calming the agitated patient and are indicated in combination with narcotic class drugs for additional chemical restraint and analgesia. Benzodiazepine agents include diazepam or midazolam. Benzodiazepines are reported to provide mild analgesia based at the spinal cord in several species. Phenothiazine tranquilizers are not considered analgesic agents with sole administration. They may be used in conjunction with other classes of analgesic agents to reduce agitation associated with pain management. Phenothiazine tranquilizers will be chosen if a longer-acting response is desired. However, they should be administered cautiously because of their tendency to produce hypotension and prolonged tranquilization.

Neuroleptanalgesia Combining opioids and tranquilizers or α_2-agonists is useful in dysphoric patients emerging from anesthesia that require profound pain management. Potent analgesia is produced by combining these drug classes; in addition, the combination may prove useful for other reasons, including behavioral aggression, to provide analgesia without dysphoria in cats, and may be useful in sedating debilitated or acutely injured patients. A full agonist opioid with a phenothiazine tranquilizer may be coadministered to produce this response. Other options include an opioid plus benzodiazepine tranquilizer, or an opioid plus α_2-agonist in exceptional cases. Profound sedative response to the combination of acepromazine and butorphanol or buprenorphine and acepromazine may be noted. Side effects include significant bradycardia.

α_2-Agonists Agents that interact with the α_2-receptors produce analgesia. The mechanism of action is inhibition of pain impulse transmission in spinal cord, thalamic, and midbrain pain pathways. Xylazine and medetomidine are the primary agents of this class. Xylazine produces profound analgesia, sedation, and muscle relaxation following administration. Adverse effects include cardiac dysrhythmias noted as bradycardia and second-degree atrioventricular (AV) block, initial hypertension followed by hypotension, emesis, respiratory depression, and myocardial sensitization. Metdetomidine shares many of these properties. The actions of these agents are reversible through specific antagonists including yohimbine, atipamezole, and 4-aminopyridine.

Nonsteroidal anti-inflammatory agents (NSAIDs) These include two distinct subclasses: the cyclooxygenase inhibitors such as aspirin, phenylbutazone, dipyrone, naproxen, meclofenamine, and flunixin meglumine. Lipoxygenase inhibitors represented by ketoprofen and carprofen produce selective blockade of leukotriene generation. NSAIDs reduce pain by inhibiting the inflammatory response that sensitizes peripheral pain receptors. Their use may be primary or supplemental in pain management. They may be considered as primary therapy in management of soft tissue pain associated with trauma or surgery; they may need supplementation in other pain etiologies.

Glucocorticoids are not generally considered for pain management but, their widespread use in neurologic disease and injury to suppress pain associated with neural swelling and inflammation suggests that they are a powerful group of analgesic drugs. Glucocorticoids are also reported to have activity at the peripheral pain receptor level. Their mechanism of action is considered to be similar to NSAIDs.

Dissociatives The dissociative drugs ketamine and tiletamine are analgesic agents that have activity in the subcortical region. They provide analgesia by inhibiting cortical recognition of pain stimuli. This effect can be obtained at ultralow doses. Evidence exists that dissociative agents activate opioid receptors in the subcortex. These actions are not entirely understood at this time.

Sedative-Hypnotics These are not analgesic per se. High doses produce analgesia by inducing anesthesia. Low doses have an adjunct role in providing sedation and sleep in disoriented, agitated patients. By reducing excitement associated with pain, the sensitivity to pain stimulus is reduced. Paradoxically, this effect occurs in combination with analgesic agents of the opioid family. Low doses of sedative-hypnotics alone increase sensitivity to pain. Therefore, they should be used in conjunction with known analgesic drugs.

...........Routes of Analgesic Agent Administration

Wound Infiltration Local infiltration of anesthetic agents in a surgical wound has been shown to reduce pain in the immediate postsurgical period. Due to the pharmacokinetics of the local anesthetic agents, 0.5% bupivacaine is generally selected based on its long duration of action.

Brachial Plexus Block Forelimb analgesia may be provided with use of a brachial plexus block technique. Generally, long-acting local anesthetic agents such as bupivicaine are selected if long-term analgesia is desired. Because of the mixed nerve function in the brachial plexus, both sensory and motor block may be anticipated. All sensory and motor function is blocked from the midhumeral and distal level. Anatomical landmarks are the shoulder joint, the cranial lateral thoracic chest wall, and the external jugular vein as it enters the thoracic cavity. Following clipping and surgical preparation of the shoulder joint area, digital palpation will identify a depression on the medial aspect of the shoulder joint just lateral to the confluence of the external jugular vein, the deep and superficial pectoral muscles, and the shoulder joint. Insert a 22-gauge 3.0-in. spinal needle for dogs and a 22-gauge 1.5-in. spinal needle for cats at this point, keeping the needle shaft parallel to the spinal column, and aiming the needle shaft approximately 15 to 20 degrees outward from the central axis of the spinal column to follow the chest wall. Insert to a depth of 2 to 3 in. Attach a syringe with the local anesthetic agent and do a trial aspiration to confirm that the needle tip is not in the brachial vessels. If no blood is obvious, begin injection of 3 mL in cats, 5 mL in small dogs, and 10 mL in large dogs of the local agent selected. As the injection is performed, withdraw the needle evenly and slowly to place the local anesthetic agent in contact with the nerve roots of the brachial plexus. We usually use 2.0% lidocaine or 0.5% bupivacaine for the administered agent.

Sciatic Nerve Block Unilateral analgesia to the hindlimb can be achieved with a sciatic nerve block. The anatomical landmarks for this block are the greater trochanter of the femur and the ischial tuberosity of the pelvis. Identify the level that corresponds with the femoral neck, and palpate the depression at a point midway between these two landmarks. Insert a 22- or 25-gauge needle for approximately 0.5 to 1.0 in., depending on the size of the animal, and inject a local anesthetic agent. Either 2.0% lidocaine or 0.5% bupivacaine may be used. Both sensory and motor blockade to the caudal, lateral, and medial portions of the upper and lower limb, except in the vicinity of the saphenous nerve, will be achieved.

Intrapleural Injection Intrapleural injection of local anesthetic agents has been shown to be a simple, effective technique for pain management in postsurgical and post-trauma patients. The technique requires administration of 1.5 mg/kg of local anesthetic agent (we commonly use 0.5% bupivacaine) into the pleural space and positioning the patient with the injured side down or in dorsal recumbency to get the agent in contact with the segmental intercostal nerves. We allow a minimum of 10 minutes following administration to produce nerve blockade. Intrapleural block has also been shown to be effective in pain management of upper abdominal pain sites, including cholecystectomy, renal surgery, pancreatitis, and cancer of this anatomical region.

Intercostal Nerve Blocks Discrete intercostal nerve blocks can provide effective analgesia for traumatic or postsurgical pain. The area of injury is identified and three segments on either side of the injury site are desensitized. The technique of desensitization is as follows. Following clipping and surgical preparation of the dorsal third of the chest wall, the intercostal space is palpated as far dorsally as possible. A 25-gauge 0.625-in. needle is inserted to strike the caudolateral aspect of the rib rostral to the intercostal space. The needle is then redirected caudally until the needle tip just "drops" off the caudal edge. This places the needle tip in proximity to the neurovascular bundle containing the intercostal nerve that runs in a groove on the caudomedial surface. A trial aspiration confirms that the needle tip is not placed in the intercostal vessels. Approximately 0.5 to 1.0 mL of local anesthetic agent is injected at each site, depending on the size of the animal. We generally use 0.5% bupivicaine for this procedure because of the long duration of action.

Epidural Analgesia Pain management of the abdominal and pelvic areas can be managed by epidural analgesia. A variety of agents, including local anesthetic agents, opioids, and α_2-agonists, have been reported to be effective in regional pain management. The technique of epidural injection is well documented in standard veterinary texts on anesthesia, but can be summarized as follows. The patient may be positioned in either ventral or lateral recumbency. The rear limbs are drawn forward to expose the lumbosacral space. The hair over the lumbosacral area is clipped and the skin is surgically prepared. The craniodorsal aspect of the ilial wings is identified and an imaginary transverse line linking the ilial wings is drawn. Approximately 1.5 cm posterior to the imaginary line, the lumbosacral space is identified by palpating the dorsal spinous processes of the caudal lumbar and cranial sacral areas. A distinct V is felt in this location because the anatomy of the dorsal spinous process of the lumbar vertebra is pointed rostrally and the dorsal spinous process of the sacral vertebra is pointed caudally. A spinal needle of appropriate size for the patient (20- to 22-gauge, 1.5 to 3.0 in.) is inserted at the midpoint of the V and advanced approximately 20 degrees from perpendicular in a rostral direction. In many cases, a distinct "pop" is felt when the needle enters the epidural space. Paresthesia in the form of tail movement or discomfort may also be noted. If firm resistance is encountered, the needle is likely contacting the spinous process or dorsal arch of the vertebra. Redirecting the needle will identify and enter the epidural space. Some trial and error may be needed for this step. Following successful entrance, a trial injection of 1 mL of air is done. No resistance to injection should be encountered. The agents chosen to be injected are then administered by slow injection, periodically pressurizing the plunger and quickly releasing pressure (barbotage) until the full dose is administered. The advantage of the epidural technique is that selective analgesia is provided for a longer duration than parenteral administration, with fewer side effects owing to the lower dose requirement. A recently reported technique for thoracic pain managment is administration of opioids through the lumbosacral epidural space. For this procedure, a traditional approach to lumbosacral epidural injection is performed, but, an epidural catheter is placed and advanced to a level of the thoracolumbar junction. The level is determined by premeasurement of the spinal length. Following placement, morphine 0.15 mg/kg diluted in 5 to 6 mL of saline is injected. Satisfactory postoperative pain management for up to 24 hours following a single dose is reported for this technique.

Oral Administration Oral administration is generally considered with NSAIDs. Tranquilizer drugs may also be administered orally if an immediate response is not mandatory. Under unusual circumstances, rapidly absorbed drugs such as ketamine and butorphanol may be considered for oral administration. They penetrate the mucous membrane and are quickly systemically absorbed.

Parenteral Administration This is the preferred route of administration for most analgesics. Traditionally, IM injection is the most common route. It is convenient and ensures complete administration of the analgesic. Many studies in humans indicate that IM injection on a fixed time basis may be inadequate if the patient is not monitored. Periods of time may occur in which therapeutic levels of the analgesic are not present. The clinician should monitor the animal after the first two or three treatments to establish the appropriate time interval for dosing. This will vary with the individual case.

SC injection may be considered with rapidly absorbed drugs. Butorphanol and ketamine demonstrate rapid absorption and may be administered by this route. Dose interval times should be similar to the IM route of administration.

IV injection ensures full dose absorption and response. Duration of action may vary with IV administration. Usually, a shorter duration of action should be expected when compared with the IM or SC routes. Individual drugs are not recommended for IV administration. Morphine and meperidine have been shown to release histamine with IV injection. This, in concert with transient delirium noted with rapid IV administration of these drugs suggests that they not be administered by this route. Other agents have lower therapeutic doses with IV administration. Opioids, ketamine, and tranquilizers may have reduced dose requirements when administered IV.

Acute Abdomen

The term "acute abdomen" is borrowed from human medicine, where it refers to any serious, acute intra-abdominal condition attended by pain, tenderness, and muscular rigidity. Although it is strictly applied only to conditions associated with abdominal pain, many veterinary clinicians also use it loosely to refer to any animal with rapidly progressive life-threatening abdominal disease. The reason for lumping this collection of conditions is related to the decision-making process. These animals often have rapidly progressive disease, and a fast decision has to be made whether or not to perform an emergency celiotomy. Another term that is commonly used is "surgical abdomen." The clinician must decide if there is enough evidence for a surgically correctable condition to warrant recommending surgery. An incorrect decision, either way, can result in the patient's death; thus much effort is expended in trying to make a correct recommendation.

...........PENETRATING ABDOMINAL TRAUMA

There are two major points regarding penetrating trauma. First, the size of the external injury bears no relation to the extent of the internal injury. Second, it takes only one hole in the bowel or gallbladder to cause peritonitis and death. One rule on penetrating injuries is that if the instrument of destruction entered the abdomen, the abdomen should be explored immediately. The rationale for this approach is that the few negative exploratory surgeries that are performed will be balanced by the lives saved by not wasting time making decisions in cases that do have injuries. A more conservative approach would be to perform peritoneal lavage on all these animals and to base the decision to perform surgery on the results of the lavage.

............Exploratory Celiotomy

The abdomen, opened from the xiphoid to near the pubis on the ventral midline, should be explored in a systematic manner. If gross contamination and peritonitis exist, irrigation of the abdominal cavity with warm, sterile lactated Ringer's solution and water-soluble antibiotics such as crystalline penicillin or kanamycin is indicated. In cases of peritonitis, the abdominal wound should not be closed but should be packed open using sterile laparotomy sponges or wound pads followed by sterile dressings and cling wrap around the abdomen. The bandage will have to be changed, because drainage soaks through; however, as the peritonitis is brought under control, drainage will be reduced and the abdomen can be closed using nonabsorbable suture materials.

■ INDICATIONS FOR EXPLORATORY CELIOTOMY

Penetrating abdominal injury
Presence of bacteria on abdominal lavage with >2000/μL white blood cells (WBCs) in the lavage fluid
Presence of >500 μL WBCs in lavage effluent, especially if degenerative neutrophils are present
Presence of food or plant materials in abdominal lavage
Presence of creatinine in the lavage effluent that has a greater concentration than the serum creatinine
Presence of bilirubin in the peritoneal lavage effluent
Presence of air in the peritoneal cavity
Continued evidence of peritoneal irritation

............BLUNT ABDOMINAL TRAUMA

The chance of life-threatening abdominal injuries being caused by blunt injury is less than with penetrating injury. The usual "surgical" injuries are continuing significant hemorrhage, ruptured urinary tract, and hernias. Rarer injuries include rupture of the biliary or GI tract, and vascular compromise of the GI tract. Look for signs that abdominal trauma may have occurred (abdominal wall bruising, blood at the vaginal, preputial, or urethral orifice, pelvic fractures, caudal rib fractures, guarding of the abdomen, abdominal wall hernias, signs associated with diaphragmatic hernia). The workup is then the same as for "nontraumatic" acute abdomens (see below), except that the focus is on the trauma-related diseases.

............ACUTE ABDOMEN WITH NO KNOWN TRAUMA

I. History: Owners vary in their observations of their pets. The animal may be "not right," lethargic, restless, adopting a "praying" position, breathing shallowly to avoid moving the abdomen, trembling, or crying out. Other signs associated with abdominal disease include anorexia, vomiting or retching, diarrhea, dyschezia, dehydration, fever, dysuria or stranguria, shock, and collapse. The owner knows the animal better than the veterinarian and owners are usually correct in the assessment that things "aren't right."

II. Physical examination: Animals with abdominal pain may cry out when

touched in the abdominal region. They splint their abdominal musculature. Use the physical examination to (1) attempt to localize pain, if present, and (2) determine if physical findings suggestive of the cause of pain are present. Lumbar spinal pain and pain due to fractured ribs may appear to localize to the abdomen, but careful palpation should allow differentiation. Physical findings other than pain that suggest abdominal disease include increased or decreased borborygmus, gas- or liquid-filled bowel, masses in the abdomen, fluid in the abdomen, inability to palpate normal structures in the abdomen, and organomegaly. Even if no obvious signs of disease, including pain, are evident on physical examination, but the animal is clearly "not right," the abdomen is still often the site of disease. Many animals with acute abdomen are in shock at the time of presentation, or develop shock rapidly. Signs of shock include pale mucous membranes, rapid thready pulse, cold extremities, and slow capillary refill time.

III. Differential diagnosis.
    A. Usually treated surgically.
        1. Gastrointestinal.
            a. Gastric dilation–volvulus.
            b. Bleeding gastric ulcer.
            c. Perforated gastric ulcer.
            d. Gastric or intestinal obstruction.
            e. Intussusception.
            f. Linear foreign body.
            g. Intestinal rupture, perforation, ulcer.
            h. Intestinal volvulus.
            i. Vascular compromise of intestine in hernia.
            j. Cecal-colic intussusception.
            k. Cecal inversion.
            l. Colonic perforation or rupture.
        2. Liver, spleen, pancreas.
            a. Liver abscess.
            b. Rupture of liver mass.
            c. Necrotizing cholecystitis (severe infection of the gallbladder).
            d. Ruptured gallbladder, bile duct.
            e. Severe obstruction of the extrahepatic biliary tract.
            f. Splenic torsion.
            g. Ruptured splenic mass.
            h. Pancreatic abscess.
        3. Urogenital.
            a. Renal abscess.
            b. Ureteral obstruction or rupture.
            c. Bladder rupture.
            d. Urethral obstruction or rupture.
            e. Prostatic abscess.
            f. Pyometra.
            g. Testicular or uterine torsion.
        4. Other.
            a. Peritonitis.
            b. Neoplasia: infection, rupture, necrosis.
            c. Sublumbar, retroperitoneal, or abdominal wall abscess.
    B. Usually treated medically.
        1. Gastrointestinal.
            a. Gastroenteritis: bacterial, viral, toxic.
            b. Hemorrhagic gastroenteritis.
            c. Obstipation.
         2. Liver, spleen, pancreas.
            a. Acute hepatitis.

        b. Cholangiohepatitis.

        c. Pancreatitis.

    3. Urogenital.

        a. Acute nephritis.

        b. Pyelonephritis.

        c. Acute prostatitis.

    4. Referred pain from intervertebral disk.

IV. Diagnostic procedures: Follow a standard protocol. Use the CBC, serum biochemistry, and urinalysis to help figure out what systems are involved and if life-threatening infection is present. Other standard tests include abdominal radiography, abdominal ultrasound, abdominocentesis, and abdominal lavage.

  A. Abdominal radiographs are often the first test used to decide if surgery is needed. Findings that might indicate the need for surgery would be:

    1. Free gas in the abdomen, indicating leakage from the GI tract.

    2. Free peritoneal fluid, which is then sampled to determine the origin.

    3. Obvious enlargement or displacement of organs, as occurs with gastric dilation volvulus, pyometra, or splenic torsion.

    4. Intestinal obstructive pattern or obvious foreign body.

    5. Bunching of intestine, associated with linear foreign body.

    6. Loss of diaphragmatic detail, stomach axis rotated forward, as occurs with diaphragmatic hernia.

  B. Abdominal ultrasound may be used in place of abdominal radiographs in many instances, but remember that the accuracy of the technique is highly operator dependent. Some indications for surgery are:

    1. Hypoechoic areas suspected to be abscesses or hematomas.

    2. Free peritoneal fluid, which is then sampled to determine the origin.

    3. Obvious enlargement or displacement of organs.

    4. Loss of blood flow to an organ.

    5. Changes in the appearance of the GI tract such as bunching (linear foreign body), intussusception, obstruction, presence of a foreign body.

    6. Severe extrahepatic biliary obstruction, dilated bile duct, and enlarged gallbladder.

  C. Abdominocentesis and lavage are often regarded as the definitive tests as to whether or not surgery is needed. The animal is placed in dorsal or left lateral recumbency (spleen down). The bladder is emptied. Lidocaine is used to block the midline area just caudal to the umbilicus. The skin is clipped and surgically prepared. If a lot of abdominal fluid is present, a needle or IV catheter directed into the abdomen may be all that is needed for sampling. In many instances, a catheter with multiple holes (peritoneal lavage catheter) is needed to sample the fluid. This is a big catheter, with a stylet; it is aimed caudally and dorsally when being pushed through the body wall, to avoid lacerating organs. If fluid does not flow readily with the catheter, 22 mL/kg of warm isotonic lactated Ringer's solution is infused in the abdomen, the animal is gently rolled back and forth, and a sample of this fluid is obtained. Findings that would indicate a need for surgery would be:

    1. A creatinine that is higher in the fluid than the serum, indicating probable urine leakage.

    2. Green staining of the fluid, indicating bile leakage.

    3. Packed cell volume (PCV) in the fluid that is similar to the PCV in the blood, and an animal that is not stabilizing with resuscitation.

    4. Vegetable fibers in the fluid, indicating bowel leakage.

    5. Bacteria in the fluid, indicating the presence of infection.

6. WBC count greater than 2000/µL, or degenerate neutrophils greater than 500/µL, indicating that severe peritoneal irritation is present.
7. An amylase or lipase concentration that is higher in fluid than in serum indicates that pancreatitis is likely. This does not usually require surgery, but if abscesses are present, they should be drained.

D. A list of common diseases and the "key facts" for each disease.
1. Continuing significant hemorrhage—known or suspected history of trauma, lack of response to adequate volume replacement and abdominal wrapping, falling PCV, positive abdominal tap or lavage. If blood is available, try transfusion first. If there is no response to transfusion or the animal is deteriorating in spite of transfusion, operate.
2. Ruptured urinary tract—no palpable bladder or a grossly distended bladder, inability to pass a urinary catheter, fluid accumulation in the abdomen or groin, loss of abdominal detail or retroperitoneal "streaking" on abdominal radiographs, decreasing level of consciousness in a traumatized animal, increasing serum blood urea nitrogen (BUN) or creatinine valves, contrast radiography demonstrating a leak, abdominal aspiration or lavage with creatinine concentration higher than the serum creatinine concentration. This condition is not a surgical emergency. Stabilize the animal, correct electrolyte abnormalities, and drain urine using a peritoneal lavage catheter or temporary tube cystostomy. When the animal is stable, perform surgery.
3. Hernias—presence of defects in the abdominal wall, groin, or perineal region; palpate irreducible abdominal contents in the hernia. Large caudal abdominal wall hernias with extensive bruising and pelvic fractures indicate the "squashed" animal syndrome. Vascular damage and urinary tract trauma are common and a guarded prognosis is warranted. Operate following initial stabilization and chest radiograph. Strangulation or obstruction usually occurs with longstanding small hernias. Operate for GI obstruction as soon as possible, and for urinary obstruction after the animal is stable. Diaphragmatic hernias may cause "acute abdomen" signs if the stomach enters the chest or strangulation or obstruction occurs. Operate as soon as the diagnosis is made.
4. Ruptured biliary tract, biliary obstruction, necrotizing cholecystitis may cause vomiting, diarrhea, abdominal pain, fever, icterus, fluid in the abdomen; generalized haze, cholecystolithiasis, or emphysema of the gallbladder on abdominal radiographs; abdominocentesis demonstrates bile or peritonitis; a CBC and blood chemistry profile demonstrate severe infection, hypoproteinemia, hypoglycemia, increased alkaline phosphatase, hyperbilirubinemia, increased alanine transferase, disseminated intravascular coagulation (DIC); ultrasound demonstrates biliary rupture or severe obstruction. If the biliary tract is ruptured, the decision is to go to surgery. Drain the bile out of the abdomen, treat sepsis, shock, and DIC, and operate as soon as possible. Biliary obstruction and necrotizing cholecystitis also require surgery as soon as the diagnosis is made, but it may be much more difficult to make the diagnosis. If the evidence suggests that the biliary tract (not the pancreas or liver) is the problem, surgery should be pursued. Always pretreat animals with biliary obstruction with a shock dose of corticosteroids before surgery because massive endotoxin release occurs once biliary obstruction is removed.

5. A perforated or ruptured GI tract is associated with a linear foreign body, sharp foreign bodies, ulcers, corticosteroid therapy, NSAIDs, and penetrating trauma. Signs are hemorrhagic diarrhea or vomiting, pain, inappetence, and depression. Abdominocentesis or lavage is usually needed to determine if perforation has occurred. If it has, perform surgery immediately.

6. Vascular compromise of the GI tract is associated with strangulation or obstruction, volvulus, intussusception, and trauma (torn mesentery). Trauma-related compromise is hardest to diagnose because the animal may show no signs for 6 to 8 hours. Abdominal aspiration or lavage may be negative for the first 3 to 4 hours. Be suspicious if a traumatized animal continues to be depressed and shows any "abdominal" signs after initial resuscitation. Immediate surgery is called for if peritoneal lavages show evidence of peritonitis or the animal shows signs of sepsis or shock.

7. Gastric dilation–volvulus is seen in the large-breed or deep-chested dog. Signs are a history of unproductive retching, "full" or obviously dilated abdomen, shock, inability to pass a stomach tube, "double-bubble" gas pattern on right lateral abdominal radiograph. Immediate surgery is necessary.

8. Intestinal volvulus is seen in large-breed dogs. Signs are a history of GI disease or splenectomy, severe colic pain, depression, anorexia, vomiting, shock, and multiple gas-filled intestinal loops on palpation and radiographs. Immediate surgery is necessary.

9. Intussusception is seen in the young dog with a history of diarrhea, a postsurgical dog that had or has peritonitis. Signs are vomiting, diarrhea (may be bloody), inappetence, palpable mass in abdomen, GI obstruction on plain or contrast radiographs. This is not an immediate crisis, but schedule surgery as soon as possible.

10. Linear foreign bodies are seen in the cat or young dog. Look for a string under the tongue or coming out the anus, intestinal "bunching" on palpation or radiographs. Some veterinarians cut the string at the level of the tongue and monitor the animal closely, operating if the patient's status declines. Others prefer to operate as soon as the diagnosis is made because of the tendency for these foreign bodies to saw through the intestinal wall. The prognosis is poorer with dogs than with cats due to extensive bowel wall necrosis often accompanying the syndrome in dogs.

11. GI obstruction is seen in the young dog or indiscriminate eater (foreign bodies), and old cat or dog (tumor). Signs are vomiting, anorexia, palpable mass in abdomen, obstructive pattern on radiographs, with contrast demonstrating obstruction. Correct acid-base and electrolyte abnormalities, then operate.

12. Cecal inversion—diarrhea, tenesmus, occasional vomiting; diagnosis is made using contrast radiographs ("coiled spring" sign), ultrasound, or endoscopy. Condition of dog dictates the need for immediate surgery.

13. Gastroesophageal intussusception—young (<3 months), male dog (German shepherd), possible history of esophageal disease, vomiting, regurgitation, dyspnea, hematemesis, abdominal discomfort, rapid deterioration, dilated esophagus on radiographs. Diagnosis is made using endoscopy or contrast radiographs. Immediate surgery is called for.

14. Hepatic abscess. Animal may present with signs ranging from elevated liver enzyme values to fully developed peritonitis and shock. Hypoproteinemia, increased alkaline phosphatase, increased alanine transferase, and mass in liver on plain films, palpation, or

ultrasound. Immediate surgery is necessary if the animal shows signs of shock or is deteriorating.

15. Splenic torsion—vomiting, depression, anorexia, polyuria or polydipsia, in a young, large-breed dog with deep chest (German shepherd). Laboratory findings include target cells, polychromasia, anemia, hemoglobinemia, hemoglobinuria, and increased alkaline phosphatase. Splenomegaly and shock may be clinically noted. Most cases in the literature are operated on on the basis of splenomegaly or rapid decline in patient's condition. Ultrasound helps confirm the diagnosis (thrombosis, twisting of splenic vessels). Immediate surgery is called for.

16. Pyometra, fetal death—older intact female, young female given mismating shot, gravid female. Signs are depression, anorexia, polyuria or polydipsia, enlarged uterus on palpation and radiographs. Vaginal discharge may or may not be present. Blood workup reveals severe infection, hypoglycemia. Unless owners understand the risk and have a valid reason for pursuing medical management of pyometra, immediate surgery is called for. (See reproductive emergencies, pp. 128 and 132.)

17. Uterine or testicular torsion are rare causes of abdominal disease. Testicular torsion usually occurs in a cryptorchid male with a Sertoli cell tumor. Look for acute pain and abdominal mass caudal to kidney. Uterine torsion usually occurs at or near parturition, particularly if breeders give too much oxytocin. Animal usually presents in shock, unable to whelp and is operated on for that reason. Immediate surgery is necessary for both conditions.

18. Prostatic abscess is seen in the older intact male dog. Signs are abdominal prostate, urinary obstruction, hematuria, urinary tract infection, palpation of "two bladders" or mass. May see pain, depression, or outright shock. Contrast urography and ultrasound will give a diagnosis of "cyst or abscess." An aspirate will tell you which it is, but it is risky. Operate based on the condition of the dog, recognizing that ruptured abscesses are an emergency. (See Urogenital Emergencies.)

19. Renal abscess—rare, associated with pyelonephritis, causes peritonitis, acute pain, often ruptures before diagnosis is made. Contrast urography and ultrasound help to localize disease to the kidney. Operate as soon as the animal is stable.

20. Ruptured intra-abdominal neoplasia. The most common is hemangiosarcoma of the spleen or liver (older German shepherd, weakness and collapse, hemoabdomen, falling PCV), but it can happen with any tumor that has a necrotic center. Usually these are older animals with palpable masses that are presented for acute depression, collapse, and shock. Abdominal aspiration or lavage reveals blood or peritonitis. Stabilize shock (transfusion) and operate immediately.

21. Peritonitis. Very painful in humans, but animals usually are presented with anorexia and depression. May be associated with ruptured GI tract, abscessed organs, penetrating wounds; occasionally no source is found. Hazy abdominal radiographs (ground-glass appearance), fluid in abdomen, severe infection on CBC, increased cells on abdominal aspiration or lavage (see p. 18.) Animals with traumatic bile peritonitis may be asymptomatic for several weeks after the injury. Most animals are presented with symptoms of lethargy, anorexia, vomiting, diarrhea, and possible abdominal pain.

   a. Treatment goals in peritonitis:

      i. Treat the cause of the contamination, which may require exploratory celiotomy. Usually indicated when the cause of the peritonitis cannot be determined or when bowel rupture, intestinal obstruction, or mesenteric tears are suspected. Penetrating abdominal injury always requires exploratory celiotomy.

      ii. Resolve the infection with broad-spectrum antibiotic therapy—ampicillin plus enrofloxacin; also possible is amikacin sulfate plus clindamycin or amikacin sulfate and metronidazole. A third-generation cephalosporin (cefotaxime sodium) can be used in gram-negative infections.

      iii. Control fluid and electrolytes; correct potassium (see pp. 588 and 600) and check blood glucose levels and correct if needed.

      iv. Treat for DIC and shock if needed (see p. 32). Administer antiprostaglandins such as flunixin meglumine.

22. Sublumbar or retroperitoneal abscess. Spay granuloma, outdoor dog (awns, hunting injuries, stick injuries), indiscriminate eater (perforating foreign body). Pain, signs of infection, sublumbar "streaking" or mass on radiographs, may have fistulous tract draining in lumbar region. Usually can operate as an elective procedure.

23. Gastroenteritis, pancreatitis, nephritis, acute liver failure, hepatitis, and acute prostatitis are treated medically. The two diseases that most commonly lead to "negative exploratories" are severe enteritis and pancreatitis. Enteritis is confusing because in severe cases numerous dilated bowel loops may be seen, pain is severe, and patient status may deteriorate quickly. Several points may help distinguish this condition: leukopenia (indicating a viral disease), severe vomiting and diarrhea (usually worse with enteritis than surgical diseases), history of other animals affected, history of garbage or toxin ingestion, no masses palpated as causes of GI obstruction, wrong breed for intestinal volvulus. Pancreatitis causes confusion because the biochemical markers used to diagnose pancreatitis are not always reliable. Many clinicians rely on signalment, radiographs, ultrasound, and excluding other diseases when amylase and lipase valves are not diagnostic.

............THERAPY

Therapy is disease-specific, but many patients need treatment for shock and sepsis. Current therapeutic recommendations include: give appropriate antibiotics, provide cardiovascular support, increase tissue oxygenation, remove the focus of infection, and manage organ failure. Appropriate antibiotics provide four-quadrant coverage. An example would be a combination of enrofloxacin (5 to 10 mg/kg IV b.i.d. and ampicillin-sulbactam 22 mg/kg IV q6h). Cardiovascular support is provided by aggressive use of colloids and crystalloids. Animals with peritonitis often have *very* high fluid needs. Early use of plasma to maintain plasma proteins improves survival. Tissue oxygenation is maintained by providing nasal oxygen supplementation, keeping the PCV above 20%, and providing respiratory support if failure occurs. The focus of infection is removed using surgical debridement or drainage, or both. Organ failure is managed by providing appropriate medical therapy for the failing organ.

REFERENCES

Davenport DJ, Martin RA: Acute Abdomen. *In* Murtaugh RJ, Kaplan PM, eds: Veterinary Emergency and Critical Care Medicine. St Louis, Mosby–Year Book, 1992, pp 153–162.
Fossum T: Small Animal Surgery. St Louis, Mosby–Year Book, 1997.

Gennari R, Alexander JW: Effects of hyperoxia on bacterial translocation and mortality during gut-derived sepsis. Arch Surg 131:57–62, 1996.

Hardie EM: Life threatening bacterial infection. *In* Emergency Medicine in Small Animal Practice. Trenton, NJ, Veterinary Learning Systems, 1997, pp 290–302.

Kirby R: Synthetic colloids. *In* Proceedings of the Fifth International Veterinary Emergency and Critical Care Symposium, San Antonio, 1996, p 884.

King LG: Postoperative complications and prognostic indicators in dogs and cats with septic peritonitis: 23 cases (1989–1992). J Am Vet Med Assoc 204:407–414, 1994.

Mann FA: Evaluation and emergency treatment. *In* Bonagura J, ed: Kirk's Current Veterinary Therapy 13. Philadelphia, WB Saunders, 2000.

Allergic Reactions

Allergic reactions that require emergency care may be divided into two main categories: anaphylactic shock and angioneurotic edema (urticaria).

............ANAPHYLACTIC (ANAPHYLACTOID) SHOCK

This is an immediate type of hypersensitivity reaction in which death may occur rapidly owing to respiratory and circulatory collapse. In animals, anaphylactic shock rarely develops without the interference of man. An exception is the condition that results from the stings of bees or wasps.

The main signs are attributable to the effect of the activation of the complement system (especially C_5a) with intensive vascular dilation of smooth muscle. The release of additional chemical mediators—histamine, slow-reacting substance (SRS), serotonin, heparin, acetylcholine, and bradykinin—increases the severity of the problem. In the dog the splanchnic viscera and liver are the major organs involved in anaphylaxis. In dogs, the most common signs are restlessness; diarrhea, which may be bloody; vomiting; circulatory collapse; epileptiform seizures; coma; and death.

In cats the respiratory system is the predominant system involved in anaphylaxis. Signs may include pruritus, ptyalism, vomiting, incoordination, bronchoconstriction, pulmonary hemorrhage, laryngeal edema, collapse, and death.

Agents that may cause anaphylaxis are penicillin, streptomycin, tetracyclines, chloramphenicol, erythromycin, vancomycin, foreign sera (antitoxins), adrenocorticotropic hormone (ACTH), insulin, oxytocin, vaccines, penicillinase, procaine, benzocaine, tetracaine, lidocaine, salicylates, antihistamines, tranquilizers, iodinated contrast media, vitamins, heparin, stinging insects, food, and allergens (hypersensitization and skin testing).

............Treatment

In severe cases, immediately administer an IV injection of 1:1000 epinephrine hydrochloride (Adrenalin), 0.01 mL/kg. If indicated, repeat in 20 to 30 minutes. Infiltrate SC the entrance site of the allergen (insect bites) with 1:100,000 epinephrine 0.3 mL.

1. Ensure a clear air passage, and administer oxygen by endotracheal tube or face mask if necessary.
2. Establish an IV line, and begin lactated Ringer's saline solution dextrose 5% in water (D5W).
3. If the reaction is mild to moderate, give 0.2 to 0.5 mL of epinephrine SC and another 0.2 to 0.5 mL by deep SC injection elsewhere. One 0.5-mL dose may be repeated in 20 minutes if manifestations of anaphylaxis have not subsided.
4. Administer an IV injection of a rapidly acting steroid, such as hydrocortisone sodium succinate (Solu-Cortef) 100 to 500 mg; prednisolone sodium succinate (Solu-Delta-Cortef) 100 to 500 mg; or dexamethasone phosphate 4 mg/kg. Repeat the injection in 3 to 4 hours if necessary.

5. Give an IV injection of an antihistamine such as diphenhydramine hydrochloride (Benadryl) 1.0 to 2.0 mg/kg slowly.
6. Hospitalize and observe the patient closely following the aforementioned procedures. If recovery occurs within 5 to 10 minutes following this intensive treatment, the prognosis is good.
7. In dogs with atopy, avoid the use of potential sensitizing drugs.

REFERENCES

Cohen R: Systemic anaphylaxis. *In* Bonagura J: Current Veterinary Therapy XII. Small Animal Practice. Philadelphia, WB Saunders, 1995, p 150.
Cowell AK, Cowell R, Tyler R, et al: Severe systemic reactions to Hymenoptera stings in three dogs. J Am Vet Med Assoc 198:1014–1016, 1991.

·········· ANGIONEUROTIC EDEMA (URTICARIA)

Angioneurotic edema, or urticaria, is characterized by swelling of the soft tissues of the head, especially around the eyes, mouth, and ears. An ocular discharge may develop, and the animal frequently rubs its mouth and eyes on the ground or with its paws. This type of allergic reaction may develop within 20 minutes after contact with the inciting allergen and is very alarming to the owner, although it seldom causes serious damage to the animal.

·········· Etiology

Food allergies, ingestion of spoiled protein material, blood transfusions, plasma transfusions, insect bites, and contact with certain chemicals are the primary causes.

·········· Treatment

1. Try to ascertain the cause, and remove the irritating substance if possible (laxatives and high colonic enemas are indicated in food allergies). Stop blood or plasma transfusions. Wash the animal free of any known chemical residues. Pretreatment with antihistamines is a good idea prior to the administration of blood or plasma transfusions.
2. Administer high doses of rapidly acting steroids and antihistamines (see Anaphylactic Shock). Administer epinephrine only if angioneurotic edema is very severe, i.e., if swelling interferes with normal respirations.

Burns

The subject of burn management is extensive. For more in-depth information than is presented here, please see the references. This section will deal with the assessment and initial therapy of the burned animal. The reader should see other texts for information on reconstructive surgery.

Fortunately, veterinarians do not encounter burned animals often even though the sources of burns in small animals are many (Table 1–2). Burns fall into the general categories of thermal, electrical, chemical, and radiation burns.

·········· THERMAL BURNS

I. Burn depth.
    A. Superficial partial-thickness burns.
        1. Epidermis involved.

Table 1–2. Causes

	Thermal Burns

Fires	Hot semiliquids (e.g., tar)
Hot hair dryers	Heat lamps
Stoves	Improperly grounded electrosurgical units
Electric heating pads*	Solar exposure
Boiling water	Heat packs
Steam	Underside of automobile motors and exhaust
Hot cooking oil	systems

Electrical Burns

Low-voltage household alternating current (chewing on electrical cords).

Chemical Burns

Oxidizing agents	Protoplasmic poisons
Reducing agents	Desiccants
Corrosives	Vesicants

Radiation Injury

Radiation therapy for neoplastic conditions.

---

*Many animals are burned after they have been placed on electric heating pads during or after surgery. The result is often massive skin loss on the dorsum or side of the animal. Circulating-water pads are much safer than electric heating pads and should be used in veterinary practice.

    2. Epidermis thickened, erythematous, then desquamates.
    3. Heals in 3 to 6 days.
    4. Usually has hair regrowth.
  B. Deep partial-thickness burns.
    1. Epidermis and varying amounts of dermis involved.
    2. Subcutaneous edema and marked inflammation.
    3. Heal by reepithelialization from deep adnexal remnants and wound edge.
    4. Rate of healing and hair regrowth is dependent on burn depths.
  C. Full-thickness burns.
    1. Entire skin thickness destroyed—eschar.
    2. Superficial subcutaneous vessels—thrombosed, deeper vessels—permeable causing subcutaneous edema, and gangrene of damaged tissue.
    3. Heal slowly by contraction and reepithelialization if not reconstructed.
II. Animal assessment and examination.
  A. Assessment for thermal shock and respiratory thermal injury.
  B. Examine eyes, ears, oral cavity, respiratory tract, urogenital tract, anus, paw pads.
  C. Assess burn depth and percent of total body surface area involvement.
  D. Decision is made as to whether:
    1. Thermal injury is minor and local therapy is needed.
    2. Local wound and systemic therapy is indicated.
    3. Burn is severe enough to warrant euthanasia.
III. Course of action criteria.
  A. Minimal supportive therapy and local wound therapy are indicated for partial-thickness burns involving less than 15% of total body surface area.

B. Emergency supportive therapy, extensive wound therapy, and reconstructive surgery are indicated for deep partial-thickness burns involving more than 15% of total body surface area.

■ PERCENT BURN ESTIMATION (RULE OF NINES)

Body Region	Percent of Body Surface Area
Head	9%
Torso	18%
Forelimb (per limb)	9%
Hindlimb (per limb)	18%

C. Euthanasia is indicated for or when:
  1. Full-thickness burns cover more than 30% to 50% of total body surface area.
  2. There are severe burns of the face and external genitalia.
  3. Reasonable return of function cannot be expected.
IV. Treatment.
  A. Neuroleptanalgesia—relieve pain and sedate (see p. 7).
  B. Catheters—jugular vein (central venous pressure), cephalic vein (fluid administration), urinary bladder (urine output monitor).
  C. Monitoring.
    1. Hct, serum protein, hemoglobin, sodium, potassium, and chloride.
    2. Albumin, BUN, creatine, blood glucose, blood gases.
    3. Vital signs, mental status, body weight, urine output.
  D. Respiratory tract evaluation and therapy.
    1. Evaluation.
      a. Facial burns, reddened oral and pharyngeal mucosa, coughing, singed vibrissae, bronchorrhea, and sooty sputum.
      b. Elevated carboxyhemoglobin.
      c. Radiography—pulmonary edema, atelectasis, and pneumonia.
      d. Bronchoscopy—edema, inflammation, necrosis, soot, and charred airways.
    2. Therapy.
      a. Tracheostomy in the presence of upper airway swelling, and severe tracheobronchial secretions.
      b. Humidified oxygen—100%.
      c. Suction of tracheal secretions every 1 to 2 hours.
      d. Antibiotics are given based on airway cultures.
      e. Expectorants and aerosolized bronchodilators.
  E. Early wound evaluation and therapy.
    1. Evaluation.
      a. With hair remaining (e.g., heating pad burn) on a deep burn the hair is easily epilated. Clip the hair.
      b. Superficial partial-thickness burn—hyperemia and may have a thin crust.
      c. Deep partial-thickness and full-thickness burns are hard to assess until eschar separates (7 to 10 days after burn), but partial-thickness burns may be painful while full-thickness burns may be anesthetic.
    2. Therapy.
      a. Application of chilled saline or water (3° to 17°C) by compress or immersion for 30 minutes early following burn. Take care not to cause hypothermia.

b. For hot tar removal apply:
   i. Polyoxyethylene sorbitan (Tween 80).
   or
   ii. Polysorbate and polyoxyethylene sorbitan (surfactant agent in antibiotic ointments).
   or
   iii. Butter in an almost liquid state on a gauze.
c. To prevent burn progression, apply an aloe vera cream (Dermaide Aloe Cream, Dermaide Research Corp.).
F. Fluid and electrolyte therapy.

Basic information on animal burn treatment is presented; however, variations and complications requiring special attention may occur with individual animals. Normal maintenance fluid levels should be considered when administering fluids.

1. First 24 hours.
   a. Four mL/kg of lactated Ringer's solution × percentage of total body surface area burned.
      i. First 8 hours—one half the amount given.
      ii. Second 8 hours—one fourth the amount given.
      iii. Third 8 hours—one fourth the amount given. (Urine production should be kept above 1 mL/kg/hr. However, during the first 24 hours fluid input exceeds urine output by a factor of 3 to 4.)
   b. During the third 8 hours, if urine output is below 1 mg/kg/hr, colloid, plasma, or 5% albumin can be given.
2. Second 24 hours—less lactated Ringer's solution.
   a. D5W at 1 to 2 mL/kg × percentage of burn area *and if needed*:
   b. Colloid or plasma at 0.3 to 0.5 mL/kg × percentage of burn area *or* 0.5% albumin at 1 g/kg/day. (Forty-eight hours after the burn, less IV fluid support is needed if the animal has begun to eat and drink. However, evaporative fluid loss must be considered.)
   c. Adjust fluids to maintain serum levels in at least the low-normal range.
      i. Serum protein 3.5 to 6.5 g/dL.
      ii. Hct 25%.
   d. If anemia develops (usually at 2 to 5 days) give whole blood.
3. Monitor and adjust potassium—the ideal range is 3.5 to 4.5 mEq/L.
   a. First 48 hours after extensive burn:
      i. There may be minimal to moderate potassium elevation. Lactated Ringer's solution (4 to 5 mEq/L potassium content) is the fluid indicated.
      ii. There may be more severe hyperkalemia (>8 mEq/L). Physiologic saline solution is the fluid indicated, and monitor electrocardiogram.
   b. After 48 hours and return of renal function:
      i. There may be increased renal potassium excretion and sodium retention, which could be life-threatening at 3 to 5 days. Potassium supplementation of 15 to 20 mEq/L added to lactated Ringer's solution is indicated.
      ii. There may be severe hypokalemia—potassium below 2.5 mEq/L. Potassium supplementation at 80 mEq/L added to lactated Ringer's solution is indicated.
      or
      iii. Use a commercially available replacement and maintenance fluids used for shock therapy—4 to 5 mEq/L and 15 to 35 mEq/L, respectively. Use them alternately in equal quantities.

4. Monitor and adjust sodium.
   a. Unreplaced evaporative water loss may result in hypernatremia (sodium 145 mEq/L and chloride 110 mEq/L). With an accompanying rise in BUN and serum and urine osmolalities, D5W or hypotonic fluids are indicated.
   b. Consumption of large water quantities before fluid therapy starts may result in hyponatremia (sodium <130 mEq/L and chloride <80 mEq/L).
      i. Limit water intake and give sodium supplementation with 3% to 5% solutions slowly over 6 to 12 hours.
5. Avoid overhydration.
   a. Watch for:
      i. Urine output approaching the fluid administration level.
      ii. Auscultation of pulmonary rales.
      iii. Radiographic signs of pulmonary edema.
      iv. Decreased urine specific gravity.
      v. Elevated serum sodium levels.
   b. Treatment.
      i. Reduce volume of fluids.
      ii. Administer diuretics.
      iii. Monitor serum electrolytes.
6. Monitor and treat acidosis.
   a. Monitoring.
      i. Monitor blood gases. Watch for decrease in pH of blood (7.35) and urine (5.5).
   b. Treatment.
      i. Improve tissue perfusion.
      ii. Improve oxygen saturation.
      iii. Careful use of sodium bicarbonate.
G. Later wound therapy.
1. Superficial and deep-partial thickness burns.
   a. Warm water or isotonic solution immersion or lavage. Between immersions or lavage, bandage with a water-soluble medication (silver sulfadiazine [Silvadene cream, Hoechst-Marion Roussel, Kansas City]).
      or
   b. Wet-to-wet bandages left in place for several hours.
   c. At bandage changes debride necrotic tissue.
   d. For large areas of burn causing difficult bandaging, apply medication and place animal in a stainless steel cage with no bedding.
   e. Other topical antimicrobials for smaller burns.
      i. Gentamicin sulfate (Garamycin ointment, Schering Corp., Liberty Corner, NY).
      ii. Povidone-iodine (Betadine ointment, Akorn, Inc., Abita Springs, LA).
      iii. Nitrofurazone (Clay-Park Labs, Bronx, NY).
   f. Systemic fluoroquinolones.
2. Full-thickness burns.
   a. Escharectomy—staged or total removal at one time.
   b. Bandage with a water-soluble medication.
   c. With burns extending to deeper tissue, debride burned tissue.
3. Wound healing or reconstructive surgery.
   a. Superficial partial-thickness burns.
      i. Open wound healing.
   b. Deep partial-thickness burns.
      i. Open wound healing.
      ii. Skin graft or flap.

      iii. Open wound healing and skin graft or flap.
   c. Full-thickness burn.
      i. Primary closure.
      ii. Reconstruction with a skin graft or flap.

(For information on reconstructive surgery procedures, the reader is referred to other texts dealing with this topic.)

REFERENCES

Cera LM, Heggers JP, Hagstrom WJ, et al: Therapeutic protocol for thermally injured animals and its successful use in an extensively burned Rhesus monkey. J Am Anim Hosp Assoc 18:633, 1982.

Cera LM, Heggers JP, Robson MC, et al: The therapeutic efficacy of aloe vera cream (Dermaide Aloe) in thermal injuries: Two case reports. J Am Anim Hosp Assoc 16:788, 1980.

Dunlop CI, Daunt DA, Haskins SC: Thermal burns in four dogs during anesthesia. Vet Surg 18:242, 1989.

Fox SM. Management of thermal burns. Part I. Compend Contin Educ Pract Vet 7:631, 1985.

Fox SM, Goring RL, Payton LC, et al: Management of thermal burns. Part II. Compend Contin Educ Pract Vet 8:439, 1986.

Johnston DE: Burns, electrical chemical and cold injuries. In Slatter DH, ed: Textbook of Small Animal Surgery. Philadelphia, WB Saunders, 1985.

Parritz DL, Pavletic MM: Physical and chemical injuries: Heat stroke, hypothermia, burns, frostbite. In Murtaugh RM, Kaplan P, eds: Veterinary Emergency and Critical Care Medicine. St Louis, Mosby–Year Book, 1992.

Pavletic M: Atlas of Small Animal Reconstructive Surgery, ed 2. Philadelphia, WB Saunders, 1999.

Pope ER: Burns: Thermal, electrical, chemical and cold injuries. In Slatter DH, ed: Textbook of Small Animal Surgery, ed 2. Philadelphia, WB Saunders, 1993.

Pope ER, Payne JT: Pathophysiology and treatment of thermal burns. In Harari J, ed: Surgical Complications and Wound Healing in the Small Animal Practice. Philadelphia, WB Saunders, 1993.

Saxon WD, Kirby R: Treatment of acute burn injury and smoke inhalation. In Kirk RW, ed: Current Veterinary Therapy XI. Small Animal Practice. Philadelphia, WB Saunders, 1992.

Swaim SF, Henderson RA: Small Animal Wound Management, ed 2. Media, Williams & Wilkins, 1997.

Tiernan E, Harris A: Butter in the initial treatment of hot tar burns. Burns 19:437, 1993.

............ELECTRICAL BURNS

  I. Etiology and assessment.
    A. Common etiology.
      1. Low-voltage household alternating current from animal chewing on electrical cords.
      2. Damage is caused as current follows the path of least resistance (i.e., small blood vessels and nerves).
        a. Heat generation.
        b. Vessel thrombosis.
    B. Assessment.
      1. Examine lips, gingiva, tongue, and palate.
        a. Early—small or large wound.
        b. Later—there may be a large wound resulting from slough of tissue with damaged vascular supply. (Slough of tissue is usually complete by 2 to 3 weeks.)

II. Treatment.
  A. Acute electrocution.
    1. Judicious fluid therapy since animals are subject to pulmonary edema—dogs more so than cats.
    2. Monitor central venous pressure and urine output.
    3. Diuretic as indicated (Furosemide Diuretic, Hoechst-Roussel Agri-Vet Co., Kansas City, MO).
    4. Morphine as indicated.
    5. Aminophylline.
  B. Wound therapy.
    1. Observe tissues over 2 to 3 weeks with staged debridement as needed.
    2. Minor wounds slough and heal within 3 weeks.
    3. Major wounds.
      a. Lip defects can be sutured or corrected with flaps.
      b. Oronasal fistulas may require reconstruction with labial advancement flaps.
      c. Tongue defects may require some salvage or reconstruction techniques.

(For more information on reconstructive surgery procedures, the reader is referred to other texts dealing with this topic.)

REFERENCES

Johnston DE: Burns, electrical, chemical, and cold injuries. *In* Slatter DH, ed.: Textbook of Small Animal Surgery. Philadelphia, WB Saunders, 1985.
Johnston DE: Skin and subcutaneous tissues-thermal injuries. *In* Bojrab MJ, ed: Pathophysiology of Small Animal Surgery. Philadelphia, WB Saunders, 1981.
Pavletic MM: Atlas of Small Animal Reconstructive Surgery, ed 2. Philadelphia, WB Saunders, 1999.
Plumb DC: Veterinary Drug Handbook, ed 3. Ames, Iowa State University Press, 1999.
Pope ER: Burns: Thermal, electrical, chemical, and cold injuries. *In* Slatter DH, ed: Textbook of Small Animal Surgery, ed 2. Philadelphia, WB Saunders, 1993.
Swaim SF, Henderson RA: Small Animal Wound Management, ed 2. Media, Pa, Williams & Wilkins, 1997.

·········· CHEMICAL BURNS

I. Etiology and assessment.
  A. Etiology.
    1. Oxidizing agents.
    2. Reducing agents.
    3. Corrosives.
    4. Protoplasmic poisons.
    5. Desiccants.
    6. Vesicants.
  B. Assessment.
    1. Observe for hard or soft eschar or coagulum over the area with underlying ulcers.
    2. Decide on feasibility of treatment based on the extent of the burn. (See Thermal Burns, III. Course of action criteria.)
II. Treatment.
  A. Initial therapy.
    1. Animal care personnel should put on protective clothing, gloves, and eyewear.
    2. Rapid dilution of the chemical agent—lavage with copious amounts of water.

3. Flush the eyes with copious physiologic saline.
4. Control the animal's head to prevent licking of the burned area.
B. Later assessment and therapy.
1. With evidence of vapor inhalation and lung involvement, do thoracic radiographs.
2. Specific neutralizing agents.
a. If used, use diluted form.
b. Apply on gauzes under a loose wrap for 20 minutes at a time as needed.
c. Use local or state poison control center for information on best neutralizing agent.
3. Staged debridement with application of a topical antibacterial agent under a bandage between debridements.
a. If wound is not debrided early enough, there will be further tissue destruction from continued chemical penetration over 24 to 72 hours.
b. If the wound is debrided too aggressively, too much tissue may be removed.
4. Wound healing or reconstructive surgery.
a. Open wound healing.
b. Secondary wound closure by tissue shifting or a skin flap.
c. Skin graft.

(For information on reconstructive surgery procedures, the reader is referred to other texts dealing with this topic.)

REFERENCES

Johnston DE: Burns: electrical, chemical, and cold injuries. *In* Slatter DH, ed: Textbook of Small Animal Surgery. Philadelphia, WB Saunders, 1985.
Pavletic MM: Atlas of Small Animal Reconstructive Surgery, ed 2. Philadelphia, WB Saunders, 1999.
Pope ER: Burns: Thermal, electrical, chemical, and cold injuries. *In* Slatter DH, ed: Textbook of Small Animal Surgery, ed 2. Philadelphia, WB Saunders, 1993.
Swaim SF, Henderson RA: Small Animal Wound Management, ed 2. Media, Pa, Williams & Wilkins, 1997.

·············RADIATION INJURY

I. Etiology, result, and assessment.
A. Etiology: Most radiation injuries in animals result from radiation therapy for neoplastic conditions.
B. Result.
1. Kills neoplastic tissue but also results in damage to normal tissue (necrosis, fibrosis, and progressive circulatory decline).
2. Radiation dermatitis, impaired surgical wound healing, and chronic nonhealing wounds.
C. Assessment.
1. First degree—cutaneous erythema.
2. Second degree—superficial desquamation.
3. Third degree—deep moist desquamation.
4. Fourth degree—dermal destruction and ulceration.
or
5. Early changes—edema, erythema, desquamation. Skin is moist or dry and scaly.
6. Late changes—pigmentation, induration, atrophy, telangiectasia, keratosis, decreased adnexal structures, and ulceration.

II. Prevention of wound healing problems.
    A. Postoperative radiation—irradiate surgical area 7 to 14 days postoperatively.
    B. Preoperative radiation—surgery 2 to 3 weeks after radiation.
    C. Begin applying hydrogel dressing containing acemannan (Carra Vet Wound Dressing, Carrington Laboratories, Inc., Irving, TX) the day radiation starts and continue for 2 weeks.

III. Treatment.
    A. Radiation dermatitis.
        1. Wash the area with warm water.
        2. Protect from self-mutilation.
        3. Apply topical medications.
            a. Acemannan-containing wound dressing gel.
            b. Silver sulfadiazine.
            c. Aloe vera cream.
    B. Acute ulcers.
        1. Staged debridement.
        2. Enzymatic debridement, (see Acute Superficial Tissue Injuries, VI. Wound debridement, B. Enzymatic debridement).
        3. Adherent bandage debridement, (see Bandaging and Splinting Techniques, Open Contaminated or Infected Wounds).
    C. Chronic ulcers.
        1. Same as acute ulcers.
        2. Submit debrided tissue for histopathologic examination.
        3. Antibacterial therapy since radiated tissue has decreased resistance to infection.
            a. Systemic antibacterials, but avoid those that sensitize to radiation, e.g., metronidazole.
            b. Topical antibacterials.
    D. Wound healing or reconstructive surgery by skin flaps.
        1. Regional flaps may have been affected by radiation therapy, which could affect healing.
        2. Distant flaps or axial pattern flaps are better choices for healing if they can be used.

(For information on reconstructive surgery procedures, the reader is referred to other texts dealing with this topic.)

REFERENCES

Dernell WS, Wheaton LG: Surgical management of radiation injury. Part I. Compend Contin Educ Pract Vet 17:181, 1995.

Dernell WS, Wheaton LG: Surgical management of radiation injury. Part II. Compend Contin Educ Pract Vet 17:499, 1995.

Laing EJ: The effects of chemotherapy and radiation on wound healing. *In* Harari J, ed: Surgical Complications and Wound Healing in Small Animal Practice. Philadelphia, WB Saunders, 1993.

McLeod DA, Thrall, DE: The combination of surgery and radiation in the treatment of cancer. Vet Surg 18:1, 1989.

Pavletic MM: Atlas of Small Animal Reconstructive Surgery, ed 2. Philadelphia, WB Saunders, 1999.

Roberts DB, Travis EL: Acemannan-containing wound dressing gel reduces radiation-induced skin reactions in C3H mice. Int J Radiat Oncol Biol Phy, 32:1047, 1995.

Swaim SF, Henderson RA: Small Animal Wound Management, ed 2. Media, P, Williams & Wilkins, 1997.

Shock

Shock is a multisystem response to an injury or insult that produces inadequate tissue perfusion and energy production. Causes of shock include severe hypovolemia, trauma, sepsis, heat stroke, hypoglycemia, heart failure, malnutrition, or any endstage visceral organ failure. Early recognition and effective monitoring and therapy are crucial to the successful clinical management of shock syndrome.

............PATHOPHYSIOLOGY

An inadequate circulating fluid volume may develop secondary to maldistribution of available blood volume (traumatic, septic, and cardiogenic origin) or as a result of absolute hypovolemia (whole blood or ECF losses). An animal normally compensates by (1) splenic and venous constriction to translocate blood from venous capacitance vessels to the central arterial circulation; (2) arteriolar constriction to help maintain diastolic blood pressure and tissue perfusion pressure; and (3) an increase in heart rate to increase cardiac output. It is important to recognize that arteriolar vasoconstriction supports brain and heart perfusion at the expense of visceral organ perfusion. If vasoconstriction is severe enough to interfere with the delivery of adequate oxygen to tissues for a sufficient period of time, the animal will die.

The presence of bacteria, viruses, rickettsiae, fungi, or protozoa in the blood constitutes septicemia. When the direct and indirect effects of the septicemia impair oxygen delivery to critical tissue beds and result in reduced tissue energy production, the animal is in septic shock, demonstrating the effects of the infectious agents as noted below.

Cardiogenic shock is the result of blood flow disturbance that produces compromised tissue perfusion. Cardiogenic shock may be a result of primary cardiac disease, acute heart failure, vascular obstruction, or pericardial fluid or fibrosis.

............RECOGNITION OF SHOCK STATES

Shock is a symptomatic disease. The hallmark of shock diagnosis is recognition of the shock state by clinical evaluation. No single variable that can be measured is adequate replacement for clinical identification. The following guidelines are based on known indicators of shock syndrome in the clinical setting.

............HISTORY AND PHYSICAL FINDINGS

Hypovolemic and Traumatic Shock A history of trauma, blood or fluid loss, coupled with the physical findings noted below (Table 1–3) suffices for a diagnosis of hypovolemic or traumatic shock.

Sepsis and Septic Shock A history of (1) a known infection, (2) an event that could cause an infection (an indwelling vascular or urinary catheter, an indwelling pleural or peritoneal tube, surgery, penetrating injury), (3) a disorder that could predispose to infection (renal failure, hyperadrenocorticism, diabetes mellitus, malnutrition, viral infections, stress), or (4) drug therapy that could predispose to infection (corticosteroids, immunosuppressants, antibiotics, IV nutrition products) in an animal that is more depressed and anorectic than expected should alert the clinician that sepsis should be high on the differential diagnosis list. An animal that is *septic* and is *responding* to the infectious process may have leukocytosis with a left shift and a few toxic neutrophils, hyperglycemia, nonspecific elevation of liver enzymes (particularly alkaline phosphatase), diarrhea, and a heart murmur. Blood oxygenation will be normal as long as pulmonary disease is not the origin of the sepsis. There should not be severe metabolic acidosis or coagulopathy. No secondary organ failure should be noted.

An animal in *septic shock* will have additional clinical signs, including depression and anorexia; a rapid fall in the leukocyte count (it may or may not

Table 1–3. Clinical Signs of Shock Syndrome

Parameter	Traumatic/ Hypovolemic	Septic	Cardiogenic
Heart rate	Increased	Increased	Increased
Pulse character	Weak	Strong early, weak late	Weak
Mucous membrane color	Pale	Injected	Pale
Capillary refill time	Increased	Increased	Increased
Respiratory rate	Increased	Increased	Increased
Core temperature	Low/normal	Elevated	Normal
Peripheral temperature	Low	Low/elevated	Low
Urine output	Low	Low	Low
Blood pressure	High early, low late	Low	Low
Central venous pressure	Low	Low	High

be leukopenic at the time that it is measured) with a left shift and many toxic neutrophils; hypoglycemia; metabolic acidosis; coagulopathies; and secondary organ failure noted as anuria, hemorrhagic diarrhea, hypoxemia, and hypotension.

Cardiogenic Shock A history of primary heart disease, trauma, heartworm disease, or other vascular obstruction in the circulation may suggest the presence of cardiogenic shock. Physical findings will be similar to other shock categories (see Table 1–3). Coexisting pulmonary abnormalities characterized by dyspnea, moist rales, and increased work of breathing are frequently noted and are magnified, compared with other causes of shock.

···········CORE SHOCK TREATMENT
···········Catheters and Catheter Placement

Hypovolemic and septic shock require aggressive fluid resuscitation. Several large-gauge catheters should be placed for volume resuscitation. A 14- to 16-gauge 5-in. catheter should be placed in a central venous location for aggressive fluid resuscitation. A minimum of one additional 18- to 20-gauge 2-in. catheter is placed in a peripheral site for drug and additional medication administration. In patients for which venous access cannot be established, fluid infusion into the intraosseous cavity of the humerus, femur, or tibia using a dedicated bone marrow infusion needle system can be lifesaving until venous access can be established. All catheters should be aseptically placed, because they may need to be maintained for several days (see p. 542).

···········Fluids

Aggressive volume resuscitation is indicated in the treatment of hypovolemic, traumatic, or septic shock (see Fluid Therapy, p. 585).

Crystalloid fluids, such as 0.9% sodium chloride, lactated Ringer's solution, or other polyionic solution (sodium, potassium, chloride, and bicarbonate in concentrations similar to normal extracellular electrolyte concentrations), should be used initially. Volumes one and a half to three times the calculated blood volume of the animal (80 mL/kg) may be required to restore cardiovascular values to acceptable levels.

Hypertonic solutions such as 7% NaCl are useful in initial shock resuscitation. A dose of 4 mL/kg of 7% saline will temporarily restore cardiovascular stability in hypovolemic shock, allowing additional therapy to achieve a resuscitation endpoint.

Artificial colloids such as high-molecular-weight (70,000) dextrans, hetastarch, and pentastarch are valuable for volume resuscitation. A dose of 10 mL/kg dextran or hetastarch over the first hour of treatment is useful for reducing administered fluid volume in the resuscitation protocol. Colloids may be administered in addition to hypertonic saline solutions.

Whole blood or plasma (or plasma substitute) should be administered in quantities sufficient to maintain the packed cell volume (PCV) above 25% and the total plasma protein concentration above 3.5 g/dL. Transfusion volume may range from 10 mL/kg to 40 mL/kg (see also p. 46).

............Oxygen (see also p. 610)

Oxygen therapy is indicated in all shock categories. Oxygen may be administered by face mask, oxygen enclosure, nasal (3 to 10 L/min), or transtracheal (0.5 to 3.0 L/min) catheter insufflation. High inspired oxygen concentrations (exceeding 60%) should not be administered for more than 12 to 24 hours for reasons of pulmonary toxicity. Oxygen therapy should be sufficient to restore mucous membrane color or partial pressure of arterial oxygen (PaO_2) values to acceptable levels ($PaO_2 > 80$ mm Hg).

............Antibiotics

Antibiotics are indicated in severe shock of any cause. Because the potential pathogens are unknown in any patient, antibiotic choices are often made on the basis of previous cultures and sensitivities. Bacteremia in companion animals is predominantly of gram-negative origin, followed in incidence by gram-positive, anaerobic, and mixed floral populations. Since the potential pathogens are unknown, it seems wise to choose antibiotics with a wide spectrum of activity and those that are most likely to be effective in the patient at hand.

In sepsis, common antibiotic choices include an aminoglycoside and a penicillin-class antibiotic given together. If the infection does not appear to respond to this combination in 12 to 24 hours, the antibiotic regimen should be changed because of preexisting bacterial resistance. A different aminoglycoside, in addition to a β-lactamase penicillin, plus metronidazole for anaerobes, may be a more appropriate combination. Chloramphenicol and clindamycin are also effective against most anaerobes. Chloramphenicol, erythromycin, and trimethoprim-sulfadiazine do not have the activity spectrum of other antibiotics and should not be used in treatment of an unknown bacteremia until sensitivity testing demonstrates that they are effective.

............CASE-SPECIFIC SHOCK MANAGEMENT

............Glucocorticosteroids

Glucocorticosteroids (Table 1–4) have beneficial effects in shock management, including improved capillary blood flow, decreased production of myocardial depressant factor, reduced intestinal absorption of endotoxin, minimized organ damage and maximized organ function, and improved survival. Their use should be supplemental to aggressive fluid management and not a substitute for rehydration and positive fluid balance necessary to support shock patients. Their role in shock subclasses remains controversial; improved response to management in cases of acute hemorrhage and sepsis has been demonstrated, but, survival outcomes have been inconclusive when comparing patients that have received glucocorticosteroid treatment with those who have not.

Table 1-4. Available Corticosteroids for Shock Therapy

Product Name	Plasma Half-Life* (min)	Biologic Half-Life* (hr)	Relative Glucocorticoid Potency*	Relative Mineralocorticoid Activity*	Equivalent Dose* (mg)	Approximate Physiologic Replacement Dose (mg/kg/day)	Pharmacologic Shock Dose (mg/kg)	Redosage Interval (hr)
Hydrocortisone Hydrocortisone sodium phosphate Hydrocortisone sodium succinate	90–180	8–12	1	2	20	0.25–0.30	300	4–6
Prednisolone Prednisolone sodium phosphate Prednisolone sodium succinate	115–252	12–36	4	1	5.0	0.05–0.10	10–30	8–12
Methylprednisolone Methyl-prednisolone sodium succinate	144–240	12–36	5	0	4.0	0.05–0.06	10–30	8–12
Dexamethasone Dexamethasone sodium phosphate	200–300	36–72	25–30	0	0.75	0.01	6–15	12–18

*American Medical Association: AMA Drug Evaluation, ed 5. Chicago, 1983, p 892.

Table 1–5. Antiprostaglandins

Aspirin	10 mg/kg b.i.d. (dog); q3d (cat)
Indomethacin	10–20 mg/kg PO (repeated once at 2 hr)
Flunixin	1–2 mg/kg IV (repeated once at 2 hr)
Ibuprofen	2–5 mg/kg PO
Phenylbutazone	20–50 mg/kg PO
Aminopyrine	25–50 mg/kg PO (repeated 10 mg/kg hr × 2 IV)
Flufenamic acid	10–20 mg/kg (repeated 10 mg/kg/hr × 2 IV)

There is no difference in antishock efficacy of succinate or phosphate esters of the commonly used corticosteroids. Adverse effects of supraphysiologic doses of corticosteroids, including immunosuppression, infection, adrenal suppression, delayed wound healing, pancreatitis, GI bleeding, tissue catabolism, and hepatopathy are not generally a problem when administration is restricted to less than 2 days. Concurrent administration of intestinal protectant agents such as H_2-receptor antagonists or oral antacid products reduces potential GI side effects.

............Antiprostaglandins

Antiprostaglandin therapy may be indicated in septic shock patients because prostaglandins are released into the systemic circulation. Prostaglandin release may cause marked systemic effects, including severe regional hypotension. Antiprostaglandins (Table 1–5) normalize hemodynamic changes and improve survival.

Antiprostaglandin therapy does not resolve the leukopenia, thrombocytopenia, acidosis, or coagulopathies that occur during septic shock. In addition, antiprostaglandins can have adverse effects including GI hemorrhage and ulceration and renal arteriolar vasoconstriction. For these reasons, use of antiprostaglandins should be limited to a single dose in the early phase of septic shock.

............Bicarbonate

Sodium bicarbonate should be administered if metabolic acidosis is severe. If the base or bicarbonate deficit is known, the dose of bicarbonate to administer can be calculated by the formula:

Base or bicarbonate deficit × 0.3 × body weight (kg)

where 0.3×kg is an estimate of extracellular fluid volume.

If the severity of metabolic acidosis is not known, replacement therapy can be administered based on an estimation of mild, moderate, or severe bicarbonate loss. Based on estimates, 1, 3, or 5 mEq/kg of bicarbonate should be administered. Bicarbonate should be administered over a period of 20 minutes or longer because it may cause hypercapnia or alkalemia, hypokalemia or hypocalcemia or both, hypotension, restlessness, vomiting, and, if severe, death.

............Glucose

Glucose should be administered if blood levels are less than 80 mg/dL. A bolus of glucose 0.1 to 0.25 g/kg IV should be administered to achieve an acceptable blood level. Blood glucose must then be maintained by a 2.5% to 10% glucose infusion (depending upon the rate of fluid infusion) titrated to the desired effect by serial glucose measurements.

...........Antiarrhythmics

Bradycardia should be treated by correcting the underlying cause. An anticholinergic agent (atropine 0.04 mg/kg IM, or glycopyrrolate 0.02 mg/kg IM) should be administered as a first order of therapy. If this is ineffective, a sympathomimetic and β-agonist should be administered (Table 1–6).

Premature ventricular contractions (PVCs) may accompany shock. The causes of PVCs are varied; however, the treatment options are similar. Treat PVCs (Table 1–7) when they are frequent in occurrence (in excess of 16 bpm), when they are increasing in frequency, when their rate would exceed 200 bpm if the paroxysmal rhythm continued for 1 minute, when they are multiform, when the ectopic beat occurs atop the T wave of the preceding complex, or when there is evidence of cardiovascular impairment.

...........Sympathomimetics

Sympathomimetic therapy is indicated when fluid resuscitation has not accomplished clinical improvement endpoints as indicated by an increased central venous pressure (CVP) (discussed below), systemic blood pressure, and tissue perfusion. Other indicators of inadequate resuscitation may include development of subcutaneous or pulmonary edema or the presence of acute heart failure.

Currently, sympathomimetic agents that predominantly enhance cardiac activity are preferred for use in shock syndromes. The first-choice drugs (see

Table 1–6. Sympathomimetics

Drug	Receptor Activity	Dosage (IV)
Dopamine (Intropin, Arnar-Stone)	Dopamine and α^{+++}, β^{+++}	5–25 µg/kg/min (blood pressure support) 1–5 µg/kg/min (diuresis)
Dobutamine (Dobutrex, Lilly)	α^+, β^{+++}	2.5–40 mg/kg/min (blood pressure support)
Mephentermine (Wyamine, Wyeth)	α^+, β^{+++}	0.1–0.75 mg/kg
Norepinephrine (Levophed bitartrate, Winthrop-Breon)	α^{+++}, β^+	0.05–0.3 mg/kg/min; 0.01–0.2 mg/kg
Metaraminol (Aramine, Merck Sharp & Dohme)	α^{+++}, β^+	0.05–0.2 mg/kg
Phenylephrine (Neo-Synephrine, Winthrop-Breon)	α^{+++}, β^0	0.05–0.2 mg/kg
Methoxamine (Vasoxyl, Burroughs Wellcome)	α^{+++}, β^0	0.05–0.2 mg/kg
Epinephrine	α^{+++}, β^{+++}	0.02–0.05 mg/kg 0.05–0.2 mg/kg/min

+ + +, Strong receptor activity; 0, no activity for that receptor; +, weak receptor activity.

Table 1–7. Antiarrhythmics Used for the Treatment of Frequently Occurring Premature Ventricular Contractions

Drug	Mechanism of Action	Dosage
Lidocaine	Fast Na$^+$ channel inhibition	1–8 mg/kg IV (dog) 25–75 μg/kg/min 0.25–1.0 mg/kg IV (cat)
Procainamide	Fast Na$^+$ channel inhibition	1–8 mg/kg IV 25–40 μg/kg min 6–20 mg/kg PO q.i.d.
Quinidine	Fast Na$^+$ channel inhibition	6–20 mg/kg PO q.i.d.
Propranolol	β-Adrenergic blocker	0.02–0.06 mg/kg IV 0.02–1.0 mg/kg PO
Verapamil	Slow Ca^{2+} channel blocker	0.05–0.15 mg/kg IV
Bretylium	Inhibits norepinephrine release	5–10 mg/kg IV over 30 min
Phenytoin	Fast Na$^+$ channel blocker	2–10 mg/kg IV 30–35 mg/kg PO t.i.d.

Table 1–6) include dopamine, dobutamine, ephedrine, and mephentermine. These drugs support myocardial contractility and arterial blood pressure, with minimal peripheral vasoconstriction.

..........Vasodilators

Vasodilators (Table 1–8) are indicated in *cardiogenic shock* to reduce vascular resistance (afterload as estimated by mean blood pressure) that the weakened heart has to pump against. They may also be useful in septic or severe hypovolemic shock to maximize tissue perfusion after fluid administration. Vasodilator therapy should be monitored carefully, since hypotension is the consequence of their injudicious use.

Morphine (0.05 mg/kg IM) primarily dilates capacitance vessels, but can also cause CNS and respiratory depression and histamine release. *Phenothiazine tranquilizers* (acepromazine 0.02 mg/kg IM) are both resistance and capacitance vessel dilators and cause CNS depression. *Furosemide* is a weak vasodilator if it is being used to treat oliguria.

..........Diuresis (see also p. 585)

Urine output reflects renal blood flow, an indirect monitor of blood pressure. Anuria or oliguria suggests inadequate renal (and visceral) perfusion, which may precipitate acute renal failure. If effective blood volume restoration does not generate an acceptable urine flow, diuretics should be administered. The diuretics listed below can be given in any order or in any combination.

Furosemide 5 mg/kg promotes renal vasodilation and is a potent loop diuretic. If urine does not flow within 10 minutes following its administration, a second dose should be administered. *Mannitol* 0.5 g/kg IV over 20 minutes acts as an osmotic diuretic. If urine does not flow within 10 minutes following the end of the infusion, another diuretic agent should be administered. *Dopamine* 1 to 5 μg/kg/min IV causes renal (and visceral) vasodilation via dopaminergic

40

Table I–8. Vasodilating Agents

Drug	Mechanism of Action	Dose and Method of Administration (Onset; Peak; Duration)	Potential Adverse Effects*
Hydralazine (Apresoline, Novartis)	Direct arteriolar smooth muscle relaxant; little effect of venous capacitance vessels	0.2–0.5 mg/kg (10–20 min; 10–80 min; 2–8 hr)	With prolonged use: systemic lupus erythematosus; neuritis; blood dyscrasias
Diazoxide (Hyperstat, Schering)	Direct arteriolar smooth muscle relaxant of primarily the resistance vessels	5 mg/kg rapid IV (immediately; 5–10 min; 30 min–10 hr)	Inhibits release: hyperglycemia
Sodium nitroprusside (Nipride, Roche)	Direct arteriolar and venular smooth muscle relaxant	3 mg (0.5–10 µg/kg/min IV); dilute in D5W IV with continuous blood pressure monitoring (immediately; 1 min; 2 min)	Light-sensitive; bottle must be covered with foil and kept for no longer than 4 hr; avoid in hepatic or renal failure; large doses may cause cyanide toxicity; keep total dose <1.5 mg/kg/2 hr; treat with sodium nitrite 0.5–0.75 mg/kg slow IV followed by sodium thiosulfate 0.2 g/kg slow IV; thiocyanate accumulation (disorientation)
Trimethaphan (Arfonad, Roche)	Postsynaptic ganglionic blocking agent (dilates resistance and capacitance vessels); direct arteriolar smooth muscle relaxant	Dilute 50 mg in 500 mL D5W 0.4–4.0 µg/kg/min	Releases histamine Parasympatholytic effects
Nitroglycerin ointment (Nitrostat, Parke-Davis)	Predominantly venous but also some arteriolar vasodilation	¼–¾-in. supracutaneously q6–8h	Tolerance
Prazosin (Minipress, Pfizer)	α-Receptor blockage; arteriolar and venous dilation	1–3 mg PO b.i.d.	GI signs
Captopril (Capoten, Squibb)	Inhibits angiotensin II–converting enzyme	0.5–2.0 mg/kg PO t.i.d.	
Enalapril (Vasotec, Merial)		0.25–0.5 mg/kg q12–24h PO	

D5W, dextrose 5% in water.
*Excessive hypotension, secondary cardiac stimulation, and renal sodium and water retention are implied adverse effects of most of the vasodilators.

receptor stimulation. The dosage should be increased in 1-µg/kg/min increments until there is acceptable urine flow or evidence of peripheral vasoconstriction (which would include renal vasoconstriction) or an increase in heart rate. If dopamine fails to induce an acceptable urine output, combination of the three diuretic groups administered simultaneously may be effective.

............Positive-Pressure Ventilation (see also p. 613)

Positive-pressure ventilation is indicated when the response to oxygen therapy is not adequate or when hypoventilation is due to pulmonary disease. The goal of positive-pressure ventilation is to provide acceptable blood oxygenation (pink color, a $PaO_2 > 60$ mm Hg) without excessive hyperventilation (a $PaCO_2 < 30$ mm Hg) and maintain pulse quality and blood pressure, which can be affected by positive-pressure ventilation. Short-term (<24 hours) airway management for positive-pressure ventilation can be accomplished via orotracheal intubation using heavy sedation to let the patient tolerate the endotracheal tube. Consideration should be given to placement of a tracheostomy tube when longer positive-pressure ventilation is attempted.

............MONITORING SHOCK (see also p. 43)

Shock monitoring should be used as a basis for evaluating the therapy used to treat shock. Multisystem monitoring is important during resuscitation and stabilization of the shock patient. The following issues are general goals for monitoring based on the identified cause of the shock state.

Monitoring of *hypovolemic shock* and *traumatic shock* should focus on the status of the cardiovascular system, the adequacy of fluid administration to restore blood volume, and maintainence of red blood cell (RBC) and protein levels.

Monitoring of *cardiogenic shock* should focus on the status of the heart and response to therapy administered to maintain cardiovascular support.

Monitoring of *septic shock* should reflect a multisystemic disease. Monitoring should include measurement of cardiovascular and pulmonary status: blood glucose, metabolic acid-base balance, coagulation, and the status of visceral organ systems such as renal, GI, hepatic, and cerebral function.

............Cardiovascular Monitoring (see also p. 202)
............*Electrical Activity*

The electrocardiogram (ECG) can be continuously monitored with an oscilloscope or intermittently with a paper recorder. Leads can be easily attached to the patient with atraumatic adhesive or fine-needle electrodes. Alligator clips should be avoided for long-term monitoring. The heart should be checked at regular intervals to make sure that the heart rate remains in an acceptable range for the species and size and to detect arrhythmias.

............*Mechanical Activity*

Auscultation The heart should be regularly auscultated for changes in heart sound intensity, heart rhythm, and for presence of murmurs. Pulse quality should be regularly evaluated as an assessment of stroke volume.

Central Venous Pressure This is valuable in monitoring the response to shock (see also p. 519). CVP should be monitored in patients with cardiogenic shock to evaluate the ability of the heart to pump venous blood and in septic shock to monitor aggressive fluid resuscitation. CVP is probably not helpful in hypovolemic and traumatic shock patients that respond well to initial fluid therapy; however, CVP should be useful to guide further fluid administration if the animal does not respond to the initial fluid therapy.

CVP measurement requires a catheter placed in the external jugular vein and positioned in proximity to the right atrium. The normal CVP is 0 to 5 cm H_2O. CVP values below 0 indicate that the animal can accommodate additional fluid volume in the vascular space, and, in conjunction with signs of vasoconstriction and hypotension, indicate hypovolemia. Fluids should be administered until the CVP is between 5 and 10 cm H_2O. CVP values above 10 cm H_2O suggest that vascular fluid volume is adequate and that further fluid therapy should be conservative. Values above 15 cm H_2O indicate that fluid therapy should stop because of excess fluid volume administration that the heart cannot pump. A high CVP value in conjunction with persistent vasoconstriction or hypotension suggests heart failure.

Arterial blood pressure measurement is helpful in evaluating response to shock therapy. Systolic arterial blood pressure is normally 100 to 160 mm Hg; mean pressure is normally 80 to 120 mm Hg. Systolic blood pressures below 80 mm Hg or mean pressures below 50 to 60 mm Hg may be associated with inadequate perfusion of the brain and heart. Systolic blood pressure can be measured with a Doppler blood flow detector; systolic, diastolic, and mean pressures can be measured with oscillometric instrumentation or by direct arterial catheterization techniques. If hypotension persists after adequate fluid therapy has been achieved, as verified by the measurement of a CVP of 5 to 10 cm H_2O, sympathomimetic therapy should be considered.

.... Peripheral Perfusion

Peripheral tissue perfusion should be evaluated at regular intervals by assessing such indices as mucous membrane color, capillary refill time, appendage temperature, core toe web temperature gradient (should be <8°C), and urinary output. Pulse oximetry is helpful in quantitating oxygen content in the capillary beds.

.... Respiratory Monitoring

.... Respiratory Rate and Ventilatory Effort

The respiratory rate may be variable but must be accompanied by appropriately sized tidal (breath) volumes to maintain adequate ventilation. Breathing effort should be free and easy; exaggerated effort or other signs suggesting increased breathing effort must be addressed. The respiratory rhythm should be regular; an irregular pattern of breathing is a sign of a central respiratory center disturbance. The lungs should be easy to auscultate over all regions of the chest; muffled or absent breath sounds suggest pleural space abnormalities or lobar lung collapse. Auscultation should reveal normal bronchovesicular sounds. Harsh, crepitant, or fluid sounds suggest parenchymal disease.

.... Tissue Oxygenation

The mucous membranes, operative sites, and arterial blood should maintain their normally pink or red coloration; dusty, dark, or cyanotic discoloration suggests an excess of unoxygenated hemoglobin. Hemoglobin oxygenation can be measured by pulse oximetry, as noted above.

.... Renal Monitoring

Visceral organ function is adversely affected in shock. Monitoring renal function indirectly monitors the status of the other visceral organs. Urinary output is used to monitor renal perfusion and function. Urinary output can be monitored by sequentially palpating the bladder or by catheterization. Normal urinary output is 1 to 2 mL/kg/hr. If there is normal urinary output, renal perfusion is probably adequate; if the animal is anuric, renal perfusion may not be adequate. Urinary catheters may predispose the patient to urinary tract infections and should be placed and maintained aseptically; collection systems must be closed (see p. 486).

...........Temperature

Temperature should be continuously monitored during shock and shock resuscitation. Core temperature may be either hypothermic or hyperthermic upon presentation and will usually normalize during shock resuscitation when adequate support has been given. Peripheral temperature at a toe web site will be low during shock (<8°C difference from core body temperature) and increase to normal gradient difference (<8°C difference from core body temperature) during shock resuscitation. An increasing core body temperature is an early index of a developing septic process. The core temperature should not be allowed to exceed 42°C (107.6°F). A temperature that decreases to below normal in a septic patient is an unfavorable prognostic sign; core temperature should be maintained in the normal range.

...........Laboratory Monitoring of the Shock Patient
...........Packed Cell Volume and Total Protein

PCV and total protein should be monitored at regular intervals. Redistribution of plasma protein and erythrocytes into extravascular tissue spaces can occur in shock. Additionally, aggressive crystalloid fluid therapy may cause excessive hemodilution. The PCV should be maintained above 25% by RBC administration and the total protein should be maintained above 3.5 g/dL by plasma or artificial colloid administration.

...........White Blood Cell Count

Leukocyte counts should be performed every 12 hours as an index to how the animal is responding to the shock syndrome and to evaluate the response of the septic patient to the selected antibiotics. An increasing WBC count generally indicates a favorable response; a decreasing WBC count indicates an unfavorable response.

...........Glucose

Glucose is commonly affected in all shock states and should be measured routinely. Hyperglycemia is a common early response to the combined effects of stress, hormonally induced glycogenolysis and gluconeogenesis, and reduced cellular glucose utilization. Hypoglycemia is a common late sign of the septic shock process. Blood glucose should be maintained between 80 and 250 mg/dL.

...........Electrolytes

Electrolytes should be measured to assess the general status of the animal's response to shock. Electrolytes that should be evaluated include sodium, potassium, chloride, calcium, magnesium, and phosphate. Specific treatment may be required if electrolyte values are not within the reference range.

...........Biochemistry Profiles (see also p. 718)

Biochemical evaluation of visceral organ function (liver and kidney) should be performed daily to evaluate the status and progress of organ damage. Biochemical values lag behind the actual organ damage. Monitoring dynamic physiologic parameters (i.e., urine output) provides a better evaluation of organ status.

...........Arterial Blood Gases (see also p. 591)

Arterial blood gas analysis can provide valuable information regarding pulmonary function and the overall acid-base status of the shock patient. Of the values reported when a blood gas sample is analyzed, oxygen and carbon dioxide levels evaluate the adequacy of respiratory gas exchange, whereas bicarbonate and carbon dioxide ($Paco_2$) are used to evaluate acid-base balance (see also p. 593).

The pH value will provide an overall assessment of the acid-base balance in the patient. A pH value of less then 7.35 indicates an acidosis; a pH value greater then 7.45 indicates an alkalosis. The origin of the pH disturbance cannot be identified solely from pH evaluation; this requires interpretation of other values that are included in the blood gas report.

Pao_2 defines the adequacy of blood oxygenation. A Pao_2 below 80 mm Hg represents hypoxemia; below 50 to 60 mm Hg, it represents life-threatening hypoxemia. Venous Po_2 reflects tissue Po_2 but bears no correlation to arterial Po_2. Venous Pao_2 is usually between 40 and 50 mm Hg. Values below 30 mm Hg may indicate reduced oxygen delivery to the tissues (hypoxemia, low cardiac output, vasoconstriction); values above 60 mm Hg (while breathing room air) suggest reduced tissue uptake of oxygen (shunting, septic shock, metabolic poisons). Venous blood must be sampled from a central vein, such as the jugular vein or anterior vena cava, or the pulmonary artery. Peripheral veins exhibit variably higher Po_2 values.

A $Paco_2$ below 35 mm Hg represents hyperventilation; a $Paco_2$ below 20 mm Hg with a pH greater than 7.55 represents severe respiratory alkalosis that may cause excessive cerebral vasoconstriction. A $Paco_2$ above 45 mm Hg represents hypoventilation; a $Paco_2$ above 60 mm Hg may be associated with hypoxemia if the patient is breathing room air, with excessive respiratory acidosis (pH<7.20), or with undesirable cerebral vasodilation in a patient with an intracranial pressure problem. Venous $Paco_2$ is usually 3 to 6 mm Hg higher than $Paco_2$ in stable states. The use of venous $Paco_2$ as an index of arterial $Paco_2$ is, in general, a satisfactory "ballpark" estimate, but can be misleading at times; the venous-arterial $Paco_2$ gradient should be determined periodically.

In addition to interpretation of the absolute values for $Paco_2$ and Pao_2, the two should be evaluated together to determine whether there is evidence of a reduced oxygenating efficiency of the lungs or venous admixture. As a simplified version of the alveolar air equation, the $Paco_2$ and Pao_2 should add up to a value of 130 to 140; a value below 120 suggests venous admixture.

Metabolic acid-base balance is determined by evaluating bicarbonate or total CO_2 levels in the blood gas sample. Normal base deficit is 0 ± 4 mEq/L; HCO_3 is 24 ± 4 mEq/L; and total CO_2 is 25 ± 4 mEq/L. Base deficit values below 10 mEq/L and HCO_3 values below 14 mEq/L warrant therapy.

...........HEMOSTATIC DEFECTS ASSOCIATED WITH SHOCK

Disseminated intravascular coagulation (DIC) is a complex syndrome resulting from inappropriate activation of intravascular coagulation. DIC produces multiple organ injury due to intravascular microthrombosis as a result of excessive consumption of platelets and clotting factors. This sequence of events results in prolonged bleeding and enhanced fibrinolysis. Several pathophysiologic mechanisms are involved in DIC. These include endothelial cell damage; platelet activation and consumption; release of tissue procoagulants; development of hypoxia; abnormal renal, cardiac, and liver function; and release of myocardial depressant factor.

■ DISORDERS ASSOCIATED WITH DIC IN THE DOG

Hemangiosarcoma
Sepsis
Immune hemolytic anemia
Pancreatitis
Electrocution
Heat stroke
Heartworm disease
Malignancies

By the time DIC is clinically evident, clotting factors are already severely depleted. Laboratory values associated with DIC include low fibrinogen levels, prolonged prothrombin time (PT) and partial thromboplastin time (PTT), and an increase in fibrin split/degradation products (FSP/FDP). Reduced levels of antithrombin III (AT III), a modulator of coagulation, are also present. The symptomatic patient requires replacement of clotting factors that have been consumed. In addition, the patient needs the administration of heparin, which is a specific coactivator of antithrombin and requires the presence of adequate levels of antithrombin to be effective.

■ DIAGNOSIS OF DIC

Regenerative anemia
Hemoglobinemia (intravascular hemolysis)
Presence of RBC fragments
Neutrophilia with left shift
Hyperbilirubinemia
Thrombocytopenia
Prolongation of the prothrombin time (PT) or activated partial
    thromboplastin time (APTT)
Hypofibrinogenemia
Positive FDP test (usually negative in cats)
Decreased AT III concentration

............Treatment of Dogs and Cats With DIC

1. Eliminate the precipitating cause.
2. Stop intravascular coagulation; administer whole blood or blood products and heparin (see p. 46). Administer the first dose of heparin in combination with blood products. Allow the heparin to remain in the blood product for 30 minutes at room temperature prior to the transfusion.

■ HEPARIN DOSAGE FOR DIC

Minidose: 5 to 10 IU/kg SC t.i.d.
Low dose: 75 to 200 IU/kg SC t.i.d.
Intermediate dose: 300 to 500 IU SC or IV t.i.d.
High dose: 750 to 1000 IU/kg SC or IV t.i.d.

---

3. Aspirin can be used to prevent platelet adhesion. Dose is 5 to 10 mg/kg orally b.i.d. in the dog and every third day in the cat.
4. Maintain parenchymal organ perfusion with good fluid balance (see p. 585).
5. Maintain adequate acid-base status, good oxygenation, and administer systemic antibiotics (see p. 893).

REFERENCES

Feldman B, Kirby R, Caldin M: Recognition and treatment of disseminated intravascular coagulation. *In* Bonagura J, ed: Kirk's Current Veterinary Therapy 13. Philadelphia, WB Saunders, 2000.
Haskins S: Therapy for shock. *In* Bonagura J, ed: Kirk's Current Veterinary Therapy 13. Philadelphia, WB Saunders, 2000.
Hauptman J, Chaudry I: Shock: Pathophysiology and management of hypovolemia and sepsis. *In* Slatter D, ed: Textbook of Small Animal Surgery, ed 2. Philadelphia, WB Saunders, 1996.
Kellerman DL, Leewis DC, Myers NC et al: Determination of a therapeutic heparin dosage in the cat. *In* Proceedings of the 14th Annual Forum of the American College of Veterinary Internal Medicine, 1996, p. 166.

Bleeding Disorders (see also p. 687)

I. **Summary**.
   A. The signalment, history, and clinical signs along with a blood smear and an activated clotting time (ACT) can be used to make a presumptive diagnosis of the most common bleeding disorders in dogs and cats.
   B. Treatment usually consists of supportive care, treatment of any underlying disease, and replacement of the deficient hemostatic factors.
II. **Initial diagnostic plan**.
   A. **History**: In addition to routine history questions, try to determine:
      1. The nature of the bleeding (sites affected, duration, previous episodes of bleeding).
      2. If the animal has had a risk of exposure to toxins, the type of toxin, amount consumed, time consumed.
      3. If any trauma has occurred and the risk of trauma (i.e., allowed to roam vs. kenneled).
      4. If any recent drug or vaccine exposure (both risk factors for thrombocytopenia).
      5. If any relatives have had a bleeding disorder.
      6. If there are any signs of concurrent illness.
   B. **Physical examination**.
      1. Try to differentiate between regional injury (e.g., disrupted vascular integrity) and a bleeding diathesis (typically persistent hemorrhage from multiple sites).
      2. Determine whether signs are most consistent with superficial bleeding (platelet problem), deep bleeding (coagulation cascade problem) or mixed (see Table 1–9).
      3. Identify concurrent illness (especially those associated with DIC,

Table 1–9. Components of Normal Hemostasis and
Clinical Signs of Disorders

Components of Normal Hemostasis	Clinical Signs When One Component Is Abnormal*	Common Disorders
Vascular integrity	Variable (usually deep bleeding)	Trauma, vessel neoplasia, vasculitis
Platelets (primary hemostasis)	Superficial bleeding (petechiae, ecchymoses, mucosal bleeding)	Decreased platelet number, immune-mediated thrombocytopenia, disseminated intravascular coagulation (DIC), decreased platelet function, von Willebrand's disease, aspirin
Coagulation cascade (secondary hemostasis)	Deep bleeding (hematomas, hemothroax, hemoabdomen, hemarthrosis); some mucosal bleeding	Anticoagulant rodenticide toxicity, hemophilia A and B, DIC
Fibrinolysis (clot lysis)	Variable (usually deep bleeding)	DIC

*Prolonged intraoperative bleeding can occur with all.

e.g., neoplasia, sepsis, pancreatitis, immune mediated hemolytic anemia, heartworm disease, heat stroke, snake bite, etc.).

C. **Activated clotting time, blood smear, PCV, total plasma protein (TPP) (see Table 1–10).**

1. ACT evaluates the intrinsic and common pathways of the clotting cascade.

   a. Procedure:

      i. Warm an ACT tube (containing diatomaceous earth) to 37°C in a heating block or water bath.

      ii. Using atraumatic venipuncture, draw 3 mL of blood into a syringe without anticoagulant. Have an assistant place gentle pressure on the site for several minutes.

      iii. Change needles and inject 2 mL of blood into the ACT tube, invert the tube several times to mix, place in the 37°C heat source, and start timing.

      iv. With the remaining blood, fill several microhematocrit tubes and make several good blood smears.

      v. Starting at 1 minute and at 5- to 10-second intervals thereafter, check the tube for a clot (remove from heat source, invert, return). Record the time when a clot (or gel) is first noted. Normal is less than 90 seconds (usually shorter in cats).

2. Use the blood smear to assess platelet number and RBC morphology.

Table 1–10. Simple Tests to Differentiate the Most Common Spontaneous Bleeding Disorders

| Disorder | Type of Bleeding | Blood Smear | | Activated Clotting Time |
		Platelet Estimate	RBC Morphology	
Thrombocytopenia	Superficial	↓ ↓ ↓	N	N (or slight ↑)
Anticoagulant rodenticide toxicity and hemophilias	Deep	N– ↓ ↓	N	↑ ↑ ↑
Disseminated intravascular coagulation	Variable	↓ – ↓ ↓	RBC fragments	↑ – ↑ ↑ ↑
von Willebrand's disease	Superficial	N	N	N

N, normal; ↑, slight increase; ↓, slight decrease; ↑ ↑, moderate increase; ↓ ↓, moderate decrease; ↑ ↑ ↑, substantial increase; ↓ ↓ ↓, substantial decrease.

    a. Platelet number:
       i. Scan the slide at low magnification, particularly the feathered edge. If there are platelet clumps, you cannot estimate the platelet count, but thrombocytopenia is not likely the cause of the bleeding.
      ii. If there are no clumps, scan many fields in the RBC monolayer area using the ×100 objective (oil immersion). The estimated platelet count equals the average number of platelets per field ×15,000. With thrombocytopenia alone, hemorrhage usually does not occur until the platelet count is less than 20,000/μL (less than two platelets per oil immersion field). If there are signs of superficial hemorrhage and more than four or five platelets per oil field, there may be a platelet dysfunction problem (e.g., DIC, von Willebrand's disease (see p. 668), aspirin-induced).
    b. RBC morphology: RBC fragments (schizocytes, keratocytes) support the diagnosis of DIC.
    c. A scan of the smear can also give an estimate of the WBC count and differential, reticulocyte count, and an assessment of other RBC changes.
  3. Measure the PCV and TPP to determine pretreatment values and identify anemia if present.
  4. Cage-side APTT monitors use smaller blood volumes and may be more accurate than the ACT; therefore they may be the preferred test if available.
D. Use the signalment, history, physical examination findings, and Table 1–10 to make a tentative diagnosis or narrow the number of potential rule-outs. Then look under the disease headings below for further diagnostic and therapeutic recommendations.
E. A CBC, **serum biochemistry analysis, and urinalysis** (voided sample) may be appropriate in any case of spontaneous bleeding to look for concurrent problems or organ dysfunction secondary to hemorrhage or

anemia. Perform additional diagnostic testing as appropriate for the clinical signs.

III. **General therapy potentially applicable in all bleeding disorders**.
  A. **Manage hypovolemia** initially with crystalloids or colloids, or both, while diagnostic testing is started and other therapies are determined and prepared (e.g., blood products).
  B. **Emergency transfusion** (rarely needed):
    1. Indications: Rapid transfusion with **fresh whole blood** (FWB) may be appropriate and lifesaving if the animal has:
      a. Hypovolemia and a pretreatment PCV less than 20%.
        or
      b. Hypovolemia that persists despite adequate crystalloid or colloid therapy regardless of PCV.
        or
      c. Had known blood loss that was extreme (>30 mL/kg in dogs, >20 mL/kg in cats).
    2. Compatibility testing (crossmatch):
      a. In dogs, if an emergency transfusion is necessary, use universal donor blood without a crossmatch.
      b. In cats, there is no universal donor. At least do a slide crossmatch (particularly in breeds where blood type B is more frequent, including British shorthair, Rex, Abyssinian, Persian, Himalayan, Scottish Fold, etc.):
        i. Collect 1 to 2 mL of blood in ethylene diaminetetraacetic acid (EDTA) from donor and recipient, centrifuge, pull off plasma into a separate tube.
        ii. Make a 4% RBC suspension of recipient RBCs (0.2 mL packed RBCs mixed with 4.8 mL 0.9% NaCl). Mix well.
        iii. Mix one drop of recipient RBC suspension with one drop of donor plasma on a slide. Rock back and forth.
        iv. Agglutination (gross or microscopic) and hemolysis indicate incompatibility. Do blood typing.
    3. Volume of FWB to transfuse = **12 to 20 mL/kg** (to start).
    4. Rate: Transfuse 50% rapidly, then reassess and adjust rate and volume to meet patient needs. If the patient is not in critical condition, but needs emergency transfusion, it is ideal to administer the transfusion at a slow rate for the first 15 to 30 minutes to identify acute transfusion reactions.
    5. Simultaneous packed RBCs and fresh frozen plasma (FFP) are an acceptable alternative to FWB, particularly if they can be prepared more quickly.
  C. **General transfusion recommendations**: transfuse based on clinical signs, dose to effect.
    1. **Cellular components**—packed red blood cells (PRBCs) or FWB.
      a. Indications (see also III.B. Emergency transfusion above):
        i. Anemia severe enough to cause tachypnea, tachycardia and weakness at rest regardless of PCV, assuming thoracic causes for these signs (e.g., hemothorax and pulmonary hemorrhage) have been ruled out.
        ii. Anemia with large expected losses (e.g., presplenectomy).
        iii. PCV less than 10% in the dog.
      b. Crossmatch (particularly in cats) (see p. 665).
      c. Volume to transfuse:
        i. Estimate:
            PRBCs: 10 mL/kg will raise PCV 10%.
            FWB: 20 mL/kg will raise PCV 10%.
          or

ii. Calculate

Milliliters of donor blood needed =

$$90 \text{ (dog) or } 66 \text{ (cat)} \times \text{BW(kg)} \times \frac{[\text{desired PCV} - \text{patient PCV}]}{\text{donor PCV}}.$$

   d. Rate: Try to transfuse the entire volume within 4 hours (start slowly to monitor for transfusion reactions). Slower rates may be appropriate if the patient cannot tolerate volume expansion (see p. 572).

  2. **FFP** contains all coagulation proteins but no viable platelets:

   a. Indication: coagulation protein deficiency or dysfunction.

     i. Associated with hemorrhage.

      or

     ii. Presurgery.

   b. Starting dose 6 to 10 mL/kg; **repeat until bleeding is controlled**.

   c. Rate is dependent on the patient's ability to handle volume expansion (e.g., very fast if hypovolemic, slow if cardiac failure). Try to transfuse FFP in less than 2 hours (coagulation proteins start to degrade as soon as the product thaws, as in vivo).

D. **Correct fluid, electrolyte, and acid-base abnormalities.**

E. **Warm the patient if hypothermic** (hypothermia impairs the function of both platelets and the coagulation cascade). Ideally, use warmed fluids even if normothermic to improve patient comfort and to prevent exacerbation of the coagulopathy.

F. **Nursing care**.

  1. Cage rest, gentle restraint, avoid neck leads, feed soft foods.

  2. If possible, give drugs PO or IV through an indwelling catheter.

  3. Avoid IM injections, use small-gauge needles, keep gentle pressure on injection sites for several minutes.

  4. Avoid medications that impair platelet function (e.g. NSAIDs, sulfa, drugs, etc.).

  5. Suture or bandage wounds (even small ones if bleeding).

............SPECIFIC COAGULOPATHIES (see also p. 607)

I. **Thrombocytopenia**.

A. Further diagnostic testing to consider:

  1. CBC or at least an evaluation of the PCV and blood smear. In animals with thrombocytopenia severe enough to cause clinical signs of hemorrhage:

   a. Normal to elevated WBC counts are more typical of immune-mediated thrombocytopenia (IMT) or Rocky Mountain spotted fever (RMSF).

   b. Low WBC counts are more typical of bone marrow production problems (chronic ehrlichiosis, aplastic anemia, myelophthisic disease, etc.).

   c. On a blood smear in the RBC monolayer area under the ×10 objective, normal dogs typically have greater than 18 WBCs per field (examine many fields, calculate average).

   d. The lowest platelet counts are typically seen with IMT (zero to two platelets per oil immersion field).

  2. Collect pretreatment serum for later analysis if desired (e.g., anti-platelet antibody titer, *Rickettsia rickettsii* titer (RMSF), *Ehrlichia* titer, etc.).

  3. Bone marrow aspirate or core biopsy to:

a. Assess megakaryocyte numbers.
b. Look for underlying diseases associated with IMT (such as lymphoma) or other causes of thrombocytopenia.
c. Obtain samples for an antimegakaryocyte antibody assay.
B. **Therapy for IMT** (See II. Initial diagnostic plan.)
1. Corticosteroids:
a. Prednisone or prednisolone 1 to 3 mg/kg PO q12h (induction dose) *or*
b. Dexamethasone 0.1 to 0.3 mg/kg IV or PO q12h (some believe dexamethasone is more effective than prednisone).
2. Stop any nonessential drugs. If drug therapy is essential, try to substitute a biochemically dissimilar drug. Potentially, any drug could be associated with hapten-mediated immune destruction (especially potentiated sulfonamides and cephalosporins) (see p. 692).
3. Transfuse to manage anemia (based on clinical signs as described above). Transfusion of platelet-containing products (FWB or platelet-rich plasma) may be appropriate if the patient needs emergency surgery or if there is life-threatening hemorrhage (e.g., hemorrhage in the brain or lungs). However, the benefit is expected to be small and transient due to the rapid rate of destruction of platelets in this disease and the very low platelet yield in these products.
4. Other medications used to treat IMT, particularly in refractory cases (efficacy not well documented in dogs):
a. Vincristine 0.01 to 0.025 mg/kg slowly IV weekly.
b. Danazol 5 mg/kg PO q12h (induction dose).
c. Azathioprine 2 mg/kg PO q24h (induction dose).
d. Cyclophosphamide 200 mg/m^2 PO or IV weekly.
II. **Anticoagulant rodenticide toxicity (and hemophilias)** (see also p. 184 and II. plan above).
A. The diagnosis of anticoagulant rodenticide toxicity can often be confirmed by the dramatic response to vitamin K therapy within 12 to 24 hours. However, it is ideal to collect plasma pretreatment for laboratory confirmation or to save for future evaluation if the animal has a poor response to vitamin K. Tests to consider:
1. Coagulation profile: APTT, PT, thrombin time (TT), FDP, fibrinogen. (See p. 687 for sample collection and interpretation.)
2. PIVKA (proteins induced by vitamin K antagonists) test to confirm vitamin K deficiency.
3. Analysis to identify the specific toxicant (contact your local diagnostic laboratory). This can be helpful in determining the appropriate dose and duration of vitamin K therapy.
4. Specific coagulation factor analysis to diagnose hemophilias.
B. Treatment:
1. Vitamin K$_1$ (phytonadione) is appropriate while diagnostic tests are pending.
a. Loading dose: 5 mg/kg SC in several sites (use a small-gauge needle).
b. Within 6 to 12 hours, follow with 2.5 mg/kg PO q12h for several days, followed by 2.5 mg/kg q24h for the expected serum life span of the toxicant (3 to 6 weeks if unknown).
c. Check the PT 2 days after stopping vitamin K. If prolonged, continue therapy 1 week, discontinue vitamin K, wait 2 days, and then recheck PT.
d. The dose schedule above is adequate for treating toxicoses with second-generation anticoagulants (currently the most common toxicoses). Lower doses may be acceptable for some of the toxi-

cants. Adjust dose and duration of therapy to the specific toxicant if known.

2. Transfusion:
   a. See emergency transfusion recommendations above.
   b. For controlling hemorrhage in severe cases, transfuse FFP or FWB.
   c. If the patient has known hemophilia A (factor VIII deficiency), cryoprecipitate is ideal.
   d. To manage both a severe anemia and control hemorrhage, consider:
      i. FWB.
      ii. PRBCs and FFP.
      or
      iii. FFP and autotransfusion (if recent hemorrhage into a body cavity).

3. Removal of stomach contents is not recommended for patients with bleeding tendencies because of the risk of hemorrhage and because anticoagulant rodenticide exposure precedes clinical signs by several days.

III. **Disseminated intravascular coagulation** (see Initial diagnostic plan above; see also p. 44).
   A. Further diagnostic testing to consider:
      1. Collect pretreatment plasma for a coagulation profile (see p. 687 for sample collection and interpretation).
      2. Based on history and physical examination, perform tests to identify the underlying cause (laboratory tests, radiographs, ultrasound, cytology, etc.).
   B. Treatment:
      1. **Treat the inciting cause**.
      2. Administer **fluid therapy** to improve tissue perfusion, inhibit vascular stasis, and dilute coagulation and fibrinolytic factors.
      3. Provide **supportive care** as described above (correct acid-base and electrolyte abnormalities, warm if hypothermic, nursing care, nutrition).
      4. Transfusion:
         a. **FFP** to supply functional coagulation proteins (repeat until bleeding is controlled).
         or
         b. If concurrent anemia warrants therapy, use FWB or PRBCs with FFP.
      5. Heparin therapy is most appropriate in cases with evidence of ongoing thrombosis or embolism or when heparin is given along with a source of AT III (transfusion of FFP or FWB). Many dose schedules are available with the lower doses suggested for those with predominant signs of hemorrhage and higher doses for those with ongoing microthrombosis:
         a. Minidose 5 to 10 IU/kg SC q8h.
         b. Low dose 75 to 200 IU/kg SC q8h.
         c. Intermediate dose 300 to 500 IU/kg SC or IV q8h.
         d. High dose 750 to 1000 IU/kg SC or IV q8h (adjust dose to prolong APTT by 1.5 to 2.0-fold normal).
         e. Add heparin to the bag prior to transfusion (2 IU/mL of plasma).

IV. **von Willebrand's disease** (vWD) see Initial diagnostic plan above).
   A. Further diagnostic testing to consider (if bleeding with a normal platelet count and normal ACT):
      1. Buccal mucosal bleeding time (BMBT)—only appropriate if the

platelet count is greater than $100,000/\mu L$ because thrombocytopenia can cause prolonged bleeding time.

a. This procedure is typically done without sedation in dogs, whereas cats are usually sedated (e.g., ketamine).

b. Using gauze around the muzzle, tie the lip so that the buccal mucosa is exposed and the veins are slightly engorged.

c. Using a template device (Simplate R, Organon Teknica, Durham, NC), make two small incisions in the buccal mucosa.

d. Without touching the incisions, periodically blot the accumulating blood.

e. Note the time from incision until hemorrhage stops. Normal is less than 3 minutes for dogs and cats.

2. If the BMBT is prolonged:

a. Consider platelet function disorders, including:

i. NSAID exposure.

ii. vWD (any breed).

iii. Congenital thrombopathies (basset hounds and otterhounds).

iv. Disorders secondary to systemic illness (severe azotemia, liver disease, malignancies).

b. Reevaluate history to rule out drug-induced thrombopathies.

c. Collect plasma for von Willebrand's factor (vWF) analysis (if there was severe hemorrhage causing hypoproteinemia, wait several weeks after the crisis to do this testing).

3. If the BMBT is normal (along with a normal ACT and platelet count), but the patient is bleeding, reexamine the bleeding areas for vascular-related problems and do a coagulation profile to further evaluate the coagulation cascade (e.g., to assess the accuracy of the ACT or identify a rare factor VII deficiency).

B. Treatment.

1. Transfusion:

a. Indications: vWD with active hemorrhage or prior to surgery.

b. Blood component therapy: cryoprecipitate or FFP.

c. Cryoprecipitate:

i. A concentrated source of vWF, factor VIII, and fibrinogen produced from 1 unit of FFP.

ii. Preferred over FFP because there is less risk of volume overload.

iii. Transfuse 1 unit/10 kg body weight; repeat until bleeding controlled.

or

d. FFP: starting dose 10 mL/kg; repeat until bleeding controlled.

2. DDAVP (1-desamino-8-D-arginine vasopressin):

a. A synthetic analogue of vasopressin with fewer pressor effects.

b. Can increase the release of vWF from endothelial cells (if there is any vWF stored).

c. Dose 1 μ/kg SC or IV (diluted with 0.9% NaCl and given slowly over 10 to 20 minutes).

d. vWF levels may increase within 10 minutes of injection and last several hours.

e. Repeated doses would not be expected to be beneficial.

f. Efficacy unproven, but this therapy appears relatively safe.

3. Thyroxine (T_4).

a. There are conflicting results in studies evaluating the association of hypothyroidism with vWD and the benefits of T_4 supplementation in vWD in dogs.

b. If you choose to supplement T_4, collect serum for analysis of thyroid status prior to treatment. The total T_4 measured at the time of the hemorrhagic episode may be low because of stress, leading to an incorrect diagnosis of hypothyroidism in some animals. The canine thyroid-stimulating hormone (TSH) level and free T_4 (measured by equilibrium dialysis) are less likely to be affected by stress than the total T_4.

4. Avoid drugs known to adversely affect platelet function, such as NSAIDs, antibiotics (e.g., sulfonamides, ampicillin, chloramphenicol), antihistamines, theophylline, phenothiazines, heparin, and estrogen.

REFERENCES

Couto CG: Spontaneous bleeding disorders. *In* Bonagura JD, ed: Current Veterinary Therapy XII. Small Animal Practice. Philadelphia, WB Saunders, 1995, pp 457–461.

Green RA, Thomas JS: Hemostatic disorders: Coagulopathies and thrombosis. *In* Ettinger SJ, Feldman EC, eds: Textbook of Veterinary Internal Medicine. Philadelphia, WB Saunders,1995, pp 1946–1963.

Lewis DC: Management of refractory immune thrombocytopenia. *In* Proceedings of the 15th Annual Forum of the American College of Veterinary Internal Medicine, 1997, pp 94–96.

Mount ME, Woody BJ, Murphy MJ: The anticoagulant rodenticides. *In* Kirk RW, ed: Current Veterinary Therapy IX. Small Animal Practice. Philadelphia, WB Saunders, 1986, pp 156–165.

Thomas JS: von Willebrand's disease in the dog and cat. Vet Clin North Am Small Anim Pract 26:1089–1109, 1996.

Cardiac Emergencies

Cardiac emergencies seldom allow the luxury of a well-pondered response. Irreversible brain damage usually occurs within 3½ to 4 minutes following cardiac arrest. Consequently, being adequately prepared is the most important step in managing a cardiac emergency.

...........PREPARATION

1. Maintain an adequately stocked emergency cart or kit (see also p. 948).
2. Know how to intubate, and begin respirations.
3. Know how to record an ECG, and be able to identify arrhythmias.
4. Be familiar with drugs used and location of equipment.
5. Know how to administer external cardiac massage.
6. Develop a system for signaling hospital staff that an emergency exists.
7. Practice the team approach until each member of the team is confident.
8. Hold regular emergency "drills" to maintain competence.
9. Have annual continuing education (CE) courses on advances in cardiac emergencies.

...........CARDIOPULMONARY RESUSCITATION (CPR)
(see also Figs. 1–1, 1–2)

...........Cardiopulmonary Arrest

Cardiopulmonary arrest (CPA) is the abrupt, unexpected cessation of spontaneous and effective ventilation and systemic perfusion.

Predisposing causes of CPA:

1. Cardiac dysrhythmia (see p. 61).
   a. Ventricular asystole.
   b. Nonperfusing rhythm.
   c. Ventricular fibrillation.

2. Respiratory system disease—is pneumonia, thoracic effusions, neoplasia, laryngeal paralysis.
3. Multisystem severe trauma.
4. Septicemia and endotoxemia.
5. Prolonged seizures.
6. Electric shock.

   Physiologic predisposing causes of CPA:

1. Vagal stimulation.
2. Cellular hypoxia.
3. Acid-base and electrolyte abnormalities.
4. Anesthetic agents.
5. Polysystemic trauma, especially involving the chest.
6. Systemic metabolic disease.

> The greatest risk factors for CPA in animals are anesthetic accidents resulting in hypoxemia and life-threatening arrhythmias. Bradycardia may be present before CPA develops.

■ DIAGNOSIS OF CARDIOPULMONARY ARREST

Absence of ventilation and presence of cyanosis

Absence of palpable pulse

Absence of heart sounds

ECG evidence of asystole or ventricular flutter or fibrillation

Dilation of pupils

##........... Goals of CPR

1. Institute artificial cardiovascular and respiratory support.
2. Identify arrhythmias and institute immediate therapy.
3. Provide continuous support to stabilize cardiovascular function.

> Rapid recognition of impending CPA and a trained team approach of at least two people to manage the CPA with CPR will provide the best results.

##........... Basic Life Support

1. Assess and establish the unresponsiveness of the airway.
   a. Check the airway for foreign material.
   b. Position the animal in ventral recumbency for preparation for intubation.
   c. Intubate with endotracheal tube.
2. Begin ventilation with an initial two long breaths (2 seconds), then go to a rate of 12 to 20/min. The preferred technique is endotracheal intubation and ventilation with an Ambu bag, the reservoir of an anesthetic machine, or a mechanical ventilator. Use 100% oxygen at flow rate of 150 mL/kg/min.
3. If two people are available for CPR (the desired approach), then begin ventilation and compression in an animal weighing less than 7 kg at 120 times per minute and in animals weighing more than 7 kg at 80 to 100

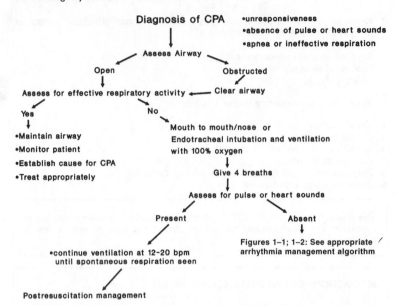

Figure I-3. Diagnosis of cardiopulmonary arrest (CPA). This general algorithm should be followed in all cases of CPA. These principles should be adhered to throughout the resuscitation attempt, including during interventions for arrhythmia management. Please refer to the relevant section of the text for a more detailed discussion. ECG, electrocardiogram, SCV, simultaneous compression ventilation. (From Miller MS, Tilley LP: Manual of Canine and Feline Cardiology, ed 2. Philadelphia, WB Saunders, 1995, p 441.)

times per minute. If one person can compress the abdomen between thoracic compressions, this will increase venous return and decrease arterial runoff during external thoracic compression.

4. If only one person is available for CPR, the ratio of ventilation to chest compression is 15:2, i.e., give 15 chest compressions, then two long ventilations.

5. Support cardiopulmonary circulation. Animals weighing less than 7 kg should be in lateral recumbency with the sternum parallel to the tabletop. Animals weighing more than 7 kg are placed in dorsal recumbency with the animal supported so that it cannot shift position. The cardiac compression-to-ventilation ratio should be 1:1. You induce breathing each time you compress the animal's thoracic wall.

6. Monitor the effectiveness of external thoracic compressions. Monitor the pulse, although it is the venous pulse that is most affected, and arterial pulse monitoring is not very effective. Use pulse oximetry to provide information about hemoglobin saturation. You should observe an improvement in oximetry values and mucous membrane color. Evaluate cardiac rhythm with ECG.

■ OPEN CHEST CARDIAC MASSAGE

1. Open chest massage requires an emergency left-sided thoracotomy, together with a pericardiotomy. The incision is made in the left lateral chest wall just behind the elbow, going ½ in. more caudal for every 5 kg of body weight. Use blunt pointed Mayo scissors to penetrate between the fifth or sixth intercostal space near the costochondral junction and penetrate the pleural space. Use a rib spreader to enlarge the opening and visualize the heart. Open the pericardium near its apex. Lift the heart out of the pericardial sac to begin massage. Initiate compression at the apex of the heart at a rate of 60 to 100 compressions per minute.
2. Following successful development of normal cardiac systole, the chest is irrigated with sterile saline and antibiotics and closed by aseptic closure.

............**Asystole** (see Fig. 1–2)

1. If unable to stimulate a heartbeat by massage alone, inject epinephrine 0.2 to 0.4 mg/kg diluted with 5 ml of sterile water via catheter through the endotracheal tube and ventilate vigorously for four to five breaths. Epinephrine 0.2 mg/kg may also be given by the IV or interosseous route. The intracardiac (IC) route of administration should be used only as a last resort. If the IC route is elected, be sure that the drug is actually injected into the lumen of the left ventricle.
2. Continue CPR, checking the lingual or femoral pulse to be sure that it is effective.
3. Establish an IV line (preferably with the catheter placed to the level of the right atrium), and begin rapid infusion of lactated Ringer's solution. Do not exceed the rate of 90 mL/kg/hr.
4. Begin abdominal compressions in between thoracic compressions, and then wrap the abdomen and pelvic limbs tightly to increase venous return and augment cerebral perfusion.
5. Reevaluate CPR and ECG findings.
6. If unable to establish a pulse or ventricular fibrillation within 5 minutes, open the chest at the left sixth intercostal space, open the pericardial sac, and begin cardiac massage. Do not incise the phrenic nerve.
   a. Cup the heart in the hand, and compress and release 80 to 100 times per minute, allowing for ventricular filling each time. Digital occlusion of the descending aorta will improve cerebral perfusion.
   b. Compress the heart from apex to base, being careful not to twist the heart on its long axis.
7. If mechanical systole returns but the heart rate is below normal, administer atropine 0.05 mg/kg IV or 0.10 mg/kg intratracheally (IT). If atropine is ineffective, use either epinephrine 0.1 μg/kg/min, dopamine 10 μg/kg/min, isoproterenol 0.01 μg/kg/min, or dobutamine, 10 μg/kg/min IV.
8. If mechanical systole returns and the heart rate is normal, administer dobutamine hydrochloride at a rate of 2.5 μg/kg/min IV by adding 250 mg (one vial) to 1000 mL of D5W at an infusion rate of approximately 1 drop/kg/min using a standard microdrip infusion system.
9. If another arrhythmia develops, continue CPR and treat as indicated (see Ventricular Fibrillation and Electromechanical Dissociation and Idioventricular Rhythm below).

............Ventricular Fibrillation (Figs. 1–4 and 1–5)

1. Initiate or continue CPR.
2. Defibrillate.
   a. Use a direct current (DC) defibrillator. If efforts are unsuccessful, double the energy dose; if still unsuccessful, repeat epinephrine and repeat defibrillation. Be sure to use adequate amounts of electrode paste on the skin. Do not use alcohol, because it is flammable. If using internal defibrillation, moisten the heart with saline.
   b. For chemical defibrillation, mix potassium chloride 1 mEq/kg with acetylcholine 6 mg/kg, and inject IC.
   c. Aggressive external massage is often sufficient to initiate a sinus rhythm in the cat, especially when fibrillation is associated with induction of anesthesia.

............Electromechanical Dissociation and Idioventricular Rhythm (Fig. 1–6)

1. Verify the rhythm. There is no pulse associated with the ECG and no mechanical systole taking place.
2. Initiate or continue CPR.
3. Administer epinephrine 0.2 to 0.4 mg/kg, diluted with 5 mL of sterile water endotracheally.
4. Administer dexamethasone sodium phosphate 2.0 mg/kg IV.
5. If there is no response, repeat epinephrine and dexamethasone.
6. If therapy is effective, proceed with postarrest procedures; if they are ineffective, proceed with thoracotomy and internal cardiac massage.

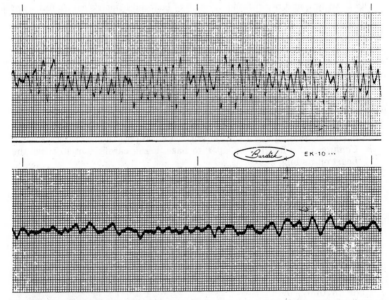

Figure 1–4. Ventricular fibrillation may be coarse, as in the upper tracing, or fine, as in the lower tracing. Patients with coarse ventricular fibrillation are easier to defibrillate.

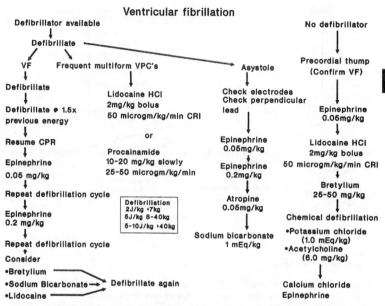

Figure 1-5. Ventricular fibrillation (VF). This algorithm for the management of VF is divided according to the availability of a defibrillator. After each intervention the electrocardiogram should be reevaluated and the next step initiated if VF is still seen. If a new arrhythmia develops, the appropriate algorithm should be selected. If sinus rhythm is seen, postresuscitation management should be instituted (see text). Please note the increasing dose for epinephrine as we progress through the algorithm. VPCs, ventricular premature complexes; CPR, cardiopulmonary resuscitation. (From Miller MS, Tilley LP: Manual of Canine and Feline Cardiology, ed 2. Philadelphia, WB Saunders, 1995, p 442.)

7. If internal cardiac massage is ineffective, try calcium gluconate 0.05 to 1.0 mg/kg IV, and continue CPR.

..........Heartbeat Following Resuscitative Efforts

1. Verify rhythm.
2. Continue respirations.

..........Postresuscitative Care

The major problems following CPR are neuronal dysfunction caused by CNS edema, hypercapnia (associated with hypoventilation), hypocapnia (hyperventilation), hypoperfusion, intracellular dysfunction, and cell membrane instability related to oxygenation and perfusion problems. Cardiac, renal, and pulmonary systems must be effectively supported. Pulmonary edema may have to be treated.

1. Support ventilation to achieve a $PaCO_2$ level of 25 to 35 mm Hg.
2. Support blood pressure using inotropic agents such as dobutamine or dopamine. Maintain a diastolic blood pressure above 60 mm Hg. If heart rate

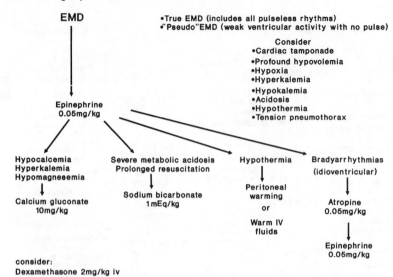

EMD

•True EMD (includes all pulseless rhythms)
•"Pseudo"EMD (weak ventricular activity with no pulse)

Consider
•Cardiac tamponade
•Profound hypovolemia
•Hypoxia
•Hyperkalemia
•Hypokalemia
•Acidosis
•Hypothermia
•Tension pneumothorax

Epinephrine
0.05mg/kg

Hypocalcemia
Hyperkalemia
Hypomagnesemia
↓
Calcium gluconate
10mg/kg

Severe metabolic acidosis
Prolonged resuscitation
↓
Sodium bicarbonate
1mEq/kg

Hypothermia
↓
Peritoneal
warming
or
Warm IV
fluids

Bradyarrhythmias
(idioventricular)
↓
Atropine
0.05mg/kg
↓
Epinephrine
0.05mg/kg

consider:
Dexamethasone 2mg/kg iv

Figure 1–6. Electromechanical dissociation (EMD). The EMD algorithm covers all rhythms where the electrocardiogram shows organized complexes but no clinically appreciable circulation is present. EMD is divided into "true" EMD, where no mechanical ventricular activity is seen, or pseudo-EMD, where weak mechanical ventricular activity is seen. Each of the many different factors that contribute to the development of EMD should be considered and managed (if recognized) when EMD is diagnosed. IV, intravenous. (From Miller MS, Tilley LP: Manual of Canine and Feline Cardiology, ed 2. Philadelphia, WB Saunders, 1995, p 443.)

slows, use atropine 0.02 mg/kg or glycopyrolate 0.01 mg/kg to increase heart rate.
3. Administer supplemental oxygen via nasal catheter (see p. 610).
4. Use therapy to reduce CNS edema (see p. 155).
5. Maintain fluid and electrolyte balance (see p. 585).
6. Antriarrhythmic therapy may be indicated with continuous rate infusion of lidocaine 50 μg/kg/min (see p. 63).
7. Control pulmonary edema (see p. 252).
8. Monitor renal function and urine output with indwelling cathether (see p. 486).

■ ADVANCED LIFE SUPPORT

Advanced cardiac life support includes the identification and correction of life-threatening arrhythmias such as ventricular fibrillation, pulseless ventricular tachycardia, and electrical mechanical dissociation.

Emergency Drugs to Have Available in Crash Cart

Epinephrine 0.1 to 0.2 mg/kg

Atropine 0.04 mg/kg IV; 0.1 mg/kg IT

(Box continued on following page)

■ ADVANCED LIFE SUPPORT *(Continued)*

Magnesium chloride 0.15 to 0.3 mEq/kg IV given over 2 to 10 minutes; 0.75 to 1.0 mEq/kg/day

Lidocaine (dogs) 2 to 8 mg/kg IV bolus followed by 50 to 100 µg/kg/min CRI (constant rate infusion)

Naloxone (dogs) 15 µg/kg IV; 30 µg/kg IV for EMD (electromechanical dissociation)

Sodium bicarbonate 0.5 to 2.0 mEq/kg IV

Methoxamine 0.1 to 0.8 mg/kg

Bretylium tosylate 10 mg/kg IV; 1 to 2 mg/min CRI

Emergency Drugs to Have Available Post Resuscitation

Dobutamine 5 to 10 µg/kg/min (dogs); 2.5 to 5 µg/kg/min (cats)

Mannitol 25% solution 0.25 to 1.0 g/kg IV

Furosemide 2 to 4 mg/kg t.i.d. to q.i.d. PO, IM, IV (dogs); 1 to 2 mg/kg b.i.d. to q.i.d. PO, IM, IV (cats)

Lidocaine (dogs) 2 to 8 mg/kg IV bolus followed by 50 to 100 µg/kg/min CRI

Verapamil 0.05 to 0.15 mg/kg IV slowly over 15 minutes; 2 to 10 µg/kg/min CRI

Sodium bicarbonate 0.5 to 2.0 mEq/kg IV

Methoxamine 0.1 to 0.8 mg/kg

Bretylium tosylate 10 mg/kg IV; 1 to 2 mg/min CRI

............OTHER CARDIAC ARRHYTHMIAS REQUIRING EMERGENCY TREATMENT

............Ventricular Arrhythmias

Ventricular arrhythmias encompass a wide range of clinical syndromes that vary greatly in their clinical significance and signs, depending on the rate, frequency, and prematurity of the arrhythmia and the severity of coexisting heart disease. It is important to emphasize that ventricular arrhythmias can occur in the absence of cardiac disease secondary to conditions such as thoracic trauma, sepsis, systemic inflammatory syndromes, pancreatitis, gastric dilation–volvulus, splenic disease, hypoxia, uremia, and acid-base and electrolyte disturbances. Common cardiac causes of ventricular arrhythmias include dilated cardiomyopathy, endstage degenerative valvular disease, infectious endocarditis, myocarditis, and cardiac neoplasia. In the cat, hypertrophic or restrictive cardiomyopathy and hyperthyroid heart disease are common causes of ventricular arrhythmias. In addition to structural heart disease or systemic diseases, arrhythmias may develop as an adverse effect of some drugs such as digoxin, dobutamine, aminophylline, and anesthetic agents (Fig. 1–7).

............Diagnosis

The physical examination finding of an arrhythmia associated with pulse deficits is worrisome for a ventricular arrhythmia. The ECG is critical to the accurate diagnosis of a ventricular arrhythmia. Ventricular arrhythmias arise from ectopic foci in the ventricles whereby the wave of depolarization is spread cell by cell rather than by the fast conduction tissue. This causes the QRS complex to be wide and bizarre. Other ECG features include a T wave polarity that is opposite the QRS, and nonrelated P waves. Ventricular arrhythmias

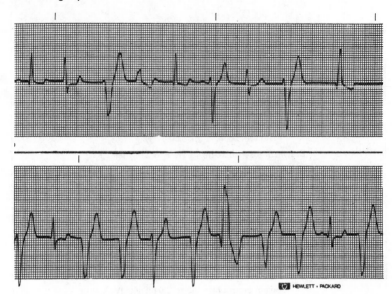

Figure I-7. Four or more ventricular premature complexes (VPCs) in succession constitute ventricular tachycardia. Multifocal VPCs are more serious than those that are unifocal.

may manifest as isolated ventricular premature complexes (VPCs), ventricular couplets or triplets, ventricular bigeminy, or ventricular tachycardia (VT). Relatively "slow ventricular tachycardia," often termed "idioventricular tachycardia," is common in the dog and may not be as hemodynamically significant as more rapid VT. Idioventricular tachycardia usually has a rate of less than 130 bpm and may alternate spontaneously with sinus arrhythmia.

.... Treatment

The decision to treat ventricular arrhythmias must factor in the hemodynamic significance and the risk of sudden cardiac death posed by the arrhythmia. Many ventricular arrhythmias, such as isolated VPCs, slow ventricular bigeminy, or idioventricular tachycardia, do not warrant specific antiarrhythmic therapy other than correcting the underlying disease process. For example, arrhythmias may be present in dogs or cats that are hypoxic secondary to severe pulmonary edema. Initial therapy in these animals should focus on management of the congestive heart failure (furosemide, oxygen) rather than an antiarrhythmic agent. Many times the arrhythmia will resolve or lessen with afterload reduction. However, if a serious arrhythmia persists, then antiarrhythmic therapy is warranted. In addition to controlling congestive heart failure and providing adequate oxygenation, severe hypovolemia, anemia, or an acid-base or electrolyte disturbance should be corrected prior to specific antiarrhythmic therapy. Serious ventricular arrhythmias causing hemodynamic compromise, such as frequent runs or sustained rapid VT (>140/min in the dog; >220/min in the cat), or frequent, multiform, R-on-T VPCs, do require immediate treatment.

Table 1–11. Antiarrhythmic Drug Therapy

Drug	Dog	Cat
Atenolol	0.25–1.0 mg/kg PO q12–24h	6.25–12.5 mg/cat PO q12–24 hr
Digoxin	0.006 mg/kg PO q12h	0.03 mg/cat PO q48h
Diltiazem	0.5–1.5 mg/kg PO q8h	7.5 mg/cat PO q8h
Lidocaine	2 mg/kg IV slowly up to 8 mg/kg by bolus Maintenance: CRI 30–80 μg/kg/min	0.25–1.0 mg/kg IV slowly over 5 min
Mexiletine	5–8 mg/kg PO q8h	None
Procainamide	4 mg/kg IV bolus slowly; up to 16 mg/kg 10 mg/kg IM q8h 8–20 mg/kg PO q6–8h CRI 25–40 μg/kg/min	None
Propranolol	0.04–0.06 mg/kg IV slowly 0.2–1.0 mg/kg PO q6–8h	0.04–0.06 mg/kg IV slowly 2.5–5.0 mg/cat PO q8h
Quinidine	6–20 mg/kg IM q6–8h 8–20 mg/kg PO q6–8h	None
Tocainide	10–20 mg/kg PO q8h	None
Esmolol	0.05–0.1 mg/kg slow IV	Same
Sotolol	40–120 mg/kg PO q12h	2 mg/kg PO q12h

CRI, constant-rate infusion.

............Dog

1. Lidocaine (without epinephrine) 2 mg/kg IV bolus. This bolus could be repeated three times within 15 minutes (total of 8 mg/kg) until control of VT is accomplished. If successful, lidocaine CRI is given at 30 to 80 μg/kg/min. Signs of lidocaine toxicity include seizures and vomiting. If lidocaine is unsuccessful, correct potassium and magnesium deficiencies or try procainamide.
2. Procainamide 4 mg/kg slow IV bolus (over 3 minutes). This bolus could be repeated three times (total 16 mg/kg) until control of VT is accomplished. If successful, procainamide CRI is given at 25 to 40 μg/kg/min. Alternatively, if the clinical setting poses difficulties in management of a CRI, procainamide 10 mg/kg IM q6h could be used.
3. The majority of ventricular arrhythmias will be controlled with either lidocaine or procainamide in addition to management of the underlying disease. However, if neither lidocaine nor procainamide control the arrhythmia, consultation with a veterinary cardiologist is recommended.
4. Chronic oral antiarrhythmic therapy may or may not be necessary after the acute management of VT. The decision to continue antiarrhythmic therapy depends on the underlying disease and expectation of the persistent arrhythmias. Oral antiarrhythmic therapy may also be appropriate in which a serious ventricular arrhythmia is recognized but the patient does not required hospitalization, such as a syncopal boxer dog with intermittent VT and no structural heart disease. It should be emphasized that asymptomatic, low-grade ventricular arrhythmias probably do not require treatment. However, if maintenance therapy for ventricular arrhythmias is needed, one of the following agents could be used. The choice of oral drug depends on

the underlying disease process, clinician familiarity, class of drug, dosing frequency, owner compliance, concurrent medications, cost, and the adverse effects of the drug.

a. Procainamide 10 to 20 mg/kg PO q6–8h.

b. Sotolol 40 to 120 mg per dog PO q12h (start low, titrate upward).

c. Mexiletine 5 to 8 mg/kg PO q8h.

d. Atenolol 0.25 to 1.0 mg/kg PO q12–24h (start low, titrate upward).

e. Tocainide 10 to 20 mg/kg PO q8h.

.... Cat

1. Lidocaine (without epinephine) should be used with extreme caution in the cat because of its susceptibility to neurotoxicity. It may also cause severe sinus bradycardia and sinus arrest. Dose is a fraction of the dog dose: 0.2 to 1.0 mg/kg slow IV over 5 minutes. If successful, CRI at 10 to 20 μg/kg/min could be continued if needed.

2. β-Blockers such as propranolol or esmolol are preferred by some in the cat for acute management of severe ventricular arrhythmias, especially if hypertrophic or restrictive cardiomyopathy or hyperthyroidism is the underlying disease.

a. Propanolol 0.02 to 0.06 mg/kg slow IV over 5 minutes.

b. Esmolol 0.05 to 0.1 mg/kg slow IV over 5 minutes.

3. For chronic oral ventricular antiarrhythmic therapy, one of the following drugs could be used:

a. Propranolol 2.5 to 5 mg PO q8h.

Table 1–12. Drugs to Treat Cardiac Arrhythmia in the Cat

Drug	Dosage and Route of Administration	Indications
Atropine sulfate	SC, IM, IV, IT: 0.04 mg/kg q4–6h	Sinus bradycardia, AV block
Calcium chloride	IC, IV: 0.05–0.10 mL of 10% solution/kg	Ventricular asystole
Digoxin (Lanoxin) 0.125 mg tablet; 0.05 mg/mL elixir	Oral: 0.005 mg/kg BW, q48h (i.e., ¼ of 0.125-mg tablet b.i.d. for 6-kg cat)	Congestive heart failure, APCs, atrial tachycardia, atrial fibrillation and atrial flutter, dilated cardiomyopathy
Isoproterenol (Isuprel 0.2 mg/ mL injectable)	IV 0.5 mg/250 mL of D5W and titrate to effect	Sinus bradycardia, complete AV block
Propranolol (Inderal) 10-mg tablet; 1 mg/mL injectable	Oral: 2.5–5.0 mg for average 5-kg cat; higher doses to effect IV: 0.25 mg diluted in 1 mL saline, given as 0.2-mL boluses to effect	Sinus tachycardia, supraventricular tachycardia, ventricular arrhythmias, preexcitation arrhythmias, with digoxin for fibrillation; secondary hyperthyroidism/HCM

IT, intrathoracic; IC, intracardiac; BW, body weight; D5W, dextrose 5% in water; AV, atrioventricular; APCs, atrial premature contractions; HCM, hypertrophic cardiomyopathy.

Table 1–13. Synthetic Inotropic Agents

Drug	Dog	Cat
Dobutamine	2.5–10 µg/kg/min IV	2.5–10 µg/kg/min IV
Dopamine	2.0–8.0 µg/kg/min IV	2.0–8.0 µg/kg/min IV
Isoproterenol	0.01 µg/kg min IV	0.01 µg/kg/min IV

b. Atenolol 6.25 to 12.5 mg PO q12–24h.
c. Procainamide 2.5 mg/kg PO q8h.
d. Sotolol 2 mg/kg PO q12h.

............Supraventricular Arrhythmias

Supraventricular (SV) arrhythmias arise from ectopic foci within the atria and are commonly associated with atrial dilation and structural heart disease such as advanced degenerative valvular or congenital heart disease, cardiomyopathies, cardiac neoplasia, or advanced heartworm disease. Occasionally, SV arrhythmias will be associated with respiratory disease or other systemic disease. Sustained SV tachycardia in the absence of structural heart disease or systemic disease (especially in a Labrador retriever) is worrisome for the presence of an accessory pathway allowing propagation of the rhythm. SV arrhythmias may manifest as isolated SV premature complexes (SVPCs or atrial premature complexes), sustained or paroxysmal SV tachycardia (SVT, or atrial tachycardia), or atrial fibrillation or flutter (AF). AF is most commonly associated with dilated cardiomyopathy in the dog. Rarely, lone AF, i.e., AF with no underlying heart disease, may occur in giant-breed dogs. AF is rare in the cat because of its smaller size but is most commonly associated with hypertrophic or restrictive or dilated cardiomyopathies (Fig. 1–8).

............Diagnosis

The physical examination finding of an arrhythmia in a patient with congestive heart failure is worrisome for an SV arrhythmia. The ECG is critical to accurate diagnosis and management. ECG features include a typically normal QRS

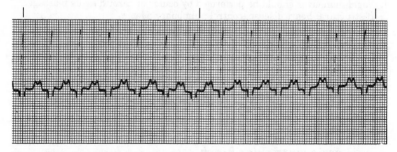

Figure 1–8. Supraventricular tachycardia usually has some degree of fusing between the T of the previous complex and the P of each succeeding complex, often forming an M-shaped configuration between R waves. The heart rate here is approximately 240 bpm. Note the very regular R–R interval.

conformation, and some evidence of atrial activity (P waves, flutter waves, or fibrillation waves).

.... Treatment

The decision to treat an SV arrhythmia depends on the ventricular rate and the hemodynamic significance of the arrhythmia. No treatment is usually required for asymptomatic isolated SVPCs, couplets, or triplets. Treatment may be warranted when the ventricular rate is high (>180/min in the dog), as ventricular filling and subsequently cardiac output is impaired. The goal of therapy many times is to slow the ventricular rate. Conversion to sinus rhythm is rarely possible in an animal with AF and congestive heart failure. However, conversion to sinus rhythm in an animal with sustained regular R–R interval SVT is entirely possible.

.... Dog

1. Vagal maneuver should be performed by ocular or carotid sinus massage.
2. If structural heart disease is present, control pulmonary edema, and if arrhythmia persists, administer digoxin 0.006 mg/kg PO q12h. Rapid oral digitalization may be accomplished by doubling the digoxin dose for 24 hours. Digoxin 0.005 mg/kg IV q1h up to four doses until effect may be used for an extremely rapid SVT in the setting of dilated cardiomyopathy and hypotension.
3. If no structural heart disease is present or if oral digoxin has not adequately controlled the ventricular rate, diltiazem 0.5 to 1.5 mg/kg PO q8h is recommended. For sustained rapid regular R–R interval SVT, diltiazem 0.1 to 0.25 mg/kg IV q2–4h as needed is recommended.
4. Alternatively, a β-blocker such as esmolol or propanolol may be used. Esmolol is an ultra-short-acting β-blocker (half-life is several minutes) which may be helpful in SVT or VT. The dose is 0.05 to 0.1 mg/kg slow IV titrated upward to effect or a cumulative dose of 0.5 mg/kg IV. IV propranolol dose is 0.04 to 0.06 mg/kg slowly.
5. If the SV arrhythmia has not responded to therapy, a sharp thump over the heart or ice water on the face may break a sustained SVT. Consultation with a veterinary cardiologist is also recommended. Misdiagnosis of the arrhythmia should be considered.

.... Cat

1. Vagal maneuver should be performed by ocular or carotid sinus massage.
2. If structural heart disease, control pulmonary edema.
3. Diltiazem 7.5 mg per cat PO q8h or propanolol 2.5 to 5.0 mg per cat PO q8h. (IV esmolol could be used at 0.05 to 0.1 mg/kg slow IV.)

.... Bradyarrhythmias

Sinus bradycardia is usually secondary to systemic disease or a result of drug therapy and thus rarely requires specific therapy. Hemodynamically significant bradyarrhythmias include high-grade atrioventricular (AV) block, sick sinus syndrome (SSS), and atrial standstill.

.... Atrioventricular Block

Complete or third-degree AV block or high-grade symptomatic second-degree AV block can be hemodynamically significant when ventricular rates are below 60 bpm/min in the dog. Typical clinical signs include weakness, syncope, leth-

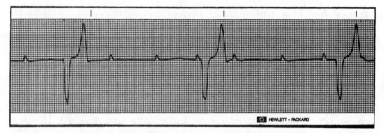

Figure 1-9. Third-degree atrioventricular heart block with a ventricular escape rhythm at 40 bpm. There is no correlation between the P waves and QRSs.

argy, anorexia, and occasionally seizures. Advanced AV block is usually caused by idiopathic degeneration of the AV node. Other less common associated conditions are digoxin toxicity, cardiomyopathy, infectious endocarditis, or myocarditis (Lyme disease). The diagnosis is made from an accurate interpretation of the ECG, which shows nonconducted P waves and ventricular escape beats. First- and low-grade second-degree AV block are not hemodynamically significant and may be normal variant (Fig. 1–9).

............Treatment

1. First- and low-grade second-degree block require no therapy.
2. Complete AV or symptomatic high-grade second-degree AV block (<60 bpm) should initially be treated with atropine 0.04 mg/kg IM. Follow-up ECG should be performed in 20 minutes. Atropine is rarely successful in complete AV block. Lidocaine should never be used for treatment of the ventricular escape rhythm associated with AV block.
3. Pacemaker implantation is the best therapy option for complete AV block secondary to idiopathic AV nodal degeneration. Consultation with a veterinary cardiologist or other specialist who implants pacemakers is recommended.

............Sick Sinus Syndrome

SSS is a disease of the sinus node most commonly recognized in the miniature schnauzer, although any dog may be affected. It usually results from an idiopathic degeneration of the sinus node in the dog. In the cat, sinus node disease is often associated with cardiomyopathy. The sinus node dysfunction may manifest as marked bradycardia with periods of sinus arrest followed by either junctional or ventricular escape complexes. A variant of SSS is the presence of bradycardia alternating with periods of SV tachycardia, often termed bradycardia-tachycardia syndrome. The most common clinical sign is syncope (rarely seizures) or exercise intolerance.

............Treatment in the Dog

1. Severe cases of SSS usually require pacemaker implantation for control of the clinical signs.
2. Less severe SSS may be managed medically, at least in the short term. Atropine 0.04 mg/kg IM is administered and a follow-up ECG is obtained 20 minutes later. If the atropine increased the heart rate and abolished the periods of sinus arrest without exacerbating any SVTs, then chronic oral

therapy may be attempted in the form of probanthine 0.5 to 1.5 mg/kg PO
q8h. Bronchodilators such as theophylline 10 mg/kg PO q8–12h or terbutaline 2.5 to 5 mg per dog PO q12h may also increase the heart rate and
could be used instead of or in addition to the probanthine. Vagolytic and
bronchodilator therapy may exacerbate the tachycardic episodes associated
with some SSSs.

............Atrial Standstill

Atrial standstill is most commonly associated with hyperkalemia. However,
occasionally it is associated with an atrial cardiomyopathy or silent atrium
syndrome. Persistent atrial standstill is most often recognized in the English
springer spaniel or the Siamese cat. Persistent atrial standstill is most effectively treated with pacemaker implantation, but atropine 0.04 mg/kg SC should
be attempted. Acute management of life-threatening hyperkalemia is reviewed
on p. 600. The ECG features of atrial standstill include a slow SV rhythm
(60 bpm in the dog; 100 bpm in the cat) with no visible atrial activity or P
wave in any lead (Fig. 1–10).

............Treatment of Atrial Standstill Secondary to Hyperkalemia (Dog or Cat)

1. Correct underlying cause if possible (e.g., relieve urethral obstruction).
2. Begin rapid IV infusion of 0.9% saline with or without D5W.
3. NaHCO$_3$ IV 1 to 2 mEq/kg slow IV over 20 minutes.
   or
4. Regular insulin IV 0.25 to 0.5 unit/kg with 2 g of dextrose per unit insulin.
   or
5. Calcium gluconate 20% 0.5 mL/kg slow IV over 10 minutes.

Regardless of the cause of the hyperkalemia, the above treatment should
improve the situation, usually within 15 to 30 minutes. The treatment of the
underlying cause of the hyperkalemia must be continued and is beyond these
emergency procedures.

............ACUTE CONGESTIVE HEART FAILURE

The majority of dogs and cats that present as emergencies with acute congestive
heart failure (CHF) have acquired heart disease, i.e., disease that develops
later in life as middle-aged or older animals. Congenital heart disease is much
less common than acquired disease, but in the dog, patent ductus arteriosus is
the most common cause of CHF. The most prevalent type of acquired heart
disease in the dog is chronic valvular disease, also known as mitral valve
disease or mitral valve endocardiosis (mitral regurgitation, MR). The AV valves
degenerate and gradually lose the ability to close effectively, which causes
abnormalities in blood flow. Typically, the degeneration of the valve is slowly
progressive, but acute exacerbation of this type of heart disease may result
when the chordae tendineae suddenly rupture or the animal ingests a big salt
load. Mitral valve disease tends to affect older, smaller breed dogs such as toy
poodles, Chihuahuas, and Cavalier King Charles spaniels. The second most
common type of acquired heart disease in the dog is dilated cardiomyopathy
(DCM), which is a primary myocardial disease in which the muscular wall of
the heart become thin and weak and the heart dilates. Contractility is diminished. There may be secondary mitral valve insufficiency because of stretching
of the valve annulus. This type of heart disease is commonly associated with
arrhythmias and affects large-breed dogs such as Doberman pinschers, Great
Danes, boxers, and Irish wolfhounds. Acute exacerbation of DCM may be

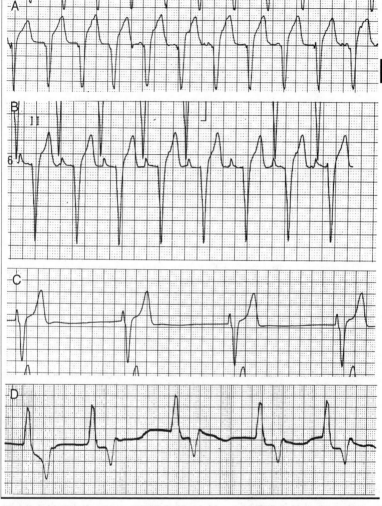

Figure 1–10. Comparison of four different electrocardiograms. A, Ventricular tachycardia. B, Sinus rhythm with right bundle-branch block. C, Persistent atrial standstill with ventricular escape rhythm. D, Probable sinoventricular rhythm with severe hyperkalemia.

related to the development of an arrhythmia. In cats, hypertrophic cardiomyopathy is by far the most common cause of heart disease. It is characterized by a stiff and noncompliant ventricle that fails to relax normally, thus causing left atrial enlargement. Other cardiomyopathies, such as restrictive or dilated, may also occur in the cat. Cats often develop acute CHF secondary to stress or arterial embolization.

The rapid diagnosis of CHF can often be made based on owner complaints, signalment, and physical examination. Owner complaints often include lethargy or weakness, tachypnea, dyspnea, and cough (rare in the cat), lack of appetite and weight loss, syncope (fainting), and abdominal distention or ascites (rare in the cat). Typical physical examination findings include a murmur or gallop sound, abnormal breath sounds, tachypnea, dyspnea, tachycardia, weak pulse quality, and pale mucous membrane color. Cardiac arrhythmias may be heard in patients with cardiomyopathies. The single most useful test to confirm CHF is a thoracic radiograph. However, the chest film should be postponed in severely dyspneic animals, especially if the diagnosis can be reached without the stress of radiology. The least stressful position for a dyspneic animal for taking radiographs is the standing lateral. Placing a severely dyspneic animal on its back for a ventral-dorsal radiograph may be life-threatening. In addition to radiography, accurate assessment of the ECG is essential to the successful management of the emergency cardiac patient. Cardiac rhythm disturbances, such as AF, SV and ventricular premature beats, and tachyarrhythmias, commonly occur in heart failure. The echocardiogram, although not essential to the diagnosis of CHF, is a useful and noninvasive method (low stress) for establishing the diagnosis.

Echocardiography can be user dependent, and the quality of the study depends not only on the experience of the sonographer but also on the quality of the echo machine. The echocardiogram is particularly useful in the diagnosis of pericardial effusion, dilated or hypertrophic cardiomyopathy, cardiac neoplasia, and endocarditis.

The medical treatment of CHF is designed to improve cardiac output and relieve clinical signs. The immediate goal of emergency therapy is to reduce abnormal fluid accumulations and provide adequate cardiac output by either increasing contractility, decreasing afterload (reducing resistance to ejection of blood), or normalizing a cardiac dysrhythmia. For acute fulminant cardiogenic pulmonary edema, some of the initial database may be postponed and administration of either IV or IM furosemide and an oxygen-rich environment (40%) is recommended. In addition to the diuretic, parenteral low-dose morphine (dog) may reduce the anxiety and provide further venodilation. Nitroglycerin, either in the form of a 2% paste or slow-release patch, may further reduce congestion. Strict cage rest is of the utmost importance.

1. Furosemide (Lasix) 2 to 4 mg/kg IV or IM q2–12 h as needed.
2. Morphine (dog only) 0.1 mg/kg IV titrated up to 0.5 mg/kg or to effect for relief of anxiety, *or* 1.0 mg/kg SQ.
3. Nitroglycerin 2% paste 0.25 in. for small dogs and cats and up to 1 in. for large dogs transdermally (inner ear pinnae, groin, or axilla) as needed q8h for the first 24 hours. Wear gloves to apply.
4. Supplemental oxygen therapy (40%).
5. Aminophylline 10 mg/kg (dog), 4 mg/kg (cat) IM or *slow* IV (dilute in D5W) q8h. This drug is primarily a bronchodilator and may assist in dyspnea by its actions on bronchodilation and strengthening muscles of respirations. This drug may promote tachyarrhythmias and may be harmful if AF or ventricular tachycardia or hypertrophic cardiomyopathy is present.

Improvement in dyspnea should occur within 30 minutes. However, if no improvement is seen, a repeat dose of furosemide is advised. Some patients will continue to be refractory to therapy despite repeated doses of the diuretic. Vasodilation should be considered in patients with CHF secondary to systolic heart failure (i.e., MR or DCM) and normal blood pressure. If the patient is severely hypotensive, vasodilation and even diuretic therapy may be detrimental. For the average CHF secondary to systolic dysfunction, angiotensin-converting enzyme (ACE) inhibitors are recommended as soon as the patient is able to take oral medications. The most commonly used ACE inhibitors in veterinary medicine are:

1. Enalapril 0.5 mg/kg PO q12–24h.
2. Benazepril 0.5 mg/kg PO q24h.

Other vasodilators that may be useful include hydralazine and sodium nitroprusside. Hydralazine is a potent afterload reducer (arterial dilator) and is available for either PO or IV administration. Hydralazine could be used in the emergency management of the normotensive CHF patient with MR or DCM and severe pulmonary edema. The patient administered hydralazine could be given it short term and then switched to an ACE-inhibitor once stable.

3. Hydralazine 0.5 to 2 mg/kg IV or PO (monitor blood pressure).

Sodium nitroprusside is a potent balanced vasodilator used for the refractory and severe CHF patient. Careful monitoring of blood pressure is required. The goal of sodium nitroprusside therapy is a mean arterial pressure of 60 to 70 mm Hg.

4. Sodium nitroprusside 1 to 10 µg/kg/min CRI.

If the patient is hypotensive and has refractory CHF despite the above therapy, then increasing cardiac output by way of increased contractility is advised. Dobutamine, primarily a β-agonist, will improve cardiac output with minimal effects on heart rate in low doses. Dobutamine must be given as a CRI with ECG monitoring. Despite minimal effects on the heart rate, sinus tachycardia may develop as well as ventricular arrhythmias and speed the ventricular rate response of AF.

Dobutamine 2.5 to 10 µg/kg/min CRI (dilute in D5W). If the patient is in atrial fibrillation, recommend digitalization prior to dobutamine. Cats are more sensitive to the effects of dobutamine than dogs.

Compared with dobutamine, the positive inotropic force of digoxin is slight. Because of its long half-life (24 hours in the dog, 60 hours in the cat), its use in the emergency management of CHF is limited. It is extremely useful in the chronic management of CHF secondary to DCM or advanced MR. The emergency clinical setting in which digoxin is useful is a patient with an SVT or AF with CHF. Digoxin may be given rapidly by way of a PO loading dose or IV, but the risk of digoxin toxicity is greater than with routine dosing.

1. Digoxin 0.006 mg/kg PO q12h. For rapid oral digitalization, double the dose for the first 24 hours (dog).
2. Digoxin 0.0005 mg/kg IV q1h for 4 hours or to effect (dog).
3. Digoxin 0.03 mg q48h in dilated cardiomyopathy (cat).

Cats with CHF often manifest with pleural effusion, in addition to pulmonary edema. If the pleural effusion is of significant quantity, the most effective immediate therapeutic maneuver is the removal of the fluid, in addition to diuretic therapy. After aseptic preparation of the skin and light sedation (if needed), a needle or catheter is inserted in the area of the seventh intercostal space just above the costochondral junction. Sometimes, both sides of the chest will need to be tapped. We prefer an 18- or 16-gauge over-the-needle catheter with multiple small side holes when performing a therapeutic thoracocentesis.

Once the diagnosis and initial urgent management of CHF have been performed, a plan for continued management and monitoring is formulated. The therapeutic plan is tailored to the individual patient based on the pathophysiology of the CHF and concurrent diseases. An important and often overlooked part of the successful emergency management of CHF is the open communication with the owner regarding his or her emotional and financial ability to deal with both the immediate and long-term management of the animal's heart disease.

............SYSTEMIC THROMBOEMBOLISM

Systemic thromboembolism is one of the most devastating complications associated with the feline heart disease. All types of feline myocardial disease (hypertrophic cardiomyopathy, restrictive cardiomyopathy, and dilated cardiomyopathy) may result in thromboembolism. A severely enlarged left atrium may be a risk factor. Systemic thromboembolism is rarely reported in the dog and is typically associated with neoplasia, sepsis, Cushing's disease, protein-losing nephropathy, or other hypercoaguable states. The most common site of embolization is the caudal aorta trifurcation (hindlegs). Other, less common sites include the front leg, kidneys, gastrointestinal tract, or cerebrum. The diagnosis is usually based on clinical findings of acute-onset paraparesis or paralysis and pain associated with absent or diminished femoral pulses and cool temperature of the hindlegs. Less commonly, a front leg may be affected. The affected footpads or nail beds may be pale or cyanotic. Vocalization and anxiety are common. Tachypnea or respiratory distress is typically present because two thirds of cats have concurrent CHF. Auscultation of a murmur, gallop sound, or arrhythmia is common.

Client education is an important part of the emergency management of systemic thromboembolism. Owners should be aware of the guarded short- and long-term prognosis. In one study of 100 cats, approximately 60% to 70% of cats were euthanized or died during the initial thromboembolic episode. The prognosis is typically better with partial or front leg embolism. The expected course of recovery is days to weeks for full recovery of function to the legs. Long-term prognosis varies between 2 months and several years; however, the average is approximately 11 months with treatment.

............Treatment

1. Treatment of the patient's heart disease should be addressed. If CHF is present, furosemide; supplemental oxygen therapy; or thoracocentesis, individually or in combination, may be beneficial. Avoid a nonselective β-blocker such as propranolol because it may enhance peripheral vasoconstriction.
2. Heparin is a relatively safe and rapid-onset anticoagulant commonly used in general practice. It has no effect on the established clot; however, it prevents further activation of the coagulation cascade. The initial dose typically is given IV, then followed with SC administrations every 8 hours. The initial IV dose is 100 to 200 units/kg and the subsequent SC dose is 200 to 300 units/kg (cat) (100 units/kg IV, then 100 units/kg SC q8h in the dog). The dose is then ideally titrated to prolong the APTT approximately twofold.
3. Thrombolytic agents such as streptokinase and tissue plasminogen activator (t-PA) are used extensively in humans and infrequently in cats. These drugs are many times prohibitively expensive and carry a significant risk for bleeding complications and thus are rarely used in general practice. Ideal use is within the first 6 hours of blood clot formation. Careful monitoring of the coagulation profile, ECG, and electrolytes is recommended. When using a thrombolytic agent, heparin therapy should be postponed until completion.
   a. Streptokinase 90,000 IU IV over 20 to 30 minutes, then a CRI at 45,000 IU/hr for 3 hours.
   b. t-PA activator 0.25 mg to 1 mg/kg/hr for a total of 1 to 10 mg/kg IV to effect.
4. Butorphanol for analgesia at 0.1 to 0.2 mg/kg SC or IV q6–8h.
5. Acepromazine for sedation and vasodilation at 0.01 to 0.02 mg/kg SC q8–12h.
6. Aspirin is theoretically beneficial during and after an episode of thromboembolism by its antiplatelet effects. The dose is 10 mg/kg every 48 hours.

7. Warfarin, a vitamin K antagonist, is the anticoagulant most widely used in humans and has recently been proposed for prevention of reembolization in cats surviving an initial episode. The initial dose is 0.25 to 0.5 mg per cat (0.1 mg/kg per dog) PO once a day. It should be overlapped with heparin therapy for 3 days. The dose is then adjusted to prolong the PT approximately two times its baseline value or to attain an international normalized ratio (INR) of 2.0 to 4.0. Because of the increased risk of bleeding, aspirin should not be used concurrently.

8. Nursing care of the affected legs is of utmost importance. No venipuncture should be performed on the affected legs. Initially, these cats may have difficulty posturing to urinate and may need to have their bladders expressed periodically to prevent overdistention of the bladder or urine scald.

··········· PERICARDIAL EFFUSION

Pericardial effusion occurs most commonly in the dog and is often caused by neoplasia in the older patient. Hemangiosarcoma, chemodectoma, mesothelioma, or metastatic neoplasia most commonly affects the pericardium. Other causes of pericardial effusion include idiopathic benign pericardial effusion, coagulopathy, left atrial rupture (dogs with chronic MR), pericardial cysts (young dogs), or infections. When the pericardial effusion becomes hemodynamically significant, signs of cardiac tamponade develop. Owner complaints usually include weakness, collapse, and anorexia. Physical examination findings include muffled heart sounds, jugular venous distention, abdominal distention (ascites), weak pulse quality, tachycardia, tachypnea, and weakness. ECG may show sinus tachycardia, low-amplitude QRS (<0.5 mV), or electrical alternans. The thoracic radiographs classically show globoid cardiomegaly. Echocardiography is extremely useful in the diagnosis of pericardial effusion. Fluid is visualized within the pericardial sac. Interrogation of the right atrium and heart base may disclose a tumor. An echocardiographic criterion for cardiac tamponade is diastolic collapse of the right atrium.

Treatment for pericardial effusion is removal of the fluid. Treatment with diuretics or vasodilators may be harmful to a patient with cardiac tamponade.

1. Sedation, if necessary. Place the animal in either sternal or left lateral recumbency (clinician preference).
2. Aseptic preparation of the skin and infusion of a local lidocaine block is performed at the site of catheter insertion. The site is typically in the area of the right fifth intercostal space just above the costochondral junction. The thoracic radiographs (and echocardiogram if available) should be used for site selection.
3. Attach ECG and monitor for ventricular premature complexes throughout the procedure. VPCs occur as the catheter or needle contacts the epicardium. IV lidocaine should be at hand but is typically not needed.
4. With sterile gloves and scalpel blade, make a couple of small 1-mm side holes in a 16-gauge 3¼- or 5¼-in. over-the-needle catheter.
5. Make a stab incision with the scalpel blade to allow smooth catheter insertion.
6. Insert catheter with a 3-mL syringe attached with constant slight negative pressure. Advance the catheter or needle stylet until a flashback of pericardial effusion is obtained. Holding the needle stylet still, advance the catheter into the pericardial space.
7. Drain fluid using an extension tube, 3-way stopcock, and syringe.
8. Cytologic analysis of the fluid should be performed, including a pH. Many times the pericardial effusion is hemorrhagic and there is concern for an intracardiac puncture. If this is a concern, a small amount of fluid is placed in a red-top tube and observed for clot formation. Hemorrhagic pericardial effusion should not clot.

Table 1–14. Differential Diagnosis of Pericardial Effusion

Type of Pericardial Effusion	Etiology	Characteristic Features
Hemorrhagic	Heart base tumors	Usually brachycephalic breeds >8 yr; blood usually nonclotting blood
	Hemangiosarcoma, metastatic neoplasia	Large-breed dogs
	Benign idiopathic pericardial effusion	Middle-aged large-breed dogs
	Physical trauma	Associated with cardiac puncture
	Left atrial rupture	Smaller breeds over 8 yr with chronic valvular disease
Transudate	Coagulopathy, congestive heart failure	Radiograph or ultrasound will demonstrate lesion
	Hypoproteinemia secondary to peritoneo-, pericardial, or diaphragmatic hernia	
Exudate (pericarditis)	Infectious pericarditis	Exudate in distemper and leptospirosis and systemic fungal infections
	Suppurative pericarditis	Foreign body or hematologic spread of inflammatory process

···········CANINE CAVAL SYNDROME OF HEARTWORM DISEASE

Caval syndrome of heartworm disease is recognized by the following signs:

1. Acute renal and hepatic failure.
2. Enlarged right atrium and posterior vena cava.
3. Ascites.
4. Hemoglobinuria.
5. Anemia.
6. Acute collapse, dyspnea.
7. DIC.
8. Jugular pulse.
9. Circulating microfilaria.
10. Tricuspid insufficiency is often present.

···········Treatment

Response to this syndrome should include:

1. Surgical removal of adult worms from the right atrium and caudal vena cava with long alligator forceps through the right jugular vein under local anesthesia.
2. Digitalization—digoxin 0.0075 mg/kg q12h.

3. Peritoneal dialysis, if needed, following normalization of circulating fluid volume.
4. Corticosteroids—dexamethasone 5 mg/kg IV.
5. Furosemide 2 to 4 mg/kg q12h, if needed.
6. Routine heartworm therapy following stabilization of the effects of postcaval obstruction.

REFERENCES

Bouvy BM, Bjorling DE: Pericardial effusion in dogs and cats. Compend Contin Educ Pract Vet 13:1117, 1991.

Bouvy BM, Bjorling DE: Pericardial effusion in dogs and cats. Compend Contin Educ Pract Vet 13:633, 1991.

Edwards NJ: Bolton's Handbook of Canine and Feline Electrocardiography, ed 2. Philadelphia, WB Saunders, 1987.

Edwards NJ: ECG Manual for Veterinary Technicians, Philadelphia, WB Saunders, 1993.

Fox PR, Sisson D, Moise NS: Textbook of Canine and Feline Cardiology: Principles and Clinical Practice, ed 2. Philadelphia, WB Saunders, 1999.

Hamlin RL: Current Uses and hazards of ventricular antiarrythmic therapy. In Kirk RW, Bonagura JD, eds: Current Veterinary Therapy XI. Small Anim Pract. Phildelphia, WB Saunders, 1992.

Kass PH, Haskins SC: Survival following cardiopulmonary resuscitation in dogs and cats. Vet Emerg Crit Care 2:57–65, 1992.

Keene BW, Rush JE: Therapy of Heart Failure. In Ettinger SJ, Feldman EC, eds: Textbook of Veterinary Internal Medicine, ed 4. Philadelphia, WB Saunders, 1995.

Kirby R, Crowe D: Emergency medicine. Vet Clin North Am Small Anim Pract. 24(6), 1994.

Kittleson MD, Kienle RD: Small Animal Cardiovascular Medicine. St. Louis, Mosby–Year Book, 1998.

Laste NJ, Harpster NK: A retrospective study of 100 cats with feline distal aortic thromboembolism: 1977–1993. J Am Anim Hosp Assoc 31:492–500, 1995.

Miller M, Tilley LP: Manual of Canine and Feline Cardiology, ed 2. Philadelphia, WB Saunders, 1995.

Miller MW, Fossum TW: Pericardial Disease. In Kirk RW, Bonagura JD, eds: Current Veterinary Therapy XI. Small Anim Pract. Philadelphia, WB Saunders, 1992.

Miller WP, Sisson DD: Myocardial diseases. In Ettinger SJ, Feldman EC, eds: Textbook of Veterinary Internal Medicine, ed 4. Philadelphia, WB Saunders, 1995.

Norotney MJ, Adams HR: New perspectives in cardiology: Recent advances in antiarrhythmic drug therapy, J Am Vet Med Assoc 189:533, 1986.

Pion PD: Feline aortic thromboembolism and potential utility of thrombolytic therapy with TPA. Vet Clin North Am Small Anim Pract 18:77–86, 1988.

Pion PD, Kittleson MD: Therapy for Feline Aortic Thromboembolism. In Kirk RW, ed: Current Veterinary Therapy X. Small Anim Pract. Philadelphia, WB Saunders, 1989.

Plumb DC: Veterinary Drug Handbook, ed 3. Ames, Iowa State University Press, 1999.

Tilley LP: Essentials of Canine and Feline Electrocardiography. Philadelphia, Lea & Febiger, 1992.

Wingfield W: Veterinary Emergency Medicine Secrets. Philadelphia, Hanley & Belfus, 1998.

Systemic Hypertension

Elevated arterial blood pressure, systemic hypertension, is now recognized as a disease in dogs and cats. Systemic hypertension remains to be fully characterized in veterinary medicine, but there is ample information and knowledge available to permit diagnosis and treatment of this emerging disease, which affects approximately 1% to 2% of the general canine population.

■ RISK FACTORS

Chronic renal disease
Hyperadrenocorticism
Hyperthyroidism
Pheochromocytoma
Diabetes mellitus
Polycythemia
Hyperaldosteronism
Hypertensive encephalopathy
Intracranial hemorrhage
CNS trauma

■ CLINICAL SIGNS ASSOCIATED WITH HYPERTENSION

Retinal detachment
Acute blindness
Intraocular hemorrhage
Epistaxis
CNS signs following intracranial hemorrhage

..........DIAGNOSIS

1. Difficult due to lack of clinical signs.
2. Reproducible measurement of high arterial blood pressure.
   a. Direct measurement by arterial catheterization is the most accurate method, but technically difficult.
   b. Indirect measurement is less accurate, but technically easy in awake patients.
      (1) Doppler ultrasound.
      (2) Oscillometric.
      (3) Dependent upon cuff placement, size, and width.
3. Normal canine blood pressure:
   a. Systolic 130 to 165 mm Hg.
   b. Diastolic 80 to 90 mm Hg.
   c. Mean 95 to 110 mm Hg.
4. Normal feline blood pressure:
   a. Systolic 150 to 190 mm Hg.
   b. Diastolic 105 to 140 mm Hg.
   c. Mean 125 to 175 mm Hg.
   d. Large variability due to difficulty of measurement without inducing stress in awake cats.
5. Patient should be considered hypertensive when blood pressure is sustained above normal values.
6. Patients suspected of having systemic hypertension should have a thorough clinical workup to determine if hypertension is a primary disease or secondary to an underlying disease process such as those mentioned above.

..........CLINICAL IMPORTANCE

1. Systemic hypertension may cause:
   a. Left ventricular hypertrophy.

   b. Cerebrovascular accident.
   c. Renal vascular injury.
   d. Ocular changes:
      (1) Early signs include optic nerve edema, retinal vascular tortuosity, intraocular hemorrhage.
      (2) Later signs include retinal hemorrhage and detachments.
   e. CNS signs:
      (1) Vomiting.
      (2) Neurologic deficit.
      (3) Coma.
   f. Excessive bleeding from cut surfaces.

··········TREATMENT OF HYPERTENSIVE DISORDERS IN DOGS AND CATS

1. Sodium restriction.
   a. Decreases intravascular volume.
   b. Gradual changes of the diet in patients with renal disease will prevent worsening of azotemia.
   c. Prescription diets are helpful.
   d. Drug therapy is necessary if salt restriction fails to reduce blood pressure adequately.
2. Diuretics: Remove sodium through urinary excretion, decreasing intravascular volume, and peripheral vascular resistance. Loop diuretics also produce vasodilation via an extrarenal prostaglandin-mediated action.
   a. Thiazide diuretics:
      (1) Chlorothiazide 20 to 40 mg/kg PO once or twice daily.
      (2) Hydrochlorothiazide 2 to 4 mg/kg PO once or twice daily.
   b. Loop diuretics:
      (1) Furosemide 2 to 4 mg/kg PO once or twice daily.
      (2) Beware of hypokalemia and volume depletion.

··········Drug Therapy

Drug therapy in addition to diuretics is indicated when salt restriction and diuretics do not alleviate hypertension (see Table 1–15).

Table I–I5. Drugs Used in the Treatment of Hypertensive Disease

Drug	Dosage	Maximum Response (min)
Acepromazine	0.05–0.1 mg/kg IV bolus	60
Adenosine	3–10 µg/kg/min	1–3
Sodium nitroprusside	1.0–3.0 µg/kg/min IV initially; maximum 10 µg/kg/min	1–2
Esmolol	25–50 µg/kg/min	1–3
Labetalol	1–2 mg/kg IV infused over 10 min (humans)	5–10
Phenoxybenzamine	0.2–1.5 mg/kg PO q12h	60–120 (?)
Hydralazine	0.5–2.0 mg/kg PO q12h	30–120
Enalapril	0.5–1.5 mg/kg PO q8–12h	60–90

1. Decrease sympathetic tone, thereby relaxing blood vessels by preventing the action of norepinephrine and epinephrine.
   a. Propranolol (nonspecific β-blocker).
      (1) Dogs: 0.21 to 1.0 mg/kg PO t.i.d.
      Cats: 2 to 5 mg PO t.i.d.
   b. Esmolol (specific β-blocker) 25 to 50 μg/kg/min IV.
   c. Acepromazine (α-blocker).
      (1) Arterial and venous dilator.
      (2) 0.05 to 0.1 mg/kg SC.
      (3) Potentially hypotensive.
   d. Phenoxybenzamine (α-blocker).
      (1) Arterial and venous dilator.
      (2) 0.2 to 1.5 mg/kg PO b.i.d.
      (3) Potentially hypotensive.
   e. Prazosin.
      (1) 0.5 to 2.0 mg PO b.i.d. or t.i.d.
      (2) Potentially hypotensive.
2. Vasodilators are indicated when patients are refractory to other therapy (Table 1–16).
   a. Hydralazine.
      (1) Arterial dilator.
      (2) 0.5 to 2.0 mg/kg PO b.i.d. (dogs).
      (3) Beware of hypotension, tachycardia, and syncope.
   b. Enalapril.
      (1) ACE inhibitor.
      (2) Dogs: 0.5 to 1.5 mg/kg PO b.i.d. or t.i.d.
      (3) Cats: 1 to 2 mg PO b.i.d. or t.i.d.
      (4) Beware of hypotension and hyperkalemia.
   c. Benazepril.
      (1) ACE inhibitor.
      (2) Effective dose in cats 0.25 mg/kg once daily.
   d. Amlodipine besylate (Norvasc).
      (1) Calcium antagonist with minimal negative inotropic effects.
      (2) Dogs: not established.
      (3) Cats: 0.625 mg/day.
   e. Adenosine.
      (1) Increases intracellular cyclic adenosine monophosphate (cAMP) in smooth muscle.
      (2) 3 to 5 μg/kg/min IV in dogs and cats.

···········HYPERTENSIVE EMERGENCIES

1. Not common, but may occur with pheochromocytoma, acute renal failure, or acute glomerulonephritis.
2. Sodium nitroprusside 1 to 10 μg/kg/min IV infusion.
3. Alternative: labetolol 1 to 2 mg/kg IV infused over 10 minutes.
4. Monitor blood pressure concurrently!
5. Beware of hypotension.

REFERENCES

Henik R: Systemic hypertension and its management. Vet Clin North Am Small Anim Pract. 27:1355, 1997.

Littman M: Treatment of hypertension in dogs and cats. *In* Kirk RW, Bonagura JD, eds: Current Veterinary Therapy XI. Small Anim Pract. Philadelphia, WB Saunders, 1992, p 838.

Table 1–16. Vasodilating Agents

Drug	Mechanism of Action	Dose	Adverse Effects
Hydralazine	Direct arteriolar smooth muscle relaxant	0.2–0.5 mg/kg	Hypotension with prolonged use; neuritis, blood dyscrasias
Sodium nitroprusside	Direct arteriolar and venular smooth muscle relaxant	0.5 mg/kg up to 2.0 mg/kg 3 µg (0.5–10 kg/min IV) Dilute in D5W IV with continuous pressure monitoring	Light-sensitive bottle must be kept covered with foil; avoid in hepatic or renal failure; large doses may cause cyanide toxicity, drug tolerance
Nitroglycerin ointments	Predominantly venous but some arteriolar vasodilation	0.25–1.0-in. transdermal q6–8h	
Prazosin	α-Receptor blockage; arteriolar and venous dilation	1–3 mg/kg q12h	GI signs
ACE inhibitors Benazapril	Inhibits angiotensin II–converting enzyme	0.5 mg/kg PO q24h	
Enalapril		0.5 mg/kg 12–24h PO	Hypotension, renal toxicity

ACE, angiotensin-converting enzyme.

79

Littman MP: Spontaneous systemic hypertension in 4 cats. J Vet Intern Med 8:79–86, 1994.

Podell M: Use of blood pressure monitors. *In* Kirk RW, Bonagura JD, eds: Current Veterinary Therapy XI. Small Anim Pract. Philadelphia, WB Saunders, 1992, p 834.

Tilley L, King JN, Droz Humbert E, et al: Benazepril activity in cats: Inhibition of plasma ACE and efficacy in the treatment of hypertension. *In* Proceedings of the 14th Annual Forum of the American College of Veterinary Internal Medicine, 1996, p 163.

Anesthetic Complications and Emergencies

Complications or emergencies during anesthesia are usually due to equipment failure, respiratory problems, cardiovascular problems, or human error.

■ EQUIPMENT FAILURE

Signs Observed With Endotracheal Tube Problems

1. Inability to keep patient anesthetized
2. Difficulty in breathing or increased breathing effort
3. Erratic breath pattern
4. Cyanosis

Possible Causes

1. Endotracheal tube placed in the esophagus
2. Cuff improperly inflated; leak in the sealing cuff
3. Bronchial intubation because endotracheal tube length is too long
4. Endotracheal tube too small
5. Obstructed or kinked endotracheal tube
6. Endotracheal tube disconnected from gas machine

Signs Observed With Vaporizer Problems

1. Inability to keep patient anesthetized
2. Excessive anesthetic depth

Possible Causes

1. No anesthetic agent in vaporizer
2. Incorrect vaporizer dial setting
3. Wrong anesthetic agent put into vaporizer
4. Calibration of vaporizer not accurate
5. Gas flow rates below minimum requirement for accurate vaporizer delivery

Signs Observed With Anesthetic Machine Problems

1. Hypoxemia or cyanosis in patient
2. Increased breathing effort or rate
3. Inappropriate plane of anesthesia

Possible Causes

1. No gas in reservoir cylinders
2. Inappropriate flowmeter settings or mechanical failure of flowmeter
3. Leaks in connection between vaporizer and other machine components
4. Breathing system leaks

(Box continued on following page)

■ EQUIPMENT FAILURE *(Continued)*

    a. Perforation of corrugated tubing or reservoir bag
    b. Worn-out gaskets or seals
    c. Incomplete seal of "pop-off" valve
    d. Poor connection to endotracheal tube
5. Exhausted CO_2 absorbent
6. Breathing circuit obstruction
    a. Unidirectional valve sticking or misassembled
    b. Misassembly of breathing circuit components

■ RESPIRATORY SYSTEM

Most anesthetic agents cause a dose-related decrease in both respiratory rate and breath volume. Because of these characteristics, respiratory rate alone is not a reliable indicator of adequate breathing (gas exchange) during anesthesia. Tidal (breath) volume or minute volume (tidal volume × respiratory rate) are more important indicators of adequate breathing than respiratory rate alone. Tidal volume can be estimated by observing excursions of the reservoir bag on the anesthetic machine and chest wall motion.

Clinical Signs of Poor Ventilation

1. Abnormal respiratory pattern
2. Sudden changes in heart rate
3. Cardiac arrhythmias
4. Cyanosis (not usually visible if inhalation agents and oxygen are used)
5. Cardiac arrest

Problems That Contribute to Decreased Breathing Effectiveness During Anesthesia

1. Anesthesia-related changes in neuromuscular function—CNS depression from anesthetic drugs, anesthesia-related respiratory muscle weakness
2. Pulmonary atelectasis—general anesthesia and surgical positioning, pneumothorax, hemothorax, pyothorax, or any disruption of alveolar stability (i.e., pneumonia, edema, emphysema, hemorrhage)
3. Anesthetic equipment—increased resistance to breathing, increased dead space from machine, improper oxygen concentration or flow rates
4. Upper airway obstruction—laryngeal edema, collapsing larynx or trachea, improper endotracheal tube position, anatomical problems associated with upper airways in brachycephalic breeds, aspiration of gastric contents.
5. Intrathoracic obstruction—hydrothorax, pneumothorax, diaphragmatic hernia

Causes of Abnormal Breathing Pattern During Anesthesia

1. Intrinsic effect of anesthetic drugs
2. Surgical positioning or maneuvers compromising ventilation
3. Improper anesthetic depth
4. Equipment malfunction or exhaustion of CO_2 absorbent
5. Thoracic wall or diaphragmatic injury
6. Injury to respiratory centers
7. Agonal breathing—death imminent

(Box continued on following page)

■ RESPIRATORY SYSTEM *(Continued)*

Causes of Postoperative Respiratory Depression

1. Residual effect of anesthetic drugs
2. Hypothermia
3. Overventilation during intraoperative support
4. Surgical techniques that compromise ventilation
5. Postoperative bandaging of the abdomen or chest
6. Increased ventilatory effort when the animal is fatigued
7. CNS injury

Causes of Postoperative Dyspnea

1. Pulmonary tissue disease or injury—pulmonary edema or respiratory distress syndrome
2. Accumulation of intrapleural air or liquid
3. Upper airway obstruction or compromise—may be anatomical abnormality, absence of muscle tone to pharynx and tongue, or intubation injury
4. Aspiration of GI contents during or following intubation

............CARDIOVASCULAR SYSTEM

Approximate normal heart rates during anesthesia are as follows:

Large dogs: 60 to 100 bpm.
Medium-size dogs: 80 to 120 bpm.
Small dogs: 90 to 140 bpm.
Domestic cats: 140 to 250 bpm.

............Bradycardia

Heart rate is below normal values noted above.

............*Common Causes of Bradycardia*

1. Anesthetic drug technique—use of narcotics, xylazine, or medetomidine.
2. Animal too deeply anesthetized—check depth evaluation parameters.
3. Increased vagal tone—give atropine or glycopyrollate.
4. Hypothermia—patient may need warming.
5. Hypoxia-bradycardia is present in advanced stage.

............Tachycardia

Heart rate is above normal values noted above.

............*Common Causes of Tachycardia*

1. Drug induced—use of vagolytic drugs such as atropine, glycopyrrolate, and ketamine; sympathomimetic drugs such as isoproterenol, epinephrine, and dopamine.
2. Anesthetic depth is inadequate for patient or for the degree of surgical stimulation.
3. Hypercapnia or hypoxemia (hypercarbia or increased CO_2 retention, hypoxia).

4. Hypotension, shock.
5. Hyperthermia.

............Hypotension

Hypotension is physiologically low blood pressure (mean blood pressure <65 mm Hg). Hypotension can result in poor tissue perfusion and oxygen delivery that can place the anesthetized patient at risk.

............Possible Causes

1. Decreased cardiac performance associated with reduced venous blood flow to the heart (preload effect). Decreased venous blood flow may result from excessive surgical manipulation of viscera, decreased circulating blood volume associated with fluid deficits during surgery, excessive bleeding at surgical site, and vasodilation of veins.
2. Decreased myocardial contractility (inotropy) associated with anesthetic agents (promazine derivatives), inhalation anesthetics, hypoxia, and toxemia.

............Recognition of Hypotension

1. Evaluation of peripheral pulse quality by palpation, mucous membrane color, and capillary refill time.
2. Oliguria or anuria.
3. Measurement of blood pressure by direct or indirect methods. The normal ranges are as follows;
   a. Systolic—100 to 160 mm Hg.
   b. Diastolic—60 to 90 mm Hg.
   c. Mean—80 to 120 mm Hg.

............Cardiac Arrhythmias (see also p. 61)

ECG monitoring is useful for early detection of cardiac arrhythmias during anesthesia. Clinical signs of cardiac arrhythmias may include irregular pulse rate or pressure, abnormal or irregular heart sounds, pallor, cyanosis, hypotension, and abnormal ECG tracing. The following should be evaluated to confirm arrhythmia:

1. Rhythm and rate of the heart.
2. Identification of P waves: Is atrial activity regular and uniform?
3. Recognition of QRS complex—morphology, rate, and uniformity. Is there evidence of ectopic beats?
4. Relationship between P waves and QRS complexes. Is the AV conduction time normal?

............Causes of Intraoperative Arrhythmias

The following factors can lead to arrhythmias during anesthesia:

1. Poor preoperative preparation, including lack of attention to fluid balance, electrolytes, and acid-base status, predispose to arrhythmias.
2. Patient management at anesthetic induction and the first 5 minutes of anesthesia. Many arrhythmias are initiated with endotracheal tube placement.
3. Sympathetic and parasympathetic nervous system stimulation. Stimulation can be induced by pain (perceived because the patient is too lightly anesthe-

tized), manipulation of extraocular muscles, tube thoracostomy, and tracheal intubation.
4. Anesthetic drugs. α_2-Adrenergic drugs (xylazine, medetomidine) are associated with sinoatrial and AV blockade producing bradycardia and bradyarrhythmias. The thiobarbiturates (thiamylal, thiopental) are arrhythmogenic and may be associated with VPCs. Lower concentrations (2.0% to 2.5%) or slower rates of administration are less likely to produce arrhythmia. Transient arrhythmias can be seen in dogs following atropine administration. Halothane can produce arrhythmias; this effect is potentiated if epinephrine is used and reduced if acepromazine is given as a preanesthetic agent.

To prevent anesthetic-related arrhythmias, the following guidelines should be observed:

1. Evaluate the preoperative patient status to detect and stabilize preexisting arrhythmias, electrolyte or acid-base disturbance, and hydration prior to anesthesia.
2. Select appropriate preanesthetic agent to allay apprehension prior to anesthesia.
3. Be aware of anesthetic drug effects on the myocardium and autonomic nervous system.
4. Ensure adequate anesthetic depth and good oxygenation prior to endotracheal intubation.
5. Ensure adequate ventilatory support during anesthesia.
6. Ensure adequate anesthetic depth prior to surgical stimulation.
7. Avoid surgical manipulation to heart or great vessels for a prolonged time period.
8. Avoid changes in anesthetic depth.
9. Avoid hypothermia.

............Therapy

Treat the underlying cause, if known, rather than indiscriminately using antiarrhythmic drugs. Correcting oxygenation, CO_2 levels, acidemia, and electrolyte balance will correct many perioperative arrhythmias. Reconfirm appropriate anesthetic depth. Ensure that adequate ventilatory support is provided. In general, the following arrhythmias may require antiarrhythmic drug therapy:

1. Atrial origin. In general, treat arrhythmias that interfere with efficient ventricular function. Examples include atrial tachycardia, fibrillation, paroxysmal atrial tachycardia, sinus bradycardia, and AV blocks.
2. Ventricular origin. Treat arrhythmias that present an R-on-T potential (ventricular fibrillation). Also resolve those that affect efficient hemodynamics.
3. Multiform ectopic ventricular beats. Therapy is necessary because of the potential for uncoordinated Purkinje system depolarization, resulting in ventricular fibrillation.
4. Ventricular ectopic beats that occur in "salvo" with three or more beats in succession. Predisposition to ventricular fibrillation is present.
5. Ventricular ectopic beats greater than 12 bpm. A parasystolic focus with repetitive depolarization occurs. There is interference with hemodynamics as well as a predisposition to more significant arrhythmias.

Antiarrhythmic drugs include the following:

1. Atropine 0.04 to 0.08 mg/kg. Half is given IV initially, and the remainder is given SC or IM for bradycardias and second- and third-degree heart blocks. Atropine can also be given via the airway, diluting the amount needed with an equal volume of sterile saline and administered through the endotracheal tube. This technique is of value if an IV catheter is not in place.

2. Lidocaine is still the drug of choice for therapy of arrhythmias of ventricular origin. The dose is 1 to 2 mg/kg IV until the effect is achieved. In cats, lidocaine should be used at 0.25 to 0.5 mg/kg IV for initial therapy. An infusion rate of 40 to 60 μg/kg/min may be used to maintain an antiarrhythmic effect. Lidocaine can also be given transtracheally (2 to 4 mg/kg, with an equal volume of saline injected into the tracheal tube using a sterile male urinary catheter to inject in the lower respiratory tract).

3. Procainamide is an effective agent for ventricular arrhythmias. It is administered IM; IV administration may be accompanied by hypotension. It may be used in conjunction with lidocaine for suppression of arrhythmia. Dose range is wide; 6 to 20 mg/kg q6h has proved effective.

4. Propanolol is an effective β-adrenergic blocking drug. Propranolol is indicated in supraventricular tachyarrhythmias and has a secondary role in ventricular arrhythmias. A lidocaine-like effect on the cell membrane depresses automaticity of ventricular tissue. Decreased cardiac output and hypotension may be noted with its use. IV administration should occur under ECG monitoring. An initial dose of 0.04 mg/kg is administered and may be repeated until desired effects are noted.

5. Potassium administration in conjunction with lidocaine may enhance antiarrhythmic activity. Rapid shifts in transcellular potassium concentration may alter automaticity, thus suppressing ectopic activity. Potassium may be safely administered at 20 to 40 mEq added to 500 mL fluids in conjunction with lidocaine. Do not give more than 0.5 mEq/kg/hr.

6. Increased oxygen support and improved ventilation may be very beneficial in severe arrhythmias.

............DEPTH EVALUATION (HUMAN ERROR)

Causes of arousal during anesthesia:

1. Postinduction hypoventilation.
2. Too low an inspired anesthetic dose.
3. Fresh gas flow too low.
4. Equipment malfunction in anesthetic machine or vaporizer.
5. Esophageal placement of endotracheal tube.
6. Undersized endotracheal tube.
7. Inadequate cuff inflation.
8. Surgical stimulus.
9. Conditions that mimic anesthetic arousal (e.g., malignant hyperthermia).

Causes of excessive anesthetic depth:

1. Interactive effects of several anesthetic agents post induction.
2. Excessive vaporizer setting and delivered concentration.
3. Vaporizer malfunction.
4. Assisted breathing by mechanical or manual means.
5. Nonrebreathing anesthetic circuits managed as a circle system.

............POSTANESTHESIA COMPLICATIONS

Reasons for delayed recovery:

1. Excessive anesthetic depth.
2. Low body temperature following anesthesia.
3. Residual action of long-acting tranquilizers, narcotics, or barbiturates.
4. Delayed metabolism of anesthetic drugs.
5. Hypoglycemia.
6. Hemorrhage.

7. Breed predisposition—e.g., sighthounds and collies.
8. Multiple doses of injectable drugs to maintain anesthesia.

Ear Emergencies

Foreign bodies within the ear canal (e.g., foxtails) may result in acute inflammation and pressure necrosis of the tissue of the external auditory meatus, causing severe pain and discomfort. Acute inflammation of the external auditory meatus or middle ear may result in sudden pain and discomfort for the animal.

Adequate examination and treatment of the ear in an animal in pain requires the use of a short-acting anesthetic or a neuroleptanalgesic agent. Examine the ear canal (see p. 313). Carefully remove visible foreign bodies with an alligator forceps. Obtain samples of pus or exudates in the ear canal and perform bacterial or fungal cultures (see pp. 466 and 476), then gently irrigate the external ear canal with warm, sterile saline, removing debris and exudates. When irrigating, do not allow excessive pressure (over 50 mm Hg) to build up, because it may rupture an inflamed tympanic membrane. After all detritus and exudate has been removed and the ear canal has been dried, inspect the tympanic membrane. Inflammation of the external ear canal requires instillation of antibiotic-steroid ointment, and the use of narcotics if pain is severe.

Characteristics of otitis media involving the inner ear are head rotation with the affected ear down, circling to the affected side, falling or rolling to the affected side, nystagmus, fever, depression, and severe pain. Most cases of otitis media are accompanied by a severe otitis externa, which must be treated simultaneously. The most common cause of otitis media is bacterial infection with *Staphylococcus, Streptococcus, Pseudomonas, Escherichia coli,* or *Proteus.* Otitis media can develop by infection spreading across the tympanic membrane from the external ear canal, through the eustachian tubes (rare), or through the blood to the middle ear. In most cases of otitis media, the tympanic membrane is ruptured. If the tympanic membrane is not ruptured but is swollen and hyperemic, a myringotomy should be performed. A culture of debris and exudate from the tympanic cavity should be obtained, and a sensitivity test should be performed. The tympanic cavity is cleaned and medicated with a combination antibiotic, antifungal, anti-inflammatory topical agent.

If otitis media persists despite initial treatment, radiographic examination of the bullae is of value in better defining the pathologic changes. Surgical drainage of the tympanic bullae may be required.

REFERENCES

Bruyette DS, Lorenz MD. Otitis externa and media: Diagnostic and medical aspects. Semin Vet Med Surg (Small Anim) 8:3–9, 1993.
Fingland RB: The ear: Medical, surgical and diagnostic aspects. Semin Vet Med Surg (Small Anim) 8:1–50, 1993.
Neer MT, Howard PE: Otitis media. Compend Contin Educ Pract Vet 4:410, 1982.
Venker-van Hagen AJ: Managing diseases of the ear. *In* Kirk RW, ed: Current Veterinary Therapy VIII: Small Animal Practice. Philadelphia, WB Saunders, 1983.

Ocular Emergencies

An ocular emergency is any serious situation that threatens or has already caused loss of vision or severe pain and deformity. The following ocular emergencies should be treated within 1 to several hours following injury:

Penetrating injuries of the globe
Proptosis of the globe

Acute corneal abrasion or ulcer
Ocular foreign bodies
Acute iritis
Hyphema
Descemetocele
Lid laceration
Pupillary block glaucoma (acute glaucoma)
Orbital cellulitis
Corneal laceration
Chemical burns

··········ASSESSMENT OF OCULAR INJURIES

A carefully performed ocular examination is necessary to assess the degree of ocular injury. Frequently, adequate sedation or a short-acting general anesthetic will be required to permit a complete examination. The following equipment is needed:

Loupe
Monocular indirect ophthalmoscope
Direct ophthalmoscope with rechargeable handle and Finoff transilluminator
Fine-toothed forceps
Lid retractors
Lacrimal probes
Sterile eyewash solution in irrigating bottle
Fluorescein-impregnated sterile strips
Methylcellulose (Weck-cel) sponges
Topical anesthetic (proparacaine 0.5%)
Culture swabs and culture media
Schiøtz tonometer
Short-acting mydriatic (tropicamide 1%)

··········Procedure

1. Obtain an adequate history. This may reveal the existence of previous eye disease, the instillation of some chemical irritant, or trauma. Try to determine when the injury occurred and whether any medication or eyewash has been used.
2. Examine the eye for any discharge, blepharospasm, or photophobia. If discharge is present, note the type. If the animal is in extreme discomfort with the eye completely closed, *do not* try to force the lids open.
3. Note the position of the globe within the orbit. If the eye is exophthalmic, there is frequently strabismus and protrusion of the third eyelid, exposure keratitis and, in cases of retrobulbar or zygomatic salivary gland inflammation, pain on opening the mouth. Note any displacement of the globe medially or temporally.
4. Note any swelling, contusions, or lacerations of the lids. Note whether the lids are able to cover the cornea. In cases of lid lacerations, try to determine the depth of the laceration. Penetrating lid lacerations may be associated with secondary injury to the globe.
5. Palpate the orbital margins, feeling for fractures, crepitus, air, and cellulitis.
6. Examine the cornea and sclera for evidence of partially penetrating or completely penetrating injuries. The use of lid retractors in these cases can be very helpful. If the wound is completely penetrating, look for loss of uveal tissue, lens, or vitreous. Do not put pressure on the globe, because intraocular herniation will result.

7. Examine the conjunctiva for hemorrhage, chemosis, lacerations, or foreign bodies. Examine the superior and inferior conjunctival cul-de-sacs for foreign bodies. Occasionally, topical anesthesia and a sterile cotton swab can be used to "sweep" the conjunctival fornix to pick up foreign bodies. Use a small, fine-toothed forceps to pick up the third eyelid, and examine its bulbar aspect for foreign bodies.
8. Examine the cornea for opacities, ulcers, foreign bodies, abrasions, or lacerations. A loupe and a good focal source of illumination are important in conducting this examination.
9. Record pupil size, shape, and response to light, both direct and consensual.
10. Examine the anterior chamber, and note its depth and the presence of hyphema, iridodonesis, or iridodialysis. Does the lens appear to be in the normal position? Luxated lenses in the anterior chamber will come into contact with the corneal endothelium, producing acute corneal edema.
11. If indicated and if the cornea is undamaged, measure intraocular pressure.
12. Examine the posterior ocular segment using a short-acting dilating agent and a direct or indirect ophthalmoscope to look for intraocular hemorrhage, retinal hemorrhage or edema formation, retinal detachment, optic nerve edema, and inflammation.

..........Conditions Producing Sudden Visual Loss

When examining an animal with an ocular emergency, the history may indicate sudden loss of vision occurring unilaterally or bilaterally. The following conditions can produce sudden loss of vision.

Hyphema or vitreous hemorrhage
Traumatic lid swelling
Extensive corneal edema or exposure keratitis
Acute congestive glaucoma
Retinal hemorrhage or extensive retinal edema
Sudden acquired retinal degeneration syndrome (SARDS)
Retinal detachment
Extensive trauma to or avulsion of the optic nerve
Intracranial damage secondary to hemorrhage, ischemia, or anoxia, resulting in the interruption of visual pathways
Proptosis of the globe

..........Instrumentation

The following basic surgical instruments should be at hand to treat ocular lacerations and other types of emergencies:

Castroviejo or Barraquer lid speculum
Bishop-Harmon tissue forceps
Stevens tenotomy scissors, standard
Castroviejo corneal scissors
Castroviejo needle holder; standard jaws with lock
Beaver knife handle and No. 64 blades
Lacrimal cannula, straight 22-gauge
Barraquer iris repositor
Foreign body spud
Enucleation scissors, medium curve
Suture material—6-0 silk, 4-0 nylon, 7-0 collagen or 6-0 ophthalmic gut, 7-0 nylon

..........INJURIES OF THE LIDS

..........Lacerations

Lid contusions and lacerations are most commonly associated with bite wounds or automobile trauma.

The lids can be considered a two-layered structure, with the anterior layer composed of skin and orbicularis muscle and the posterior layer composed of tarsus and conjunctiva. The openings of the meibomian glands in the lid margin form the approximate line separating the lids into anterior and posterior segments. Splitting the lid into these two components facilitates the use of sliding skin flaps to close wound defects.

Gentle cleansing and careful and thorough irrigation are necessary preoperative routines before correcting lid lacerations. Use sterile IV saline to irrigate the wound. The conjunctival sac is also irrigated, and foreign bodies are removed. A 1% solution of povidone-iodine can be used on the skin. Draping the wound with eye drapes (3M Steri-drape) is necessary to prevent further contamination.

In lid lacerations, ragged wound margins should be trimmed and very conservative tissue debridement should be performed. However, *as much tissue as possible should be saved* to minimize wound contracture and lid deformity.

Close small wounds of the lid margin with a figure-eight or two-layered simple interrupted suture of 6-0 gut or collagen in the conjunctiva and 4-0 or 5-0 silk, polypropylene, or nylon in the skin. The lid margins must be absolutely apposed to prevent postoperative lid notching.

..........Ecchymosis of the Lids

Because of the excellent vascular supply to the eyelids, direct blows may cause ecchymosis. Associated ocular injury such as orbital hemorrhage, proptosis, or corneal laceration may occur. Trauma, allergic reactions, and internal or external hordeolum may also result in lid ecchymosis.

Treat lid ecchymosis initially with cold compresses, followed later by warm compresses. Resorption of blood may occur in from 3 to 10 days. Ocular allergies respond to topical and systemic administration of corticosteroids, such as dexamethasone ointment t.i.d. or q.i.d., plus the application of cold compresses. Ecchymosis associated with allergic reactions should be treated with systemic corticosteroids and epinephrine if the inflammation is acute and severe (see p. 23).

..........CONJUNCTIVAL LACERATIONS

The conjunctiva may have to be carefully dissected away from the underlying sclera to provide a better view of any abnormalities. Undue pressure should not be placed on the globe when performing this dissection to prevent herniation of intraocular contents through a scleral wound.

Repair of large conjunctival lacerations can be accomplished by the use of 6-0 gut or collagen using an interrupted or continuous suture pattern. The margins of the conjunctiva should be carefully approximated to prevent inclusion cysts from forming. When large areas of conjunctiva have been damaged, conjunctival advancement flaps may be used to close the defect.

..........SUBCONJUNCTIVAL HEMORRHAGE

Subconjunctival hemorrhage is a common sequela to head trauma. In itself, it is not a serious problem. However, it may indicate the presence of more severe intraocular damage; therefore, a complete eye examination is indicated.

Subconjunctival hemorrhage also may be associated with various types of blood dyscrasias and systemic diseases, including thrombocytopenia, autoimmune hemolytic anemia, hemophilia, leptospirosis, severe systemic infections, and difficult or prolonged labor (dystocia).

Uncomplicated subconjunctival hemorrhage usually clears within 14 days. If the conjunctiva is exposed because of the hemorrhage, use a protective ophthalmic antibiotic ointment.

............CHEMICAL INJURIES

Chemical injuries of the eye are arbitrarily classified as toxic, acid, or alkali. The severity of ocular burns from chemical injury is dependent on the concentration of the chemical, the duration of exposure, and the pH of the solution.

Weak acids do not penetrate biologic tissues very well. The hydrogen ion precipitates protein on contact, providing some protection to the corneal stroma and intraocular contents. Precipitation of the epithelial proteins produces a ground-glass appearance of the cornea.

Alkalis (and very strong acids) penetrate tissues rapidly, saponify plasma membranes, denature collagen, and cause vascular thromboses in the conjunctiva, episclera, and anterior uvea.

The severe pain, blepharospasm, and photophobia accompanying chemical ocular injury results from direct stimulation to free nerve endings located in the epithelium of the cornea and the conjunctival lining. Severe burns with alkalis produce a rise in intraocular pressure; intraocular prostaglandin release; increase in aqueous humor pH; alteration in the blood-aqueous barrier and secondary uveitis; and intraocular uveitis with secondary synechia formation, eventual chronic glaucoma or phthisis, secondary cataract, and corneal perforation.

Early repair of epithelial defects is accomplished by sliding and increased mitosis of epithelial cells. Healing of the epithelial surface is usually accompanied by vascularization. Severe corneal stromal burns heal by degradation and removal of necrotic debris and replacement of collagenous matrix and cells. A polymorphonuclear neutrophil (PMN) response can result in degranulation of these cells with release of agents, such as collagenase, endopeptidases, and cathepsins, and serve to further break down the corneal stroma. In very severe corneal burns, only PMNs may be present in the corneal stroma, and fibroblasts may never invade the stroma.

............Initial Treatment

All chemical burns should receive copious lavage with any clean aqueous solution available. Remove any sticky paste or powder (e.g., lime) from the conjunctival sac with cotton-tipped applicators that can be soaked in EDTA 0.01M solution.

In very severe burns with alkali, paracentesis of the anterior chamber and replacing fluid with balanced salt solution may help bring the pH back toward normal.

Begin mydriasis and cycloplegia with topical atropine 1% drops or ointment. Begin antibiotic therapy with gentamicin ointment four or five times a day. Secondary glaucomas can be treated with carbonic anhydrase inhibitors. Analgesics are needed for pain. Keep the conjunctival cul-de-sacs free of proteinaceous exudate to avoid fibrinous adhesions and symblepharon formation.

Persistent epithelial erosions can be treated with a conjunctival flap left in place for 3 to 4 weeks. Additionally, porcine collagen contact lenses can be used. Topical antibiotics, mydriatics, and lubricants such as Adapt drops or Lacrilube ointment should be used.

Corneal stromal loss is most likely to develop in eyes burned with strong alkali or strong acids. Although the type of treatment is controversial, the use of acetylcysteine, 10% (Mucomyst), or EDTA 0.2M solution dropped onto the cornea five times a day is used to inhibit mammalian collagenase activity.

The use of topical steroids after the ocular chemical burn is very controversial. The advantage of steroid use, such as prednisolone acetate 1% drops topically, is to reduce intraocular inflammation. The disadvantage is the retardation of wound healing by inhibiting fibroblast formation. It is best to avoid topical steroids if possible, especially 7 to 10 days after an alkali burn.

···········CORNEAL ABRASIONS

Corneal epithelial abrasions are exceedingly painful and are characterized by intense blepharospasm, lacrimation, and photophobia. Movement of the eyelids or third eyelid seems to cause more discomfort. Animals in such discomfort are difficult to examine until effective relief from pain is achieved. Topical use of 0.5% proparacaine hydrochloride will permit relaxation of the lids so that the eye can be examined. Using a focal source of illumination and an eye loupe, examine the inferior and superior conjunctival fornices and medial aspect of the membrana nictitans for foreign bodies. Place a drop of sterile saline on a sterile paper strip impregnated with fluorescein and touch the superior conjunctiva. Irrigate the excess fluorescein from the eye with sterile saline. Areas of corneal epithelial damage will remain green.

In epithelial erosions, loose epithelial margins must be mechanically debrided back to a point where no further loose epithelial tissue is present. Debridement can be accomplished with a fine cotton swab (Q-Tip) and topical anesthesia. Barring complications, minor corneal epithelial abrasions heal rapidly. A cycloplegic (1% atropine) is used to make the eye more comfortable and to reduce the effects of the secondary iridocyclitis that usually develops. A broad-spectrum antibiotic ointment is used six times a day to prevent secondary infections. The animal is kept out of bright light, and an analgesic is administered if pain is severe. The use of a corneal contact lens placed over the affected cornea may make the animal more comfortable. Porcine collagen bandage lenses can be used to make the animal more comfortable. The lenses will disintegrate in approximately 4 days. The eye is reexamined in 48 hours and again after 1 week.

···········ACUTE INFECTIOUS KERATITIS

Acute infection of the cornea with bacterial agents is characterized by:

- Mucopurulent ocular discharge
- Rapid progression of epithelial and corneal stromal loss
- Inflammatory cellular infiltrates into the corneal stroma
- Secondary uveitis often characterized by hypopyon formation

Confirmation of infectious keratitis can be based on corneal scrapings that are stained with a Gram stain. Initial treatment of bacterial keratitis should involve appropriate systemic antibiotics and the topical use of ciprofloxacin 0.3% eyedrops or ointment (Ciloxan, Alcon Laboratories, Fort Worth, TX).

···········PENETRATING CORNEAL LACERATIONS

Penetrating corneal lacerations may result in prolapse of intraocular contents. Frequently, pieces of uveal tissue or fibrin effectively but temporarily seal the wound and permit the anterior chamber to re-form. Manipulation of these wounds should be avoided until the animal has been anesthetized. Care should be used in anesthetizing an animal with a corneal laceration, because struggling or excitement during administration of anesthesia may result in loss of the temporary seal in the corneal laceration and extrusion of intraocular contents.

Superficial corneal lacerations need not be sutured. However, if the laceration extends through 50% or more of the cornea or if it is more than 3 to 4 mm in length, sutures are required to close the wound.

Use of magnification by the surgeon is advantageous in placing sutures in the cornea properly. Silk sutures, 7-0 or 8-0; collagen sutures, 7-0 or 8-0; or fine sutures, 8-0 to 9-0 nylon, all with micropoint spatula-type needles, are effective in closing corneal wounds. Sutures are tied individually and are left in place for a minimum of 3 weeks. Many corneal wounds are jagged in appearance or the cornea is edematous and tight closure is not possible. In these cases, a thin conjunctival flap is pulled down (or up) over the corneal wound to help seal it and prevent aqueous loss. Sutures must never be placed through the entire full thickness of the cornea but should cross into the middle third of the stroma.

Following closure of the corneal wound, the anterior chamber must be re-formed to prevent synechia formation and the resulting secondary glaucoma. Taking care to avoid injury to the iris, insert a 25- or 26-gauge needle into the anterior chamber at the limbus. Gently instill sterile saline solution to re-form the anterior chamber. Defects in the suture line will be recognized by leakage of fluid and they should be repaired.

Incarceration of uveal tissue in corneal wounds presents a difficult surgical problem. Persistence of incarcerated uveal tissue predisposes to a chronic filtering wick in the cornea, shallow anterior chamber, chronic irritation, edema and vascularization of the cornea, and intraocular infection, leading to panophthalmitis.

Occasionally, the use of a mydriatic agent (e.g., 1% atropine or 10% phenylephrine, or both) permits removal of a small tag of uveal tissue from a corneal wound. This is only possible soon after the injury, before synechiae have formed (usually within 24 to 48 hours).

Incarcerated uveal tissue (usually iris) can be surgically removed from a corneal wound in several ways. The uveal tissue can be trimmed from the corneal wound using an electroscalpel or scissors and the wound swept with a blunt cyclodialysis spatula to free further adhesions. Repair the corneal wound as previously described.

Conjunctival flaps can be used in the correction of large corneal lacerations and in deep stromal ulceration or perforation.

............OCULAR FOREIGN BODIES

The most common foreign bodies associated with ocular injuries in small animals are birdshot, BB pellets, and glass. The site of intraocular penetration of these foreign bodies may be obscured by the eyelids.

A foreign body entering the eye may penetrate the cornea and fall into the anterior chamber or become lodged in the iris. Foreign bodies may penetrate the anterior capsule of the lens, producing cataracts. Some metallic, high-speed foreign bodies may pass through the cornea, iris, and lens to lodge in the posterior wall of the eye or in the vitreous cavity.

Direct visualization of a foreign body is the best means of localization. Examination of the eye with the biomicroscope or indirect ophthalmoscope may prove invaluable in locating foreign bodies.

Indirect demonstration of the intraocular foreign body may be achieved by radiographic techniques. At least three radiographic views should be taken.

In addition to radiography, the more refined technique of ultrasonography may be used to locate foreign bodies.

When considering removing any foreign body from an eye, weigh the dangers of leaving the foreign body in the eye against the surgical difficulty of removing it. Foreign objects in the anterior chambers are much easier to remove than nonmagnetic ones. Attempted removal of foreign bodies from the vitreous cavity of animals has consistently produced poor results. In many cases, the eye has been enucleated.

...........OCULAR TRAUMATIC INJURIES

Blunt trauma to the eye can result in luxation or subluxation of the lens. The subluxated lens may move anteriorly, thus shallowing the anterior chamber. Trembling of the iris (iridodonesis) may be noticed when the lens is subluxated. In complete luxation, the lens may come to lie in the anterior chamber, thus causing obstruction to aqueous outflow, or it may be lost in the vitreous cavity. Luxation of the lens is almost always associated with rupture of the hyaloid membrane and herniation of the vitreous through the pupillary space.

Emergency surgery for lens dislocation is required if the lens is entirely within the anterior chamber or incarcerated within the pupil, thus causing a secondary pupillary block glaucoma. This elevation of intraocular pressure can result in severe visual loss within 48 hours; thus, lens removal should be accomplished as quickly as possible.

...........Severe Trauma to the Globe

Severe trauma to the globe or a direct blow to the head can result in retinal or vitreous hemorrhage. There may be large areas of subretinal or intraretinal hemorrhage. Subretinal hemorrhage usually assumes a discrete, globular form, and the blood appears reddish-blue in color. The retina is detached at the site of hemorrhage. Superficial retinal hemorrhage may assume a flame-shaped appearance, and preretinal or vitreal hemorrhage assumes a bright-red amorphous appearance, obliterating the underlying retinal architecture. Retinal and vitreous hemorrhage associated with trauma usually resorbs spontaneously over a 2- to 3-week period. Unfortunately, vitreous hemorrhage, as it organizes, can produce vitreous traction bands that may eventually produce retinal detachment.

Expulsive choroidal hemorrhage can occur at the time of injury and usually leads to retinal detachment, severe visual impairment, and total visual loss.

Treatment of retinal and vitreous hemorrhage involves rest and the correction of factors that may predispose to intraocular hemorrhage. Veterinary ophthalmologists may be able to help in the more complicated cases by performing a vitrectomy.

...........Hyphema

Hyphema refers to blood in the anterior chamber of the eye. Its most common cause is trauma resulting from automobile injuries. Hyphema may also be present secondary to penetrating intraocular wounds.

Blood within the eye may come from the anterior or posterior uveal tract. Trauma to the eye may result in iridodialysis or a tearing of the iris at its root, permitting excessive bleeding from the iris and ciliary body.

Usually, simple hyphema resolves spontaneously in 7 to 10 days and does not cause visual loss. Loss of vision following bleeding into the anterior chamber is associated with secondary ocular injuries, including glaucoma, traumatic iritis, cataract, retinal detachment, endophthalmitis, or corneal scarring.

Treatment of hyphema must be individualized. There are, however, several general principles of treatment:

1. Arrest continuing bleeding and control recurrent bleeding.
2. Aid in the elimination of blood from the anterior chamber.
3. Control secondary glaucoma.
4. Treat associated injuries, including traumatic iritis.
5. Detect and treat late complications of hyphema.

Unfortunately, little can be done to arrest and prevent rebleeding in the eye.

In cases of early hyphema, it is advisable to keep the affected animal confined and to prohibit active exertion. If the hyphema is so extensive that it may produce a secondary glaucoma, observe the animal while it is hospitalized.

Rebleeding may occur within the first 5 days following injury. The intraocular pressure should be closely observed.

After 5 to 7 days, the blood in the anterior chamber changes from a bright-red color to a bluish-black color (eight ball hemorrhage). If the total hyphema persists and an elevation in ocular pressure is evident despite medical therapy, surgical intervention is indicated.

Primary escape of RBCs from the anterior chamber is via the anterior drainage angle, with iris absorption and phagocytosis accounting for minor removal of blood elements. Because of the associated traumatic iritis in hyphema, topical corticosteroids such as 1% prednisolone acetate should be used to control anterior segment inflammation. In addition, a cycloplegic agent such as 1% atropine should be used.

The formation of fibrin in the anterior chamber of the eye secondary to bleeding can produce adhesions of the iris and secondary glaucoma from blockage of the trabecular meshwork. The use of t-PA injected into the anterior chamber has been proved to be helpful in cases of hyphema. Altepase (Activase, 20-mg vial, Genentech, San Francisco) is used as the source of recombinant t-PA. The t-PA is reconstituted to make a 250-µg/mL solution, which is then frozen to $-70°C$ in 0.5-mL aliquots. The warmed reconstituted t-PA is injected into the anterior chamber.

The hyphemas secondary to retinal detachment (e.g., collie ectasia syndrome) and endstage glaucoma are extremely difficult to treat medically and have a poor prognosis.

...........Glaucoma Secondary to Hyphema

Control of glaucoma secondary to hyphema may prove extremely difficult. Carbonic anhydrase inhibitors such as acetazolamide or dichlorphenamide decrease aqueous secretion and may effectively reduce intraocular pressure if the trabecular outflow system is still functioning at 40% of capacity. An eye with glaucoma and a completely blocked trabecular outflow system will respond poorly to a carbonic anhydrase inhibitor. Osmotic agents, such as oral glycerol or IV mannitol may be helpful in controlling glaucoma secondary to hyphema. Reduction in vitreous volume deepens the anterior chamber and may increase aqueous fluid outflow.

Evacuation of blood or blood clots from the anterior chamber is not advisable unless there is secondary glaucoma that cannot be controlled medically or if there is no indication over a prolonged period that blood resorption is occurring. The use of t-PA injected into the anterior chamber may be helpful in lysing blood clots and in preventing extensive fibrin formation (see Martin et al.).

It is important to emphasize that surgical intervention and blind probing of the anterior chamber in an attempt to remove blood or blood clots may cause serious surgical complications such as rebleeding, luxated lens, extensive iris damage, and damage to the corneal epithelium.

...........Proptosis of the Globe

Proptosis of the globe secondary to trauma is common, especially in brachycephalic breeds. Proptosis of the globe in the dolichocephalic breeds requires a greater degree of initiating contusion than in the brachycephalic breeds. Therefore, secondary damage to the eye and CNS associated with proptosis of the globe may be far greater in the collie than in the Pekingese.

In a case of proptosis of the globe, careful evaluation of the cardiovascular system for evidence of shock and examination of the respiratory and nervous systems should be carried out. Establish an adequate airway, treat shock, control overt bleeding, and so on, before replacing the eye in the orbit. While the initial examination and treatment are being carried out, protect the proptosed globe against further exposure and drying. This can be accomplished by using sponges soaked in cold, hypertonic solution (hypertonic 10% dextrose) to reduce ocular edema and prevent corneal drying.

Proptosis of the globe can be associated with severe intraocular problems such as iritis, chorioretinitis, retinal detachment, luxation of the lens, and avulsion of the optic nerve.

Surgical replacement of the proptosed globe should be carried out under general anesthesia. Carefully evaluate the patient to determine whether general anesthesia can be tolerated. Make a lateral canthotomy incision to widen the palpebral fissure.

Using gentle pressure applied to the globe with a moistened, sterile sponge, replace the globe in the orbit. Do not probe the retro-orbital space with a needle or attempt to reduce intraocular pressure by paracentesis. When the eye is replaced in the orbit, place a nictitating membrane flap in position. Three nonpenetrating mattress sutures are placed in the lid margins but not drawn taut. Gently replace the eye in the orbit and tighten the nictitating membrane and lid sutures. Use small pieces of rubber tubing under the sutures to prevent pressure necrosis of the skin overlying the lids. The nictitating membrane sutures are also tied over a piece of rubber tubing.

After replacing the eye in the orbit, inject 2 to 4 mg of methylprednisolone acetate into the retrobulbar space to aid in reducing inflammation.

Postoperative treatment is aimed at controlling traumatic iritis and the extensive corneal damage that is associated with proptosis and exposure keratitis. Systemic broad-spectrum antibiotics are indicated. One percent atropine is used t.i.d.; 1% prednisolone acetate drops and gentamicin ophthalmic ointment are used six times a day. If it is believed that trauma to an eye has been extensive, the topical steroids will be supplemented with systemic steroids for a 1-week period.

Leave the sutures in place until intraorbital swelling is markedly reduced—usually 10 days to 2 weeks. After this time, remove the sutures and inspect the globe. If proptosis recurs, replace the sutures and reevaluate after an additional 2 weeks.

Extraocular muscle injury and resultant strabismus are very commonly seen following proptosis. The most frequent deviation observed is upward and outward, indicating possible paralysis or rupture of the medial rectus, superior oblique, and inferior rectus muscles, or an overaction of the lateral superior rectus muscles. The strabismus is most noticeable immediately following removal of the lid sutures.

............ACUTE GLAUCOMA

Acute glaucoma is a rise in intraocular pressure not compatible with normal ocular function. The cardinal signs of glaucoma are sudden onset of pain, photophobia, lacrimation, deep episcleral vascular engorgement, an edematous ("steamy") and insensitive cornea, shallowing of the anterior chamber depth, a dilated and unresponsive pupil, and loss of visual acuity.

Most forms of clinical glaucoma in dogs are secondary, meaning that the pressure increase is associated with other ocular problems. Some breeds of dogs such as the basset hound, cocker spaniel, Samoyed, and Bouvier des

Flandres may be affected with an abnormality in drainage angle development, namely mesodermal dysgenesis predisposing these animals to angle-closure glaucoma. In several of the terrier breeds of dogs such as the Jack Russell terrier, Sealyham terrier, Manchester terrier, Boston terrier, Cairn terrier, and fox terrier may be predisposed to lens subluxation, often following cyclitis, with resultant pupil blockage or angle blockage, narrowing of the iridocorneal angle, and secondary glaucoma. Other commonly observed causes of glaucoma are severe anterior uveitis and cyclitis, and intumescent or swollen lenses secondary to the rapid development of cataract formation, especially observed in diabetic dogs.

It is important to recognize the underlying cause of the rise in intraocular pressure and, if possible, to correct this while simultaneously beginning treatment to reduce intraocular pressure. Those cases presented in which the affected eye has already become buphthalmic (chronically enlarged) have resulted in permanent damage to the optic nerve and retina, producing permanent visual impairment. Treatment recommendations are for emergency management. Referral of cases of glaucoma is suggested.

............Treatment of Acute Glaucoma Eye Is Visual and Not Buphthalmic

Intraocular pressure may be reduced by three medical methods:

1. Improving the facility of aqueous outflow.
2. Reducing ocular volume by the use of osmotic agents.
3. Reducing aqueous formation.

............Improving Drainage

Most cases of acute congestive glaucoma in the dog are associated with a narrowed drainage angle and, in many cases, beginning anterior synechia secondary to anterior uveitis or severe cyclitis. The topical use of pilocarpine on an emergency basis in most of these cases will be of little benefit and, in the case of uveitis or lens subluxation, may make the condition worse.

If angle-closure glaucoma is secondary to forward displacement of the lens, as occurs in lens subluxation, miotic therapy is contraindicated, because it may worsen the glaucoma by increasing pupillary block and further narrowing the angle.

Most cases of glaucoma with angle alteration such as intumescent lenses, lens subluxation, and iris bombé with broad-based synechia formation require referral to an ophthalmic specialist for emergency surgery.

............Reducing Ocular Volume

Osmotic agents can be used to reduce the size of the vitreous body and the amount of aqueous present. These agents create an osmotic gradient between intraocular fluids and the vascular bed, thus acting independently of the aqueous outflow and inflow system.

1. Oral glycerol 50% 1.4 g/kg (0.6 mL/kg) q8h, can be used to effectively reduce intraocular pressure. Oral glycerol may induce vomiting. Glycerol should be avoided in the diabetic patient.
2. Mannitol 20% 1 to 2 g/kg IV within 1 hour reduces intraocular pressure. Administer mannitol through a filtered IV set and examine the mannitol for crystal formation before administering.

If the filtration mechanism is open and working, pressure may be controlled medically. If increased intraocular pressure rapidly recurs following osmotic therapy, there is extensive obstruction to the aqueous drainage mechanism and referral to an ophthalmologist for surgical intervention is indicated.

..........Reducing Aqueous Secretions

1. Carbonic anhydrase inhibitors are used to reduce aqueous production (see dichlorphenamide, methazolamide, and acetazolamide). This method is not very effective because secretory inhibition by carbonic anhydrase inhibitors is incomplete, reducing aqueous production by only 50% to 60%. If the aqueous drainage apparatus is so severely damaged that it cannot handle 40% of its normal drainage function, the carbonic anhydrase inhibitors will not be able to control intraocular pressure effectively. Prolonged administration of systemic carbonic anhydrase agents in dogs will produce metabolic acidosis. Recently, a new topical carbonic anhydrase inhibitor, dorzolamide (Trusopt, Merck Co., Rahway, N.J.), has become available that does not produce the systemic side effects that systemic drugs do.
2. Adrenergic agents: β-Adrenergic antagonists decrease the production of aqueous humor (e.g., timolol 0.25% 0.5% solution t.i.d). Other available β-blockers are metipranolol, levobunolol, and betaxolol.

REFERENCES

Bistner SI: Ocular emergencies and trauma. *In* Slater D, ed: Textbook of Small Animal Surgery, ed 2. Philadelphia, WB Saunders, 1993, p 1276.
Catlano RA: Ocular Emergencies. Philadelphia, WB Saunders, 1992.
Deutsch TA, Feller D: Paton and Goldberg's Management of Ocular Injuries, ed 2. Philadelphia, WB Saunders, 1985.
Freeman HM: Ocular Trauma. Norwalk, Conn, Appleton-Century-Crofts, 1979.
Gelatt KN: Veterinary Ophthalmology, ed 3. Philadelphia, Lippincott Williams & Wilkins, 1999.
Gilger BC, Hamilton HL, Wilkie DA, et al: Traumatiic ocular protrusion in dogs and cats: 84 cases: J Am Vet Med Assoc 206(8):1186–1189, 1995.
Kural E, Lindley D, Krohne Sl: Canine glaucoma. Compend Contin Educ Pract Vet 17:1017–1026, 1253–1264.
Martin C, Kaswan R, Gratzek A, et al: Ocular use of tissue plasminogen activator in companion animals. Prog Vet Com Ophthalmol 3:29, 1993.
Pfister RR: Chemical injuries of the eye. Ophthalmology 90:1246, 1983.

Environmental Exposure

..........COLD INJURIES
..........Frostbite

Local freezing is most commonly experienced in peripheral tissue (ears, tail) that may be sparsely covered with hair, poorly vascularized, or previously traumatized by cold.

Immediate treatment includes slow rewarming by moist heat applications at 29.5°C (85°F) or by immersion in warm baths. Analgesics may be needed to alleviate pain, and administration of prophylactic antibiotics must be considered. The injured areas should be dried gently and protected from trauma.

Do not rub or apply pressure dressing or ointments. Do not use corticosteroids, and do not be in a hurry to amputate or debride the frozen area. Many tissues recover that do not appear to be viable on first examination. Because intravascular coagulation is a common problem, this problem must be addressed (see discussion of disseminated intravascular coagulation above).

............Hypothermia

Chilling of the entire body from exposure results in a decrease in physiologic processes that becomes irreversible at a body temperature of about 24°C (75°F). Mild hypothermia can be 32° to 37°C, moderate hypothermia from 28° to 32°C, and severe hypothermia below 28°C. The duration of exposure and the animal's physical condition influence its ability to survive.

■ SIGNS ASSOCIATED WITH HYPOTHERMIA

1. Shivering, vasoconstriction
2. Mental depression, hypotension, sinus bradycardia, depressed respiration, increased blood viscosity, muscle stiffness without shivering
3. Atrial irritibility, ventricular premature contractions, ventricular fibrillation
4. Decreased level of consiousness, markedly decreased oxygen consumption, metabolic acidosis, later production of respiratory acidosis
5. Prolongation in blood coagulation times, possible DIC

............*Treatment*

1. If the animal is breathing, supply warm, humidified supplemental oxygen at four to ten times a minute.
2. Hypoventilation may require intubation and positive pressure ventilation (see p. 613).
3. Establish IV line and begin warmed fluid solutions. Add dextrose to the maintenance fluids if blood glucose is less than 60 mg/dL.
4. Monitor core body temperature and ECG.
5. Institute appropriate methods of rewarming such as hot-water bottles, recirculating warm water blanket covering the patient, or radiant heat. Apply external rewarming to the thoracic area. *Do not bring excessive heat into contact with patient lest the patient develop burn injury.*
6. Severe hypothermia may require core rewarming. An effective mechanism to warm a very cold patient is via peritoneal dialysis, 20 mL/kg of lactated Ringer's solution warmed to 39.4°C (103°F), and repeating dialysis at 30-minute intervals until the body temperature is 36.6° to 37.7°C (98° to 100°F). The body temperature always increases slowly. Because the body's response to drugs is unpredictable, medications should be avoided, if possible, until the body temperature approaches normal.
7. Complications encountered during rewarming include DIC, shock, cardiac dysrhythmias, pneumonia, pulmonary edema, acute respiratory distress syndrome, CNS edema, and renal failure.

............HEAT INJURIES
............Heat Stroke

Heat stroke occurs in dogs exposed to a high environmental temperature and placed under stress (such as confinement in an enclosed space or overexertion). Brachycephalic breeds, obese dogs, and older dogs with cardiovascular disease are particularly affected. Hyperthermia is indicated by a rectal temperature of 41° to 43°C (105° to 110°F). Dogs presenting with hyperthermia have congested mucous membranes and tachycardia and are panting rapidly. Other clinical signs may include collapse, vomiting, ataxia, hypersalivation, diarrhea, loss of conciousness, seizures, and muscle tremors. Heat stroke can be associated with alterations of all organs and systems of the body. There is generalized cellular necrosis associated with heat denaturization of cellular proteins. Severe hypotension may develop, and renal failure and hypotensive shock may be seen. The most frequently seen signs are panting, tachycardia, hyperemic and dry mucous membranes, vomiting, diarrhea, dehydration, oliguria, and proteinuria. More profound changes, such as shock, DIC, and coma, develop rapidly.

Dogs with heat stroke will pant excessively, leading to respiratory alkalosis. As the respiratory exertion continues, metabolic acidosis develops. These abnormalities of blood and tissue pH can lead to cerebral edema and death. Severe electrolyte abnormalities develop, including hypernatremia and hypokalemia due to excess water loss from the respiratory tract. Ventricular arrhythmias are detected more in severely affected dogs. Additionally, hypophosphatemia and hypocalcemia develop later. A marked increase in packed cell volume (PCV) also occurs with heat stroke.

·············Treatment

Immediate treatment is aimed at lowering the patient's temperature. This can be accomplished by immersion of the animal in cold water or spraying the body with cold water. Attempt to produce a temperature of 39°C (102°F) in 30 to 60 minutes of cooling therapy. Monitor the rectal temperature because hypothermia can develop rapidly. Start an IV drip of lactated Ringer's solution. Determine the acid-base status by a study of blood gases; however, if this is not feasible, IV administration of fluids coupled with supportive care often proves beneficial in controlling pH abnormalities (see p. 591). Insert a urethral urinary catheter with a closed system of drainage and monitor urine output (see p. 486). Caution must be used in administering fluids if oliguria is present. Furosemide can be used to induce diuresis. Evidence of progressive primary renal disease may develop following correction of the acute temperature rise. Obtain baseline laboratory tests including CBC, platelet count, coagulation profile, BUN, creatinine, glucose, and liver enzyme valves. Look for evidence of DIC, such as hemorrhagic diathesis and melena, and begin treatment (see p. 44). Determining the level of conciousness is important because severe abnormalities in mentation such as coma and seizures portend a poorer prognosis. An ECG is indicated looking for ventricular arrhythmias.

Following initial emergency treatment, keep the affected animal in a well-ventilated cool room and confine it so it does not become overactive. If available, a cool (22°C, or 71.6°F) oxygen chamber can be used for small dogs, provided that excessive CO_2 buildup does not develop (see Oxygen, p. 610). Anticipate delayed effects, including hemorrhagic bowel disease and DIC. Dogs that are going to die as a result of heat stroke usually do so within the first 25 hours after initial evaluation.

REFERENCES

Ahn A: Approach to the hypothermic parient. In Current Veterinary Therapy XII. Small Animal Practice. Philadelphia, WB Saunders, 1995, p 157.
Dhupa N: Hypothermia in dogs and cats. Compend Contin Educ Pract Vet 17:61, 1995.
Drobatz K, Macintire D: Heat induced illness in dogs: 42 cases (1976–1993). J Am Vet Med Assoc 209:1894, 1996.
Fettman MJ: Fluid and electrolyte metabolism during heat stress. Compend Contin Educ Pract Vet 8:391, 1986.
Holoway SA: Heatstroke in dogs. Compend Contin Educ Pract Vet 14:1598–1605, 1992.
Schall WD: Heatstroke. In Kirk RW, ed: Current Veterinary Therapy VIII: Small Animal Practice. Philadelphia, WB Saunders, 1983.
Zenoble RD: Accidental hypothermia. In Kirk RW, ed: Current Veterinary Therapy VIII. Small Animal Practice. Philadelphia, WB Saunders, 1983.

............MALIGANT HYPERTHERMIA SYNDROME

Malignant hyperthermia syndrome is a pharmacogenetic disease involving the uninhibited flow of calcium into the muscle substance. Unfortunately, the disease entity is usually diagnosed only when an animal is placed under general anesthesia. The signs of malignant hyperthermia are massive muscle fasciculations or spasm, supraventricular tachycardia, unstable blood pressure, metabolic and respiratory acidosis, very elevated temperature (42.2° to 43.3°C or 108° to 110°F), increased rate and depth of ventilation, and cardiac arrest. If malignant hyperthermia is not immediately controlled, cellular death results.

Predisposing and aggravating factors in malignant hyperthermia include hypercarbia or hypoxia, hyperthermia caused by infections, high ambient temperatures, high sympathetic activity, muscle trauma, and the use of depolarizing muscle blocking agents (e.g., succinylcholine hydrochloride). There is a genetic predisposition to the development of malignant hyperthermia; this has been demonstrated in the dog.

............Treatment

Malignant hyperthermia syndrome is treated using the following procedures:

1. Surgery must be immediately stopped. Discontinue all anesthetic gases and muscle blocking agents.
2. Hyperventilate the patient with 100% oxygen.
3. Begin cooling with cold packs, give an ice bath, bus stop cooling when the animal's temperature is down to 38.8°C (102°F).
4. Administer dantrolene sodium 1 to 2 mg/kg IV. This decreases the permeability of the sarcoplasmic membrane to calcium ion.
5. Give procainamide 1 g in 500 mL of D5W, if needed for cardiac arrhythmia, or IV lidocaine (see p. 63).
6. Administer IV solutions; fluids can be 0.9% NaCl, lactated Ringer's solution, or D5W. Add 10 to 50 mL of 50% dextrose (depending on size) because of the increased metabolic demands during hyperthermia. Correct the base deficit with sodium bicarbonate (see p. 603).
7. Following an acute episode, dantrolene sodium 2.2 mg/kg q8h for 24 hours can be used.

Fractures and Musculoskeletal Trauma

The majority of musculoskeletal emergencies are the result of external trauma, most commonly from motor vehicle accidents. Injury to multiple organ systems is the rule, rather than the exception.

Massive musculoskeletal injuries must be assigned a relatively low priority in any triage of treatment. A rapid survey physical examination and immediate lifesaving treatment must often be performed simultaneously. This is best accomplished through adherence to A CRASH PLAN, or the ABCs of resuscitation (see p. 3).

In spite of the low priority initially assigned to musculoskeletal injuries, the degree of recovery from these injuries or from complications associated with them is often a critical factor, if not the deciding factor, in the patient's long-term prognosis for a useful life.

Furthermore, the *initial* emergency management of these injuries is often far more important in ensuring maximal early recovery with the fewest complications than is the eventual definitive fracture fixation. This is particularly true if the injuries include spinal cord compromise, open fractures, multiple fractures, open joints, articular fractures, physeal fractures, concomitant ligamentous disruption, or neurovascular compromise in conjunction with a fracture or luxation.

During or immediately following stabilization of the patient, a more thorough physical examination and treatment of the less critical injuries are indicated.

The patient should be protected from further injury or contamination during initial diagnosis and treatment by:

1. Gentle handling and the judicious use of sedation to minimize pain and to prevent displacement at fracture sites, which causes further damage to adjacent soft tissues and may result in conversion of a closed fracture to an open fracture. Additional displacement in cases of vertebral fractures or luxations may be catastrophic. Narcotic sedatives work well for the trauma patient as their effects are dose-related and can be reversed. Particular care needs to be taken with patients potentially sustaining traumatized spinal column injury. Heavy sedation in these patients can cause relaxation of the paraspinal musculature endangering further trauma to the spinal column as the result of routine handling.
2. Immediate (preferably prior to hospitalization) bandaging of open fractures or joints to minimize hemorrhage, contamination by hospital pathogens, and exposure desiccation of bone and cartilage. Clean disposable diapers are vastly preferable to no bandage at all. Initial bandages should be left in place until the patient is moved to clean (if not sterile) surroundings (see p. 549).
3. Application of temporary immobilization devices to fractures distal to the stifle or elbow. The modified Robert Jones bandage is ideally suited to this application.
4. Minimizing palpation of fractures and ligamentous injuries and maximizing radiographic diagnosis of the exact nature and extent of the injury. Localization of the injury can be determined by motion in abnormal locations or directions, swelling due to hemorrhage or edema, vocalization during gentle palpation or manipulation, deformity, angular change, or significant increase or decrease in the normal range of motion of joints. Crepitus should not be intentionally produced. Excessive palpation is inappropriate, as it increases adjacent tissue trauma, hemorrhage, pain, nerve damage, and may convert a closed fracture with a good prognosis to an open fracture with a guarded prognosis. Sedation facilitates efforts to localize the injury, comparison with the opposite extremity, examination of adjacent joints or wounds, and further adjustment of appropriate external fixation devices. It also expedites high-quality radiographic examination (at least two views, frequently with comparison views of the opposite extremities, and stress films), and further facilitates patient positioning without struggling or forcible restraint.

···········PHYSICAL EXAMINATION

Patients predisposed to multiple injuries include animals suffering from falls from high places, vehicle or gunshot injuries, and the "big dog–little dog" encounter. In multiply injured or depressed patients, search meticulously for areas of injury to the spinal column or limbs. Helpful physical signs include swelling, contusion, abnormal motion, or crepitus. If the patient is alert, look carefully for areas of tenderness. All potentially multiple-injury patients will need radiographs evaluating the thorax, abdomen, and the entire injured limb(s). Unconscious or immobile patients must have radiographic evaluation of the spinal column following stabilization and support. In the depressed patient, repeat a thorough examination when the patient becomes more alert. Injuries are missed frequently during the initial examination because of the early response to attenuation of pain.

Once the diagnosis of a limb fracture or luxation is confirmed, look for evidence of associated skin lacerations or punctures. In long-haired breeds, clip the hair to identify signs of open injuries. A fracture is classified as open whether the fracture is grossly open with bone protruding through the soft tissue, or there is only a pinpoint break in the skin.

The clinician should examine the neurologic and vascular status of the limb before and after treatment. The vascular status of the limb is determined by checking the color and temperature of the limb, the state of the distal pulses, and the degree of bleeding from a cut nail bed. Reduction of the fracture or luxation or straightening of gross deformities may return normal vascularity to the limb. Examine both sensation and motor function of the limb when checking neurologic status. Swelling may increase pressure on nerves as they run through osteofacial compartments, resulting in attenuated sensory and motor function. Diminished function often returns once swelling subsides.

There is a high incidence of multiple organ injury with musculoskeletal trauma. A high index of suspicion must be maintained with these cases. The more occult injuries (such as diaphragmatic hernia or perforated bowel) are identified by serial physical evaluations and by appropriate diagnostic tests.

..........INITIAL MANAGEMENT

After the initial examination has been completed, splint the fracture to reduce pain and swelling, prevent further soft tissue damage and self-induced trauma, and to simplify movement. When the fracture or luxation is below the elbow or stifle joint, apply a temporary support splint. Temporary immobilization of fractures above this region is difficult and sometimes dangerous due to leverage on the fracture from the splint. Immobilize these fractures by using an over-the-shoulder or over-the-hip coaptation splint.

■ CLASSIFICATION OF SKELETAL TRAUMA

Group I—Critical

Immediate treatment, within a few hours
Compressive fractures of the skull, fracture or dislocation of the spine, open fracture or luxation

Group II—Semicritical

Early treatment, within 2 to 5 days; otherwise, may result in delayed healing, complications after treatment, and poor long-term results
Articular fractures, physeal fractures, joint subluxations or luxations, slipped capital epiphysis

Group III—Noncritical

Delayed treatment, within several days
Scapular and pelvic fractures, greenstick fracture, and closed fracture of the shafts of the long bones

---

..........OPEN MUSCULOSKELETAL INJURY

Wounds associated with musculoskeletal trauma are common and include injury to bone, joints, and tendons. Two major problems may be associated with these cases:

1. Extensive soft tissue trauma makes wound closure hazardous or impossible and produces the potential for acute infection.
2. Chronic deep infection can develop in traumatized tissues. This is common when avascular bone and cartilage are in the wound.

■ CHARACTERISTICS OF OPEN MUSCULOSKELETAL INJURY

Bone penetration
Fat droplets or marrow elements in blood coming from the wound
Air in soft tissues or joints on radiographs
Lacerations in the area of a fracture (assume that a laceration communicates with
   the fracture, especially the tibia, radius, or ulna)

Early and careful treatment of the wound is necessary to restore function and prevent infection. Immediately protect wounds with a sterile covering. Splint an open fracture or luxation without pulling the exposed bone back into the soft tissue. Do not probe the wound. Do not push or force the extruded soft tissue and bone back into the wound. Do not soak the wound. Nosocomial microorganisms (hospital bacteria) contaminate exteriorized material and will contaminate deeper recesses if replacement into the wound is attempted. Probing, flushing, or replacing tissues at this time will only serve to contaminate deeper tissues and is performed at the time of formal debridement after the patient is physiologically stable.

Immediately start bactericidal antibiotic therapy. Begin antibiotic therapy early to obtain adequate concentration of antibiotics in the fracture hematoma. To avoid side effects to antibiotics such as superinfections, limit the duration of antibiotic therapy to 2 or 3 days.

■ CLASSIFICATION OF OPEN WOUNDS BY DEGREE OF SOFT TISSUE
   INJURY

Type I Wound

Has minimal of soft tissue trauma and devitalization. When associated with a fracture, a type I wound is often created from the inside-out characterized by penetration of bony fragments through the skin or is the result of a low-energy gunshot. There is simple or comminuted fracture pattern, with good stability of the two main bone segments. The treatment and prognosis of a type I wound is similar to that of closed injuries if debrided and stabilized within 6 to 8 hours of injury.

Type II Wound

Has a moderate amount of soft tissue contusion and devitalization. When associated with a fracture, type II wounds are created from the outside-in. It has major deep injury with considerable soft tissue stripping from bone and significant muscle damage. There may be a simple or comminuted fracture pattern. Prognosis is good if debridement is performed within 4 to 6 hours of injury and there is rigid stabilization with a bone plate or external skeletal fixator.

Type III Wound

Results from major external force. There is a great deal of damage and necrosis to the skin, subcutaneous tissue, muscle, and bone, commonly together with nerve, tendon, and artery injuries. The soft tissue damage may vary from crush injury of the whole extremity, to a major regional crush injury produced by an automobile, to a major shearing-type injury associated with dog bites. These injuries require immediate and extensive debridement and initial rigid stabilization with an external skeletal fixator. These injuries can require prolonged healing times constituting a guarded prognosis.

...........Treatment

Treatment of the open musculoskeletal injury involves three considerations: inspection and wound debridement, stabilization and repair, and wound bandaging.

...........Inspection and Wound Debridement

1. Anesthetize the patient and remove the temporary splint.
2. Leave the wound covered and shave the surrounding skin.
3. Remove the covering, fill the wound with sterile K-Y jelly, and then shave the hair to the margin of the wound. Wash away any entrapped hair and the K-Y jelly. Complete an antiseptic scrub of the surrounding skin.
4. If the wound is a small puncture (often seen with gunshot injuries or bites), probe the hole with a sterile hemostat. Do a thorough debridement if tissues deep to the hole are cavitated. If not deep, then open the hole to allow drainage.
5. Flush the wound with a balanced electrocyte solution and remove any detached tissue or debris.
6. Debride the wound from outward to inward. Cut away damaged areas of skin and deeper tissues to "open up" underlying cavitations and tissue injury.
7. Continuously irrigate the wound with warm physiologic electrocyte solution. The stream must be strong enough to flush debris out from the bottom of the wound (7 psi delivered from a 35-mL syringe attached to a 20-guage needle or catheter). Excise obviously devitalized tissue.
8. Do not remove bone fragments that are firmly attached to soft tissue. Do not cut into healthy soft tissue to find and remove bullet fragments, unless the bullet may cause injury to joints or nerve tissue.
9. Do a primary repair of damaged tendons and nerves if the wound is type I and recent (within the first 8 hours of the accident). If the wound is too severe or if there is obvious infection, tag the ends of damaged nerves and tendons with sutures for later repair.

...........Stabilization and Repair

It is best to stabilize open fractures immediately, provided adequate fixation is possible. If inadequate stabilization may present a problem because of the inexperience of the surgeon or inadequate equipment, it is best to perform wound management and place a temporary splint on the patient until definitive repair can be properly performed.

...........Wound Bandaging (see p. 549)

...........ARTICULAR CARTILAGE INJURY

Injuries to joint structures are common, involving not only ligament damage, but occasionally articular cartilage trauma. Cartilage does not heal well and may have significant loss of function and degenerative joint disease (osteoarthritis) following injury. Cartilage injuries that are superficial (no penetration below the tidemark) evoke only a short-lived metabolic and enzymatic response. This response fails to provide sufficient numbers of new cells or matrix to repair even the nominal defect. Superficial lesions remain as defects and do not evolve to chondromalacia or osteoarthritis. Deep lacerations that extend to subchondral bone produce an exuberant healing response from the cells of the underlying cartilage. In many circumstances this material undergoes degeneration and leads to osteoarthritis. Impact injuries to surface cartilage can cause chondrocyte and underlying bone injury. These lesions rapidly to progress to osteoarthritis; however, they may be partially or totally reversible.

..........LIGAMENT INJURIES

> ■ CLASSIFICATION OF LIGAMENT INJURIES
>
> Grade I sprain: A portion of the ligament is ruptured with minimum lengthening. Anatomical and mechanical integrity is preserved.
> Grade II sprain: A portion of the ruptured ligament is stretched, leaving the ligament longer but still in continuity.
> Grade III sprain: The ligament is completely disrupted.

..........Treatment

Grade I injuries require short-term coaptation splints and have a good prognosis. Grade II tears need surgical treatment with a suture stent and consistent postoperative coaptation splints to heal and maintain good function. Grade III injury healing can be a problem. Surgical reapproximation or suture stents are indicated. Failure to immobilize joints that are frequently flexed (elbow and stifle can result in late complications of ligament repair. Ligament injuries to joints, especially collateral ligaments of the stifle, elbow, and hock, and hyperextension injuries of the carpus are commonly missed.

..........FRACTURES IN THE IMMATURE ANIMAL

Fractures in immature animals differ from those in adults in that young puppies and kittens have a striking potential for remodeling bone. Remodeling is dependent upon the age of the patient and the location of the fracture. The younger the puppy or kitten and the closer the fracture to the epiphysis or the growth plate, the greater the potential for remodeling of angular deformities. The long-limbed breeds of dogs can remodel more effectively than the short-limbed breeds. Fractures through the growth plate in immature animals may potentially cause angular deformities, joint dislocations, and osteoarthritis. This form of injury is commonly observed in the distal ulnar growth plate and proximal and distal radial growth plates.

..........HIGH-RISE SYNDROME IN CATS

This syndrome is used to identify cats that fall from a height usually greater than 30 ft. The problem is most frequently observed in urban areas where cats lie on window ledges and, when suddenly startled, fall out of the window.

The most frequently observed lesions in cats falling from these heights are thoracic trauma characterized by thoracic injuries and fractures, pulmonary contusions and pneumothorax; facial and oral trauma, including fractures of the jaws, fractures of the hard palate, and avulsion of the skin and lips from the lower or upper jaw; limb and spinal cord fractures or luxations; fractures of the radius and ulna (reported in 92% of cases); and abdominal trauma, diaphragmatic hernias, and urinary tract trauma.

Cats suffering from high-rise syndrome must:

1. Be treated for shock and stabilized (see p. 32).
2. Have a chest radiograph and an ECG.
3. Make sure the bladder is intact and the cat is able to effectively urinate.
4. Make sure that respirations are normal.
5. Have the hard palate examined for any evidence of fractures.
6. Have all the external limbs checked for evidence of soft tissue damage and fractures.
7. Receive a neurologic examination (see p. 330).

REFERENCES

Aron DN: Emergency management of the musculoskeletal trauma patient. *In* Emergency Medicine and Critical Care in Practice. Trenton, NJ, Veterinary Learning Systems, 1992, p 241.

Gastrointestinal Emergencies

.... FOREIGN BODIES

.... Oral Cavity

Clinical Signs These result from irritation or pain, from the sensation of having an object lodged in the mouth or oropharynx, or from difficulty swallowing or breathing.

1. Pawing at the mouth or attempting to put a foot in the mouth is common when bones or sticks are lodged in the roof of the mouth.
2. Drooling may result from salivation caused by irritation, from inability to close the mouth, or from blockage of the oropharynx. Concurrent trauma to mucous membranes may cause the saliva to be blood-tinged.
3. Cyanosis can result from foreign bodies that obstruct the glottis. Oxygen deprivation may be severe enough to cause syncope, cardiovascular collapse, and death. The most common foreign bodies causing airway obstruction are rubber or synthetic balls small enough to enter the pharynx but too large to be expelled.
4. Oral foreign bodies present for more than a few days are associated with halitosis and drooling.

Diagnosis Often the owner witnesses the foreign body being ingested. Many incidents occur in a recreational setting (e.g., fetching sticks or catching a ball). Cats may ingest string or thread that loops around the base of the tongue and extends into the intestines (see p. 108). Otherwise, the diagnosis of oral foreign body is suspected from clinical signs and verified by direct examination.

1. Sedation or anesthesia may be required for examination and removal. Acepromazine 0.05 to 0.1 mg/kg IV, maximum total dose of 3 mg, or oxymorphone, 0.1 mg/kg IV is suitable for restraint. However, beware of sedating or anesthetizing animals with balls lodged in the pharynx. These animals usually present with marginal respiratory function. Inattentive anesthesia in a hypoxic animal may cause acute cardiovascular collapse.
2. Many affected animals are anxious when presented and panic when attempts are made to open the mouth. Owners can experience multiple (inadvertent) bite wounds while trying to remove oral foreign bodies from their pets. These owners should be encouraged to seek medical attention.

Treatment Bones lodged transversely in the palate may have to be cut into fragments. Ham bones or other ring-shaped foreign bodies that encircle the tongue (like some dog toys) have to be cut to be removed because of massive edema of the tongue distal to the foreign body. Animals with oropharyngeal foreign bodies require anesthesia or heavy sedation to remove the object, even though the animal may be hypoxic.

1. All instruments required should be prepared prior to anesthesia.
2. Preparation for a tracheostomy should be made prior to anesthesia or sedation.
3. An open venous line should be established.
4. An assistant should be available to hold the mouth open.
5. A light plane of anesthesia, sedation, or neuroleptanalgesia is induced IV. Just enough drug is given for immobilization.
6. The mouth is quickly opened and the foreign body is grasped firmly with sponge forceps and extracted. Rubber, plastic, or latex balls become very slippery and are difficult to grasp securely.
7. During the extraction process, the cardiorespiratory status of the animal should be closely monitored. Severe respiratory distress accompanied by poor mucous membrane perfusion, cyanosis, ventricular arrhythmias, or bradycardia is reason for immediate tracheostomy.
8. Once the foreign body is removed, tracheal intubation and the administration of oxygen are desirable. Corticosteroids (dexamethasone sodium phosphate 0.5 mg/kg IV) help to reduce pharyngeal edema. Diuretics should be avoided, because they increase the viscosity of oral saliva and mucus by dehydration. Secretions thus become sticky and difficult for the patient to clear.

.... Esophagus

Clinical Signs Observation of the foreign body ingestion by the animal's owner is helpful. The most common clinical signs are drooling secondary to excess salivation, gulping, and regurgitation after attempts to eat. Some animals make repeated swallowing motions (see Dysphagia). A "sawhorse" stance with reluctance to move is common immediately after foreign body ingestion and esophageal entrapment.

Diagnosis

Radiography Common esophageal foreign bodies, such as bones, are radiodense. The most common sites for foreign bodies to lodge are the base of the heart and just orad to the esophageal hiatus. Pleural effusion or pneumomediastinum can be associated with perforation.

Endoscopy Preremoval and postremoval esophagoscopy is recommended to assess the integrity of the esophagus. Focal perforations are caused by sharp-edged bones. Foreign bodies that fill the lumen of the esophagus may cause pressure necrosis of the mucosa and submucosa, leading to subsequent stricture formation or perforation.

Treatment Attempts should be made initially to retrieve the foreign body by flexible fiberoptic esophagoscopy if available. Rigid tube esophagoscopy can also be done. If the foreign body is firmly lodged or if perforation has already occurred or occurs during retrieval, esophagotomy or esophageal resection must be done. Occasionally, smooth foreign bodies that cannot be easily grasped can be pushed into the stomach and removed by gastrotomy. After removal, the traumatic esophagitis should be treated with protectants (sucralfate 0.5 to 1.0 g per dog), antacid (famotidine 5 mg/kg PO q24h), and NPO (nothing by mouth) for 36 to 48 hours. Owners should be warned of the potential for stricture development in the esophagus.

............Stomach

Clinical Signs The most common clinical sign is persistent vomiting. Vomiting results from irritation of gastric mucosa or from obstruction of gastric outflow.

Diagnosis Initially based on clinical signs and the lack of response to standard empirical treatments for vomiting (NPO, protectants, antiemetics). Plain films and contrast radiography are helpful for detecting the presence of radiopaque and radiolucent objects.

Treatment Remove the foreign object either by gastroscopy or gastrotomy. Although most animals with uncomplicated gastric foreign bodies are relatively healthy, those with foreign bodies that cause outflow obstruction may have serious fluid and electrolyte imbalances needing correction prior to surgery (see p. 585).

............Small Intestine

Clinical Signs Severity of clinical signs depends on the location of the object in the bowel and the degree of the obstruction. *The more orad the obstruction, the worse the clinical signs and the more acute their onset.* Complete obstructions are worse than partial obstructions.

The most significant clinical signs in an animal with complete small bowel obstruction are depression, dehydration, and vomiting. Early clinical signs may consist only of depression and anorexia. Eventually, all patients with intestinal obstruction vomit. Animals with proximal, complete obstruction are usually extremely sick. Functional fluid loss (into distended bowel) and actual fluid loss (from vomiting) cause rapid dehydration and electrolyte imbalances. Obstructions proximal to the common bile duct and pancreatic papillae result in loss of gastric acid, leading to hypochloremic alkalosis. Obstruction caudal to the common bile duct and pancreatic papillae results in loss of all electrolytes and in mixed deficits. Linear foreign bodies (e.g., string, thread, pantyhose, cloth strips) should be suspected in any vomiting patient. String or thread often loops around the base of the tongue and can be visualized by oral examination. The base of the tongue can be viewed orally by opening the cat's mouth while pressing the thumb onto the intermandibular space.

Linear foreign bodies cause bowel obstruction and eventual perforation of the bowel along the mesenteric border. The foreign material becomes entrapped proximally (commonly around the base of the tongue or at the pylorus) while the remainder is passed into the bowel by peristalsis. The bowel "climbs" the stationary string and becomes plicated, producing obstruction. Eventually, continued peristalsis causes the string to saw through the mesenteric border, and multiple perforations result. Once perforation occurs, peritonitis ensues and the prognosis becomes poor.

Diagnosis Any vomiting patient that does not respond promptly to symptomatic treatment should be evaluated. Any vomiting patient that is also dehydrated, depressed, or anorectic should not be treated symptomatically. Intestinal masses may be palpable on physical examination.

Radiography or ultrasound is the most useful diagnostic aid. Plain radiographs may be diagnostic when the foreign body is radiodense or when there is pathologic dilation of the small bowel in a symptomatic patient. Ultrasound will often demonstrate nonradiopaque foreign bodies. Contrast radiography is indicated when confirmation of the suspected diagnosis is absolutely necessary (dogs or cats with concurrent illnesses that might be worsened by unnecessary surgery) or when plain films are not typical. Diagnostic celiotomy is sometimes necessary when an intestinal foreign body is suspected but cannot be confirmed by other means.

■ CLINICAL SIGNS OF INTESTINAL OBSTRUCTION

High Small Bowel

Rapid onset
Rapid progression
Frequent vomiting
Large-volume vomitus
No tenesmus
Minimal abdominal distention
Diarrhea

Low Small Bowel

Subacute onset
Slow progression
Vomiting less frequent
Smaller-volume vomitus
No tenesmus
Abdominal distention present
Diarrhea

Large Bowel

Subacute to chronic
Slow progression
Vomiting occasional
Scant-volume vomitus
Often tenesmus
Abdominal distention
Diarrhea

Treatment As a general rule, all intestinal foreign bodies in the small intestine should be removed. An exception is the ingested sewing needle that does not have thread attached. Needles can be treated expectantly and will often be passed in the feces. Linear foreign bodies sometimes pass but should never be treated expectantly in symptomatic animals.

The timing of surgery is critical. Once the probability of a small intestinal foreign body is established, the only definitive treatment is removal. However, many animals are severely ill and dehydrated and have electrolyte imbalances, endotoxemia, or peritonitis.

An attempt should be made to partially correct fluid and electrolyte imbalances. Specific deficits should be corrected if known. Otherwise, balanced electrolyte solutions in quantities sufficient to correct dehydration are begun. Fluid therapy is continued for 1 to 2 hours as long as the patient's clinical condition is stable or improving. If the patient is deteriorating in spite of supportive therapy, enterotomy or resection and anastomosis is performed as soon as possible.

............Large Intestine

Clinical Signs Signs of foreign bodies in the large bowel are usually nonexistent. Objects that traverse the small intestine usually pass through the large bowel without incident. Penetrating foreign bodies (usually needles) may cause localized or generalized peritonitis or local abscess formation. Vomiting and abdominal pain are the most common signs of peritonitis or abscess. Hematochezia may occur when foreign bodies abrade or lacerate mucosa.

Diagnosis Symptomatic patients should be evaluated radiographically. Colonoscopy is indicated when radiographic survey films are suggestive of colonic obstruction or perforation.

Treatment Most foreign bodies in the large intestine of asymptomatic patients can be treated expectantly. Surgery is indicated to remove obstructions or to treat perforations, peritonitis, or abscesses.

..........Rectum and Anus

Foreign bodies result from ingestion (bones, needles) or external insertion. Ingested bones and needles can traverse the entire digestive system, only to lodge in the anal ring.

Clinical Signs The most common clinical sign is dyschezia with or without hematochezia.

Diagnosis Animals in pain should be sedated, narcotized, or anesthetized. Acepromazine 0.05 to 0.1 mg/kg IV or oxymorphone 0.1 mg/kg IV may be given. Cautious digital examination of the rectum will usually enable the object to be detected. Radiography is helpful in locating needles that have penetrated the rectum and have lodged in perirectal or perianal tissues. Proctoscopy can be done to inspect the rectal mucosa; to identify other causes of rectal pain or straining, such as tumors or perineal hernias; and to visualize areas that cannot be palpated.

..........GASTRIC DILATION–VOLVULUS COMPLEX IN THE DOG

Acute gastric dilation with or without volvulus occurs primarily in large, deep-chested dogs such as the Great Dane, Weimaraner, Saint Bernard, Gordon setter, Irish setter, and standard poodle. The risk of bloat increases with age, with dogs over 7 years of age being twice as likely to bloat as dogs 2 to 4 years of age. Deep, narrow-chested dogs are more likely to bloat than dogs with wider chests. Recent studies have shown that the overall mortality for surgically treated gastric dilation is 18%, with most deaths occurring in dogs undergoing splenectomy and partial gastric resection.

Clinical Signs Early in the course of disease, it is difficult or impossible to distinguish volvulus from dilation on the basis of clinical signs. Abdominal distention occurs and is often the first sign noted by the owner. The animal makes repeated nonproductive retching motions. There may be a history of being fed a large meal minutes to hours before signs appear. There may be a history of postprandial water engorgement or of excessive postprandial activity.

Diagnosis

Physical Examination The animal is in various stages of weakness and lethargy, with a distended abdomen, poor mucous membrane perfusion, weak and rapid pulse, grunting, and anxiety.

Stomach Tube Stomach tubing can be a diagnostic aid. However, inability to pass a tube does not rule out dilation, nor does ability to pass the tube eliminate the possibility of volvulus.

Radiography The right lateral recumbenty position is helpful. Dogs with volvulus have a characteristic "double-bubble" gas pattern. The stomach is distended with gas and appears to have a dorsal compartment and a ventral compartment divided by a partial horizontal septum. Displacement of the pylorus can also be identified. Dogs with simple dilation have gaseous distention of the stomach, but the radiographic anatomy of the gastric gas pattern is normal.

Treatment

(*Note*: Affected patients should be treated immediately.)

1. If there is assistance, catheters for IV fluids should be started while the animal's stomach is being intubated. Infusion of a colloid solution (heta-starch 5 to 10 ml/kg) and lactated Ringers solution up to 90 mL/kg/hr is begun. If chemical restraint or sedation is required, use ketamine 8 mg/kg plus diazepam 0.1 mg/kg IV.

2. A role of 2-in. tape is placed in the dog's mouth with holes rostral and caudal. The jaws are then encircled with 1-in. tape to hold them closed. Most dogs readily tolerate this maneuver.

3. A lubricated silicone (Silastic) stomach tube (1 to 1½ in. diameter) is passed through the roll of tape and guided into the esophagus by gentle twisting and pushing. If the tube enters the stomach, a container should be ready to catch the effluent.

4. After the stomach is decompressed, lavage may be done with several liters of tap water.

5. The dog is then radiographed in right lateral recumbency to determine if volvulus is present. If no volvulus is present, conservative care may be elected.

6. The animal is observed closely for at least 24 hours.
   a. NPO.
   b. IV fluids and antibiotics are administered until cardiovascular status is stable.
   c. The ECG is monitored. Ventricular arrhythmias are common and may require treatment with medication. These arrhythmias commonly appear 6 to 24 hours after presentation. Prior to antiarrhythmic therapy, it should be determined that the dog's perfusion is adequate and that serum electrolyte levels (especially potassium) are normal. Antiarrhythmic therapy is initiated with an IV bolus of lidocaine hydrochloride 2 mg/kg. If the arrhythmia responds, begin a lidocaine drip at a rate of 40 to 60 μg/kg/min. The infusion is prepared by removing 50 mL of lacatated Ringer's solution from a 1-L bag. Fifty milliliters of 2% lidocaine hydrochloride *(without epinephrine)* is injected into the bag to make a solution with a concentration of 1 mg lidocaine for each milliliter of solution. Infusion of this solution at a rate of 30 mL/kg/day will deliver the proper amount and rate of lidocaine. If the lidocaine is either ineffective or transiently effective, procainamide hydrochloride 3 to 8 mg/kg IM t.i.d. or q.i.d. may be added. Quinidine gluconate 6 to 12 mg/kg IM t.i.d. or q.i.d is an alternative to procainamide. If these drugs are not successful, a test dose of diazepam 5 mg IV is given. If the arrhythmia improves, propranolol 0.04 to 0.06 mg/kg IV slowly may be given.

7. If the stomach tube cannot be passed or if gastric distention recurs within hours of decompression, it should be assumed that a gastric volvulus is present. Radiographs may be taken in right lateral recumbency to confirm volvulus, or the patient may be taken directly to surgery for repositioning of the stomach and gastropexy.

Immediate Postoperative Care

1. NPO for 36 hours.

2. Supportive therapy with balanced electrolyte solutions and colloid solutions is continued.

3. Serum electrolytes must be measured; there are no "characteristic" imbalances.

4. Monitor the cardiac rate and rhythm. Medications are begun or continued as indicated. Most arrhythmias are transient and improve as the animal's overall conditions improves.

5. Antibiotic therapy is controversial, but may be justified to counteract enterotoxemia or sepsis.

Long-Term Postoperative Care

1. Small amounts of clear liquids are begun PO 36 hours postoperatively
2. If liquids are well received, small amounts of baby food are given hourly.
3. If baby food is tolerated, frequent small meals of moistened dog food may be given throughout the day.
4. Upon the patient's release from the hospital, owners are counseled to divide the day's ration into at least three feedings, to prevent water engorgement after eating, and to prevent excessive postprandial activity.

............SMALL INTESTINAL OBSTRUCTION

Intestinal obstruction may be caused by foreign bodies, tumors, intussusception, volvulus, or strangulation within hernias. Regardless of the cause, complete intestinal obstruction results in the following pathophysiologic sequence:

1. Fluid and electrolytes are secreted into the lumen of the obstructed bowel. The secretory function is among the last of the physiologic processes to cease.
2. The bowel distends proximal to the site of the obstruction. Obstructive ileus ensues.
3. Intraluminal pressure increases and reduces venous and lymphatic drainage from the bowel wall. Edema of the bowel wall results; this further complicates venous circulation.
4. Eventually, the bowel wall becomes ischemic and may rupture.

The most common clinical signs of bowel obstruction are vomiting and dehydration. The more orad the obstruction, the more acute the onset of clinical signs and the more severe the physiologic derangement. Fluids are lost to the body in the vomitus and in the dead space created by the distended gut. Therefore, supportive treatment consists of attempts to correct fluid and electrolyte deficits before, during, and after removal of the obstruction.

............Obstruction by a Foreign Body (see p. 108)

............*Acute Intussusception*

Intussusception is the invagination of one segment of bowel (the intussusceptum) into another (the intussuscipiens). The proximal segment always invaginates into the caudal segment of bowel. Puppies and kittens (<1 year of age) are most commonly affected. Although intussusception may be idiopathic, any condition that produces bowel irritation and hypermotility (parasites, viral enteritis, distemper) can presumably induce it.

Clinical Signs Clinical signs include abdominal discomfort, hemorrhagic diarrhea, and vomiting. Hemorrhagic diarrhea is often the earliest noticeable sign. Obstruction is usually partial at first, but progresses to complete obstruction with time. Initial signs are often mild, since most intussusceptions occur in the distal small bowel; the distal jejunum, ileum, ileocecocolic and junction are the most common locations.

Diagnosis Diagnostic findings include pain on abdominal palpation. A sausage-shaped mass may be palpable. Plain radiographs show dilation of bowel. This may be segmental or generalized, depending on the duration of illness. Contrast radiographs provide a definitive diagnosis, but are seldom necessary. Differential diagnosis includes hemorrhagic gastroenteritis, parvovirus enteritis, parasitic enteritis, intestinal foreign body, and any of the myriad causes of vomiting.

Treatment Treatment is supportive (correction of fluid deficits) and definitive (reduction or removal of the intussusception followed by enteroplication of the small intestine prevent recurrence).

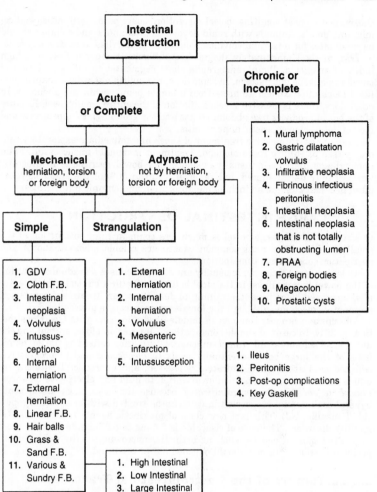

Figure I–11. This schematic drawing depicts the classification of intestinal obstructions. F.B., foreign body; PRAA, persistent right aortic arch; GDV, gastric dilation volvulus; Key Gaskell, autonomic ganglionopathy. (From Lippincott L, et al: Surgical case report: Intestinal obstructions. Pulse 35:13, 1993.)

............Small Intestinal Volvulus

Volvulus of the small intestine occurs when the intestine twists around the root of the mesentery. The problem occurs in young large-breed dogs with a median age of 2.6 years. Predisposing causes may be pancreatic atrophy, GI disease, splenectomy, or trauma. The jejunum is most commonly affected. The problem is rare in cats.

Clinical Signs The major presenting signs are endotoxic shock, hematochezia, acute-onset vomiting, bowel distention, acute pain, peritonitis, septicemia, and death. Animals with rapid development of shock and collapse should be candidates for intestinal volvulus. Vomitus and diarrhea are extremely fetid.

Diagnosis Unfortunately, diagnosis is difficult. It depends first on a high index of suspicion. Plain radiographs show segmental to diffuse dilation of bowel in palisade gas pattern. In some dogs, the multiple teardrop-shaped, gas-filled loops often appear to arise from a single point within the abdomen. In other dogs, there is massive gaseous dilation of the entire small bowel. Rupture of the bowel produces free abdominal gas and the ground-glass appearance and lack of detail characteristic of peritonitis.

Treatment Supportive treatment of shock and immediate exploratory celiotomy (see p. 16) are recommended. Treatment is usually unsuccessful. Fetid hemorrhagic diarrhea is usually evidence that bowel necrosis is in progress. Surgery may be attempted, but removal of up to 80% of the small bowel is often necessary. Sequelae include malabsorption and chronic unthriftiness.

............LARGE INTESTINAL OBSTRUCTION

Obstruction of the large bowel is much less common than obstruction of the small intestine. The most common causes are colonic adenocarcinoma and obstipation (obstructive constipation).

Colonic adenocarcinoma is usually annular and causes a gradual stricturing of the bowel lumen. Blood in the stool is usually the first clinical sign. Eventually, increased bleeding and straining to defecate occur. Treatment consists of segmental colectomy, although the long-term prognosis is guarded.

Obstipation is most common in middle-aged and older cats (see Constipation, p. 391). In cases of simple constipation, rehydration of the animal and the use of stool softeners and bran is sufficient. Obstipation caused by the adynamic ileus of the large bowel eventually leads to *megacolon* and is progressive. Affected cats are often dehydrated, depressed, and anorectic. Treatment requires rehydration, with particular attention to fluid and electrolyte balances. *Phosphate enemas are contraindicated* because they can cause fatal, acute hyperphosphatemia. Megacolon in cats can be treated with cisapride (Propulsid, Titusville, NJ). This is a new class of prokinetic agents used to treat GI motility disorders. The dose of cisapride is 2.5 mg to 5.0 b.i.d. to t.i.d. for most cats. Predisposing causes, such as arthritis, narrowing of the pelvic canal, perineal hernia, or tumor, should be ruled out or corrected.

............Tumors of the Gastrointestinal Tract

Emergency treatment is required only when chronic partial obstruction eventually becomes acutely complete or when severe hemorrhage occurs from the tumor or the effects of the tumor.

............Adenocarcinoma

Adenocarcinoma is the most common neoplasm causing partial to complete obsturction. Adenocarcinomas tend to be annular and constricting. Adenocarcinoma occurs most commonly in the small intestine of older Siamese cats. In the dog, the colon is the most common site.

Clinical Signs Signs are both chronic and acute. Weight loss and progressively severe vomiting are common and may occur over weeks or months. Eventually, complete obstruction develops. Effusion may be present if metastases to peritoneal surfaces have developed.

Diagnosis Diagnosis is usually based on surgical exploration after viewing radiographs characteristic of bowel obstruction (diffuse dilation of bowel) or of peritoneal effusion.

Treatment Treatment of small intestinal adenocarcinoma consists of resection and anastomosis of the affected segment. The prognosis for long-term survival of cats after surgery is good if no evidence of metastasis is seen. Median survival is 15 to 30 weeks. Lymph nodes, hepatic metastases, or peritoneal metastases shorten survival.

..........Leiomyomas and Leiomyosarcomas

These tumors may cause partial obstruction of bowel. Chronic blood loss anemia is also common because these tumors tend to bleed into the lumen of the bowel. Hypoglycemia has also been associated with these tumors.

..........Strangulated Hernias

Incarceration of a loop of bowel into congenital or acquired defects in the body wall may cause bowel obstruction. Pregnant females and young animals with congenital hernias are most at risk. Rarely, older male dogs with perineal hernias and animals of any age with traumatic hernias are affected.

Clinical Signs Signs are those of obstruction (i.e., pain, vomiting, and dehydration).

Diagnosis The diagnosis can often be made on physical examination. Simple hernias with nonstrangulated contents are usually not symptomatic. Radiography can be used to confirm bowel distention orad to hernia.

Treatment Treatment is supportive (correction of fluid balance) and definitive (reduction or resection of compromised bowel and closure of the hernia).

..........BOWEL PERFORATION

The potential for injury to bowel should be suspected anytime there are penetrating injuries (knife, gunshot, or stick wounds). Injuries resulting in bowel rupture can also occur with blunt trauma. Avulsion of mesenteric attachments to a sufficiently long segment of bowel will cause ischemic necrosis of that segment with eventual rupture. Perforating ulcers of the upper GI tract have been associated with administration of NSAIDs and liver disease.

Diagnosis The diagnosis first depends on alertness to the possibility that bowel may have been perforated or penetrated. As a general rule, all penetrating abdominal injuries should be investigated by laparotomy. Clinicians skilled in the procedure and in interpretation of diagnostic lavage may wish to modify the rule. When any bluntly traumatized animal (e.g., those suffering from an automobile injury) either does not respond to treatment for shock or responds initially and then deteriorates, this should arouse suspicion that structural injury has occurred to abdominal viscera. Abdominal radiographs show free peritoneal gas, loss of detail, and the homogenous appearance characteristic of peritoneal effusion. Abodominocentesis may show extracellular and intracellular bacteria, inflammatory cells, and debris characteristic of bowel contents. Contrast radiography is usually contraindicated because the procedure delays surgery.

Treatment Treatment consists of:

1. IV fluids and electrolytes.
2. Antibiotics.
3. Surgery, the definitive measure. In most cases, it is safer to remove perforated segments than to attempt debridement and closure.

..........RECTAL PROLAPSE

Affected dogs and cats are usually immature animals younger than 6 months of age. The cause is frequently indeterminable, but chronic parasitism has been incriminated. Older animals with rectal prolapse usually have a source of irritation, such as a tumor or other mucosal lesion.

Diagnosis Diagnosis is made by physical examination. Prolapse must be distinguished from intussusception of the small bowel. In rare instances, the intussusception can invaginate through the large bowel, rectum, and anus. These are differentiated by inserting a thermometer or blunt probe into the cul-de-sac formed by the junction of the prolapsed mucosa and the mucocutaneous junction at the anal ring. Inability to insert the probe signifies that the rectal mucosa is prolapsed. Passage of the probe indicates that the prolapsed segment is actually the intussusceptum.

Treatment Acute prolapses can be reduced. A loose purse-string suture is applied and left in place for 48 hours. Prognosis with the purse-string method is guarded to poor. Inability of a purse-string suture to effect a permanent correction, or the presence of severely ischemic or necrotic tissue requires surgical intervention:

1. If the prolapsed portion is viable, colopexy can be done. Through a laparotomy, sufficient tension is applied to the colon to reduce the prolapse and the colon is sutured to the peritoneum of the lateral abdominal wall with two or three rows of 2-0 or 3-0 monofilament suture material.
2. If the prolapsed portion is nonviable, it must be amputated. Four stay sutures are placed at 90-degree intervals through the wall of the prolapse at the mucocutaneous junction. The prolapse is resected distal to the stay sutures, and rectal continuity is reestablished by suturing the seromuscular layers together in one circumferential line and mucosal layers together in the other. The sutured incision is replaced in the anal canal.
3. Postoperatively, a stool softener is given with food. Analgesic gel can be given per rectum to reduce irritation and straining. An investigation for the inciting cause ensues.

...........ACUTE GASTRITIS

Hemorrhage from the mouth—especially with highly fermentable, poorly digestible foods—can precipitate acute gastritis. Eating of foreign materials, such as bone and other garbage, is frequently seen in puppies. Diarrhea often develops following gastritis and may be hemorrhagic. Severe hemorrhagic gastroenteritis may precipitate a shocklike syndrome, with a rapidly rising hematocrit level. Various toxins, such as heavy metals, arsenic, thallium, or ethylene glycol, may also produce severe gastric irritation. Gastritis is characterized by pain in the anterior abdomen, vomiting, excessive water drinking, depression, and dehydration.

■ CAUSES OF ACUTE GASTRITIS

Dietary indiscretions
Food allergies
Drugs
Toxic chemicals
Bacterial toxins
Infectious diseases
Stress and trauma
Brain lesions
Renal failure
Hepatic failure

The differential diagnosis in acute gastritis must eliminate other acute problems such as pancreatitis, hepatitis, intestinal obstructions, and toxicities.

Table 1–17. Drugs to Control Vomiting

Drugs (Proprietary Name)	Suggested Dosages*
Phenothiazines	
Chlorpromazine	0.2–0.5 mg/kg IM q8h, 0.05 mg/kg IV
(Thorazine)	q4h, 1.0 mg/kg rectal q8h (dog)
Prochlorperazine	
(Compazine)	0.1 mg/kg IM q6h, 0.5 mg/kg IM, IV q8h
Triethylperazine (Torecan)	0.25 mg/kg IM q8h (dog), 0.5 mg/kg rectal q8h (dog), 0.125 mg/kg IM q8h (cat)
Others	
Metoclopramide (Reglan)	0.2–0.5 mg/kg SC q8h, 1.0–2.0 mg/kg IV
Trimethobenzamide (Tigan)	drip over 24 hr, 3 mg/kg IM q8h (dog)

*All doses apply to dog *and* cat unless otherwise noted.

Diagnosis A careful history and examination of the vomitus may be helpful in arriving at a differential diagnosis (see Vomiting, p. 447). Persistent severe vomiting can be very debilitating and may lead to severe dehydration and electrolyte imbalances. The following supportive steps are helpful until a more conclusive diagnosis can be reached:

1. Withhold oral fluids and solids for the first 24 hours. Do not give drugs PO.
2. Correct fluid and electrolyte imbalances (see p. 585).
3. Control vomiting with antiemetics (Tables 1–17 and 1–18) such as prochlorperazine, chlorpromazine, perphenazine, and trimethobenzamide.
4. With severe vomiting, especially when disruption of the mucosal wall of the stomach is suspected, high doses of systemic antibiotics are indicated to treat both aerobic and anaerobic bacteria.
5. Antacids t.i.d. or q.i.d. can reduce gastric activity and irritation. Anticholinergics are not effective either in inhibiting the vomiting reflex or in reducing gastric acidity.
6. In gastritis associated with azotemia (see p. 122), increased secretion of gastrin and H_2-receptor stimulation, the use of cimetidine is indicated (see p. 955). Ranitidine 1 mg/kg PO q12h has H_2-receptor antagonism. Sucralfate 250 mg q.i.d. to a 15-kg animal may help to stop vomiting.
7. Locally acting medication containing bismuth subsalicylate (Pepto-Bismol) 0.25 mL/kg q.i.d. may be helpful in reducing gastric irritation associated with prostaglandin release.
8. When oral fluids and food can be tolerated, a bland diet should be given in small quantities.

Table 1–18. Narcotic Antiemetics

Drug	Dosage
Meperidine	10 mg/kg, IV, IM, SC (dog)*
Paregoric	0.05–0.06 mg/kg b.i.d. or t.i.d. PO (dog and cat)
Diphenoxylate	0.05–0.01 mg/kg q.i.d. PO (dog)
Loperamide	0.08 mg/kg q.i.d. PO (dog)
	0.1–0.3 mg/kg once daily or b.i.d. PO (cat)

*Give slowly IV to prevent hypotension.

..........HEMORRHAGIC GASTROENTERITIS

Hemorrhagic gastroenteritis (HGE) is an acute GI upset usually seen in small-breed dogs (e.g., poodles, dachshunds, miniature schnauzers) 2 to 4 years of age. The history usually reveals that the dog has been in good health and is well cared for. Signs develop rapidly and include vomiting, fetid diarrhea with hemorrhage, and jamlike consistency of stool. Dehydration may be severe, and Hct values may range from 55% to 70%. The patient is depressed and hypovolemic; it strains when defecating but shows no marked abdominal pain. Fluid and electrolyte abnormalities develop if the diarrhea is prolonged. Bleeding may be associated with the development of DIC.

The definitive cause of this condition is unknown but an association with high concentrations of clostridial organisms in the intestine has been noted. Acute, fulminating diarrhea associated with coronavirus or parvovirus may mimic these signs. Mechanical obstruction of the GI tract causing vascular stasis, sepsis, hepatic cirrhosis, and severe shock must be ruled out.

Treatment The aim is to restore fluid and electrolyte balance and eliminate invasion by bacterial organisms that can produce septicemia or more severe enteritis. Treatment is usually given for at least 48 hours and includes the following steps:

1. Correct fluid deficits with IV fluids administered via catheter (see also p. 585).
2. Allow no oral food for 72 hours. If vomiting is controlled, small amounts of electrolyte solutions can be given PO in small, divided amounts.
3. Use antibiotics providing four quadrant coverage, such as ampicillin-sulbactam 22/mg/kg IV q6h and gentamicin 6 mg/kg q24h or amikacin 20 mg/kg q24h.
4. Carefully observe the animal for DIC and treat with systemic heparin if indicated (see p. 44).
5. When systemic signs are controlled, return oral food to the diet very gradually. Cooked white rice and cottage cheese plus very small amounts of cooked lamb are acceptable.

..........ACUTE PANCREATITIS

Pancreatitis occurs most frequently in dogs and is often associated with the feeding of a meal high in fat content and in animals with fasting hypertriglyceridemia. Pancreatitis can also be drug-induced. Glucocorticoids are the drugs most incriminated. Glucocorticoids can increase the viscosity of pancreatic secretions and may induce ductal proliferation, thus narrowing the pancreatic duct lumen, resulting in obstruction. Pancreatitis can also occur following penetrating or blunt trauma, ischemia of the pancreas, duodenal reflux, biliary tract disease, and hyperadrenocorticism.

Acute necrotizing pancreatitis in cats is associated with anorexia, lethargy, hyperglycemia, and icterus. A rapidly fatal course often occurs. The chronic form of pancreatitis is more common in cats, resutling in intermittent vomiting, anorexia, weight loss, and depression. Numerous predisposing causes have been described: pancreatic flukes, viral infection, hepatic lipidosis, drugs, and organophosphate poisoning.

Clinical Signs Acute pancreatitis usually produces sudden severe vomiting, abdominal pain, marked depression, hypotension, and a shocklike syndrome. It must be remembered that pancreatitis can also occur as a subclinical entity in which clinical signs are minimal. Vascular damage to the pancreas resulting in ischemia can produce acute inflammation. Hypovolemic shock and DIC can contribute to vascular alteration. The blood supply to the pancreas is critical in determining whether edematous pancreatitis progresses to hemorrhagic necrotic pancreatitis. Embolization of blood vessels supplying the pancreas leads to necrosis. Diarrhea can follow vomiting and is associated with duodenal irritation. Pain may be very acute, especially on palpation of the right upper abdominal quadrant. Some dogs show only minimal pain on abdominal palpation. The major differential diagnosis is the same as that for acute abdomen (see p. 15).

Complications The most common complications of pancreatitis are fluid and electrolyte abnormalities, profound hypotension, and peritonitis. Hypotension results from the actions of bradykinin, phospholipase A and elastase release, vomiting and diarrhea, endotoxic shock, DIC, and release of vasoactive polypeptide myocardial depressant factor. Complement activation, which subsequently activates the clotting cascade, activates platelets, causes release of serotonin and histamine, and produces vasodilation and shock. *Myocardial depressant factor* can further lead to shock, hyperemia, cardiomyopathy, and cardiac arrhythmia. Toxins produced by intestinal bacteria, especially if there is ileus, can lead to shock and toxemia. Electrolyte imbalances can develop because of persistent vomiting; potassium loss by this mechanism can be severe. Localized chemical peritonitis can develop, producing intestinal ileus and diarrhea. Hepatic lesions, characterized by hepatic necrosis, fatty infiltration, congestion, and less-than-normal hepatic architecture, may be profound. Diabetes mellitus is a potential complication of acute pancreatitis. Patients with recurring episodes of pancreatitis should be monitored for hyperglycemia and glucosuria.

Laboratory Findings Laboratory examination may help in confirming the diagnosis, but laboratory tests are often unreliable when it comes to interpreting the results of serum lipase and amylase levels. Determination of serum amylase performed by the amyloclastic method and lipase are the tests of choice (see pp. 720 and 732). Both serum amylase and lipase are excreted in the urine, and renal insufficiency can result in elevations of both. Additionally, intestinal foreign bodies may elevate serum lipase levels. Amylase values are *not* as specific for acute pancreatitis as are lipase values. Serum amylase levels rise to abnormal levels (two to six times greater than normal) early in the course of the disease. Serum lipase levels also become elevated, and the amylase and lipase tests can be run concurrently. Hypotension and prerenal azotemia result in an elevated BUN. Hyperlipemia and hyperglycemia may occur. Hypocalcemia and hypoproteinemia may be observed in acute pancreatitis. Coagulation function tests may be abnormal, including platelet counts, complement, and antithrombin III concentrations. Increases in fibrinogen and plasminogen concentrations and prolongations of PTT and PT levels may be present.

Radioimmunoassay looking for increased levels of canine trypsin-like immunoreactivity (TLI) also may prove helpful in diagnosis (see p. 764) The results of this test take time to obtain and animals must be treated prior to obtaining test results. Plasma trypsinogen is excreted by glomerular filtration, and altered renal function can lead to elevated levels of plasma TLI.

Urinalysis and a urine specific gravity are obtained to determine whether azotemia is renal or prerenal in origin. A hemogram usually reveals to mild to moderate leukocytosis, with stress response. Hemoconcentration is usually present, despite extensive fluid therapy.

Diagnosis Diagnostic peritoneal lavage can be an aid in acute pancreatitis. Abdominal amylase concentrations that are higher than serum values indicate chemical peritonitis. WBC counts greater than 1000/mm^3 and the presence of bacteria or toxic neutrophils indicate septic pancreatic necrosis (e.g., pancreatic abscess). Exploratory celiotomy is available is usually required.

Ventrodorsal and lateral radiographic views should be taken. The following radiographic changes may be seen:

1. Increased density, diminished contrast, and granularity in the right cranial abdomen.
2. Stomach displaced toward the left or pyloric antral border.
3. Mass medial to the proximal descending duodenum or duodenal displacement toward the right flank.
4. Gastric gas pattern in or thickened walls of the descending duodenum.
5. Static gas pattern in or caudal displacement of the transverse colon.

Ultrasound may show edema and enlargement of the pancreas, dilation of the pancreatic ducts, poor blood flow to the pancreas, or the presence of pancreatic abcess.

Treatment Therapy in acute pancreatitis is designed to correct hypovolemia, prevent or reverse shock, provide symptomatic relief, and reduce inflammation. The most critical period in the course of the disease is 24 to 48 hours after the onset of pancreatitis. Treatment should include the following measures:

1. Restrict all oral intake of food and liquid.
2. Correct shock, fluid, electrolyte, and acid-base abnormalities (see p. 32).
3. Administer plasma (fresh or frozen) to replace alpha-macroglobulins.
4. Administer systemic trimethoprim-sulfadiazine or ampicillin-sulbactam and an aminoglycoside.
5. Suppression of pancreatic secretion can be accomplished by complete restriction of all oral intake, including food, water, and medications. As the clinical condition improves, confine oral intake to nutrients that will stimulate pancreatic secretion the least (e.g., boiled rice as a carbohydrate source and cottage cheese or cooked eggs as a source of high biologic value proteins).
6. Anticholinergic drugs (e.g., atropine) to control pancreatic secretion are not indicated. Anticholinergics may reduce intestinal motility in an already atonic intestinal tract with ileus. Vomiting can be controlled with antiemetics, such as prochlorperazine or chlorpromazine, but should not be used in hypovolemic patients. Administer metoclopramide hydrochloride 0.2 to 0.4 mg/kg SC q6–8h or 1 mg/kg/day by continuous IV infusion.
7. To reduce pain give an analgesic such as oxymorphone (0.05 to 1.0 mg/kg IV q3–4h).
8. Animals with a chronic course of pancreatitis (>5 days) are treated with placement of a jejunal feeding tube and are fed well below the level of the pancreas.

Cats with acute pancreatitis may have more subtle signs, with little or no vomiting. Lipid abnormalities precipitating acute pancreatitis in the cat appear to be uncommon. More common causes in cats appear to be Feline Infectious Peritonitis (FIP), trauma, toxoplasmosis, and parasites.

............ACUTE HEPATIC FAILURE

Acute hepatic failure can be associated with a wide variety of hepatotoxins, including mushrooms, algae, organic chemicals and drugs. The most frequently observed signs are vomiting, diarrhea, anorexia, jaundice, bleeding, and CNS signs. Physical examination may reveal hepatomegaly, abdominal pain, jaundice, ascites, hemorrhage, and cerebral encephalopathy.

Differential Diagnosis (Table 1–19)
Treatment

1. Treat shock with crystalloid and colloid therapy. Plasma or albumin is the colloid of choice.
2. Treat hemorrhage with injectible vitamin K_1 2 to 5 mg/kg SC q24h and fresh whole blood.

Table 1–19. Causes of Acute Liver Failure

Hepatotoxins	*Infectious Agents*
Exogenous drugs	Infectious canine hepatitis virus
Acetaminophen (cat)	*Leptospira* spp.
Arsenicals	*Salmonella* spp.
Halothane	Feline infectious peritonitis virus
Ketoconazole	*Toxoplasma gondii*
Mebendazole	*Bacillus piliformis* (Tyzzer's disease)
Methoxyflurane	*Others*
Phenazopyridine (cat)	Pancreatitis
Phenytoin	Septicemia
Sulfonamides (trimethoprim-	Inflammatory bowel disease
sulfadiazine), tetracycline	Acute hemolytic anemia
Environmental toxins	
Aflatoxin	
Carbon tetrachloride	
Dimethylnitrosamine	
Heavy metals, herbicides	
Pesticides	
Phosphorus	
Pyrrolizidine alkaloids	
Selenium	
Endogenous	
Bacterial endotoxins	

From Sherding RG: Medical Emergencies. New York, Churchill Livingstone, 1985.

3. Treat gastric bleeding with cimetidine 5 mg/kg IV q4–6h.
4. Treat hypoglycemia with IV glucose administration. Monitor closely.
5. Treat sepsis with IV broad-spectrum antibiotics, such as ampicillin-sublactam plus a quinolone.
6. Treat hepatic encephalopathy with lactulose enemas.
7. Monitor for cerebral edema (deteriorating neurologic signs, changes in pupillary light reflexes, increase in muscle tone of the limbs, hyperventilation, decerebrate posture). At the first sign of progression, treat with mannitol 1 g/kg IV over 30 minutes, repeated q4h as needed, and furosemide 1 to 2 mg/kg q8h for two to three doses.

REFERENCES

Bagley RS, Levy JK, Malarky DE: Hypoglycemia associated with intra-abdominal leiomyoma and leiomyosarcoma in six dogs. Am Vet Med Assoc 208:69–71, 1996.

Basher A, Fowler D: Conservative versus surgical management of gastrointestinal linear foreign bodies in the cat. Vet Surg 16:135, 1987.

Brourman JD, Schertel ER, Allen DA, et al: Factors associated with perioperative mortality in dogs with surgically managed gastric dilation–volvulus. 137 cases (1988–1993). J Am Vet Med Assoc 208:1855–1864, 1996.

Burrows CF, Ignaszewski LA: Canine gastric dilation–volvulus. J Small Anim Pract 31:495, 1990.

Edwards KF, et al: Pancreatic masses in seven dogs following acute pancreatitis. J Am Anim Hosp Assoc 26:189–198, 1990.

Hall JA, Macy DW, Husted PW: Acute canine pancreatitis. Compend Contin Educ Pract Vet 10:403–417, 1988.

Hardy R: Hepatic encephalopathy. *In* Kirk RW, Bonagura JD, eds: Current Veterinary Therapy XI-Philadelphia, Saunders, 1992.

Hess RS, Saunders M, Van Winkle TJ, Shofer F, Washbau R: Clinical, clinicopathologic, radiographic, and ultrasonographic abnormalities in dogs with fatal acute pancreatitis: 70 cases (1986–1995). J Am Vet Med Assoc 213(5):665, 1998.

Hill RC, Van Winkle TJ: Acute pancreatitis in the cat. *In* Proceedings of the eighth Annual Forum of the American College of Veterinary Internal Medicine, 1990, pp 329–331.

Kirby R: GI emergencies: Acute hemorrhagic diarrhea. *In* Proceedings of the Sixth Annual Forum of the American College of Veterinary Internal Medicine, 1988, pp 564–566.

Kosovsky JE, Matthiesen DT, Patnaik AK: Small intestinal adenocarcinoma in cats: 32 cases (1978–1985) Am Vet Med Assoc 192:233–235, 1988.

Lantz GC: Treatment of gastric dilitation volvulus syndrome. *In* Bojrab MJ, ed: Current Techniques in Small Animal Surgery, ed 3. Philadelphia, Lea & Febiger, 1989.

Leib MS, Konde LJ, Wingfield WE, et al: Circumcostal gastropexy for preventing recurrence of gastric dilatation–volvulus in the dog: An evaluation of 30 cases. J Am Vet Med Assoc 180:245–248, 1985.

Murtaugh RJ: Acute pancreatitis: Diagnostic dilemmas. Semin Vet Med Surg (Small Anim) 2:282–295, 1987.

Nemzek JA, Walshaw R, Hauptman JG: Mesenteric volvulus in the dog: A retrospective study. J Am Anim Hosp Assoc 29:357–362, 1993.

Schaer M: Acute pancreatitis in dogs. Compend Cointin Educ Pract Vet 13(2):1769, 1991.

Schulman AJ, Lusk R, Lippincott CL, et al: Muscular flap gastropexy: A new surgical technique to prevent recurrences of gastric dilation–volvulus syndrome. J Am Anim Hosp Assoc 22:339–346, 1986.

Shealy P, Henderson R: Canine intestinal volvulus. Vet Surg 21:15–19, 1992.

Simpson KW:Current concepts of the pathogenesis and pathophysiology of acute pancreatitis in the dog and cat. Compend Contin Educ Pract Vet 15(2):247–253, 1993.

Washabau R: Acute gastrointestinal hemorrhage. Part I. Approach to patients. Compend Contin Pract Vet 18:1317, 1996.

Washabau R: Acute gastrointestinal hemorrhage. Part II. Causes and therapy. Compend Contin Pract Vet 18:1327, 1996.

Willard MD: Pancreatitis. *In* Proceedings of the 11th Annual Forum of the American College of Veterinary Internal Medicine, 1993, 230.

Urinary Emergencies

·············UREMIC CRISES

············Definitions

Azotemia—Defined as an increased concentration of nonprotein nitrogenous compounds in blood, typically BUN and serum creatinine.

Prerenal Azotemia—A condition due to reduced renal perfusion.

Postrenal Azotemia—A condition due to interference with excretion of urine from the body (e.g., obstruction or uroabdomen caused by rupture of the urinary tract).

Primary (Intrinsic) Renal Azotemia—A condition due to parenchymal renal disease.

Uremia—The constellation of clinical signs and biochemical abnormalities associated with a critical loss of functional nephrons, including the extrarenal manifestations of renal failure.

Renal Failure—The clinical syndrome that occurs when the kidneys are no longer able to maintain their regulatory, excretory, and endocrine functions, resulting in retention of nitrogenous solutes and derangements of fluid, electrolyte, and acid-base balance.

Renal Disease—The presence of morphologic or functional lesions in one or both kidneys, regardless of extent.

············Azotemia (see also p. 721)

Azotemia occurs when 75% or more of the nephron population is nonfunctional. The magnitude of azotemia alone cannot be used to determine whether the azotemia is prerenal, renal, or postrenal, or to determine whether the disease process is acute or chronic, reversible or irreversible, and progressive or nonprogressive.

............Treatment

The approach to the azotemic patient is as follows:

1. Localize the azotemia. This requires an evaluation of the history, physical examination findings, urine specific gravity prior to fluid therapy, and response to fluid therapy. For example, an azotemic patient with a history of fluid loss (e.g., vomiting, diarrhea), dehydration on physical examination, and a urine specific gravity greater than 1.045 is likely to have prerenal azotemia. The azotemia likely will be resolved after rehydration. As another example, an azotemic patient with a history of polyuria and polydipsia, dehydration and a large bladder without obstruction on physical examination, and urine specific gravity of 1.007 to 1.015 before fluid therapy is likely to have abnormal kidneys. If the azotemia resolves with fluid therapy, the patient had prerenal azotemia and has renal disease. If the azotemia improves but does not resolve after rehydration, the patient had both prerenal and primary renal azotemia. Dogs with hypoadrenocorticism may have prerenal azotemia and urine specific gravity values in the isosthenuric range, possibly as a result of medullary washout of solute. Drugs such as corticosteriods and diuretics can cause prerenal azotemia and urine specific gravity values in the isosthenuric range in the absence of intrinsic renal disease as a result of interference with the urinary concentrating mechanism.
2. Estimate dehydration as a percentage of body weight, and calculate the amount of fluid necessary for rehydration (1 L = 1 kg) and maintenance (40 to 60 mL/kg/day) over the next 24 hours. Place an IV catheter, and begin rehydration with a balanced electrolyte solution (e.g., lactated Ringer's solution).
3. Diagnose and treat any underlying disease process responsible for prerenal azotemia (e.g., shock, hypoadrenocorticism, congestive heart failure).
4. Monitor urine output during rehydration. *Oliguria* is defined as less than 1.0 to 2.0 mL/kg/hr in dogs and cats. Urine output should return to normal as rehydration occurs in patients with prerenal azotemia. If the animal remains oliguric after rehydration, consider the possibility of oliguric acute intrinsic renal failure (AIRF) and administer additional fluid carefully based on urine output, central venous pressure (CVP), or serial body weight determinations (see also p. 124).

............Prerenal Azotemia

Prerenal azotemia results from conditions that reduce renal perfusion, such as hypovolemic shock, severe dehydration, hypoadrenocorticism, CHF, cardiac tamponade, cardiac arrhythmias, and general anesthesia. Initially, the kidneys are normal and can resume normal function when adequate perfusion is restored. In animals with intact renal autoregulation, mean systemic blood pressure must fall below 80 mm Hg before the glomerular filtration rate (GRF) decreases. In some diseases, however, autoregulation may be impaired. Also, azotemia can result from passive reabsorption of urea from tubular fluid during states of low tubular flow rate (e.g., dehydration) even if the GFR is not markedly decreased. If renal hypoperfusion is allowed to persist, the animal may progress from prerenal disease to AIRF. Prerenal azotemia also may coexist with renal azotemia in animals with primary renal disease as a result of vomiting and ongoing polyuria in the absence of any oral fluid intake. The treatment of prerenal azotemia is described above.

..........Acute Intrinsic Renal Failure

AIRF is characterized by an abrupt decline in renal function of sufficient magnitude to cause azotemia and inability to regulate solute and water balance. Patients with AIRF may be oliguric or polyuric. The most common causes of AIRF in small snimals are ischemia and nephrotoxins. Nephrotoxic AIRF is more common in dogs and cats than is ischemic AIRF.

..........Phases

There are three phases of AIRF: induction, maintenance, and recovery.

Induction Phase The induction phase occurs between the time of renal insult and the development of azotemia, defective concentrating ability, and oliguria or polyuria. Clinical intervention at this time may prevent progression to the maintenance phase. Clinically, the induction phase is characterized by a progressive loss of concentrating ability, progressive azotemia and a progressive increase in the numbers of renal epithelial cells and casts observed in the urinary sediment. Glucosuria also may be observed.

Maintenance Phase The maintenance phase develops after a critical amount of irreversible nephron injury. Removal of the inciting factor and correction of prerenal azotemia at this point do not result in a return to normal. The extent of nephron injury probably is greater in AIRF patients with oliguria than in those with polyuria. The maintenance phase may last several weeks, and recovery of renal function may not occur if injury was severe. In oliguric patients, the most serious complications are overhydration and hyperkalemia.

Recovery Phase The patient enters the recovery phase if sufficient renal healing occurs. Azotemia may resolve, but concentrating defects may remain. If the patient was oliguric in the maintenance phase, a marked diuresis develops during the recovery phase and may be accompanied by fluid and electrolyte losses. The recovery phase may last for weeks or months.

..........Treatment

The principles of treatment of AIRF are as follows:

1. Rule out obstruction and uroabdomen.
2. Determine from the history whether there has been any exposure to nephrotoxic drugs or chemicals.
3. If there is a history of recent exposure to ethylene glycol (<4 to 6 hours), induce vomiting by administration of apomorphine 0.02 mg/kg IV. Give activated charcoal 5 g/kg by stomach tube. The minimum lethal dose of ethylene glycol in the dog is approximately 5.0 mL/kg and 1.5 mL/kg in the cat. Administer 5.5 mL/kg of a 20% ethanol solution IV of q4 h for five treatments and then q6 h for four treatments. Ethanol treatment is not likely to be effective if ingestion occurred more than 24 hours prior to presentation. In dogs, consider 4-methylpyrazole as an alternative to ethanol for inhibition of alcohol dehydrogenase (see p. 200). The dosage of 4-methylpyrazole in dogs is 20 mg/kg IV followed by 15 mg/kg at 12 and 24 hours and 5 mg/kg at 36 hours. It is not effective in cats. If marked hypocalcemia is present, administer 2 to 10 mL of a 10% calcium gluconate solution IV. Give sodium bicarbonate 1.0 to 2.0 mEq/kg IV if metabolic acidosis is severe (pH <7.2, serum bicarbonate <12 mEq/L). Calcium gluconate and sodium bicarbonate must not be given simultaneously because calcium carbonate crystals form and the solution becomes turbid.
4. Rule out chronic renal failure by determining the presence or absence of polyuria and polydipsia and nonregenerative anemia. Evaluate radio-

graphic renal size. Normal renal size is 2.5 to 3.5 times the length of L2 in dogs and 2.4 to 3.0 times the length of L2 in cats.

5. Weigh the animal, and continue to monitor body weight serially (twice or three times a day) throughout the course of treatment. Use extreme care to avoid overhydration (a 1-kg decrease or increase in body weight implies a 1-L deficit or excess of body fluid).

6. Estimate dehydration, and replace the hydration deficit over the first 6 to 8 hours. If dehydration is not clinically apparent, administer a volume of fluid equivalent of 3% to 5% of body weight to cause mild volume expansion.

7. After rehydration has been established, give an amount of fluids equal to insensible needs (14 to 20 mL/kg/day) plus a volume equal to the volume of urine produced each day. An indwelling urinary catheter should be used only during the first 24 hours to document oliguria. After the first 24 hours, urine output can be monitored by collecting all voided urine. If urine output cannot be monitored, serial measurement of body weight and CVP can be used to evaluate fluid balance and prevent overhydration.

8. Attempt to increase urine output. Give furosemide 2 to 4 mg/kg IV. Double the dosage and repeat if no response. If furosemide fails, administer mannitol 0.25 to 0.5 g/kg. Do not repeat if there is no response. If diuretics fail, administer dopamine 2 to 10 μg/kg/min (40 mg added to 500 mL lactated Ringer's solution). Dopamine 2 to 10 μg/kg/min and furosemide 1 mg/kg/hr may be synergistic. Management is facilitated if polyuria can be established, since there is less risk of overhydration and hyperkalemia.

9. Manage hyperkalemia with 0.5 to 1.0 mEq/kg sodium bicarbonate IV.

10. Monitor acid-base balance and administer sodium bicarbonate 0.5 to 1.0 mEq/kg to correct severe metabolic acidosis (pH <7.2, serum bicarbonate <12 mEq/L).

11. If unsuccessful in establishing polyuria and controlling hyperkalemia, begin peritoneal dialysis (see p. 614).

12. Monitor for infections, and treat with appropriate antibiotics.

13. Consider phosphorus binders (e.g., Amphogel [aluminum hydroxide gel] 30 to 90 mg/kg/day). Their effectiveness in anorectic animals is limited, but treatment may coat uremic GI ulcers and reduce vomiting.

14. Administer cimetidine 10 mg/kg IV, followed by 5 mg/kg IV b.i.d. to reduce gastrin-mediated acid production. Consider ranitidine 2 mg/kg b.i.d. (or famotidine 0.5 mg/kg q24 h) to avoid adverse drug interactions with cimetidine and in patients with liver disease.

15. Use prochlorperazine 0.5 to 1.0 mg/kg SC to centrally inhibit intractable vomiting.

16. Avoid all nephrotoxic drugs and genral anesthesia if possible.

17. Consider enteral (i.e., nasogastric tube) or parenteral nutrition to improve the catabolic state.

18. A renal biopsy may be needed to establish a diagnosis and prognosis (see p. 502).

19. If the animal enters the recovery phase and diuresis occurs, prevent dehydration and electrolyte imbalance (e.g., hypokalemia, hyponatremia) by adequate parenteral fluid and electrolyte replacement (see Table 1–20 for guidelines for potassium supplementation).

...........Postrenal Azotemia

Postrenal azotemia results from obstruction of the excretory pathway or uroabdomen owing to rupture of the urinary tract. Complete urinary tract obstruction or uroabdomen is fatal within 3 to 5 days if untreated. In the dog, urinary tract obstruction usually is caused by urethral calculi or tumors. In the male cat, feline urologic syndrome (FUS) is the most common cause of urethral

Table I-20. Guidelines for Intravenous Potassium Supplementation in Dogs and Cats in Renal Failure*

Serum Potassium (mEq/L)	Potassium Chloride to Add to 250-mL Fluids (mEq)	Maximum Fluid Infusion Rate (mL/kg/hr)
<2.0	20	6
2.1–2.5	15	8
2.6–3.0	10	12
3.1–3.5	7	16

*Do *not* exceed 0.5 mEq/kg/hr. Method of Dr. R.C. Scott, Animal Medical Center, New York.

From Muir WW, DiBartola SP: Fluid therapy. *In* Kirk RW, ed: Current Veterinary Therapy VIII. Small Animal Practice. Philadelphia, WB Saunders, 1983, p 38.

obstruction. Ruptured bladder is the most common cause of uroabdomen, and most cases are caused by blunt trauma.

...........Urinary Tract Obstruction

Clinical signs include dysuria, hematuria, inability to urinate or initiate a good stream of urine, and a distended bladder. Late signs are those of postrenal uremia and include dehydration, lethargy, anorexia, and vomiting. These signs progress to coma and death within 5 days of complete obstruction.

...........*Treatment*

The immediate treatment is to relieve the obstruction. This often can be accomplished in dogs by passing a well-lubricated, small-diameter (3.5 F) polypropylene catheter past the obstruction or by hydropropulsion (see References). If these methods fail, the bladder should be decompressed by cystocentesis using a 23-gauge needle. The next priority is correction of fluid, electrolyte, and acid-base disturbances by appropriate fluid therapy. A postobstructive diuresis lasting 2 to 5 days may occur following relief of obstruction. It is importnat to prevent excessive fluid and solute losses (e.g., potassium, sodium) during this time. Definitive treatment ultimately necessitates surgery in most cases (e.g., calculi removal, tumor removal).

...........Feline Lower Urinary Tract Disease (FLUTD)

A complete discussion of FLUTD is beyond the scope of this section (see References for additional information). Cases involving a short duration of obstruction (<36 hours) are considered *uncomplicated*, whereas those associated with a longer duration of obstruction (<36 hours) are considered *complicated*. The following approach may be used in the management of cats with urethral obstruction due to FLUTD.

1. Draw blood for diagnostic tests if indicated (complicated obstruction).
2. Place an IV catheter, and begin fluid therapy with 0.9% saline or lactated Ringer's solution if indicated (complicated obstruction).
3. Treat hyperkalemia if indicated (complicated obstruction) based on ECG findings or serum potassium concentration by IV administration of 0.5 to 1.0 mEq/kg $NaHCO_3$. Insulin, regular insulin 0.1 to 0.25 units/kg IV and glucose 0.5 to 1.5 g per unit of insulin IV as an infusion over 2 hours, or calcium gluconate 0.2 mL/kg of a 10% solution IV, is used less often.

4. If the obstructing material (urethral plug) is visible at the external urethral meatus, it sometimes may be dislodged by gentle massage of the penis.

5. If sedation is required, give ketamine 5 to 10 mg IV and atropine 0.05 mg IV. Additional sedation can be achieved by adding diazepam 0.5 mg IV. Muscle relaxation and analgesia will last 20 minutes. Inhalation anesthesia utilizing the "fish tank" method is also effective and nontraumatic in these patients.

6. Relieve the obstruction by aseptically passing a well-lubricated 3.5 F open-end polypropylene catheter to the level of the obstruction, occluding the tip of the penis around the catheter, and irrigating the urethra with a sterile, cold, balanced electrolyte solution (e.g., lactated Ringer's solution) to distend the urethra while advancing the catheter into the bladder.

7. Decompress the bladder by removing all urine, and irrigate the bladder with warm sterile saline until the flushing fluid is clear of blood and sediment.

8. If the obstruction cannot be relieved, consider cystocentesis with a 23-gauge needle to decompress the bladder. Relief of obstruction should be tried again after bladder decompression.

9. Decide whether or not an indwelling catheter should be placed (Sovereign open-end Tom Cat catheter, Sherwood Medical Industries, St. Louis, MO). Criteria for placing an indwelling catheter include prolonged obstruction (complicated case), severe hematuria, considerable trauma during relief of obstruction, or poor urine stream after relief of obstruction. The indwelling portion of the catheter should be at least 9 to 12 cm to provide adequate bladder drainage.

10. Secure the catheter in place by means of a butterfly adhesive strip and two sutures. Attach the urinary catheter to a closed collection system if possible.

11. Place an Elizabethan collar on the cat. Keep the cat warm. Uremic cats are often hypothermic.

12. Promote diuresis by IV administration of a balanced electrolyte solution (e.g., lactated Ringer's solution).

13. Monitor the urine sediment for evidence of bacterial infection (e.g., pyuria, bacteriuria), and use antibiotics as needed.

14. Prevent fluid and electrolyte (e.g., potassium, sodium) disturbances during the period of postobstructive diuresis (2 to 5 days) by careful attention to amount and composition of parenteral fluids administered. This can be done by measuring urine output or weighing the cat frequently (twice or three times a day) to ensure adequate fluid therapy. Supplement potassium as needed (see Table 1–20 for guidelines).

15. Remove the urinary catheter *after* 24 to 48 hours (uncomplicated obstruction) or after postobstructive diuresis subsides (complicated obstruction). Palpate the bladder frequently to detect recurrence of obstruction.

16. Instruct owners regarding the long-term management of FUS at the time of release (i.e., water always available, canned food, salt).

...........Ruptured Bladder (see p. 19)

...........Renal Trauma, Ruptured Ureter, and Ruptured Urethra (see pp. 19, 20)

...........DRUG ADMINISTRATION IN RENAL FAILURE

Many drugs are eliminated from the body primarily by renal excretion, and such drugs may accumulate in patients with renal failure unless modification is made in the dosage regimen. The dosage regimen can be modified by one of two methods: decreased dosage (D) or increased interval (I).

The reduced dosage method results in decreased peak and increased trough concentrations of the drug, whereas the initial loading dose is unchanged. This method is useful for bacteriostatic antibiotics but should be avoided with nephrotoxic drugs:

$$D\ (renal\ failure) = D\ (normal) \times [Cr\ Cl\ (patient) / Cr\ Cl\ (normal)]$$

where D = dosage and Cr Cl = creatinine clearance.

The increased interval (in hours) method results in peak and trough concentrations similar to those observed with regular use of the drug in patients with normal renal function:

$$I\ (renal\ failure) = I\ (normal) \times [Cr\ Cl\ (normal) / Cr\ Cl\ (patient)].$$

If the creatinine clearance (Cr Cl) is unknown, the following formulas may be substituted: $D\ (renal\ failure) = D\ (normal) \times (1/serum\ creatinine)$ or $I\ (renal\ failure) = I\ (normal) \times (serum\ creatinine)$

See references for additional information.

REFERENCES

Barasanti JA, Finco DR, Brown A: Feline urethral obstruction: Medical management. *In* Kirk RW, ed: Current Veterinary Therapy XI. Small Animal Practice. Philadelphia, WB Saunders, 1992, p 883.

Chew DJ: Fluid therapy during intrinsic renal failure. *In* Dibartola S, ed: Fluid Therapy in Small Animals. Philadelphia, WB Saunders, 1992.

DiBartola SP: Clinical approach and laboratory evaluation of renal disease. *In* Ettinger SJ, Feldman EC, eds: Textbook of Veterinary Internal Medicine, ed 4. Philadelphia, WB Saunders, 1995.

Kirby R: Acute renal failure as a complication in the critically ill animal. Vet Clin North Am Small Anim Pract 19:189–1208, 1989.

Lulich JP, Osborne CA, Carlson M, et al: Nonsurgical remval of urocystoliths in dogs and cats by voiding urohydropulsion. J Am Vet Med Assoc 203:660–663, 1993.

Osborne CA, Finco DR: Canine and Feline Nephrology and Urology. Baltimore, Williams & Wilkins, 1995.

Stone EA, Barsanti JA: Urologic Surgery in the Cat and the Dog. Philadelphia, Lea & Febiger, 1992.

Emergencies of the Male Reproductive Tract and Genitalia

............Scrotal Trauma

In the dog and cat, scrotal trauma is most likely to be the result of direct scrotal injury sustained during fights with other animals or during accidents in which extensive abrasion occurs to the genitalia. At the time of initial evaluation, injuries should be categorized as (1) superficial or (2) penetrating.

Superficial injuries to the scrotum should be cleansed with a mild or diluted surgical soap, dried thoroughly, and treated with a topical antimicrobial as needed until the pain and inflammation subside. Extreme swelling of the scrotum may develop within 24 hours of an abrasive injury, requiring administration of anti-inflammatory doses of corticosteriods (e.g., prednisolone 0.5 to 1.0 mg/kg PO q12h) for 2 to 4 days. Additionally, some dogs and most cats will require an Elizabethan collar during the convalescent period. The prognosis for recovery is excellent. The owner should be cautioned that scrotal inflammation and subsequent increased scrotal temperature may alter semen quality for months post injury.

Penetrating injuries to the scrotum may be associated with severe swelling,

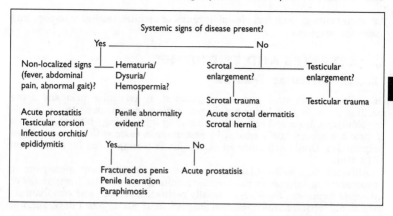

pain, and secondary infection. As such, wounds should be surgically debrided as necessary and systemic antimicrobials administered. Animals with severe penetrating wounds, particularly those involving the testicle, or full-thickness abrasions are best treated by castration and scrotal ablation.

...........Acute Scrotal Dermatitis

Traumatic scrotal dermatitis subsequent to abrasion, either self-induced (licking) or direct physical or chemical injury, is common among intact male dogs. Allergic contact dermatitis, defined as type IV hypersensitivity, is regarded as far less common and clinically difficult to confirm. In affected dogs, the scrotum can become extremely swollen, erythematous, and painful. Physical evidence of pyotraumatic dermatitis may develop if left untreated.

Treatment Treatment is directed at removing offending chemicals, if any, from the scrotal skin by thorough bathing and alleviating the pain by suppressing inflammation and managing secondary infection. Although topical medications are generally effective in treating superficial scrotal abrasions, many topical products, or the vehicle in which they are contained, may actually cause or aggravate the dermatitis (e.g., neomycin, tetracaine, tar shampoos, and petrolatum). Therefore, oral or parenteral administration of corticosteroids at anti-inflammatory doses for 24 to 72 hours is recommended in patients with uncomplicated infections.

An attempt should be made to establish the presence of underlying disorders that could predispose to scrotal dermatitis. For example, the widespread vasculitis associated with *Rickettsia rickettsii* (Rocky Mountain spotted fever) may lead to scrotal edema, hyperemia, and pain with subsequent secondary traumatic dermatitis. Scrotal irritation is also described as a clinical finding in dogs infected with *Brucella canis*. Arbitrary treatment with corticosteroids could, in fact, complicate primary infections, and treatment with antibiotics may confound ability to diagnose specific infectious agents.

...........Scrotal Hernia

Scrotal hernias are defined as those inguinal hernias in which the contents (intestines, mesentery, omentum, fat) protrude through the inguinal canal into the scrotum. As with inguinal hernias, scrotal hernias are surgical emergencies only if intestinal incarceration or venous obstruction has occurred. Rule-outs for scrotal enlargement include epididymitis or orchitis, testicular torsion, and testicular neoplasia.

............TESTES AND EPIDIDYMES
............Testicular Trauma

In addition to physical evidence of penetration, testicular pain and acute swelling of one or both testes are characteristic signs of trauma to the testicle or epididymis. Dogs and cats with penetrating injuries (e.g., bite wounds) to a testicle are appropriately treated by castration in cases with trauma-induced pulpefaction. Orally administered amoxicillin is recommended for a minimum of 10 days.

Although rare, acute enlargement of the scrotum may occur subsequent to nonpenetrating injuries to the testicle, resulting in testicular hemorrhage or hydrocele formation. Swelling is usually peritesticular, soft, and compliant on palpation. If spontaneous resolution does not occur within 5 to 7 days, surgical exploration and drainage are indicated.

Treatment Application of cool compresses to the scrotum over the injured testicle can be beneficial if treatment is started soon after the injury. Corticosteroids are recommended initially to reduce testicular inflammation following trauma. The owner should be cautioned that testicular inflammation and subsequent increased scrotal temperature may alter semen quality for months post injury.

............Testicular Torsion (Torsion of the Spermatic Cord)

Rotation of the testicle on the cord is most likely to involve an enlarged, neoplastic testicle retained in the abdomen, but is also seen in nonneoplastic scrotal testes. Pain, the predominant clinical sign, results from venous congestion and swelling. Additional signs, such as anorexia, vomiting, and acute abdominal pain, may resemble acute intestinal obstruction. An intra-abdominal mass may be palpable. Ultrasonography, preferably with color flow Doppler, of the spermatic cord near the testicle may be useful in confirming a diagnosis of torsion. Surgical removal of the involved testicle is recommended.

............Infectious Orchitis and Epididymitis

Infectious orchitis or epididymitis in the dog is most often caused by ascending infection by aerobic bacteria that are normal preputial or urethral flora. These include *Escherichia coli*, *Staphylococcus* spp., *Streptococcus* spp., and *Mycobacterium canis*.

B. canis is also capable of causing orchitis or epididymitis in the dog. (It may also induce licking the scrotum and acute dermatitis.) Rocky Mountain spotted fever (*R. rickettsii*) is reported to cause epididymal pain and enlargement in male dogs.

Dogs with orchitis or epididymitis have testicular enlargement with acute pain, and are reluctant to walk. They are often febrile, and may exhibit licking or chewing at the affected region of the scrotum. Diagnostic tests should include an attempt at ejaculation for semen culture, or collection of specimens by needle aspirate of the affected organ(s) for culture and cytology, and *B. canis* serology.

Treatment Specific antibiotic therapy should be administered for 3 weeks followed by quantitative culture of the semen to demonstrate eradication of the etiologic agent. Castration is often necessary in patients that do not respond. Dogs infected with *B. canis* may be treated with minocycline 50 mg/kg b.i.d. for 14 days and doxycycline 5 mg/kg PO, b.i.d. for 7 days, which is reported to suppress but not eradicate the infection. The owner should be cautioned that testicular inflammation and subsequent increase in scrotal temperature may alter semen quality for months post injury.

............ACUTE PROSTATITIS

Clinical Signs Acute prostatitis is characterized by fever, caudal abdominal pain, blood in the ejaculate or dripping from the penis, hematuria, difficulty in defecation, and occasional dysuria. Associated signs include depression, anorexia, vomiting, and postural changes attributable to pain. On physical examination, the patient may be febrile; evidence of sepsis may be present in severely affected dogs. Prostatic enlargement may be symmetric or asymmetric (abscess formation). Pain may be manifested during rectal palpation of the prostate. Bacterial infection, particularly with gram-negative organisms (e.g., *E. coli, Proteus* spp., *Pseudomonas* spp., and *Mycoplasma* spp.), is the most commonly reported cause of acute prostatitis. Less common causes include anaerobic bacteria or fungi such as *Blastomyces dermatitidis.* If a prostatic abscess ruptures, acute diffuse peritonitis, shock, and death may occur within 2 days.

Diagnosis Bacterial prostatitis is confirmed on the basis of presenting signs, neutrophilic leukocytosis with or without a left shift, and positive culture results. Samples for culture may be obtained from the prostatic portion of the ejaculate, fluid collected by prostatic massage, urine, urethral discharge, or, less commonly, fine-needle aspirate of the prostate. Although semen culture and sensitivity are quite helpful, dogs with acute bacterial prostatitis may be unwilling to ejaculate. Radiography may reveal the presence of an enlarged prostate gland, but this alone does not confirm the diagnosis of acute prostatitis. Ultrasonography often reveals the presence of prostatic abscessation and aloows for collection of culture samples from apparently affected areas of the prostate gland, if desired. Be aware that aspiration of infected prostatic tissue may lead to iatrogenic formation of extraprostatic septic tracks.

Cytologic examination of an ejaculate or prostatic washes from a dog with acute prostatitis reveals abundant inflammatory cells (exudate) and may contain organisms.

Treatment Immediate treatment of acute prostatitis is directed at correcting complications associated with an enlarged prostate, especially dysuria and constipation. Enrofloxacin (Baytril) appears to be particularly effective against gram-negative infections and mycoplasmas, and moves well into prostatic tissue. Enrofloxacin 5 mg/kg PO, is administered b.i.d. for at least 10 days. Trimethoprim or chloramphenicol is an appropriate alternative to enrofloxacin, assuming that the therapy prescribed is administered daily for a minimum of 2 to 3 weeks.

Since hyperplasia may be a predisposing factor in the development of acute prostatitis, castration is recommended as adjunctive therapy with the purpose of preventing recurrence. Castration should not be performed, however, until after the patient has received antibiotics for at least 1 weeks, so as to prevent the surgical complication of scirrhous cords. Concurrent medical therapy with megestrol acetate (Ovaban) 1 mg/kg PO once daily or the antiandrogen finasteride (Proscar 1 mg/kg PO once daily may cause a decrease in prostate size during the time of antibiotic therapy, until the castration can be performed. If prostatic abscess is confirmed, marsupialization or surgical drainage may be indicated because antimicrobial therapy is unlikely to be totally effective in these patients. Surgical therapy is associated with a high degree of complications, including incontinence, chronically draining stomas, septic shock, and death.

...........PENIS
...........Fractured Os Penis

This is an uncommon condition encountered in male dogs. Although fractures of the os penis occur with minimal soft tissue injury, dysuria and hematuria are signs usually observed by the owner. On physical examination, crepitus and urethral obstruction may be present. A lateral radiograph will usually confirm the extent of injury to the penis.

Treatment Conservative treatment is recommended. Immobilization of simple fractures is not required. Severe fractures, particularly those involving injury to the urethra, can be immobilized with a urethral catheter positioned beyond the fracture site, and maintained for 7 days. Systemic antimicrobial therapy should be administered to prevent secondary urinary tract infection.

Fractures of the os penis that are comminuted or severe enough to prevent effective urination may require open reduction and fixation with a finger plate to stabilize. For extensive trauma to the urethra, partial penile amputation or a prescrotal urethrostomy may be required.

...........Laceration

Because of its rich vascular supply, even small lacerations of the penis may bleed extensively. Dogs and cats with penile lacerations tend to lick the exposed penis and may thereby prevent effective clot formation. Depending on the extent and location of the laceration, sedation or general anesthesia will be required to evaluate the lesion. To facilitate identification of the laceration, the penis should be thoroughly examined under a gentle stream of cold, sterile water or saline after placement of a urethral catheter.

Treatment Assuming that the patient does not have a coagulopathy, hemorrhage from small lacerations should be managed by a cold compress and pressure. Persistent bleeding may be managed by placement of one or more absorbable sutures, although extensive suturing is not recommended. Erection in patients with penile bleeding should be minimized by isolation from estrous females, use of sedation, and application of an Elizabethan collar to dogs that lick or self-traumatize the penis at the site of the lesion. Systemic therapy with antibiotics should be instituted to prevent secondary infection.

...........Paraphimosis

The inability of male dogs or cats to withdraw the penis into the prepuce defines paraphimosis, a condition that usually develops in male dogs during erection (physiologic and therefore not a true emergency), in young male dogs, and in dogs after coitus.

Treatment Treatment includes cold water soaks and lubrication of the penis and prepuce using water-soluble or petrolatum-based products. The base of the penis should be examined for the presence of hair rings. In severe cases, general anesthesia may be required to effect replacement of the penis within the prepuce; less often, surgery may be indicated to enlarge the diameter of the preputial orifice. Failure to correct paraphimosis may result in severe penile injury, desiccation, necrosis, and urethral obstruction, which ultimately would necessitate amputation of the penis.

Emergencies of the Female Reproductive Tract and Genitalia
...........UTERUS
...........Uterine Prolapse

Prolapse of the uterus is a serious postparturient emergency that occurs more often in the bitch than in the queen; immediate intervention is indicated. The

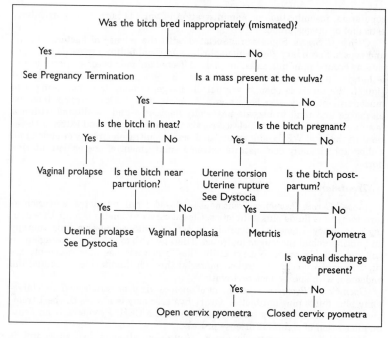

Was the bitch bred inappropriately (mismated)?

- Yes → See Pregnancy Termination
- No → Is a mass present at the vulva?
  - Yes → Is the bitch in heat?
    - Yes → Vaginal prolapse
    - No → Is the bitch near parturition?
      - Yes → Uterine prolapse (See Dystocia)
      - No → Vaginal neoplasia
  - No → Is the bitch pregnant?
    - Yes → Uterine torsion / Uterine rupture (See Dystocia)
    - No → Is the bitch post-partum?
      - Yes → Metritis
      - No → Pyometra → Is vaginal discharge present?
        - Yes → Open cervix pyometra
        - No → Closed cervix pyometra

cause is usually linked to excessive straining during or following parturition; therefore, the patient should be examined carefully for evidence of a retained fetus.

Treatment General anesthesia for physical replacement of the prolapsed organ is required. If the uterus is edematous, physical replacement may be difficult or impossible. Applying a hypertonic solution of glucose or saline to the exposed endometrium, in addition to gentle massage and lubrication, may facilitate replacement if the uterine tissue is healthy and viable. To ensure proper replacement and position within the abdominal cavity and to minimize recurrence, laparotomy and hysteropexy are required. Ovariohysterectomy is indicated if feasible. Postoperatively, oxytocin 5 to 20 units IM should be given to contract the uterus. If uterine contraction is accomplished, it is not generally necessary to suture the vulva. Recurrence is uncommon even subsequent to future pregnancies. Postoperatively, 7 to 10 days of antibiotic therapy is indicated.

If severe uterine edema exists, exposed tissue is devitalized, or if the prolapsed uterus has been physically traumatized to the extent that replacement would pose additional risk to the patient, an ovariohysterectomy should be performed. In some instances, it is not necessary to replace the uterus prior to removal.

···········Pyometra

Pyometra occurs in both dogs and cats. The disease process involves infection overlying irreversible cystic endometrial hyperplasia (CEH), which develops under the influence of progesterone. Pyometra is a progressive, recurrent disorder, exacerbated after each estrous cycle. It may occur spontaneously during the 2-month luteal phase of the cycle that follows estrus, or subsequent to copulation, insemination, or administration of various hormones, particularly estradiol or progesterone.

Clinical Signs Signs are associated with the release of bacterial toxins and sepsis. Secondary glomerulonephritis and renal failure are serious complications occurring in untreated animals. Affected animals become anorectic and lethargic; in some cases, polydipsia may be the predominant early clinical sign. If the cervix is open, a vaginal discharge, ranging from blood-tinged to mucopurulent, may also be present. Animals with a closed cervix have no discharge and tend to become physically depressed and debilitated within a few days. In patients with a closed cervix pyometra, sepsis and extreme elevations in the total WBC count occur; furthermore, ultrasonography or abdominal radiographs usually demonstrate extreme enlargement of one or both uterine horns.

Treatment

Closed Cervix Pyometra Treatment of closed cervix pyometra is ovariohysterectomy plus fluids plus antibiotics. Closed cervix pyometra is a life-threatening emergency. Immediate ovariohysterectomy with aggressive fluid therapy and antimicrobial therapy is indicated. Therapy with oxytocin or prostaglandin will not reliably promote cervical dilation, and their use may cause uterine rupture or movement of purulent material through the uterine tubes into the abdomen, with subsequent peritonitis.

Open Cervix Pyometra Treatment of open cervix pyometra is ovariohysterectomy plus fluids plus antibiotics. Ovariohysterectomy is always the best treatment since the bitch has underlying irreversible CEH. Pyometra is an acute manifestation of a chronic disease process.

Medical therapy (prostaglandin $F_{2\alpha}$, Lutalyse), although less successful, is an alternative to surgery in selected patients and may be the only alternative in some breeding animals. The most widely used medical therapy for both the bitch and queen is the administration of prostaglandin $F_{2\alpha}$ ($PGF_{2\alpha}$). This drug is not approved in the United States for use in the bitch or queen.

1. Determine uterine size.
2. Collect specimens of the vaginal discharge for aerobic culture and sensitivity. Institute empirical therapy with ampicillin 10 mg/lb PO t.i.d. pending sensitivity results.
3. Treat with $PGF_{2\alpha}$ 250 µg/kg SC s.i.d. for 2 to 7 days, until uterine size nears normal. If the bitch is in diestrus, evidenced by serum progesterone concentration, 2 ng/mL b.i.d. may be indicated as it will induce luteolysis and a subsequent decline in serum progesterone, which may be exacerbating the disease.

$PGF_{2\alpha}$ is an abortifacient and therefore should not be administered to pregnant animals (see Pregnancy Termination in the Bitch and Queen). Reactions subsequent to $PGF_{2\alpha}$ administration are common and may be expected within 5 to 60 minutes. A reaction in the bitch may last 20 to 30 minutes; in the queen, it may last from 2 to 20 minutes. Reactions include restlessness, hypersalivation, vomiting, panting, defecation, tachycardia, abdominal pain, fever, and vocalization (in cats). Death can occur in a very ill bitch.

Efficacy of treating open cervix pyometra with $PGF_{2\alpha}$ is based on limited studies in dogs and cats. The likelihood of complete resolution of uterine infection is 90% in bitches (30% require two treatments) and 100% in cats. The future fertility of those responding to therapy varies inversely with the severity of endometrial disease. The affected bitch may be placed on (mibolerone) drops to prevent estrus until the heat period in which she is to be bred, and should undergo ovariohysterectomy as soon as her breeding life is over.

............Acute Metritis

Typically presenting within 7 to 14 days following parturition, acute metritis is a severe bacterial infection of the uterus, usually caused by *E. coli*, which may progress rapidly, leading to toxemia or sepsis. Clinical signs include inability to nurse, a foul-smelling purulent or sanguinopurulent vulvar discharge, anorexia, lethargy, and vomiting. Acute collapse may occur in septic females.

On physical examination, affected dogs are usually febrile (40°C or 104°F). The patient may be dehydrated. Abdominal palpation may reveal a turgid and enlarged uterus. Cytologic examination of the vulvar discharge confirms septic inflammation. Abdominal ultrasonography or radiographs usually demonstrate an enlarged uterus.

Treatment Therapy is directed at stabilizing the patient with IV fluid therapy and antibiotics. Dogs with gram-negative infections can be treated PO using a quinolone antimicrobial if the patient is not vomiting. Definitive therapy is surgical; ovariohysterectomy should be performed as soon as the patient is stable and able to undergo general anesthesia. Medical treatment becomes an option (1) when the patient is a valuable breeding bitch and (2) when surgery can be safely delayed while medical treatment is pursued. Medical therapy includes 5 to 10 units of oxytocin q3h for three injections or administration of $PGF_{2\alpha}$, 250 µg/kg/day SC for 2 to 5 days, which can be administered to evacuate the uterine exudate and increase uterine blood flow. Either drug should be used in conjunction with antimicrobial therapy.

............Uterine Torsion

Uterine torsion is an uncommon condition, although it is reported in both dogs and cats. Torsion of both gravid and nongravid uterine horns have been reported in the dog and cat. The onset of signs associated with uterine torsion is usually acute and therefore may present as an emergency. Abdominal pain predominates, although the bitch or queen may crouch and strain as if in labor and may attempt to defecate. There may have been prior history of delivery of a live or dead fetus. A vaginal discharge may be present. Ultrasonographic or radiographic examination of the abdomen often discloses a large air-filled or fluid-filled tubular structure.

Treatment Treatment of uterine torsion is ovariohysterectomy. If there are viable fetuses present, a cesarean section may be performed first. Preoperative evaluation of affected patients is critical, since they are predisposed to large losses of fluids and vascular obstruction.

............Uterine Rupture

Rupture of the gravid uterus in the dog and cat is rare, although it may occur spontaneously during parturition or as a result of severe abdominal trauma. Fetuses expelled into the peritoneal cavity may be resorbed or may cause peritonitis. If fetal circulation is not disturbed, the fetuses may live to term.

Treatment Treatment of acute uterine rupture is surgical. Ovariohysterectomy with surgical removal of extrauterine puppies and membranes is recommended. A unilateral ovariohysterectomy is indicated when the rupture involves only one uterine horn and when it is desirable to preserve the breeding ability of the animal. If the ruptured uterus is a pyometra, extensive peritoneal contamination and subsequent peritonitis are likely. Copious saline lavage and careful suctioning during laparotomy are essential. At least 10 to 14 days of antibiotic therapy is indicated.

..........VAGINA

..........Vaginal Prolapse

Vaginal prolapse is an uncommon clinical emergency and is generally considered to result from proliferation of the vaginal mucosa, possibly an exaggerated response of the vagina to increased estrogen levels during proestrus. The hyperplastic vaginal tissue may recede during diestrus, only to recur on subsequent heat cycles. This condition may be confused with vaginal neoplasia; the latter is more likely to occur in older bitches and does not vary with stage of the estrous cycle.

   Clinical Signs Signs include a mass protruding from the vagina, dysuria, stranguria, and anuria. Persistent vaginal discharge and licking of the vulva may also be seen. During breeding, the bitch may not allow penetration by the male, or the male and bitch are unable to establish a copulatory lock ("tie").

   Treatment Treatment is generally not required if the hyperplastic tissue is within the vagina. However, mildly affected dogs are unlikely to be presented as an emergency. Dogs presented with dysuria or anuria should be treated as an emergency. Surgical therapy is indicated for extremely large prolapses when devitalized tissue is evident and when the patient is dysuric. An indwelling urinary catheter should be placed in the urethra prior to resection of the hyperplastic tissue. Retention sutures should be placed in the vulva postoperatively for no more than 7 to 10 days.

   Medical therapy is indicated only in mild cases. Antibiotics can be applied topically several times daily along with regular cleansing with saline washes. Systemic hormonal therapy is not effective.

..........EMERGENCIES OF PREGNANCY AND PARTURITION

..........Dystocia

Difficult parturition can occur in the dog and cat but is far more common in the dog. Several conditions can result in a diagnosis of dystocia:

1. No puppies born within 4 to 6 hours from the onset of labor.
2. More than 2 hours since the last pup was born.
3. Weak or infrequent labor contractions.
4. No puppies born 2 to 3 hours after the amniotic-allantoic membranes have ruptured.
5. Depression, weakness, and signs of toxemia are present.
6. No puppies born by the 72nd day of gestation (days counted from breeding) or 65th day post ovulation.

   Dystocia may be either maternal or fetal. Maternal dystocia can include primary and secondary uterine inertia, hypocalcemia, pelvic abnormalities, psychological disturbances, inguinal herniation, and uterine torsion. Fetal dystocia includes oversized fetuses and abnormal presentation (*Note*: Both anterior and posterior presentations are normal in dogs and cats.)

   Once dystocia is diagnosed, the perineum should be clipped, cleaned, and thoroughly rinsed. Using a sterile glove and abundant lubricant jelly, perform digital exploration of the pelvic canal to assess the position of the fetus. Lateral abdominal radiographs are invaluable in helping to determine fetal size and number. Ultrasonography is required to assess fetal viability.

   Treatment "Feathering" or massaging the dorsal vaginal wall with a gloved finger may stimulate labor in very early, uncomplicated dystocia. The treatment course varies with findings on the digital vaginal examination and lateral abdominal radiograph. Begin treatment with oxytocin 2 to 20 units IM. Ensure that the dystocia is nonobstructive before administering oxytocin. Repeat oxytocin at 20- to 30-minute intervals for up to three doses if necessary. Ten percent calcium gluconate 1 mL (100 mg/5 kg) of body weight IV may potentiate the action of oxytocin, especially in bitches experiencing fatigue of uterine smooth muscle. If labor has not progressed to the birth of a puppy after multiple injections of oxytocin, cesarean section is indicated.

.... Pregnancy Termination in the Bitch and Queen
.... Ovariohysterectomy

Of the several treatment options available for terminating the pregnancy of a mismatched bitch, ovariohysterectomy is still the best option, since it is safe, relatively inexpensive, and eliminates the risk of future pregnancies.

.... Estrogens

Oral diethylstilbestrol (DES) is not an effective pregnancy termination agent in the bitch. Estradiol cypionate (ECP) has traditionally been used as a "mismate shot" to cause early termination of an unwanted pregnancy. The most effective regimen is 0.02 mg/lb ECP IM, given one time in late estrus or diestrus. This treatment is, however, associated with significant side effects, most notably open cervix pyometra and bone marrow suppression. Estradiol cypionate is not approved for use in the dog in the United States, and is not recommended for use in the queen.

.... Prostaglandin $F_{2\alpha}$

Naturally occurring $PGF_{2\alpha}$ is consistently effective as an abortifacient in the bitch if the treatment is started more than 5 days after onset of cytologic diestrus (a noncornified vaginal smear). $PGF_{2\alpha}$ is administered at a dose of 250 μg/kg SC q12h for 4 days (eight injections). Side effects that occur 10 to 60 minutes following treatment include hypersalivation, vomiting, panting, urination, and defecation. These signs, which decrease in severity with each injection, appear milder in bitches that are walked for 20 to 30 minutes following treatment. Concurrent administration of atropine 100 to 500 μg/kg SC) may also decrease the severity of side effects. Bitches treated in the first half of pregnancy usually resorb their embryos; those treated in the second half of pregnancy usually abort fetuses within 5 to 7 days of onset of treatment. $PGF_{2\alpha}$ causes lysis of the corpora lutea, and decline in serum progesterone concentrations to less than 2 ng/mL. Serum progesterone concentrations should be measured at the end of treatment to document completeness of luteolysis. $PGF_{2\alpha}$ is not approved for pregnancy termination in the bitch.

After day 4 of gestation, $PGF_{2\alpha}$ can terminate pregnancy in the queen. Its use should be limited to healthy queens. Treatment consists of 100 to 250 μg/kg SC once daily for 2 days. Side effects in queens are similar to those in the bitch but normally last only 2 to 20 minutes. Treatment with $PGF_{2\alpha}$ does not preclude rebreeding at a future date. $PGF_{2\alpha}$ is not approved in the United States for use in cats.

.... Spontaneous Abortion

Spontaneous abortion is the expulsion of one or more fetuses prior to term. It is possible for dogs and cats to abort one or more fetuses but retain others to term and deliver normally. Clinical signs include abdominal contractions and vaginal discharge. The actual expulsion of a fetus may be observed, or a remnant of aborted tissue may be found. Infection, particularly with *B. canis*, should be suspected whenever a bitch aborts 45 to 55 days into pregnancy. However, several other infectious agents—e.g., herpesvirus, feline coronavirus (FIP), feline leukemia virus (FeLV), and toxoplasmosis (dogs only)—have been associated with abortion. Trauma, hormonal factors, environmental pathogens, drugs, and fetal factors represent other possible causes.

Metabolic Emergencies

Emergency treatments for hyperglycemia (diabetic ketoacidosis), hypoglycemia, puerperal tetany (canine eclampsia), adrenocortical insufficiency, and acidosis are discussed below:

...........DIABETIC KETOACIDOSIS

Diabetic ketoacidosis (DKA) is a potentially fatal consequence associated with the terminal result of insulin insufficiency and possible glucagon excess. The overproduction of acetoacetic acid and β-hydroxybutyrate dehydrogenase by the liver occurs in diabetes mellitus owing to a deficiency of insulin and relative excess of glucagon. The liver is shifted from its normal role in esterification of fatty acids into triglycerides into the production by beta oxidation of fatty acids into keto acids. Early in the disease, patients exhibit the typical signs of diabetes mellitus. DKA is characterized by vomiting, dehydration, hypotension, oliguria, severe depression, epigastric pain, a strong odor of acetone on the breath, diarrhea, weight loss, and coma.

The initial physical examination reveals:

1. Dehydration (in 4% to 12% of patients).
2. Prerenal azotemia. (BUN 40 to 60 mg/dL).
3. Severe depression, possibly progressing to coma.
4. Fever (not always).
5. Shock, hypovolemia.
6. Blood glucose usually greater than 300 mg/dL, urine glucose 4+, urine ketones 4+, elevated BUN (prerenal), urine specific gravity 1.030 or greater (see p. 122).
7. Hyperosmolarity of the serum (>330 mOsm kg).
8. Plasma may be lipemic.
9. Plasma sodium is usually increased (>145 mEq/L).
10. Deficit in total body potassium is present. There may be a normal serum potassium, because acidosis results in translocation of intracellular potassium to extracellular space (see p. 728). Plasma phosphorous is decreased in cats (1 to 2 mg/dL).
11. Acute pancreatitis may be present (see p. 118).
12. Liver enzymes may be elevated, associated with altered glucose metabolism and fatty liver.
13. Metabolic acidosis is present with elevated levels of β-hydroxybutyric acid. Respiratory compensation for the metabolic acidosis may result in Kussmaul-type respiratory pattern.
14. A large anion gap is present, along with the metabolic acidosis. Hypokalemia and hypophosphatemia may be present.
15. Diabetics are more susceptible to infections; thus, cystitis, pyelonephritis, and metritis may be present. Urine should be cultured.

···········Treatment of Diabetic Ketoacidosis

Treatment is aimed at:

1. Providing adequate amounts of insulin to normalize metabolism.
2. Correcting fluid and electrolyte losses.
3. Correcting acidosis.
4. Identifying additional precipitating causes of ketoacidosis.
5. Providing carbohydrates that may be needed during insulin administration.

Draw blood for hemogram, glucose, and BUN. Monitor blood pH, bicarbonate, sodium, potassium, and chloride, if possible. Collect urine for specific gravity, glucose, pH, ketones, and urine culture. Maintain an adequate airway passage and, if necessary, insert an endotracheal tube.

Place an indwelling catheter in either the jugular or cephalic vein. Start an IV infusion of 0.9% NaCl or 2.5% fructose in 0.45% NaCl. If serum sodium is over 155 mEq/L, use 0.45% saline. Replace 50% of the calculated fluid loss over the first 12 hours; however, do not give fluids faster than 70 mL/kg/hr, so that the vascular compartment can adjust and until renal perfusion and renal output are adequate. Add 10 to 20 mEq of sodium bicarbonate per liter of fluid if bicarbonate levels cannot be measured. The potassium deficit can be estimated at 3 mEq/kg, and plans should be made to replace the deficit over a 24-hour period. Do not exceed more than 40 mEq/L (see also p. 600). Phosphorus replacement should be initiated in cats. Supplement phosphorus when phosphorus is <20 mg/dL with 0.01 to 0.03 mmol/kg/h. Quantify urine production and balance losses with replacement fluid therapy. It may be necessary to catheterize the bladder (see p. 486) and attach a catheter to a closed collection system for urine.

Attempt to measure the acid-base balance. Ideally, $Paco_2$ and pH should be measured; however, if not available, total carbon dioxide can be measured (see p. 591). Animals with total carbon dioxide or arterial bicarbonate concentrations of less than or equal to 11 mEq/L require bicarbonate therapy.

In patients with DKA, insulin administration begins by either the *low-dose IV* or *low-dose IM* method. In the low-dose IV method, begin insulin administration by continuous infusion. Add 5 units of regular insulin to 250 mL of lactated Ringer's solution. Administer insulin, using a pediatric infusion drip, at a rate of regular insulin 0.5 to 1.0 units/kg/hr for dogs and 0.1 to 0.2 units/kg/hr for cats. Insulin binds to plastic; therefore, once insulin has been added to the fluids, run out the first 50 mL of fluid through the IV line. This provides insulin saturation into the plastic. More rapid administration of noninsulin solutions is performed by using a second vein to maintain hydration. When the blood glucose begins to fall, do not administer more insulin until the full effect of the last dose is known (Table 1–21). Monitor blood glucose concentration every 30 to 60 minutes. Maintain blood glucose concentration in a range of 200 to 300 mg/dL until the patient is stable. A 5% dextrose solution can be used if the blood glucose levels fall below 200 mg/dL.

In the low-dose IM method, administer regular insulin 0.22 unit/kg IM, followed by 0.1 unit/kg IM every hour (Table 1–22). Blood glucose levels should be determined hourly. The goal is to slowly reduce blood glucose levels to 150 to 250 mg/dL. This usually takes 8 hours, and ketone reduction may take 1 to 4 hours. Blood glucose should be evaluated every 2 hours. When blood glucose levels reach 200 to 250 mg/dL, add 50% dextrose to IV solutions to maintain blood glucose concentration at 200 to 300 mg/dL. Begin to administer regular insulin 0.1 to 0.4 units/kg q4–6h until the animal stabilizes. Continue to monitor blood glucse every 4 hours. Administer these doses of insulin until the blood glucose level fails from 250 mg/dL or higher to 150 mg/dL. Then change fluids to 5% dextrose, with 4 to 8 mEq/L of potassium chloride added. If the blood sugar is 150 to 250 mg/dL, give fluids and potassium chloride as previously,

Table 1-21. Insulins

	Estimated Time Until Maximum Effect (hr)		Estimated Duration of Effect (hr)	
	Dog	Cat	Dog	Cat
Regular and NPH (isophane)	2–10	2–8	6–24	4–12
Lente	2–10	2–10	8–24	6–10
Ultralente	4–16	4–12	8–28	7–18

- Beef-pork insulins are 70% beef and 30% pork.
- Pork insulin is identical to insulin of dogs. Human preparations are also OK.
- Cat insulin is closer to beef insulin. Human insulin is not close to cat insulin.
- Insulin is commercially available in 40, 100, and 500 units/mL.
- U-40 is no longer commercially available in the United States.
- Must purchase exact syringe for insulin.
- U-100 syringes are available in 0.3-, 0.5-, and 1-mL capacity.
- Lilly Pharmaceutical has discontinued production of Ultralente Iletin I beef-pork insulin. For cats, the Ultralente beef source is manufactured by Novo Nordisk. Cats may undergo a trial of human Ultralente at 75% of beef insulin dosage.

From Peterson M: Insulin and insulin syringes. *In* Kirk RW, ed: Current Veterinary Therapy XI. Small Animal Practice. Philadelphia, WB Saunders, 1992, p 357.

but add regular insulin 0.5 units/kg SC until the animal is stabilized (i.e., animal is eating, electrolytes are normalized, vomiting has stopped, and metabolic abnormalities are under control), then begin therapy as for an uncomplicated diabetic with an intermediate or long-acting insulin preparation.

Measure blood glucose, urine volume, urine pH, glucose, and ketones every hour. Perform an ECG or take blood samples to assess potassium needs. As urine volume increases, replace losses with lactated Ringer's solution IV.

As the animal begins to respond to insulin, carefully monitor for hypoglycemia, hypokalemia, and hypophosphatemia. Insulin facilitates movement of potassium from the extracellular fluid compartment into the cell, and hypokalemia may result. Potassium supplementation will be needed, and in most cases the oral route, being safe, is preferred. Potassium gluconate can be given PO q6h if the urine output is adequate. In severe cases of hypokalemia, potassium 30 mEq can be added to each liter of IV fluids administered only if renal function is reestablished. IV potassium should not be given at a rate exceeding 1 mEq/kg/hr. Signs of acute hypophosphatemia include rapid hemolysis, muscle weakness, and rhabdomyolysis, and decreased cerebral function leading to seizures, stupor, and coma. Up to 25% of cats may develop hypophosphatemia (<2.0 mg/dL) following therapy. Phosphorus can be supplemented as

Table 1-22. Low-Dose Intramuscular Administration of Insulin

Body Weight (kg)	Initial Dose	Hourly Dose
<10	2 units (total)	1 unit
>10	0.25 units/kg	0.1 unit/kg

potassium phosphate at a dose of 0.03 to 0.12 mmol/kg/hr followed by repeated phosphate determinations every 12 to 24 hours. Two to four treatments of phosphates at 6-hour intervals may be required.

··········· Major Complications of Treatment

- Infections, especially of lower urinary tract—obtain bacterial culture if possible.
- Acute renal failure due to poor renal perfusion; can use dopamine 1 to 3 μg/kg/min IV and furosemide 1 mg/kg/hr IV to increase renal perfusion (see also p. 122).
- When plasma bicarbonate concentration is 11 mEq/L or less, bicarbonate should be given IV during the first 6 hours of treatment. Bicarbonate deficit can be calculated using

$$0.4 \times kg\ weight \times (15 - measured\ HCO_3) = HCO_3\ deficit.$$

Hypokalemia caused by insulin and bicarbonate administration. A low normal or low serum potassium level is less than 4.5 mEq/L. ECG may be helpful in evaluation of animals with suspected potassium abnormalities (see also p. 728).

Serum Potassium	Potassium Added to 250 mL Fluids
<2.0 mEq/L	20 mEq/250 mL
2.0–2.5 mEq/L	15 mEq/250 mL
2.5–3.0 mEq/L	10 mEq/250 mL
3.0–3.5 mEq/L	7 mEq/250 mL

- Iatrogenic hypoglycemia or insulin shock.
- Hypophosphatemia can be a major problem in DKA, especially in cats. Hypophosphatemia can lead to reduced concentrations in erythrocyte adenosine triphosphate (ATP) resulting in hemolysis.
- If phosphate has to be supplemented, give 0.01 to 0.03 mmol/kg/hr. Both sodium phosphate and potassium phosphate are available.
- Since hypokalemia commonly exists with hypophosphatemia, the potassium form is used most frequently. The dose of phosphate is calculated from the potassium phosphate solution:

Total mEq potassium to be replaced over 24 hours − mEq K derived from KPO_4 replacement solution = mEqK derived from KCl.

When the blood glucose has decreased to below 200 mg/dL and urine ketones have decreased, NPH (neutral protamine Hagedorn) (H) insulin can be administered. After the patient has been stabilized, maintenance therapy for chronic diabetes mellitus can be initiated (see p. 142).

1-mL Tuberculin Syringes Can Be Substituted for Insulin Syringes According to the Following:

$$\frac{Desired\ amount\ of\ drug}{Strength\ on\ hand} = \frac{unknown\ quantity\ (x)}{= known\ quantity\ drug}$$

Cats are very sensitive to insulin, especially when in DKA. In the severely dehydrated cat that is hypotensive, initial insulin treatment should be crystalline zinc insulin administered via slow infusion in fluids, using a pediatric drip set to give 0.25 to 1.0 unit/hr. Monitor blood glucose until levels are between 200 and 300 mg/dL.

Two acceptable long-acting insulins are Humulin U Ultralente human insulin (recombinant [extended zinc suspension], Eli Lilly Co., Indianapolis, IN) and Ultralente (beef) (Novo Nordisk Pharmaceuticals, Princeton, NJ). Initial dose should be 1 to 3 units of Ultralente once daily initially in the morning. Many cats will eventually require twice-daily insulin treatment. In about 20% of cats, Ultralente insulin is poorly absorbed and these cats may require Lente insulin b.i.d. Cats are maintained on Ultralente for 3 days and can then be evaluated with repeated blood samples every 2 hours and serum glucose levels measured.

............Uncomplicated Diabetes Mellitus in the Dog

Uncomplicated diabetic cases involve those animals with serum fasting blood glucose greater than 200 mg/dL that are not ketonuric, although they are glycosuric. They are not severely ill with their diabetes, i.e., not ketoacidic or hyperosmolor. The following points are important in regulating these diabetic cases with insulin:

1. Insulin (usually NPH) is administered early in the morning, so that peak insulin activity occurs in the late afternoon and mild hyperglycemia is present in the morning.
2. The dose of insulin administered to dogs is variable, depending on the size, activity, diet (type and caloric intake), and environmental stress. Generally, the larger the dog, the smaller the dose of insulin needed on a per-kilogram basis. Animals require 2 to 4 days to equilibrate insulin, and repeated blood glucose determinations should be made over a 24-hour period after a 3-day equilibration period.
3. NPH insulin in the dog is initially administered at ½ to ⅔ unit/kg SC once or twice daily. Blood glucose should be serially monitored to establish an effective dose. At peak insulin activity, the plasma glucose content should not be lower than 125 to 150 mg/dL.

............Problems Encountered in Regulating the Diabetic Dog

Commercially available insulin preparations may be a combination of beef and pork insulin, pork insulin, beef insulin, or recombinant human insulin. Canine insulin most closely resembles pork insulin. The duration of action of pork and human recombinant insulin is shorter than that of beef/pork insulin in the dog. Insulin zinc suspension of beef–pork is therefore initially used in the dog. Pork insulin or human recombinant insulin is used if it is suspected that the animal is developing resistance to the use of beef–pork insulin. Pork insulin is usually administered twice a day.

Insulin-induced hypoglycemia typically develops during the peak action of insulin. Additional glucose can be administered by using oral Karo syrup or, in a hospitalized animal, beginning an IV drip of 10% dextrose and water. In the unconscious patient, 50% dextrose 1 mL/kg IV, can be administred as a bolus, and then an IV dextrose drip of 5% to 10% can be maintained as needed (see p. 144).

Widely fluctuating blood glucose levels may develop in some dogs being given insulin. When the blood glucose levels are taken infrequently and found to be abnormally elevated, increased levels of insulin are administered. These

increased insulin levels cause an outpouring of glucagon, cortisol, and epinephrine during the hypoglycemic phase, resulting in a paradoxic hyperglycemic
response. This syndrome (Somogyi effect) occurs most often when insulin administration exceeds I.O.U/pound by body weight.

When there appear to be widely fluctuating blood glucose levels or the
Somogyi effect is suspected, serial measurements of blood glucose (glucose
curve) should be measured every 2 hours from the time of insulin administration until it is peaked. This can be done using a blood glucose analyzer.

If insulin administration is *not effective* in lowering blood glucose levels, the
following should be considered:

- Inappropriate insulin administration technique
- Insulin underdose
- Very short duration of insulin effect
- Increased blood glucose levels associated with increased stress levels dur-
  ing sampling
- Hyperadrenocorticism (Cushing's disease)
- Poor absorption of insulin from injection sites
- Somogyi effect
- Insulin resistance

Demonstration of hypoglycemia (<60 mg/dL) followed by hyperglycemia confirms the diagnosis of the Somogyi effect. Treatment for this problem is reduction in insulin administration to achieve a blood glucose nadir not less than
80 mg/dL, with 1+ urine glucose in the morning.

■ DIFFICULTIES IN REGULATING THE DIABETIC CAT (see also p. 648)

Etiology of Diabetes in the Cat

There are several unique characteristics of diabetes, its diagnosis, and its regulation
as it affects the cat. Cats with abnormal elevations of blood sugar can be categorized
into insulin-dependent diabetes mellitus (IDDM) (type I) and noninsulin dependent
diabetes (NIDDM) (type II). NIDDM is found in 30% to 50% of cats initially presented
with abnormal elevations of blood glucose. In diabetic cats 50% to 70% are classified
as having IDDM. In these cats, clinical signs of diabetes are mild, there is no DKA,
there is a close association with obesity as well as islet-specific amyloid deposit,
there is impaired glucose tolerance, and there may be treatment response to oral
hypoglycemic agents such as glipizide (Glucotrol, Roerig, New York, NY) 5 to 15 mg
b.i.d. and dietary management (high-fiber diet).

Helpful Steps in Evaluating Regulation of Diabetes in the Cat

Use of Glucose Tolerance Curve: In cats that have IDDM, once that affected
animal is on a maintenance level of insulin with either Ultralente or Lente insulin, a
glucose tolerance test should be performed:
Obtain a blood glucose level early in the morning before insulin administration
  or feeding.
Determine blood glucose every 2 hours to determine the following:
  Time lapse until peak insulin effect.
  Blood glucose concentration at peak insulin effect.
  Is the blood glucose level likely to rise above 200 to 300 mg/dL?
  Does rebound hyperglycemia occur?
If insulin therapy is effective in the diabetic cat, the clinical signs of diabetes should
be eliminated. If the cat has normal water intake, normal urine output, and normal

(Box continued on following page)

■ DIFFICULTIES IN REGULATING THE DIABETIC CAT (Continued)

appetite and body weight, then the insulin is effective. If repeated blood glucose levels are greater that 300 mg/dL with no clinical signs of diabetes, the cat may be suffering from stress-induced hyperglycemia.

The initial choice of insulin for the cat is Ultralente insulin of human recombinant origin at a dosage of 1 to 3 units per cat in a single morning injection. Most cats will eventually require Ultralente insulin b.i.d. Ultralente is ineffective in about 20% of cats. These cats should be switched to Lente insulin b.i.d. The duration of Lente insulin in the cat is 6 to 14 hours and Lente must be administered q12h.

Is the client administering insulin correctly? Is the proper insulin dose being administered? Is the insulin stored correctly? Are proper syringes being used? Are dosing intervals being followed? Is there any insulin incompatibility (beef-pork insulin vs. human recombinant insulins)? The amino acid sequence of feline insulin is similar to bovine insulin and different from pork and recombinant human insulin.

Is the feeding regimen or diet for the cat proper?

Is the cat in a household where more than one cat is present?

Is the owner able to observe the diabetic cat effectively?

Is the diabetic cat spayed?

Is the diabetic cat obese?

Does the diabetic cat have additional systemic diseases that may affect control of diabetes? Hyperadrenocorticism, hyperthyroidism, growth hormone production (acromegaly). *Have any exogenous corticosteroids or megesterol acetate been administered to the diabetic cat?*

Monitoring serum fructosamine concentrations is helpful in monitoring long-term glucose regulation in treated diabetic cats (see p. 730).

·········· HYPEROSMOLAR, NONKETOTIC DIABETIC COMA

Coma can develop secondary to increased serum osmolality associated with extreme hyperglycemia. In diabetes, the hyperosmolality can be associated with severe hyperglycemia and hypernatremia. Normal canine serum osmolality is approximately 300 mOsm/L of serum, and hyperosmolality is suspected when serum osmolality is above 340 mOsm. If equipment for determining serum osmolity is not available, serum osmolality can be estimated from the formula:

$$\text{Serum osmolality (mOsm/L)} = 2(\text{Na} + \text{K}) + \frac{\text{blood gluscose}}{18} + \frac{\text{BUN}}{2.8}.$$

Patients with severe dehydration, hyperglycemia, and hyperosmolality without ketosis may experience cerebral edema. The treatment should be aimed at lowering glucose levels slowly and gradual rehydration.

Hypotonic fluids, such as half-strength saline or 2.5% dextrose in water, should be used in the therapy of hyperosmolar DKA. Start potassium supplementation using conservative dosage after the initial rehydration period.

·········· HYPOGLYCEMIA

Hypoglycemia is a manifestation of various systemic abnormalities that can involve the intestinal absorption of nutrients, hepatic production of glucose, normal function of liver enzymes, and adequate peripheral glucose utilization.

The clinical manifestations center around the dependency of the brain on glucose oxidation for energy, its inability to store quantities of glucose, and increased secretion of catecholamine (i.e., epinephrine). Clinical signs can be extremely variable and may include weakness, tremors, nervousness, polyphagia, tachycardia, ataxia, muscular twitching, incoordination, visual disturbances, generalized seizures, and other neurologic abnormalities. Blood glucose levels of 45 mg/dL or lower may precipitate clinical signs of hypoglycemia. The coupling of clinical signs just described, a low blood glucose, and relief of symptoms by the administration of glucose is known as *Whipple's triad*.

Several factors are important to consider when evaluating hypoglycemia: (1) age of onset, (2) nature of the hypoglycemia episode (transient, persistent, or recurrent), and (3) the pattern, as indicated by the patient's history (e.g., Is it induced by stress, fasting, or physical exertion?).

■ CAUSES OF HYPOGLYCEMIA

Accelerated Glucose Removal	**Failure of Glucose Secretion**
Insulin overdosage	Functional hypoglycemia (nonrecognizable
Ethanol poisoning	lesion)
Salicylate ingestion	Neonatal hypoglycemia
Propranolol	"Toy breed hypoglycemia"
Functional islet cell tumor (see p.	"Hunting dog hypoglycemia"
649)	Starvation
Toxicity or oral hypoglycemic agents	Hepatic enzyme deficiencies
Renal glycosuria	Adrenal insufficiency (see p. 149)
Hepatoma	Hepatic insufficiency (see p. 120)
Endotoxemia, septic shock	Malabsorption and starvation (see p. 764)
	Large mesodermal tumors that use larger
	quantities of glucose than can be main-
	tained with gluconeogenesis
	Sepsis
	Increased extrahepatic utilization of glucose
	substrates
	Hematomas
	Hepatic abscesses
	Renal failure
	Extrapancreatic tumors

.... Treatment

Treatment of acute hypoglycemia includes the following measures. Each case of hypoglycemia requires individualized treatment aimed at correcting the underlying cause.

1. Fluids—half-strength lactated Ringer's solution 0.45% NaCl, 5% dextrose.
2. Give 2 to 4 mL/kg of 50% glucose IV or 20 mL/kg of 10% glucose orally.
3. Monitor hypokalemia with the ECG. Prolongation of the Q-T interval to greater than 0.22 second in the dog and greater than 0.16 second in the cat is suggestive of hypokalemia.
   a. *Mild hypokalemia* (serum K = 3.0 to 3.5 mEq/L): give KCl 1 to 3 mEq/kg body weight over 24 hours.
   b. *Moderate hypokalemia* (serum K = 2.5 to 3.0 mEq/L): give KCl 3 to 5 mEq/kg body weight over 24 hours.
   c. *Severe hypokalemia* (serum K <2.5 mEq/L): give KCl 5 to 10 mEq/kg body weight over 24 hours.
4. Potassium supplementation for moderate or severe hypokalemia, using potassium chloride added to fluids. If supplementation is given, do not give more than 0.25 mEq/kg/hr potassium. (See also p. 141.)

5. *Do not rush* into potassium supplementation aggressively. Stabilize the animal first.
6. When the patient recovers, begin frequent administration of food.
7. Watch closely for relapse.
8. Schedule the patient for tests to determine the cause of hypoglycemia.

··········PUERPERAL TETANY

The history and clinical signs of puerperal tetany are usually diagnostic and result from serum calcium level below 8.0 mg/dL in dogs and 7.0 mg/dL in cats. Clinical signs are not usually evident until levels fall to below 6.5 mg/dL. Because the disease is seen primarily in small, excitable dogs, a stress factor may be involved in the etiology. Puerperal tetany is usually observed 1 to 3 weeks post partum in bitches. Hypophosphatemia may accompany hypocalcemia.

Severe hypocalcemia has been associated with the administration of hypertonic phosphate enemas to small animals. Clinical signs can include muscle fasciculations, tetany, tachycardia, hypotension, cyanosis, acidosis, hyperthermia or hypothermia, and coma. Treatment involves the administration of calcium and glucose solutions. The most common cause in cats is hypoparathyroidism secondary to thyroidectomy in hyperthyroidism.

■ CLINICAL SIGNS ASSOCIATED WITH HYPOCALCEMIA

Muscle tremors, fasciculations	Fever
Panting	Stiff gait
Restlessness	Seizures
Aggression	Tachycardia
Hypersensitivity to the environment	ECG alterations
Disorientation	Polydipsia, polyuria
Muscle cramping	Respiratory arrest

··········Treatment

Treatment of puerperal tetany involves the following steps:

1. Administer calcium gluconate IV as a 10% solution at dosage of 15 mg/kg (0.15 mL/kg) over 30 minutes. This dose provides 0.68 mEq/kg body weight of calcium. Low-dose calcium can be administered IV at a dose of 5 to 10 mg/kg/hr.
2. If tetany persists, sedate the patient with diazepam or barbiturates given IV.
3. If hyperthermia is present, cool the patient (see p. 99).
4. Administer oral calcium carbonate therapy (see p. 147). Calcium carbonate (40% elemental calcium) can be administered by giving Tums tablets, one to two tablets per day in divided doses t.i.d.

··········HYPOCALCEMIA—WITHOUT ECLAMPSIA
(see p. 723)

··········HYPERCALCEMIA (see p. 724 for etiology)

The renal, GI, and nervous systems are most severely affected by hypercalcemia. Hypercalcemic values of greater than 16.0 mg/dL coupled with hypokalemia and hyperphosphatemia cause the most severe systemic disease. Soft tissue mineralization develops when the serum calcium level multiplied by the serum phosphate level exceeds 70.

Hypercalcemia produces muscle weakness, vomiting, seizures, coma, and

Table 1-23. Treatment of Hypocalcemia

Drug	Preparation	Available Calcium	Dosage	Comments
*Parenteral Calcium**				
Calcium gluconate	10% solution	9.3 mg/mL	a. Slow IV to effect (0.5–1.5 mL/kg IV) b. 5–15 mg/kg/hr IV c. 1–2 ml/kg diluted 1:1 with saline SC t.i.d.	Stop if bradycardia or shortened Q–T interval occurs; infusion to maintain normal Ca; may be given SC
Calcium chloride	10% solution	27.2 mg/mL	5–15 mg/kg/hr IV	Only given IV, as extremely caustic perivascularly
Oral Calcium†				
Calcium carbonate	Many sizes	40% tablet	25–50 mg/kg/day	Most common calcium supplement
Calcium lactate	325-, 650-mg tablets	13% tablet	25–50 mg/kg/day	
Calcium chloride	Powder	27.2%	25–50 mg/kg/day	May cause gastric irritation
Calcium gluconate	Many sizes	10%	25–50 mg/kg/day	
Vitamin D			Time for Maximal Effect to Occur	Time for Toxicity Effect to Resolve
Vitamin D₂ (ergocalciferol)	Capsules, syrup, parenteral (IM)	—	*Initial:* 4000–6000 units day; *Maintenance:* 1000–2000 units/kg once daily to once weekly	5–21 days · 1–18 wk
Dihydrotachysterol	Tablets, capsules, oral solution	—	*Initial:* 0.02–0.03 mg/kg/day; *Maintenance:* 0.01–0.02 mg/ kg q24–48h	1–7 days · 1–3 wk
1,25-dihydroxyvitamin D₃ (calcitriol)	Capsules	—	2.5 mg/kg/day	1–4 days · 2–14 days

*Do not mix calcium solution with bicarbonate-containing fluids, as precipitation may occur.
†Calculate dose on elemental calcium content.
From DiBartola SP: Fluid Therapy in Small Animal Practice. Philadelphia, WB Saunders, 1992, p 169.

147

muscle twitching. Cardiac conduction abnormalities include prolongation of the P–R interval, shortening of the Q–T interval, and ventricular fibrillation.

Severe hypercalcemia (>14 mg/dL) can progress rapidly to acute renal failure when the calcium-phosphorus product exceeds 60 to 80 mg/dL because of mineralization of renal tissue. Renal complications can be very serious and include defects in renal concentrating ability, polyuria-polydipsia, elevated BUN and creatinine, and decreased GFR and renal blood flow. GFR and renal blood flow are most compromised at calcium levels of 20 mg/dL or greater. The extent of the renal lesions namely, the degree of renal mineralization, the presence of adequate numbers of functional nephrons, and the presence of intact tubular basement membrane, determine whether the renal lesions are reversible (see p. 122).

########## Treatment

Emergency treatment is indicated with severe renal decompensation, cardiac disease, and systemic disease associated with hypercalcemia in the 15- to 20-mg/dL range and if calcium×phosphorus is greater than 60. Removal of the underlying cause of the hypercalcemia is the treatment of choice. This is not always possible, and while this form of treatment is being evaluated, emergency treatment to reduce serum calcium levels must be undertaken. Regimens of emergency treatment must be tailored to each patient.

1. Give fluids to increase extracellular fluid (ECF) volume and to increase GFR. The fluid of choice is 0.9% NaCl, but potassium supplementation may be needed (see p. 600). Initial fluid volume is aimed at supplying two to three times maintenance needs (120 to 180 mL/kg/day).
2. Search for the underlying cause of hypercalcemia, and decide whether to treat it. The most common cause is paraneoplasic syndrome (lymphosarcoma), but it may be difficult to determine the primary tumor focus (anterior mediastinal, intestinal, bone marrow; see p. 178 for further discussion of calcium metabolism).
3. Begin diuretic therapy with a diuretic that is calciuretic. Furosemide is the drug of choice. Give an initial IV bolus at 2 to 5 mg/kg with IV fluid maintenance. Observe the urine volume, and ensure that the patient is well rehydrated.
4. Glucocorticoids reduce calcium levels by decreasing calcium loss from bone, decreasing intestinal absorption of calcium, and increasing renal excretion of calcium. Do not use high doses of steroids (unless absolutely necessary) before performing a biopsy and looking for the source of lymphosarcoma.
5. Calcitonin 4 units/kg IM q12h in cats and 8 units/kg SC q24h in dogs may be given until the calcium normalizes.

■ STEROID—RESPONSIVE HYPERCALCEMIAS

Lymphomas, leukemia
Multiple myeloma
Thymoma
Vitamin D toxicity
Granulomatous disease
Hyperadrenocorticism

---

6. Toxicosis caused by cholecalciferol (vitamin D_3) rodenticide results in severe, prolonged hypercalcemia. Treatment with salmon calcitonin as adjunct treatment is helpful. The dose is variable. The extrapolated dose from human patients is 4 units/kg IV initially, followed by 4 to 8 units/kg SC once or twice daily. A more aggressive scheme of dosage in cholecalciferol poison-

ing is 8 IU/kg SC once daily, 5 IU/kg SC q.i.d., and 4 to 7 IU/kg SC q6–8h. Side effects of treatment are vomiting and anorexia. (See Dougherty et al. in References.)

⋯⋯⋯⋯ACUTE ADRENOCORTICAL INSUFFICIENCY

Hypoadrenocorticism is a disease seen most frequently in young and middle-aged female dogs. The major clinical signs are associated with deficiencies of both aldosterone and cortisol. The signs seen with adrenal insufficiency may develop slowly; adrenal gland reserve function is not lost until the point at which 90% or more of the adrenal glands are nonfunctional and complete adrenal collapse (addisonian crisis) can develop. Lack of aldosterone results in impaired ability to conserve sodium and excrete potassium (see p. 728).

The most significant clinical signs associated with hypoadrenocorticism are (1) depression and lethargy, (2) weakness, (3) anorexia, (4) shaking and shivering, (5) vomiting, (6) diarrhea (may be hemorrhagic), (7) weight loss, (8) abdominal pain, (9) polydipsia and polyuria, (10) weakness, (11) weak pulse and bradycardia, and (12) dehydration.

⋯⋯⋯⋯Diagnosis

Hyperkalemia Serum potassium levels may be greatly elevated (6.0 to 9.5 mEq) and produce typical cardiovascular changes (see p. 68).

Hyponatremia The serum sodium levels are greatly reduced (115 to 130 mEq). A decrease in the sodium-potassium ratio from 33:1 (normal) to 25:1 or below is usually diagnostic.

Cardiovascular Changes Changes include (1) bradycardia (<60 bpm), (2) weak pulse, (3) an elevated, spiked T wave, (4) decreased amplitude of P waves and atrial arrest, and (5) a widening of the QRS complex (normal or slow heart rate in the face of circulatory shock).

⋯⋯⋯⋯Treatment of Addisonian Crisis

Treatment involves the following steps:

1. Establish a patent IV catheter.
2. Obtain blood samples for electrolyte levels. Record an ECG. Use IV aqueous corticotropin 0.5 unit/kg. Obtain serum samples at 0 and 1 hour (see p. 630).
3. Begin a rapid IV infusion of 0.9% sodium chloride or 2.5% glucose in 0.45% sodium chloride (see p. 35). Inject 10 mg/kg of prednisolone sodium succinate. Add dexamethasone 1 to 2 mg/kg to the IV fluids being administered. A wide variety of glucocorticoids are available in the crisis situation, although the hydrocortisone sodium hemisuccinate and prednisolone sodium succinate work most rapidly.
   a. Hydrocortisone sodium hemisuccinate 10 to 20 mg/kg IV.
   b. Prednisolone sodium succinate 11 to 30 mg/kg IV.
   c. Dexamethasone sodium phosphate 2 to 4 mg/kg IV.
   d. Prednisolone acetate 0.1 to 0.2 mg/kg IM q8–12h.
   e. Hydrocortisone acetate 0.1 to 0.2 mg/kg IM q8–12h.
4. Continue therapy until blood pressure rises and urine output has returned to normal.
5. Administer the mineralocorticoid, desoxycorticosterone pivalate (DOCP) (Percorten-V, Novartis Animal Health, Greensboro, NC) 1 to 2 mg/kg IM, or fludrocortisone acetate (Florinef, Apothecon, Princeton, NJ) 0.1 to 0.6 mg PO q24h. Give fludrocortisone acetate as follows:
   a. Small dog: 0.1 to 0.2 mg/day PO.
   b. Medium-sized dog: 0.2 to 0.3 mg/day PO.

    c. Large dog: 0.4 to 0.6 mg/day PO.

    d. Giant breed: 0.6 to 1.2 mg/day PO.

6. Continue desoxycorticosterone acetate (DOCA) injections daily, and monitor serum sodium and potassium levels. Give hydrocortisone acetate IM q12h. Adding salt to the diet may be healthful if tolerated. As an alternative to DOCA injections, microcrystalline DOCA can be given at 1 to 2 mg/kg by deep IM injection and repeated on days 25 and 50.

7. Obtain an ECG tracing. If serum electrolyte levels and ECG tracings indicate severe hyperkalemia (>8.0 mEq/L), rapid lowering of potassium levels by the use of IV glucose and insulin should be considered (see p. 68).

8. Evaluate the acid-base status of the patient (see p. 591). If the total venous carbon dioxide or the serum bicarbonate concentration is less than 12 mEq/L, conservative bicarbonate therapy is indicated (see p. 604).

9. If hypoglycemia is present, administer dextrose 50 % solution 1 mL/kg IV and maintain on a 2.5% dextrose and 0.9% saline IV fluid drip. When the crisis has been controlled and the serum electrolytes are normal, begin therapy for chronic adrenal insufficiency.

10. All dogs should receive GI protectants: misoprostol 2 to 5 μg/kg PO t.i.d. or ranitidine 2 mg/kg IV or PO b.i.d.

Iatrogenic secondary adrenocortical insufficiency is a potential sequela to glucocorticosteroid therapy in the dog. The primary problem is the development of ACTH insufficiency secondary to either the sudden withdrawal of long-term exogenous glucocorticosteroids or the presence of acute stress reaction in an animal that has been on low-dose daily maintenance glucocorticosteroids. The normal mineralocorticoid function of the zona glomerulosa of the adrenal gland is not affected (see Hyperthyroidism in Cats, p. 640); therefore, the signs of Addison's disease are not seen. Failure to compensate for stress, marked hypotension, weakness, and collapse can characterize the clinical signs. These animals require IV glucocorticoids. For more chronic forms of treatment, oral replacement of hydrocortisone, 0.2 to 0.5 mg/kg once daily between 7 and 10 A.M. is the treatment of choice.

··········THYROTOXICOSIS (see Hyperthyroidism in Cats, p. 640)

Thyrotoxic crisis manifested as severe hypermetabolism may be observed in cats with hyperthyroidism. The clinical signs may be characterized by fever, tachycardia, pulmonary edema, or congestive heart failure. GI signs, characterized by anorexia, vomiting, and marked hypotension and collapse, can occur.

··········Emergency Treatment

1. Antagonize adrenergic mediated aspects of peripheral thyroid hormone action. Large doses of dexamethasone may inhibit thyroxine (T_4) release from the thyroid.

2. Cardiac manifestations should be treated using β-blockers such as propranolol 0.02 mg/kg/hr or esmolol 25 to 50 μg/kg/min by continuous IV infusion.

3. Begin medical control with methimazole (Tapazole) 15 mg/day q8–12h.

REFERENCES

Bertoy EH, Newlson RW, Feldman EC: Effect of Lente Insulin for treatment of diabetes mellitus in 12 cats; J Am Vet Med Assoc 206:1729–1731, 1995.

Carothers M, Chew D: Management of cholecalciferol rodenticide toxicity. Compend Contin Pract Vet 13:1058, 1991.

Chew DJ, Nagode LA, Carothers M: Disorders of calcium. *In* Dibartola Sp, ed: Fluid Therapy in Small Animal Practice. Philadelphia, WB Saunders, 1992.

Dibartola SP, ed: Fluid Therapy in Small Animal Practice. Philadelphia, WB Saunders, 1992.

Dougherty SS, Center S, Dzanis DA: Salmon calcitonin as adjunct to treatment for Vitamin D toxicosis in a dog. J Am Vet Med Assoc 196:1269–1272, 1990.

Feldman EC, Nelson R: Canine and Feline Endocrinology and Reproduction. Philadelphia, WB Saunders, 1987.

Feldman EC, Nelson RW: Diagnosis and management of diabetic ketoacidosis in dogs and cats. *In* Proceedings of the Waltham Symposium, 1991, pp 73–85.

Feldman EC, Nelson RW: Feline diabetes mellitus. *In* Kirk RW, ed: Current Veterinary Therapy IX. Small Animal Practice. Philadelphia, WB Saunders, 1986, pp 1000–1005.

Fooshee SK, Forrester D: Hypercalcemia secondary to cholecalciferol rodenticide toxicosis in two dogs. J Am Vet Med Assoc 196:1265–1268, 1990.

Ford S: NIDDM in the cat: Treatment with oral hypoglycemic medication, glipzide. Vet Clin North Am Small Anim Pract 25:599, 1995.

Greco D: Endocrine emergencies. Parts 1 and 2. Compend Contin Educ Pract Vet, 19:15–23, 27–39, 1997.

Greco D, Broussard J, Peterson ME: Insulin therapy. Vet Clin North Am Small Anim Pract 25:677, 1995.

Hoenig M: Pathophysiology of canine diabetes. Vet Clin North Am Small Anim Pract 25:140,637, 1995.

Ihle SL, Nelson RW: Insulin resistance and diabetes mellitus. Compend Cont Pract Vet 13:197, 1991.

Kintzer P, Peterson M: Treatment and long-term follow-up of 205 dogs with hyperadrenocorticism: J Vet Intern Med 11:43, 1997.

Leifer CE, Peterson ME, Matus RE: Insulin secreting tumors: Diagnosis and medical and surgical management in 55 dogs. J Am Vet Med Assoc 188:60–64, 1986.

Lutz T, Rand J: Pathogenesis of feline diabetes mellitus. 527. Vet Clin North Am Small Anim Pract 25:141,637, 1995.

Lynn RC, Feldman BC, Nelson RW: Efficacy of microcrystalline desoxycorticosterone pivalate for the treatment of hypoadrenocorticism in dogs. J Am Vet Med Assoc 202:392, 1993.

Macintire D: Emergency therapy of diabetic crises: Insulin overdosage, diabetic ketoacidosis, and hyperosmolar coma. Vet Clin North Am Small Anim Pract 25:639, 1995.

McMillan F, Feldman EC: Rebound hyperglycemia following overdosing of insulin in cats with diabetes mellitus. J Am Vet Med Assoc 188:1426, 1986.

Miller E: Long-term monitoring of the diabetic dog and cat: Vet Clin North Amer Small Anim Pract 25:571, 1995.

Nelson R: Insulin resistance in diabetic dogs and cats. *In* Bonagura J: Current Veterinary Therapy. Small Anim Pract. Philadelphia, WB Saunders, 1995 p 122.

Nelson RW: Diabetes mellitus. *In* Ettinger SJ, Feldman EC, eds: Textbook of Veterinary Internal medicine, ed 4. Philadelphia, WB Saunders, 1995, pp 1510–1537.

Nelson RW: Disorders of the endocrine pancreas. *In* Nelson RW, Cook XX, eds: Essentials of Small Animal Internal Medicine. St Louis, Mosby–Year Book, 1992.

Nelson RW: Feline diabetes mellitus. Vet Med Rep 3(1):4–12, 1991.

Nelson RW, Feldman EC: Insulin therapy for diabetic dogs and cats. *In* Proceedings of the Waltham Symposium, 1991, pp 87–92.

Nelson RW, Feldman EC, DeVries SE: Use of Ultralente insulin in cats with diabetes mellitus. J Am Vet Med Assoc 200:1828, 1992.

Nelson RW, Feldman EC, Ford SL, et al: Effect of an orally administered sulfonylurea, glipizide, for treatment of diabetes mellitus in cats. J Am Vet Med Assoc 6:821, 1993.

Nichols R, Crenshaw K: Complications and concurrent disease associated with diabetic ketoacidosis and other severe forms of diabetes, mellitus. *In* Bonagura J: Current Veterinary Therapy XII. Small Animal Practice. Philadelphia, WB Saunders, 1995, p 384.

Nosworthy GD: The difficulties in regulating diabetic cats. Vet Med 88:342–348, 1993.

Peterson M, Sampson G: Insulin and insulin syringes. *In* Bonagura J: Current Veterinary Therapy XII. Small Animal Practice. Philadelphia, WB Saunders, 1995, p 387.

Peterson ME: Diagnosis and management of insulin resistance in dogs and cats with diabetes mellitus. Vet Clin North Am Small Anim Pract 25:691, 1995.

Peterson ME: Endocrine diseases. *In* Sherding RG, ed: The Cat, Diseases and Clinical Management, ed 2. New York, Churchill Livingstone, 1994, pp 1465–1470.

Peterson ME: Hypoparathyroidism and other causes of hypocalcemia in cats. *In* Kirk RW:

Current Veterinary Therapy XI. Small Animal Practice. Philadelphia, WB Saunders, 1992, p 376.

Struble A, Nelson R: Non–insulin-dependent diabetes mellitus in cats and humans. Compend Contin Educ Pract Vet 19:935, 1997.

Wallace MS, Kirk CA: The diagnosis and treatment of insulin-dependent and non-insulin dependent diabetes mellitus in the dog and cat. Probl Vet Med 2:573–590, 1990.

Willard MD, Zerbe CA, Schall WD, et al: Severe hypophosphatemia associated with diabetes mellitus in six dogs and one cat. J Am Vet Med Assoc 190:1007–1010, 1987.

Wolfsheimer KJ: Problems in diabetes mellitus management. Probl Vet Med 2:591–601, 1990.

Neurologic Emergencies

Neurologic emergencies can seriously jeopardize an animal's life. In this section, four conditions that constitute neurologic emergencies are discussed: (1) head injuries, (2) injuries of the spinal cord and vertebral column, (3) coma, and (4) seizures.

..........HEAD INJURIES

Head injuries may include skin and superficial lacerations, concussions, fractures (including extracranial, linear, and depressed intracranial), and extracranial and intracranial hemorrhage (including extradural, subdural, subarachnoid, and intracerebral).

..........Immediate Care

The animal must be handled carefully so that it does no harm to the handler or further injury to itself. The anxious animal is reassured and handled gently to enhance compliance during the examination. Sedative drugs should be avoided. Tranquilizers (in minimal dosages) may have to be administered if the animal cannot be evaluated without chemical restraint. A rapid-acting, short-duration, reversible agent can be used if sedation is required (e.g., for skull radiographs). Oxymorphone 0.1 mg/kg IV can be used judiciously, because it depresses respiration and vital signs in an animal that is already severely depressed owing to injury to the CNS.

Hypoxia is one of the most common causes of death following severe head trauma. An adequate airway and exchange of air must therefore be maintained. In the comatose animal, an endotracheal tube should be inserted and oxygen administered. Hyperventilation is very helpful in maintaining cerebral oxygenation and helping to prevent hypercarbia with consequent vasodilation and CNS edema. Repeated sampling of blood gases to check $Paco_2$ and Pao_2 is warranted. If severe head trauma has resulted in laryngeal edema or marked dyspnea associated with blockage of the upper airway, a tracheostomy will have to be performed. An intermittent positive-pressure mechanical respirator may be necessary to assist respiration. Oxygen may also be administered by the use of a face mask, oxygen tent, nasopharyngeal tube, or transtracheal catheter (see p. 610). The level of oxygenation of the brain may be reflected in the state of consciousness of the animal.

Control any bleeding and treat shock (see p. 32).

Frequently examine and elicit vital signs such as pulse, respirations per minute, depth of respiration, and temperature, and evaluate the neurologic status, including the state of consciousness, size and response of pupils, perception of noxious stimuli, and voluntary motor activity. Progressively dilating pupils usually indicates brain stem edema or hemorrhage. Any deterioration of the aforementioned neurologic data usually indicates progressive brain stem compression or edema. With an initial rapid rise in intracranial pressure, the pulse and respirations become slowed and the temperature is elevated. If intracranial pressure continues to rise and reduced cerebral circulation leads to progressive hypoxia, vital signs may become reversed, producing a rapid pulse, rapid respirations, and an elevated temperature. Cheyne-Stokes respirations occur with diencephalic lesions. Central neurogenic hyperventilation follows mesencephalic lesions. Irregular or ataxic respirations occur with medullary lesions and precede arrest.

............Initial Examination

In order to follow the animal's course, a baseline neurologic assessment must be made as soon as possible and the neurologic status must be continually reevaluated.

The initial neurologic examination should include evaluation of the following:

............State of Consciousness

Examine the animal's state of consciousness and elicit the response to commands, to noxious stimuli such as a toe pinch, and to movement of people in the room. The various levels of consciousness may be described as:

1. Coma (unconscious with no response to noxious stimuli).
2. Semicoma (unconscious but responsive to noxious stimuli).
3. Delirium.
4. Confusion.
5. Depression.
6. Alertness. Initial consciousness followed by unconsciousness generally indicates severe brain stem injury. In dogs, hemorrhages into the midbrain and pons may produce coma and decerebrate rigidity. Brain stem compression can also be associated with compressed skull fractures, extradural or subdural hematomas, or cerebral edema with herniation.

............Pupil Size and Response

Bilateral mydriatic pupils that are nonresponsive to bright light in an unconscious animal are a very grave sign and indicate severe midbrain contusion and usually an irreversible condition. Bilateral miotic pupils with normal nystagmus and ocular movements occur with diffuse cerebral or diencephalic lesions. Miotic pupils that become mydriatic indicate a progressive midbrain lesion and a poor prognosis. Unilateral, slowly progressing pupillary abnormalities in the absence of direct ocular injury are characteristic of brain stem compression or herniation caused by progressive brain swelling. Asymmetric pupils occur with rostral brain stem lesions and can change rapidly. A change from dilated to constricted to normal pupils indicates a favorable prognosis. Unresponsive pupils that are fixed in midposition occur with lesions extending into the medulla and are a grave sign. Examine the eyes because the pupillary dilation may be due to ocular lesions and not the brain stem.

............Vision

Vision deficits are common in intracranial injury. Less severe lesions limited to the cerebrum will produce contralateral menace deficits with normal pupil response to light. Bilateral cerebral edema will cause blindness with normal pupillary response to light if the midbrain is not disturbed. A severely depressed recumbent animal may not respond to menacing gestures, even though visual pathways are intact. Ocular, optic nerve, chiasm, or optic tract lesions will interfere with vision as well as pupillary responses to light. Brain stem contusion and cerebral edema may produce blindness and dilated unresponsive pupils from oculomotor neuronal disturbance.

...........Other Cranial Nerves

Initial evidence of cranial nerve abnormality indicates direct contusion or laceration of the neurons within the brain stem or where they pass through the skull. Cranial nerves that initially are normal and subsequently lose their function indicate a progressive expanding lesion. Prognosis must be guarded when specific cranial nerve deficits are present.

Petrosal bone or cerebellomedullary lesions commonly produce signs of vestibular neuron disturbance with rolling to one side or torsion and head tilt to one side and abnormal nystagmus. Petrosal bone fractures often cause bleeding and cerebrospinal fluid (CSF) otorrhea from the external ear canal. If the lesion is limited to the membranous labyrinth, the loss of balance will be toward the injured side and the quick phase of the nystagmus will be toward the opposite side.

Normal physiologic nystagmus requires a pathway to be intact from the peripheral vestibular neurons to the pontomedullary vestibular nuclei to the nuclei of the cranial nerves that innervate the extraocular muscles (III, IV, VI). Severe brain stem lesions will disrupt this pathway. This is indicated by the inability to produce a normal nystagmus on moving the head from side to side. Occasionally, this cannot be elicited in severely depressed animals.

...........Posture and Motor Function

Loss of normal oculocephalic reflex activity is an early sign of brain stem hemorrhage and a late sign with brain stem compression and herniation. Opisthotonos and extensor rigidity of all four limbs indicate a severe caudal midbrain or pontine lesion or rostral cerebellar lesion. Opisthotonos, with extended forelimbs and hindlimbs extended forward with the hips flexed, occurs with rostral cerebellar lesions. Tetraplegia indicates a pontomedullary or cervical spinal cord lesion. Be aware that the intracranial injury may be accompanied by a cervical vertebral fracture and spinal cord injury. These animals must be handled with care. If uncertain, obtain a radiograph of the cervical vertebrae before manipulating the patient. Hemiplegia usually indicates an ipsilateral pontomedullary or cervical spinal cord lesion. Hemiparesis can be caused by acute lesions in the opposite rostral brain stem or cerebrum. With the latter lesions, the hemiparesis usually resolves in 1 to 3 days. Severe neck torsion or turning of the head and neck to one side may accompany contralateral midbrain-pontine tegmental lesions.

Evaluation of cranial nerve function at frequent intervals may reveal an initial nerve injury or the presence of a progressive, expanding lesion of the brain (see p. 155). Signs of severe vestibular disorientation, marked head tilt, and abnormal nystagmus can also occur with contusion of the membranous labyrinth, which is usually associated with a fracture of the petrosal bone. Hemorrhage and CSF otorrhea may occur from the external ear canal. Rolling movements usually indicate a cerebellar-medullary vestibular system lesion.

Alterations in respirations may be present with head injuries. Cheyne-Stokes respirations are seen in diencephalic lesions, hyperventilation in mesencephalic lesions, and irregular respirations with medullary lesions.

Seizures following head injury may be associated with intracranial injury, hemorrhage, and an expanding intracranial mass. Medical treatment to control the convulsive state should be instituted. If necessary, give IV injections of diazepam 5 to 10 mg for sedation, if needed. IV pentobarbital should be administered to produce light general anesthesia (see p. 164).

...........*Special Studies*

Special studies useful in the management of animals with head injuries include radiographic examination of the head and chest. Radiographic studies of the skull should be taken only after all other emergency procedures have been initiated. If the animal is not cooperative, and if sedation and the use of a short-acting anesthetic are contraindicated, radiographs should be delayed until diagnostic films can be safely obtained. Oxymorphone 0.1 mg/kg IV can be used for sedation, if needed. Radiographs of both skull and cervical vertebrae are indicated in traumatic injuries of the head.

If possible, brain imaging should be performed in animals with severe or deteriorating neurologic signs. Computed tomography (CT) and magnetic resonance imaging (MRI) can help detect edema and hemorrhage in the brain and brain stem. Because brain stem hemorrhage is most often irreversible, early detection can improve the accuracy of prognosis and may alter the course of therapy. A CSF tap is contraindicated in animals with head trauma because it may induce brain herniation.

...........Treatment of Specific Head Injuries

1. The hysterical, delirious animal may be sedated with diazepam or phenobarbital. Seizures may occur, associated with intracranial lesions, and should be treated with IV diazepam 5 to 10 mg. IV pentobarbital should be administered to produce a light, general anesthesia, or diazepam can be added to the IV fluids at the rate of 5 to 20 mg/hr (see p. 164). IV administration of phenobarbital has been recommended, but its effect is often delayed. Phenobarbital 2 to 4 mg/kg is used for all subsequent injections as the animal recovers from the initial dose of pentobarbital.
2. Brain edema commonly occurs with intracranial injury. The disruption of vascular endothelium produces vasogenic edema, which is extracellular and predominantly in the white matter. The use of glucocorticosteroids in the management of head-injured animals is controversial. Experimental evidence suggests that they may help if administered before the trauma occurs, but clearly this is seldom of practical value. Experimental data indicate that methylprednisolone sodium succinate at an initial dose of 30 mg/kg IV followed by 15 mg/kg IV at 6-hour intervals for 24 to 48 hours may help treat vasogenic edema that may attend head trauma. The GI tract should be protected with misoprostol PO during the administration of corticosteroids. Dimethyl sulfoxide (DMSO) has been effective experimentally in reducing of preventing vasogenic edema without some of the side effects of glucocorticoids. The dose is 2 g/kg IV, diluted 1:1 with 5% dextrose in saline and administered slowly over 30 minutes. This can be repeated two to three times in the first 24 hours. This drug is not approved for veterinary use, and client permission should be obtained. Hypoxia that occurs secondary to the vascular compromise and vasogenic edema causes cytotoxic edema with neuronal and glial swelling. Furosemide 0.5 to 2.0 mg/kg IV q48h is administered. This is followed by low levels of mannitol 0.1 to 0.25 g/kg IV, using a 20% solution over 60 minutes. This can be repeated once at 3 to 4 hours. If there has been extensive blood loss or intracranial hemorrhage is apparent from epistaxis, if there is bleeding from the ear canal, or if there are palpable skull fractures, mannitol should be avoided.
3. Keep the animal in an oxygen-rich environment. Maintain PaO_2 over 60 mm Hg. Avoid increasing CO_2 levels. Administer oxygen by methods that avoid stimulating the respiratory passageways to promote cough reflex. Use adequate sedation with narcotic thiopental to maintain tolerance of the endotracheal tube. Use IV lidocaine 1 mg/lb to decrease cough reflex.
4. If there are skull fractures or evidence of meningeal breach (i.e., CSF

otorrhea or CSF rhinorrhea), broad-spectrum antibiotics should be administered. Examples include ampicillin 10 mg/kg q6h IV, or trimethoprim-sulfadiazine 15 mg/kg q12h IM.

5. Maintain adequate blood flow to the brain tissue that is edematous without giving crystalloid solutions or lactate-containing solutions, which will make the edema worse. The use of 7.5% hypertonic saline and hetastarch has been suggested to maintain cerebral blood flow without increasing intracranial pressure. The dose is 4 mL/kg IV in dogs and 2 mL/kg in cats. Combination solution is 25% saline and 75% hetastarch.

6. Maintain blood glucose between 100 and 200 mg/dL.

7. If the animal is hyperthermic, cold water baths and cool enemas should be used to lower the temperature to normal or slightly subnormal.

8. If possible, keep the head elevated (approximately at a 45-degree angle) and prevent obstruction of venous return to the heart. Insert an indwelling catheter into the bladder to avoid bladder distention, which may occur during unconsciousness.

9. Maintain the animal's metabolic requirements with oral alimentation with nasogastric tube (see p. 537). The vital and neurologic signs should be monitored closely every few hours. If the signs worsen, more vigorous medical therapy is indicated, decompressive surgery can be considered, or fragments of the fractured calvaria can be gently removed.

Surgery is usually limited to depressed fractures of the calvaria that compress the brain. These can be diagnosed by careful palpation and radiography. When the patient is stabilized on medical therapy, surgery to remove this compression can be performed. Surgery to decompress the brain where fractures are not apparent and clinical signs are severe or progressing is rarely performed because of the poor prognosis and results. The surgery involves making several 1- to 2-cm diameter openings into the cranial cavity over the cerebrum (burr holes or gently removing fragments from the fractured calvaria). Blood clots can be removed through these openings. If needed, the cranial defect can be enlarged with rongeurs or by creating a bone flap. The bone window should be enlarged to visualize normal brain tissue. If possible, the frontal sinus and dorsal sagittal sinus should be avoided. Replacement of the bone flap is optional unless the frontal sinus is entered. In some instances brain swelling may preclude bone flap replacement. The dura mater must be sutured if the frontal sinus is involved. A fascial graft from the masseter muscle can be used to close any defect if the remaining dura is inadequate.

The most common lesion present in animals that are presented initially with severe brain stem signs is contusion, with laceration and hemorrhage in the midbrain and pons. This is irreversible, and the prognosis is hopeless. Subdural or extradural hemorrhages with space-occupying blood clots are uncommon. If the hemorrhage slowly accumulates in these sites, repeated neurologic examinations will reveal a deteriorating animal. If the signs can be lateralized to one cerebrum or noticed in CT or MRI studies, burr holes or bone flap surgery can be performed to relieve the hemorrhage.

...........Prognosis of Head Injuries

1. The prognosis is always initially guarded.

2. Initial care (first 30 minutes) is most critical in preventing severe cerebral edema.

3. Head trauma patients may require extensive nursing care over a prolonged period of time (months) before recovery is seen. Remarkable recovery from severe cerebellar vestibular signs may occur. Often, owners do not give animals enough time to recover before deciding in favor of euthanasia.

4. Early cerebral decompression is important if progressive loss of consciousness is developing.

............SPINAL CORD INJURIES

Spinal cord injuries are usually associated with disk ruptures, fractures, and dislocations of the vertebral column.

............Handling and Management

Move animals suspected of having vertebral injuries with extreme care and caution. All animals rendered unconscious following an injury are regarded as having cervical or thoracolumbar injury until ruled out by radiographs. They should be moved on a wide board or a rolling cart, and flexion, extension, or torsion of the vertebral column should be avoided. The vertebral column should be kept as immobile as possible from the time of injury to the time of repair.

Sedation with tranquilizers and pain relievers may be required before the animal can be moved safely. Narcotics should be used in amounts necessary only to relieve pain, because if more than minimal amounts are used, respiration and other vital signs may also be depressed.

Treat shock, respiratory embarrassment, and open wounds immediately, as required.

............Thoracolumbar Disk Disease

Protrusion of the disk implies that the intervertebral disk is bulging into the vertebral canal resulting from dorsal shifting of the disk nuclear material. Disk extrusion refers to rupture of the outer disk membrane and extrusion of the nuclear material into the vertebral canal. There are 36 intervertebral disks in the canine and feline spinal column. Breeds of dogs predisposed to endochondral ossification and "disk disease" are called chondrodystrophoid and include dachshunds, beagles, Pekingese, French bulldogs, basset hounds, Welsh corgis, American spaniels, Shih Tzus, and Lhasa apsos.

............Examination

In the initial examination, try to identify the location and evaluate the extent of the spinal cord lesion and establish an initial prognosis.

The presence of pain, edema, hemorrhage, or a visible deformity may localize an area of vertebral injury.

Identifying the location of spinal cord injuries necessitates a neurologic examination (see p. 330). This examination should be carried out without excessive manipulation of the animal.

Good radiographic visualization of the area of spinal cord injury is essential to achieve an early diagnosis and to institute treatment. In almost all cases, the animal must receive a short-acting anesthetic so that good radiographs can be taken without causing further injury. Lateral and cross-table dorsoventral (DV) or ventrodorsal (VD) projections require less manipulation of the animal compared with standard DV or VD projections. The entire spine should be radiographed. Myelography may be needed to delineate the area of spinal cord injury more clearly (see p. 533).

Prognosis in spinal cord injury depends on the extent of the injury and the reversibility of the damage. Perception of noxious stimuli on the part of the animal when stimulus is applied caudal to the level of the lesion is a good sign. For a noxious stimulus, apply firm pressure to a toe with hemostatic forceps. Flexion of the limb is a spinal reflex. Movement of the head or vocalization is evidence of perception of the noxious stimulus. Absence of such a response following recovery from spinal shock (1 to 2 hours) portends a very poor prognosis.

Focal lesions in one or more of the spinal cord segments from T3 to T4 may cause complete dysfunction of the injured tissue from concussion, contusion, or laceration. The degree of structural damage cannot be determined from the neurologic signs. Transverse focal lesions result in paraplegia, with intact pelvic limb spinal reflexes and analgesia of the body and limbs caudal to the lesion.

These lesions are usually associated with vertebral fractures and displacements of the vertebral canal. The most common site is the caudal thoracic and cranial lumbar region. Lesions here often result in the Schiff-Sherrington syndrome, which is characterized by rigidly extended hypertonic thoracic limbs and flaccid hypotonic paralyzed analgesic pelvic limbs with intact spinal reflexes. The thoracic limbs have normal voluntary motor function, despite their marked hypertonia. They can perform all the postural reactions; spinal reflexes and sensory perception are normal.

Severe injury to the spinal cord from the T4 through the caudal segments causes a flaccid paraplegia, with atonia, areflexia, and analgesia of the pelvic limbs, anus, and tail. Injuries to the spinal cord from the C6 to the T2 segments cause tetraparesis or tetraplegia, with depressed spinal reflexes from the thoracic limbs and hyperactive spinal reflexes from the pelvic limbs. Horner's syndrome (miosis, protruded third eyelid, smaller palpebral fissure, and enophthalmos) occurs with lesions in the T1–3 segments. Injuries craniad to the C6 segment will cause spastic tetraparesis or tetraplegia, with hyperactive reflexes in all four limbs. If the injury is severe, death will occur from respiratory failure. Assess the patient for respiratory function, and supplement, if necessary. Care should be taken in handling animals with fractures because displacement of fractures may cause deterioration of neurologic signs.

............Therapy

The injured animal is examined for any life-threatening conditions, especially pneumothorax, hemorrhage, or hypovolemic shock, and treated appropriately. The specific treatment for spinal cord injury is the same as for brain injury (see p. 155). If there is palpable or radiographic evidence of a vertebral lesion compressing the spinal cord, surgery is indicated unless the vertebral displacement has compromised most or all of the vertebral canal. Displacements through 50% to 100% of the vertebral canal are associated with a poor prognosis, especially if deep pain is absent in the limbs caudal to the lesion. In the absence of a radiographic lesion and the persistence of severe neurologic deficit, exploratory surgery is indicated. The objectives of surgery are to (1) provide spinal cord decompression by hemilaminectomy or laminectomy with removal of blood clots, disk material, etc.; (2) realign and stabilize the vertebral column; and (3) perform a meningotomy, if necessary. Meningotomy is indicated to help decompress the spinal cord following severe trauma. In addition, if myelomalacia is present, the spinal cord parenchyma may exude from the meningotomy defect, signaling a poor to hopeless prognosis for neurologic recovery.

Prior to surgical stabilization of the injured vertebrae, it is important to restrict any movement of the vertebral column by using a padded back brace or splint taped around the body and over the vertebral column. All activity of the animal must be severely restricted.

An animal with severe spinal cord injury must receive special care with respect to bowel and bladder function. Retention of urine develops quickly after many spinal cord injuries and may not cause any distress to the animal because of associated loss of sensory perception from the bladder. Urinary retention leads to bladder infections and loss of the normal tonicity of the bladder wall. Frequent manual expression of the urine and washing of the hindquarters with warm water may be enough to keep the bladder empty. Repeated catheterizations (two or three times daily), especially in males, may be necessary to prevent urinary retention. This often predisposes to infection; thus, these animal should receive appropriate antibiotic and urinary antiseptic therapy.

Indwelling catheters of soft rubber should be used. Povidone-iodine (Betadine) ointment should be placed in the prepuce and on the penis at the entry site of the catheter. The catheter should be stabilized in the urethra by suturing the end of the preputial orifice, and a collar should be placed on the dog so that the catheter cannot be pulled out. A collecting vessel or plastic bag should be attached to the catheter, and urine should be prevented from flowing back into the catheter.

Paralytic ileus and fecal retention are also frequent complications of spinal cord injury. The correction of fluid and electrolyte imbalances, together with the ingestion of small amounts of highly digestible foods, will help to relieve the ileus. Mild enemas will help to control the fecal retention. A nasogastric tube may be needed to prevent gas retention in the stomach.

High-dose glucocorticosteroid should only be used for the initial 48 hours of treatment. Prolonged treatment of these dogs with glucocorticosteroid may precipitate bloody diarrhea, vomiting, GI ulceration, colonic ulceration, peritonitis, and death. This form of GI complication has been estimated to occur in 15% to 20% of all dogs with intervertebral disk extrusions treated with dexamethasone. When GI complications are noted, glucocorticosteroid therapy should be stopped immediately. Cimetidine 10 mg/kg q8h PO, a commonly used H_2-antagonist, can be administered to reduce GI complications.

■ CORTICOSTEROID DOSAGE IN ACUTE SPINAL TRAUMA

Acute spinal cord injuries of less than 8 hours are initially treated with sodium prednisolone succinate or methylprednisolone:
Initial dose 20 to 30 mg/kg IV; T 3 hours, 10 to 15 mg/kg IV; T 6 hours, 10 to 15 mg/kg IV; T 9 hours to T 33 hours, 2 mg/kg/hr IV.
T, time following the initial dose.
Data from Shores A: Spinal trauma. Vet Clin North Am Small Anim Pract 22:859, 1992.

Special care of the skin is also required in spinal cord injuries. Areas of decubital ulceration may develop rapidly and lead to ischemic necrosis of dermal and muscle tissue. Place the injured animal on an air mattress, waterbed, or foam rubber pad, and change the body position frequently. Preventing excessive moisture such as urine from accumulating on the skin over pressure points will also help to prevent decubital sores. Following bowel movement, enemas, expression of urine, or catheterization of the bladder, clean and dry the perineum or preputial area. The use of a warm whirlpool bath may be exceedingly valuable by providing hydromassage in paralytic animals and by keeping the skin clean. However, if vertebral instability is suspected, whirlpool treatment is contraindicated.

Management of ruptured intervertebral disk depends on the severity of the disk rupture and degree of injury to the spinal cord.

If the vertebral canal is displaced at the site of the injury, realignment or laminectomy should be performed. If there is a complete discontinuity of the vertebral canal, nothing can be done for the animal to recover the lost neurologic function. Displacements of 50% to 100% of the vertebral canal, especially if deep pain is absent in the limbs caudal to the lesion, are associated with a very poor prognosis.

········· INJURIES TO THE PERIPHERAL NERVOUS SYSTEM (see also p. 330)

········· Radial Nerve

The radial nerve innervates all the extensors of the elbow, carpus, and digits. The radial nerve supplies the only sensory innervation to the distal cranial and lateral surface of the forearm and dorsal surface of the forepaw. Injuries to the radial nerve at the level of the elbow result in inability of the animal to extend its carpus and digits; the animal walks supporting its weight on the dorsal surface of the paw. Additionally, there is loss of cutaneous sensation. Injuries of the radial nerve in the shoulder area result in inability of the animal to extend the elbow and bear weight on the affected limb.

...........Brachial Plexus

Injuries to the brachial plexus (roots C6–T2) are involved predominantly with signs of radial nerve paralysis. Other nerves may also be injured, resulting in the following signs: (1) musculocutaneous (inability to flex the elbow); (2) axillary or thoracodorsal (dropped elbow); and (3) median and ulnar nerves (loss of flexor ability of carpal and digital muscles and loss of sensation from the caudal surface of the forearm and the palmar and lateral surfaces of the forepaw).

Contusion or avulsion of the roots of the brachial plexus may involve C8–T1 (radial, median, and ulnar nerves) or C6 and C7 (musculocutaneous, suprascapular, and axillary). Horner's syndrome can be seen associated with damage to the area of C7–T3.

...........Sciatic Nerve (L6–S1)

The sciatic nerve innervates the caudal thigh muscles, which primarily flex the stifle and extend the hip. Its tibial nerve branch innervates the caudal leg muscles that extend the tarsus and flex the digits. The tibial nerve provides the sole cutaneous sensory nerves to the plantar surface of the paw. The peroneal branch of the sciatic nerve innervates the cranial leg muscles, flexors of the tarsus, and extensors of the digits. The peroneal nerve is the sole cutaneous innervation to the dorsal surface of the paw. With sciatic nerve injury, there is decreased stifle flexion, the hock is overflexed (tibial), and the animal walks on the dorsal surface of the paw (peroneal). Sciatic nerve injury occurs with pelvic fractures, especially those that involve the body of the ilium at the greater ischiatic notch, or with sacroiliac luxations that contuse the L6 and L7 spinal nerves, which pass ventral to the sacrum to contribute to the sciatic nerve.

The signs of tibial or peroneal nerve deficit follow femoral fractures, with displacement of fragments caudally, or the inadvertent injection of drugs in or around the nerve in the caudal thigh muscles.

...........Femoral Nerve (L4–L6)

The femoral nerve innervates the extensors of the stifle, and its saphenous nerve branch supplies the sole cutaneous innervation to an area on the medial side of the distal thigh, the leg, and the paw. The nerve is protected by muscles and rarely is injured by pelvic fractures. Clinical signs of injury are inability to support weight on the pelvic limb, absence of the patellar reflex, and analgesia in the area of sole cutaneous innervation.

REFERENCES

Bunch S: Anticonvulsant therapy in companion animals. *In* Kirk RW, ed: Current Veterinary Therapy 8: Small Animal Practice. Philadelphia, WB Saunders, 1983.
Chrisman CL: Problems in Small Animal Neurology. Philadelphia, Lea & Febiger, 1982.
deLahunta A: Veterinary Neuroanatomy and Clinical Neurology, ed 2. Philadelphia, WB Saunders, 1983.

Dewey CW, Budsberg S, Oliver JE: Principles of head trauma management in dogs and cats. Compend Contin Educ Pract Vet 14:199, 1992.

Hopkins AL: Head trauma. Vet Clin North Am. Small Anim Pract, 26:875, 1996.

Johnson J, Murtaugh M: Craniocerebral trauma. *In* Bonagura J, ed: Kirk's Current Veterinary Therapy 13. Philadelphia, WB Saunders, 2000.

Kirby R: Severe head injuries: Prog Vet Neurol 5:72, 1994.

Kraus K: Medical management of acute spinal cord disease. *In* Bonagura J, ed: Kirk's Current Veterinary Therapy 13. Philadelphia, WB Saunders, 2000.

Meintjes E, Hosgood G, Daniloff J: Pharmaceutic treatment of acute spinal cord trauma. Compend Contin Educ Pract Vet 18:625, 1996.

Oliver JE, Hoerlein BF, Mayhew IG: Veterinary Neurology. Philadelphia, WB Saunders, 1989.

Seim III HB: Thoracolumbar disk diseases: Diagnosis, treatment and prognosis. Canine Pract 20:8–13, 1995.

Shores A: Development of a coma scale for dogs: Prognostic value in cranio-caudal trauma. *In* Proceedings of the 6th Annual Forum of the American College of Veterinary Internal Medicine, 1988, pp 251–252.

Shores A: Spinal trauma. Vet Clin North Am Small Anim Pract 22:859, 1992.

Toombs JP: Colonic perforation in corticosteroid-treated dogs. J Am Vet Med Assoc 88:145, 1986.

············ COMA

Coma is the complete loss of consciousness, with no response to noxious stimuli (see p. 389). In some animals presented in a stuporous or comatose state, the cause will be apparent. However, in most instances, a careful diagnostic workup must be performed. A coma scale has been devised to assist in the clinical evaluation of the comatose animal (Table 1–24).

············ Treatment

For initial treatment of coma:

1. Maintain a clear airway and provide respiratory assistance if needed; treat systemic shock and control existing hemorrhage.
2. Take as complete a history as possible from the owner, especially noting the presence of trauma or previous seizures or comatose episodes.
3. Begin the physical examination by taking the animal's temperature, pulse, and respiration.
   a. An elevated temperature suggests a systemic infection such as pneumonia or hepatitis, or a brain lesion with loss of normal temperature control. Very high temperatures associated with signs of shock are indicative of heat stroke. A lowered body temperature is seen in barbiturate intoxication and circulatory collapse.
   b. Slow breathing can be seen in barbiturate intoxication or with elevated intracranial pressure.
   c. A rapid respiratory rate may indicate pneumonia, diabetic or uremic acidosis, or brain stem injury.
4. Examine the skin and note any bruises, ecchymoses, swellings, or lacerations that may signify a traumatic incident.
5. Examine the mucous membranes, noting the presence of pallor, indicative of possible internal hemorrhage, or the presence of icterus, indicative of possible liver disease.
6. Smell the breath for the odor of spoiled fruit, indicative of diabetic acidosis; for uremic odor; or for the musty odor associated with hepatic coma.
7. Following the initial examination, a more complete physical examination, including neurologic evaluation, should be conducted. Any indication of asymmetric neurologic signs suggests an intracranial structural lesion such

Table 1–24. Small Animal Coma Scale (SACS)*

Motor Activity	
Normal gait, normal spinal reflexes	6
Hemiparesis, tetraparesis or decerebrate activity	5
Recumbent, intermittent extensor rigidity	4
Recumbent, constant extensor rigidity	3
Recumbent, constant extensor rigidity with opisthotonus	2
Recumbent, hypotonia of muscles, depressed or absent spinal reflexes	1
Brain Stem Reflexes	
Normal pupillary light reflexes and oculocephalic reflexes	6
Slow pupillary light reflexes and normal to reduced oculocephalic reflexes	5
Bilateral unresponsive miosis with normal to reduced oculocephalic reflexes	4
Pinpoint pupils with reduced to absent oculocephalic reflexes	3
Unilateral, unresponsive mydriasis with reduced to absent oculocephalic reflexes	2
Bilateral, unresponsive mydriasis with reduced to absent oculocephalic reflexes	1
Level of Consciousness	
Occasional periods of alertness and responsive to environment	6
Depression or delirium, capable of responding to environment but response may be inappropriate	5
Semicomatose, responsive to visual stimuli	4
Semicomatose, responsive to auditory stimuli	3
Semicomatose, responsive only to repeated noxious stimuli	2
Comatose, unresponsive to repeated noxious stimuli	1

*Neurologic function is assessed for each of the three categories and a grade of 1 to 6 is assigned according to the descriptions for each grade. The total score is the sum of the three category scores. This scale is designed to assist the clinician in evaluating the neurologic status of the craniocerebral trauma patient. As a guideline and according to clinical impressions, a consistent total score of 3 to 8 represents a grave prognosis, 9 to 14 a poor to guarded prognosis, and 15 to 18 a good prognosis. (Modified from the Glasgow Coma Scale used in humans.)

From Shores A: Craniocerebral trauma. *In* Kirk RW, ed: Current Veterinary Therapy X. Small Animal Practice. Philadelphia, WB Saunders, 1989, p 849.

as an injury, acute hemorrhage, or neoplasm. Toxicities and metabolic disease will not produce asymmetric signs, and cerebral signs predominate. Pupils are usually normally responsive in metabolic encephalopathy and in most toxicities.

8. The following laboratory tests may be of value:
   a. A urinalysis, which should include tests for specific gravity, sugar, acetone, and albumin. Urine of high specific gravity, glycosuria, and acetonuria is indicative of diabetic coma. Urine of low specific gravity with an elevated protein content is found in uremia together with high fevers. Urine may be saved for specific tests such as determining barbiturate intoxication. Urine sediment should be examined for evidence of ammonium urate or oxalic acid crystalluria.
   b. A venous blood sample should be obtained for a WBC count, differential,

hematocrit, hemoglobin, glucose, sodium, BUN, amylase or lip
Paco$_2$, HCO$_3$, plasma osmolality, potassium, and chloride. Also con
measuring blood ammonia concentrations and checking for lead levels.
c. A sample of CSF should be obtained (see p. 516) and examined (see p.
517), and the cerebrospinal pressure should be determined.

············Care of the Comatose Animal

Therapy should be aimed at finding and eliminating the cause of coma; however, there may be no specific therapy for some disease processes. If direct, specific therapy is not possible, supportive measures must be instituted.

············Diabetic Coma (see also p. 138)

In the uncontrolled diabetic animal, disorientation, prostration, and coma can result. Evidence indicates that abnormalities in serum osmolality (hyperosmolarity) can markedly alter the level of consciousness. Plasma osmolality can be estimated by the formula:

$$\text{Plasma osmolality (mOsm/L)} = 2(Na + K) + \frac{\text{blood glucose}}{18} + \frac{\text{BUN}}{2.8}$$

Signs of a hyperosmolar state can occur with serum osmolality levels over 340 mOsm/L.

Treatment of diabetic acidosis is accomplished by reducing keto acid production, stimulating carbohydrate utilization, and impeding peripheral release of fatty acids. During ketosis, a marked insulin resistance may be present. IV rehydration with Ringer's solution or sodium chloride should be carried out. Cerebral edema may develop if initial volume replacement is too rapid. Therefore, fluid replacement should be over a period of 24 to 48 hours. In severe acidosis, give sodium bicarbonate 1 mEq/kg over 15 minutes, then another 1 to 2 mEq/kg over a period of 3 hours.

············Hepatic Coma (see also p. 120)

Hepatic encephalopathy is characterized by an abnormal mental state and neurologic abnormalities associated with severe hepatic insufficiency. Congenital portocaval shunts are the most common cause of hepatic encephalopathy in dogs and cats. Acute hepatic destruction caused by toxins, drugs, or infection can also lead to hepatic encephalopathy. The treatment of very severe cases of hepatic encephalopathy can be considered a medical emergency. The following treatment rationale can be used:
1. Prevent ammonia and other nitrogenous substances from entering the blood through the GI tract by:
   a. Restricting dietary proteins: The recommended dietary protein intake on a dry matter basis is 15% to 20% for dogs and 30% to 35% for cats. Caloric requirements are met with carbohydrates and fats. The source of the dietary protein should be vegetable if possible (soybeans). There are numerous diets available (see p. 813).
   b. Using cleansing enemas to rid the colon of residual material.
   c. Beginning antibiotic therapy to reduce the bacterial population in the GI tract. Administer neomycin by high-retention colonic enema 15 mg/kg q6h and metronidazole 7.5 mg/kg PO b.i.d. or t.i.d.
2. Begin general supportive care to restore fluid and electrolyte balance (see p. 585)
3. Stop administration of all drugs such as diuretics, tranquilizers, barbiturates, and others that may be extensively metabolized through the liver.

...atic ...athy	Clinical Signs
	Listlessness, depression, mental dullness Personality changes Polyuria
	Ataxia Disorientation Compulsive pacing or circling, head-pressing Apparent blindness Personality changes Salivation Polyuria
3	Stupor Severe salivation Seizures
4	Coma

4. Administer lactulose 2.5 to 5 mL for cats or 2.5 to 1.5 mL for dogs PO t.i.d. (Cephulac syrup, Hoechst-Marion Roussel, Kansas City, MO). This drug will cause the animal to have two or three soft stools a day. Do not administer to a comatose amimal. Lactulose causes a decrease in blood ammonia concentration and reduces the degree of hepatic encephalopathy. Bacterial degradation of lactulose in the colon acidifies the colonic contents, resulting in the retention of ammonia in the colon. Lactulose syrup therapy reduces blood ammonia levels by 25% to 50%. Lactulose acts as a laxative; diarrhea should be expected.

............SEIZURES (see also p. 432)

(see also p. 432)

A seizure or convulsion is a transient disturbance of brain function that is sudden in onset, ceases spontaneously, and has a tendency to recur. Most seizures are generalized and involve the loss of consciousness and severe involuntary contraction of skeletal muscles, causing tonic and clonic limb activity and opisthotonos. Mastication, salivation, pupil dilation, and excretions are common. Partial seizures vary from limited limb activity, to facial muscle twitching, to episodic behavioral abnormalities, to brief loss of consciousness.

............Immediate Measures

Most seizures are of short duration and may have subsided by the time the animal is presented for treatment. It is important, however, to prevent the patient from injuring either itself or a bystander. Confinement in a blanket may be useful in this regard.

In beginning treatment of the animal that has seizures, it is important to evaluate the possibility of coexisting systemic diseases that can predispose the animal to seizures, such as uremia, hepatic disorders, insulin-secreting tumors of the pancreas, electrolyte imbalances, hypoglycemia, lead poisoning, carbon monoxide poisoning, organophosphate poisoning, chlorinated hydrocarbon poisoning, cyanide poisoning, strychnine poisoning, and thiamine deficiency in cats. Treatment of these disease entities will help to control the seizures. (Table 1–25).

Status epilepticus (continuous seizures) is an emergency situation in which there is usually no time for an extensive diagnostic workup. The seizures must be controlled as quickly as possible.

Table I-25. Drugs, Dosages, Advantages, and Disadvantages of the Most Commonly Used Anticonvulsant Drugs

Drug	Indications/Uses	Dose Availability	Dose Range	Advantages	Disadvantages
Phenobarbital	Generalized major motor seizures, minor motor seizures, and behavioral seizures	Tablets: 15 mg 30 mg Liquid Injectable: 30–60 mg/mL Injectable: 0.5–1.0 g/mL	2–6 mg/kg q6–12h or to effect Cats 1 mg/kg q12h Therapeutic serum concentration 6 hr after oral administration Effective serum level in dogs is peak level* 30–40 μg/mL and trough level 25–40 μg/mL†	High efficacy Rapid action, few hrs Low toxicity in animals Can be administered (IV, IM, or PO) Generally the most effective drug in status epilepticus Low cost Drug of choice in cats	Sedative effects Restricted drug Long-term prescription not honored Polyphagia, polydipsia, polyuria Reverse effects, irritability, and restlessness Length of sedation precluding a neurologic examination, following IV, IM, and PO administration, is often several hr
Primidone	Generalized major motor seizures, minor motor seizures	Tablets: 50 mg scored 250 mg scored Suspension: 250 mg/5 mL	5–10 mg/kg t.i.d. (therapeutic range 15–45 μg/mL) Use in dogs only; may be administered with phenobarbital	High level of efficacy Rapid action Useful in most clinical seizure disorders Widely available 85% of effect associated with phenobarbital	Controlled substance Sedation dramatic and severe in many animals; sedation may be transient as the patient becomes accustomed to the medication Great variability in dose tolerances Only one form available; no parenteral form Only two size tablets available (50 and 250 mg) Occasionally hepatotoxic

Table continued on following page

165

Table 1-25. Drugs, Dosages, Advantages, and Disadvantages of the Most Commonly Used Anticonvulsant Drugs *Continued*

Drug	Indications/Uses	Dose Availability	Dose Range	Advantages	Disadvantages
Diazepam	Control of exacerbation of seizures Control of status epilepticus Feline status epilepticus	Tablets: 2.5 mg 5 mg 10 mg Injectable: 5 mg/mL in 2-mL vials	2.5–100 mg IV, or IM to effect *or* 5–15 mg PO t.i.d. (dog) 2.5–5.0 mg PO t.i.d. (cat)	Effective in stopping status epilepticus and other generalized seizure disorders Rapid action Safety Relative brevity of action; neurologic evaluation can be done shortly afterward Useful in cats, parenteral or oral Can be used as tranquilizer	Relatively short action; often needs to be repeated several times in status epilepticus management May not control status epilepticus Relatively expensive Controlled substance Seldom used for oral prevention and control Reverse effects sometimes seen, restlessness, viciousness
Diphenylhydantoin, phenytoin (Dilantin)‡	Generalized major motor seizures, minor motor seizures, and behavioral seizures Not for cats	Capsules: 30 mg 100 mg 100 mg with 0.25 g phenobarbital	Usually 10–20 mg/kg b.i.d. or t.i.d. (therapeutic range 10–20 µg/mL)	Absence of sedation Low toxicity and absence of many side effects noted in humans Low cost Worldwide availability In combination with phenobarbital, is not a controlled substance	Transient ataxia Rapid metabolism, difficulty in maintaining adequate blood levels, possibly poorly absorbed in dogs Some polyphagia, polydipsia, polyuria Relatively toxic in cats; generally not desirable as an anticonvulsant in cats Does not stop initial ictal discharge Occasionally, liver toxicity

Valproic acid§	In controlled seizures, used alone or in combination with other anticonvulsants Potassium bromide (see Principles of Anticonvulsant Medication, p. 168) in large-breed dogs	Oral solution: 250 mg/5 m² Capsules: 250 mg	Up to 200 mg/kg t.i.d.; lower doses if combined with other anticonvulsant	Long-term side effects are unknown	Not evaluated in cats
Potassium bromide (KBr)	Generalized major motor seizures, minor seizures; may be used alone or in combination with phenobarbital	There are no products labeled for use in dogs/cats; must use USP grade or reagent (ACS) grade powder: 25 g dissolved in 100 mL distilled water; for oral administration only	30 to 4 mg/kg PO q24h; a loading dose of 300 mg/kg (total) may be administered over 3 days	Inexpensive; fewer known side effects than phenobarbital	Dogs may experience transient lethargy/mild sedation for up to 3 weeks following the onset of therapy.

*Samples taken 4 to 6 hours after drug administration for highest (peak) level and 11 hours after drug administration for lowest (trough) level.
†In dogs that do not respond to adequate levels of phenobarbital, clonazepam 0.5 mg/kg PO b.i.d. or t.i.d. may be added to the treatment regimen.
‡Pharmacologic studies in dogs do not show that this drug develops an effective anticonvulsant blood level.
§Not approved by the Food and Drug Administration for use in dogs or cats.
From Sherding RG: Medical Emergencies. New York, Churchill Livingstone, 1985.

An IV line should be established, and antiseizure medication can be administered through this route. Collect laboratory samples prior to initiation of therapy. All animals on systemic phenobarbital should have a phenobarbital level determined.

1. Administer thiamine 25 mg IV or B complex vitamins IV for cats and 25 to 100 mg IV for dogs.
2. Administer dextrose 1 g/kg of 10% dextrose IV over a 35-minute period.
3. Start IV fluid maintenance dose.
4. If seizures have not been controlled with glucose, start on short-acting antiepileptics: to stop the seizures, give diazepam 0.7 to 3.0 mg/kg IV. If this regimen fails to control status epilepticus, administer pentobarbital IV to anesthetize the patient if necessary. Immediately begin supportive treatment with fluids, and collect blood, urine, and CSF samples for diagnostic workup. Careful attention should be given to blood glucose and calcium levels; if needed, dextrose or calcium gluconate should be provided.
5. If the patient has not been on phenobarbital, initiation of phenobarbital levels can be carried out in conjunction with the initial dose of diazepam: phenobarbital can be given slowly at a dose level of 12 to 36 mg/kg. Onset of action will take 15 to 30 minutes. To calculate the loading dose of phenobarbital:

   Desired serum level phenobarbital × (body weight [kg] × 0.8) = loading dose.

6. In refractory seizure patients who continue to have seizure clusters, start a diazepam drip administered at a rate of 0.1 mg/kg/hr in a D5W 0.9% saline drip
7. Protracted cases of seizures may have to be treated for cerebral edema (see p. 155).
8. These patients must be supported with adequate oxygen, with repositioning every 2 hours and use of soft bedding to avoid pressure sores: urine may have to be periodically expressed from the bladder, the temperature monitored, and the ECG recorded. Monitor blood glucose and maintain hydration.
9. Home therapy of dogs with idiopathic epilepsy and generalized cluster seizures can be administered with per rectal doses of diazepam 0.5 mg/kg.

Seizures in cats are often associated with structural brain disease. The occurrence of partial seizures is unequivocal evidence of focal cerebral lesion and acquired structural brain disease. An intial high frequency of seizures is a good indicator of structural brain disease. In cats, seizure activity may be characterized by mild generalized seizures and complex partial seizures. Seizures are often accompanied by other evidence of generalized neurologic disturbances. Seizures in cats may be associated with systemic diseases such as feline infectious peritonitis, cryptococcosis, toxoplasmosis, lymphosarcoma, meningiomas, ischemic encephalopathy, and thiamine deficiency.

Thiamine deficiency in the cat may present as a neurologic emergency characterized by dilated pupils, ataxic gait, cerebellar tremor, abnormal oculovestibular reflex, and seizures. Treatment consists of administration of thiamine 50 mg/day for 3 days.

■ PRINCIPLES OF ANTICONVULSANT MEDICATION

■ Try to stay with one drug; change only if the drug fails to control seizures at the maximum dosage or if the toxicity level is reached.

■ If the first drug fails, administer the second-choice drug; maintain on the first drug at therapeutic levels; withdraw the first drug gradually and evaluate the blood levels on the second drug.

(Box continued on following page)

■ **PRINCIPLES OF ANTICONVULSANT MEDICATION** *(Continued)*

■ All barbiturates induce pharmacologic tolerance.

Phenobarbital Is the Antiepileptic of Choice

■ Phenobarbital is eliminated primarily by hepatic biotransformation.

■ The elimination half-life in the dog is about 40 hours.

■ Initial dose is 5 mg/kg/day in divided doses.

■ Maintenance dose is based on serum levels and clinical effects.

■ Principal adverse effect is sedation.

■ Most animals develop a tolerance to the sedative effect.

■ Forty percent of dogs may become hyperexcitable or restless on phenobarbital.

■ Sudden withdrawal of the drug may cause seizures.

Potassium Bromide Is an Inexpensive Second-Line Anticonvulsant for Refractory Seizures in Dogs

■ The drug must be custom-compounded, since no pharmaceutical grade is available in the United States.

■ It can be formulated as the inorganic salt, potassium bromide, as a 200 mg/mL solution in double-distilled water.

■ With patients already on phenobarbital, suggested dose is 22 to 40 mg/kg/day divided q12h given in food. Taper dose of phenobarbital to lowest dose that will control the seizures.

■ When administered as a single agent, loading dose is 70 to 80 mg/kg.

■ Therapeutic monitoring is carried out after 1 month, at 4 months, and at 6-month intervals. Therapeutic range is 1000 to 2000 mg/mL. Steady-state trough concentrations desired are 25 μg/mL.

■ Bromide is not approved for use in dogs. It should be dispensed in child-proof containers.

REFERENCES

Brown SA: Anticonvulsant therapy in small animals. Vet Clin North Am Small Anim Pract 8:1199–1216, 1988.

Bunch SE: Anticonvulsant drug therapy in companion animals: *In* Kirk RW, ed: Current Veterinary Therapy VII. Small Animal Practice. Philadelphia, WB Saunders, 1986.

deLahunta A: Veterinary Neuroanatomy and Clinical Neurology, ed 2. Philadelphia, WB Saunders, 1983.

Forrester SD, Boothe DM, Troy GC: Current concepts in the management of canine epilepsy. Compend Contin Educ Pract Vet 11:811–822, 1989.

Knowles J; Seizures disorders in the pediatric animal patient. Semin Vet Med Surg (Small Anim) 9:108–115, 1994.

Lane B, Bunch SE: Medical management of recurrent seizures in dogs and cats. J Vet Intern Med 4:26–39, 1990.

Munana Kn: Encephalitis and meningitis. Vet Clin North Am Small Anim Pract 6:857, 1996.

Oliver JE Jr, Lorenz MD: Handbook of Veterinary Neurology, ed 2. Philadelphia, WB Saunders, 1993.

Parent JM: Clinical management of canine seizures. Vet Clin North Am Small Anim Pract 18:947–964, 1988.

Parent J. Quesnel A: Seizures in cats. Vet Clin North Am Small Anim Pract 6:811, 1996.

Pearce LK: Potassium bromide as an adjunct to phenobarbital for the management of uncontrolled seizures in dogs. Prog Vet Neurol 1:95, 1990.

Podell M: Seizures In dogs. Vet Clin North Am Small Anim Pract 6:779, 1996.

Podell M, Fenner WR: Use of bromide as an antiepileptic drug in dogs. Compend Contin Educ Pract Vet 16:767–772, 1994.

Quesnel A, Parent J, McDonell W: Clinical management and outcome of cats with seizure disorders: 30 cases (1991–1993). J Am Vet Med Assoc 210:72, 1997.

Quesnel A, Parent J, McDonell W, et al: Diagnostic evaluation in cats with seizure disorders: 30 cases (1991–1993). J Am Vet Med Assoc 210:65, 1997.

Selcer RB, Selcer E: A practical approach to seizure management in dogs and cats. Prog Vet Neurol 1:147, 1990.

Taboida J, Dimski D: Hepatic encephalopathy: Clinical signs, pathogenesis and treatment: Vet Clin North Am Small Anim Pract 25:337, 1995.

Trepanier LA: Pharmokinetics and clinical use of bromide. In Proceedings of the 11th Annual Forum American College of Veterinary Internal Medicine, 1993, p 878.

Electrocution (Electric Shock)

Electric shock is usually the result of a young animal chewing an electric cord. Other causes are contacting defective electrical equipment or being struck by lightning. Electric current passing through the body can produce several major abnormalities:

1. Electrophysiologic abnormalities producing ventricular tachycardia and first- and third-degree heart block.
2. Tissue destruction by heat and electrothermal burns (see p. 24).
3. Acute pulmonary edema.

The likelihood of ventricular fibrillation developing depends on the intensity of the current, the duration of contact, and the path of the current (whether or not the heart is in the pathway). (See pp. 4–5 for treatment of ventricular fibrillation.)

Clinical Signs Signs include acute onset of dyspnea, with moist rales, and localized burns, with necrosis of lips and tongue. Caudal lung lobes may have alveolar infiltration (radiographs). Additional signs are muscular contractions, loss of consciousness, pulmonary edema, and ventricular fibrillation. The first 12 hours are the most critical for the patient; then the prognosis improves.

Treatment (see also p. 3) Administer oxygen 40% to 60%; support respiration with positive pressure if needed; treat shock (see p. 62); and administer diuretics (furosemide IV), bronchodilators (aminophylline IV), and antibiotics prophylactically for possible pneumonia. If pulmonary congestion is severe, consider performing a phlebotomy and remove up to 10% of the blood volume (see Pulmonary Edema, p. 252). Sedate the animal with oxymorphone IV for anxiety only if needed.

Oncologic Emergencies (see also p. 713)

..........NEOPLASTIC SYNDROMES

Many clinical conditions that present as emergencies may be due in part or wholly to the presence of a neoplasm. Prompt identification of the neoplasm combined with knowledge of treatment and prognosis can aid owners and practitioners in making appropriate treatment decisions.

..........Hemorrhage or Effusion

- Can occur in any body cavity.
- Can occur with benign or malignant tumors.
- Hemorrhage is a result of rupture of a neoplasm or invasion of a neoplasm into a major vascular structure.

- Effusion is a result of direct fluid production by the mass or obstruction of lymphatic or venous flow.

............*Abdominal Cavity*

............Hemorrhage

1. Most commonly, hemorrhage is associated with a splenic or hepatic tumor; hemangiosarcoma and hepatocellular carcinoma are the most common.
2. Clinical signs are similar to those seen with acute hemorrhage—pale mucous membranes, tachycardia, anemia, acute collapse, and shock.
3. Treatment is aimed at stabilization:
   a. IV fluids, whole blood, or packed RBC transfusions; monitor for cardiac arryhthmias, abdominal pressure bandage.
   b. Surgery is indicated when the patient is stabilized.
   c. Emergency surgery is indicated if the patient cannot be stabilized or becomes acutely destabilized.

Hemangiosarcoma

1. Spleen or liver.
2. Presence of free blood in the abdomen—80% chance a malignant tumor is present.
3. No free blood in the abdomen—50% chance that a malignancy is present.
4. Abdominal paracentesis.
   a. Free blood that does not clot.
   b. Analysis usually nondiagnostic—consistent with free blood.
   c. Packed cell volume—same or higher than peripheral packed cell volume.
5. Poor prognosis with hemangiosarcoma—median 83-day survival.
6. Good prognosis with hematoma or hemangioma.
7. Other tumor types—lymphoma, mast cell tumor, leiomyosarcoma, fibrosarcoma, malignant fibrous histiocytoma.

Hepatocellular Carcinoma

1. Usually one lobe is involved; the left lobe most commonly.
2. Surgery is the treatment of choice.
3. Greater than 300-day survival with complete surgical excision.
4. Poor prognosis with diffuse disease.

............Effusion

1. Mesothelioma, lymphoma, carcinomatosis, or any tumor causing venous or lymphatic obstruction.
2. Clinical signs are usually not as severe as with acute abdominal hemorrhage, dyspnea, and abdominal distention.
   a. Treatment is aimed at identification of the underlying cause.
   b. Fluid analysis with cytology will many times elucidate the causative tumor type.
   c. Therapeutic abdominal paracentesis is indicated only if the patient is severely dyspneic; it can create secondary hypovolemia and shock.
   d. Abdominal ultrasound is indicated to determine the degree of tumor spread.
   e. Tumor aspiration can be performed under ultrasound guidance.

Mesothelioma

1. Rare tumor type, associated with asbestos exposure, more common in urban environments.
2. Generally a diffuse disease.

3. Sometimes difficult to differentiate reactive mesothelial cells from malignant mesothelial cells.
4. Treatment is aimed at controlling malignant effusion.
    a. Intracavitary cisplatin—good control rates.

Lymphoma

1. Effusion may emanate from any affected tissue.
2. Fluid usually contains abundant lymphoblasts.
3. Treatment is recommended with multiagent chemotherapy protocols.

Carcinomatosis

1. Diffuse seeding of abdominal cavity with malignant carcinomas.
2. May occur de novo or as a result of metastasis from a primary tumor.
3. Treatment is similar to that for mesothelioma.

.... Thoracic Cavity

.... Hemorrhage

1. Rare in association with a neoplastic condition.
2. Generally associated with hemangiosarcoma of the lungs or rupture of a right auricular hemangiosarcoma.
3. Hemorrhage may be confined to the pericardium showing a globoid heart on thoracic radiographs.
4. Surgery relieves signs of right heart failure but metastatic disease generally develops soon afterward.
5. Hemorrhage can also result when a primary lung tumor erodes a major vessel. Clinical signs are dyspnea, collapse, shock, and anemia.

.... Effusion

1. More common than hemorrhage.
2. Mesothelioma, lymphoma, carcinomatosis, thymoma.
3. Clinical signs are dyspnea, cyanotic mucous membranes, and sometimes coughing.
4. Fluid analysis with cytology will identify the underlying cause in many cases therapy is aimed initially at stabilization.
    a. Therapeutic thoracocentesis.
    b. Supplemental oxygen.
    c. Supportive fluids—crystalloids and colloids if indicated.
5. Following identification of a cause, definitive therapy may be undertaken.

Mesothelioma

1. Rare, more common in urban environments in association with asbestos exposure.
2. Generally a diffuse serosal disease; surgery not indicated.
3. Can affect pleural or pericardial cavities.
4. More common in dogs than cats.
5. Treatment is aimed at controlling effusion.
    a. Intracavitary cisplatin controls effusion an average of 241 days (three dogs treated).
    b. Intracavitary carboplatin—anecdotal responses in cats.
    c. Intracavitary talc or doxorubicin results in chemical pleurodesis; the technique is more important than the agent; variable results in the canine patient.

Lymphoma

1. Effusion is seen often with a cranial mediastinal mass.
2. T-cell immunohistochemical subtype is associated with the presence of a cranial mediastinal mass in dogs.
   a. Poorer response to therapy and shorter remission times than in dogs with B-cell lymphoma.
3. Combination chemotherapy is recommended for treatment in dogs and cats.
   a. Dogs—6-month to 1-year survival.
   b. Cats—4- to 9-month survival.
4. Treatment with prednisone alone for greater than 2 weeks is not recommended if combination chemotherapy is to be undertaken. It results in a poorer response to therapy with shorter remission times.

Carcinomatosis

1. Diffuse disease in the pleural cavity is often a result of a metastasis from a primary pulmonary or mammary adenocarcinoma.
2. Treatment is similar to that for mesothelioma.
3. Treatment is aimed at controlling effusion and delaying its recurrence.

Thymoma

1. Dogs are more commonly presented with a cough, cats more commonly with dyspnea and effusion.
2. A cranial mediastinal mass is seen on radiographs.
3. Aspiration of primary mass reveals a malignant epithelial tumor with small lymphocytes and mast cells.
4. The treatment of choice is surgery. Small encapsulated tumors carry a good prognosis with complete excision.
5. Paraneoplastic syndrome of myasthenia gravis is reported in dogs and cats. If megaesophagus is present, it carries a poor prognosis because of high rate of complications.

·········· Obstruction

·········· Urinary Tract

1. Extramural—intra-abdominal, pelvic, or retroperitoneal.
2. Intramural—urethral, bladder, or urethral wall.
3. Transitional cell carcinoma (most common bladder tumor), prostatic adeno-carcinoma, or lymphoma affecting sublumbar lymph nodes.
4. Treatment is aimed at relieving obstruction, then identifying cause.
   a. Attempt passage of urinary catheter.
   b. Cystocentesis if unable to pass catheter.
   c. Supportive therapy to normalize electrolytes.
   d. Plain film radiographs, ultrasound, and double contrast cystography are useful in localizing mass.
   e. Biopsy or surgery is indicated when the patient is stabilized.

·········· Transitional Cell Carcinoma

1. Good prognosis with complete surgical excision and with benign tumors.
2. Poor prognosis with incomplete excision; most tumors are trigonal and complete excision is unlikely.
3. With incomplete excision, a 4-month median survival is reported.
4. Piroxicam is helpful in relieving clinical signs (7-month median survival).
5. Cisplatin and carboplatin may have some activity.

.... Prostatic Adenocarcinoma

1. Prostatic tumors are always malignant.
2. Equal frequency of occurrence in castrated and uncastrated dogs.
3. Diagnosis is via ultrasound or transrectal aspiration or biopsy.
4. Surgery, chemotherapy, and radiation therapy are generally unrewarding;
5. Palliative radiation therapy can relieve clinical signs for 2 to 6 months.

.... *Gastrointestinal Tract*

1. Luminal—primary GI tumors causing obstruction.
2. Extraluminal—adhesions or strangulation causing obstruction.
3. Perforation.
   a. Occurs when a tumor erodes through the gastrointestinal wall.
   b. Occurs in patients with mast cell tumors secondary to elevated histamine levels.
4. Treatment is initially aimed at stabilization followed by surgical exploration for adenocarcinoma, leiomyosarcoma, and lymphoma.

.... Gastric and Intestinal Adenocarcinoma

1. Most common tumor type in dogs.
2. Usually also a history of vomiting, anorexia, and weight loss.
3. Ultrasound-guided biopsy is frequently diagnostic; can also evaluate regional lymph nodes.
4. Endoscopy may be inconclusive if mucosa is not involved. Many tumors are not surgically resectable and metastases are common (70% of cases).
5. Dogs with small tumors that are completely resectable may have longer survival times.

.... Leiomyosarcoma

1. Carries a better prognosis than adenocarcinoma; low rate of metastases.
2. Paraneoplastic syndrome of hypoglycemia.
3. With complete surgical excision, average survival is greater than 1 year.

.... Lymphoma

1. Most common tumor type in cats, rare in dogs.
2. Recommended treatment is combination chemotherapy.
3. Treatment responses are often poor.
4. Dogs with full-thickness disease are at risk for bowel perforation and peritonitis.

.... Mast Cell Tumor

1. GI tract ulceration is present in 35% to 83% of patients.
2. Bowel perforation is a rare complication.
3. Results from increased gastric acid secretion secondary to circulating elevated histamine levels.
4. Treat with H_2-blockers (cimetidine, ranitidine, famotidine).

.... PARANEOPLASTIC SYNDROMES
.... Neutropenia and Sepsis

Decreased levels of circulating neutrophils or immunosuppression leaves many cancer patients susceptible to a wide variety of infections. The most life-threatening of these is when overwhelming bacterial infection or sepsis occurs. It is imperative that veterinarians identify a causative agent and begin immediate therapy once a diagnosis of sepsis is established. Sepsis is frequently fatal unless appropriate therapy is undertaken.

.... Common Causes

1. Neutropenia can occur in lymphoma with bone marrow involvement, multiple myeloma, leukemias, and secondary to chemotherapy administration.
2. Cellular immune dysfunction is associated with abnormal immunoglobulins produced in lymphoma and multiple myeloma, and administration of prednisone and certain antineoplastics.
3. Iatrogenic causes include indwelling urinary or IV catheterization, prolonged hospitalization, inadequate or poor nutritional status.
4. Bacterial agents are generally skin or enteric in in origin.
   a. Gram-negative—*E. coli*, *Klebsiella* sp., *Pseudomonas* sp., *Enterobacter* sp.
   b. Gram-positive—*Staphylococcus epidermidis*, *Staphylococcus aureus*.

.... Clinical Signs

1. Circulatory collapse—hypotension, peripheral vasodilation, splanchnic vascular pooling.
2. Fever—not always present in the severely granulocytopenic patient.
3. Acute renal failure.
4. Vomiting, diarrhea, lethargy, melena.

.... Treatment

1. Aggressive crystalloid and colloid therapy. (See p. 596.)
2. Broad spectrum antibiotic combinations.
   a. Gentamicin and ampicillin
   b. Amikacin and cephalothin
   c. Enrofloxacin and ampicillin
3. Lactate-containing solutions may be contraindicated in patients with lymphoma as many of these patients have a preexisting lactic acidosis.

.... Thrombocytopenia

Thrombocytopenia is a frequent complication associated with neoplasia. The danger of spontaneous bleeding occurs when the platelet count is less than $50,000/\mu L$. Treatment of the underlying cause is necessary to resolve the condition.

.... Causes

1. Decreased production.
   a. Primary bone marrow disease—leukemia, lymphoma.
   b. Chemotherapy-related bone marrow suppression—all drugs except vincristine, bleomycin, and cytoxan.
   c. Hyperestrogenism—usually associated with a Sertoli cell tumor.
2. Increased use.
   a. Disseminated intravascular coagulation (DIC)—can occur with any tumor type.
   b. Microangiopathic disease—destruction of platelets as they circulate through abnormal tortuous vessels in tumors.
   c. Hemangiosarcoma, thyroid carcinoma, inflammatory carcinoma.
3. Increased loss or lysis.

4. Tumor-associated bleeding.
   a. Primary GI tumors.
   b. Mast cell tumor–associated gastric ulcers.
5. Secondary immune-mediated.
   a. Coating of platelets by abnormal tumor-associated proteins.
   b. Destruction by hemophagocytic system.
   c. Lymphoma, multiple myeloma.

............Anemia

Anemia is the most common hematologic disorder in cancer patients; it may be the result of an acute or chronic condition.

............Causes

1. Chronic disease.
2. Blood loss or destruction.
   a. Primary GI tumors—adenocarcinoma, lymphoma.
   b. Microangiopathic disease—hemangiosarcoma, thyroid carcinoma.
   c. DIC—any tumor type.
   d. Immune-mediated destruction—lymphoma, multiple myeloma.
3. Decreased production.
   a. Primary bone marrow disease—leukemia, lymphoma.
   b. Chemotherapy-related bone marrow suppression (rare).

............Treatment

1. Blood transfusion for acute loss or for chronic loss when packed cell volume is less than 15% (see p. 46).
2. Treatment of underlying disease process

............Erythrocytosis

Erythrocytosis is a rare complication associated with neoplasia. Many patients are presented as an emergency because of clinical signs associated with an elevated RBC count. Erythrocytosis may also be an incidental finding without associated clinical signs.

............Causes

1. Erythropoietin produced directly by the tumor causing increased RBC release from the bone marrow.
   a. Renal cell carcinoma, lymphoma.
2. Erythropoietin produced by the kidney in response to tumor hypoxia.
3. Increased erythropoietin release from the kidney in response to tumor-releasing factors.
4. Primary polycythemia vera—myeloproliferative disorder with a clonal proliferation of RBCs precursors; results in an increased release of RBC from the bone marrow independent of erythropoietin concentration.

............Clinical Signs

1. Signs are generally referable to increased viscosity of blood and decreased flow through small capillaries.
2. Lethargy, dementia, vomiting, renal azotemia.

............Treatment

1. Identify and treat the underlying neoplastic condition.
   a. May require therapeutic phlebotomies initially.
   b. Hydroxyurea is effective for polycythemia vera.

............Acute Tumor Lysis Syndrome

Acute tumor lysis syndrome is a rare occurrence but reported in dogs with lymphoma and leukemia. The syndrome appears to occur most frequently in debilitated animals with a large tumor burden following cytolytic therapy.

............Clinical Signs

1. Signs are referable to acute tumor cell death and release of intracellular contents.
   a. Hypocalcermia hyperkalemia, and hyperphosphatemia.
   b. Bradycardia with decreased P-wave amplitude and spiked T waves.
   c. Acute collapse and shock, possibly with GI signs.

............Treatment

1. Aggressive crystalloid therapy (see p. 596).
2. Careful monitoring of electrolyte and cardiac status

............Disseminated Intravascular Coagulation (see also p. 44)

1. DIC occurs in a wide variety of conditions.
2. Increased risk associated with hemangiosarcoma, thyroid carcinoma, inflammatory mammary carcinoma, lymphoma.
3. Thrombosis with or without DIC is associated with an elevated glucocorticoid levels in dogs; can be endogenous (pituitary or adrenal tumor) or exogenous (prednisone as part of a chemotherapy protocol).

............Treatment

1. Address the underlying condition.
2. Heparin, fresh frozen plasma colloids (see p. 46).

............Hypergammaglobulinemia (see also p. 703)

Hypergammaglobulinemia is also known as M component or hyperviscosity syndrome. Patients have an elevated total protein with a monoclonal gammopathy. The syndrome occurs when neoplastic cells secrete abnormal immunoglobulins.

............Causes

1. Associated with plasma cell neoplasms or multiple myeloma 75% of the time.
2. Other tumors—lymphoma, lymphocytic leukemia, and as a primary macroglobulinemia.

............Clinical Signs

1. Signs are related to the "sludging" of blood in small capillaries due to increased serum viscosity.

a. Ocular—dilated retinal vessels, hemorrhage, retinal detachment.
b. Neurologic—CNS hypoxia, dementia, seizures.
c. Renal—azotemia, polydipsia, polyuria.
d. Hemorrhagic diathesis—coating of platelets by the abnormal proteins resulting in inhibition of the clotting cascade.
e. Immunologic—myeloma proteins are thought to suppress lymphocyte and macrophage functions; many patients are prone to occult or overt secondary infections.

.... Treatment

1. Chemotherapy—melphalan and prednisone result in good long-term response in many patients (>500-day survival).
2. Antibiotic therapy if secondary infections are present.

.... Hypercalcemia (see also p. 146)

Hypercalcemia is the most common metabolic emergency in oncology.

.... Causes

1. Results when a parathyroid hormone—related peptide is released by the tumor.
   a. Increase in osteoclast activity
   b. Increased release of calcium from bone
2. Peptide release is found with lymphoma, apocrine gland anal sac adenocarcinoma, mammary adenocarcinoma, and parathyroid adenoma or adenocarcinoma.
3. Rarely associated with tumor destruction of bone causing direct calcium release.

.... Clinical Signs

1. Vomiting, dehydration, constipation, bradycardia, hypertension, stupor, weakness, seizures.
2. Elevated serum calcium when corrected for serum albumin level.

.... Treatment (see also p. 148)

1. Aggressive saline diuresis.
2. Loop diuretics.
   a. Furosemide.
   b. Well-hydrated patients only.
   c. Prevents calcium resorption from the loop of Henle.
   d. Never use thiazide diuretics.
3. Biphosphonates.
   a. Directly inhibit osteoclast activity.
4. Gallium nitrate.
   a. Binds to and decreases the solubility of hydroxyapatite crystals.
   b. Concentration-dependent decrease in osteolytic response to parathyroid hormone.
5. Mithramycin.
   a. Decreases osteoclast number and activity.
   b. Directly inhibits further bone resorption.
6. Salmon calcitonin.
   a. Use in refractory cases.
   b. Rapid onset of action.
   c. Directly inhibits bone resorption.

7. Corticosteroids.
   a. Block bone resorption by inhibiting osteoclast activation.
   b. Increase urinary calcium excretion.
   c. Inhibit vitamin D metabolism.
   d. Tissue diagnosis needs to be made prior to initiation of therapy as it may cause a partial to complete response making definitive diagnosis difficult.
8. Treat underlying condition.

···········Hypoglycemia (see p. 144)

Clinical signs of hypoglycemia occur when blood glucose is less than 45 mg/dL. Hypoglycemia may be related to direct factors released by a tumor or secondary to conditions created by a tumor or its treatment. Hypoglycemia causes endogenous release of catecholamines, growth hormone, glucocorticoids and glucagon as compensatory mechanisms.

···········Causes

1. Tumor release of insulin or insulin-like hormone or increased glucose utilization by the tumor.
2. Functional pancreatic beta cell tumor, leiomyosarcoma, oral melanoma, hemangiosarcoma, salivary gland adenocarcinoma.
3. Hypoglycemia in face of normal to elevated insulin levels associated with pancreatic tumors.
4. Hypoglycemia with normal to low insulin levels associated with extrapancreatic tumors.
5. Tumor-associated organ dysfunction; lack of glycogenolysis or gluconeogenesis by the liver.
   a. Hepatoma, hepatocellular carcinoma.
6. Sepsis.
   a. Treatment-related due to neutropenia.
   b. Disease-related—neutropenia secondary to leukemia.
7. Insulin overdose.

···········Clinical Signs

1. The brain is a highly glucose-dependent organ—seizures, dementia.
2. Ataxia, weakness, muscular fasiculations.

···········Treatment

1. Surgical removal of the tumor.
2. Glucose-containing fluids.
   a. May trigger more insulin release by the tumor.
   b. Constant rate infusion preferred to bolus.
3. Prednisone.
   a. Induces hepatic gluconeogenesis.
   b. Decreased peripheral utilization of glucose.
   c. Attempt to confirm diagnosis prior to beginning prednisone.
4. Diazoxide.
   a. Directly inhibits pancreatic insulin secretion and tissue uptake of glucose.
   b. Enhances catecholamine-induced glycogenolysis.
   c. Increases rate of mobilization of free fatty acids.
5. Hydrochlorothiazide.
   a. Potentiates diazoxide's hyperglycemic effects.

6. Propranolol.
   a. Blocks insulin release from pancreatic beta cells.
   b. Insulin release is also inhibited through membrane stabilization.
   c. Somatostatin inhibits insulin release.
7. Octreotide acetate.
   a. Long-acting somatostatin analogue agent.
8. Streptozocin.
   a. Chemotherapeutic.
   b. Selectively cytotoxic to pancreatic cells.
   c. Extremely nephrotoxic.
9. L-Asparaginase.
   a. Can secondarily inhibit insulin synthesis by inhibiting protein synthesis.
   b. Short-acting.

............CHEMOTHERAPY-RELATED TOXICITIES

Chemotherapeutic agents have their greatest effect on rapidly dividing cells—both normal and neoplastic cells. Normal tissues that are commonly affected are the bone marrow, gastric and intestinal epithelium, skin and hair follicles, and reproductive organs. Some drugs have unique organ-specific toxicities that must be monitored. Knowledge of expected complications and anticipation of these problems can decrease their severity and alleviate clinical symptoms.

............Bone Marrow Toxicity

- Most common toxicity seen with chemotherapy for neutropenia
- Usually the dose-limiting cytopenia; rapid marrow transit time and short circulating half-life (3 to 8 hours); lowest neutrophil count varies with drug and route of administration but often occurs 5 to 10 days after treatment.
- Bone marrow recovery within 36 to 72 hours

............Causative Agents

1. **Severe myelosuppression** at 7 to 10 days post administration—doxorubicin, cyclophosphamide, vinblastine.
2. **Moderate myelosuppression** 7 to 10 days post administration—melphalan, cisplatin, mitoxantrone, actinomycin D.
3. **Mild to no myelosuppression**—L-aspariginase, corticosteroids, low-dose vincristine.

............Treatment

1. Most common complication is sepsis—a neutropenic febrile patient is an emergency (for treatment, see p. 32).
2. For an afebrile patient with a neutrophil count of less than 2000/μL, prophylactic antibiotics are recommended.
3. Trimethoprim-sulfadiazine is the drug of choice, because it is broad-spectrum but spares the anaerobic gastrointestinal flora.
4. Colony-stimulating factors (CSFs)—granulocyte CSF, granulocyte-monocyte CSF.
   a. Recombinant human product.
   b. Stimulates increased release of neutrophils from the bone marrow.
   c. Will shorten time for recovery from a myelosuppressive drug.
   d. Dogs and cats will develop neutralizing antibodies to the product within 21 to 28 days.
   e. Costly.

5. Lithium.
   a. Utilized in humans as a myelostimulant.
   b. Dogs—no consistent benefit shown.
   c. Cats—neurotoxic, myeloid and erythroid hypoplasia.

············Prevention

1. Reduce chemotherapeutic agent dose by 25%.
2. Increase interval between treatments.
3. Avoid overlapping myelosuppressive agents.

············Gastrointestinal Toxicity (see also p. 116)
············Acute

1. Occurs within 6 to 12 hours of chemotherapy administration.
2. Related to direct stimulation of the chemoreceptor trigger zone.
3. Cisplatin, actinomycin D.
4. Treat with centrally acting antiemetics such as metoclopramide, butorphanol, or prochlorperazine.

············Delayed

1. Occurs 3 to 5 days following treatment.
2. Doxorubicin, actinomycin D, methotrexate, cytoxan.
3. Vomiting and diarrhea are a result of damage to intestinal crypt cells causing malabsorption.
4. Treat with antiemetics, IV fluids, and highly digestible diets.

············Unique Gastrointestinal Toxicities

1. Hemorrhagic colitis—doxorubicin, 5 to 7 days post drug administration, generally treated with bismuth subsalicylate.
2. Paralytic ileus—vincristine, 2 to 5 days post drug administration; treat with metoclopramide when obstruction has been ruled out.

············Cardiotoxicity (see also p. 68)

Cardiotoxicity is primarily associated with doxorubicin administration, but can occur with high-dose cyclophosphamide administration.

············Acute

1. Transient arrhythmias during drug administration.
2. Development of arrhythmias does not correlate with development of chronic cardiotoxicity.

············Chronic

1. Dilated cardiomyopathy (DCM).
2. Can occur with cumulative doses as low as 100 to 150 mg/m^2.
3. Most commonly occurs at cumulative doses greater than 240 mg/m^2.
4. Once damage occurs to the myocardium the lesions are irreversible.
5. When DCM is established, it will progress to congestive heart failure and death.

············Treatment

1. Treat heart failure.
   a. Diuretics if indicated (furosemide).

b. Administer appropriate cardiac drugs dependent on patient's status—digoxin, enalapril, propranolol, milrinone, diltiazem.
2. Discontinue doxorubicin in all dogs with evidence of decreased myocardial contractility.
3. Substitute mitoxantrone or liposome-encapsulated doxorubicin in dogs with abnormal echocardiograms prior to doxorubicin chemotherapy.
4. Cardioprotectants.
   a. Vitamin E, selenium, and N-acetylcysteine also show promise as cardioprotectants.

...........Prevention

1. Prolonged infusion time—decreases peak plasma concentration of drug which is associated with decreased cardiotoxicity.
2. Pretreatment echocardiography for dogs at increased risk of cardiotoxicity.
   a. Predisposed DCM breeds—Doberman pinschers, boxers, giant-breed dogs—dogs with prior heart disease or heart murmurs.
   b. Echocardiogram for all dogs when a cumulative dose of 240 mg/m^2 is reached.

...........Nephrotoxicity (see also pp. 122, 124)

...........Causes

1. Doxorubicin.
   a. May be a dose-dependent nephrotoxicity.
   b. Cats may be more sensitive than dogs.
2. Cisplatin.
   a. Most nephrotoxic drug.
   b. Characteristic lesions of reduced GFR and damage to renal tubular epithelium.
   c. Administration requires use of 1- to 24-hour saline diuresis protocol.
   d. When given without diuresis will result in renal failure in most patients.
3. Methotrexate.
   a. Eliminated by the kidneys.
   b. Associated with rare nephrotoxicity.

...........Predisposing Factors

1. Use of other nephrotoxic drug—aminoglycosides, antifungals.
2. Dehydration.
3. Urinary tract obstruction—transitional cell carcinoma.
4. Preexisting renal disease.
5. Decreased cardiac output.

...........Diagnosis

1. Elevated BUN and creatinine with isosthenuric or minimally concentrated urine.
2. Vomiting, diarrhea, oral ulcers may also be present.
3. Glucosuria, proteinurias, and tubular or epithelial casts may be present in the urine.

...........Treatment

1. Discontinue all nephrotoxic drugs.
2. Begin on IV fluid therapy, correct dehydration, and induce diuresis.

3. Monitor urine output and ensure that it remains adequate.
4. Correct any acid-base abnormalities.

.... Prevention

1. Do not give nephrotoxic drugs to patients with prior existing renal disease.
2. Give cisplatin with an adequate diuresis protocol.

.... Urinary Bladder Toxicity
.... Causes

1. Cyclophosphamide.
   a. Sterile hemorrhagic cystitis.
   b. Hematuria, stranguria, pollakiuria.
   c. Metabolite of both drugs is acrolein which concentrates in the urinary bladder causing damage to bladder mucosa and arterioles.

.... Treatment

1. Discontinue drug.
2. Collect urine for culture and sensitivity as secondary infections are common.
3. Induce diuresis and administer anti-inflammatory drugs such as prednisone.
4. If signs persist, can treat with intravesical medication.
   a. Dimethyl sulfoxide 25% solution instilled into the bladder for 20 minutes.
   b. Formalin 1% solution in sterile water into the bladder for 20 minutes.
   c. Will cauterize bladder and decrease bleeding.
5. Severe, refractory cases may require surgical debridement and electrocautery of the bladder mucosa.

.... Prevention

1. Administer drugs in the morning and allow frequent emptying of the urinary bladder.
2. Induce polyuria and polydipsia with concurrent administration of prednisone.
3. Administer Mesna in conjunction with drugs.
   a. Sulfhydryl drug that binds acrolein in the urinary bladder.
   b. Must be given before drug administration.
   c. Does not appear to decrease drug efficacy.
4. Substitute chlorambucil for cyclophosphamide when hemorrhagic cystitis occurs.

.... Anaphylactoid Reactions
.... Causes

1. L-asparaginase.
   a. Enzyme acts as a foreign protein.
   b. Likelihood of reaction increases with repeated administration.
   c. Some animals will react at first administration.
2. Doxorubicin.
   a. Can cause acute mast cell degranulation.
3. Etoposide and paclitaxel.
   a. Drug vehicle results in mast cell degranulation and anaphylaxis.

.... Treatment

1. Life-threatening reaction.
2. Requires immediate intervention.

3. IV corticosteroids and epinephrine.

............*Prevention*

1. Route of administration.
   a. SC administration is less likely to cause a reaction than the IM or IV route.
2. Rate of administration.
   a. Rapid infusion of doxorubicin, etoposide, or paclitaxel is more likely to result in a reaction.
3. Pretreatment with diphenhydramine 2.2 mg/kg IM will decrease the likelihood of an anaphylactoid reaction.

............**Species-Specific Toxicities**

1. Cisplatin.
   a. Fatal, irreversible pulmonary edema in cats.
   b. Occurs even at low doses.
   c. High protein exudate in alveoli that is nonresponsive to conventional therapies.
2. 5-Fluorouracil.
   a. Severe neurotoxicity in cats.
   b. Seizures, ataxia.

REFERENCES

Cotter SM, Kanki PJ, Simon M: Renal disease in five tumor bearing cats treated with Adriamycin. Am Anim Hosp Assoc 21:405–411, 1985.

Couto CG: Management of complications of cancer chemotherapy. Vet Clin North Am Small Anim Pract 4:1037–1053, 1990.

Johnson KA, Powers BE, Withrow SJ, et al: Splenomegaly in dogs: Predictors of neoplasia and survival after splenectomy. J Vet Intern Med 3:160–166, 1989.

Kosovsky JE, Manfra-Marretta S, Matthiesen DT, et al: Results of partial hepatectomy in 18 dogs with hepatocellular carcinoma. J Am Anim Hosp Assoc 25:203–206, 1989.

Mauldin GE, Fox PR, Patnalk AK, et al: Doxorubicin-induced cardiotoxicosis: Clinical features of 32 dogs. J Vet Intern Med 6:82–88, 1992.

Moore AS, Rand WM, Berg J, et al: A randomized evaluation of butorphanol and cyproheptadine for prevention of cisplatin-induced vomiting in the dog. J Am Vet Med Assoc 205: 441–443, 1994.

Ogilvie GK, Moore AS: Managing the Veterinary Cancer Patient. A Practice Manual. Trenton, NJ, Veterinary Learning Systems, 1995.

Withrow SJ, Macewen EG, eds: Small Animal Clinical Oncology ed 2. Philadelphia, WB Saunders, 1996.

Poisonings

............GENERAL PRINCIPLES OF POISONS MANAGEMENT

............Overview

The first several pages are a text-based discussion of both the preliminary and inpatient management of poisonings. Various checklists are included here which can assist both the practitioner and technician. The text outlines the six essential steps in the management of poisonings, and discusses the various therapeutic strategies which may be used. Each therapeutic strategy is identified by a number and letter (e.g., 3b. Gastric Lavage). These alphanumeric codes appear later in the tables sections, as appropriate to the various poisons.

Table I–26. Therapeutic Strategies

1a. Maintain respiration
1b. Maintain cardiovascular function, control arrhythmias, electrolytes, and acid-base balance
1c. Control CNS excitation
1d. Control body temperature
2a. Obtain history
2b. Evaluate patient
3a. Emetics
3b. Gastric lavage
3c. Enemas
3d. Cathartics
3e. Adsorbents
3f. Ion exchange resins
3g. Precipitating, chelating, and diluting agents
3h. Eliminating poison from the skin
3i. Eliminating poison from the eyes
 4. Antidotes
5a. Diuresis
5b. Urine acidification
5c. Urine alkalinization
6a. Maintenance of renal perfusion, beware of oliguria
6b. Gastrointestinal protectants
6c. Antiemetics
6d. Analgesics
6e. Nutritional support

For a specific poison, refer to the tables to find the active ingredients, therapeutic strategies, and specific antidote names. The box below is an index to tables. Table 1–26 is a summary list of 22 possible therapeutic strategies which might be used in the management of poisonings. The numbering of therapeutic strategies corresponds to their numbering in the general text, if an explanation or elaboration is required. Tables 1–27 through 1–31 are the Poisons Tables. Table 1–32 contains all doses of drugs to be given, both for therapeutic strategies and antidotes.

■ Index to Tables

············How to Use This Article:

■ Poison ingested = acetaminophen

■ Look in the Index to Tables above to see where it might be (probably in Table 1–30, Medications and other Drugs).

■ Turn to Table 1–30, and locate acetaminophen in the alphabetic listing. You

Text continued on page 216

Table I–27. Pesticides, Insecticides, and Herbicides*

Generic Name	Brand Names or Description	Toxic Dose†	Mechanism and Actions	Therapeutic Strategies	Antidotes and Comments
Algacides	See Triazines and Dipyridyl Compounds				
Amitraz	Acaricide (antitick product), Mitaban, Taktic	10–20 mg/kg	α-Adrenergic agonist; signs similar to effects of xylazine; CNS depression, ataxia, bradycardia, hypotension, emesis, and mydriasis	1b, 3a/3b, 3d, 3e, 4	Yohimbine
Arsenic, inorganic (arsenic trioxide, sodium arsenite, sodium arsenate)	Ant killer	Sodium arsenate: 100–150 mg/kg; sodium arsenite: 1–25 mg/kg; arsenic trioxide less toxic; cats more susceptible	Interferes with cellular respiration by combining with sulfhydryl enzymes; severe gastroenteritis; muscle weakness, renal failure, capillary damage; acute onset usually	3g, then 3a/3b, 4, 1a, 1b, 6a, 6b, 6d	3g: Sodium thiosulfate or sodium bicarbonate solution 4: Dimercaprol
Boric acid, borate	Ant, roach killer	Dog: 1–3 g/kg → vomiting	Mechanism unknown; presumed cytotoxic to all cells; vomiting, gastroenteritis; blue-green vomitus and stools; renal damage; CNS excitation, then depression	3a/3b, 3d, 6a, 6b, 3e not useful	

Carbamates	Agricultural, home and garden insecticides Examples: carbofuran, aldicarb, propoxur, carbaryl, methiocarb	Varies	Cholinesterase inhibition; CNS excitation; muscarinic ACh overload: salivation, lacrimation, miosis; vomiting, diarrhea; nicotinic ACh overload: muscle tremors	1a, 1c, 1d, 3a/3b, 3c, 3d, 3e, 4	Atropine: 2-PAM not useful
Chlorinated hydrocarbons	DDT, methoxychlor, lindane, dieldrin, aldrin, chlordane, chlordecone, endosulfan	Varies	Mechanism unknown; appears much like organophosphates symptoms; myocardial sensitization to epinephrine	1c, 1d, 3b, 3d, 3e, 3h, 5a	No antidote; protracted clinical course
Chlorophenoxy derivatives	2,4-D; 2,4,5-T, MCPA, MCPP, Silvex	2,4-D: LD_{50} = 100 mg/kg; toxic dose lower; $t_{1/2}$ = 18 hr	Mechanism unknown; causes gastroenteritis and muscle rigidity	1b, 1c, 3b, 3e, 3h, 5a, 5c, 6b	No antidote; good prognosis
Diethyltoluamide (DEET)	Insect repellent (Off, Cutters, Hartz Blockade)	Cat: lethal dose: 1.8 g/kg dermally, much less if oral exposure; small dogs: toxic dose: 7 g/kg dermally	Lipophilic neurotoxin; 5–10 min post exposure in cats: aimless gazing, hypersalivation, chewing motions, muscle tremors → seizures; mentation normal, appears to be cerebellar dysfunction; 30 min: recumbency, death	1a, 1c, 3a/3b, 3d, 3e, 3h	—

Table continued on following page

Table 1–27. Pesticides, Insecticides, and Herbicides* Continued

Generic Name	Brand Names or Description	Toxic Dose†	Mechanism and Actions	Therapeutic Strategies	Antidotes and Comments
Dipyridyl Compounds					
Paraquat	Paraquat	$LD_{50} = 25$–50 mg/kg	Initially CNS excitation and renal failure; metabolism of dipyridyl compounds causes free radical production; concentrates in alveolar cells → pulmonary interstitial fibrosis in one third; respiratory failure, death	1b, 1c, 3e, 5a, 6a	3e: preferable to use kaolin or bentonite; free radical scavengers under investigation; oxygen therapy contraindicated; hemoperfusion may be useful if early; grave prognosis
	Dichlone (Phygone)	LD_{50} (rats) = 1500 mg/kg	CNS depressant; reacts with thiol enzymes → possible methemoglobinemia; hepatorenal damage	1a, 1b, 3a/3b, 3d, 3e, 6a	—
	Diquat	$LD_{50} = 25$–50 mg/kg	CNS excitation; gastroenteritis with high volume loss; renal failure	1b, 1c, 3e, 5a, 6a	*3e: preferable to use kaolin or bentonite; grave prognosis
Fipronil	Flea product (Frontline, Merial)		GABA inhibitor, may cause CNS excitation	1c, 1d, 3e	
Glyphosate	Round-up, Kleen-up	Low toxicity if applied properly	Irritant, gastroenteritis, CNA depression	3a/3b, 3d, 3e, 3h, 6b	—

Agent	Source/Use	Toxicity	Signs/Mechanism	Treatment	Atropine or 2-PAM
Imidacloprid	Flea product (Advantage, Bayer)	Rat oral LD_{50} = 1732–1943 mg/kg	Nicotinic cholinergic agonist; neuromuscular excitation followed by collapse; may include respiratory paralysis	1a, 1c, 3c, 3d, 3h	of no use
Lawn herbicides *d*-Limonene, linalool	See Carbamates Citrus oil extracts; used in flea control products	Unknown, but cats recognized to be sensitive	Hypersalivation, muscle tremors, ataxia, hypothermia	1d, 3e, 3h	—
Lufenuron	Flea product (Program, Novartis)	Dog: >200 mg/kg; Cat: >300 mg/kg	Insect growth regulator, benzoylphenylurea compound; mammalian effects unknown		
Melaleuca oil (tea-tree oil)	Herbal-origin flea repellent; toxic principle: monoterpenes	Unknown	Neuromuscular weakness, ataxia	3d, 3e, 3h	
Metaldehyde	Snail bait	LD_{50} = 210–600 mg/kg	Probable GABA inhibition → CNS excitation; muscle tremors, hyperthermia	1c, 1d, 3a/3b, 3c, 3d, 3e	—
Methiocarb	Snail bait (Baysol, Bayer)	Toxic dose: 0.5–1.0 mg/kg LD_5 = 900 mg/kg	As for carbamates, acetylcholinesterase inhibition	1a, 1c, 1d, 3a/3b, 3c, 3d, 3e, 4	Atropine; 2-PAM not useful
Naphthalene	See Mothballs, Table 1–29				

Table continued on following page

Table 1–27. Pesticides, Insecticides, and Herbicides* *Continued*

Generic Name	Brand Names or Description	Toxic Dose†	Mechanism and Actions	Therapeutic Strategies	Antidotes and Comments
Organophosphates	Flea rinses, agricultural insecticides, home and garden insecticides; examples: chlorpyrifos, coumaphos, diazinon, dichlorvos, malathion	Varies	Cholinesterase inhibition; CNS excitation; muscarinic ACh overload: salivation, lacrimation, miosis, excessive bronchial secretions, vomiting, diarrhea; nicotinic ACh overload: muscle tremors, respiratory paralysis	1a, 3a/3b, 3e, 3h, 4	Atropine for muscarinic signs; 2-PAM if within 12 h, perhaps longer; diphenhydramine for nicotinic signs
Paraquat	See Dipyridyl compounds				
Pennyroyal oil	Herbal-origin flea repellent; toxic principle: menthofuran	Unknown	Hepatotoxic; may cause GI hemorrhage, coagulopathies	3d, 3e, 3h	
Piperonyl butoxide	Used in conjunction with pyrethrins, organophosphates to prolong their $t_{1/2}$		Cytochrome P-450 inhibitor; inhibits hepatic microsomal enzymes; will prolong $t_{1/2}$ life of various drugs, similarly to cimetidine	See Pyrethrins	

Pyrethrins and pyrethroids	Based on insecticidal extract from chrysanthemums; examples: allethrin, decamethrin, fenpropanthrin, flucythrinate, permethrin, resmethrin	Oral toxicity low; inhalant and dermal toxicity significant	Depolarization and blockade of nerve membrane action potential; CNS excitation, dyspnea, paralysis; contact dermatitis	1a, 1c, 3d, 3e, 3h, 5a	Contact dermatitis: vitamin E ointment
Rotenone	Garden insecticide, also delousing agent	Fish and birds very susceptible	Inhibits mitochondrial electron transport; topical or ingested exposure: tissue irritation; hypoglycemia; inhaled exposure: depression, seizures, guarded prognosis	3b, 3d, 3e, 3h	—
Triazines					
	Atrazine, Prometone	LD_{50} = 200–1000 mg/kg generally	Mechanism unknown; salivation, ataxia, and muscular spasms, dyspnea; death	1a, 1b, 1c, 5a	—
	Monuron (Telvar)	LD_{50} (rats) = 1500 mg/kg	Dermatitis, ataxia, hyporeflexia, hepatorenal damage	1b, 3a/3b, 3d, 3e, 3h, 6a	—

ACh, acetylcholine; 2-PAM, 2-pyridine aldoxine methylchloride; MCPA, 2-methyl-4-chlorophenoxy-acetic acid; MCPP; LD_{50}, median lethal dose; $t_{1/2}$, half-life; GABA, α-aminobutyric acid.

*Solvents used in many of these products are low-molecular-weight hydrocarbons and alcohols which may also cause signs of toxicity, generally CNS excitation and neuromuscular tremor.

†The toxic dose may be much less than the LD_{50}.

Table 1–28. Rodenticides

Generic Name	Brand Names or Description	Toxic Dose*	Mechanism and Actions	Therapeutic Strategies	Antidotes and Comments
α-Naphthylthiourea (ANTU)	White or blue-gray bitter-tasting powder	Dogs: 10–40 mg/kg (younger dogs are more resistant) Cats: 75–100 mg/kg	Strong emetic, increased permeability of pulmonary capillaries → pulmonary edema	1a, 3a/3b, 6b, 6d	Guarded prognosis; survival >12 hr → more favorable prognosis
Bromethalin	Assault, Vengeance, Trounce; 0.01% in green or tan pellets; packaged in 16–42.5-g place packs	Minimum toxic dose of bait: Dogs: 16.7 g/kg Cats: 3 g/kg	Uncouples oxidative phosphorylation; acute/high-dose syndrome: like strychnine, within 24 hr post ingestion; delayed/low-dose syndrome: hindlimb neurologic deficits, CNS depression, coma, 3–7 days post ingestion	Acute syndrome: 1c, 3a, 3b, 3d, 3e Delayed syndrome: 1c, 6e	1c: treat cerebral edema 3d: magnesium-based cathartics contraindicated 3e: repeated q6h × 3 days, activated charcoal and sorbitol
Cholecalciferol (vitamin D₃)	Quintox, Rampage; 0.075% cholecalciferol in 25–30-g packs	2–3 mg/kg LD₅₀ reported = 88 mg/kg	Increases serum calcium, leads to dystrophic calcification in renal, hepatic, GI tissues 1–2 days post ingestion	3a, 3d, 3e, 4, 5a, 6a	4: calcitonin; also prednisolone, dexamethasone, aluminum hydroxide
Coumarins	See Vitamin K antagonists				

192

Sodium fluoroacetate (1080, 1081)	Colorless, odorless, tasteless	Dogs and cats: 0.05–1.0 mg/kg	Uncouples oxidative phosphorylation, causes massive CNS excitation, seizures	1a, 1b, 1c, 3a/3b	Guarded prognosis
Strychnine	0.3% bait (3 mg/g)	Dogs: 0.75 mg/kg; Cats: 2 mg/kg	Antagonizes spinal inhibitory neurotransmitters; severe muscle tremors, extensor rigidity, seizures, precipitated by noise, light, touch; mydriasis, respiratory paralysis	1a, 1c, 3b, 3d, 3e, 5a, 5b	3b: tannic acid or potassium permanganate Caution: no morphine
Vitamin K antagonists	Grain-based baits or impregnated wax blocks (Talon, Bromakil, etc.)	Toxic dose and $t_{1/2}$ vary; see References	Inhibition of clotting factors II, VII, IX, and X; latent period of 2–7 days before clinical signs; anemia, internal hemorrhages into various body spaces	3a for acute ingestion; if symptomatic, then 1a, 4	Vitamin K_1, possibly fresh whole blood or cryosupernatant transfusion; duration of vitamin K therapy; depends on class of anticoagulant
Zinc phosphide	Gray-black powder, used at 2%–5%	20–50 mg/kg; faint fish or acetylene odor	Gastric acid + zinc phosphide → release of phosphine gas; leads to respiratory distress; also GI, renal, hepatic damage; peracute onset <4 hr	1a, 1b, 1d, 3b, 6b, 6d	3b: $NaHCO_3$ by lavage and PO for next 24 hr; NPO × 24 hr

*The toxic dose may be much less than the LD_{50}.

193

194

Table 1–29. Household Compounds, Chemicals, and Plants

Common Name	Active Ingredient	Toxic Dose,* Exposure, or Potential	Mechanism and Actions	Therapeutic Strategies	Antidotes and Comments
Acids, corrosives	Hydrochloric sulfuric, nitric or phosphoric acid	Contact	Localized coagulative necrotic lesions, usually not full-thickness; contact painful	Not 3a, 3b; 1b, 3g, 3h, 3i, 6b, 6d	Do not give NaHCO₂ PO 3g: 4 egg whites in qt of warm water, or 15 mL of milk of magnesia, or magnesium oxide in water 1:25 solution 3h: 5% NaHCO₃ OK dermally; steroids and antibiotics indicated
Alcohols			Ingestion: disruption of neuron membrane structure; impaired motor coordination, CNS excitation; then depression, stupor, arrest; inhalation: ocular, mucosal damage; dermal: irritation, cutaneous hyperemia	1a, 1b, 1c, 1d, 3a, 3e, 3h	—
Alcohol, drinking	Ethanol	Dog: 5.5–8.0 g/kg PO	CNS depressant	See Alcohols	—
Alcohol, rubbing	Isopropyl alcohol	Dog: 4.1 g/kg PO	CNS depressant	See Alcohols	—
Alcohol, methyl	Methanol	Dog: 4–8 g/kg PO	CNS depressant; hepatotoxicity	5c, 6a; see Alcohols	

Alkalis, caustics	Sodium or potassium hydroxide	Contact	Deep liquefactive necrosis, often full-thickness; esophageal burns common	Not 3a/3b; 1b, 3g, 3h, 3i, 6b, 6d	3g; 4 egg whites in qt of warm water, then vinegar or lemon juice in water 1:4 solution 3h: vinegar OK dermally; endoscopy within 24 hr —
Ammonia, cleaning	Ammonium hydroxide	Contact	See Alkalis, Caustics; Inhalation: Pulmonary edema, Pneumonia See Ethylene glycol	See Alkalis, Caustics	
Antifreeze	95% ethylene glycol				
Aquarium algacides	Triazines or Diquat	—			
Barbecue lighter fluid	Petroleum distillates	—			
		Ingestion: low toxicity; inhalation: 1 mL	Severe aspiration pneumonitis; see Fuels		
Batteries, automotive	Sulfuric acid	Contact	See Acids, Corrosives		
Batteries, dry cell	Sulfuric acid	Contact	See Acids		
Batteries, "button"	Sodium or potassium hydroxide	Contact if chewed	See Alkalis, Caustics		
Bleaches					
Chlorine	Sodium hypochlorite (household: 3%–6%; industrial or swimming pool: 50%)	Serious toxic potential	Contact irritant and tissue destruction, according to concentration (household: mild; industrial: severe)	Not 3a/3b; 3g, 3h, 3i, 6b	3g; milk or eggs PO; milk of magnesia PO; aluminum hydroxide PO

Table continued on following page

195

Table 1–29. Household Compounds, Chemicals, and Plants *Continued*

Common Name	Active Ingredient	Toxic Dose,* Exposure, or Potential	Mechanism and Actions	Therapeutic Strategies	Antidotes and Comments
Nonchlorine (color-fast)	Sodium peroxide, sodium perborate	Moderate toxic potential	Sodium peroxide → GI gas distention; sodium perborate as sodium peroxide + boric acid in Table 1–27	1a, 3a/3b 3e, 3h	—
Boric acid Carbon monoxide	See Table 1–27 Carbon monoxide	Serious toxic potential	Competes with oxygen for binding sites on hemoglobin; mucous membranes bright red early, cyanotic at higher concentrations; respiratory embarrassment	1a	Oxygen
Chocolate	Theobromine; $t_{1/2}$ in dogs = 17.5 hr	Dog: 100–150 mg/kg	See Caffeine in Table 1–30	1a, 1b, 1c, 3a/3b, 3d, 3e	3e: repeat q6h × 4 days; catheterize bladder to reduce reabsorption from urine
Milk chocolate	Theobromine 44 mg/oz (154 mg/100 g)	Low toxic potential	See Caffeine in Table 1–30		
Semisweet chocolate	Theobromine 150 mg/ oz (528 mg/100 g)	Moderate toxic potential	See Caffeine in Table 1–30		
Baking chocolate	Theobromine 390 mg/ oz (1365 mg/100 g)	Serious toxic potential	See Caffeine in Table 1–30		
Cresol	Aromatic hydrocarbon	—	See Hydrocarbon, aromatic		

Product	Composition	Toxic potential	Signs/Symptoms	Treatment codes	Additional treatment
Deicer, automotive	Ethylene glycol and isopropanol	Serious toxic potential	See Ethylene glycol and Alcohol, rubbing		—
Denture cleaners	Sodium perborate	Serious toxic potential	Direct irritant, may be CNS depressant; see also Bleaches, nonchlorine and Boric acid, borate (Table 1–27)	3e, 3h, 6b, 6c	
Deodorants	Aluminum chloride, aluminum chlorhydrate	Moderate toxic potential	Oral irritation or necrosis, gastroenteritis, nephrosis	3b, 6b	—
Detergents (anionic)	Sulfonated or phosphorylated forms of benzene; example: dishwashing liquid	1–5 g/kg	Mucosal damage and edema, GI irritation, CNS depression, seizures; possible hemolysis	1a, 1c, 3b, 3e, 3d, 3g, 3h, 6b	3g: milk or calcium-containing solutions
Detergents (cationic), disinfectants	Quaternary ammonium with alkyl or aryl substituent groups; also ethanol or isopropanol; example: Nolvasan	Serious toxic potential	Irritant, corrosive to mucous membranes and skin; neuromuscular signs similar to those of anticholinesterase compounds; may cause methemoglobinemia	Not 3a; 1a, 1c, 3d, 3e, 3g, 3h, 3i	3g: milk, egg whites, water 3h: neutralize with ordinary soap dermally

Table continued on following page

Table 1-29. Household Compounds, Chemicals, and Plants *Continued*

Common Name	Active Ingredient	Toxic Dose,* Exposure, or Potential	Mechanism and Actions	Therapeutic Strategies	Antidotes and Comments
Detergents (nonionic)	Alkyl and arylpolyether sulfates, alcohols or sulfonates, alkyl phenol, polyethylene glycol; may contain phenols; example: Pinesol	Phenols toxic to cats, puppies particularly; moderate toxic potential	Gastroenteritis, or topical irritation most common; potentially metabolized to glycolic and oxalic acid, causing renal damage; see also Ethylene Glycol, Phenols	3e, 3g, 3h, 6a	Milk or water
Diaper soaks	Cationic detergents, bleach		See Detergents (cationic), and Bleaches		
Dishwasher (electric) detergents	Alkaline detergents (anionic)		See Detergents (anionic) and Alkalis, caustic; may also cause hypocalcemia		
Dishwashing (liquid) detergents	Anionic detergents		See Detergents (anionic)		
Drain cleaners	Sodium hydroxide, possibly sodium hypochlorite	Contact	Contact tissue destruction; see Alkalis, caustics, and Bleaches		
Dry-cleaning fluids	1,1,1-trichloroethane	Adult human: fatal dose = 5 mL ingestion or inhalation	CNS depression, ventricular fibrillation; hepatorenal damage	Not 3a/3b; 1a, 1b, 3e, 6a	

	Carbon tetrachloride	Adult human: fatal dose = 3–5 mL by ingestion or inhalation	Gastroenteritis initially, then CNS and respiratory depression; ventricular arrhythmias, hepatorenal damage	1a, 1b, 3e, 6a
Ethylene glycol	Toxic metabolites: glycolate, glyoxylate, oxalate	Dogs: 6.6 mL/kg Cats: 1.5 mL/kg	1–12 hr: CNS signs; 12–24 hr: nonspecific; 24–72 hr: renal failure	3a/3b, 3e, 4, 5c, 6a; 4: ethanol 20%; 4-methylpyrazole, thiamine
Fabric softener liquids	Cationic detergents		See Detergents (cationic)	
Fertilizer	Urea/ammonium salts; nitrates (N), phosphates (P), potash (K); possibly metal salts	Moderate toxic potential	Gastroenteritis, acidosis, diuresis; urea of low toxicity to monogastrics	1b, 3b, 3d, 3e, 6b, 6c
Fire extinguisher (liquid)	Chlorobromomethane, methyl bromide	Serious toxic potential	Dermal or ocular irritation; metabolized to methanol; pulmonary edema, CNS signs, hepatorenal damage	Not 3a/3b; 1a, 3h, 3i, 6a
Fireplace colors	Heavy metal salts (copper, rubidium, cesium, lead, arsenic, antimony, barium, selenium, zinc)	Moderate toxic potential	Gastroenteritis, renal insult; other signs vary with metal involved	3d, 3e, 3g, 6b, 6c

Table continued on following page

Table 1-29. Household Compounds, Chemicals, and Plants *Continued*

Common Name	Active Ingredient	Toxic Dose,* Exposure, or Potential	Mechanism and Actions	Therapeutic Strategies	Antidotes and Comments
Fireworks	Oxidizing agents (nitrates, chlorates); metals (mercury, antimony, copper, strontium, barium, phosphorus)	Moderate toxic potential	Gastroenteritis, possibly hemorrhagic; possible methemoglobinemia	3a/3b, 3e, 3g, 6b, 6c	Treat methemoglobinemia; for specific metals if known
Flux (solder)	Acids (hydrochloric, glutamic, salicylic, boric)	Moderate toxic potential	Corrosive; skin, mucosal damage, gastroenteritis	See Acids, corrosives	
Fuels	Petroleum hydrocarbons, kerosene, gasoline	Moderate toxic potential	Early CNS depression, mucosal irritation; aspiration pneumonia (proportional to volatility) within minutes to hours; hepatorenal damage; seizures possible; transient corneal irritation	Not 3a, 3b; 1a, 1c, 3e, 3g, 3h, 3i, 6b	3g: milk or egg whites
Furniture polish	Mineral spirits (a petroleum distillate)	Moderate toxic potential	See Fuels		
Gasoline	Petroleum distillates	Moderate toxic potential	See Fuels; transient corneal irritation see Fuels		
Glues, adhesives	Aliphatic or aromatic hydrocarbons, toluene	Moderate toxic potential			
Children's glue (Elmer's)	Polyvinyl acetate	Low toxic potential	Pneumonitis if inhaled; otherwise negligible toxicity		

Superglue	Methyl-2-cyanoacrylate				Leave to exfoliate naturally
Hexachlorophene	Phenol derivative		As for Detergents (nonionic) and Phenols; in pups: vacuolation of brain white matter and spinal cord	Not 3h; 3a	
Hydrocarbons, aromatic	Phenols, cresols, toluene, naphthalene	Moderate toxic potential	CNS depression, hepatorenal damage, muscle tremors, pneumonia, possible methemoglobinemia, hemolysis	Not 3a; 1a, 1c, 3b, 3e, 3g, 3h, 6b	3g: milk or egg whites
Iron, iron salts		LD_{50} rats = 5 g/kg Humans: 1–2 g only can be lethal	Severe gastroenteritis, myocardial toxicity, hepatic damage	1b, 3a/3b, 3d, 3g, 4, 6b	3g: $NaHCO_3$ PO 4: deferoxamine; radiographs may be helpful
Kerosene	Petroleum distillates	Moderate toxic potential	Aspiration pneumonitis, severe; see also Fuels; minimal ocular injury	1a, 3h, 3i, 6b	
Laundry detergent	See Detergents (anionic)				
Lead		>3 mg/kg toxic, 10–25 mg/kg lethal	Inhibits sulfur-containing enzymes, increases RBC fragility, CNS damage	1c, 3b, 3c, 3e, 3g, 4	3g: magnesium sulfate; surgery if lead object in GI tract 4: calcium EDTA ± penicillamine

Table continued on following page

I

Table 1–29. Household Compounds, Chemicals, and Plants *Continued*

Common Name	Active Ingredient	Toxic Dose,* Exposure, or Potential	Mechanism and Actions	Therapeutic Strategies	Antidotes and Comments
Matches "Strike-anywhere"	Inert phosphorus, potassium chlorate	Low toxic potential	Gastroenteritis; possible methemoglobinemia	3a, 3b, 3d, 3e	As for methemoglobinemia
Safety matches	Potassium chlorate	Low toxic potential	Gastroenteritis; possible methemoglobinemia		
Matchbook cover (striking surface)	Red phosphorus (50%)	Nontoxic			
Metal cleaners	Acids, sodium or potassium hydroxide/aliphatic hydrocarbons and chlorinated solvents	Serious toxic potential	See Acids, corrosives; Alkalis, caustics; Fuels		
Mineral spirits	Petroleum distillates	Inhalation: serious; ingestion: moderate	Aspiration pneumonitis; severe; see Fuels	5c	
Mothballs	Naphthalene	Moderate toxic potential	See Hydrocarbons, aromatic		
Oil (lubricating, fuel, mineral)	Petroleum distillates	Dermal: moderate toxic potential	See Fuels		
Onions, garlic, chives	Contain sulfoxide compounds	Moderate toxic potential	Hemolysis, Heinz body anemia, methemoglobinemia	1b, 3a/3b, 3d, 3e	
Oven cleaners	Sodium or potassium hydroxide and petroleum distillates	Serious toxic potential	see Alkalis, caustics; Fuels		
Oxalic acid	Oxalic acid	Serious toxic potential	Renal damage	3a/3b, 3g, 6a	3g: chalk or other calcium salts PO

Paint and varnish removers	Benzene, methanol, toluene, acetone (10%–75%)		See Fuels	
Paints, varnishes	Petroleum distillates, aromatic hydrocarbon solvents, lead		See Hydrocarbons, aromatic, and Lead	
Paraffin wax	Petroleum distillate	Nontoxic	See Fuels	
Pencils	Graphite and wood		Potential foreign body	
Pennies	See Zinc, Zinc Oxide			
Pens, marker and ink	Commonly contain xylene (a petroleum distillate) and boric acid		See Hydrocarbons, Aromatic and Boric acid, Borate (Table 1–27)	
Petroleum distillates	Hydrocarbons		See Fuels	
Perfumes	Perfume essence containing various volatile oils (savin, rue, tansy, juniper, cedar)	Moderate toxic potential	Dermal, ocular irritation; CNS signs, hepatorenal damage	3b, 3d, 6b	3b: 5% bicarbonate solution
Phenols	Aromatic alcohol derivative of coal tar	Serious toxic potential; worse in puppies and cats	Denatures and precipitates cellular proteins; corrosive burns; hepatic, renal damage; methemoglobinemia	1a, 1b, 3g, 3d, 3e, 3h, 4, 6a	3g: milk or egg white 3h: glyerol or polyethylene glycol, then dish detergent, then water; can apply 0.5% NaHCO$_3$-soaked dressings to dermal sites; 4: N-acetylcysteine

Table continued on following page

203

Table 1-29. Household Compounds, Chemicals, and Plants *Continued*

Common Name	Active Ingredient	Toxic Dose,* Exposure, or Potential	Mechanism and Actions	Therapeutic Strategies	Antidotes and Comments
Photographic developer	p-Methylaminophenol		See Phenols		—
Pine oil disinfectants	Pine oil 5%–20%, phenols 2%–6%; also alcohols and soaps	Serious toxic potential; LD_{50} for pine oil = 1.0–2.5 mL/kg; less in cats	Mucous membrane and ocular irritation; gastroenteritis, CNS depression; pneumonitis; hemoglobinemia; hepatic and renal necrosis; see also Phenols	Not 3a/3b; 3g, 3d, 3e, 1b, 6a, 3h, 3i	3g: milk or egg whites
Plants	Various toxic principles	Varies	Generally: GI irritation, tremors, potential renal and hepatic damage	1b, 1c, 3a/3b, 3d, 3e, 6a, 6b	
Radiator cleaners	Oxalic acid (40%–100%)	Serious toxic potential	Corrosive acid, gastroenteritis; hypocalcemia; oxalate-induced renal failure	1a, 3g, 4, 6a	4: calcium gluconate IV; calcium hydroxide PO
Rubbing alcohol	Ethyl or isopropyl alcohol		See Alcohols		
Rust removers	Acids (hydrochloric, phosphoric, fluoric, oxalic)	Serious toxic potential	Corrosive; see Acids, corrosives	Not 3a/3b; 3g/3h	3g: milk of magnesia PO 3h: bicarbonate paste topically after rinsing Egg whites PO
Salt, thawing	Calcium chloride	Moderate toxic potential	Strong local irritant; gastroenteritis, ulcers	1a, 3b, 3e, 3h, 6b, 6c	

Product	Ingredient	Toxic potential	Effects	Code	Treatment
Shampoos, antidandruff					
Zinc-based	Zinc pyridinethione	Serious toxic potential	GI irritation; progressive blindness, retinal detachment, exudative chorioretinitis	3a/3b, 3d, 3e	3g: egg whites, milk of magnesia PO
Coal tar-based	Cresol	Moderate toxic potential	See Hydrocarbons, aromatic		
Selenium sulfide	Selsun Blue	Low toxic potential	Possible GI irritation	3b, 3g	
Shampoo, nonmedicated	Lauryl sulfates and triethanolamine dodecyl sulfate; usually <5% concentration	Moderate toxic potential	Ocular, mucosal, and GI irritation; see also Detergents (anionic)	3d, 3e, 3h, 3i	
Shoe polish	Aniline dyes (3%) in some; small amounts of nitrobenzenes or terpenes	Moderate toxic potential	See Hydrocarbons, aromatic; methemoglobinemia		
Silver polish	Sodium carbonate (an alkali) and cyanide salts	Serious toxic potential	Sodium carbonate results in rapid vomiting; potential for cyanide poisoning → rapid death; see also Alkalis, caustics	1a, 1b, 3b, 3e, 4	4: sodium nitrite IV followed by sodium thiosulfate IV
Soaps					
Bath, bar soap	Salts of fatty acids	Low toxic potential	GI irritation	3g, 6b	3g: milk or water
Hexachlorophene	See Hexachlorophene				

I

Table continued on following page

205

Table 1–29. Household Compounds, Chemicals, and Plants *Continued*

Common Name	Active Ingredient	Toxic Dose,* Exposure, or Potential	Mechanism and Actions	Therapeutic Strategies	Antidotes and Comments
Solvents	See Hydrocarbons, aromatic				
Styptic pencil	Potassium alum sulfate	Low toxic potential	Corrosive due to release of sulfuric acid during hydrolysis of the salt	3g, 3h	3g: milk of magnesia
Sunscreen, fluoro	Zinc oxide	Acute: low toxic potential	See also Zinc	3a/3b	
Suntan lotion	Shampoo-type emulsifiers, solvents, alcohol, (PABA, aloe vera)		See Shampoo, nonmedicated; Alcohols, rubbing		
Tar	Petroleum distillates		See Fuels		
Toilet bowl cleaner	Acids		See Acids, corrosives		
Turpentine	Hydrocarbon distillate of pine oil		See Fuels		
Window cleaners	Ethylene glycol monobutyl ether (10%), ammonia		See Ethylene glycol, Ammonia, cleaning		
Zinc, zinc oxide	Found in pennies, metal nuts, sunscreen ointments	Serious toxic potential; normal serum [Zn] = 1 ppm†	Gastroenteritis, hemolytic anemia, renal failure	3g, 3a, 4, 6a, 6b, 6c	4: Dimercaprol and calcium EDTA; remove any ingested object
Zephiran	Cationic detergents	—	See Detergents (cationic)		

PABA = para-aminobenzoic acid.

*Toxic dose may be much less than LD_{50}.

†Use plastic containers or tubes specifically labeled for trace element analysis for collection of samples for zinc analysis. Red-top Vacutainers or EDTA tubes may contain extraneous zinc.

Table 1–30. Medications and Other Drugs

Generic or Class Name	Mechanism and Actions*	Therapeutic Strategies	Antidotes and Comments
Acetaminophen	Oxidant to RBCs and hepatocytes → methemoglobinemia; severe respiratory distress; hepatotoxicity	1a, 1b, 3a/3b, 3e, 4, 6a	4: acetylcysteine, ascorbic acid; not methylene blue in cats; in humans: marked prolongation of prothrombin time or acidosis after day 4 are indicators of impending hepatic failure
Alcohol (methanol, ethanol, isopropyl)	See Alcohols in Table 1–29		
Amphetamine	Neurosynaptic stimulation: CNS, GI, neuromuscular excitation	1c, 1d, 3a/3b, 3d, 3e, 5a, 5b	Sedatives
Arsenic, organic (caparsolate, arsanilic acid)	Severe gastroenteritis, garlic odor, cyanosis	1a, 1b, 4, 6a, 6b, 6d	4: dimercaprol
Aspirin	Prostaglandin inhibition, metabolic acidosis, GI ulceration, decreased platelet aggregation, hypophosphatemia	3a/3b, 3d, 3e, 5c, 6b	
Asthma medications	See β-Adrenergic agonists		
Atropine	Parasympatholytic (muscarinic)	1b	Physostigmine
β-Adrenergic agonists (terbutaline, albuterol, metaproterenol)	Muscle tremors, tachycardia, agitation; effects usually transient	1b, 1c	
Barbiturates	GABA mimetics; cause CNS depression	1a, 1b, 1d, 3a, 3e, 3d, 5c	
Benzoyl peroxide (Clearasil)	Hydrogen peroxide production; topically: blistering; ingested: gastric dilation	Not 3a; 3b, 6b,	3d: do not use Mg²⁺-based cathartics
Bisacodyl (Carter's Little Pills, Ducolax)	Stimulant/irritant laxative; diarrhea	1b	
Bismuth subsalicylate (Pepto-Bismol)	Salicylic acid; see Aspirin		

Table continued on following page

207

Table I–30. Medications and Other Drugs *Continued*

Generic or Class Name	Mechanism and Actions*	Therapeutic Strategies	Antidotes and Comments
Caffeine	Phosphodiesterase inhibition; CNS and skeletal/cardiac muscle stimulation, diuresis, GI ulceration; lethal dose in dogs = 140 mg/kg; $t_{1/2}$ = 4.5 hr	1a, 1b, 1c, 3a/3b, 3e, 6b	
Cardiac drugs	Consult pharmaceutical reference		
Cascara sagrada (Nature's Remedy)	Stimulant/irritant laxative; diarrhea	1b	
Castor oil	Stimulant/irritant laxative; diarrhea	1b	
Chlorpheniramine	H_1-receptor blocker; sedation	3a, 3e	
Cocaine	CNS and cardiovascular stimulation; street concentrations 12%–60%; Freebase 90% pure; dog LD_{50} = 25–40 mg/kg PO	a, 1b, 1c	Phenylephrine if severe hypotension Sedatives, muscle relaxants
Cough syrups; see also ingredients by generic name	Any combination of antihistamine, decongestant, antitussive, expectorant, NSAID, alcohol or caffeine	1b, 1c, 3c, 3e	
Dextromethorphan	Opioid derivative but without analgesic or addictive effects; antitussive; mild sedation	3e	
Diphenhydramine	H_1-receptor blocker; antimuscarinic effects; sedation	1a, 3a, 3e	
Docusate sodium (dioctyl sodium succinate) (Colace)	Stool softener, laxative	1b, 3e	
Doxylamine	Antihistamine	1b, 3a, 3e	
"Ecstasy"	3,4-methylenedioxy-methylamphetamine; in humans: fulminant hyperthermia, convulsions, disseminated intravascular coagulation, rhabdomyolysis, acute renal failure, and hepatotoxicity	1b, 1c, 1d, 6a	

Flea products	See Table 1–27		
Hashish	See Marijuana		
Ibuprofen	Prostaglandin inhibition, GI ulceration, renal failure; see NSAIDs	3a/3b, 3d, 3e, 6a, 6b	3e: repeatedly
Ivermectin	GABA agonist: collies, Old English sheepdogs; ataxia, hypersalivation, CNS deficits; microfilaria-positive dogs: fever, shock, ataxia; cats: CNS deficits	1b, 3a, 3d, 3e, 6e	No antidote established
Laxatives; see also ingredients by generic names	Variety of mechanisms, depending upon substance; effects: diarrhea, abdominal pain	1b	
Loperamide	Antidiarrheal opioid derivative; constipation, nausea, sedation	3a/3b, 3c, 3d, 3e, 4	Naloxone
LSD	Hallucinogen	1c	Give sedatives to effect
Marijuana	CNS depression, bradycardia, mydriasis, hypothermia	1b, 1d, 3b, 3d, 3e	
Mineral oil	Lubricant laxative; diarrhea	Not 3a; 1b	
Morphine	Opioid agonist; CNS depression or excitation, respiratory depression, increased GI motility	1a, 1c	Naloxone
Nicotine	Low doses stimulate autonomic ganglia; high doses block autonomic ganglia and myoneural junction	1c, 3a/3b, 3d, 3h	3b: gastric lavage with 1:2000 KMnO$_4$ solution; later in curse: stimulants may be required
NSAIDs (ibuprofen, ketoprofen, carprofen, diclofenac, naproxen, etc.)	Inhibit cyclooxygenase, resulting in decreased production of certain prostaglandins; acute renal failure, nephrotic syndrome, GI ulceration, decreased platelet function, hepatotoxicity	1b, 3a/3b, 3d, 3e, 6a, 6b	3e: repeat q2h
Paracetamol	See Acetaminophen		
Phencyclidine ("angel dust")	Weak base; ketamine-like CNS depression and excitation, decreased cardiovascular function	1a, 1b, 1c, 3e, 5a, 5b	3e: repeat q2h

Table continued on following page

Table 1-30. Medications and Other Drugs *Continued*

Generic or Class Name	Mechanism and Actions*	Therapeutic Strategies	Antidotes and Comments
Phenobarbital	See Barbiturates		
Phenolphthalein (Ex-Lax)	Stimulant/irritant laxative; diarrhea; intestinal cramping	1b	Dx: add sodium bicarbonate to urine sample; phenolphthalein if present turns alkaline urine pink
Phenylephrine	α-Adrenergic agonist; decongestant	1b	Prazosin, propanolol
Phenylpropanolamine	α- and β-Adrenergic agonist; decongestant	1b	Prazosin, propanolol
Pseudoephedrine	α- and β-Adrenergic agonist; decongestant	1b, 1c	Prazosin, propanolol
Piperazine	GABA agonist; cervical/truncal ataxia, tremors; also seizures in cats	1b, 1c, 3a, 3d, 3e, 5b	No antidote established
Psyllium (Metamucil)	Bulk-forming laxative; diarrhea	1b	
Quinine	60 mg/L in tonic water; child's toxic dose <20 mg/kg; in humans: visual deficits, cardiovascular collapse	1a, 1b, 3a/3b, 5a, 5b, 6a	
Salicylates	See Aspirin		
Tricyclic antidepressants (amitriptyline, amoxapine, desipramine, doxepin, imipramine, nortriptyline, protriptyline, trimipramine)	Quinidine-like cardiovascular effect → reentry ventricular arrhythmias; CNS, excitation and then norepinephrine depletion; also anticholinergic properties; 15 mg/kg ingestion is potentially fatal; $t_{1/2}$ = 10–80 hr	1a, 1b, 1c, 3b, 3d, 3e	3b: do not induce vomiting, may trigger seizures 3d: do not use Mg^{2+}-based cathartics 3e: repeat q4-6 h
Vitamin tablets	Vitamin A, vitamin D, and iron toxicity potentially; see also Iron, Iron salts, in Table 1–29	3a/3b, 3d, 6a	Monitor hepatic enzymes, calcium, phosphate
Xanthines	See Caffeine		

GABA, γ-aminobutyric acid; NSAID, nonsteroidal anti-inflammatory drug; LSD, lysergic acid diethylamide.
*The toxic dose may be much less than the LD_{50}.

Table I-31. Bacterial and Fungal Toxins

Clinical Diagnosis	Common Source and Route	Mechanism and Actions	Therapeutic Strategies	Antidotes and Comments
Aflatoxin	Moldy feed grains, esp. corn	*Aspergillus flavus*; GI signs, hepatic damage	3e, 6e	Beware of liver failure
Botulism	Carrion, food, garbage, environment; ingestion	*Clostridium botulinum* neurotoxin; generalized cholinergic blockade of spinal and cranial nerves → LMN signs, including respiratory paralysis; signs usually within 6 days post ingestion	1a, 1d, 6a, 6b, 6e	Antitoxin of no proven value; supportive care only
Ingesta-borne enterotoxemia	Garbage, compost, rotten food; ingestion	*Staphylococcus, Streptococcus, Bacillus, Clostridium perfringens* toxins; *Escherichia coli* or *Salmonella* overgrowth; cause gastroenteritis and some gas distention of the abdomen, shock, sometimes CNS excitation; 2–8 hr post ingestion	1c, 3a/3b, 3c, 3d, 3e, 6b	Ampicillin or trimethoprim-sulfadiazine
Mycotoxins	Moldy foods, cream cheese, walnuts	*Penicillium* spp.; GABA inhibition → CNS excitation	1c, 3d, 3e	
Tetanus	Soil, feces; anaerobic wound infection	*Clostridium tetani*; neurotoxin inhibits the spinal inhibitory neurons causing motor neuron excitation; 5–8 days incubation period	1a, 1c, 4, 6e	4: tetanus antitoxin (only effective against that toxin not yet in the CNS); penicillin G IV initially, then procaine penicillin daily

LMN, lower motor neuron; GABA, γ-aminobutyric acid.

Table 1–32. Drug and Antidote Doses

Generic Name	Concentration or Brand Name	Usage	Dose
N-acetylcysteine	Mucomyst	Antidote in oxidant injuries, acetaminophen toxicity	140 mg/kg IV initially, then 70 mg/kg PO q6h × 3 days
Activated charcoal		Adsorbent	2–5 g/kg PO
Aluminum hydroxide	Amphojel	Enteric phosphate binder, neutralizing bleach	10–30 mg/kg PO q8h
Ammonium chloride	Acidurin	Urinary acidification	Dog: 25–50 mg/kg PO q6h Cat: 10 mg/kg PO q6h
Ampicillin sodium		Bacterial enteritis	10 mg/kg IV, IM q6h
Apomorphine		Emetic in dogs	0.4–0.8 mg/kg IV/IM or subconjunctivally
Ascorbic acid	Vitamin C	Methemoglobinemia	30 mg/kg PO q.i.d. × 48 hr
Atropine		Relief of muscarinic stimulation in anticholinesterase toxicity	0.05–0.1 mg/kg IM, repeat q4h or as needed to minimize muscarinic signs; avoid atropine toxicity
Buprenorphine	Temgesic	Analgesia	10–20 µg/kg IM/IV q6–8h
Butorphanol	Torbugesic	Analgesia	0.1–0.4 mg/kg IM/IV q4–6h
Calcitonin, salmon		Hypercalcemia	4–6 IU/kg SC q2h
Calcium EDTA	Versenate	Lead toxicity	25 mg/kg in D5W q6h SC for 2–5 days
Calcium gluconate	10%	For hypocalcemia, various causes	2–10 mL slow IV: monitor ECG
Copper sulfate	0.2% solution	For gastric lavage	500 mL–2 L
Deferoxamine		Iron chelator	10 mg/kg IM at 0 and 2 hr; if urine then clear, discontinue; if urine then reddish-orange, continue 10 mg/kg IM q8h × 24 hr; total dose not to exceed 80 mg/kg in 24 hr
Dexamethasone		Promotes diuresis	0.25 mg/kg SC q6h
Dextrose	50%	Osmotic diuretic	Give 1 g/kg initially
Diazepam		Sedation	0.25–0.5 mg/kg IV initially, up to 5 mg/kg for severe seizures

Drug	Preparation	Indication	Dosage
Diazepam-ketamine	5 mg/mL and 100 mg/mL respectively	Short-term anesthesia	Mix 50:50 in same syringe; *of the mix,* give 1 mL/10 kg IV for induction; top up with additional 0.5–1.0 mL boluses; do not exceed 3 mL/10 kg.
Dimercaprol	BAL: 10% solution in oil	Arsenic and other heavy metal toxicities	4 mg/kg IM q4h × 4 doses maximum
Diphenhydramine	Benadryl	Relief of nicotinic stimulation in organophosphate toxicity	1–4 mg/kg PO t.i.d.
Dopamine		Renal perfusion support	1–3 µg/kg/min IV CRI
Egg whites		As binding agent	Separate yolk from white, administer whites PO
Ethanol	20%	In ethylene glycol toxicity	Dog: 0.5 g/kg IV q4h × 24 hr, then 16h × 24 hr Cat: 0.5 g/kg IV q6h × 30 hr, then q8h × 32 hr
Furosemide	50 mg/mL	Diuretic	Dog: 2–4 mg/kg IV q8h Cat: 1–2 mg/kg IV q12h
Glycerol guaiacolate (guaifenesin)		Muscle relaxation	100 mg/kg IV to effect
Hydrogen peroxide	3%	Emetic in dogs	5 ml PO
Mannitol	20%	Diuresis or treatment of cerebral edema	0.5 g/kg slow IV in first hour; if successful, begin infusion of 5% mannitol at 10 mL/kg/hr
Magnesia, milk of		Demulcent, GI protectant	1–15 mL PO
Magnesium sulfate		Cathartic, also in precipitation of barium and lead compounds	2–25 g (10–125 mL)
Methocarbamol	Robaxin, 10% solution	Muscle relaxation	150 mg/kg IV to effect
Methylene blue	1% solution (maximum)	Nitrite- or chlorate-induced methemoglobinemia	9 mg/kg slow IV; beware hypotension
4-Methylpyrazole	Antizol-Vet	Ethylene glycol toxicity	Dog: 20 mg/kg IV initially, then 15 mg/kg IV at 12 and 24 hr, then 5 mg/kg IV at 35 hr; not for use in cats
Naloxone	Narcan	Opioid antagonist	0.04–0.1 mg/kg IV, IM q1h or as needed
Oxymorphone	Numorphan	Short-term anesthesia	Dog: 0.1–0.2 mg/kg IV, maximum 3 mg
2-PAM (pralidoxime chloride)		In organophosphate toxicity	20 mg/kg IV b.i.d.

Table continued on following page

213

Table 1-32. Drug and Antidote Doses *Continued*

Generic Name	Concentration or Brand Name	Usage	Dose
D-penicillamine	Cuprimine	Oral chelating agent in heavy metal toxicities	10–15 mg/kg q12h PO × 7 days; premedication with antiemetic; should be given 30 min before feeding so as not to bind essential dietary minerals; contraindicated if allergic to penicillin
Penicillin G		Initial treatment of tetanus	10⁶ units IV; see also Procaine penicillin G
Phenobarbitone		Medium/long-term control of seizures	4–8 mg/kg IV q8–12h; approximately 30 min lag time to effect
Phenylephrine hydrochloride	Neo-Synephrine HCl 1:2000 solution	CNS stimulant	0.15 mg/kg IV every 15 min
Potassium permanganate		In strychnine poisoning	5 mL/kg as lavage solution
Pralidoxime	See 2-PAM		
Prazosin	Minipress	Treatment of drug-induced hypertension	1 mg/15 kg PO q8h
Prednisolone		Promotes diuresis	1–2 mg/kg PO q8h
Procaine penicillin G		Daily treatment of tetanus	20,000–40,000 units/kg q24h
Propranolol	Inderal	Treatment of drug-induced supraventricular tachycardia	0.02–0.06 mg/kg slow IV; 0.2–1.0 mg/kg PO q8h
Sodium bicarbonate	8.4% solution = 1 mEq/mL	Urine alkalinization	1–2 mEq/kg IV q4h

Sodium chloride		Hastens excretion of bromide compounds	0.5–1.0 g PO t.i.d. × 7 days
Sodium nitrite	1% solution	Cyanide poisoning	16 mg/kg IV
Sodium sulfate	Glauber's salts, GoLYTELY	Cathartic	0.25 g/kg PO
Sodium thiosulfate	20% solution	Arsenic toxicosis, also cyanide toxicity	40–50 mg IV t.i.d.
Sorbitol	70%	Cathartic	3 mL/kg PO
Syrup of ipecac	7%	Emetic	Dogs: 1–2 mL/kg PO Cats: 3 mL/kg PO
Tannic acid	+ 2% solution (tea)	Various poisons	500–2000 mL as lavage solution
Tetanus antitoxin (not toxoid)		Initial treatment of tetanus	Test dose: 0.1–0.2 ml SC, observe for 30 min for anaphylaxis; if OK, then 30,000–100,000 units IV over 30 min, once only
Thiamine		In ethylene glycol toxicity, to facilitate conversion of glyoxylate to nontoxic metabolites	10–100 mg PO q24h
Trimethoprim-sulfadiazine		Bacterial enteritis	15 mg/kg PO, IM/IV q 12h
Vitamin K₁	Konakion	Vitamin K antagonists (rodenticides)	1–5 mg/kg PO b.i.d. × 5 days to 4 wks, depending on toxin; warfarin: 5 days; bromadialone: 4 wks; monitor therapy with PT or ACT times

BAL, British antilewisite; CRI, constant-rate infusion; PT, prothrombin time; ACT, activated clotting time.

will see under Mechanisms and Action "oxidation of RBCs and hepatocytes." The therapeutic strategies listed are 1a, 1b, 3a, 3b, 3e, 4, 6a, and antidotes are acetylcysteine and ascorbic acid. Copy these.

■ Turning to Table 1–26 we find that 1a is "Maintain respiration"; 1b is "Maintain cardiovascular function"; 3a is "emesis"; 3b is "Gastric lavage"; 3e is "Activated charcoal"; 4 is "Antidote" and 6a is "Maintain renal perfusion". These are the specific interventions appropriate for treatment of acetaminophen intoxication. Further explanations of each are found in the general text section under the corresponding number.

■ Check Table 1–33, Drug and Antidote Doses, for dose rates and intervals of acetylcysteine and ascorbic acid. Give the drugs accordingly.

Poisoning cases benefit from a rapid, organized approach. Key points in this approach are giving appropriate advice over the telephone (Section 1), being able to access information resources (Section 2), and providing appropriate treatment (Section 3).

There are just a few classes of poisons that account for the majority of toxicities in dogs and cats. In dogs, the top 10 most frequently reported toxicities reported to the ASPCA National Animal Poisons Control Center in 1997 were insecticides, rodenticides, NSAIDs, fertilizers, chocolate, cleaning products, plants, human medications, cosmetics, and veterinary medications. In cats, the most frequently reported toxicities were insecticides, plants, physical agents (ingested objects), NSAIDs, veterinary medications, rodenticides, cleaning products, fertilizers, aspirin or acetaminophen, and corrosives.

These incidence figures remain largely unchanged from previous years, and it behooves every veterinarian to develop familiarity with the clinical management of rodenticides and insecticides and to be prepared for them with antidotes at hand. Beyond these most common toxins, the spectrum of possibilities is endless and a veterinarian must rely on a good set of information resources. It is suggested that every veterinarian keep some comprehensive pharmaceutical and plant identification references on hand. Other information resources are discussed in Section 2.

Remarkably, though a veterinarian may encounter many different poisonings, there are in fact only a few specific antidotes that are commonly used in veterinary medicine. Because of the lack of specific antidotes, the veterinarian must also be a master of general poisons management and basic critical care. These principles are outlined and discussed in Section 3.

············Section I. Advising Clients Over the Telephone

The first step in managing patients actually begins before the patient arrives. The checklist below. Telephone Advice for the Client, can serve as a useful reminder for staff who are fielding client enquiries.

■ Telephone Advice for the Client

I. *Questions to ask the Client*

■ What is the suspected substance?

■ How much did the animal have?

■ How long ago was the exposure?

■ Was it swallowed or is it on the animal's skin or eyes?

■ How is the patient acting?

■ How long has the patient been acting that way?

(Box continued on following page)

■ Telephone Advice for the Client *(Continued)*

2. *Give first aid instructions as applicable*
   a. Induce vomiting* and save the vomitus. The owner may have the following emetics available:
      Table salt: 1–3 tsp in dogs

Syrup of ipecac: 1–2 mL/kg in dogs; 3.3 mL/kg in cats

Hydrogen peroxide (3% w/v†) 5 mL

   b. If the animal has had skin or ocular exposure to toxic or corrosive material, the owner should be advised to immediately begin rinsing the eye or skin with unlimited volumes of warm water and to continue this for as long as possible during transport to the veterinary hospital.
   c. If the patient is excited or having convulsions, advise the owner to try to protect the animal from injuring itself. Also remind the owner *not* to worry about the animal "swallowing its tongue," in the interests of owner safety.

3. *Remind the owner to bring a sample* of the vomitus or the container of the suspected poison to the hospital with the patient.

4. *Advise the owner to transport* the animal as rapidly as possible to the veterinary hospital.

*Do not induce vomiting if it appears that the animal has ingested corrosive substances, such as strong acid or alkali, or petroleum-based substances such as kerosene or turpentine. Instead, give milk or water to dilute the poison.
†Hydrogen peroxide is also sometimes sold as 30% w/v for hairdressing purposes; this concentration is not suitable for oral administration.

..........Section 2. Accessing Resources

With thousands of potentially toxic substances on the market today, it is important that every practice have access to a database of information on toxic substances. At the time of this writing, the following resources are available to veterinarians. The ASPCA National Animal Poisons Control Center provides access to qualified veterinary toxicologists. For additional information, you may contact them, or call your nearest veterinary school or emergency center.

ASPCA National Animal Poison Control Center
1717 S. Philo Road, Suite #36
Urbana, IL 61802
Inside the United States:
1-800-548-2423 or 1-888-426-4435 : flat fee of $30 per case, including follow-up calls. Payable by Visa, Mastercard, Discover, or American Express
1-900-680-0000 : charges billed to your telephone bill; $20 for first 5 minutes, $2.95 for each additional minute, $20 minimum; follow-up calls are not included.
Outside the United States:
1-2173375030: flat fee of $US30 per case, payable by credit card at the time of calling. See above.
Be ready to provide the following information:
   Your name, address, and telephone number
   Information concerning the exposure
   Species, breed, age, sex, weight, and number of animals involved
   Information on the agent involved, if known
   Clinical signs
Useful information for clients is provided on the ASPCA website—
http://www.napcc.aspca.org

.... *Textbooks*

There are several excellent veterinary textbooks which can provide more detailed information on specific poisons.

- Gfeller R, Messonier S: Handbook of Small Animal Toxicology and Poisoning. St Louis, Mosby-Year Book, 1997.

- Kirk RW, Bonagura JD, eds: Current Veterinary Therapy, Editions IX–XIII. Small Animal Practice. Philadelphia, WB Saunders. These volumes have a cumulative index which includes many key articles on specific poisons.

- Lorgue G, Lechenet J, Riviere A: Clinical Veterinary Toxicology. Cambridge, Massa, Blackwell Science, 1996.

- Murphy Michael J: A Field Guide to Common Animal Poisons. Ames, Iowa State University Press, 1996.

- Osweiler GD: Toxicology. Baltimore, Williams & Wilkins, 1996.

.... *Human Poison Control Centers*

Check your local telephone book for a poisons control telephone number among the list of Emergency numbers which is usually found inside the front cover. Although these numbers are for human poisonings, they do have access to an extensive poison and toxin database and can provide useful information for veterinarians. Human poison control centers can be useful sources of information, particularly regarding antidotal substances suitable for out-of-the-ordinary toxins and human medications.

All available information on the toxic ingredients in thousands of medicines, insecticides, pesticides and other registered commercial products has been placed confidentially by the government in these poison control centers. As new products are marketed, information regarding the toxic ingredients is forwarded to the centers.

.... *Internet*

Various e-mail discussion lists can serve as an informative resource for practitioners, but generally require an initial subscription and may have delayed response times. They are most useful for ideas on medium- and long-term therapy, but not emergency stabilization. Contact your local veterinary association or Internet service provider for guides to accessing veterinary lists.

.... *Manufacturers*

Many manufacturers operate an information service on their products. If the product label or name is available, check it for a telephone number which may route you to specialist advice.

.... Section 3. Essential Steps of Treatment

There are six essential steps in treating toxicities.* They are:

1. Stabilize vital signs.

---

*Modified from: Beasley VR, Dorman DC: Management of Toxicoses. Vet Clin North Am Small Anim Pract 20:307–377, 1990.

2. Obtain history and evaluate patient.
3. Prevent continued absorption of the toxin.
4. Administer antidotes if available.
5. Facilitate clearance or metabolism of absorbed toxin.
6. Supportive and symptomatic care.

Each of these steps is discussed in the following pages and identified alphanumerically by its listing in the poisons Tables 1–26 through 1–31.

............Step 1. Stabilize Vital Signs

When the patient is presented to the veterinarian, the client can be asked to complete a Toxicologic History Form while the animal is initially assessed and stabilized.

■ TOXICOLOGIC HISTORY FORM

DATE:
TIME:
A.M. P.M.

Patient Information

Name of Animal:
Age:
Breed:
Male or Female?
Neutered?
Weight:
Vaccinations given within the last year?
Any current medications (including routine medicines such as heartworm preventive)?

Today's Problem

When did you first notice anything wrong with your pet?
How long before that had you seen your pet acting normally?
What was the first thing you noticed?
What other symptoms developed, if any? How soon?
Have the symptoms become better or worse since you first noticed them? Over
    what time span?

Information on any Suspected Poison

What is the name of the product?
Is it a liquid concentrate, diluted spray, or solid?
Do you still have the container?
How long ago do you think your pet was exposed to the poison?
Where do you think it happened?

Your Pet's Recent Activity

Did your pet eat his/her food as usual last night or this morning?
What is he/she normally fed?
Anything different lately?
Has your pet been off your property within the last 24 hours?
Has your pet had any antiflea products applied within the last week?

(Box continued on following page)

■ TOXICOLOGIC HISTORY FORM (Continued)

Your Pet's Environment

Is your pet normally kept inside or outside the house? Or both? Different during
  day or night?
Is your pet kept in a fenced-in area? Or tied up?
Any access to neighboring properties (even for a short time)?
Where has your pet been in the last 24 hours?
Has your pet been to rural areas within the last week?

Your Household's Recent Activity

Has there been any gardening work done lately?
Any compost, fertilizer, or weed killers used within the last week?
Any construction work or renovations underway?
Any mouse/rat baits present in the house/garage/shed/barn?
Any cleaning products used inside or outside the house within the last 48 hours?
  Which?

Any Other Comments or Information?

Stabilization of vital signs should have four major goals of treatment:

1a. Maintain Respiration Provide an immediate oxygen source if the patient demonstrates any degree of respiratory compromise. For immediate short-term oxygen supply, a mask, oxygen hood, or percutaneous tracheal cannula is appropriate. For longer-term oxygen supply, an intranasal cannula, endotracheal intubation, or an oxygen cage is suitable. Ventilatory assistance may become necessary and should be employed if needed. Irritant or corrosive substances may cause such damage to the oropharyngeal mucosa that a tracheostomy may be required. Arterial blood gases or pulse oximetry, or both, should be used to monitor ventilatory status. (See also p. 612.)

1b. Maintain Cardiovascular Function An IV catheter should be placed immediately and used for administration of fluid therapy, inotropes, and antiarrhythmics as applicable. Lactated Ringer's solution is the initial fluid of choice; adjustments to fluid therapy can be made later based on serum electrolytes and chemistries. Some toxins can cause severe arrhythmias and any critically ill patient is at increased risk for arrhythmias. ECG monitoring should be employed routinely and arrhythmias managed according to standard therapy. Some toxins cause hemolysis or methemoglobinemia; some cause coagulopathies; whole blood, packed RBCs, cells and frozen plasma should be available and used if necessary. Methemoglobinemia is generally treated by administration of ascorbic acid and methylene blue. (See also p. 612.)

1c. Control CNS Excitation Diazepam is the drug of choice for initial control of CNS excitation, but may need to be followed shortly with muscle relaxants such as guaifenesin or methocarbamol (see Table 1–32 for doses). Animals who are in status epilepticus subsequent to poisoning should be classified as high-risk and the clinician should realize that they may not require the usual full dose of anesthetics or sedatives. IV phenobarbital can be used to maintain longer-term control of seizures, but, clinicians must ensure that the toxic material is being effectively eliminated from the body before using long-acting sedatives which may mask the continued presence of the poison.

1d. Control Body Temperature Animals may present as either hypo- or hyperthermic, depending upon the toxin ingested and the stage of toxicity. Hypothermia can be managed with heating pads and hot-water bottles to provide a source of warmth, and by using "space blankets" or bubble wrap packing material to provide insulation. Hyperthermia can be managed by quickly bathing the animal in lukewarm water until the rectal temperature reaches 39.5°C (103°F). If sedatives or anesthetics have been used, initial hyperthermia will rapidly resolve due to the loss of thermoregulatory control, and bathing should not be performed. (See also p. 97.)

............*Step 2. Obtain History and Evaluate Patient*

2a. Obtain History When initial stabilization of vital signs has been accomplished, the veterinarian can then discuss the patient history with the owner. Use of the Toxicologic History Form on p. 219 can be helpful in obtaining a complete scenario and all relevant information.

Initially, in urgent situations, the veterinarian needs to know:

- When was the animal last seen as normal?
- What was the progression of symptoms?
- How fast did it all happen?

In questioning the owner, make sure to cover the basic areas of:

- Onset of clinical signs
- Animal's activity
- Owner's activity
- Access to poisonous substances

The time elapsed since the animal was last seen in a normal state provides the veterinarian with a time frame in which the poison was probably accessed, allowing differentials to be ranked in some order of probability by rate of onset.

In eliciting a history from the owner about the animal's access to poisons, it is important not to take anything for granted. Many owners do not realize how poisonous common substances can be, such as insecticidal products, garbage, and cleaning chemicals. Many owners will deny that their dog or cat could have eaten any such thing, not wanting to believe that the source of toxin might be from within their own household or property. It is useful to phrase questions in a neutral fashion. e.g., "Is the (substance) present on the premises?" rather than asking, "Could the dog have eaten (substance)?" This approach serves to minimize any bias or preconceptions.

When questioning the owner about recent events, it is useful to realize and acknowledge that disruption in household routine is a distinct risk factor for accidents, including poisonings. Examples of such disruptions are moving house, family member illness or hospitalization, and renovations or new construction. These events all too often result in doors or gates left open, animals outside instead of usually inside (or vice versa), and different people watching the animal—all of which mean that the safeguards of a normally careful owner may have been disrupted. Once the owners are made aware of the importance of assessing access and risk, they are often able to provide insight into otherwise baffling circumstances.

2b. Evaluate Patient Patient evaluation should normally consist of three elements:

1. Physical examination.
2. Minimal laboratory database.
3. Sample collection for analysis.

Physical Examination It is important to systematically evaluate the patient's physical status, focusing particularly on clues associated with common poisons in veterinary medicine, such as organophosphate toxicity and anticoagulant rodenticides or those poisons common to a geographical region, such as snail bait or an insect or spider venom. The checklist below is useful.

■ PHYSICAL EXAMINATION CHECKLIST

EENT (Eyes, Ears, Nose, Throat)

Pupil size?
Ocular examination normal?
Sensitivity to sound?
Nose—moist, dry, bubbling, caked with dirt?
Throat—any characteristic odors on breath?
Any traces of foreign material on tongue or in crevices of molars or gums?

CARDIOVASCULAR

Mucous membrane color?
Capillary refill time—rapid, slow?
Heart rate—increased or decreased?
Femoral pulse strength—bounding, normal, faint? Pulse deficits?
Heart rhythm—auscultation, ECG

RESPIRATORY

Rate—fast, slow?
Character—shallow, labored, agonal?
Auscultation—pulmonary congestion, harsh airway sounds?

GASTROINTESTINAL, HEPATIC

What is the rectal temperature?
Any excessive salivation?
Evidence of vomiting?
Abdominal palpation—painful?
Intestinal loops liquid- or gas-filled or ropy?
Feces—color character, consistency?

UROGENITAL

Bladder palpable?
Urine production?
Urine color?

MUSCULOSKELETAL, NEUROLOGIC

Gait: Walking or recumbent? Weak? Ataxic? Hypermetric? Muscle fasciculations?
    Increased extensor tone?
Attitude: Score the animal's level of consciousness on a simple scale:
    Alert
    Responds to voice
    Responds to touch
    Responds to pain
    Doesn't respond—unconscious

INTEGUMENT

Any wet patches that smell of foreign substances?
Any erythematous regions on the skin?

PERIPHERAL LYMPH NODES

Should be normal in poisonings

Minimum Database Much information useful in the initial management of toxicities can be obtained from a simple minimal database that can be done in-house.

- Packed cell volume and total protein
- Urine specific gravity and dipstick analysis
- Serum urea and glucose (dipsticks available)

Use the information obtained from the minimum data base to evaluate for:

- Dehydration
- Hemoconcentration or anemia
- Azotemia and source (prerenal, renal postrenal)
- Hypo- or hyperglycemia

Samples should also be drawn for panels that may require outside laboratory analysis:

- Serum electrolytes
- Blood gases
- Serum osmolality
- Complete hemogram
- Serum chemistry profile

Samples of serum, urine, and any vomitus should be obtained as well, in case toxicologic analysis is required later.

............Step 3. Prevent Continued Absorption of the Toxin

The veterinarian may have to employ a variety of methods to remove poisons from the GI tract, such as emesis, gastric lavage, cathartics, or enemas. For certain toxins, adsorbents, ion exchange resins, or precipitating or chelating agents can be used. Removal of toxic substances from body surfaces may also be necessary, depending upon the toxin. These procedures are discussed below. Both emesis and gastric lavage are fading from use in human emergency medicine because of the risk of aspiration and some doubt about their efficacy. Currently, management of poisonings in human medicine relies heavily upon the use of activated charcoal combined with sorbitol as a cathartic where appropriate, and supportive critical care. However, this approach should be taken in the context that the vast majority of poisonings in humans relate to drug overdoses, illicit or otherwise, which have a relatively small volume and rapid absorption. Furthermore, adoption of this approach rests upon the availability of a hospital intensive care infrastructure, which is not always available in veterinary practice.

3a. Emetics

Principles of Usage Use emetics only if the animal's physiology is stable, i.e., not seizuring, not in mental or respiratory depression. Do not give the same emetic more than twice. If it doesn't work after two doses, switch to a different emetic or go to gastric lavage. *Emetics are strictly contraindicated for petroleum products and corrosives because the risk of aspiration and further damage to the esophagus is too great.* Emetics may also be of little value if poisons with antiemetic properties have been ingested, such as the benzodiazepines and tricyclic antidepressants.

Various emetics used in veterinary medicine are listed below. Apomorphine remains the standard, but is less useful in certain situations, i.e, with poisons that cause CNS stimulation, and in cats. Other emetics include syrup of ipecac, ordinary table salt, and xylazine.

■ EMETICS

Apomorphine

Supplied: 6.25 mg tablets, soluble.
Dose: 0.02–0.04 mg/kg IV, IM, or place part of the tablet in the conjunctival fornix (SC route not recommended; onset and duration of effect are unnecessarily prolonged).
Onset: 5 minutes.
Mechanism: Stimulates dopaminergic receptors in chemoreceptor trigger zone. Causes both CNS depression and stimulation, usually more stimulation. Some respiratory depression.
Adverse effects: Respiratory depression, protracted vomiting. Undesirable CNS excitation in snail bait poisonings sometimes. Not recommended for use in cats.

Syrup of Ipecac (7%)

Dose: Dogs:1–2 mL/kg PO; cats: 3.3 mL/kg PO.
Onset: 10–30 minutes.
Mechanism: Gastric irritant and chemoreceptor trigger zone stimulation.
Adverse effects: Cardiotoxicity $\Rightarrow$ arrhythmias.
Notes: (1) Not to be confused with fluid extract of ipecac, which is concentrated form; (2) out-of-date syrup of ipecac can still be used; (3) cats hate the taste.

Hydrogen Peroxide (3% Solution)

Dose: 1–2 mL/kg PO, can be repeated once
Onset: 10 minutes
Mechanism: Presumably gastric irritation
Adverse effects: None known.

Xylazine

Dose: 0.5–1.0 mg/kg IM
Onset: 5–10 minutes
Mechanism: Centrally acting α_2 agonist
Adverse effects: Respiratory depression, bradycardia, sedation

Sodium Chloride (Table Salt) (for owners at home)

Dose: 1–3 tsp.
Onset: 5–10 minutes.
Mechanism: Gastric irritant.
Adverse effects: Hematemesis. Theoretically, hypernatremia if vomiting does not occur. Beware usage in young animals easy to overdose. Follow successful emesis with ad lib water.

3b. Gastric Lavage If done within 1 to 2 hours of poison ingestion, gastric lavage can be very effective. It is messy, but even if a poisons table is not available the procedure can and should be performed for those toxins that warrant it (outdoors, if necessary). The box below provides a quick checklist of equipment needed for gastric lavage. Several prerequisites are needed for maximum effectiveness. The patient should be unconscious or lightly anesthetized. Diazepam and ketamine or oxymorphone provides, short-duration anesthesia of the appropriate depth (refer to Table 1–32 for doses). Pass a cuffed endotracheal tube to prevent aspiration of gastric contents. Pass a large-bore stomach tube (same diameter or bigger than the endotracheal tube) to serve as an egress tube for the lavaged material. Then pass a second *small-bore* stomach tube to serve as a fluid ingress tube. This method sets up a circuit of fluid flow, allowing rapid and complete emptying of the stomach. Avoid passing the stomach tubes too far and avoid using too much water pressure. Keep one hand on the animal's abdomen to monitor gastric filling and do not overdistend the stomach with water.

■ EQUIPMENT NEEDED FOR GASTRIC LAVAGE

Large-bore stomach tube, with extra fenestrations at one end
Small-bore stomach tube, with flared end or funnel attached
Endotracheal tube, cuffed
Hose-faucet connections
Water source (warm)
Small amount of obstetrical lubricant
Mouth gag

The lavage should be repeated until the lavage fluid runs clear. This will require at least 5 to 10 mL/kg of water or saline. In some cases where solid material has been ingested, the lavage volume required will be much more than this. Keep the animal's head lowered during the lavage procedure. It is sometimes helpful to put the animal in both right and left lateral recumbency during the lavage to help ensure that the stomach is well emptied.

At the end of the lavage, remove the small ingress tube and double-check that the endotracheal tube is still in place and appropriately cuffed. Then administer a slurry of activated charcoal (see Table 1–32 for dose) through the large-bore egress tube if desired. Then kink off the large-bore tube and remove it. Do not remove the endotracheal tube immediately; leave it in place until the animal is semiconscious so as to minimize the risk of aspiration.

3c. Enemas Enemas are useful in facilitating the action of cathartics and in cases where the poison is a solid material, such as compost, garbage, or snail bait. It is best to simply use lukewarm water. Commercial phosphate enema solutions can cause severe electrolyte (hypernatremia, hypocalcemia, hypomagnesemia) and acid-base (metabolic acidosis) disturbances in small dogs and cats and should not be used for those toxins which place renal function at risk, due to aggravation of hyperphosphatemia.

The fluid volume required will depend upon the size of the animal and the state of its lower GI tract. As with gastric lavage, the objective is to continue the procedure until the water runs clear. If difficulty is encountered with emptying the lower GI tract, it is better to repeat the enema in 1 to 2 hours than to be overzealous on the first attempt.

■ EQUIPMENT NEEDED FOR ENEMA ADMINISTRATION

Tubing

Cats: Soft IV tubing, or dog urinary catheter. Melt sharp edges with a match to round them.
Dogs: Soft rubber tubing, about 1 cm in diameter

Obstetrical Lubricant

Use nonsterile water-soluble lubricant.

(Box continued on following page)

■ EQUIPMENT NEEDED FOR ENEMA ADMINISTRATION *(Continued)*

Fluid Reservoir

Cats: Use an old IV fluid bag
Dogs: Need approximately 1 L

Fluid

Warm water, with or without soap

3d. Cathartics Cathartics are useful for hastening GI elimination of undesirable substances and are particularly useful for most ingested solid toxicants, such as compost, garbage or snail baits. They can be used in conjunction with activated charcoal. Magnesium-based cathartics should not be used in CNS-depressant toxicoses because hypermagnesemia may further exacerbate CNS depression.

■ CATHARTICS

Sodium Sulfate (Glauber's Salts, GoLYTELY)

Dose: 250–500 mg/kg in 10 × volume of water

Sorbitol (70%)

Dose: 3 mL/kg PO

Magnesium Sulfate (Epsom Salts)

Less effective than sodium sulfate and may produce clinical signs of hypermagnesemia

Mineral Oil (Paraffin Oil)

Dose: 5–15 mL per dog; 2–6 mL per cat
Is not normally absorbed across intestinal wall. Do not use in conjunction with dioctyl sodium sulfosuccinate as emulsification may cause accumulation of indigestible oil in the liver. *No longer recommended* for organochlorine insecticide and other organic compound ingestions.

Vegetable Oil

Not recommended due to its absorption across the intestinal wall. Increases absorption of oil-soluble toxicants; pancreatitis is a possibility.

Note: All cathartics should be given approximately 30 minutes after administration of activated charcoal.

3e. Adsorbents
Activated charcoal is the safest and to date most effective adsorbent for ingested toxins. It can be administered following emesis or gastric lavage, or can be administered as a sole treatment. Various preparations are available on the market, including dry powder, compressed tablets, granules, and liquid suspensions. Vegetable-origin activated charcoal is the most efficient adsorbent and binds compounds with weak, nonionic bonds. Some preparations are combines with sorbitol to provide simultaneous administration of an adsorbent and cathartic; this combination has been shown to be efficacious. Repeated

administration of activated charcoal every 4 to 6 hours has been shown to be beneficial in management of toxicoses by interrupting enterohepatic recycling. Administration of an oily cathartic in conjunction with activated charcoal will serve only to reduce the absorptive surface of activated charcoal and they should not be used together. There are some substances that are not well adsorbed by activated charcoal—generally, substances that are highly soluble and readily absorbed, such as alkalis, nitrates, mineral acids, ethanol, methanol, ferrous sulfate, ammonia, and cyanide.

Whatever preparation is used, the dose of activated charcoal remains at 1 to 4 g/kg of body weight. The high end of the dose range should be used whenever possible. Activated charcoal powder can be effectively mixed for easy administration if the powder is put first into the mixing container, followed by a small amount (10 to 20 mL) of a viscous liquid such as Kaopectate or (radiographic) barium sulfate. Once the charcoal is mixed with the viscous liquid, a suitable amount of water can then be successfully added to create a pourable slurry. One cup of activated charcoal powder weighs approximately 75 g. The compressed tablets are somewhat less effective than the powder and should definitely be given at the higher end of the dose range. The tablets commonly contain 300 mg each of activated charcoal; at that strength one would need to give *at least* four tablets per kilogram.

Kaolin and *bentonite* are both clays that have been used as adsorbents. Both are generally less effective than activated charcoal. The clays, however, are reported to be better adsorbents than activated charcoal for the herbicide paraquat.

3f. Ion Exchange Resins Ion exchange resins can ionically bind certain drugs or toxins. Cholestyramine is one such resin, commonly used in human medicine to bind intestinal bile acids and thereby lower cholesterol absorption. Its application in toxicology extends to the absorption of fat-soluble toxins such as organochlorine and certain acidic compounds such as digitalis. Ion exchange resins have also been used to delay or reduce the absorption of phenylbutazone, warfarin, chlorothiazide, tetracycline, phenobarbital, and thyroid preparations.

3g. Precipitating, Chelating, and Diluting Agents These agents are used primarily in the management of heavy metal intoxications, but also for some plant toxic principles, such as alkaloids or oxalates. They work by binding preferentially to the metal ion and creating a more soluble complex which is amenable to renal excretion. Those chelating agents in common usage are calcium EDTA (ethylenediaminetetraacetic acid), deteroxamine, and D-penicillamine. Calcium EDTA and deferoxamine should both be kept in stock, as they are necessary for zinc and iron toxicity, respectively, both of which have a short window of opportunity for therapeutic intervention. D-penicillamine has wide application for a number of metal toxicities, but tends to be used more for long-term chronic therapy since it can be administered orally.

Various agents can be used for nonspecific dilution of toxins. Milk of magnesia and egg whites, while old-fashioned, still have wide application in many cases where low-grade irritants have been ingested.

3h. Eliminating Poison From the Skin Bathing the animal is an important aspect of treatment for topical exposures to toxins such as insecticidal products, petroleum-based substances, and aromatic oils. A cautionary note: bathing an ill animal is not an innocuous procedure. Care must be taken to avoid hypothermia and shock by using <u>warm</u> water at all times. Active drying should be performed to further minimize any risk of hypothermia. Rubber gloves and plastic aprons should be used to avoid exposure of the person bathing the animal.

For most substances, a mild dishwashing detergent is appropriate. Medicated or antibacterial shampoos are less appropriate in this situation. For petroleum-based substances particularly, mechanics' hand cleaners or coconut oil-based soaps are recommended in preference to dishwashing detergent. As a general principle, best results are obtained by barely wetting the patient until the detergent is worked well into the hair, keeping the amount of water in the hair coat at a minimum until ready for the rinse.

Oil-based paint is best removed by clipping rather than by attempting removal with solvents, since the solvents are also toxic.

3i. Eliminating Poison From the Eyes For ocular exposures, a minimum of 20 to 30 minutes of irrigation with warm (body temperature) normal saline is recommended. The use of neutralizing agents is generally not recommended. Following adequate irrigation, chemical burns to the eyes should be treated with lubricant ointments and possibly a temporary tarsorrhaphy. Atropine may be indicated as a cycloplegic agent. Daily follow-up examinations are required because epithelial damage may be delayed, especially with alkali burns, and it is difficult to predict the final extent of ocular damage. Topical corticosteroids should be used only if the corneal epithelium is intact; however systemic NSAIDs can and should be employed to reduce the ocular inflammatory response. (See also p. 86.)

............Step 4. Administer Antidote if Available

Refer to Tables 1–27 through 1–30 for the names of antidotes appropriate to a specific toxin. Refer to Table 1–32 for doses of antidotes.

There are three categories of agents used in the management of poisonings. The first category is specific antidotes, of which in fact there are only a few. Current recommendations for the use of these antidotes are noted in Table 1–32. There are some "classic" toxins and antidotes, now considered to be rare, such as curare and physostigmine, thallium and prussian blue, and fluoride and calcium borogluconate. These and a few others have been omitted from the tables. The second, broader category of antidotes is those drugs used in symptomatic management of clinical signs and which are part of our routine veterinary therapeutic stock. Drugs such as atropine, sedatives, and steroids fall within this category. These drugs are also listed in the tables where applicable. The third category comprises nonspecific decontaminants, such as activated charcoal, cathartics, and emetics. These have been discussed earlier and are included in the tables where appropriate.

............Step 5. Facilitate Clearance or Metabolism of Absorbed Toxin

Many patients can benefit from efforts to enhance clearance or metabolism of absorbed toxins. Some specific therapies have been developed with this in mind, such as 4-methylpyrazole in ethylene glycol toxicity and specific antibodies such as Digibind (digoxin immune Fab [ovine]) for digitalis toxicity. More generally, other strategies may be aimed at promoting renal excretion. Renal excretion strategies include diuresis, ion trapping, and peritoneal or hemodialysis. The first two are applicable to a large number of toxins and are discussed in more detail below. Those toxins to which diuresis, urine acidification, or urine alkalinization apply have the notation 5a, 5b, or 5c, respectively.

Enhancing renal excretion of substances is most useful for those organic substances that are present in significant concentrations in the plasma. Substances that are nonionic and primarily lipid-soluble, such as some of the herbicides, are likely to be little affected by attempts at renal elimination.

Before commencing any diuresis or ion trapping, IV fluid therapy should be adequate as indicated by normal central venous pressure, urine output, and mean arterial pressure. If any of these valves are less than normal, other measures should first be employed to ensure adequate renal perfusion, including, but not limited to, a constant-rate infusion of dopamine.

5a. Diuresis Simple fluid diuresis is of some influence on the excretion of certain substances. The use of mannitol as an osmotic diuretic will reduce passive resorption of toxic substances in the proximal convoluted tubule by reducing water resorption there. Dextrose (50%) can also be used as an osmotic diuretic. Furosemide can be used to promote diuresis, but, again, is no substitute for fluid therapy. Care should be taken to avoid patient dehydration when using any diuretic; central venous pressure monitoring is strongly recommended.

5b and 5c. Urine Acidification and Alkalinization

Ion trapping is based on the principle that ionized substances do not cross renal tubular membranes easily and are not well resorbed. If the urinary pH can be changed so that the toxin's chemical equilibrium shifts to its ionized form, then that toxin is "trapped" in the urine. Alkaline urine favors the ionization of acidic compounds, and acidic urine favors the ionization of alkaline compounds. Those toxins amenable to ion trapping are mostly weak acids and weak bases.

5b. Urine Acidification Use ammonium chloride (see Table 1–33). Contraindications to the use of ammonium chloride include preexisting metabolic acidosis, hepatic or renal insufficiency, and hemolysis or rhabdomyolysis leading to hematuria or myoglobinuria. Signs of ammonia intoxication include depression and coma. Monitor serum potassium concentration and urine pH frequently.

5c. Urine Alkalinization Use sodium bicarbonate (see Table 1–32). Contraindications to the use of sodium bicarbonate include metabolic alkalosis (particularly a risk with concurrent use of furosemide), hypocalcemia, and hypokalemia. As with urine acidification, monitor the serum potassium concentration and urine pH frequently.

···········Step 6. Supportive and Symptomatic Care of the Poisoning Patient

The five major steps in management of poisonings must be accompanied by application of the fundamentals of critical care. Respiratory and cardiovascular support have been discussed in earlier. Renal function, GI function, and analgesia are also particularly relevant to the poisoning patient, and are discussed below.

6a. Maintenance of Renal Perfusion This is a priority in the poisoning patient. Fluid balance and electrolyte and acid-base control must be accurate. These patients are generally all at high risk for renal damage and acute renal failure, whether by a primary toxic insult to the renal parenchyma or by acute or prolonged renal hypoperfusion. For this reason, a protocol which aims to prevent oliguria and ensuing acute renal failure is one of the therapeutic strategies which should be routinely employed.

This protocol consists of:

- IV fluid therapy at maintenance rates, using balanced electrolyte solution
- Urinary catheterization and collection
- Monitoring urine output hourly
- Monitoring serum creatinine and urea q6h
- Monitoring serum electrolytes q6h
- Monitoring central venous pressure q2h
- A *rapid* response to a drop in urine production to less than 1 mL/kg/hr

1. Initial fluid challenge with colloid of dextran 70 or a similar 5 mL/kg IV colloid.
2. If no response within 30 minutes, then dopamine at a constant-rate infusion.
3. If no response within 30 minutes, consider mannitol 0.5 g/kg IV.
4. If no response to mannitol within 1 hour, consider furosemide.
5. If no response to furosemide, peritoneal dialysis is indicated immediately.

6b. Gastrointestinal Protectants These may be required for the management of those poisons which are GI irritants or ulcerogenic. Cimetidine, ranitidine, sucralfate, and misoprostol may all be helpful. Refer to p. 955 for dose information.

6c. Antiemetics These may be necessary to suppress intractable vomiting. Metoclopramide is commonly used, as it is the drug of choice for centrally induced nausea. However, antiemetics that work by different mechanisms may be used in combination as necessary. Examples are dopamine$_2$-receptor antagonists such as prochlorperazine and droperidol, 5-hydroxytryptamine antagonists such as ondansetron, and H$_1$-antagonists such as diphenhydramine. Refer to p. 955 for further information on antiemetics.

6d. Analgesics Analgesics are more commonly appropriate in poisoning patients than was once thought. Common effects of poisons such as severe gastroenteritis or topical burns and ulcerations may warrant the use of analgesics. Longer-acting narcotic agonist-antagonists, such as butorphanol or buprenorphine, are particularly useful. See Table 1–33 for dose information.

6e. Nutritional Support This may be necessary in many of these patients, since they commonly have GI damage or may need to be sedated for long periods. Endoscopy may be helpful in judging the degree of esophageal and gastric damage, particularly after ingestion of alkalis or other corrosives. Enteral and parenteral nutrition may be necessary. See p. 537 for information on these techniques.

REFERENCES

Bailey EM Jr, Garland T: Toxicologic emergencies. *In* Murtaugh RJ, Kaplan PJ, eds: Veterinary Emergency and Critical Care Medicine. St Louis, Mosby–Year Book, 1992, p 427.

Beasley VR, ed: Toxicology of selected pesticides, drugs and chemicals. Vet Clin North Am Small Anim Pract 20:1990.

Dorman DC: Diagnosing and treating toxicoses in dogs and cats. Veterinary Medicine, February and March 1997.

Dumonceaux GA: Household toxicoses in exotic animals and pet birds. *In* Kirk RW, Bonagura JD, eds: Kirk's Current Veterinary Therapy XI. Small Animal Practice. Philadelphia, WB Saunders, 1992. p 178.

Firth AM: Recommendations for antidotes and therapeutics used in management of toxicities. *In* Bonagura JD, ed: Kirk's Current Veterinary Therapy XIII. Small Animal Practice. Philadelphia, WB Saunders, 1998.

Knight MW, Dorman DC: Selected poisonous plant concerns in small animals. Veterinary Medicine, March 1997, pp 260–272.

Osweiler GD, Carson TL: Toxicology. *In* Morgan RV ed: Handbook of Small Animal Practice, ed 3. Philadelphia, WB Saunders, 1997, p 1247.

..........SNAKE BITES
..........Nonpoisonous Bites

Identify the offending reptile, if possible.

..........Clinical Signs

1. The bite wound is usually multitoothed and relatively painless.
2. Local reaction is usually negligible. Bites by large pet snakes, boas and pythons, can cause marked trauma, and bone fractures are possible.

3. Bites appear as superficial scratches and do not produce signs of envenomation. Several species of colubrids (the "typical" snakes) have been documented to produce moderate to severe envenomations; therefore, these "nonpoisonous" snakes may be more hazardous than previously assumed.

.... Treatment

1. Clip the hair, clean the wound carefully with surgical soap, and, if needed, apply a sterile, dry dressing.
2. Because of the extensive bacterial flora of snake mouths, broad-spectrum systemic antibiotics are indicated.
3. All snakebite victims should be observed closely for 4 to 6 hours following the bite. This is extremely important when the identity of the offending reptile is in question.
4. Modify treatment appropriately if signs of envenomation appear (see the next section, Poisonous Bites).

.... Poisonous Bites

There are two groups of venomous snakes in North America: pit vipers and coral snakes.

All venomous snakes are dangerous; however, the severity of any given bite is dependent upon several factors. These include (1) toxicity of the venom, (2) the amount of venom injected, (3) the site of envenomation and medical intervention.

.... Pit Vipers

The vast majority of reptile envenomations in the United States are inflicted by pit vipers. Included in this group are the water moccasin (cottonmouth), copperhead, and numerous species of rattlesnakes. Pit vipers are characterized by a deep pit located between the eye and nostril, elliptic pupils, and retractable front fangs (Fig. 1–12).

Signs Local signs of pit viper envenomation may include the following:

1. Presence of bleeding puncture wounds (i.e., one fang is capable of severe envenomation, or local edema may close puncture wounds).
2. Immediate severe pain.
3. Edema, petechiae, and ecchymosis. These usually develop rapidly; however, severe envenomation may occur without marked local signs.
4. Decreased sensitivity. With time, the area becomes less sensitive.
5. Subsequent tissue necrosis.

Systemic signs of pit viper envenomation may include the following:

1. Marked hypotension and shock.
2. Coagulopathies.
3. Lethargy and weakness.
4. Muscle fasciculations.
5. Lymphangitis.
6. Rhabdomyolysis.
7. Neurologic signs, such as respiratory depression, especially with some Mojave and canebrake rattlesnake envenomations (several species of rattlesnakes have subpopulations identified with venoms containing a potent neurotoxin—Mojave toxin A).

Clinical signs of severe envenomation may take several hours to appear; therefore, all suspected victims should be hospitalized and monitored for 24

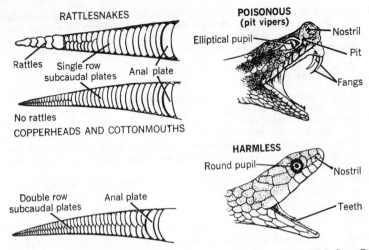

Figure I–12. Characteristics of poisonous snakes. (From Parrish, HM, Carr CA: Bites by copperheads *(Ancistrodon contortrix)* in the United States. JAMA 201:927, 1967.)

hours. The severity of envenomation cannot be judged solely by the degree of local tissue reaction.

Diagnosis Obtain a laboratory baseline upon presentation: CBC, PTT, PT, platelet count, creatine kinase (CK), BUN, and urine hemoglobin and myoglobin. These should be repeated in 6 hours and thereafter as necessary. Any abnormal value is an indicator of moderate to severe envenomation. Platelet counts can be sensitive indicators, along with prolonged clotting times, of the severity and progressiveness of some severe envenomations and should be repeated as needed.

Measure the circumference of the affected body part above, below, and at the bite site. Measurements should be recorded at set intervals. This will allow objective assessment of the progression of tissue swelling.

Treatment Pit viper venom consists of multiple fractions; thus envenomation should be approached as a complex poisoning.

Treatment should be initiated as early as possible. First-aid measures are of little value, and rapid transport to a medical facility is the best advice for owners.

1. Give diphenhydramine 10 mg for small dogs and cats; for large dogs, give up to 25 mg IV or SC. This drug has no effect upon venom; however, it aids in calming the victim and pretreating a possible reaction to antivenin.
2. Give IV fluids: lactated Ringer's solution or 0.9% NaCl. Give aggressive fluid therapy, as the majority of deaths are due to cardiovascular collapse from marked vascular leakage and pooling of blood.
3. Administer antivenin (Wyeth-Ayerst, Philadelphia).
   a. Administer a minimum of one vial, with dosage dependent upon clinical signs and laboratory values. Smaller patients may require larger doses of neutralizing antibody. This will make them more susceptible to delayed serum sickness 7 to 14 days post administration.
   b. Antivenin must be mixed with a swirling action to prevent foaming.
   c. IV administration is slow to prevent complement-mediated reaction to

foreign proteins, is easiest to mix in with IV fluids, and should be in such a volume to allow complete administration within 1 hour.

d. Skin testing is highly unreliable.

e. Monitor inner pinna for hyperemia while administering antivenin as an indicator of a possible allergic reaction; also look for nausea or pruritus.

f. Epinephrine should be available but is rarely needed. The incidence of true anaphylaxis to antivenin is less than 2%. If a reaction occurs, stop infusion of antivenin and give antihistamine. Wait 10 minutes, and re-start antivenin infusion slowly. If the reaction recurs, stop the infusion and seek consultation.

g. The earlier antivenin is given, the more effective its action. Antivenin can correct snake venom–induced clotting abnormalities even 72 hours post envenomation.

h. Bite site or IM administration of antivenin should be avoided, as uptake is markedly delayed.

i. Low platelet counts may recur 3 to 4 days post antivenin administration. The significance of this phenomenon is unknown, as clinical bleeding usually does not develop. Additional antivenin should be considered if platelet levels are lower than 50,000 μL or if petechiae or ecchymoses develop.

Note: Corticosteroids should be avoided, as they may increase the severity of toxicity. They also alter important laboratory values necessary for monitoring the status of the patient. Cryotherapy is contraindicated.

············ Coral Snakes

Coral snakes are characterized by fixed front fangs and brightly colored bands fully encircling the body, with black and red bands separated by yellow bands. Types include the eastern coral, Texas coral, and Sonoran coral snakes.

Signs Local signs of coral snake envenomation may include:

1. Small puncture wounds.
2. Transient initial pain.

Systemic signs may be delayed as long as 18 hours. These signs include:

1. Fasciculations.
2. Weakness.
3. Difficulty swallowing (aspiration is a common complication).
4. Pinpoint pupils.
5. Bulbar paralysis with respiratory collapse (primary cause of death).
6. Severe hemolysis (monitor hemoglobinuria).

Treatment

1. If coral snakebite is highly suspected, start early and aggressive antivenin administration before onset of clinical signs (use a minimum of two vials). Therapeutic benefits may not be obtained if antivenin is given after the onset of clinical signs. Although the onset of clinical signs may be delayed, once they develop, they progress with alarming rapidity.

2. If respiratory paralysis occurs, it can be managed with respiratory support. It usually will subside within 48 to 72 hours.

3. Aspiration pneumonia is the primary complication and is due to pharyngeal paralysis. The clinician should be prepared to prevent this via intubation.

4. Several weeks may be necessary for complete recovery.

Note: Antivenin (Elapidae) (Wyeth) is not effective against Sonoran coral snake venom, and treatment consists of supportive care. Coral snake antivenin is of equine origin. See discussion of antivenin under Pit Vipers for administration precautions.

............OTHER VENOMOUS BITES

............Gila Monster* *(Heloderma suspectum)* and Mexican Beaded Lizard *(Heloderma horridum)* Bite

The lizards of the family Helodermatidae are the only two poisonous lizards in the world. They are found in the southwestern United States and Mexico. The venom glands are located on either side of the lower jaw. These heavy-bodied lizards are lethargic and nonaggressive, and animal poisonings are therefore rare. The lizards do not have fangs per se but rather grooved teeth. These lizards hold tenaciously onto the victim and, with chewing movements, increase the quantity of envenomation. The vast majority of victims are dogs bitten on the upper lip. Bites by these lizards are extremely painful.

............Treatment

There are no proven first-aid measures. The lizard can be disengaged by using a prying instrument between the jaws and pushing against the back of the mouth. A flame to the underside of the lizard's jaw seems to be very effective. The teeth of the lizard are very brittle and often will break off in the bite wound. Topical irrigation (not infusion) with lidocaine and probing with a needle will help to find these teeth. The bite wounds bleed profusely and should be cleaned and mild pressure applied until the hemorrhage subsides. IV fluids should be started, and the patient should be monitored for the onset of hypotension. The degree of envenomation correlates well with the duration of the bite. There is no antivenin, and treatment thus is supportive. Antibiotic therapy is indicated.

............Brown Spiders (Fiddleback, Brown Recluse, Arizona Brown, *Loxosceles* spp.)

The small brown nonaggressive spider has a violin-shaped marking on the cephalothorax (the neck of the violin points toward the abdomen) and three sets of eyes. Brown spiders are found primarily in the southern half of the United States.

The venom has a potent enduring dermonecrotic effect, starting as a classic "bulls-eye" lesion. This is followed by enlarging indolent ulceration into dependent tissues. The ulcer formation may take several days to become evident and may take several months to heal. It often leaves a disfiguring scar. Ulceration is mediated by polymorphonuclear neutrophils (PMNs) and complement influx into the bite area. General systemic reactions are rare but may include hemolysis, thrombocytopenia, fever, weakness, and joint pain. Fatalities are possible.

............Treatment

There is no specific antidote. Dapsone has been recommended at a dose of 1 mg/kg for 14 days. The remaining ulcer should then heal as any open wound. Surgical excision has been advocated in the past; however, the ulcer must be at its full size or excised in the very early stages to be effective. Corticosteroids

---

*See Russell in the references for an excellent chapter on the Gila monster.

may be of value if used within 48 hours of the bite. Unfortunately, the diagnosis in veterinary patients is extremely difficult until the full ulcer is formed (7 to 14 days following the bite). Antibiotic therapy is advised with large or deep ulcerations.

............Black Widow Spider (*Latrodectus* spp.)

The adult female may be recognized by an hourglass-shaped marking, red to orange, on the underside of her globose, shiny, black abdomen. It is equally important to identify the immature female with a colorful pattern of red, brown, and beige on the dorsal surface of her abdomen, as she has the same potential for envenomation. As a result of his small size, the male is unable to penetrate the skin. These spiders are found throughout the United States and Canada.

The venom is neurotoxic and acts presynaptically, releasing large amounts of acetylcholine and norepinephrine. There is seasonal variation in venom toxicity, lowest in spring and highest in fall. The spider controls the amount of venom it injects.

In dogs, envenomation results in hyperesthesia with dull progressive muscle pain, hypertension, fasciculations, and intense excitability. Muscle rigidity (often abdominal) without tenderness is a hallmark. Tonic-clonic convulsions are rare but may occur.

Paralytic signs are particularly marked in cats and appear early. Cats are extremely sensitive to the toxin. Increased salivation, possible diarrhea, and vomiting occur. The body loses tonus and becomes adynamic. Afflicted cats often lose up to 20% of their body weight in the first 24 hours following envenomation.

............Treatment

Antivenin (Wyeth-Ayerst, Philadelphia) is available and should be administered as soon as possible. One vial IV is usually sufficient. Pretreatment with antihistamines and monitoring for systemic reactions to horse serum are advised. If antivenin is not available, a slow IV infusion of 10% calcium gluconate while carefully monitoring cardiac rate and rhythm will aid in antagonizing the effects of the venom.

REFERENCES

Kitchens CS, Van Mierop LHS: Envenomation by the eastern coral snake *(Micrurus fulvius fulvius)*: A study of 39 victims. JAMA 258:1615–1618, 1987.
Marks S, Mannella C, Schaer M: Coral snake envenomation in the dog: Report of 4 cases. J Am Anim Hop Assoc 26:629, 1990.
Rauber A: Black widow spider bites. J Toxicol Clin Toxicol 21:473–485, 1983–1984.
Rees RS, Altenbern DP, Lynch JB, et al: Brown recluse spider bites: A comparison of early surgical excision versus dapsone and delayed surgical excision. Ann Surg 202:658, 1985.
Russell FE: Snake Venom Poisoning. Great Neck, NY, Scholum International, 1983.

Respiratory Emergencies

Respiratory emergencies threaten the patient by producing severe hypoxia and hypercarbia. The conditions most often encountered result in air flow obstruction, prevention of normal expansion of the lungs, interference with alveolar gas exchange (ventilation-perfusion abnormalities), and alteration of pulmonary circulation.

............INITIAL EVALUATION OF THE PATIENT IN RESPIRATORY DISTRESS

............General Signs of Respiratory Distress

Animals in respiratory distress have a rapid respiratory rate (>30 breaths per minute). With increasing distress they become anxious and open mouth–breathe. They become reluctant to move from a sternal position with the neck extended and the elbows abducted. Cyanosis of the mucous membranes indicates extreme decompensation.

Animals with acute exacerbation of a more chronic problem may have a history of cough, noisy respirations, or exercise intolerance.

............Localization of Disease

Localization of the cause of respiratory distress is essential to successful management. It is essential to attempt to localize the cause of the respiratory distress by rapid assessment of the patient. Primary cardiac failure (see p. 54) and decreased oxygen-carrying capacity of the blood—e.g., severe anemia (see p. 656), carbon monoxide poisoning (see p. 612), and methemoglobinemia (see p. 612)—must be considered, in addition to primary respiratory diseases.

Respiratory disorders can usually be localized to the upper airway, pleural cavity, or pulmonary parenchyma by observing the pattern of respirations and through careful auscultation (see p. 353). Such localization is extremely useful in the initial stabilization of the patient. The pattern of respiration should be confirmed by placing a hand on the chest wall to be sure that the periods of inspiration and expiration have not been confused due to marked abdominal excursions.

............Upper Airway Obstruction

The *upper airway* is defined herein as the pharynx, larynx, and extrathoracic trachea. Marked inspiratory efforts with a prolonged inspiratory time are typical. Inspiratory wheezing audible without a stethoscope, stridor, is often heard. Auscultation of the larynx and trachea reveals more subtle obstructions to normal air flow. Lung sounds are normal. The neck is palpated for mass lesions, tracheal collapse, or subcutaneous emphysema (suggestive of a tracheal tear). Historic voice change suggests laryngeal involvement.

Rule out: laryngeal paralysis, brachycephalic airway syndrome, laryngeal edema, laryngeal collapse, tracheal or pharyngeal foreign body, tracheal collapse, fracture of laryngeal or tracheal cartilages (traumatic), nasopharyngeal polyp, neoplasia, obstructive laryngitis, granuloma, and abscess.

............Pleural Cavity Disease

Marked inspiratory efforts are also typical but may be of short duration, often with a marked abdominal component. Expiration is effortless. No abnormal upper airway sounds are heard or auscultated. Lung sounds are typically muffled or absent ventrally and enhanced dorsally. There is decreased resonance by percussion with effusion, and increased resonance with pneumothorax (see p. 242). Decreased compressibility of the anterior thorax may be present in cats with mediastinal masses. Pneumothorax and diaphragmatic hernias are commonly associated with evidence of trauma, with or without rib fractures. Respiratory distress due to hemothorax is exacerbated by blood loss (anemia, hypovolemia).

Rule out: pleural effusion, pneumothorax, neoplasia, and diaphragmatic hernia.

...........*Pulmonary Disease*

Pulmonary disease can involve the intrathoracic airways, alveoli, interstitial space, or pulmonary vasculature. Marked expiratory efforts are present with airway obstructive disease, such as acute bronchitis in cats. Increased expiratory and inspiratory efforts may be seen with other diseases. Crackles or wheezes are generally auscultable.

Rule out: cardiogenic and noncardiogenic edema, feline asthma, lung contusions, aspiration pneumonia, pulmonary thromboembolism, and severe infection, especially bacterial, protozoal, or mycotic. Decompensation of chronic disease, such as neoplasia, chronic bronchitis, and parasitic disease, can also result in an acute presentation.

...........ASSESSMENT OF OTHER ABNORMAL BREATHING PATTERNS

1. Tachypnea: Alone, in the absence of other signs of distress, tachypnea can be a normal response to a nonrespiratory problem such as pain, hyperthermia, or stress.
2. Minimal thoracic excursions: Motor unit diseases (see p. 330) can interfere with normal function of respiratory musculature. If adequate ventilation cannot be maintained by the patient, ventilatory assistance is indicated.
3. Kussmaul's respiration (not commonly observed in dogs): Deep sighing movements secondary to metabolic acidosis, especially diabetic acidosis and renal failure.
4. Cheyne-Stokes respiration: Normal or hyperventilation following periods of apnea or hypoventilation; disorders that affect the respiratory center or respiratory control.
5. Diaphragmatic breathing: The diaphragm assumes almost all the control of ventilatory movement; lower cervical cord damage or damage to the respiratory centers of the CNS may be present.

...........INITIAL MANAGEMENT OF THE PATIENT IN RESPIRATORY DISTRESS

...........All Patients

1. Minimize stress. Generally benign procedures such as thoracic radiography, blood collection, and catheter placement can be fatal in animals in respiratory distress. Stabilization should precede further diagnostic evaluation. Sedation may be beneficial in some cases
2. Increase inspired oxygen concentration. All patients in distress may benefit, but it should not replace immediate thoracocentesis in animals with suspected pleural effusion or pneumothorax.
3. Treat shock (see p. 32).

...........Upper Airway Obstruction

Reestablish airflow and consider the following:

1. Sedation: especially laryngeal paralysis, brachycephalic airway syndrome, laryngeal edema, laryngeal collapse, and tracheal collapse.
2. Rapid-acting corticosteroids: especially laryngeal edema, brachycephalic airway syndrome, laryngeal paralysis, laryngeal collapse, and tracheal collapse.
3. Bypassing obstruction: endotracheal tube, transtracheal catheter, and tracheostomy.
4. Removing obstruction: especially foreign bodies.

...........Pleural Cavity Disease

Allow expansion of lungs.

1. Thoracocentesis (see p. 620).
2. Chest tube: if thoracocentesis alone is inadequate (see p. 621).

...........Pulmonary Disease

1. Increase inspired oxygen concentration: all cases (see p. 610).
2. Fluid therapy: with caution if edema suspected (see p. 589).

Consider:

1. Bronchodilators:bronchial asthma, acute bronchitis, allergic bronchitis, thromboembolism postadulticide therapy for heartworm disease, aspiration pneumonia, and smoke inhalation. Consider especially if expiratory wheezes are auscultated.
2. Diuretics: edema only.
3. Rapid-acting corticosteroids:bronchial asthma, acute bronchitis, overwhelming inflammation. (*Note*: long-acting products should not be administered until a diagnosis has been obtained.)
4. Antibiotics: bacterial pneumonia. (*Note*: whenever possible, specimens should be obtained for cytologic and microbiologic analysis prior to the administration of antibiotics.)
5. Positive-pressure ventilation: inadequate response.

...........INCREASING INSPIRED OXYGEN CONCENTRATION (see p. 610)

1. Face mask: allows access to the patient, but is often stressful; 50% to 60% oxygen can be achieved with a flow rate of 8 to 12 L/min.
2. Oxygen cage: least stressful method of administration. Patient inaccessible; 60% oxygen can be achieved with flow of 2 to 3 L/min once the cage has been filled. Expensive to maintain high oxygen levels in cage.
3. Nasal catheter (see also p. 613): Placement may be too stressful until the patient is stabilized. Once catheter is in place it is well tolerated. Excellent method to deliver oxygen while maintaining patient accessibility. Can achieve 50% oxygen with flow of 6 to 8 L/min.
4. Transtracheal catheters: Jugular catheter can be placed into the trachea using sterile technique, as for a tracheal wash. Useful for stabilization of patient with upper airway obstruction; 30% to 40% oxygen can be delivered with flow of 1 to 2 L/min.
5. Endotracheal tube (see also p. 613). allows maximum control of oxygen delivery and positive-pressure ventilation. May be able to bypass upper airway obstruction. Awake patients will not tolerate presence of tube. Oxymorphone and diazepam combination may be adequate for some patients. Pentobarbital IV is added if necessary; 100% oxygen can be delivered with flow of 0.2 L/kg/min.
6. Tracheostomy tube (see also p. 623): provides same advantages as endotracheal tube, but is tolerated by awake patients. Placement requires anesthesia. Frequent care is necessary to prevent obstruction of tube with secretions (initially, every 30 to 60 minutes). High-volume, low-pressure cuffs are recommended.
7. Plastic tents with high-flow oxygen.

..........HUMIDIFICATION OF ADMINISTERED OXYGEN

Oxygen is anhydrous and will result in drying of the airways. If endotracheal or tracheal tubes or catheters are used for delivery, sterile saline can be instilled directly at a rate of 0.4 mL/kg/hr. Nebulization is also effective. Pass-over or bubble-through humidifiers can increase the moisture content, but are inadequate when used as the sole means of hydration except with nasal catheters. Maintaining adequate systemic hydration is also critical.

..........VENTILATION THERAPY (see also p. 610)

Positive-pressure ventilation is indicated for patients who have not responded adequately to increased inspired oxygen concentrations and treatment directed at the underlying problem. Prolonged exposure to inspired oxygen concentrations of greater than 50% is detrimental to the patient. Positive-pressure ventilation is indicated if a PaO_2 of at least 60 mm Hg cannot be maintained with an inspired oxygen concentration of 50% or less. Ventilation therapy is also needed for patients with neurologic or muscular disorders that are not able to ventilate adequately on their own. A $PaCO_2$ of greater than 60 mm Hg is an indication for ventilatory support.

..........Further Diagnostic Evaluation

Blood gas measurement (p. 591).
Thoracic radiography (p. 360).
Tracheal wash (p. 499).
Cardiac evaluation (p. 282).
See also Respiratory System (p. 353).

..........MAJOR RESPIRATORY EMERGENCIES
..........Upper Airway Obstruction

Obstructions from laryngeal paralysis, anatomical abnormalities, trauma, foreign bodies, intraluminal masses, and extraluminal masses are found in small animals. All are serious, and those that are of an acute onset require immediate care.

Clinical Signs In most cases, the animal's extreme efforts to inhale air past the obstruction result in marked negative pressures within the extrathoracic airways and worsening of signs may result through collapse of the airways. The development of inflammation and mucosal edema can further add to the obstruction.

Therapy Interrupting this vicious cycle is frequently successful in the initial stabilization of these patients. Tranquilizers are administered (e.g., acepromazine 0.05 mg/kg IV, SC), the animal is kept cool and calm, and when possible the animal is placed in an oxygen cage so the inspired oxygen concentration can be increased with minimal stress. Rapid-acting corticosteroids can be administered to decrease secondary edema and inflammation (prednisolone sodium succinate 10 to 20 mg/kg IV).

If the obstruction is extremely severe or there is no response to the above therapy, bypassing the obstruction is indicated. Rapid control of ventilation can usually be achieved by administering a short-acting anesthetic agent and intubating the patient. Most obstructions can be bypassed using a long, narrow endotracheal tube. Once the patient is stabilized, a tracheal tube can be inserted using sterile technique if necessary.

Another technique for rapidly bypassing most obstructions in an emergency is to pass a jugular catheter into the trachea using the technique described for transtracheal washing—100% oxygen is administered through the catheter. Hypercapnia may persist, and once the patient is stabilized a tracheal tube can be placed if necessary.

Rarely is an emergency tracheostomy needed to stabilize these patients. The majority of cases can be stabilized first and the tracheostomy performed under controlled, sterile conditions.

...........Laryngeal Paralysis

Intrinsic laryngeal muscles receive their motor and sensory innervation from branches of the vagus nerve. Laryngeal paralysis results when there is interruption in the transmission of impulses through the recurrent laryngeal nerves, resulting in degeneration of the intrinsic laryngeal muscles. With denervation, the vocal folds and arytenoid cartilage move to a paramedian position rather than abduct, resulting in upper airway obstruction. Laryngeal paralysis may be partial or complete, unilateral or bilateral, and congenital or acquired.

Congenital laryngeal paralysis is seen in the Siberian husky, Bouvier des Flandres, and bull terrier. Acquired laryngeal paralysis is more commonly found in Saint Bernards, Labrador retrievers, Irish setters, and Siberian huskies. Acquired laryngeal paralysis can be idiopathic, a component of systemic neuromuscular disease or secondary to disruption of the recurrent laryngeal nerve due to masses or trauma of the anterior thorax or ventral neck. Laryngeal paralysis is rare in cats.

Clinical Signs In addition to signs of upper airway obstruction, a change in bark may be reported. Laryngeal paralysis may be associated with signs of systemic polyneuropathy.

Once the patient is stabilized, diagnostic evaluation is performed to confirm the diagnosis and to rule out acquired causes of paralysis and systemic neuropathies. Definitive diagnosis is based on laryngoscopy, with the dog lightly anesthetized with short-acting barbiturates. Just enough drug should be administered to allow visualization of the larynx to avoid anesthetic depression of motion. Absent or paradoxical laryngeal motion is observed (closed during inspiration, slightly open during expiration).

Permanent correction of laryngeal paralysis may involve (1) arytenoid lateralization (2) partial laryngectomy, (3) castellated laryngofissure. These procedures predispose the animal to aspiration pneumonia.

...........Brachycephalic Airway Syndrome and Laryngeal Collapse

Brachycephalic breeds of dogs, and rarely cats, have multiple anatomical abnormalities that result in great resistance to air flow through the upper airways. The negative pressures created within the airways to overcome this resistance exacerbate the obstruction over time. Stress, exercise, or high ambient temperatures can cause sudden decompensation and require emergency intervention. The anatomical abnormalities associated with this syndrome include stenotic nares, elongated soft palate, everted laryngeal saccules, laryngeal collapse and, in English bulldogs, hypoplastic trachea.

Components of this syndrome can occur in any combination, and individual abnormalities (such as elongated soft palate) can occur in other breeds as well. Specific abnormalities are identified during laryngoscopy performed under general anesthesia.

Animals presenting in distress are stabilized as previously described. Treatment requires surgical correction of the anatomical abnormalities. With laryngeal collapse, surgical correction may not be possible.

Elongated soft palate or stenotic nares can often be identified prior to the development of clinical signs. Surgical correction should be performed to improve air flow and decrease negative intra-airway pressures necessary to move air past these obstructions.

··········· Tracheal Collapse

Tracheal collapse is common in middle-aged toy and small-breed dogs. A chronic cough is reported and is readily induced by applying digital pressure to the trachea. Diagnostic confirmation is obtained by cervical and thoracic (lateral view during both inspiration and expiration) radiography. Acute decompensation is uncommon, but can occur in severely affected dogs due to stress, exercise, or high ambient temperatures.

Therapy Acute management involves sedation, increased inspired oxygen concentrations, a cool environment with minimal stress, and rapid-acting corticosteroids as described previously. Cough suppressants, e.g., Hycodan (hydrocodone bitartrate–homatropine methylbromide) 0.25 mg/kg q8–12h PO, or butorphanol 0.5 mg/kg q6–12h PO, are also useful in these patients. It is difficult to bypass the obstruction because the collapse often involves the entire length of the trachea.

··········· Trauma

Crushing or biting injuries of the neck can result in fractures of laryngeal or tracheal cartilages that may obstruct the airway. Bypassing the obstructed area may be necessary until the patient is stable and can undergo surgical correction of the injury. Neck injury can also result in damage to the recurrent laryngeal nerve and laryngeal paralysis.

··········· Foreign Bodies

Foreign bodies most commonly lodge in the nasal cavity where they cause acute sneezing and possibly pawing at the face. If not removed, the sneezing subsides and chronic nasal discharge ensues. Respiratory distress is not expected. Pharyngeal and tracheal foreign bodies can cause obstruction to air flow and respiratory distress. A diagnosis of foreign body is usually suspected based on the history and auscultation findings. Many foreign bodies are not apparent radiographically.

Treatment Foreign bodies can often be removed from the nose or pharynx with an alligator forceps. General anesthesia is usually needed. Retrieval of nasal foreign bodies is greatly assisted with a small endoscope (rhinoscope, arthroscope, or bronchoscope). If not available, an otoscope can be used. Foreign objects lodged in the trachea may be small and function like a ball valve, causing episodic collapse or anoxia. In attempting to remove these objects, suspend the patient with the head down. Removal can usually be achieved with alligator forceps using a laryngoscope to assist in visualization. Foreign bodies that are lodged within the trachea or bronchi require bronchoscopic removal.

··········· Intraluminal Masses

Nasopharyngeal polyps (feline), tumors, obstructive laryngitis, granulomas, abscesses, and cysts can cause upper airway obstruction. The onset of signs is usually gradual. They are identified by careful laryngoscopic examination performed under general anesthesia. The nasopharynx above the soft palate is included in the evaluation. Pedunculated masses and cysts are excised at the time of evaluation. Biopsy of diffusely infiltrating masses is always indicated for histologic examination. It is impossible to distinguish obstructive laryngitis from neoplasia based on gross appearance alone. Material should be collected from abscesses and granulomas for cytologic examination and bacterial culture and drainage performed where possible.

...........Extraluminal Masses

Masses compressing the upper airways usually result in slowly progressive signs. Masses are generally identified by palpation of the neck. Enlarged mandibular lymph nodes, thyroid tumors, and other neoplasms may be present. Radiography and ultrasonography can be used to better characterize the lesion. A diagnosis is obtained by fine-needle aspirate or biopsy of the mass.

...........PLEURAL CAVITY DISEASE

The inside of each hemithorax is covered by parietal pleura, whereas the surface of the lobes of the lungs is covered by visceral pleura. These two surfaces are in close contact and are contiguous with each other at the hilum. Pneumothorax refers to air accumulation in the pleural space, between the parietal and visceral pleurae. The general term "pleural effusion" means a collection of liquid in the pleural space, but does not indicate what kind or how much is present. The mediastinal reflections of pleura are thin in dogs and cats, and bilateral involvement is common. Respiratory compromise results from the inability of the lungs to expand because of the presence of fluid or air.

...........Pneumothorax

Pneumothorax is classified as (1) open (an open chest wound), (2) closed (tears in the visceral pleura), and (3) tension (air entering the pleural cavity during inspiration through a valvelike lesion in the lung or chest wall that closes during expiration).

Pneumothorax is frequently traumatic in origin. Spontaneous pneumothorax occurs with rupture of cavitary lesions of the lung that may be either congenital or acquired from prior trauma, airway disease (emphysema), paragonimiasis, neoplasia, heartworm disease, or lung abscess. Pneumothorax is rarely a result of esophageal tears; it is usually secondary to esophageal foreign bodies.

Pneumothorax following traumatic injury to the chest may be associated with several conditions that can lead to the rapid development of respiratory and circulatory insufficiency: (1) open pneumothorax, (2) tension pneumothorax, (3) rib fractures, (4) airway obstruction, (5) hemothorax, (6) lung contusions, (7) cardiac arrhythmias (8) cardiac tamponade, (9) hypovolemia, and (10) shock. These patients must be quickly assessed and emergency therapy initiated.

Diagnosis Pneumothorax is generally detected by physical examination and confirmed with immediate thoracocentesis. Following stabilization, thoracic radiography can be performed. Pneumothorax is indicated by (1) elevation of the cardiac silhouette above the sternum, (2) increased density of the pulmonary tissue, (3) free air between the parietal and visceral pleura, and (4) absence of vascular shadows in the peripheral portions of the thorax. The lungs are best evaluated for parenchymal lesions after as much air as possible has been removed from the pleural space to allow maximum expansion of the lungs. Left and right lateral views and either dorsoventral (DV) or ventrodorsal (VD) views are indicated. Standing lateral views are useful for the identification of cavitary lesions that contain both air and fluid. If underlying pulmonary disease is suspected as a cause of spontaneous pneumothorax, further pulmonary testing such as tracheal wash, bronchoscopy, heartworm tests, and fecal examination for parasitic ova may be indicated.

Treatment   Thoracocentesis is performed immediately in all patients suspected of having pneumothorax (see p. 620). Usually the mediastinum is disrupted and air can be removed from either side; however, it is prudent to attempt to remove air from both sides to allow for maximal expansion of the lungs. All penetrating chest wounds should be treated as open or sucking wounds until proved otherwise. Wounds should be immediately closed with a pressure dressing while the animal is stabilized.

If air continues to accumulate within the pleural space during stabilization, chest tube placement is indicated. A chest tube is also placed if thoracocentesis must be performed more than twice in 24 hours while the animal is undergoing strict cage rest (see p. 621).

Most cases of traumatic pneumothorax resolve over time, necessitating only strict cage rest and the maintenance of negative intrathoracic pressures until healing can occur. Thoracotomy is indicated if the volume of air accumulating within the pleural cavity does not decrease after several days of management or if foreign material from a penetrating wound is present. Dogs with spontaneous pneumothorax can also be managed conservatively with cage rest and thoracocentesis. However, most dogs with spontaneous pneumothorax ultimately require thoracotomy to control continuous or intermittent accumulation of air. Thoracotomy may also be indicated for diagnostic purposes, or for primary treatment of the disease (e.g., neoplasia or abscess).

Chest Tubes   Chest tubes must be placed using surgical technique and maintained using sterile technique. Local anesthesia may be adequate if the patient can be easily restrained. Pediatric chest tubes or feeding tubes can be used. In general, the tube should be the largest diameter that will fit comfortably between the ribs. Extra side holes must be added to feeding tubes, being careful not to destroy the strength of the tubing. Have a three-way stopcock, any necessary adaptors, and a tube clamp ready. The length of tube to be passed into the chest should be measured to just reach the thoracic inlet.

To place the tube, clip and surgically prepare the entire chest wall. Place the animal in lateral recumbency. Grasp the skin along the lateral chest wall, and pull the skin forward. Place a 1% lidocaine local block into the seventh intercostal space just caudal to the seventh rib. Make a small incision in the skin and subcutaneous tissue over the seventh intercostal space. Use a Metzenbaum scissors and bluntly dissect a small opening to the pleura. The incision is just large enough to allow passage of the tube.

Use Kelly or Carmault forceps to clamp the tip of the chest tube or use an internal stylet and introduce the chest tube into the incision and through the pleura. Pass the tube into the pleural space in a cranial and ventral direction. The skin is released; it moves caudally back to its natural position, creating a skin-subcutaneous tunnel over the tube. Immediately suction any air or fluid out of the pleural space and clamp the tube. Close the skin around the tube with a purse-string suture. Secure the tube to the skin adjacent to the entry site using either a Chinese finger trap suture pattern or by suturing the skin to a piece of butterfly tape placed securely around the tube. Cover the opening with antiseptic ointment and gauze pad and apply a chest wrap. Placement of the tube and adequacy of drainage are evaluated radiographically (two views).

The end of the chest tube can be attached to (1) a three-way stopcock for intermittent aspiration, (2) a three-bottle suction system, or (3) a bedside pediatric suction unit. A Heimlich valve can be used in large dogs. All openings of three-way stopcocks are covered with sterile caps when not in use, and should be wiped with hydrogen peroxide before being used.

An Elizabethan collar is placed on all animals and the tube carefully secured against any disruption. Animals can die quickly and quietly of pneumothorax from a leak in the system.

The presence of the tube itself can result in formation of a nonseptic effusion at a low rate of less than 2 mL/kg/day.

............Cardiovascular Changes Associated With Thoracic Trauma

Cardiac injury is a frequent complication of nonpenetrating thoracic trauma.

Often myocardial injury leads to arrhythmias that can be characterized by (1) multiple premature systoles, (2) ventricular tachycardia, (3) abnormal S–T segment elevation or depression, (4) atrial fibrillation, and (5) evidence of myocardial infarction and cardiac failure (see Cardiac Emergencies, p. 54).

............Rib Fractures and Flail Chest

Rib fractures are characterized by localized pain and painful respiratory movements. Radiographs are helpful in confirming the diagnosis; however, careful and gentle palpation may reveal crepitus and instability of the ribs. Pneumothorax is a commonly associated problem. Other associated problems can include lung contusions, pericardial laceration, contusion of the heart (traumatic myocarditis), diaphragmatic hernia, and splenic rupture.

Severe chest injuries can result in multiple rib fractures that produce a "floating segment" of the thoracic wall known as flail chest. The floating segment moves paradoxically with respiration: medially during inspiration and laterally during expiration. Respiratory distress is primarily the result of underlying lung contusions. Decreased ventilation due to pain and paradoxical wall movements also contribute.

Therapy Stabilization of the animal is generally achieved by strict cage rest and increased inspired oxygen concentration. Positive-pressure ventilation is needed for unresponsive cases. The animal must be carefully monitored for pneumothorax. Although controversial, positioning the animal with the flail side up may reduce pain and improve ventilation of the underlying lung. Chest wraps are not likely to stabilize the flail segment and can further restrict ventilation. Reduction of pain can be accomplished with small doses of narcotics (such as oxymorphone 0.05 mg/kg IV or IM in dogs to effect; in cats butorphanol 0.1 mg/kg IV, IM, or SC to effect; and in dogs and cats, buprenorphine 0.005 mg/kg IV or IM to effect) and may be helpful in allowing the animal to ventilate more normally.

Following stabilization of the animal, the flail segment is surgically stabilized by the use of a large piece of orthoplast. The orthoplast is anchored to the fractured ribs and the adjacent normal ribs using nonabsorbable sutures.

............Pleural Effusions

Pleural fluid cytologic analysis is indicated for all patients with pleural effusion prior to initiation of antibiotics

The general term *pleural effusion* means a collection of liquid in the pleural space between the parietal and visceral pleurae but does not indicate what kind of fluid or how much is present.

Clinical signs associated with pleural effusion depend on how much fluid accumulates and how rapidly. Severe signs are dyspnea, reluctance to lie down, labored breathing with marked abdominal lift, cough, and lethargy. Auscultation may reveal muffled heart and lung sounds ventrally and increased lung sounds dorsally. There may be decreased resonance with percussion.

The presence of pleural effusion is confirmed radiographically in stable patients. Thoracentesis is performed immediately in patients in respiratory distress, because positioning for radiography may decompensate the animal. Radiographic confirmation should include films taken in right and left lateral recumbency and ventrodorsally. Use DV and standing lateral views to minimize stress of the patient. When large amounts of fluid are suspected, a standing lateral view is indicated so that fluid collected in the costrophrenic recess will be visualized.

Caution. Positioning for radiography may decompensate the animal.

When attempting to explain pleural effusions, one must think of (1) an imbalance of transpleural or hydrostatic osmotic forces or protein osmotic forces, (2) changes in the permeability of membranes, (3) a decrease in the rate of reabsorption fluid, and (4) combinations of these mechanisms (see Table 1–33).

Pathologic involvement of the pleura is almost always a secondary complication except for primary bacterial pleuritis and pleural mesotheliomas.

■ CAUSES OF PLEURAL EFFUSION IN THE CAT

Pyothorax

Feline infectious peritonitis (FIP)

Congestive heart failure (feline cardiomyopathy)

Intrathoracic neoplasia (lymphoma, thymoma, mesothelioma)

Chylothorax

Heartworm disease

Hemothorax

Hypoalbuminemia

Lung lobe torsion

Diaphragmatic hernia

Diagnosis Thoracic radiography can be used to confirm the presence of fluid in the stable animal and to determine if the effusion is unilateral or bilateral. Effusions in dogs and cats are usually bilateral. The cardiac silhouette and lung parenchyma cannot be effectively evaluated until most of the fluid has been removed from the pleural space. Left lateral, right lateral, and VD or DV views are indicated following thoracocentesis.

Pleural fluid cytologic analysis is indicated for *all* patients with pleural effusion. Specimens should always be collected *prior to* the initiation of antibiotics because treatment with antibiotics can cause septic inflammation (pyothorax) to appear cytologically as a nonseptic condition. The remainder of the diagnostic evaluation and the treatment are based on the type of fluid present (see Table 1–33). Fluid may be a (1) transudate—pericardial disease, right heart failure, bypoalbuminemia, intrathoracic neoplasia, or diaphragmatic hernia; (2) nonseptic exudate—suggesting FIP, neoplasia, hernia, lung lobe torsion, or septic effusion in an animal treated with antibiotics prior to specimen collection; (3) septic exudate—idiopathic pyothorax or pyothorax secondary to trauma or foreign body; (4) chylous effusion—usually idiopathic or congenital, but possibly secondary to trauma, neoplasia, cardiac disease, pericardial disease, dirofilariasis, lung lobe torsion, or diaphragmatic hernia; (5) hemorrhagic effusion—suggesting trauma, systemic coagulopathy, neoplasia, or lung lobe torsion; or (6) neoplastic—especially malignant lymphoma in cats. Further diagnostic evaluation is based upon the appropriate differential diagnoses.

Ultrasonographic examination of the thorax can be helpful in identifying intrathoracic masses, hernias, lung lobe torsions, and for cardiac abnormalities. Unlike radiography, ultrasonography is facilitated by the presence of fluid in the thorax.

Common causes of respiratory emergencies are pyothorax, chylothorax, and hemothorax. See pp. 68 and 73 for management of right heart failure and pericardial effusion.

.... *Pyothorax*

Pyothorax is treated with anitibiotics and drainage.

Pyothorax refers to septic effusion of the pleural cavity. The infection is

Table 1–33. Analysis of Pleural Effusions

	Transudates	Exudates					
		Modified Transudates	Nonseptic Exudates	Septic Exudates	Chylous Effusions	Hemorrhagic Effusions
Color Transparency	Pale yellow Clear	Yellow-pink Clear to cloudy	Yellow-pink Cloudy	Yellow Cloudy to flocculent	White-pink Opaque	Red Opaque
Protein (g/dL) RBCs	<2.5 Absent to rare	<3.5 Variable	>3.0 Variable	>3.0 Variable	>2.5 Variable	>3.0 Acute: high number Chronic: moderate number
Nucleated cells/mL	<500	<5000	>5000	>5000	400–10,000	>1000
Neutrophils	Rare	Variable number	Moderate	Moderate to high number	Acute: low number Chronic: moderate number	Variable number
		Nondegenerative	Nondegenerative	Nondegenerative to degenerative	Nondegenerative	Nondegenerative
Lymphocytes	Rare	Variable	Variable	Variable	Acute: high number Chronic: low number	Variable

Macrophages	Occasional	Variable	Increased number Contain ingested debris	Increased number	Present	Chronic: moderate number Contain ingested RBCs
Mesothelial cells	Occasional	Occasional	Rare	Rare	Occasional	Chronic: present
Fibrin	Absent	Absent	Present	Present	Chronic: present	Variable
Bacteria	Absent	Absent	Absent	Present intra- and extracellularly	Absent	Absent
Lipid	Absent	Absent	Absent	Absent	High triglycerides relative to serum low cholesterol; positive to lipotrophic stains	Absent
Etiology	Right heart failure Hypoproteinemia	Chronic transudates Diaphragmatic hernia Neoplasia Right heart failure Pericardial disease	Neoplasia Feline infectious peritonitis Chronic diaphragmatic hernia Lung torsions Pyothorax	Foreign body Penetrating wound Idiopathic pyothorax	Idiopathic Congenital Lymphangiectasia Trauma Neoplasia Cardiac disease Pericardial disease Dirofilariasis	Trauma Neoplasia Bleeding disorders Lung torsions

generally the result of a combination of aerobic and anaerobic bacteria. Rarely, fungal organisms are present. The source of organisms is often undetermined, particularly in cats, but can be from penetrating wounds through the chest wall, esophagus, or bronchi; from migrating foreign bodies (especially grass awns); or from primary lung infections. The most common organisms associated with pyothorax in the cat are *Pasteurella, Bacteroides*, and *Fusobacterium*. In addition to signs of effusion, fever is often present. Septic shock can occur.

Diagnosis The diagnosis is based on cytologic analysis (see Table 1–33). Bacterial cultures are indicated for antibiotic selection but can be negative in some cases. Prior treatment with antibiotics can obscure the diagnosis by causing the fluid to appear cytologically as a nonseptic exudate even though the effusion continues.

Therapy Emergency management consists of thoracocentesis, shock therapy, and IV antibiotics. Portions of fluid obtained by thoracocentesis should be evaluated cytologically and submitted for both aerobic and anaerobic culture. Gram stains of the fluid can assist in the initial identification of bacterial organisms. Ampicillin or chloramphenicol are reasonable antibiotics to initiate prior to obtaining results of cultures. Using ampicillin or amoxicillin with a β- lactamase inhibitor (i.e., amoxicillin-clavulanate or ampicillin-sublactam) increases activity against Bacteroides spp. Antibiotics are initially administered IV.

As soon as the animal is stabilized a chest tube must be placed to allow for continued drainage of this intrathoracic "abscess" (see p. 621). Inadequate drainage will result in treatment failure. Usually one tube is adequate, but success of drainage must be based on radiographic evaluation following tube placement and every 24 to 48 hours thereafter. Ideally, fluid is removed every 2 hours initially, with the interval increasing as the recovered volume decreases. Lavage of the thoracic cavity can be performed twice daily with 10 mL/kg of warmed saline. Recovery is expected to be about 75% of the infused volume. Exploratory thoracotomy is indicated to remove a suspected nidus of infection, if adequate drainage cannot be achieved, or if there is incomplete response to medical therapy after 1 week (based on the character and volume of fluid retrieved). Antibiotics are continued for 4 to 6 weeks after removal of the chest tube.

Early diagnosis and aggressive treatment allow for a good prognosis for the majority of animals with pyothorax.

............Chylothorax

Chylothorax refers to the abnormal accumulation of lymphatic fluid (chyle) in the pleural cavity from the thoracic duct. The cisterna chyli is the dilated collecting pool of the lymphatics located within the abdominal cavity that leads into the thoracic duct cranially. The thoracic duct enters the chest through the aortic hiatus; however, numerous collateral ducts exist. The lymphatic vessels deliver triglycerides and fat-soluble vitamins from the intestines, lymphocytes, and proteins to the venous circulation.

True chylous effusions are those in which the pleural fluid cholesterol is less than the serum cholesterol and the pleural triglycerides are greater than the serum triglycerides. *Psedochylous effusions* are those in which the pleural fluid cholesterol is greater than the serum cholesterol and pleural fluid triglyceride is less than the serum triglyceride.

Disease processes resulting in leakage of chyle include thoracic neoplasia (especially lymphoma in cats), lung lobe torsion, venous thrombi, heart disease, pericardial disease, heartworm disease, diaphragmatic hernia, and trauma. Trauma may be surgical or nonsurgical. Heart disease may be secondary to hyperthyroidism in cats. Idiopathic chylothorax is common in dogs and cats, and Afghan hounds are predisposed. Thoracic lymphangiectasia may be present.

Thoracic duct rupture is not a common cause of chylothorax in the dog and cat. The more common condition is thoracic lymphangiectasia with multiple, dilated lymphatic vessels located in the cranial mediastinum. The chyle leaks transmurally.

Signs are usually chronic. In addition to signs of effusion, weight loss, anorexia, and cough occur.

Diagnosis The diagnosis is based on thoracocentesis and the removal of a milky, often blood-tinged, chylous fluid. Shaking of chyle with ether after alkalinization usually clears the fluid. The typical cytologic characteristics are described in Table 1–33. Fluid recovered should be placed in an EDTA tube for cytologic examination. Confirmation of chyle requires measurement of triglyceride concentrations of the fluid and serum collected concurrently (readily available from commercial laboratories). Chylothorax is confirmed when triglycerides of the fluid are higher than those of serum. Lymphangiography can be performed to visualize the thoracic duct, but it is generally not necessary unless surgical ligation is to be performed. The diagnostic evaluation includes a careful search for the underlying causes listed above.

Therapy Emergency stabilization depends on thoracocentesis. Medical management consists of direct treatment of any underlying disease, intermittent thoracentesis as needed to control signs, and a low fat diet to minimize lymphatic flow. The last is achieved by parenteral nutrition or, less aggressively, a low fat diet. Attention must be paid to electrolyte balance, and fluid therapy is often necessary initially. Surgical treatment of nonresponsive cases includes ligation of the thoracic duct and all identifiable collateral vessels, and placement of pleuroperitoneal or pleurovenous shunts.

Pleurodesis is attempted in refractory cases.

In the absence of trauma or a correctable underlying problem, the long-term prognosis for animals with chylothorax is fair to guarded. In addition to persistent effusion, pleural fibrosis can occur, particularly in cats.

............Hemothorax

Extensive bleeding into the thoracic cavity can lead to severe respiratory distress due to sudden hypovolemia and anemia, as well as interference with expansion of the lungs. Hemothorax can be associaed with (1) trauma (lung laceration or rupture of intercostal vessels), (2) systemic coagulopathy, (3) lung lobe torsions, or (4) erosive lesions within the thorax (usually neoplasia).

Diagnosis The diagnosis is made by thoracocentesis. Hemorrhagic effusion is differentiated from systemic blood collected inadvertently during thoracocentesis by the following criteria (unless the hemorrhage is peracute): (1) blood with the pleural cavity is rapidly defibrinated and will not clot; (2) the packed cell volume (PCV) of effusion is less than that of venous blood; and (3) macrophages present in effusions contain hemosiderin and RBCs (erythrophagocytosis). Hemorrhagic effusions often contain relatively higher proportions of WBCs than peripheral blood.

Hemothorax can be the sole presenting sign of animals with intoxication from warfarin or other vitamin K antagonists. The systemic clotting abilities of the animal should be immediately assessed with an activated clotting time (ACT) (see p. 688) and examination of a blood smear for platelets. Further evaluation of coagulation is performed as indicated by clinical signs (see p. 687).

Therapy Emergency management primarily addresses the acute blood loss. IV fluid therapy is indicated for volume replacement. Blood transfusions to replace RBCs, coagulation factors, and platelets are administered as needed. Blood is evacuated from the pleural cavity by thoracocentesis to the extent necessary to alleviate respiratory distress due to the presence of the fluid.

Fluid that remains can be reabsorbed to assist in recovery. Autotransfusion can also be performed. Massive, uncontrolled bleeding into the chest necessitates exploratory thoracotomy.

............Diaphragmatic Hernia

Diaphragmatic hernia is a protrusion of abdominal viscera through the diaphragm, often secondary to trauma. Associated traumatic lesions may be rib fractures, pneumothorax, hemothorax or other effusions, lung contusions, and shock. Respiratory distress can be the result of all these factors in addition to displacement of lung by abdominal contents. Commonly herniated abdominal organs include liver, small intestines, and stomach.

In addition to signs of respiratory distress and trauma, rarely, auscultation may reveal peristaltic sounds within the chest, and an absence of normal contents may be noted on abdominal palpation.

Diagnosis The diagnosis of diaphragmatic hernia is based on history (especially that of trauma), clinical signs, and radiographs (see p. 353). Ultrasonography or positive contrast peritoneography may be necessary to confirm the diagnosis. Contrast radiographs following the oral administration of barium may show the presence of intestines within the thorax; however, the intestines are not always involved. Hyperoxygenation of patients with suspected diaphragmatic hernias is helpful prior to the stress of radiography.

Treatment Animals with chronic diaphragmatic hernias due to previous trauma or congenital abnormalities can be minimally symptomatic in spite of the presence of abdominal organs within the thoracic cavity. Signs of respiratory distress are usually due to the concurrent problems of lung contusion, pneumothorax, pleural effusion, rib fractures, pain, and shock. These problems are addressed as described elsewhere in this article. Positive-pressure ventilation is rarely necessary. Surgical correction of the hernia is postponed until after the animal is fully stabilized. (*Note*: Emergency surgery is indicated for the repair of hernia if the stomach has entered the thoracic cavity.)

............PULMONARY DISEASES

............Feline Bronchitis (Feline Bronchial Asthma)

- Bronchial asthma
- Acute bronchitis
- Chronic bronchitis
- Chronic asthmatic bronchitis
- Chronic bronchitis with emphysema

Cats with disease of the lower airways may present in severe distress. Historically, the disease of such cats was termed feline bronchial asthma; however, several different types of bronchial disease can occur in cats. Cats with acute episodes of distress may have acute bronchitis, chronic bronchitis, chronic bronchitis with asthma, chronic bronchitis with emphysema, or bronchial asthma.

All of these bronchial syndromes are associated with lower airway obstruction. Respiratory emergencies usually result from the reversible problems of bronchoconstriction (asthma) in conjunction with inflammation. Cats with acute bronchitis generally have reversible changes contributing to obstruction, including (1) increased intraluminal mucus, (2) intraluminal inflammatory exudate, (3) inflammatory infiltration of the airway walls, and (4) bronchoconstriction. Cats with chronic bronchitis, with or without emphysema, have permanent airway damage (fibrosis) in addition to potentially reversible inflammatory changes. Such cats have a history of respiratory signs but can present in critical condition during an acute exacerbation. Underlying causes of bronchial disease include allergy, bacterial infection, parasitic infection (lungworms, dirofilariasis), and exposure to inhaled irritants. Some cases are idiopathic.

Signs Respiratory distress is typically characterized by prolonged expiratory efforts with auscultable expiratory wheezes. Thoracic radiography, tracheal or bronchial washings (for cytologic and microbiologic examination), heartworm tests, and fecal examinations for pulmonary parasites are indicated following stabilization. Consideration is given to inhalant allergen or irritant exposure in the home environment (e.g., smoke, litter dust, perfumes).

Immediate stabilization can usually be achieved by administering prednisolone sodium succinate 10 to 20 mg/kg IV, or IM if necessary, and placing the cat in a stress-free, oxygen-enriched environment. Bronchodilators can also be used, such as aminophyline 5 mg/kg PO or slow IV or terbutaline 0.01 mg/kg SQ, repeated once in 5 to 10 minutes, if needed.

Therapy following stabilization is dependent on the underlying cause. Bacterial bronchitis is treated with antibiotics. Pulmonary parasites are treated directly. Management of feline heartworm disease is discussed (see p. 756). The presence of airborne allergens is eliminated, if possible, from the environment. Allergic and idiopathic bronchitis is managed with a combination of oral prednisone and bronchodilators (theophylline products or β-agonists).

·········· Pulmonary Contusions

Contusions of the lung are frequently present following trauma. Hemorrhage into the interstitial and alveolar spaces can significantly interfere with oxygenation. Respiratory distress is often compounded by other traumatic damage such as pneumothorax, hemothorax, rib fractures, or diaphragmatic hernia. Shock and hypovolemia may also be present.

The diagnosis is based on historic evidence of trauma, signs of respiratory distress localized at the pulmonary parenchyma, and, following stabilization, radiographic confirmation of patchy interstitial and alveolar densities. Radiographic signs may be delayed for up to 24 hours following the traumatic event.

Treatment Treatment of contusion consists of general supportive care. Increased inspired oxygen concentration may be necessary. Concurrent problems associated with the trauma are also addressed.

The animal is monitored clinically and radiographically for signs of complications. Possible sequelae include secondary bacterial infection, abscessation, lung lobe consolidation, and development of cavitary lesions.

·········· Aspiration Pneumonia

Aspiration pneumonia occurs in animals with abnormal laryngeal and pharyngeal reflexes. Aspiration pneumonia may be associated with vomiting during states of altered mentation, as during general anesthesia or recovery from anesthesia. It can occur with regurgitation due to megaesophagus or other esophageal disorders. Systemic neuromuscular disease such as polyneuropathy, polymyopathy, or myasthenia gravis, or localized oropharyngeal defects, such as cleft palate in neonates, laryngoplasty, cricopharyngeal motor dysfunction, and occasionally brachycepahalic airway syndrome, can predispose the patient to aspiration pneumonia. Iatrogenic causes include improper placement of nasogastric feeding tubes, overly aggressive force feeding, and oral administration of mineral oil. Aspiration compromises pulmonary function through mechanical obstruction, bronchoconstriction, chemical damage, and infection. Severe edema and inflammation are common; hemorrhage and necrosis can occur.

Diagnosis Diagnosis is based on clinical signs of pulmonary parenchymal disease, a history consistent with vomiting or other predisposing causes, and thoracic radiographs demonstrating bronchoalveolar infiltrates in the dependent regions of the lungs (usually the cranial and middle lobes). Tracheal wash is useful for bacterial culture and sensitivity testing.

Treatment Severe respiratory distress secondary to aspiration is treated with increased inspired oxygen concentration, IV fluids, and bronchodilators (aminophylline: dog, 11 mg/kg IV *slowly* or PO t.i.d.; cat, 5 mg/kg IV *slowly* or PO b.i.d.). Positive-pressure ventilation may be necessary in some cases. Dehydration is avoided.

Suctioning of aspirated material blindly or with a bronchoscope is effective only if performed immediately following aspiration. Rapid-acting corticosteroids (prednisolone sodium succinate 10 to 20 mg/kg IV) are indicated in the treatment of shock. Their use to diminish the inflammatory response is controversial because they interfere with the lungs' normal defense mechanisms. If the animal is sufficiently stable, thoracic wash fluid is collected, then antibiotic therapy is initiated. Deterioration after several days may indicate development of a secondary infection, even if antibiotics have been given. Antibiotics to consider in the absence of sensitivity data include amoxicillin-clavulanate, trimethoprim-sulfadiazine, cephalexin, or chloramphenicol. More agressive antibiotic therapy is reserved for patients with resistant infections. If large airway obstruction is suspected, removal of foreign material with bronchoscopy is helpful. Unfortunately, this condition is difficult to recognize. Management of animals with aspiration pneumonia must also include consideration of the underlying disease process.

............Pulmonary Edema

Pulmonary edema refers to the accumulation of excessive amounts of fluid within the lung. It initially forms within the interstitium, then progresses to fill the alveoli, and ultimately the airways. Hypoxia results from ventilation-perfusion abnormalities.

Pulmonary edema is associated with increased capillary hydrostatic pressure (vascular overload), decreased plasma oncotic pressure, obstruction of lymphatic drainage, and increased capillary permeability. Multiple factors can occur simultaneously.

Causes The most common cause of edema is increased hydrostatic pressure secondary to left-sided heart failure (see p. 68). Decreased plasma oncotic pressure occurs with profound hypoalbuminemia (usually <1 g/dL), possibly secondary to GI disease, glomerulopathy or liver failure. Overzealous fluid administration can contribute to edema through both increased hydrostatic pressure and decreased oncotic pressure. Obstruction to lymphatic drainage is usually caused by neoplasia.

Many diseases can lead to increased capillary permeability and the formation of edema with relatively high protein concentration (acute or adult respiratory distress syndrome, ARDS. The differential diagnosis includes severe trauma, sepsis, smoke inhalation, aspiration, oxygen toxicity, snake envenomation, electrocution, pancreatitis, uremia, and disseminated intravascular coagulation (DIC).

Other causes of edema include pulmonary thromboembolism, severe upper airway obstruction, seizures, and head trauma.

Diagnosis Animals are presented with signs of pulmonary disease. Crackles are common on thoracic auscultation. Fulminant edema may be evident by the presence of blood-tinged foam around the mouth. Following stabilization, thoracic radiographs demonstrate interstitial and alveolar densities. Cardiogenic edema is often most severe in the perihilar regions in dogs, but can have patchy distribution in cats. Pulmonary vasculature and cardiac size are also assessed. Further diagnostic testing is performed as needed to determine the underlying cause.

Table I–34. Initial Treatment for Emergency Management of
Pulmonary Edema

All Animals

1. Oxygen supplementation (see p. 610)
   a. Oxygen cage or tenting over the head
   b. Nasal catheter
   c. Endotracheal or tracheal tube with suction
   d. Positive-pressure ventilation
2. Sedation
   a. Dogs: morphine sulfate 0.1 mg/kg IV boluses, to effect
   b. Cats: Acepromazine 0.05 mg/kg IV or SC to effect
3. Cage rest
4. Bronchodilators
   a. Aminophylline (dog: 11 mg/kg PO or slow IV q8h; cat: 5 mg/kg PO slow IV q12h)

Heart Failure (see p. 68)

Fluid Overload

1. Discontinue fluids and reevaluate type of fluids—think about use of colloids (see also p. 597)
2. Diuretics, if needed, with caution
   a. Furosemide 2.2 mg/kg IV or SC

Hypoalbuminemia

1. Replace albumin; plasma transfusion (see also p. 46)
2. Diuretics, with caution

Increased Vascular Permeability

1. Recommendations for All Animals above
2. Corticosteroids for shock (see also p. 36)
3. Use osmotic colloids as IV fluids (see also p. 597)
4. Address underlying problems

Treatment   In all cases, increased oxygen supplementation, minimal stress, and sedation can be helpful (see Table 1–34). Bronchodilators may be helpful through mild diuretic effects and decreased ventilatory muscle fatigue. Airway suction and positive-pressure ventilation are indicated for severe edema. The clinician should try to determine whether the edema is likely to be a result of heart failure, volume overload, hypoalbuminemia, or increased permeability.

Heart failure is managed with diuretics and possibly vasodilators and positive inotropes (see p. 68). Volume overload is managed by discontinuation of fluids and the administration of diuretics. Hypoalbuminemia is addressed by replacing albumin through plasma transfusions. Diuretics may be helpful in initial stabilization, but can contribute to hypovolemia.

Edema secondary to increased permeability is usually poorly responsive to diuretic treatment. Care should be taken to avoid dehydration of the animal, which can be particularly detrimental to animals with many of the underlying diseases associated with this form of edema. Corticosteroids are administered for shock. Their usefulness as a direct treatment for ARDS is controversial.

............Pulmonary Thromboembolism

A diagnosis of pulmonary thromboembolism (PTE) is difficult to make, and a high index of suspicion must be maintained to avoid underdiagnosis of this condition.

Hypercoagulable states of the blood and vessels may be associated with blood vessel endothelial injury, alterations in blood flow with increased blood stasis, and altered blood coagulability.

Clinical conditions in the dog that may predispose to thrombogenesis include (1) catheterization of blood vessels, (2) DIC, (3) bacterial endocarditis, (4) hyperviscosity syndromes, (5) hyperadrenocorticism, (6) protein-losing nephropathy, (7) diabetes mellitus, (8) heat stroke, (9) hemorrhagic pancreatitis, (10) inflammatory bowel disease, and (11) immune-mediated hemolytic anemia.

Diagnosis Diagnosis of PTE is difficult, and is predicated on a high degree of suspicion based on clinical signs consistent with PTE, presence of an associated condition, and radiographic findings. Confirmation is obtained with angiography or nuclear imaging, when available.

Tachypnea is a fairly consistent sign of PTE, usually of acute onset. With increased severity, dyspnea, orthopnea, and cyanosis can occur. The distress may be poorly responsive to oxygen supplementation. The heart is carefully auscultated for a prominent or split heart sound, associated with pulmonary hypertension. Signs of right heart failure occur rarely.

Normal thoracic radiograph in the face of respiratory distress is highly suggestive of PTE. Potential radiographic abnormalities include dilated, tortuous, or blunted pulmonary arteries; wedge-shaped opacities in the lungs distal to an obstructed artery due to hemorrhage or edema; or interstitial or alveolar opacities. The right heart may be enlarged.

Echocardiography can show right heart enlargement, pulmonary hypertension, or evidence of underlying heart disease, possibly with thrombi in the atria.

Definitive diagnosis requires pulmonary angiography or nuclear perfusion scans (ideally, in conjunction with nuclear ventilation scans).

Measurement of antithrombin III (AT III) concentrations can be useful in identifying hypercoagulable states associated with nephrotic syndrome, DIC (see p. 45), or liver disease. Treatment of any animal with AT III deficiency should include plasma transfusions to replace this protein, particularly if heparin is administered.

Treatment

1. In acutely decompensated patients, treat cardiovascular shock, provide oxygen therapy, and administer a high dose of a rapid-acting corticosteroid (prednisolone sodium succinate 10 to 20 mg/kg IV). Such treatment is often sufficient for PTE following heartworm adulticide treatment.
2. Oxygen supplementation is provided to produce pulmonary vasodilation.
3. Animals with PTE and a persistent condition resulting in hypercoagulability are treated with anticoagulant therapy.
   a. Heparin is administered initially. Patients deficient in AT III should also receive plasma.
      Initial dosage: 200 to 300 units/kg SC q8h.
      Monitor activated partial thromboplastin time (APTT) before and 2 hours post injection.
      Adjust dosage to achieve an APTT that is 1.5 to 2.0 times normal.
   b. Long-term anticoagulation is achieved with warfarin sodium (Coumadin). Frequent monitoring and dosage adjustments are required, and drug interactions are common. This drug is used with caution.
      Initial dosage: 0.1 to 0.2 mg/kg PO q24h in dogs, and 0.5 mg *total dose* in cats
      Monitor prothrombin time (PT) or international normalized ratio (INR). The INR is calculated from the PT and adjusts for differences in the strength of reagents used to measure the PT. It is a safer index of therapy and can be calculated by the laboratory.
      Adjust dosage to achieve an INR that is 2.0 to 3.0, or a PT that is 1.5 to 2.0 times normal.

Stabilization of INR or PT can require up to 5 days of therapy.
Initially, monitor every 24 hours.
Gradually increase the interval if results are consistent. The maximum interval should be 4 to 6 weeks.
4. Eliminate underlying disease.

............Smoke Inhalation

Animals trapped in building fires may be presented with thermal burns (see p. 24), but more commonly they are presented with signs of severe respiratory distress associated with burns of the respiratory tract and carbon monoxide and smoke toxicity.

Carbon monoxide results in hypoxia because it combines with hemoglobin and displaces oxygen in the transport system. The percentage of carboxyhemoglobin in the blood depends on the amount of carbon monoxide in the inspired air and the time length of exposure. Carboxyhemoglobin concentrations of 40% to 80% in the blood result in cyanosis, nausea, collapse, respiratory failure, and death.

Smoke toxicity is caused by excessive heat severely damaging the mucous membranes of the upper respiratory tract, including the larynx, leading to laryngeal edema. Inhalation of incomplete products of combustion can enter the bronchi and bronchioles and combine with mucus to produce noxious acids and alkalis, damaging the bronchioles. Specific noxious fumes may damage lungs when plastics, rubber, or other synthetic products burn. Pulmonary edema due to ARDs and secondary bacterial infection can be serious complications.

Physical Examination The initial physical examination of an animal that has been trapped in a fire should include:

1. Examination of the mouth and pharynx to detect evidence of burns.
2. Careful examination of the respiratory system (rate, rhythm, and auscultation for crackles or wheezes).
3. Measurement of carboxyhemoglobin concentrations, and arterial blood gas analysis for acid-base status and pulmonary function. Caution must be used in interpreting PaO_2 levels in carbon monoxide poisoning, because blood oxygen may be normal, even though carboxyhemoglobin levels may be very elevated.
4. Radiographs can be helpful, although severe lung changes do not usually develop until 16 to 24 hours after inhalation damage. Radiographs may reveal edema, atelectasis, or evidence of beginning pneumonia. Pleural effusion may develop.
5. More accurate evaluation of upper respiratory injury can be achieved by bronchoscopy (see p. 521). However, caution must be used in passing the scope or endotracheal tubes through inflamed larynx and trachea. Further risks associated with anesthesia may be too great in many patients.

Treatment The initial treatment of smoke inhalation includes the following procedures:

1. If severe laryngeal edema is present and an endotracheal tube (even a small one) cannot be inserted, a tracheostomy is indicated (see p. 623). Positive-pressure ventilation can be begun, if needed. The trachea should be suctioned of mucus and debris.
2. Treatment of carbon monoxide poisoning is begun immediately with the administration of 100% oxygen. The half-life of carboxyhemoglobin is 4 hours in room air and ½ hour in 100% oxygen. If there is not severe respiratory difficulty, the patient can be placed in an oxygen cage (see p. 610). and 40% oxygen that has adequate humidity can also be placed in the cage.

3. Treat fluid loss and electrolyte needs. While hydration must be maintained, overhydration is avoided.
4. Evaluate for further injury, and begin treatment for pulmonary edema, if indicated (see p. 252).
5. If signs deteriorate after 24 to 48 hours, reevaluate the animal for secondary bacterial pneumonia.

............MISCELLANEOUS

............Epistaxis

Epistaxis can be caused by facial trauma, foreign body, neoplasia, nasal fungal infection, systemic clotting disorder, ehrlichiosis, or hypertension. Acute, severe bilateral hemorrhage without exudate is suggestive of a systemic disorder. A history of chronic nasal discharge is suggestive of a nasal disorder. Acute, unilateral hemorrhage can occur from nasal or systemic disease.

In most cases, cage rest is adequate to diminish the loss of blood. Sedation may be beneficial. Acepromazine 0.05 mg/kg IV or SC is often effective because of its tranquilizing and hypotensive effects. The hypotensive effects are essentially harmful if volume loss is severe. Volume is replaced with IV fluid therapy.

Rapid assessment of systemic clotting ability is performed (ACT and examination of a blood smear for platelets). Continued bleeding from a clotting disorder may require blood transfusion for treatment.

Persistent bleeding due to intranasal disease can be treated by dripping dilute epinephrine 1:100,000 into the nasal cavity with the nose pointed toward the ceiling to induce vasoconstriction. If this fails, the animal can be anesthetized and umbilical tape packed into the nasal cavity from both the external naris and the caudal nasopharynx. Continued bleeding is exceedingly rare, but if necessary the external carotid artery on the side of hemorrhage can be ligated.

REFERENCES

Baty CJ, Hardie EM: Pulmonary thromboembolism: Diagnosis and treatment. *In* Kirk RW, ed: Current Veterinary Therapy XI. Small Animal Practice. Philadelphia, WB Saunders, 1992.

Boudreau PJ, Muir WW: Pathophysiology of traumatic diaphragmatic hernias in dogs. Compend Contin Educ Pract Vet 9:379–386, 1987.

Forrester D, Fossum TW, Rogers KS: Diagnosis and treatment of chylothorax associated with lymphoblastic lymphosarcoma in four cats. J Am Vet Med Assoc 198:291–294, 1991.

Fossum,TW: Chylothorax — New perspectives and cardiovascular implications. *In* Proceedings of the 15th Annual Forum of the American College of Veterinary Internal Medicine, 1995, pp 314–317.

Fossum TW. Feline chylothorax. Compendium Contin Educ Pract Vet 15:549–567, 1993.

Fossum TW, Birchard SJ: Chylothorax. *In* Kirk RW, ed: Current Veterinary Therapy X. Small Animal Practice. Philadelphia, WB Saunders, 1989.

Gaber CE, Amis TC, LeCouter A: Laryngeal paralysis in dogs: A review of 23 cases. J Am Vet Med Assoc 186:377–380, 1985.

Harpster N: Pulmonary edema. *In* Kirk RW, ed: Current Veterinary Therapy X. Small Animal Practice. Philadelphia, WB Saunders, 1989.

Hawkins EC: Respiratory diseases. *In* Nelson RW, Couto CG, eds: Essentials of Small Animal Internal Medicine. St Louis, Mosby–Year Book, 1992.

Holtisinger RH, Beale B, Bellah J: Spontaneous pneumothorax in the dog: A retrospective analysis of 21 cases. J Am Anim Hosp Assoc 29:195–210, 1993.

Moise NS, Wiedenkeller D, Yeager AE, et al: Clinical radiographic, and bronchial cytologic features of cats with bronchial disease: 65 cases (1980–1986). J Am Vet Med Assoc 194:1467–1473, 1989.

Moon PF, Concannon KT: Mechanical ventilation. *In* Kirk RW, ed: Current Veterinary Therapy XI. Small Animal Practice. Philadelphia, WB Saunders, 1992.

Nelson TE: Malignant hyperthermia in dogs. J Am Vet Med Assoc 98:989, 1991.

Peterson SW, Rosin E, Bjorling PE: Surgical options for laryngeal paralysis in dogs: A consideration of partial laryngectomy. Compend Contin Educ Pract Vet 13:1531, 1991.

Riley P: Nasopharyngeal grass foreign bodies in eight cats. J Am Vet Med Assoc 202:299–300, 1993.

Saxon WD, Kirby R: Treatment of acute burn injury and smoke inhalation. *In* Kirk RW, ed: Current Veterinary Therapy XI. Small Animal Practice. Philadelphia, WB Saunders, 1992.

Steyn PF, Wittum TE: Radiographic, epidemiologic and clinical aspects of pleural and peritoneal effusions in dogs and cats. J Am Vet Med Assoc 202:307–312, 1993.

Sullivan M, Reid J: Management of 60 cases of diaphragmatic rupture. J Small Anim Pract 31:425–430, 1990.

Sweet DC, Waters DJ: Role of surgery in management of dogs with pathologic conditions of thorax, part II. Compend Contin Educ Pract Vet 13:1671, 1991.

Turner WD, Breznock EM: Continuous suction drainage for management of canine pyothorax: A retrospective study. J Am Anim Hosp Assoc 24:485–494, 1988.

Acute Superficial Soft Tissue Injuries

·········· CLASSIFICATION OF SUPERFICIAL INJURIES
(see Table 1–35)

Wounds have been classified in several ways. These include (1) tissue integrity, (2) etiologic force, (3) degree of contamination and infection, and (4) degree of contamination (Table 1–35). There are also unique causes of wounds such as burns, psychogenic dermatoses, frostbite, pressure sores, and snake bites.

·········· TREATMENT (see Table 1–36)

I. Animal transport.
  A. Protect animal care personnel from bite wound, e.g., muzzle dog.
  B. Pack wound firmly with dry gauze or clean linen.
    1. Protects.
    2. Prevents further contamination.
    3. Helps attain hemostasis.
  C. Open fractures—splint without replacing exposed bone back in the wound.
    1. Avoids soft tissue injury from bone fragment movement.
    2. Helps prevent contamination of deeper tissue.
  D. Transport animal on a firm flat surface if spinal fracture is suspected.
II. Initial assessment and care.
  A. History.
    1. Animal's general health and current medications.
    2. Circumstances of wounding.
    3. Emergency therapy already administered.
  B. Patient evaluation.
    1. ABC (*a*irway, *b*reathing, and *c*irculation) assessment.
    2. Level of consciousness assessment.
    3. Resuscitation and stabilization of the animal.
    4. Detailed physical examination.
    5. Ancillary tests—hematologic, biochemical, radiographic ultrasonographic, and electrophysiologic.
  C. Wound management—when there has been a delay in wound assessment.
    1. Obtain culture and sensitivity samples, if this testing is to be done.
    2. Apply a wound support bandage. It may have water-soluble antibiotic ointment or a nonirritating antimicrobial solution, e.g., 0.05% solution of chlorhexidine diacetate (Nolvasan) or gluconate (Chlor-Hexiderm).

Table 1–35. Superficial Wounds

Classification	Characteristics
Tissue Integrity	
Open	Lacerations or skin loss
Closed	Crushing injuries and contusions
Etiologic Force	
Abrasion	Loss of epidermis and portions of dermis; usually due to shearing between two compressive surfaces
Avulsion	Tearing of tissue from its attachment due to forces similar to those causing abrasion but of greater magnitude
Incision	Created by a sharp object; wound edges are smooth and minimal tissue trauma is present in surrounding tissue
Laceration	Irregular wound caused by tearing of tissue with variable damage to superficial and underlying tissue
Puncture	Skin penetration by a missile or sharp object; superficial damage may be minimal; damage to deeper structures may be considerable; contamination by hair and bacteria with subsequent infection is common
Degree of Contamination and Duration	
Class I	0–6 hr duration with minimal contamination
Class II	6–12 hr duration with significant contamination
Class III	≥12 hr with gross contamination
Degree of Contamination	
Clean wound	Surgically created under aseptic conditions; no invasion of respiratory, alimentary, or genitourinary tracts, or of oropharyngeal cavities
Clean contaminated wound	Minimal contamination, and contamination can be effectively removed; includes operative wounds involving respiratory, alimentary, and genitourinary tracts
Contaminated wound	Open traumatic wound with heavy contamination and possibly foreign debris; includes operative wounds with major breaks in aseptic technique, and incisions in areas of acute nonpurulent inflammation adjacent to inflamed or contaminated skin
Dirty/infected wound	Old traumatic wounds and wounds with clinical infection or perforated viscera

Modified from Swaim SF, Henderson RA: Small Animal Wound Management, ed 2. Media, PA, Williams & Wilkins, 1997.

    3. Administer systemic antibiotics.
  D. Wound evaluation.
    1. Limb wounds—assess neural, vascular, and orthopedic structures.
    2. Wounds on other body areas—assess structures deep to the superficial wounds.
  E. Microbial evaluation and systemic therapy.

Table 1–36. Potential Problems With Superficial Wounds

Circumstance	Primary Potential Problem(s)
Improper handling of animal transport (e.g., improper limb or spine immobilization)	Further tissue damage may occur
Inadequate assessment of animal's general condition or wounded tissues	Animal's condition may worsen or it may succumb, or tissue injuries may be overlooked
Inadequate wound protection during assessment, resuscitation, or stabilization procedures	Further wound contamination at veterinary facilities
Inadequate wound protection while preparing the surrounding area	Further wound contamination with hair and debris
Insufficient analgesia of wound tissues by local analgesia	Difficult debridement following surgical invasion of the area with sensation
Insufficient wound lavage	Wound infection
Hydrogen peroxide wound lavage	Little bactericidal activity and it may cause tissue emphysema
Povidone-iodine wound lavage	Short residual activity, absorption with acidosis (esp. in large wounds), and possible thyroid problems
Overly aggressive initial layered debridement	May result in removal of tissue that may still be viable
En bloc debridement	Results in removal of large amounts of tissue and a large defect for closure
Use of drains	Potential for bacteria to ascend along drain, animal molestation with drain breakage in the wound or premature drain removal, and possible tissue emphysema with air being sucked into the wound by movement (e.g., in the axillary and inguinal area)
Tube-type drains	May cause postoperative discomfort and fenestrations may become occluded to stop intraluminal drainage
Deeply placed sutures in the presence of a drain	May incorporate the drain to impair drain removal
Active drains	High negative pressure may cause tissue injury and highly productive wounds may necessitate changing the evacuated blood tubes several times daily with constructed drains

1. Microbial evaluation (when performed) on recent contaminated wounds.
   a. Swab wound for culture and sensitivity.
   b. Results may confirm or alter antibiotic therapy.
2. Microbial evaluation of older infected wounds.
   a. Gram stain of an impression smear—bacterial population.
   b. May help in selection of systemic antibiotic.
3. Systemic antibiotics.

       a. Begin early—preferably in the first 3 hours.

       b. Possibilities—cephalosporins, amoxicillin or clavulanate potassium (Clavamox), trimethoprim and sulfadiazine (Tribrissen), amoxicillin, or ampicillin. With gram-negative flora—aminoglycosides. For a broader spectrum—enrofloxacin (Baytril).

       c. Administer for 5 to 7 days unless a change of antibiotic therapy is indicated.

III. Wound protection and surrounding area preparation.

  A. Protection of the wound.

    1. Pack the wound with saline moistened sterile gauze sponges.

      or

    2. Pack the wound with water-soluble lubricating gel (K-Y jelly, Johnson & Johnson, Arlington, TX) or a sterile lubricating gel that contains chlorhexidine gluconate (Surgilube, E. Fougera Co., Melville, NY).

      or

    3. Apply a thin coat of gel to hold a sterile gauze sponge on the wound.

  B. Preparation of the surrounding area (usually done after general anesthesia or neuroleptanalgesia).

    1. If the animal's hair coat is covered with dirt and debris, bathing with the animal on a grate over a tub is indicated.

    2. Clip hair for an ample distance around wounds.

    3. Remove gauze sponges or lavage gel from the wound and replace with a new gel or gauze sponges.

    4. Scrub the skin with antiseptic detergent (Nolvasan Surgical Scrub, ChlorhexiDerm, Solvahex, or Betadine [povidone-iodine]), and apply a corresponding antiseptic soltuion.

IV. Anesthesia and analgesia. (See also p. 7.)

  A. General anesthesia for animals in good physical condition.

    1. Neuroleptanalgesia (premedication) prior to general anesthesia.

      a. Butorphanol and acetylpromazine or diazepam.

        or

      b. Oxymorphone and acetylpromazine or diazepam.

    2. General anesthesia induction and endotracheal intubation.

      a. Halothane or isoflurane, mask.

        or

      b. Thiopental sodium, IV.

        or

      c. Propofol IV.

    3. General anesthesia maintenance.

      a. Halothane or isoflurane.

      b. Intermittent or continuous IV infusion with propofol or thiopental.

  B. Neuroleptanalgesia followed by local or regional analgesia for animals in questionable physical condition.

    1. Neuroleptanalgesia (usually done before preparation of the area around the wound).

      a. See Neuroleptanalgesia (premedication) prior to general anesthesia.

        or

      b. Meditomidine and butorphanol.

    2. Local analgesia (usually injected after preparation of the area around the wound).

      a. Halothane or isoflurane, mask.

        or

      b. Thiopental sodium, IV.

or
   c. Propofol IV.
  3. General anesthesia maintenance.
    a. Halothane or isoflurane.
    b. Intermittent or continuous IV.
 C. Neuroleptanalgesia followed by local or regional analgesia for animals in questionable physical condition.
  1. Neuroleptanalgesia (usually done before preparation of the area around the wound).
    a. See Neuroleptanalgesia (premedication) prior to general anesthesia.
    or
    b. Meditomidine and butorphanol.
  2. Local analgesia (usually injected after preparation of the area around the wound).
    a. One percent or 2% lidocaine without epinephrine injected into undamaged tissue parallel to the wound's perimeter.
    b. Warm the lidocaine if it has been refrigerated, and mix sodium bicarbonate 0.1 mL with each milliliter of lidocaine to make the injection more comfortable.
  3. Regional analgesia (usually done after preparation of the area surrounding the wound).
    a. Ring block on a limb—circumferential skin-to-bone lidocaine injection.
    b. Injection is proximal to the wound.
 V. Wound lavage.
  A. Drape the wound area.
  B. Remove gauze sponges or gel from wounds.
  C. Lavage the wound with copious quantities of lavage solution.
   1. Pressure delivery of lavage solution.
    a. Lavage solution container, 30-mL syringe, IV administration set, three-way stopcock valve, and 18-gauge needle.
    b. Plastic squeeze bottle with small fluid delivery aperture.
    c. Plastic bottle with trigger-type delivery apparatus.
   2. Lavage solutions—warmed.
    a. Tap water—use one time in grossly contaminated wounds.
    b. Hydrogen peroxide—use one time in grossly contaminated wounds without pressure delivery.
    c. Isotonic saline, lactated Ringer's, or Ringer's solution.
    d. Chlorhexidine diacetate or gluconate solution 0.05% solution.
    e. Povidone-iodine 1.0% solution.
VI. Wound debridement.
  A. Staged layer debridement.
   1. Obviously nonviable tissue and tissue that is not attached are excised leaving viable and questionable tissue.
    a. Skin.
      i. Remove extremely dark or white segments.
      ii. Retain questionable and viable segments.
      iii. Wait 48 to 72 hours to trim questionable skin edges.
    b. Subcutaneous tissue and panniculus muscle—attached to skin flaps.
    c. Excise fat contaminated with debris and blood stains.
    d. Excise loose ragged fragments of fascia.
    e. Ligate severed blood vessels if collateral circulation is intact.
    f. Cleanse and cover exposed intact nerves with tissue or bandage; if cleanly severed without trauma, anastomose. If severed with trauma and contamination, defer definitive anastomosis

until healthy tissue is present. Perform temporary anastomosis and immobilize limb.

g. Muscle.

    i. Friable, no hemorrhage, no contraction with stimulation, ground-in dirt, dark or pale—excise until hemorrhage or contraction occur.

    ii. Retain questionable muscle and reevaluate in 24 hours.

    iii. Cat muscle normally appears pale.

h. Tendons.

    i. Contaminated and denuded of paratenon—cleanse and cover with tissue or bandage.

    ii. Cleanly severed without trauma—anastomose.

    iii. Severed with trauma and contamination—defer definitive anastomosis until healthy tissue is present. Perform temporary anastomosis and immobilize limb.

    iv. Severed and frayed ends not identifiable, with large gaps—trim frayed ends.

i. Joints containing debris, clots, and cartilage fragments.

    i. Lavage thoroughly.

    ii. Discard small fragments, replace large fragments.

    iii. Smooth sharp edges.

    iv. Suture joint capsule and ligaments partially or totally when possible.

    v. Remove bullets or metal fragments.

    vi. Subcutaneous tissue and skin left open—delayed primary closure.

    vii. Immobilize joint.

j. Bone.

    i. With periosteal covering—cover with bandage or tissue.

    ii. Ground-in dirt—remove with brush, curet, or rongeur.

    iii. Dirt in broken end—remove with curet or cut bone end off.

    iv. Fragments—retain fragments; immobilize fractures.

2. Bandage wound, reevaluate tissues at bandage change every 24 hours, and debride as needed.

B. Enzymatic debridement.

1. Enzymatic debriding agent (Granulex-V, Pfizer Animal Health, New York, NY) is applied to the wound under a bandage. (See also p. 549.)

2. Uses.

a. When animal is a poor anesthetic or surgical risk.

b. With staged debridement for removal of small amounts of necrotic tissue and debris between bandage changes.

c. When excision might jeopardize vital structures.

C. Adherent bandage debridement.

1. Apply dry or wet wide-mesh gauze sponges, intermediate layer and outer layer, (see Bandaging and Splinting Techniques, Open Contaminated and Infected Wounds).

2. Uses.

a. With staged debridement for removal of small amounts of necrotic tissue and debris between bandage changes.

b. When excision might jeopardize vital structures.

D. En bloc debridement.

1. Complete excision of the wound without entering the wound cavity.

2. Used on badly infected wounds without signs of systemic infection avoids breaking barriers around the wound to prevent systemic infection.

3. Technique.

a. Use only for areas with sufficient surrounding tissue to allow such debridement.

b. Use only where there are no vital vessels, nerves, and tendons.

c. Pack wound with gauze and close it with several sutures or paint the wound surface with sterile methylene blue.

d. Dissect the entire wound with a margin of normal tissue, never entering the wound cavity.

VII. Open wounds—those to be managed by healing by second intention, delayed primary closure, or secondary closure.

A. Systemic antibiotics (See also p. 893.)

B. Topical medications (See also p. 540.)

1. Antibiotic and antibacterial agents—choice may be governed by results of culture and sensitivity or Gram stain of an impression smear.

a. Bacitracin, neomycin, polymixin (triple antibiotic)

b. Silver sulfadiazine 1% (SSD) (Hoechst-Marion Roussel, Kansas City, MO).

c. Nitrofurazone (Clay Parks, Bronx, NY).

d. Gentamicin sulfate (Garamycin ointment 0.1%) (Schering Corp., Liberty Corner, NJ).

2. Hydrophilic agent—healing stimulant.

a. d-glucose polysaccharide—maltodextrin.

b. Used to cleanse and promote healing.

c. Proposed to provide energy for cell metabolism.

d. Promotes chemotaxis of polymorphonuclear cells, macrophages, and lymphocytes.

3. Enzymatic agent (See also p. 549.)

4. Hydrogel wound dressing—healing stimulant.

a. Topical hydrogel wound dressing (Carravet Wound Dressing, Carrington Laboratories, Inc., Irving, TX).

b. Contains acemannan—stimulates macrophage production of tumor necrosis factor and interleukin-1.

c. Promotes fibroblast proliferation, neovascularization, epidermal growth, and collagen deposition.

VIII. Closed wounds—sutures, drains, and bandages.

A. Primary wound closure.

1. Consider when:

a. There has been short time lapse since infliction.

b. There is minimal contamination and trauma.

c. Thorough debridement and lavage have been done.

d. There is good hemostasis, no tissue tension, or dead space.

2. Closure technique.

a. Eliminate dead space with 2-0 or 4-0 simple interrupted sutures of absorbable multifilament or monofilament or nonabsorbable or monofilament material.

b. Use the smallest diameter and fewest sutures that are still effective.

c. Avoid inclusion of major vessels and nerves in sutures.

d. Close subcutaneous tissues with similar suture materials in a simple continuous pattern.

e. Skin closure is with 2-0 to 4-0 nonabsorbable suture in one of several suture patterns.

3. Passive drains.

a. Place at the time of closure if any doubt exists about tissue status.

b. Use a passive drain of thin latex rubber (Penrose drain) rubber, or plastic tubing.

  c. One end of the drain is anchored in the proximal aspect of the wound with a simple interrupted nonabsorbable suture. The suture is passed through the skin, the drain, and back out through the skin. The suture is tied. Removal of this suture frees the drain for removal.

  d. Exit the drain below the distal end of the wound closure, anchoring it with a simple interrupted suture at the exit hole.

  e. Close subcutaneous tissue over a drain before skin closure.

  f. During wound closure, check the mobility of the drain to avoid drain incorporation in a suture.

  g. Remove the drain when drainage becomes minimal (as revealed by fluid absorbed in a bandage).

 4. Active drains.

  a. Technique 1 (constructed drain).

   i. Indicated in wounds that are free of necrotic tissue and foreign material that may plug the drain.

   ii. Use a butterfly scalp needle apparatus and a 5- or 10 mL. evacuated blood collection tube.

   iii. Remove the syringe adaptor from the apparatus and fenestrate the tubing.

   iv. Place the tubing in the wound via a small stab incision distal to the wound.

   v. A purse-string suture is placed around the tubing at this exit point for a tight seal.

   vi. After wound closure, the needle of the apparatus is inserted in the collection tube to pull fluid into the tube.

   vii. The tube is incorporated in a bandage and replaced as needed when it becomes full.

  b. Technique 2 (constructed drain).

   i. Remove the needle from the butterfly scalp needle apparatus and fenestrate the tubing.

   ii. Place and secure the tubing in the wound as with technique 1.

   iii. The wound is closed and the syringe adaptor of the tubing is connected to a plastic syringe.

   iv. The syringe plunger is withdrawn enough to create the desired negative pressure without collapsing the tubing.

   v. A metal pin or 16 to 18 gauge needle is inserted through the plunger at the top of the barrel to hold it at the desired level.

   vi. The suction apparatus is incorporated in a bandage and replaced as needed when it becomes full.

  c. Technique 3 (commercially available drains).

   i. Install as per manufacturer's recommendations.

 5. Delayed primary closure.

  1. Consider when:

   i. There is heavy contamination, purulent exudate, residual necrotic or questionable tissue, edema, erythema, lymphangitis, and skin tension.

   ii. It has been 3 to 5 days since the wound infliction and the above abnormalities have been controlled by open wound therapy.

  2. Technique.

B. Secondary wound closure.

 1. Consider when:

  a. Infection and tissue trauma necessitate open wound management beyond 5 days.

    b. After the wound has formed a healthy bed of granulation tissue.
    c. A wound has disrupted and has formed granulation tissue.
 2. Technique.
    a. Technique 1 (early secondary closure).
       i. Done when wound edges can still be manipulated into apposition (have little granulation tissue) and epithelialization has not begun.
      ii. Cleanse the wound surface with antiseptic solution.
     iii. Wound edges are apposed and sutured.
    b. Technique 2 (later secondary closure).
       i. Done when wounds have considerable granulation tissue and edges cannot be manipulated into apposition, and epithelialization has started.
      ii. Cleanse the wound surface with antiseptic solution.
     iii. Remove the epithelium from the wound edges.
     iv. Suture the remaining wound edges over the granulation tissue.

    Complicating factors involved in managing soft tissue wounds are depicted in Table 1–36.

REFERENCE

Swaim, SF, Henderson, RA: Small Animal Wound Management, ed 2. Media, Pa, Williams & Wilkins, 1997.

Section 2

PATIENT EVALUATION AND ORGAN SYSTEM EXAMINATION

2

· ·

PATIENT EVALUATION

Making the Diagnosis

Every new case is a challenge for diagnosis. Everything is keyed to the proper and complete answer to the question: What is wrong with the patient? Only when the question is answered can one plan the proper treatment and forecast the results with reasonable accuracy. Experienced clinicians often "eyeball" the patient, or arrive at possible diagnoses almost by intuition, but this approach to medicine is dangerous. Important, even vital, information is almost always missed.

One must collect and analyze clinical evidence methodically and accurately so that no diagnostic possibility is overlooked. Diagnosis necessitates two basic steps: (1) collecting the facts and (2) analyzing the facts.

............DATABASE

Collecting the facts involves four steps: (1) obtaining a complete clinical history, (2) performing a thorough physical examination, (3) using ancillary methods for further evaluation (e.g., radiographs, ultrasound exams, laboratory data, endoscopy), and (4) observing the course of the illness.

The first three points are discussed in the following pages. The fourth point, however, deserves comment here. In many cases, a diagnosis is not immediately evident, even after a careful case workup. Patients may be hospitalized "for observation," or the patient may be seen at appropriate intervals, serial tests performed, and consultation with special colleagues arranged. As a disease progresses, more evidence becomes available, and eventually the diagnosis becomes a reality. There should be no stigma attached to delay in reaching a definitive diagnosis, but many veterinarians feel that there is; thus, they fail to use one of the most important aids to diagnosis: observing the course of the illness.

............Clinical History

It requires skill to elicit an unbiased history of their pet's illness from most owners. Some owners are good observers and can supply important information, whereas others either do not notice things or may purposely withhold information. It is important to impress upon the owner how important it is that he or she help you to help the pet. When talking to the pet owner, one should use a vocabulary commensurate with his or her intelligence, background, and formal education. Ask neutral questions—ones that will not prejudice the owner's answers—such as, "Tell me about your dog's water consumption." Direct or leading questions can be asked, provided that one realizes that bias may be introduced. Comments such as "Anything else?," "How do you mean?," or "Tell me about that" are helpful in inducing the owner to elaborate. Do not belittle the owner's opinion of the illness or its cause.

If the same sequence of history taking and physical examination is followed each time, the procedure gradually requires less time and important facts will not be glossed over or omitted.

............The Chief Complaint

The complaint is the reason the patient is being presented. What should be recorded is a sign (diarrhea), not a diagnosis (enteritis) that may have been made by the owner or another clinician. It is important to record the duration of the sign; e.g., diarrhea for 3 months.

########### *Present Illness*

No exact description can be given because of the variety of presenting complaints. It is important, however, to record data in sequence *by date*. Record the type of onset and possible exposure to other sick animals. Determine whether other persons or animals have become infected by contact with the patient.

If the present illness has progressed in attacks separated by intervals of good health, obtain a history of a typical attack (onset, duration, signs, and treatment). Both positive and negative data about disturbances to organic and systemic functions are important.

########### *Past History*

The past history of the animal should include whether it has experienced any of the following:

1. *Infectious diseases*: distemper, hepatitis, leptospirosis, panleukopenia, and pneumonitis
2. *Major illnesses*: dates of infections or severe illness, treatment, complications, and sequelae
3. *Allergies*: contact, atopy, and food and drug reactions
4. *Accidents*
5. *Operations*
6. *Pregnancies*: number of offspring whelped and weaned from each delivery
7. *Immunizations*: panleukopenia, pneumonitis, distemper, hepatitis, leptospirosis, rabies, and dates of immunization and the products used

########### *Environmental History*

The animal's present or past environment may be obscure, but information about the present health of the parents, siblings, and offspring may be of interest. Find out when and where the animal was born and raised; the environments it has been exposed to during travel and with different owners; whether it is a working animal or a house pet; and the kind of shelter, care, diet, grooming, and medications it routinely receives.

########### **Routine Physical Examination**

A routine physical examination should include determining the state of the following:

1. *Vital signs*: Temperature, pulse, respiration, and weight.
2. *General appearance*: Conformity, state of nutrition, apparent age, degree of grooming care, type of disposition, mental alertness, gross deformities, and striking findings (e.g., severe dyspnea, weakness, and depression).
3. *Skin*: Inspect and palpate. Note the color, texture, degree of moisture or oil present; amount, texture and distribution of hair, pattern of alopecias, ease of epilation; presence of parasites; and types and distribution of primary and secondary skin lesions.
4. *Lymph nodes*: Palpate all superficial nodes and the spleen. Note enlargement, consistency, mobility, and pain.
5. *Eyes*: Examine the conjunctiva and sclera for injection, exudation, and petechiae. Elicit the pupillary reflex. Perform an ophthalmoscopic examination (cornea, iris, lens, and retina).
6. *Ears*: Look for discharge and perform an otoscopic examination for exudates or parasites. Note the appearance of the tympanic membranes.

7. *Nose*: Look for evidence of discharge and patency.
8. *Mouth and throat*: Smell the breath; note any discharges or excess saliva; and observe the color and appearance of mucous membranes, the pharynx, and the tonsils.
9. *Neck and back*: Assess the extent of rigidity or limitation of motion, deformities, and pain.
10. *Thorax*: Evaluate for conformity, symmetry, and free respiratory movements. Percuss and auscultate systematically from the dorsal to the ventral aspects.
11. *Heart*: Palpate, noting the intensity of apex beat and the presence of thrills. Evaluate rate, rhythm, quality of sounds, bruits, or rubs. Record the auscultated heart rate and femoral pulse rate if they are different. Carefully auscultate all four valvular areas.
12. *Abdomen*: Determine the conformity, symmetry, masses, gases, fluids, rigidity, or splinting. Auscultate for peristalsis and palpate deeply.
13. *Genitalia*: In the male, palpate and inspect the testes and penis; in the female, palpate and inspect the vulva and the mammary glands.
14. *Rectum*: Palpate the confines of the pelvic canal; check the prostate for size, conformity, and consistency.
15. *Extremities*: Watch the animal walk. Inspect and palpate the legs and joints. Note the presence of pain, heat, swelling, deformities, or limitation of motion.
16. *Neurologic*: Watch the animal walk. From dorsal recumbency, allow it to right itself and perform coordinate tasks. Palpate muscles and compare tonus and balance with opposite numbers. Check tendon reflexes and sensory responses.

..........Routine Laboratory Procedures—The Minimum Database

Although more testing may be needed, the screening tests described here are usually done as part of a complete physical examination.

- Complete blood count
- Biochemical profile
- Urinalysis—to include:
    Urine biochemistries
    Microscopic examination of sediment
    Urine specific gravity
- Fecal examination for parasite ova by:
    Flotation
    Direct examination
- Heartworm antigen
- Feline leukemia virus (FeLV) antigen
- Feline immunodeficiency virus (FIV) antibody

..........Problem List

The problem list can be considered as a table of contents listing all the animal's problems, past as well as present. At presentation of an ill animal, the clinician must strive to develop a working problem list from which a logical diagnostic plan evolves. A patient's problems are defined as (1) the client's interpretation of the patient's problem(s), (2) abnormal physical findings, and (3) abnormal laboratory or diagnostic test results. To reach a clinical diagnosis, the veterinarian must rely heavily on interpretive skills and experience to construct a problem list effectively and to subsequently determine the nature of the patient's illness.

..........Initial Plan

For each problem, there should be (1) plans for the collection of further data in order to establish a diagnosis or facilitate management, (2) plans for treatment with specific drugs, and (3) plans to educate the owner of the animal about existing problems. The plans should be dated when initiated, and the goals of therapeutic plans should be stated briefly.

..........Progress Notes

The progress notes are the follow-up mechanism for a problem. It is necessary to evaluate each aspect of the treatment plan carefully and to note this assessment in the record.

2

REFERENCES

Ettinger SJ: Pocket Companion to Textbook of Veterinary Internal Medicine. Philadelphia, WB Saunders, 1993.
Ford RB: The study of clinical signs. *In* Ford RB, ed: Clinical Signs and Diagnosis in Small Animal Practice. New York, Churchill Livingstone, 1988, pp 1–8.
Nelson RW, Couto G: Essentials of Small Animal Internal Medicine. St Louis, Mosby–Year Book, 1993.

....

ORGAN SYSTEM EXAMINATION

Alimentary System

Diseases of the oral cavity and gastrointestinal (GI) tract are common afflictions of small animals. Careful examination with a systematic approach is necessary to evaluate the alimentary system completely. History taking and acquiring answers to the following questions are extremely important:

1. What is the duration of the clinical illness?
2. What is the animal's vaccination history?
3. Where did the animal come from and what is its travel history?
4. Is vomiting part of the syndrome, and what is its relationship to eating? Is it projectile?
5. What is the diet? Is the appetite affected? What is the sequential relationship of the GI abnormality to the animal's eating pattern?
6. Has the animal been examined for endoparasites?
7. Have any treatments already been instituted?
8. Has the animal had previous illness or surgery? Is the animal losing weight?
9. Is halitosis present?

Before proceeding to examination of specific areas of the alimentary system, carefully observe the general physical status of the animal, particularly noting any evidence of emaciation, abdominal enlargement or asymmetry, the position of the animal at rest, and body carriage while moving (tucked up abdomen, stiffness, etc.).

............ORAL EXAMINATION

In most animals, a routine examination of the mouth can be done without anesthesia or tranquilization. Gently retract the lips, and examine the teeth and gums (see also p. 278).

............Dentition in the Dog

Formula for deciduous dentition:

$$2(\text{Di}\frac{3}{3}\,\text{Dc}\frac{1}{1}\,\text{Dm}\frac{3}{3}) = 28$$

Formula for permanent dentition:

$$2(\text{I}\frac{3}{3}\,\text{C}\frac{1}{1}\,\text{P}\frac{4}{4}\,\text{M}\frac{2}{3}) = 42$$

Eruption dates are shown in Table 2–1.

The deciduous dentition should be in place by 7 to 8 weeks. Permanent teeth begin to replace the deciduous teeth at about 4 months of age. All permanent teeth should be in place at about 7 months. In some breeds all the permanent teeth are not erupted until about 1 year of age.

............Dentition in the Cat

Formula for deciduous dentition:

$$2(\text{Di}\frac{3}{3}\,\text{Dc}\frac{1}{1}\,\text{Dm}\frac{3}{2}) = 26$$

Formula for permanent dentition:

$$2(\text{I}\frac{3}{3}\,\text{C}\frac{1}{1}\,\text{PM}\frac{3}{2}\,\text{M}\frac{1}{1}) = 30$$

Eruption dates are shown in Tables 2–1 and 2–2.

Table 2–1. Eruption Dates of Deciduous and Permanent Teeth—Canine

Teeth	Age at Eruption	
	Deciduous (wk)	Permanent (mo)
Incisor 1	4–5	4–5
Incisor 2	4–5	4–5
Incisor 3	5–6	4–5
Canine	3–4	5–6
Premolar 1	—	4–5
Premolar 2	—	5–6
Premolar 3	—	5–6
Premolar 4	—	5–6
Molar 1	4–6	4–5
Molar 2	4–6	5–6
Molar 3	6–8	6–7

Table 2–2. Eruption Dates of Deciduous and Permanent Teeth—Feline

| | Age at Eruption | |
Teeth	Deciduous (wk)	Permanent (mo)
Incisor 1	2–3	3½–4
Incisor 2	2–4	3½–4
Incisor 3	3–4	4–4½
Canine	3–4	5
Premolar 1	—	—
Premolar 2	—	4½–5*
Premolar 3	—	5–6
Premolar 4	—	5–6
Molar 1	—	4–5
Molar 2	4–5*	—
Molar 3	4–6	—

*Upper only.

The normal oral mucosa is pink or partially pigmented, depending on the breed of animal. Discharge from the mouth is usually not evident. The oral cavity should be moist.

Examine the gums for color; petechiae or gross hemorrhage; hypertrophy or recession of the gums; any discharge around the base of the teeth; or any inflammation, swelling, or growth. Examine the hard palate for the presence of foreign bodies, an oronasal fistula, or palatoschisis. Inflammation of the mucous membranes of the mouth is called stomatitis and can be associated with a variety of primary pathogens, as well as being secondary to systemic diseases. Stomatitis may be associated with plant foreign bodies; uremia; diabetes mellitus; heavy metal poisoning (such as thallium); viral infections (especially those of the respiratory system in the cat); mycotic infections associated with *Candida albicans (Monilia)*; and chemical, thermal, or electrical burns.

Examine the teeth for caries; faulty enamel; exposure of roots; deposition of tartar; periodontitis; and loose, crooked, or sharp-edged teeth. Determine the apposition of the upper and lower jaws for prognathism (undershot jaw) or brachygnathism (overshot jaw).

Cats with FeLV or FIV infection and suppression of the immune system may have gingivitis and stomatitis with ulceration of the tongue and oral mucous membranes. Several endocrine abnormalities, including hypothyroidism, diabetes mellitus, and hypoparathyroidism, can produce oral ulcers.

·········· Tooth Terminology (Fig. 2–1)

Crown—Portion above the gum line and covered by enamel.
Neck—Construction of the tooth located at the gum line where the enamel ends and the dentin covered by cementum begins.
Root—Portion below the gum line and covered by cementum.
Furcation—Space between roots of a multirooted tooth.
Apex—Most terminal portion of the root.
Apical delta—Numerous small openings found at the apex allowing the nerves and vessels of the tooth to enter.
Enamel—Outer covering of the crown; very shiny, hard substance. It is the hardest substance in the body and is made up of less than 5% of organic material.

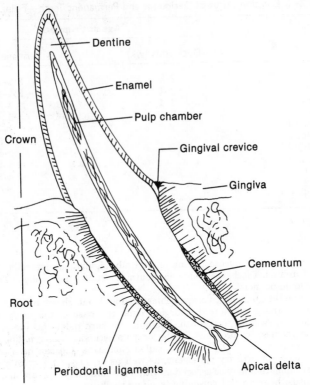

Figure 2–1. The canine tooth.

Dentin—Dense, bonelike material underlying the enamel and making up the substance of the tooth. It can be sensitive to heat and cold and is made up of 26% to 28% of organic material. It continues to be formed in the healthy tooth by odontoblasts, cells which line the pulp chamber.

Cementum—Layer of bony tissue that covers the root of the tooth and is attached to the alveolar bone by the periodontal ligament fibers.

Pulp—The soft tissues of the tooth: the nerves, which contain sensory fibers only, and the vessels coming in through the apical delta extending through the length of the tooth in the root canals.

Periodontal ligaments—Network of fibrous connective tissue that attaches the tooth to the alveolar bone and to other teeth and the gingiva to the alveolus.

Gingiva—Gums.

..........Surfaces of the Tooth

Buccal (vestibular)—The surface toward the cheek (molars).

Labial (vestibular)—The surface toward the lips (incisors, canines, premolars).

Lingual—The surface toward the tongue, lower jaw.

Palatal—The surface toward the tongue, upper jaw.

Occlusal—The surfaces that face the antagonist in the opposite jaw. There are no true occlusal surfaces in carnivores such as cats.
Contact—The surface that faces adjacent teeth.
Mesial—The surface closest to the midline.
Distal—The surface most distant from the midline.

·············Record Forms

Like all medical disciplines, dentistry has its special forms. Diagnostic and therapeutic procedures should be carefully recorded. Figures 2–2 and 2–3 are examples of dental record forms.

·············Formation of Teeth

The teeth of small animals are fully developed (erupted) into their adult form by the time the animal is 6 to 7 months of age usually. Teeth have both an epithelial and a mesenchymal precursor. Cells that produce the enamel of the tooth are called *ameloblasts*. The enamel organ of the developing tooth is in the shape of a crown, and the columnar cells lying next to the ameloblast are the odontoblast cells which produce the dentin of the tooth. The nerves and vessels are in the center of the tooth.

·············Occlusion and Dentition

The major malocclusion defects that are inherited are brachygnathism and prognathism. In brachygnathism, the upper jaw is longer than the lower (overshot). In prognathism, the mandible is longer than the maxilla (undershot). This condition is the breed standard for brachycephalic breeds, including boxers, bulldogs, and Pekingese, but it is not anatomically normal. Any occlusion other than the normal "scissors" occlusion predisposes the patient to dental disease. There can be crowding or rotation of teeth (early onset of periodontal disease) in the short jaw and trauma to the soft tissues or teeth in the long and short jaw (abnormal attrition).

Supernumerary teeth occur occasionally in the maxilla and mandible and should be extracted if they are causing problems. Oligodontia (too few teeth) can be diagnosed in large or small breeds. Radiographs should be taken to confirm tooth absence. Enamel hypoplasia may occur during the ameloblastic phase (2 to 5 months of age). Those are commonly called "distemper teeth" and are usually rough and dark-staining. Tetracyclines or tetracycline derivatives should be avoided in pregnant patients and patients less than 5 months old. Yellow staining of deciduous or permanent teeth can result following 10 or more days of consecutive treatment.

·············Periodontal Disease

Periodontal disease is the most common oral disease in dogs and cats. Eighty-five percent to 95% of all small animals 2 years old or older have periodontal disease. It is completely preventable. Periodontal disease has two phases: gingivitis (reversible) and periodontitis (irreversible, but usually controllable). It is caused by the accumulation of plaque on teeth. Plaque is a soft, sticky, bacteria-ladened film of saliva and debris. The bacteria and bacterial byproducts cause soft tissue inflammation. Plaque mineralizes to form calculus, which then migrates into the gingival sulcus, causing further inflammation, periodontal ligament loss, bone loss, and, eventually, tooth loss. The general health, as well as the dental health, of a periodontal disease patient declines.

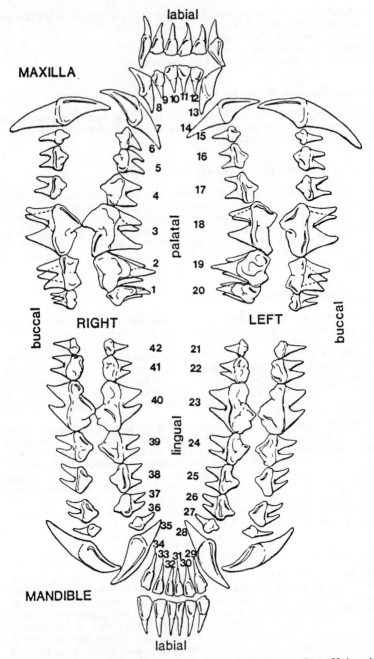

Figure 2–2. Canine dental chart. (Courtesy of North Carolina State University, Veterinary Teaching Hospital, Raleigh.)

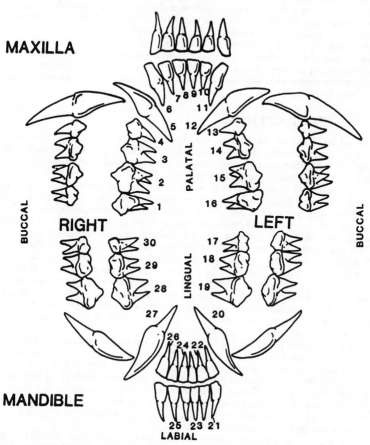

Figure 2–3. Feline dental chart. (Courtesy of North Carolina State University, Veterinary Teaching Hospital, Raleigh.)

··········ABSCESSED TEETH

Abscessed teeth are often associated with advanced periodontal disease. A periodontal probe is inserted into the gingival sulcus to locate periodontal pockets, where tissue and bone have been lost. Loose teeth can sometimes be salvaged using techniques such as root planing and subgingival curettage. If only one root of a multirooted tooth is involved, a dental bar in a high- or low-speed dental handpiece can be used to section the tooth. The affected root is removed and a pulpotomy performed on the remaining tooth. This is an especially useful procedure for small old dogs with one root of the lower first molar involved and the other root healthy.

··········FRACTURED TEETH

Fractured teeth with an exposed pulp chamber often form periapical abscesses. An infraorbital abscess indicates a problem with the upper fourth premolar.

This problem will not resolve permanently unless endodontic therapy or extraction is performed. A fractured lower first molar may drain into the oral cavity or through the ventral aspect of the mandible. A fractured upper canine tooth may drain into the nasal cavity or through a fistulous tract at the level of the upper first or second premolar. An inapparent (the tooth is in place) oronasal fistula may also be present (this is seen often in old small-breed dogs secondary to periodontal disease). A fractured lower canine tooth may drain internally or externally. Endodontic therapy and crown restoration have returned many patients to dental health.

............EXTRACTIONS

Not all teeth can or should be saved. Teeth that are loose or fractured, such that root canal therapy is not suitable, should be removed. Retained deciduous teeth or teeth that are crowded and predisposing a canine or carnassial tooth to periodontal disease, should be extracted.

If the tissues around the tooth are healthy and the tooth is not loose, the gingival margin should be freshened and the epithelial attachment to the tooth severed using a scalpel. A No. 301 or larger dental elevator, sharpened on the convex side, is positioned between bone and tooth. The elevator is rotated gently and held for a count of 30, repositioned, and the procedure repeated. This allows blood to accumulate within the alveolus to help push the tooth from the socket. The periodontal ligaments begin to fatigue and the tooth gradually loosens. It can then be removed using a dental forceps. Root tip elevators are used to remove deciduous teeth or fractured root tips. Multirooted teeth should be sectioned using a cutting burr in a high-speed dental handpiece.

To extract a canine tooth from healthy bone, incise the gingiva on the labial side down to the alveolar bone and gently move the gum away from the side wall of the alveolar bone with a periosteal elevator. *Incise the periosteum at the base of the flap to prevent oronasal fistula formation!* Use a dental cutting burr to cut the buccal cortical plate. Extend the line to about two-thirds the depth of the root. Position a dental elevator in the grooves, first on one side of the tooth, and then on the other, and rotate and hold for a count of 30 to fatigue the periodontal fibers. Extract the loosened tooth using forceps. Suture the flap of gum closed using polyglycolic acid suture. *Do not* lever the canine tooth laterally, because this rotates the tip of the root medially, forcing the root through the bone into the nasal cavity.

During and following extraction, the exposed dental socket should be irrigated with sterile 0.2% chlorhexidine solution (1:10 dilution of chlorhexidine and water).

............The Tongue

Examine the tongue for the presence of any abnormal discoloration, membrane or pseudomembrane, foreign bodies, inflammation, ulcers, growth, or hyperplasia. Note whether the tongue protrudes normally and whether both halves are bilaterally symmetric. The underside of the tongue should be examined for ulcers, foreign bodies such as string wrapped around the base of the tongue (in cats), hyperplasia, indicating a gum chewer syndrome, and swelling of the lingual frenulum.

............Palate, Pharynx, and Buccal Mucosa

The ability of the animal to swallow effectively should be tested by stimulating the pharyngeal area. Dysphagia refers to difficulty in swallowing and can be asociated with localized diseases of the oropharynx or central nervous system (CNS) diseases (see p. 330).

Careful examination of the palate, pharynx, and cheeks requires sedation or a short-acting anesthetic. A focal source of illumination and a tongue depressor or laryngoscope are also needed. Material may be cultured (see p. 466) and a biopsy of tissue may be done to obtain useful information.

Retropharyngeal tumors or abscesses may produce a ventral displacement of the pharynx and larynx. Careful digital exploration of the retropharyngeal area may reveal an undiagnosed mass. Fractures of the hyoid bone may occasionally occur and lead to difficulty in swallowing. Palpation of the posterior pharyngeal area may reveal crepitus and swelling. Inspiratory stridor in brachycephalic breeds of dogs is often associated with an elongated soft palate, weakened laryngeal cartilages, and evagination of the laryngeal ventricles.

In the dog, malignant melanoma, squamous cell carcinoma, and fibrosarcoma are the most common oral and pharyngeal neoplasms. Thoracic radiographs should always be taken to check for lung metastases. In cats, squamous cell carcinoma and fibrosarcoma are the most common oral tumors.

............Tonsils

Inspect the oral mucous membranes for changes in color, hemorrhage, inflammation, abrasions, ulceration, abnormal discharges, membranes or pseudomembranes, and abnormal growths. The tonsils should be examined for size, color, and consistency; the surrounding tissue should be examined for any abnormality. Conclusive diagnosis of the cause of tonsillar enlargement may depend on the results of a biopsy. Examine the uvula and note its length. Foreign bodies may lodge at the opening of the posterior nares, and the uvula must be pulled down and forward and the posterior nares visualized. Examine the hard and soft palate with a dental mirror for the presence of tumors or foreign bodies. Fractures of the hard palate are frequently seen in cats that fall from high elevations.

............Odors

Smell the breath. Mouth odors may be caused by bad teeth, ulcerations of the lip folds or the mucous membranes, and tonsillitis. Uremia produces an ammoniacal odor; diabetic ketosis, a smell of acetone; and suppurative conditions of the lungs, a putrid odor.

............EXAMINATION OF THE ESOPHAGUS

The esophagus starts in the posterior pharynx dorsal to the cranial portion of the trachea and continues in a caudal direction slightly dorsal and to the left of the trachea to the thoracic inlet. Just caudal to the thoracic inlet, the esophagus becomes more ventral in position and further to the left of the trachea. At the base of the heart, the esophagus is dorsal to the bifurcation of the trachea. The esophagus then continues caudally to the diaphragm and empties into the fundus of the stomach.

Examination of the esophagus depends on the use of either a gastroscope or radiographic techniques. It is important, however, to know whether the animal can swallow normally. The signs of esophageal disease are general and include regurgitation, abnormal or painful swallowing, and weight loss associated with a caloric deficit. Regurgitation is the act of ejecting undigested food through the mouth; vomiting indicates the expulsion of gastric contents. Physical findings in esophageal disease may include distention of the cervical esophagus by food, liquid, foreign body, or tumor, and filling of the esophagus with air when the hindlegs are elevated. Dogs with regurgitation associated with an esophageal lesion frequently have aspiration pneumonia and pharyngitis.

Disorders of the esophagus can be divided into the following categories:

1. Impaired function—dilation, constriction or obstruction, abnormal peristalsis, gastric reflux
2. Irregular contour—mucosal and submucosal disease, intramural disease with secondary mucosal alteration
3. Abnormal position—diaphragmatic or hiatal hernia, periesophageal mass, pneumothorax

...........EXAMINATION OF THE ABDOMEN

...........Observation

Stand the animal on a table, its head facing away from you. Step back and inspect the abdomen for general contour and for swelling or retraction. Swelling can be either localized or general. The most common cause of localized swelling is a neoplasm. General swelling can be caused by fat, fluid, flatus, or fetus.

Note whether the abdominal walls move normally during respiration. Abnormal movement may reflect pain from peritonitis. Decide whether the abdominal musculature seems tense, the abdomen "tucked up." The animal will frequently stand with the hindlegs drawn forward well under the body, so that its back appears to be arched. When in severe abdominal pain, some animals will assume a "praying position" (lie down with front legs, stand up on hindlegs). Look for soft tissue edema, as well as abnormal venous distention of the abdominal wall, indicating circulatory interference.

...........Palpation

Following visual inspection, palpate the abdomen. Stand behind the animal while an assistant gently restrains the animal's head. In order to gain the animal's confidence, move the hands lightly over its entire abdomen. When performing palpation, avoid using the fingertips; instead, use the metacarpophalangeal joints, with the hand placed flat on the abdominal wall. Begin with a very light, systematic palpation of the entire abdomen, and note any localized or general rigidity and tenderness. Next, palpate the deeper structures. Palpate the liver by pressing the fingers inward and forward around the costal arches on either side. The normal dog liver is not easy to palpate. Enlargement, however, causes it to protrude beyond the costal margins and facilitates palpation. Note the amount of distention beyond the costal margins, and determine whether the edge of the liver is sharp or rounded. The spleen can be palpated in the anterior left lateral region of the abdomen.

The spleen is a tongue-shaped organ resting against the left rib cage at the level of the 11th to 12th ribs. In the normal dog or cat with an empty stomach, the nonengorged spleen is entirely within the intrathoracic portion of the abdominal cavity. The degree of distention of the stomach and engorgement of the spleen with blood must be known in order to evaluate the position of the spleen. Abnormal position of the spleen is present if the proximal extremity and body of the spleen are not in contact with the left lateral abdominal wall or are caudal and lateral to the fundus of the stomach. Abnormal position of the spleen may occur in patients with diaphragmatic herniation, gastric torsion, splenic enlargement or torsion, and intra-abdominal tumors.

The kidneys are palpable in certain dogs. The right kidney lies ventral to the L1–3 vertebrae; the left kidney is ventral to the L2–4 vertebrae. In the normal cat, the liver and kidneys can be palpated. Do not confuse the kidneys of a cat with a fetus or tumor.

The stomach of the dog and cat cannot normally be palpated. Large tumors of the gastric wall and gastric torsion may cause the stomach to be displaced and palpable.

The small bowel is located in the midventral portion of the central abdomen. In the dog, the small intestine is approximately 3.5 times the body length. The duodenum passes caudad from the pylorus on the right side, lateral to the ascending colon and cecum. The jejunum occupies the right ventral quadrant of the abdomen. The ileum approaches the cecum from the left and joins it at the cecocolic junction. The cecum is usually ventral to the L2–3 vertebrae and is in the middle of the right half of the abdomen. Palpate the descending duodenum and the ileocecocolic junction on the right by pressing them dorsally against the sublumbar muscles and rolling them from medial to lateral.

The large bowel of the dog and cat includes the cecum, colon, rectum, and anus. The cecum is a diverticulum of the colon near the ileocolic junction. The cecum is located to the right of the midline, approximately at the level of L3. The proximal colon passes from right to left in front of the root of the mesentery. The descending portion extends from the splenic flexure to the level of L5 or L6, parallels the left lateral abdominal wall, and then enters the pelvic canal to become the rectum. The descending colon can be palpated on the left and is more prominent when the dog is constipated. Intussusception often begins at the ileocecocolic junction. The bladder is located within the posterior portion of the abdomen and is capable of distention as far craniad as the umbilicus.

If an abnormal mass is felt while palpation is being carried out, note its position, associated pain, degree of mobility, and consistency, if possible. Masses such as lipomas may seem to be in the abdomen upon palpation when they are actually in the abdominal musculature.

·········· Percussion

Following palpation, percuss the abdomen. The normal abdomen yields a tympanitic note throughout except over a solid viscus such as the liver, spleen, or a full bladder. Increased accumulations of air in the stomach or abdomen will give a larger area of tympanitic sound.

Free fluid in the peritoneum (ascites) may shift as the patient is moved. When ascites is suspected, place one hand on one side of the abdomen over the lumbar area and, with the other hand, "flick" or tap the opposite abdominal wall. A distinct impact is felt from one hand to the other if fluid under tension is present.

·········· Auscultation

Carry out auscultation in a quiet room and determine whether the peristaltic sounds are normal, increased, decreased, or absent.

·········· RECTAL EXAMINATION

The rectum is an elongated tube, 5 to 6 cm in length. Its diameter varies with the breed and size of the animal. The rectum traverses the pelvic canal and ends at the anal canal. Innervation to the anorectal area is supplied by the pudenal nerve (formed by S1, S2, and S3), which also provides motor nerves to the external anal sphincter and to the skin of the anus and perianal region. The rectum and internal anal sphincter are supplied by nerves from the pelvic plexus.

Tenesmus and dyschezia are the primary signs in anorectal diseases. Carefully examine the external anal area and perineum for evidence of inflammation, swelling, neoplasms, and crypts at the mucocutaneous line.

Conclude the examination of the intestinal tract by performing a rectal examination. Use a rubber glove or a finger cot lubricated with a water-soluble gel or petroleum jelly. Digital examination will reveal the color and consistency of the stool in the rectum, any narrowing of the rectum, the possibility of a fractured pelvis, the size of the pelvic canal, impaction or tumors of the anal glands, and the presence of rectal polyps. In males, always check the size of the prostate gland. Little discomfort should accompany this examination. Following digital examination of the rectum, direct visualization of the rectal canal can be accomplished by use of a proctoscope (see p. 524) or an anoscope. This procedure may be performed under sedation or a light plane of anesthesia.

A careful examination of the alimentary tract and abdomen may indicate that further diagnostic work is needed. Passage of a stomach tube (see p. 538), esophagoscopy, radiography (see p. 526), ultrasonography, test meals, proctoscopy (see p. 524), or clinicopathologic tests may be required. Do not hesitate to perform tests that may help in arriving at a definitive diagnosis.

REFERENCES

Ettinger SJ, Feldman EC, eds: Textbook of Veterinary Internal Medicine, ed 4. Philadelphia, WB Saunders, 1995.
Guilford WG, Center SA, Strombeck DR, et al, eds: Strombeck's Small Animal Gastroenterology, ed 3. Philadelphia, WB Saunders, 1996.
Harvey CE, Emily PP: Small Animal Dentistry. St Louis, Mosby–Year Book, 1993.

Cardiovascular System

Evaluation of the cardiovascular system should encompass assessment of all of its parts by inspection, palpation, percussion, and auscultation of not only the heart but also the arteries and veins. Familiarity with normal and confirmational variations between breeds and species will allow the veterinarian to appreciate the abnormal.

............History

Certain key questions are helpful in defining the cardiac patient's problems:

1. *Is there intolerance to exercise?* Most patients with significant cardiac disorders have exercise intolerance at some level of exertion, be it walking, running, prolonged play, or prolonged physical effort.
2. *Is either coughing or dyspnea present?* If so, under what circumstances? The most frequent presenting complaint associated with heart disease is a cough, which may be aggravated by exercise or excitement.
3. *When was the onset, and what is the duration of signs?* In most instances, cardiac disease begins somewhat insidiously, with a slow progression over a period of several months to years.
4. *Are the problems progressively worsening?* Cardiac disease, although usually progressive, may be characterized by short periods of clinical stability or even improvement without therapy.
5. *Is weakness or syncope present?* Weakness usually implies a significant decrease in cardiac function that results in tissue hypoxia. Syncope may signify the presence of an arrhythmia.
6. *Are medications currently being administered?* If so, for how long? At what levels? Have they been effective? The knowledge of a prior response or lack of response to therapy is invaluable in formulating an effective therapeutic plan for the cardiac patient.
7. *What is the current diet and feeding regimen of the patient?* Sodium and caloric restrictions are frequently part of the management plan for canine and feline cardiac patients.
8. *What is the medical history of the parents and siblings of the patient?* A positive genetic history of cardiac disease in previous generations or littermates is a common finding when such information is available.

Table 2–3. Breed Predilections in Dogs With Congenital Heart Disease

Airedale terrier	Pulmonic stenosis (PS)-2
Beagle	PS*
Bichon frisé	Patent ductus arteriosus (PDA)-2
Boxer	Aortic stenosis (AS)-3
Boykin spaniel	PS*
Bull terrier	Mitral dysplasia (MD)*
Chihuahua	PS,* PDA*
Cocker spaniel	PDA-1, PS-1
Collie	PDA-1
Doberman pinscher	Atrial septal defect (ASD)*
English bulldog	PS-3, Ventricular septal defect (VSD)-3, AS-1, Tetralogy of Fallot (TF)*
English springer spaniel	PDA-2
German shepherd	Tricuspid dysplasia (TD)-3, AS-1, persistent right aortic arch (PRAA)-2, MD,* PDA*
German shorthair pointer	AS*
Golden retriever	AS-3, TD*
Great Dane	AS-1, PRAA-3, MD,* TD*
Irish setter	PRAA*
Keeshond	PDA-2, TF*
Kerry blue terrier	PDA-3
Labrador retriever	TD-3
Maltese	PDA-3
Mastiff	PS-3
Miniature schnauzer	PS-2
Newfoundland	AS-3
Pomeranian	PDA-3
Poodles, toy and miniature	PDA-2
Rottweiler	AS-3
Samoyed	PS-3, AS-1, ASD*
Scottish terrier	PS-2
Shetland sheepdog	PDA-3
West Highland white terrier	PS-3
Weimaraner	TD,* peritoneopericardial hernia*
Yorkshire terrier	PDA-1

Data from Veterinary Medical Data Base at Purdue University 1987–1989: 1320 dogs with congenital heart disease out of 154,233 dogs. Numbers 1–3 identify predisposed breeds represented by four or more affected dogs in which relative risk for the indicated abnormality was significantly elevated in this series ($P < .05$ to $P < .0001$). −1, mild increased risk (odds ratio 1.5–2.9 times all other dogs); 2, moderate risk (odds ratio 3.0–4.9 times others); 3, marked risk (odds ratio > 5 times others). Sex predominances: PDA, females 3:1; PS in English bulldogs, males 4:1; MD and TD, males 2:1.

*Breed-associated diseases not confirmed in this study but suggested or confirmed by others.

Modified from Buchanan JW: Changing breed dispositions in canine heart disease. Canine Pract 18:13, 1993.

9. *Do other problems exist?* Cardinal signs of illness should be investigated in the cardiac patient as in any other patient. These signs include anorexia, polydipsia, polyuria, vomiting, diarrhea, and previous illness. It is well known that cardiac disease may affect the kidney and the liver; thus, dysfunctions of these organs must always be investigated in the medical evaluation of the cardiac patient.

............PHYSICAL EXAMINATION
............Observation

Before the animal is placed on the examination table, it should be observed for its gross appearance, attitude, body condition, and breathing pattern.

Body Condition Note if the patient is overweight or underweight. Animals with advanced heart disease can be very thin (cardiac cachexia). Also note if abdominal distention is present. Abdominal effusion (ascites), hepato- and splenomegaly may be present in animals with right heart failure.

Respiratory Rate Observe the animal's respiratory rate. A normal respiratory rate (eupnea) is somewhat variable and factors such as excitement, fear, and a ride in a overheated car may increase the rate (tachypnea).

Normal dog respiratory rate: 10 to 30/min
Normal cat respiratory rate: 20 to 30/min

Respiratory Character Observe the animal for ease or difficulty in breathing. A normal animal should not use its abdominal muscles for breathing. Dyspnea is difficult or labored breathing. An animal cannot tell us that it is experiencing dyspnea, but changes in respiratory rate and effort suggest dyspnea. A dysneic animal may breathe with its mouth open and may recruit its abdominal muscles to aid in respiration. It may also have an anxious facial expression with eyes bulging, nostrils flaring, and head and neck extended. There are several types of dyspnea, depending on which phase of respiration is most prolonged. Inspiratory dyspnea is characterized by a longer than normal inspiratory phase, usually accompanied by stridor (noisy breathing). Inspiratory dyspnea is suggestive of upper airway obstruction, such as laryngeal paralysis or brachycephalic syndrome. Expiratory dyspnea is characterized by forced, abdominal respirations during the expiratory phase. This type of breathing pattern suggests asthma or chronic obstructive pulmonary disease. Dyspnea throughout inspiration and expiration is typical of pulmonary diseases and pulmonary edema.

Dyspnea—difficult or labored breathing
Hyperpnea—increased rate and depth of respiration
Orthopnea—inability to breath unless in a sitting or standing position, often with elbows abducted

Body Posture and Gait Cats with cardiomyopathy may present with systemic arterial thromboembolization (saddle thrombus), resulting in acute onset and painful paraparesis. (weakness in the hindlegs). Animals with saddle thrombus will also have an absent or diminished femoral pulse and have cool, pale, or cyanotic footpads.

............Palpation
............The Neck

Palpate the trachea in an animal that presents with cough to assess its sensitivity. Animals with collapsing trachea and tracheobronchitis (kennel cough) will usually have a cough induced by tracheal palpation. Beware, even a normal animal will cough with excessive tracheal palpation. Palpate the neck for a thyroid nodule in cats over 6 years of age, especially if it has a heart murmur or tachycardia.

............The Jugular Vein

Assess the jugular vein for distention and pulsation. *Jugular venous distention* suggests increased central venous pressure (CVP) and is a sign of right heart failure. Jugular venous distention may occur with conditions causing tricuspid regurgitation or impaired filling of the right heart such as pericardial effusion, constrictive pericarditis, or a mass lesion in the right heart or cranial thorax. All animals with ascites should have the jugular vein carefully evaluated and a hepatojugular reflex performed. A positive *hepatojugular reflex* suggests right heart failure and occurs when the jugular vein becomes distended with upward compression of the cranial abdomen. Also observe for jugular venous pulsation. A *jugular pulse* traveling more that one-third the way up the neck is abnormal and is generally associated with tricuspid valve insufficiency (i.e., congenital tricuspid valve dysplasia, or tricuspid valve insufficiency caused by chronic degeneration, pulmonary stenosis, heartworm disease, and pulmonary hypertension). An arrhythmia causing atioventricular (AV) dissociation, such as a ventricular premature complex and second- or third-degree AV block, may also cause a jugular pulse. The atria contract against a closed AV valve causing the pulsation. In thin animals, beware of the carotid pulse beneath the jugular vein, which may be confused with a jugular pulse.

2

.... *The Thorax*

In a standing position, palpate the thorax for any trauma or deformities. One may also assess the compressibility of the chest in a cat. *Compressibility* is quite variable even in a normal cat but this physical examination maneuver may be helpful in cats with space-occupying lesions such as pleural effusion, which will cause decreased compressibility. Cats with cranial mediastinal masses will have reduced compressibility in the cranial thorax.

Palpate the precordium (area of chest wall next to the heart) for the *apex beat*. The palm of the hand, ventral surface of the proximal metacarpals, as well as the fingertips, should be used for optimal appreciation of the precordium. The apex beat is the point of maximum intensity of the heartbeat. The normal location is at the left fifth intercostal space around the costochondral junction. *Displacement of the normal apex beat may result from right heart enlargement or a thoracic mass.* The intensity of the apex beat may be decreased or increased. An increased apex beat may occur in thin animals, hyperdynamic states (anemia, hyperthyroidism), mitral valve regurgitation (or other volume-overloaded state with maintained myocardial contractility), and hypertrophic cardiomyopathy. Decreased intensity of the apex beat may occur in dilated cardiomyopathy and pleural or pericardial effusion.

Precordial thrill is the vibration felt on the surface of the chest caused by a murmur. The location of the thrill is always the point of maximum intensity of the murmur.

Thoracic percussion may be helpful in animals with restrictive breathing patterns and quiet breath sounds. This technique may not be helpful in obese animals. First, the flat part of a fingertip is placed in the intercostal space. Then the fingertip (usually the middle finger) of the other hand briskly strikes the finger on the intercostal space producing a resonating sound. Percussion of the chest should be done systematically from dorsal to ventral, evaluating the entire chest. The sound produced by percussion may be increased or hyperresonant in pneumothorax or asthma. The resonance may be decreased with pleural effusion, consolidated lung (lung filled with fluid or exudate), or a thoracic mass.

.... *The Abdomen*

Palpate for ascites and hepatic or splenic enlargement which may accompany right heart failure in the dog. Ascites is an uncommon sign of right heart failure in the cat. *Ballottement* is a palpation technique used to help determine if abdominal distention is caused by fluid. One taps the abdomen (once or twice) with the fingertips to evaluate a fluid wave or rebound of an abdominal organ floating in fluid.

...........Mucous Membranes

The color of the mucous membranes is usually assessed in the mouth, but some animals have pigmented gums and the vulva, penis, or conjunctiva should be examined. The normal mucous membrane color is pink. Alterations in color may suggest various conditions pertinent to the cardiopulmonary systems such as the following:

Cyanosis (blue discoloration) suggests hypoxia as a result of a congenital right-to-left shunting defect (tetralogy of Fallot) or as a result of respiratory disease (upper airway obstruction or pulmonary disease). If cyanosis is suspected in the oral mucous membrane, the caudal mucous membrane should also be observed for differential cyanosis. Animals with a reverse (right-to-left) patent ductus arteriosus (PDA) will have more cyanosis in the caudal mucous membrane (penis or vulva) vs. the oral mucous membrane (differential or caudal cyanosis).

A pale mucous membrane (light pink or white discoloration) suggests anemia or poor perfusion, usually associated with low cardiac output.

Hyperemia of the mucous membrane (bright red) suggests peripheral vasodilation as seen in septic shock or exercise.

Capillary Refill Time (CRT) Press a finger against a mucous membrane and cause it to blanch. The CRT is the time required for the pink color to return. Prolonged CRT indicates poor peripheral perfusion or low cardiac output.

...........The Arterial Pulse

Assessment of the pulse, usually the femoral pulse, is a basic and important part of the cardiovascular physical examination. The normal pulse should feel full, with a rapid rise and fall. Femoral pulses may be difficult to assess in normal cats and obese dogs and cats. Evaluate the pulse quality as well as the rate. Do they correlate with the heartbeat?

...........Abnormal Arterial Pulses

Pulse Deficits Pulse deficits—fewer pulses than heartbeats—typically occur with arrhythmias such as ventricular premature complexes or atrial fibrillation.

Hyperkinetic Pulse (other terms are bounding, BB-shot or water-hammer) This is a strong pulse, which rises quickly and decays quickly. Associated conditions include PDA and aortic insufficiency (wide pulse pressure because of diastolic runoff) or hyperdynamic conditions such as anemia, fever, and hyperthyroidism.

Hypokinetic Pulse (other terms are weak or thready) This pulse is hard to feel and barely perceptible. The weak pulse is usually associated with diminished stroke volume such as left heart failure (dilated cardiomyopathy or mitral regurgitation), cardiac tamponade, or a sustained tachyarrhythmia or hypotension caused by extracardiac diseases. *A weak and late rising pulse (pulsus parvus et tardus) is characteristic of severe aortic stenosis.*

Pulses Paradoxus This is defined as a marked decrease in pulse pressure during inspiration and is associated with cardiac tamponade caused by pericardial effusion.

...........Cardiac Auscultation

The Stethoscope The main components of the stethoscope are the bell, diaphragm, tubing, and earpieces. The bell transmits both low-frequency and high-frequency sounds. The diaphragm attenuates low-frequency sounds and selectively transmits the high-frequency sounds. The diaphragm also transmits louder sounds than the bell by virtue of its size. The tubing should not be too long because sounds attenuate in the longer tubing. The earpieces should fit comfortably without entering the ear canals. A properly fitted stethoscope is the first step to successful auscultation. In addition to a good stethoscope, a *quiet room and properly restrained patient* are essential. Whenever possible, perform auscultation with the animal in a standing position. Control respirations if necessary by holding the mouth closed or occluding a nostril transiently. Sometimes, if the animal is overly excited, auscultate again after the animal relaxes. Purring in cats may interfere with auscultation and running tap water or the smell of alcohol may stop the purring. Care should be taken not to confuse respiratory sounds, shivering, or rubbing of the hair for heart sounds.

Proper use of the bell and diaphragm is also important for accurate auscultation. The majority of the auscultation should be performed with the diaphragm firmly placed on the chest. The bell is used to hear low-frequency sounds such as gallop sounds or low-frequency murmurs. The bell should be used with light pressure; too much pressure on the bell tightens the skin and creates a diaphragm. Auscultation with the bell should be used in animals with an extra heart sound (auscultated with the diaphragm), all cats (to screen for gallop sounds), and dogs suspected of cardiomyopathy or with congestive heart failure.

Develop a *systemic approach to auscultation*. Determine heart rate and rhythm and correlate it with the femoral pulse. *Auscultate over all valve areas* for any abnormal heart sounds.

···········Normal Heart Rate and Rhythm

Certainly heart rate can vary in a normal animal depending on the state of excitement and fitness. Sometimes true resting heart rates can only be determined in the home environment by the owner. In general, the heart rate increases (tachycardia) with excitement, pain, shock, hyperdynamic states (anemia, fever, hyperthyroidism), and congestive heart failure of various causes. Slow heart rates (bradycardia) may be noted in athletic animals, hypothyroidism, increases in vagal tone, or a conduction abnormality of the heart (sick sinus syndrome, advanced AV block).

Normal heart rate (dog)
Large dogs: 60 to 100 bpm
Medium-size dogs: 80 to 120 bpm
Small dogs: 90 to 140 bpm
Normal heart rate (cat)
Domestic cats: 140 to 250 bpm

Heart rhythm is typically regular in cats and dogs. However, *many normal dogs (especially brachycephalic breeds) have respiratory sinus arrhythmia.* In respiratory sinus arrhythmia, the heart rate increases with inspiration and decreases with expiration.

···········Areas for Cardiac Auscultation

There are four main areas for cardiac auscultation (Fig. 2–4):

1. **Mitral valve (left AV valve).** The left fifth intercostal space around the costolchondral junction—in the normal animal, the area of the apex beat. Usually in the standing animal, the area opposite to the point of the elbow. First heart sounds are heard better at the mitral valve.
2. **Aortic valve.** The left fourth intercostal space dorsal to the mitral valve

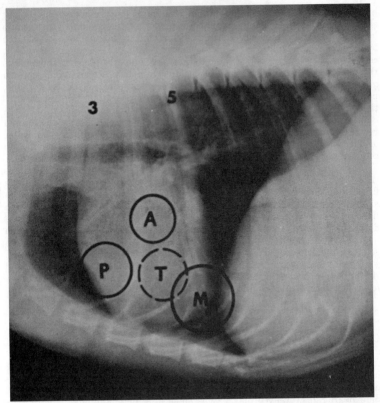

Figure 2–4. Left lateral radiograph of the canine thorax. Circles identify the valve areas: M, mitral valve area; P, pulmonic valve area; A, aortic valve area; T, tricuspid valve area. Because the tricuspid valve area is located on the right side of the thorax, it is indicated by a broken circle. The numbers represent the third and fifth ribs. (From Ettinger SJ, Suter PF: Canine Cardiology. Philadelphia, WB Saunders, 1970.)

(usually the level of the point of the shoulder). The second heart sound is heard better at the aortic and pulmonary valves.

3. *Pulmonary valve*. The left third intercostal space at the sternal border (usually at the axilla).

4. *Tricuspid valve (right AV valve)*. The right third to fourth intercostal space at the costochondral junction.

...........Normal Heart Sounds

The intensity of normal heart sounds may be increased with conditions such as a thin body, young age, and hyperdynamic states (anemia, fever, hyperthyroidism). The intensity may also be decreased with obesity or in a heavily muscled animal, in addition to pathologic conditions such as pericardial effusion or pleural effusion.

The *first heart sound (S₁)* is associated with closure of the AV valves ("lubb") and is typically loudest over the mitral and tricuspid valve areas. Pulse occurs just after S₁.

The *second heart sound (S₂)* is associated with closure of the semilunar valves (pulmonary and aortic valves) ("dupp") and is typically loudest over these valve areas.

.... Transient Heart Sounds

These are short-duration extra heart sounds and include:

Split S₁: Asynchronous closure of the AV valves. May be a normal variant in a large-breed dog. Other causes include a ventricular premature complex or bundle-branch block.

Split S₂: Asynchronous closure of the pulmonic and aortic valves. Associated conditions include heartworm disease or other causes of pulmonary hypertension, pulmonic stenosis, aortic stenosis, and atrial septal defects.

Midsystolic click: A high-frequency sound in the middle of systole usually associated with early mitral valve disease. May precede a murmur in some animals.

S₃ gallop: A low-frequency, diastolic sound associated with rapid ventricular filling. Abnormal in the small animal patient and represents ventricular stiffness. A common associated condition is dilated cardiomyopathy.

S₄ gallop: A low-frequency, diastolic sound associated with atrial contraction. Abnormal in the small animal and represents ventricular stiffness. A common associated condition is hypertrophic cardiomyopathy.

.... Heart Murmurs

A heart murmur is produced by an interruption of laminar blood flow, in other words, turbulent blood flow. The majority of heart murmurs are caused by a lesion in the heart causing turbulence. However, some murmurs may be physiologic such as murmurs associated with severe anemia or shock. Murmurs are classified by their timing in the cardiac cycle, intensity, location (or point of maximum intensity, PMI), quality (subjective), phonographic configuration, and frequency.

.... Timing

Systolic murmur occurs during systole (with pulse). These murmurs are heard between S₁ and S₂. Most murmurs are systolic and associated conditions include mitral and tricuspid valve insufficiency, aortic or pulmonary stenosis, and ventricular septal defect (VSD).

Diastolic murmur occurs during diastole (after the pulse), after S₂. Diastolic murmurs are rare and occur most commonly with aortic insufficiency.

Continuous murmur occurs throughout systole and diastole. PDA is the most common cause of a continuous murmur.

One could further classify the timing of the murmur by commenting on the duration and position in the cardiac cycle such as holosystolic (entire systole), vs. early-, mid-, or late-systolic murmurs.

.... Intensity

Intensity is a subjective determination of the loudness of the murmur. In most cases, murmur intensity does not correlate with the severity of heart disease. Murmurs are usually graded on a scale of I to VI

Grade I—very faint murmur requiring concentration and a quiet room to be heard

Grade II—soft murmur that is consistently auscultated over only one valve area

Grade III—moderate-intensity murmur, readily auscultable, usually radiating to another valve area

Grade IV—loud murmur without a precordial thrill, usually radiating to both sides of the chest

Grade V—loud murmur with a precordial thrill

Grade VI—loud murmur with a precordial thrill and still audible with the stethoscope off the chest wall

...........Location

Note the valve area where the murmur is heard best or the PMI. Also note where the murmur radiates. In some cases of severe subaortic stenosis, the murmur can radiate up the carotid arteries.

...........Quality

Regurgitant-quality (**plateau**-shaped) murmurs are the most common and are associated with AV valve insufficiency.

Ejection-quality (**crescendo-decrescendo** or **diamond**-shaped) murmurs are associated with aortic and pulmonary stenosis.

Machinery-quality murmur is a continuous murmur most commonly associated with PDA.

Decrescendo murmur is most commonly associated with VSD or AV valve insufficiency.

...........Frequency

Low—30 to 80 cps, low rumbling sound (usually aortic insufficiency, PDA)

High—120 cps (aortic or pulmonary stenosis)

Mixed—80 to 120 cps (usually AV valve insufficiency)

...........Murmur Classification (see also Table 2–4)

<u>Mitral valve insufficiency (regurgitation)</u>—early systolic to holosystolic regurgitant (plateau) or occasionally decrescendo murmur with PMI over the left apex (mitral valve area). This is the most commonly heard murmur and is usually associated with chronic degenerative mitral valve disease in the older small-breed dog.

<u>Tricuspid valve insufficiency (regurgitation)</u>—systolic regurgitant murmur heard loudest in the tricuspid valve area (right apex).

<u>Patent ductus arteriosus</u>—usually a loud continuous machinery murmur with PMI at the left heart base (pulmonary and aortic valve areas). PDA is the most common congenital defect in the dog.

<u>Pulmonary stenosis</u>—usually a loud, high-frequency, harsh holosystolic crescendo-decrescendo ejection murmur with a PMI at the left heart base (pulmonary valve area). The murmur usually peaks in midsystole and radiates well caudally and to the right.

<u>Subaortic Stenosis</u>—usually a loud, harsh mixed or high-frequency holosystolic crescendo-decrescendo ejection murmur with a PMI at the left heart base. Sometime the PMI is the right heart base. The murmur radiates well to the right side and up the thoracic inlet and up the carotids. It is sometimes associated with aortic insufficiency.

<u>Ventricular septal defect</u>—usually a holosystolic murmur with PMI at

Table 2-4. Summary Characterization of Common Murmurs

	Mitral Insufficiency	Patent Ductus Arteriosus	Aortic Stenosis	Pulmonic Stenosis	Ventricular Septal Defect	Anemic Murmur	Physiologic (Functional) Murmur
Timing Duration	Systolic Holosystolic	Continuous Holosystolic, holodiastolic	Systolic Midsystolic (crescendo-decrescendo diamond-shaped murmur)	Systolic Midsystolic (crescendo-decrescendo diamond-shaped murmur)	Systolic Holosystolic	Systolic Early systolic	Systolic Early systolic
Pitch	Early—high frequency Later—mixed frequency	Mixed frequency with low-frequency components	Harsh mixed frequency, with some high-frequency components	High frequency	Mixed frequency	High frequency	High frequency
Intensity	Usually moderate to loud	Usually loud	Usually loud	Usually loud	Usually loud	Usually very soft; may wax and wane	Very soft; may wax and wane; usually disappears by 8 wk of age
Valve area	Mitral valve area	Anterior on chest in area of pulmonary and aortic valve areas; may have PMI on ventral sternum cranial to left foreleg	Aortic valve area	Pulmonic area on left	Mitral area on left; anterior midthorax on right	Mitral area Aortic area	Mitral area Aortic area
Radiation	Rightward, cranioventral, or dorsal	Craniodorsal	Cranial and rightward; thoracic inlet	Tends not to radiate beyond thoracic inlet; radiates to right	Heard on both sides of chest, but PMI is on right side	None	None

PMI, point of maximal intensity.

291

the right side near the sternum. VSD is the one of the most common congenital defects in the cat.

SPECIAL EXAMINATION AND DIAGNOSTIC PROCEDURES

Indirect Blood Pressure Monitoring (see also p. 75)

The following definitions are pertinent to blood pressure monitoring:

Diastolic pressure—Minimal pressure prior to next ejection cycle
Mean pressure—Average pressure (one-third the difference between systolic and diastolic)
Pulse pressure—The difference between systolic and diastolic
Systolic pressure—The maximal pressure obtained with each cardiac ejection

It is possible to have a weak pulse in a normotensive patient if the heart rate is fast and stroke volumes are small.

Indirect blood pressure monitoring can be accomplished in the dog and cat by using ultrasonography and the Doppler principle of arterial wall motion detection. The Doppler cuff is placed on top of a shaved skin area over the cranial tibial artery. A small amount of gel is applied between the skin and transducer. The 4.0-cm neonatal cuff is used for medium-size to large dogs, and the 2.5-cm premature infant cuff is used for cats and smaller dogs. When an occlusive cuff is placed around the distal tibia and inflated to a pressure greater than the systolic blood pressure, the cranial tibial artery is compressed, no motion of the arterial wall occurs, and there is no sound. When the cuff pressure is reduced to a level just below systolic pressure but above diastolic pressure, the artery opens rapidly during the peak of the pulse pressure wave and an ultrasound frequency is produced. When the cuff pressure drops below diastolic pressure, the artery rhythmically expands and collapses with the passing pulse waves. The systolic pressure is interpreted as the point at which Doppler sounds are first heard; diastolic pressure is the point at which the Doppler sounds change in character or intensity.

Normal blood pressures in the dog as recorded with the indirect Doppler technique and sphygmomanometry have been estimated to be 155 ± 27 mm Hg for systolic and 73 ± 14 mm Hg for diastolic, and 147 ± 15 mm Hg systolic, 87 ± 8 mm Hg diastolic, and 102 ± 9 mm Hg mean.

Indications

Indirect blood pressure monitoring is helpful in identifying the hypertensive patient and in monitoring the response to therapy. It is also helpful in monitoring the cardiovascular state under anesthesia with particular reference to hypotension as an early sign of cardiovascular problems.

Interpretation

Hypertension in the dog is defined as a systolic blood pressure greater than 180 mm Hg or a diastolic pressure greater than 95 mm Hg. *Hypotension* in the dog is defined as a systolic blood pressure less than 100 mm Hg or a diastolic pressure less than 70 mm Hg. Left ventricular dysfunction associated with hypertrophy occurs secondarily to hypertensive states in patients with renal disease, hyperadrenocorticism, diabetes mellitus, pheochromocytoma, hyperthyroidism, or hypothyroidism.

Table 2–5. Criteria for Normal Electrocardiogram*

	Dog	Cat
Heart Rate (bpm)		
Adult	70–160	90–240
Giant breeds	60–140	
Toy breeds	70–180	
Puppies	70–220	
Rhythm		
Normal sinus rhythm		Normal sinus rhythm
Sinus arrhythmia		Sinus tachycardia (excitement)
Wandering pacemaker		
Axis		
+40 to +100 degrees (toy breeds: +40 to +90 degrees)		+0 to ±180 degrees (mean electrical axis in frontal plane not valid in many cats)
Measurements (Maximum Values)		
P wave: 0.04 s × 0.4 mV		P wave: 0.04 s × 0.2 mV
P–R interval: 0.06–0.13 s		P–R interval: 0.05–0.09 s
QRS complex: 0.05 s × 2.5 mV (toy breeds); 0.06 s × 3.0 mV (larger breeds)		QRS complex: 0.04 s × 0.9 mV
S–T segment: elevation, <0.15 mV; depression, <0.1 mV		S–T segment: elevation, <0.1 mV; depression, <0.1 mV
T wave: may be positive, negative, or biphasic; should be positive in CV_5RL and negative in V_{10} (except Chihuahua); amplitude generally <25% of the corresponding R wave		T wave: may be positive, negative, or biphasic maximum; amplitude <0.3 mV
Q–T interval: 0.15–0.25 s		Q–T interval: 0.12–0.18 s†

s, seconds (width); mV, millivolt (amplitude).
*Measured in lead II, unless otherwise noted.
†Q–T intervals and, to a lesser extent P–R interval, will vary inversely with heart rate.

·········· Electrocardiography

The electrocardiograph (ECG) provides the clinician with a fast, efficient way to obtain considerable data about a patient's cardiovascular status. Electrocardiography is a clinical test and must be correlated with clinical findings (Table 2–5). It should be kept in mind that an ECG measures only electrical activity of the heart as seen on the body surface at any one instant.

·········· Indications

The ECG is used for the following purposes:

1. It may detect enlargement of any of the cardiac chambers.
2. It is used to diagnose cardiac arrhythmias.
3. It detects electrolyte imbalances.
4. It monitors response to therapy (digitalis therapy for heart failure, antiarrhythmic therapy, treatment of metabolic diseases that cause electrolyte imbalances, and pericardiocentesis).

5. It is useful in the diagnosis of nonspecific diseases (myocarditis, endocarditis, metabolic diseases, neoplasia).
6. It helps to establish prognosis (estimated severity of enlargement and of arrhythmia; serial ECGs are helpful in determining the rate of change).

...........Interpretation

Each ECG should be read using a definite system. Begin by examining the lead II rhythm strip: Is there a P for every QRS? Is there a QRS for every P? Do all the P waves look alike? Do all the QRS complexes look alike? Are the P and QRS consistently related to each other?

If the answer to any of these questions is no, proceed to identify the abnormality. Next, determine the rate, rhythm, and measurements of the P wave, P–R interval, and QRS complex. Evaluate the S–T segment and T wave and the Q–T interval. Use all leads to determine the axis and any miscellaneous criteria.

...........Heart Rate

Normal heart rate is 70 to 160 bpm, up to 180 bpm in toy breeds, and 220 in puppies. The normal heart rate for the awake cat is 110 to 240 bpm (mean = 195 bpm).

Determination of Heart Rate There are small linear marks at the top of the ECG paper. At a paper speed of 50 mm/second, the time between adjacent marks is 1.5 seconds. By counting two of these divisions and multiplying by 20, the heart rate is calculated (Fig. 2–5). Heart rate may also be determined

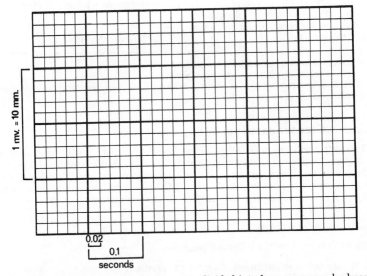

Figure 2–5. Electrocardiographic paper is divided into larger squares by heavy vertical and horizontal lines at 5-mm intervals. Within each large square are twenty-five 1-mm² boxes. At the standard amplitude of 1 mV and a paper speed of 50 mm/second, each box is equal to 0.1 mV on the vertical axis and 0.02 second on the horizontal axis; five boxes equal 0.1 second.

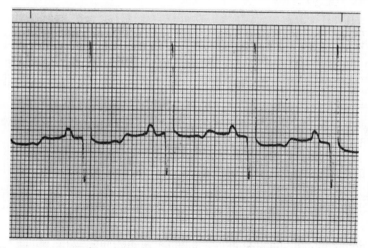

Figure 2–6. Using the electrocardiogram to determine heart rate: The distance between R waves is 20 small boxes, 3000/20 = 150 bpm. (Paper speed = 50 mm/second.)

by counting the number of small squares between R waves (50 mm/second paper speed) and dividing into 3000 (Fig. 2–6).

............Heart Rhythm

The normal heart rhythm is sinus in origin. There is a P wave for every QRS complex (Fig. 2–7). The P waves are related to QRS complexes (P–P interval is constant). Sinus arrhythmia, sinus arrest, and wandering pacemaker are all normal rhythm variations. In sinus arrhythmia, the P–P interval is irregular. The pauses are never longer than twice the usual P–P interval (Fig. 2–8). A wandering pacemaker means that the P waves vary in height and may even be negative temporarily (Fig. 2–9). *Sinus arrest* is defined as a prolongation of the P–R interval longer than twice the usual P–P interval.

............Normal Electrocardiogram Measurements

P Wave The normal P wave is 0.04 second × 0.4 mV (two boxes wide × four boxes tall) for the dog and 0.04 second × 0.2 mV for the cat. In P mitrale (left atrial enlargement), the P wave is wider than 0.04 second. In P pulmonale (right atrial enlargement), the P wave is taller than 0.4 mV for the dog and 0.2 mV for the cat.

P–R Interval The P–R interval is measured from the beginning of the P wave to the beginning of the QRS complex. The normal interval is 0.06 to 0.13 second (3 to 6.5 boxes wide) for the dog and 0.06 to 0.08 second for the cat. In first-degree AV heart block, the P–R interval is prolonged. The P–R interval is sometimes useful in monitoring the effects of digitalis therapy.

QRS Complex The QRS complex duration is measured from the beginning of the Q wave to the end of the S wave. Normal duration is up to 0.04 second in cats, 0.05 second in small dogs, and 0.06 second in large dogs. A QRS complex that is too wide indicates left ventricular enlargement (Fig. 2–10). An R wave that is too tall indicates left ventricular enlargement. The amplitude

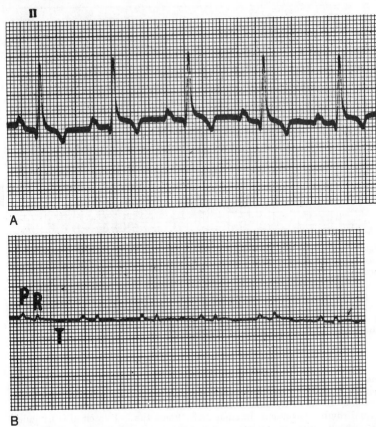

Figure 2–7. Normal sinus rhythm in the dog (A) and the cat (B). (From Edwards NJ: Bolton's Handbook of Canine and Feline Electrocardiography, ed 2. Philadelphia, WB Saunders, 1987.)

is measured from the baseline to the top of the R wave (Fig. 2–11). The normal R wave can be up to 0.8 mV tall in cats, 2.5 mV in small dogs, and 3.0 mV in large dogs.

S–T Segment The S–T segment is between the end of the S wave and the beginning of the T wave. Normally, it lies on the baseline and then dips into the T wave. Slurring of S–T indicates left ventricular enlargement and is seen when the S wave slurs into the T wave and no S–T segment is discernible (see Fig. 2–11). The S–T segment is elevated if it lies more than 0.1 mV (one box) above the baseline (>0.2 mV in CV_6LL and CV_6LU). Elevation of the S–T segment may occur with hypercalcemia or myocardial hypoxia. The S–T segment is depressed if it lies more than 0.1 mV (one box) (>0.2 mV in CV_6LL and CV_6LU) below the baseline. Depression of S–T may be seen with myocardial ischemia, hypoxia, or hypocalcemia.

Q–T Interval The Q–T interval is measured from the beginning of the Q wave to the end of the T wave. The normal interval is 0.14 to 0.22 second (7 to

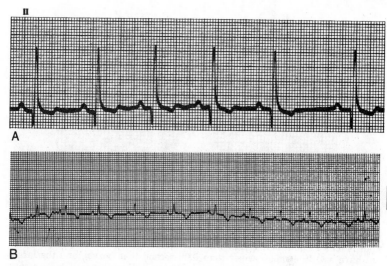

Figure 2–8. A, Mild sinus arrhythmia in a dog. There are P waves for every QRS complex, and the P waves are related to the QRS complexes, which make this a sinus rhythm. It can also be seen that the R–R intervals vary. An irregular sinus rhythm is a sinus arrhythmia. B, Sinus arrhythmia in the cat. (From Edwards NJ: Bolton's Handbook of Canine and Feline Electrocardiography, ed 2. Philadelphia, WB Saunders, 1987.)

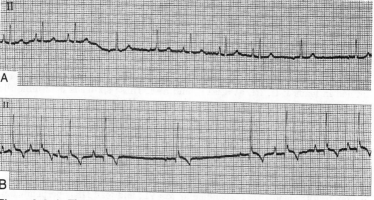

Figure 2–9. A, The wandering pacemaker in this recording is suggested by the slightly negative P waves in some of the complexes. Negative P waves of this nature result from vagal depression of the sinoatrial node and the development of a junctional atrioventricular nodal rhythm. B, Marked sinus arrhythmia and a wandering pacemaker result in a decreased heart rate (increased R–R interval) and negative P waves in the fifth complex. As the pacemaker returns to the sinoatrial node, the rate increases, and positive P waves of varying amplitude result in the sixth and seventh complexes.

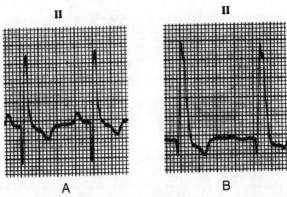

Figure 2–10. In these two examples of left ventricular enlargement the QRS complexes have normal configuration but are too wide. A, This QRS from a miniature poodle is 0.07 second (three boxes) wide; B, This QRS from a Doberman is 0.09 second (four boxes) wide. A small dog such as the poodle should not have a QRS complex wider than 0.05 second (two boxes), and the larger dog's QRS complex should not exceed 0.06 second (three boxes). Because each dog's QRS complex is too wide, left ventricular enlargement is diagnosed in both cases. The Doberman has no P waves because he is in atrial fibrillation. (Paper speed = 50 mm/second, 1 cm = 1 mV.) (From Edwards NJ: Bolton's Handbook of Canine and Feline Electrocardiography, ed 2. Philadelphia, WB Saunders, 1987.)

11 boxes wide) in dogs and up to 0.16 second in cats. A lengthened Q–T interval may be seen with hypokalemia or hypocalcemia. The Q–T interval varies with heart rate and tends to be prolonged when bradycardia occurs. A decreased Q–T interval may be seen with hypercalcemia.

.... Axis Determination

The mean electrical cardiac axis measures the direction (vector) of the cardiac ventricular impulse during depolarization. Therefore, the QRS complex is examined in leads I, II, III, aVR, aVL, and aVF. These six leads determine the axis. They are arranged in a manner known as *Bailey's hexaxial lead system* (Fig. 2–12). The procedure is as follows:

1. Find an isoelectric lead; i.e., a lead for which the total number of positve (upward) and negative (downward) deflections of the QRS complex is equal to zero (Fig. 2–13). When there is no perfectly isoelectric lead, the one that comes closest is used.
2. Find the lead that is perpendicular to the isoelectric lead: lead I is perpendicular to aVF; lead II is perpendicular to aVL; and lead III is perpendicular to aVR (see Fig. 2–13).
3. Determine whether the perpendicular lead is positive or negative on the patient's ECG. If it is negative, the axis is at the negative end of that lead (each lead has a plus and a minus pole marked; see Fig. 2–12). If it is positive, the mean electrical axis is at the positive end of the perpendicular lead. For example, if aVL is isoelectric (normally it is), lead II is its perpendicular. If lead II is positive on the ECG, the axis is +60 degress. If lead II is negative on the ECG, the axis is −120 degrees.

II

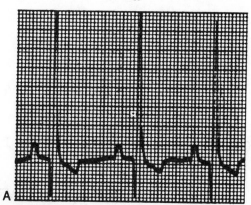

A

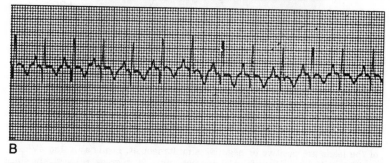

B

Figure 2–11. A, In this tracing, the R wave averages 3.8 mV (38 boxes). The R wave should not be taller than 3.0 mV (30 boxes) in any dog. A tall R wave indicates left ventricular enlargement. The measurement is made from the baseline (not from the bottom of the Q wave) to the top of the R wave. Two other criteria that indicate left ventricular enlargement are present. The QRS complex is 0.07 second (three boxes) wide and S–T slurring is present, because the S–T segment moves into the T wave without straightening out along the baseline. (Paper speed = 50 mm/second, 1 cm = 1 mV.) B, Left ventricular enlargement in a cat. This lead II electrocardiogram was recorded from an aged cat suffering from hyperthyroidism. Thyroxine levels were 9.9 mg/dL. Note the tall R waves (>0.9 mV). (Paper speed = 50 mm/seconds 1 cm = 1 mV.) S–T slurring is characterized by the slurring of the downstroke of the R wave into the T wave, with no discernible S–T segment. This occurs because of ischemia secondary to wall strain in cardiac enlargement. (Courtesy of Dr. N.S. Moise, New York State College of Veterinary Medicine, Cornell University, Ithaca, N.Y.) (From Edwards NJ: Bolton's Handbook of Canine and Feline Electrocardiography, ed 2. Philadelphia, WB Saunders, 1987.)

··········· *Significance*

Normal axis for the dog is +40 to +100 degrees; for the cat it is more variable, ±0 to ±180 degrees. Right axis deviation (axis over +100) indicates right ventricular enlargement in the dog (Fig. 2–14). Left axis deviation (axis 0 to

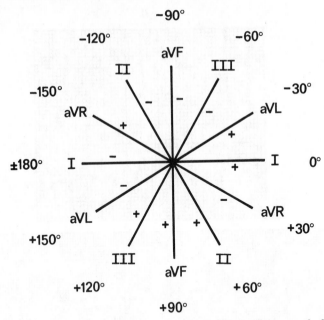

Figure 2–12. Bailey six-axis reference system. The lead axes are marked in 30-degree increments from 0 degrees to 180 degrees and from 0 to −180 degrees. The six leads are marked with a + at the positive electrode and a − at the negative electrode. Note that for leads I, II, III, and aVF the polarity and angle of the leads are positive or negative simultaneously. Leads aVR and aVL are positive at the positions of −150 degrees and −30 degrees, respectively, since the positive electrodes for those leads lie in the negative 0 to −180 degrees zone. (From Ettinger SJ, Suter PF: Canine Cardiology. Philadelphia, WB Saunders, 1970.)

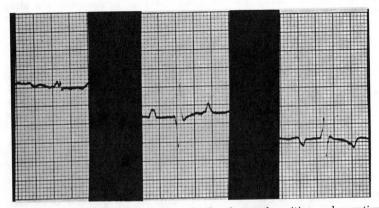

Figure 2–13. In each of these three leads, the total positive and negative deflections equal zero. Each is considered an isoelectric lead.

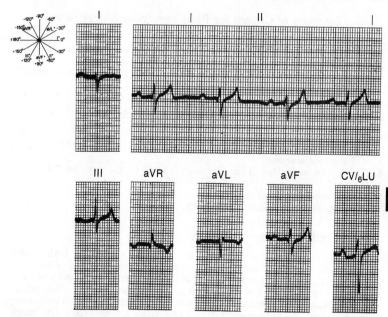

Figure 2–14. The mean electrical axis in the frontal plane of this electrocardiogram recorded from a wire-haired fox terrier with pulmonic stenosis is approximately +165 degrees. (From Edwards NJ: Bolton's Handbook of Canine and Feline Electrocardiography, ed 2. Philadelphia, WB Saunders, 1987.)

+40 degrees) indicates left ventricular enlargement in the dog. When there is biventricular enlargement, the axis usually remains normal.

Axis determinations are of less value in the cat because the normal range is so wide.

............Rhythm Disturbances

The most useful and dependable indication for electrocardiography is an abnormal heart rhythm. Rhythm disturbances and their significance are covered elsewhere in this book (see p. 63).

............Miscellaneous Criteria for Ventricular Enlargement

............Summary of Criteria for Left Ventricular Enlargement

1. Left axis deviation (dog)
2. QRS complex too wide (but has normal configuration)
3. R wave too tall
4. S–T slurring
5. May be associated with P mitrale, because the left atrium and ventricle tend to enlarge together

............Summary of Criteria for Right Ventricular Enlargement

1. Right axis deviation (dog and cat)
2. Presence of an S wave in leads I, II, and III ($S_1S_2S_3$ pattern; dog only)
3. S wave deeper than 0.7 mV in lead CV_6LU (V_4) in the dog
4. May be associated with P pulmonale, because the right atrium and ventricle tend to enlarge together

............Summary of Criteria for Biventricular Enlargement

1. Tall R wave
2. Wide QRS complex
3. S–T segment slurring
4. Deep Q waves in lead II: deeper than 0.3 mV for the cat and 0.5 mV for the dog
5. Normal mean electrical axis
6. P and mitrale or P pulmonale, or both

............Radiography

Lateral and dorsoventral radiographs are valuable in assessing both cardiac enlargement and pulmonary changes that may have occurred (Figs. 2–15 through 2–19). Thus, radiographs assist in diagnosis, treatment, and prognosis.

Changes in lung vasculature may be evident on radiographs. With pulmonary congestion, the pulmonary veins are engorged with blood. With pulmonary overcirculation, the pulmonary arteries and veins are engorged. On lateral radiographic films, the veins appear indistinct and tortuous and are seen emanating from the area of the left atrium. On the other hand, the pulmonary arteries appear straight and branching, like a tree. On the dorsoventral view, veins are medial and arteries are lateral to each bronchus. Decompensated mitral insufficiency causes pulmonary venous congestion; heartworm disease, chronic lung disease, and congenital left-to-right shunt pulmonary artery enlargement.

The mediastinum is a compartment of the thorax between the medial aspects of the two pleural sacs. The mediastinal pleural layers are thin, and disease processes such as pneumothorax and pleural effusion seldom remain unilateral. Signs related to abnormalities in the mediastinal area may be dysphagia, regurgitation, coughing and dyspnea, syncope, head and neck edema, thoracic pain, abdominal breathing. Horner's syndrome, and emphysema.

............*Disease Processes That Alter Mediastinal Position*

1. Unilateral pleural or pulmonary masses
2. Unilateral pneumothorax or pleural effusion
3. Lung lobe collapse, agenesis, hypoplasia, or resection
4. Pleural adhesions
5. Hypostatic congestion of a lung

............*Diseases That Result in Mediastinal Widening*

1. Accumulation of mediastinal fat or fluid
2. Inflammation secondary to tracheal or esophageal puncture
3. Hemorrhage
4. Tumor formation (lymphosarcoma, thymoma)
5. Heart base tumors
6. Enlargement of tracheobronchial lymph nodes

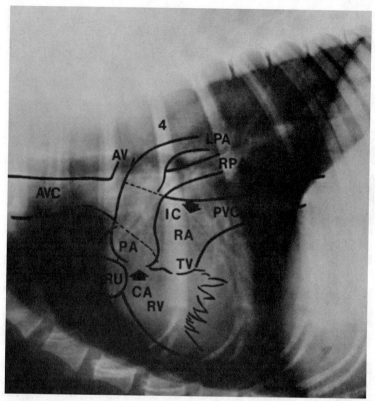

Figure 2–15. Left lateral radiograph of dog. Tracing delineates the structures of the right heart. The details for the tracing were obtained from angiocardiograms. AVC, cranial vena cava; AV, junction of the azygos vein with the AVC; RU, right auricle; RV, right ventricle; CA, conus arteriosus, or right ventricular outflow tract, extending to the tricuspid valve *(arrow)*; PA, main pulmonary artery; LPA, left pulmonary artery, RPA, right pulmonary artery; RA, right atrium, divided dorsally by the intervenous crest (IC); the arrow caudal to the IC points to the foramen ovale; PVC, caudal vena cava; 4, fourth rib. (From Ettinger SJ, Suter PF: Canine Cardiology. Philadelphia, WB Saunders, 1970.)

The intrathoracic trachea is about three times the width of the proximal third rib but increases in diameter on inspiration and decreases on expiration. Normal trachea enters the thoracic inlet in the dorsal third of the inlet. The intrathoracic trachea may collapse on expiration, which may extend to the carina and main stem bronchi.

Congenital tracheal hypoplasia is seen in the English bulldog. Tracheal compression or left main stem bronchus compression may be associated with enlargements of tracheobronchial lymph nodes or of the left atrium.

··········· Survey Radiographs of the Heart

1. The normal canine heart is on a 45-degree angle with the sternum.
2. The heart extends from T1 to T8.

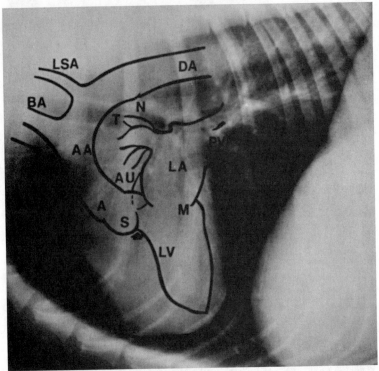

Figure 2–16. Lateral radiograph of dog. Tracing delineates the structures of the left heart. The details for the tracing were obtained from angiocardiograms. BA, brachiocephalic artery; LSA, left subclavian artery; AA, aortic arch; A, ascending aorta; S, sinus of Valsalva (*arrow* points to the aortic valve); AU, small portion of the left auricle; T, tracheal bifurcation; N, notch in the descending aorta (DA), indicating the area of the ligamentum arteriosum; LV, left ventricle; M, mitral valve; LA, left atrium; PV, pulmonary veins. (From Ettinger SJ, Suter PF: Canine Cardiology. Philadelphia, WB Saunders, 1970.)

3. Breed variation can greatly affect the appearance of the cardiac silhouette, as can the respiratory and cardiac cycle.
4. Thoracic radiographs should be taken at the height of inspiration.
5. The heart of the cat assumes a more elongated and elliptic position than that of the dog; the feline heart occupies 2 to 2 1/2 intercostal spaces, and the caudal border is separated from the diaphragm by one or two intercostal spaces.
6. In ventrodorsal (VD) and dorsoventral (DV) positions, the canine heart has a curved right border and a straight left border with the long axis oriented at a 30-degree angle to the spine and to the left of the midline.
7. The feline heart is more oval in appearance in the VD position; in the DV view, the cardiac apex is just to the left of the midline; the ratio of the longitudinal axis to the transverse axis is 1.4:1.

Radiograph evaluation of the cardiovascular system and lungs is important

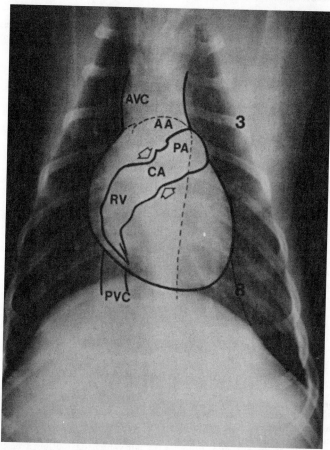

Figure 2–17. Dorsoventral radiograph of dog. Tracing delineates the right ventricle. Details for the tracing were obtained from angiocardiograms. AVC, cranial vena cava; AA, aortic arch; PA, main pulmonary artery, so-called pulmonary artery segment; CA, conus arteriosus, or right ventricular outflow tract; RV, right ventricle; PVC, caudal vena cava. Numbers 3 and 8 indicate the respective ribs. (From Ettinger SJ, Suter PF: Canine Cardiology. Philadelphia, WB Saunders, 1970.)

in the differential diagnosis of cardiovascular disease. It is especially important to evaluate (1) enlargement of cardiac chambers; (2) dilation of great vessels; (3) increased or decreased pulmonary circulation; (4) venous congestion, pulmonary edema, and pleural effusion; and (5) mediastinal space.

When viewing thoracic radiographs to determine whether there is evidence of cardiovascular disease concomitant with clinical findings, ask the following questions:

1. Is the cardiac silhouette larger or smaller than normal?
2. Is the cardiac apex pointing to the right or left?

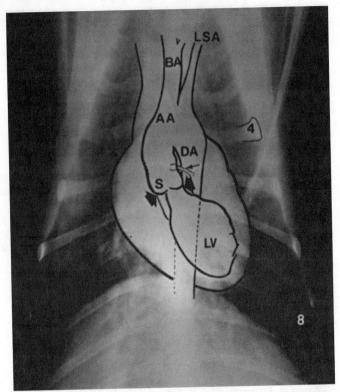

Figure 2-18. Dorsoventral radiograph of dog. Tracing delineates the structures of the left ventricle and aorta. Details of the tracing were obtained from angiocardiograms. LSA, left subclavian artery; BA, brachiocephalic artery; AA, aortic arch; DA, descending aorta; S, sinus of Valsalva; LV, left ventricle. Large arrows point to the muscular lining of the left ventricular outflow tract; small arrow indicates the origin of the left coronary artery, which is indicated by broken lines. Numbers 4 and 8 indicate the respective ribs. (From Ettinger SJ, Suter PF: Canine Cardiology. Philadelphia, WB Saunders, 1970.)

3. Are cardiac chamber shapes normal or abnormal?
4. Are there changes in size, shape, or position of cardiac or intrathoracic vessels or of trachea and bronchi?
5. Is there evidence of pleural fluid accumulation?
6. Is there evidence of pulmonary edema?
7. Is there evidence of intrathoracic disease other than cardiovascular in origin?
8. Is the mediastinum normal or abnormal?

When interpreting changes in cardiac size and shape, note the consistency of the radiographic technique. Short radiographic exposure times of 1/60 or 1/120 second with radiographs taken at full inspiration give the best results.

Enlargement of Right Atrium Right atrial enlargement is usually associated with right ventricular enlargement.

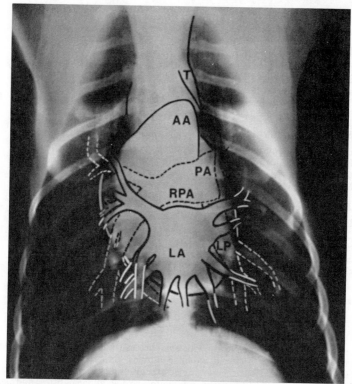

Figure 2–19. Dorsoventral radiograph of dog. Tracing outlines pulmonary arteries and the confluence of the pulmonary veins at the left atrium. Solid lines represent veins and the left atrium; broken lines indicate the pulmonary arteries. Details of the tracings were obtained from angiocardiograms. T, thymus seen only in growing dogs; AA, aortic arch; PA, pulmonary artery; RPA, right pulmonary artery; LP, left pulmonary artery; LA, left atrium. (From Ettinger SJ, Suter PF: Canine Cardiology. Philadelphia, WB Saunders, 1970.)

1. Bulging cranial heart border on lateral view
2. Bulging at 9- to 11-o'clock position on VD (DV) view

Right Ventricle

1. Cranial border of heart is more rounded with increased sternal contact (>3 sternebrae), and the heart may be elevated dorsally on lateral view.
2. Overall width of heart is increased.
3. Elevation of trachea, cranial to tracheal bifurcation.
4. VD (DV) view: heart rounded from 6- to 11-o'clock position.
5. Distance between right heart border and thoracic wall is decreased.

Left Atrium

1. Bulging caudal dorsal heart border on lateral view
2. Loss of caudal waist on lateral view
3. Elevation of trachea, compression of main stem bronchi

4. Bulging at 2- to 3-o'clock position on VD (DV) view
5. Increased size of pulmonary veins

Left Ventricle

1. Elongation of cardiac silhouette on either lateral or VD (DV) view.
2. Elevation of trachea.
3. Rounded caudal border of the heart.
4. Distance between left heart border and thoracic wall is decreased on VD (DV) view.

Biventricular Enlargement

1. Heart appears rounded on both views.
2. Increased sternal contact on lateral view, with elongation and widening of the heart shadow.
3. May mimic pericardial effusion if uniform and severe.

Decrease in Size of Cardiac Silhouette

1. Heart elevated off the sternum
2. Increase in ratio of longitudinal axis to transverse axis to more than 1.4:1
3. Shifting of heart away from midline
4. Small caudal vena cava
5. Seen in Addison's disease, hypothyroidism, shock, and pneumothorax

..........Significance

..........Differential Diagnosis Based on Survey Radiographs (Table 2–6.)

A severe degree of cardiomegaly with evidence of right heart failure suggests advanced mitral and tricuspid valvular fibrosis, dilated cardiomyopathy, of pericardial effusion. Nonselective angiocardiography can be helpful in distinguishing between cardiomyopathy, congenital cardiac abnormalities, and pericardial effusion.

..........Radiographic Appearance of the Lungs in Left-Sided Heart Failure

1. *Pulmonary congestion*—engorgement and distention of pulmonary veins, especially at the junction of the veins with the left atrium. Pulmonary radiodensity is unchanged.
2. *Pulmonary interstitial lung edema phase*—pulmonary radiodensity is increased, and lungs appear hazy. Accumulated fluid in perivascular spaces makes the vascular markings appear hazy.
3. *Alveolar edema*—fluid enters the alveoli and peripheral bronchioles, creating alveolar radiodensity and air bronchograms. Alveolar radiodensity is most severe in the perihilar area.

The lung fields should also be carefully reviewed for evidence of vascular changes compatible with heartworm disease or pulmonary embolism.

..........Ancillary Radiographic Signs Associated With Heart Disease

1. Ascites
2. Liver enlargement
3. Increased size of portal venous circulation
4. Decreased pulmonary circulation
5. Increased venous congestion of the intestines

Table 2–6. Typical Radiographic Findings in Heart Disease

Lesion	RA	RV	LA	LV	Aorta	MPA	Circ	PV	VC	Other Features
Mitral insufficiency	N	N↑	↑	↑	N	N	N	↑	N	Can be secondary to cardiomyopathy, endocarditis, or left-to-right shunt
Aortic lesion	N	N↑	N↑	↑	N↑	N	N	N↑	N	Widened mediastinum is common
Aortic insufficiency	N	N↑	↑	↑	N	N	N	N↑	N	Caused by endocarditis or congenital disease
Tricuspid insufficiency	↑	↑	N	N	N	N	N	N	↑	Can be secondary to cardiomyopathy, heartworm disease, or pulmonary stenosis
Pulmonary stenosis	↑	↑	N→	N→	N	↑N	N	N	N↑	Apex displacement mimics LVH
Tetralogy of Fallot	N↑	↑	N↓	N↓	N	N↓→	N→	N→	N	Aortic position is cranial and may widen the mediastinum; apex shift is common
Atrial septal defect	↑	↑	N↑	N	N	N↑	↑	N	N↑	Generalized cardiomegaly if VSD is present
Dirofilariasis	↑	↑	N	N	N	↑	↑	N	↑	Enlarged pulmonary arteries, pulmonary infiltrates
Patent ductus arteriosus	N	↑	↑	↑	↑	↑	↑	↑	N↑	Pulmonary edema is common
Ventricular septal defect (VSD)	N	↑	↑	↑	↑	N↑	↑	N↑	N↑	Findings vary; may be part of endocardial cushion defect in cats
Hypertrophic cardiomyopathy	↑	↑	↑	N↑	N	N	N	↑	N↑	Valentine-shaped heart, apex shift, pulmonary edema, or pleural effusion
Congestive (dilated) cardiomyopathy	↑	↑	↑	↑	N↓	N	N↓	↑	↑	Pleural effusion, pulmonary edema are common
Pericardial disease	↑	↑	↑	↑	N↓	N	N↓	↑	↑	Globoid silhouette

RA, right atrium; RV, right ventricle; LA, left atrium; LV, left ventricle; MPA, main pulmonary artery; Circ, pulmonary vascular circulation; PV, pulmonary veins; VC, caudal vena cava; N, normal; ↑, enlarged or increased; ↓, smaller or decreased; LVH, left ventricular hypertrophy.

From Myer CW, Bonagura JD: Survey radiography of the heart. Vet Clin North Am Pract Vet 12:223, 1982.

2

6. Pleural effusion, pericardial effusion
7. Increased size of cranial and caudal vena cava
8. Splenic enlargement

Cardiac Catheterization

Indications

Cardiac catheterization is most helpful in identifying and quantifying congenital cardiac abnormalities and their associated pressure or shunt flows.

Interpretation

Evaluation of catheterization pressure data involves comparison with normal values (Table 2–7) and assessment of pressure gradients across stenotic or diseased valves. In general, systolic pressure gradients of more than 30 mm Hg across either the pulmonary or aortic valve are clinically significant. Assessment of blood gas values obtained by cardiac catheterization is helpful in evaluating intracavitary shunting of blood. Evaluation of angiographic data produced by catheterization is helpful in defining the presence of anatomical abnormalities of the heart and vessels. Angiographic data often aid in defining the location of congenital defects but frequently are insensitive in predicting the severity of the defect, especially in the pediatric patient.

Significance

The analysis of pressure gradient data is helpful in assessing whether to manage a particular defect (usually pulmonary stenosis or aortic stenosis) by surgery, balloon dilation, or medically. Blood gas assessment is also important in determining the proper course for left-to-right and right-to-left shunting defects (VSD, atrial septal defect, tetralogy of Fallot, PDA). With the utilization of two-dimensional and Doppler echocardiography to assess congenital heart defects noninvasively, the use of cardiac catheterization for this purpose has declined.

Procedure

Cardiac catheterization may be either selective or nonselective in type. Selective catheterization consists of passing a catheter into the right side of the heart, through either the femoral or jugular veins, and into the left-sided cardiac chambers, through the femoral or carotid arteries, under fluoroscopic guidance. Injection of contrast media, either by hand or with a mechanical pressure injector, will selectively outline individual chambers and major vessels. Individual chamber and vessel pressures may be obtained (Fig. 2–20 and Table 2–7). Blood gas analysis can be performed on blood withdrawn from selected cardiac chambers.

Table 2–7. Normal Cardiac Chamber Pressures (mm Hg)

	PA	RV	RA	AO	LV	Wedge (LA)
Systolic	15–30	15–30	3–5	100–180	100–180	6–10
Diastolic	10	0–5	3–5	60–90	0–10	6–10

PA, pulmonary artery; RV, right ventricle; RA, right atrium; AO, aorta; LV, left ventricle; LA, left atrium.

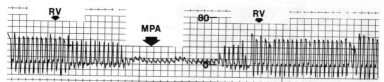

Figure 2–20. Pressure tracing recorded from a dog with mild pulmonic stenosis. The pressure gradient between the right ventricle (RV) and the main pulmonary artery (MPA) is approximately 34 mm Hg. The catheter is initially in the right ventricle, is advanced into the pulmonary artery, and is withdrawn across the valve.

Nonselective catheterization is limited to angiographic evaluation of cardiac chambers and major vessels. A bolus of contrast medium is injected by hand through a large-bore (16- to 18-gauge) catheter placed in one of the jugular veins. Because of the length of time needed to make the bolus injection, the technique is best accomplished in patients who weigh less than 15 kg (33 lbs).

Time	Structures Opacified
1 to 3 seconds post injection	Superior vena cava, right atrium, right ventricle, and pulmonary arteries
4 to 8 seconds post injection	Pulmonary veins, left atrium, left ventricle, and aorta

In the cat, the radiographic film should be large enough that emboli can be detected in the renal arteries, distal aorta, and femoral arteries.

In dogs with valvular pulmonary stenosis, a cardiac catheterization is done for diagnosis and therapy. Once the defect has been defined and pressures measured, a special balloon catheter can be placed and the opening dilated. Pressure measures are taken after the procedure to evaluate the success of the balloon dilation.

............Echocardiography

Echocardiography is the technique of displaying the image of the heart and its structure by transmitting and receiving ultrasound waves as they are reflected from cardiac structures. The techniques of M-mode, two-dimensional, and Doppler echocardiography are used. These techniques provide valuable diagnostic information without risk to the patient.

Note: It is beyond the scope of this article to detail the vast amount of information concerning echocardiography; however, to introduce the reader to the possibilities of echocardiography some classic examples of common cardiac diseases are shown in Figures 2–21, 2–22, and 2–23.

REFERENCES

Edwards NJ: ECG Manual for the Veterinary Technician. Philadelphia, WB Saunders, 1993.

Fox PR, Sisson D, Moise MS: Textbook of Canine and Feline Cardiology: Principles and Clinical Practice, 2nd ed. Philadelphia, WB Saunders, 1999.

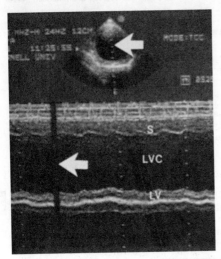

Figure 2-21. With the cursor *(arrow)* positioned in the left ventricle, an M-mode echocardiogram is derived from the two-dimensional image. S, interventricular septum; LVC, left ventricular chamber; LV, left ventricular wall.

Figure 2-22. Long-axis two-dimensional echocardiogram recorded from the right hemithorax of a dog with pericardial effusion. Pericardial fluid and pleural fluid are seen as hypoechoic areas on either side of the pericardium *(arrow)*. S, interventricular septum; LV, left ventricle.

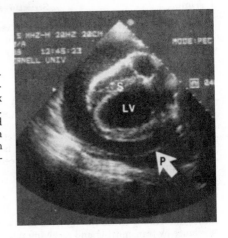

Kittleson MD, Kienle RD: Small Animal Cardiovascular Medicine. St. Louis, Mosby–Year Book, 1998.

Miller M, Tilley LP: Manual of Canine and Feline Cardiology, ed 2. Philadelphia, WB Saunders, 1995.

Morgan JP: Techniques in Veterinary Radiography, ed 5. Ames, Iowa State University Press, 1993.

Myer W, Bonagura JD: Survey radiographs of the heart. Vet Clin North Am Small Anim Pract 12:213, 1982.

Penninck D: Ultrasonography. Vet Clin North Am Small Anim Pract 28: 1998.

Pion PR, Kittleson MD: Therapy for feline aortic thromboembolism. *In* Kirk RW, ed: Current Veterinary Therapy X. Small Animal Practice. Philadelphia, WB Saunders, 1989, pp 295–301.

Smith FWK: Rapid Interpretation of Heart Sounds, Murmurs, and Arrhythmias (Sound Recording): A Guide to Cardiac Auscultation in Dogs and Cats. Philadelphia, Lea & Febiger, 1992.

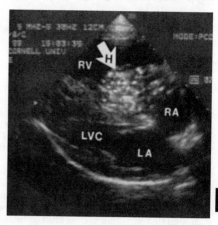

Figure 2–23. Long-axis two-dimensional echocardiogram recorded from the right hemithorax of a dog with severe heartworm disease. Speckled echodensities representing the heartworms *(arrow)* are seen in the inflow tract of the right ventricle. The right ventricle is enlarged. LVC, left ventricular chamber; LA, left atrium; RA, right atrium; RV, right ventricle.

2

Thrall DE. Textbook of Veterinary Diagnostic Radiology, ed 3. Philadelphia, WB Saunders, 1998.

Tilley LP: *In* Tilley LP, Smith WK, Miller MS, eds: Cardiology: Pocket Reference, ed 2. Denver, American Animal Hospital Association, 1993.

Tilley LP. Essentials of Canine and Feline Electrocardiography: Interpretation and Treatment, ed 3. Philadelphia, Lea & Febiger, 1992.

Tilley LP, Smith WK: The 5 Minute Veterinary Consult; Canine and Feline. Baltimore, Williams & Wilkins, 1997.

Ware WA: Acquired valvular and endocardial diseases. *In* Nelson RW, Cuoto CG, eds: Essentials of Small Animal Internal Medicine. St Louis, Mosby–Year Book, 1992, pp 107–113.

Ware WA: Disturbances of cardiac rhythm. *In* Nelson RW, Cuoto CG, eds: Essentials of Small Animal Internal Medicine. St Louis, Mosby–Year Book, 1992, pp 59–77.

Eye and Ear

............EYE

............External Examination

............*Inspection of the Globe and Neuromuscular Examination*

A general inspection of the globe and external ocular structures should be conducted before any detailed examination of the eye is undertaken. Inspect the globe in normal daylight or room light and observe the relationship of the globe to the orbit and the eyelids. Note whether the eyes are in the same visual axis or whether atropia is present. Observe any undue prominence of either or both eyes. Note the presence of any other facial lesions (e.g., facial paralysis) that may affect the symmetry of the orbit. Inspect the external ocular structures (lids, conjunctiva, cornea, sclera, and lacrimal apparatus). Note the position of the eyelids; the size of the palpebral aperture; the position of the nictitating membrane; and the presence of nystagmus, unequal pupils, blepharospasm, lagophthalmos, or ocular discharges.

The tonic eye reflexes are used in the determination of extraocular muscle function and localization of lesions in the CNS. Cranial nerves III (oculomotor), IV (trochlear), and VI (abducent) innervate the extraocular striated muscles and are examined together. Cranial nerve IV innervates the m. obliquus dorsalis; cranial nerve VI innervates the m. rectus lateralis and part of the m. retractor bulbi; and cranial nerve III innervates the m. rectus medialis and m.

rectus ventralis, m. obliquus ventralis, and m. levator palpebrae superioris. Pupillary dilation is controlled by preganglionic neurons in the first three thoracic spinal cord segments, the cranial thoracic and cervical sympathetic trunks, and by postganglionic neurons in the cranial thoracic and cervical trunks, and in the cranial cervical and sympathetic nerves that course through the middle ear to reach the orbit and the m. dilator pupillae. Parasympathetic fibers in cranial nerve III innervate the sphincter pupillae muscle.

The integrity of cranial nerve III may be evaluated by examining (1) the size of the pupil; (2) the reaction of the pupil to light; (3) the presence or absence of ptosis (drooping of the upper eyelid) because of paralysis of the levator palpebrae superioris muscle; and (4) the medial deviation of the eye, which occurs in oculomotor nerve palsy (different from humans), possibly because the m. obliquus dorsalis is stronger than the m. rectus lateralis. In oculomotor nerve palsy with a normal pupillary response, if all the extraocular muscles innervated by cranial nerve III are affected, an intracranial lesion should be suspected. If individual extraocular muscles are involved, a peripheral nerve lesion may exist. If an oculomotor nerve palsy exists in association with a dilated pupil, an intraorbital or intracranial lesion should be suspected.

Paralysis of the trochlear nerve produces a transient strabismus and results in a slight upward deviation of the eye (rarely seen). The affected animal may compensate for this by developing a head tilt.

Paralysis of the abducent nerve results in a medial deviation of the affected eye with inability to gaze laterally.

It is important to check tonic neck and eye reflexes when evaluating the extraocular muscles. When the nose is elevated, the forelimbs extend and the hindlimbs flex. As the nose is elevated, the eye should remain focused within the center of the palpebral fissure. Deviating the head to one side results in increased extensor tonus on that side. Normally, nystagmus should be observed on lateral deviation of the head (with the quick phase toward the side of the deviation). Normal tonic eye reflexes signify a healthy brain stem and peripheral vestibular system and motor efferent pathways to the eyes. Tonic eye reflexes are not dependent on vision.

Cranial nerve II (optic) has its origin in the retina at the optic disk. About 66% of the optic nerve fibers in the cat and about 75% in the dog decussate at the optic chiasm. The optic nerve has two components: one is composed of the fibers that pass to the pupillary centers within the brain stem; the other is composed of fibers that synapse in the thalamus and project impulses to the visual cortex of the brain. Shine a light in the temporal portion of each eye. Note the pupillary response. Test the consensual pupillary response by shining a focal source of light in one eye and noting the effects in the opposite eye. The normal pupillary response requires that nerves II and III be intact and involves only brain stem connections.

............Assessment of Visual Function (See also p. 443)

Veterinarians must depend on objective signs and reflexes to estimate vision. A test often used to assess vision is the "menace reaction." This test involves passing the hand or an object in front of the animal's eyes and noticing the presence or absence of a blink reflex.

An obstacle course can also be valuable in assessing visual function. Styrofoam cylinders mounted on a platform can be used to create the course. The light intensity in the examining room can be varied, and alternate patching of the eyes can be helpful in detecting lesions.

............Examination of the Orbit

Observe the orbit for size. Look for swelling, depression, fistulas, or laceration of the orbital margin. If the orbit is enlarged, note whether the swelling is hard or soft, painful or nonpainful. Retrobulbar abscesses produce exophthalmos accompanied by pain, immobility of the eye, chemosis, edema of the eyelids, and pain on opening of the mouth. Orbital tumors may not be painful. Orbital retrobulbar hemorrhage or orbital fracture may occur following severe head trauma from automobile accidents. Enophthalmos may result from shrinkage of orbital contents (as in pthisis bulbi following ocular injury), from paralysis of the sympathetic nerve in Horner's syndrome, or from loss of retrobulbar fat in emaciation and dehydration.

...........Examination of the Eyelids

Note any inflammation along the margins of the eyelids and any inability to close the lids (lagophthalmos). The eyelids should touch the globe, thus preventing accumulation of tears and debris. The cilia or eyelashes on the dog's upper eyelids are arranged in three irregular rows. The lower eyelids of dogs and both eyelids of cats are devoid of cilia. When examining the lids for the presence of entropion or ectropion, do not manipulate the head because this may distort the normal lid-globe relationship. The lids of dogs and cats have a very poorly developed tarsal plate, which makes manipulation relatively easy. Observe the edges of the lids for signs of entropion, ectropion, trichiasis, or distichiasis. Observe the eyelids for symblepharon or for swelling, edema, redness, or localized inflammation, which may indicate an internal or external hordeolum. Examine the lid margins for indication of any growths. The most common or benign, epithelial growth observed on the lids of older dogs is the papilloma. The most common benign, adnexal-derived growth observed in older dogs is the sebaceous gland adenoma.

...........Examination of the Eye Using Focal Illumination

Use a focal source of illumination and a condensing lens with an ophthalmic loupe or magnifying glass to illuminate and examine various structures of the eye. A halogen, illuminated Finoff transilluminator on a rechargeable 3.5-V handle* works well.

...........Examination of the Conjunctiva

Note whether the conjunctiva is pale, injected, pigmented, hemorrhagic, or jaundiced. The inferior or ventral conjunctiva normally is more hyperemic than the upper conjunctiva. Pigmentation is occasionally present, especially on the superior bulbar conjunctiva. Usually, a few follicles are present on the conjunctival surface, especially that of the third eyelid.

Note whether the conjunctiva is relatively smooth and dry, excessively moist, or abnormally congested. Note any lacerations or erosions of the conjunctiva. Lacerations or erosions may be demonstrated using fluorescein. After initial inspection of the conjunctiva, additional tests may be required, such as the Schirmer tear test, culture, cytologic examination, or the use of stains.

When presented with "red eye" as a result of conjunctival vascularization, the clinician must decide whether it is a superficial ocular condition with conjunctival congestion or a problem deeper within the eye, producing ciliary congestion. Tables 2–8 and 2–9 may be helpful in differential diagnosis.

The palpebral (outer) and bulbar (inner) surfaces of the nictitating membrane should be inspected. The anterior surface of the membrane is normally

---

*Welch Allyn, Inc, Skaneateles Falls, N.Y.

Table 2–8. Differentiation of Deep and Superficial Congestion

Signs	Ciliary Congestion	Conjunctival Congestion
Pain	Usually present	Usually absent
Photophobia	Usually marked	Usually absent
Location of congested area	More intense circumcorneally	More marked in fornices and tarsal conjunctiva
Course of vessels	Straight, radiating limbus	Irregular and tortuous
Mobility of vessels	Cannot be moved	Easily moved
Blanching by vasoconstriction	Not blanched	May be blanched
Discharge	Absent	May or may not be present
Pupil size	Usually contracted	Unaffected
Iris	Usually congested	Unaffected

Table 2–9. Differential Diagnosis of Acute Conjunctivitis, Acute Iritis, and Acute Glaucoma

	Acute Conjunctivitis	Acute Iritis	Acute Glaucoma
Onset	Gradual	Acute	Acute
Pain	None to mild irritation	Fairly severe	Fairly severe
Discharge	Mucopurulent or purulent	Tearing	None
Vision	Unaffected	Slightly reduced	May be markedly reduced
Conjunctiva	Superficial congestion	Deep circumcorneal and ciliary congestion	Deep conjunctival, episcleral, and ciliary congestion
Cornea	Clear	Keratic precipitates may be present	Steamy and insensitive
Iris	Unaffected	Muddy and congested; posterior synechiae may be present	Congested and displaced forward
Pupil	Normal	Contracted	Dilated
Anterior chamber	Unaffected	May contain cells, opacities, and exudates	Shallow
Tenderness	Absent	Present over ciliary body	Usually absent
Intraocular pressure	Unaffected	Lower than normal	Increased
Constitutional signs	Absent	Slight	Slight to moderate

smooth, and the leading edge is frequently pigmented. The bulbar surface can be examined by placing a few drops of topical anesthetic (proparacaine hydrochloride) in the eye and gently using a small, atraumatic thumb forceps to evert the third eyelid. The bulbar surface usually contains a few small follicles. The following abnormalities are frequently associated with the third eyelid: eversion of the cartilage, hypertrophy, protrusion, inflammation and hypertrophy of the gland of the third eyelid, foreign bodies, and neoplasia.

............Conjunctival Smears, Scrapings, and Cultures

In performing conjunctival scrapings, use a platinum spatula (Kimura spatula) whose tip has previously been sterilized in the flame of an alcohol lamp and allowed to cool. Scrape the inferior conjunctival cul-de-sac, preferably without prior topical anesthesia, because anesthetics may distort the cells. Place the material on two glass slides. Fix one slide in acetone-free 95% methanol for 5 to 10 minutes; then stain with Giemsa stain. Heat-fix the other slide, and apply Gram stain.

To culture the conjunctiva, use sterile cotton applicators, fluid thioglycollate medium, and blood agar medium. Evert the palpebral conjunctiva of the lower lid, and pass one side of a sterile cotton applicator, previously moistened with sterile broth or thioglycollate medium, over the palpebral conjunctival surface. Streak the swab onto a sterile blood agar plate; then place it in a tube of thioglycollate broth. No topical anesthesia is used prior to culturing because preservatives present in anesthetics can inhibit the growth of bacteria.

............Examination of the Lacrimal System

Look for excessive tearing or hypofunction of tear secretion. Note any swelling, redness, or pain in the area of the lacrimal puncta and the lacrimal sac. When excessive tearing exists, it must be determined whether the tearing is due to (1) partial or complete obstruction of the excretory mechanism; (2) increased lacrimal secretion from chronic ocular irritation, as in distichiasis or trichiasis; or (3) physiologic increase in tear production, as may occur with uveitis.

To perform a primary dye test, place a drop of fluorescein dye from a sterile fluorescein strip into the eye. After 2 to 5 minutes, examine the external nares with the aid of a cobalt blue filter or Wood's light for the presence or absence of fluorescein dye. If dye is present, the lacrimal excretory system is patent and functioning. If epiphora exists but the primary dye test indicates that the lacrimal excretory system is patent, hypersecretion of tear fluid may be implicated as the cause of the epiphora.

Irrigation of the nasolacrimal system is indicated if the primary dye test is negative. In the dog, the nasolacrimal puncta are located 1 to 3 mm from the medial canthus on the mucocutaneous border of the upper and lower lids. In the dog, a 20- to 22-gauge (in the cat, a 23-gauge) nasolacrimal cannula should be used, often under topical anesthesia. A 2-mL syringe is filled with saline, and the lacrimal cannula is attached and passed into the lacrimal puncta of the upper lid.

Several points should be made about evaluating the nasolacrimal system. Brachycephalic breeds of dogs and cats may occasionally have a negative primary dye test, although no blockage in the nasolacrimal system exists. In flushing the nasolacrimal system of some animals, fluid may not appear at the nose; however, the animal may gag and exhibit swallowing movements, indicating that the fluid has entered the mouth and the system is patent.

Basic tear secretion comes mainly from the tarsal and conjunctival glands and the accessory tarsal glands. The reflex tear secretors are the main lacrimal gland and accessory lacrimal glands. The production of normal lacrimal secretion can be tested by using the Schirmer test with the paper in the eye for 1 minute. In normal dogs, wetting of Schirmer test papers ranges from 10 to 25 mm in 1 minute.

...........Examination of the Sclera

Note the color of the sclera, and look for nodules, hemorrhages, lacerations, cysts, and tumors. Normal sclera is white to blue-white. The sclera may appear blue when it is abnormally thinned and the uveal tract shows through. Look for staphylomas and for any injection of the scleral vessels and accompanying edema. Episcleritis can produce local scleral inflammation, whereas deep-seated ocular diseases such a glaucoma and uveitis produce generalized scleral vessel injection.

...........Examination of the Cornea

The cornea should be smooth, moist, free of blood vessels, and transparent. Note any ulceration or opacity of the cornea. Slight opacities are termed nebulae; dense ones are called leukomas. In puppies, the cornea tends to be hazy, which restricts ophthalmoscopic examination until the animals are 4 to 6 weeks of age. Diseases of the cornea, such as corneal inflammation, pigmentation, degeneration, trauma, and neoplasia, frequently may alter its transparency. Test the corneal sensitivity by touching the cornea with a wisp of dry cotton.

External ophthalmic stains help in diagnosing lesions of the cornea. Any break in the epithelial barrier permits rapid penetration of fluorescein into the stroma or even into the anterior chamber. When the epithelial surface has regenerated, the green color disappears.

Rose bengal dye stains cells and their nuclei. The dye selectively stains devitalized corneal and conjunctival epithelium a readily visible red. The main use of this dye has been in the identification of corneal and conjunctival lesions caused by keratitis sicca.

If an ulcer is present, note whether the borders are regular or irregular and whether the ulcer is superficial or deep. With ulcers that are progressive and deep, the prognosis is guarded. It is advisable to culture deep ulcers and to take scrapings of their borders. The scrapings should be stained with Giemsa, and the type of cells should be determined. If the ulcer appears to be deep, look for evidence of anterior synechiae, prolapsed iris, iridocyclitis, cataract, extrusion of the lens, fistula, or hemorrhage.

Note the presence of blood vessels in the cornea. The depth at which vascularization is taking place is usually directly related to the cause of the vascularization. Superficial vascularization is commonly associated with superficial keratitis, superficial ulcers, or pannus. Deep vascularization usually indicates a deep corneal stromal lesion, uveitis, or glaucoma.

Look for deposits on the posterior surface of the cornea (keratic precipitates). These precipitates vary in size and shape, but they are usually indicative of a disease of the uveal tract.

...........Internal Examination
...........Examination of the Anterior Chamber

Examine the anterior chamber, and observe its depth; note changes in the transparency of the ocular media, such as hypopyon, hyphema, fibrin, or foreign bodies. Look for anterior synechiae, and make sure the lens is in the normal position.

The anterior drainage angle cannot be visualized readily in the dog without the use of a contact lens. Large tumors and some anterior synechiae can be visualized with a loupe and a focal light source.

...........Examination of the Iris

The color of the iris in each eye may vary. Observe the shape and size of the iris. An iris that is thickened and muddy in color indicates an infiltration of the uveal tract. Look for the presence of atrophy, tears, synechiae, persistent pupillary membranes, iridodonesis, iridodialysis, nodules, tumors, cysts, or colobomas. Examine the pupillary border of the iris for signs of atrophy or posterior synechiae to the anterior lens capsule. Complete posterior synechia results in iris bombé and secondary glaucoma.

Examine the pupil of each eye by diffuse and focal illumination. Note the size and shape of the pupil and its direct and consensual response to light. Note any inequalities between the two pupils. Check to see whether the pupils are dilated. Find out from the owner whether the patient has had a mydriatic placed in its eye. Determine whether the pupils, when dilated, constrict when light is applied. The pupil may be dilated because of trauma, a mydriatic, fear, stimulation of the cervical sympathetic nerve, or irritation of the third cranial nerve.

Note whether the pupil of one eye is equal in size to the pupil of the other and whether the size remains equal with changes in the degree of illumination. Inequality of pupil size (anisocoria) may be caused by physiologic or pathologic factors.

...........Examination of the Lens

The pupil must be dilated to examine the lens. The lens may be examined with a focal source of illumination, an ophthalmoscope, or a biomicroscope. Examine the lens for the presence of pigment, adhesions, opacities, the position of the lens (subluxation or luxation), or absence of the lens (aphakia). Normal changes of the lens with aging can be observed in dogs over 7 years and in cats over 8 years of age. This condition is called *nuclear sclerosis* and appears as a cloudy, white, or light-blue pupil. True opacities of the lens are called *cataracts*.

...........Ophthalmoscopy
...........Examination of the Retina

For complete visualization of the fundus, dilate the iris with 1% tropicamide solution.

Examine each fundus in a dark room. To examine the right fundus, hold the ophthalmoscope in the right hand and view the fundus with the right eye. Starting with the ophthalmoscope at 0 setting, hold the ophthalmoscope about 20 in. from the patient's eye. Observe the pupil and the tapetal reflex. Bring the ophthalmoscope to within 1 in. of the patient's eye, and place the setting on −1 to −3 (negative 1 to 3) to view the optic disk and retina. If the disk is not seen immediately, follow the retinal vessels back to the disk. Inserting more positive (+) lenses into the ophthalmoscope focuses the instrument on more anterior structures within the eye.

The fundus is the portion of the inner eye that includes the optic disk or papilla, retinal vessels, tapetum lucidum, and nigrum.

...........Specialized Diagnostic Techniques in Ophthalmology
...........Tonometry

Glaucoma is an increase in intraocular pressure incompatible with normal ocular and visual functions. One method used to measure intraocular pressure is tonometry, in which the tension of the outer coat of the eye is assessed by measuring the impressibility, or applanability, of the cornea. Because the measurements based on tonometry involve calculations that have a wide base of variations, tonometry readings are always approximations.

Schiøtz Tonometry The Schiøtz tonometer consists of a corneal footplate, plunger, holding bracket, recording scale, and 5.5-, 7.5-, 10.0-, and 15.0-g weights. The principle of the Schiøtz tonometer is that the amount that the plunger protrudes from the footplate is related to the indentability of the cornea, which in turn is related to the intraocular pressure. The plunger is connected to a scale so that 0.05-mm protrusion of the plunger equals one scale unit (Table 2–10).

The dog is placed in the sitting or dorsal recumbent position. Topical anesthesia is instilled, and the eyelids are held open by the fingers, which are placed quite far away from the lid margins. The footplate must be placed vertically on the central aspect of the cornea. Three readings are taken in each eye and then averaged. Normal intraocular tension with the Schiøtz tonometer in dogs is 15 to 25 mm Hg (see Table 2–10).

Applanation Tonometry In applanation tonometry, a very small area of the cornea is flattened by a known force. The advantage of this technique over the indentation (Schiøtz) method is that the errors resulting from ocular rigidity and corneal curvature are greatly reduced.

..........Gonioscopy

Glaucoma can be caused by many different disorders that elevate intraocular pressure. In many types of glaucoma, there is an abnormality in the anterior angle of the eye (filtration angle). Gonioscopy permits one to visualize and examine the iridocorneal angle, which cannot be seen without the use of a contact lens.

The Koeppe gonioscopic lens seems to be well suited to dogs and cats. It is available in 17-, 19-, and 21-mm sizes. The lens can be inserted into the eye following the application of topical anesthesia. The gonioscopic lens can be filled with 1% methylcellulose or saline. The inside of the lens is illuminated with a Barkan lamp, otoscope head, or binocular indirect ophthalmoscope. Magnification suitable for visualization of the angle can be provided by an otoscope head, indirect ophthalmoscope, or Haag-Streit goniomicroscope.

REFERENCES

deLahunta A: Veterinary Neuroanatomy and Clinical Neurology, ed 2. Philadelphia, WB Saunders, 1983.
Gelatt KN: Veterinary Ophthalmology, ed 2. Philadelphia, Lea & Febiger, 1991.
Millichamp NJ, Dziezyc J: Vet Clin North Am Small Anim Pract 20:1990.
Noden DM, deLahunta A: The Embryology of Domestic Animals. Baltimore, Williams & Wilkins, 1985.
Peiffer R: Small Animal Ophthalmology: A Problem Oriented Approach, ed 2. Philadelphia, WB Saunders, 1996.
Rubin LF: Inherited Eye Diseases in Purebred Dogs. Baltimore, Williams & Wilkins, 1990.
Slatter DH: Fundamentals of Veterinary Ophthalmology, ed 2. Philadelphia, WB Saunders, 1990.

..........EAR

..........General Examination

Among the most important aspects of the ear examination is careful observation of the patient at rest. Physical evidence of a painful ear, e.g., loss of hair around the ear, frequent head-shaking, or head tilt, may facilitate localizing which ear, and which part of the ear, is affected. Compare one ear with

Table 2–10. Schiøtz Tonometer—Calibration Table for the Canine Eye

Schiøtz Scale Reading	Intraocular Pressure (mm Hg)		
	5.5 g Weight	7.5 g Weight	10.0 g Weight
0.5	52.6	71.2	93.6
1.0	49.3	67.0	88.3
1.5	46.3	63.1	83.3
2.0	43.4	59.4	78.6
2.5	40.8	55.9	74.1
3.0	38.3	52.6	69.6
3.5	36.0	49.6	66.0
4.0	33.9	46.7	62.2
4.5	31.9	44.0	58.7
5.0	30.1	41.6	55.4
5.5	28.4	39.2	52.3
6.0	26.9	37.1	49.4
6.5	25.5	35.1	46.7
7.0	24.2	33.2	44.2
7.5	23.0	31.5	41.8
8.0	21.9	29.9	39.6
8.5	21.0	28.5	37.5
9.0	20.1	27.1	35.6
9.5	19.3	25.9	33.8
10.0	18.6	24.8	32.1
10.5	18.0	23.8	30.6
11.0	17.4	22.8	29.1
11.5	17.0	22.0	27.8
12.0	16.6	21.3	26.6
12.5	16.3	20.6	25.5
13.0	16.0	20.0	24.5
13.5	15.8	19.5	23.6
14.0	15.7	19.1	22.8
14.5	15.7	18.8	22.0
15.0	15.7	18.5	21.4
15.5	15.8	18.3	20.8
16.0	15.9	18.1	20.3
16.5	16.1	18.0	19.9
17.0	16.4	18.0	19.5
17.5	16.8	18.1	19.2
18.0	17.2	18.2	19.0
18.5	17.7	18.4	18.8
19.0	18.3	18.7	18.7
19.5	19.0	19.0	18.6
20.0	19.7	19.4	18.7

the other. Observe the skin for signs of inflammation (swelling, redness, or desquamation of the epithelium). Movement and handling of the normal pinna should not produce pain. Look for pus or blood emanating from the external ear canal.

··········Otoscopic Examination

An otoscope is required to examine the auditory canal. Use a clean, preferably sterile, otoscope head. Do not examine a noninfected ear with the head that

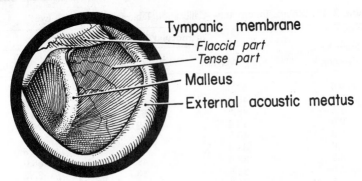

Figure 2–24. Canine tympanic membrane. (From Habel RE, deLahunta A: Applied Veterinary Anatomy. Philadelphia, WB Saunders, 1986.)

was used for an infected ear, and always examine the noninfected or normal ear first.

To examine the right ear, hold the otoscope in the right hand and the pinna between the thumb and first two fingers of the left hand. Reverse the procedure for the left ear. Draw the ear flap caudally. Insert the otoscope cone carefully in a rostroventral direction, but always watch the progress of the tip by looking through the otoscope. When the angle of the meatus is encountered, draw the ear laterally and turn the tip of the instrument medially to straighten the meatus. Otoscopes are usually provided with several specula, and visualization of the ear canal is easier if the largest one that will fit the canal is used.

The eardrum is a thin membrane with a white curved bone (the malleus) running from the dorsal margin postventrally (Fig. 2–24). The tympanic membrane consists of a small upper portion, the pars flaccida, and a large lower part, the pars tensa. The membrane separates the horizontal portion of the external auditory canal from the tympanic cavity. The posterior portion of the pars tensa is the part that is usually visualized to the greatest extent with the otoscope. The tense part of the tympanic membrane is dark, because the dark cavity of the middle ear is seen through it. The flaccid part is opaque white with red blood vessels.

The eardrum can usually be seen in normal dogs younger than 1 year of age. It may be difficult to visualize the eardrum in older dogs, because the meatus is narrowed, the tense part of the eardrum is obscured by the flaccid part, the lining of the meatus obscures the eardrum, or the eardrum is ruptured, a common occurrence in dogs with chronic otitis externa.

Any abnormal changes in the tympanic membrane, such as swelling, redness, loss of translucency, or absence of the membrane, should be recorded. If the tympanic membrane has recently ruptured, a small amount of blood-stained discharge may be seen around the membrane.

..........Cleaning the Ear Canal

In otitis externa, the external canal is frequently blocked with cerumen, exudate, and tissue debris. In many breeds, but especially poodles, Bedlington terriers, and Kerry blue terriers, the canal contains hair that frequently obscures the view. If the canal is plugged with wax, the hair must be removed first. Instill warm olive oil or a ceruminolytic agent (trolamine polypeptide oleate-condensate, Ceruminex) to soften the wax. Cotton applicators may be used to wipe the wax gently from the outer part of the external meatus. If the animal resents the cleaning, administer a short-acting general anesthetic or tranquilizer. Any deep cleaning of the ear canal should be done very cautiously and, preferably, under magnification. The patient should be adequately restrained or, preferably, anesthetized. For all but very simple external cleaning, it is best to use gentle irrigation with warm-water solutions to clean the canal thoroughly and enable a complete otoscopic examination. Cotton applicators can be dangerous and may pack debris into the canal.

If the canal contains pus or other exudates, a culture should be taken to determine antibacterial sensitivity. Before the canal can be examined visually, the discharges must be removed. The advent of the pulsating water dental hygienic apparatus has made irrigation and careful cleansing of the ear canal a much easier process. Five milliliters of povidone-iodine (Betadine, Purdue Frederick) or chlorhexidine (Nolvasan) is added to each 8 to 12 oz of warm water. The irrigation stream is kept parallel to the external ear canal and is applied with a rotating motion. The excess water and debris can be caught in a sink or basin. The canal can then be reinspected and carefully dried with cotton or by using an aspirator.

This technique should not be used in cases of acute otitis media or if the tympanic membrane has been ruptured.

REFERENCES

August JR: Diseases of the ear canal. Vet Clin North Am Small Anim Pract 18:1988.

Bruyette DS, Lorenz MD: Otitis externa and otitis media. Semin Vet Med Surg 8:3–10, 1993.

Murtaugh RJ: The ear: Medical, surgical and diagnostic aspects. Semin Vet Med Surg 8:1993.

Complete Manual of Ear Care. Trenton, NJ, Veterinary Learning Systems. 1986.

Reproductive Organs

···········EVALUATION OF THE MALE

···········History and General Examination

General information includes age, breed, history of breedings and breeding problems, body condition, vaccination, and comments on specific disease problems. Also determine the environmental setting, feeding, management practices, fertility, and breeding data about related animals. The degree of inbreeding may be important in evaluating sexual function. Previous information related to reproduction is particularly important and should include dates and results of all matings (especially for the previous year). Include comments about libido, breeding techniques, previous fertility and therapy, number of pups born, number weaned, and any abortions or deaths.

···········Special Examinations Related to Reproduction

Inspection and palpation of the genital organs is the first procedure. A thickened scrotal wall may produce testicular degeneration from increased temperature. Palpate the spermatic cord and testes for size, symmetry, and consistency (firm resilience), and note whether the testes are both located in the scrotum. Small, soft testes indicate degeneration or hypoplasia; firm masses may be the result of inflammation, fibrosis, or tumors. Testicular tumors are relatively common in dogs and may produce estrogens or testosterone, with impact on reproductive function. The epididymis, dorsal to the testis, may be prominent or firm because of fibrosis or ascending infection.

The penis, sheath, and external urethral orifice should be checked for congenital malformations. Look for frenula, hypospadias, phimosis, balanoposthitis, and neoplasia.

Naturally occurring canine transmissible venereal tumors (TVTs) can be found on the external genitalia of dogs of both sexes. The exfoliated tumor cells are transplanted into vaginal or penile tissue during coitus. Contact of infected genital discharge with the eye, mouth, or skin wounds may produce tumors at the sites. In the male, TVTs are usually located around the glans penis and result in preputial discharge. In the female, TVTs are often located in the vagina, where they assume a cauliflower appearance. The tumors may ulcerate, and bleeding from the vagina may develop. Spread of tumor tissue may be from the vagina to the uterus and uterine tubes and then to the internal iliac lymph node.

The prostate is the only accessory sex gland in the dog. Examine the prostate by rectal palpation. The prostate should be smooth, bilaterally symmetric, nonpainful, and, in most dogs, usually smaller than 3 cm in diameter. Nodules, fixation, and pain are found in carcinomas; nonpainful symmetric enlargements (often so large as to pull the organ into the abdomen) are seen with cysts or benign prostatic hypertrophy. The four major causes of prostatomegaly are benign hypertrophy; prostatitis, including abscessation of the prostate; prostatic cysts; and primary or secondary prostatic tumors. The appearance of an enlarged prostate on survey radiographs, combined with positive contrast retrograde urethrography and prostatic ultrasonography, can be helpful in the differential diagnosis. Hyperplastic and inflammatory prostatic diseases result in more symmetric prostatomegaly than do cystic, neoplastic, or prostatic abscess processes. Signs of acute bacterial prostatitis include urethral discharge, constipation, tenesmus, stilted gait, fever, depression, abdominal pain, dysuria, and leukocytosis. Chronic bacterial prostatitis may include signs associated with recurrent urinary tract infection, and the use of radiography, prostatic fluid evaluation, cultures, and biopsy may be necessary to establish a diagnosis.

Numerous additional testing procedures can be used in evaluating the animal with prostatic disease, including ejaculation and microscopic evaluation (see p. 461); prostatic biopsy (see p. 505); and prostatic aspiration and massage.

Testicular biopsy is a most important procedure indicated in azoospermic dogs that provides histologic evidence of infertility. While the patient is under general anesthesia, make a small incision over the lateral wall of the scrotum. Using a No. 11 blade, cut the tunica albuginea with three connecting incisions. With compression of the testis, a small triangular plug of tissue will protrude from the incision. The tissue is sliced off with a razor-sharp blade and placed in Bouin's solution (not formalin) for prompt transportation to the laboratory. If testicular abnormalities are palpated, it is best to perform testicular ultrasonography prior to surgery; in addition, the scrotum may be opened more liberally so that the entire testis can be examined carefully.

Semen collection and evaluation are described on p. 461. This analysis is the most important aspect of the evaluation of male breeders. Semen volume, sperm concentration, motility, and morphology, and results of seminal plasma bacterial culture should be within normal ranges for good fertility. If a dog has not ejaculated for a long period of time, the first semen sample collected may contain much debris; the second sample, collected a day or two later, may be a more reliable indicator of true semen quality. Abnormal semen samples may indicate testicular hypoplasia or degeneration, hypothyroidism, other hormonal interferences, or senility, or may be caused by toxic agents, nutritional factors, obstructive lesions in the efferent tubules, severe stress, acute immune disease, or even extreme cold. If infection is present in the reproductive tract, the pH of one of the three semen fractions may be abnormal. Culture and sensitivity studies of semen or prostatic fluid may be necessary for proper microbiologic evaluation. All male dogs should have blood tested for evidence of *Brucella canis*, which may produce acute or chronic orchitis and epididymitis. Positive rapid card test sera should be confirmed by laboratory tube tests or blood culture. With the tube agglutination test (TAT), canine sera are usually screened at 1:50 dilution; positive sera should be retested with the 2-mercapto-ethanol tube agglutination test (2ME-TAT). Positive results in the TAT test and negative results in the 2ME-TAT test for the same animal are considered suspicious. A titer of 1:200 with the 2ME-TAT test is considered presumptive evidence of canine brucellosis infection. Other organisms that may cause genital infection in males include *Escherichia coli*, *Proteus vulgaris*, *Streptococcus*, *Staphylococcus*, and *Mycoplasma* spp.; fungi such as *Blastomyces dermatitidis*; and various rickettsial organisms. Distemper infection causes epididymitis, and ascending urine via the vas deferens following trauma may cause a sterile epididymitis.

...........EVALUATION OF THE FEMALE
...........History and General Examination

With breeding problems, the history is particularly important, and is often neither detailed nor reliable. General data should include age, breed, body condition, vaccination, and comments on specific disease problems. Highly nervous or shy bitches frequently have reproductive problems. Determine the environmental setting, feeding, breeding, and other management practices concerning the animal and the fertility and breeding data for related animals. The stud dog's records should also be examined. Pedigrees should be examined to determine inbreeding or possible genetic defects. Obtain information about the age at first estrus; number and frequency of estrous cycles; breedings; pregnancies; parturitions; urogenital problems; litters whelped; and numbers of pups born and weaned, with causes of abortions or deaths, if known. Treatments and prophylactic measures, especially if they involve sex hormones, should be investigated.

...........Special Examinations Related to Reproduction

Inspection and palpation of the genital organs furnish much valuable information. The vulva is usually small and wrinkled, with good tone and almost no discharge. Note the size and condition of the clitoris. The vulva swells during proestrus and has a serosanguineous discharge; during estrus an odorless bloody or mucoid discharge is present. Exudates at other times, especially if fetid, may be suggestive of infections, tumors, or endocrine problems (pyometra). Digital examination of the vestibule and caudal vagina and abdominal palpation of the uterus should be performed in all bitches. Contrast vaginography and hysterography and ultrasonographic examination of the uterus and ovaries may be indicated when disease processes have been localized to these organs. More details about examination of the vagina and evaluation of vaginal smears may be found on p. 480. Cytologic studies of vaginal smears are very important in evaluating female breeders.

The mammary glands should be palpated and inspected for the presence of mastitis or tumors. Acute infections are hot, painful, and swollen; usually involve only one gland; and produce a purulent secretion. Chronic mastitis involves several glands; the glands are enlarged, firm, and nodular on palpation.

Mammary gland tumors constitute about half of all neoplasms in the intact bitch, and about half of these are malignant. The median age of affected bitches is 10.5 years, and mammary gland tumors are multicentric in about 50% of bitches. Of the benign tumor forms, the most frequently recognized histologic patterns are fibroadenomas (benign mixed tumors), 45%; simple adenomas; and benign mesenchymal tumors. Of the malignant tumors in the dog, the most common histologic types are solid carcinomas, tubular adenocarcinomas, papillary adenocarcinomas, anaplastic carcinomas, and sarcomas.

In malignant tumors that metastasize, tumor cells from glands 4 and 5 drain to the inguinal lymph nodes and via the thoracic duct to the lungs. The iliac lymph nodes may also be involved with metastasis. Tumor cells from glands 1 and 2 drain to the axillary lymph nodes and to the lungs and may involve the intrathoracic lymph nodes. Gland 3 appears to drain more commonly to the axillary lymph nodes. Hematogenous spread of mammary tumors with no lymph node involvement is also possible. Many malignant mammary tumors of the bitch metastasize widely and may affect abdominal as well as thoracic organs.

Fine-needle biopsy and cytologic examination may be helpful in distinguishing benign from malignant cell types. Multiple mammary gland tumors, which are present in 50% of dogs, may have different tumor types; thus, all tissues and regional lymph nodes should be sectioned.

Mammary gland neoplasia in the bitch is *almost 100% preventable* if ovariectomy is performed prior to the first estrous cycle. The incidence of mammary gland neoplasia can be *markedly reduced* if ovariectomy is done before the animal is 2½ years old or prior to the first four estrous periods. Pharmacologic doses of progestational compounds have been associated with the development of mixed mammary gland tumors.

Mammary tumors occur more frequently in cats than in any other domestic animal except the dog. Ninety percent of the tumors observed are malignant. The tumors are usually adenocarcinomas and are seen most commonly in cats 7 years of age or older. The tumors usually ulcerate early in their development. The cat normally has four pairs of mammary glands. The cranial two glands on each side have a common lymphatic system and drain into the axillary lymph nodes. The caudal two mammary glands also have a common lymphatic system and drain into the superficial inguinal lymph nodes.

Bacteriologic examination of mammary secretion, vaginal smear or culture, and intrauterine culture (collected at laparotomy) is very important if infectious processes are suspected. All breeding bitches should be tested for brucellosis; a positive rapid slide test plate should be confirmed by laboratory tube tests or blood cultures.

Infertility, abortion, premature births, stillbirths, or neonatal deaths can be caused by many infectious agents, such as β-hemolytic streptococci, *E. coli*, *B. canis*, *Staphylococcus*, *Proteus*, *Pseudomonas*, and *Mycoplasma* spp.; canine distemper; adenovirus; and herpesvirus. Fetal resorption, mummification, and abortion may be caused by any of the infectious agents just listed or by numeric chromosomal abnormality, inherited metabolic disease, maternal endocrine abnormality (thyroid insufficiency), lack of uterine space, trauma, placental hemorrhage, hormone deficiency (progesterone), exogenous estrogen, myometrial cysts, hyperplasia, and endometritis. In evaluating these problems, supplement the bacteriologic examination with maternal serology and hormone analysis, pedigree studies of the sire and dam, and, particularly, aggressive diagnostic evaluation of the dead fetus(es) (karyotype, culture, histopathology, metabolic screening).

Radiographic examination of the uterus can be performed easily if the organ is enlarged (pyometra, pregnancy, tumors). Radiopaque dye injected through the cervix during proestrus or estrus may help delineate problems that involve little change in organ size (cystic hyperplasia, myometrial cysts). Pneumoperitoneal contrast radiography or ultrasonic examination may also reveal pathologic changes. *Peritoneal laparoscopy* is a technique that may be useful for direct observation of abdominal organs such as the uterus. The ovaries are embedded in fatty bursae and thus are difficult to visualize unless the examiner is skilled at incising the bursae. *Exploratory laparotomy* is sometimes necessary to complete examination of the genital organs. One can directly view and palpate the uterus, oviducts, and ovaries for malformations and pathologic changes that cannot be delineated in other ways. Placental sites or corpora lutea can counted to determine embryonic death, and microbiologic samples and biopsy material can be obtained for laboratory evaluation. At the same time, surgical or medical measures may be performed for treatment of abnormalities.

···········Pregnancy Examination

Palpation of the uterus through the abdominal wall is the most practical method of pregnancy examination. At 20 to 22 days following ovulation, the uterus has distinct swellings 2 cm in diameter. After 28 days, these swellings have increased to about 3 to 5 cm in diameter, and this is the optimal time for diagnosis. (Diagnosis in the queen is easiest within 18 to 24 days and is difficult after 30 days.) By 35 days, the uterine swellings become confluent and diagnosis becomes more difficult. As pregnancy continues, individual fetuses may be palpated per rectum or through the abdominal wall.

Mammary glands enlarge at about 35 days of gestation, and the teats become enlarged and turgid. The nipples of a primiparous bitch are often quite red in color. Milk can be expressed from the teats during the last week of pregnancy.

Radiographs first show calcified fetal skeletons between 43 and 54 days after the first breeding in the bitch. Radiographs may be especially helpful if only one or two fetuses are present.

Other methods of pregnancy diagnosis include ultrasonography, which may reveal the presence of viable fetuses by the detection of fetal heart beats at 24 to 28 days post breeding.

···········NORMAL BREEDING—PHYSIOLOGY AND BEHAVIOR

···········Canine Female

The puberal estrus in the bitch usually occurs between the ages of 6 and 12 months: reproductive life of the female dog is 8 to 10 years. The canine female is seasonally monestrous and ovulates spontaneously. The interval between estrous cycles ranges from 4 to 12 months, depending on the size and breed of the animal (e.g., basenji, once a year; small breeds, two or three times a year; and large breeds, one or more times a year). For cellular characteristics of vaginal smears, see p. 480.

Proestrus lasts for 3 to 17 (mean = 9) days, during which time serum estradiol concentrations increase. Other characteristics are a bloody discharge from the vagina and a swollen vulva. The bitch attracts males but will not accept mating. Plasma estrogens reach a maximum level at the end of proestrus and then decrease.

Estrus lasts from 3 to 21 (mean = 9) days. Proestrus and estrus periods combined are called the "heat" period. The character of the discharge usually changes from bloody (during proestrus) to straw-colored (during estrus) but may remain sanguineous without an adverse effect on fertility. The vulva is less turgid. The bitch is receptive and courts the male through foreplay, jumping, and trying to mount the male. The canine female presents the perineum in a lordosis-like posture and reflexively deviates the tail to one side. The bitch first refuses mating by the male at a variable time after the onset of estrus (usually 6 to 15 days). Ovulation usually occurs early in estrus (within the first

3 days), but some normal bitches may ovulate several days before to 11 days after onset of estrus. The ovum is not ready for fertilization until 48 hours later, after the second polar body has been extruded. The ovum lives 4 to 5 days, the transit time to the uterus being 4 to 10 days. Implantation occurs in 18 to 20 days, and an endotheliochorial deciduate zonary placenta forms. The gestation cycle is 58 to 71 days from a single breeding or 62 to 64 days from ovulation.

Luteinizing hormone (LH) surges within 24 hours of the estrogen peak and causes ovulation. Progesterone increases gradually during estrus and is the cause of "behavioral" estrus. Serum progesterone concentration rises to about 2 ng/mL on the day of the LH surge; best reproductive performance (conception rate and litter size) occurs when the bitch is bred 4 days after the LH surge, which is also 2 days after ovulation. Progesterone reaches a maximum 25 to 30 days after the LH surge and then gradually decreases to less than 1 mg/mL at parturition in the pregnant bitch. The progesterone decline is the cause of the temperature drop just before parturition. After ovum implantation, the hematocrit falls from 40% to 45% to 30%, which is probably a reflection of plasma volume expansion in the pregnant bitch; nonpregnant luteal-phase bitches also show a decline in hematocrit level from anestrous values but do not show the magnitude of decline seen in pregnancy.

Diestrus (2 months) is the period when the corpus luteum produces progesterone, which is present in the bitch's serum in concentrations exceeding 2 ng/mL. Diestrus begins on the first day of a predominantly noncornified vaginal smear and ends when serum progesterone declines to less than 2 ng/mL. Both pregnant and nonpregnant bitches have periods of diestrus lasting approximately 2 months.

During *anestrus* (approximately 4 months), the genital organs are relatively quiescent; the uterine lining is sloughed and regenerates.

·········· Canine Male

Puberty in the canine male occurs between 6 to 12 months of age (see p. 461 for data about normal sperm).

Follicle-stimulating hormone (FSH) initiates spermatogenesis; LH increases the testosterone secretion of Leydig cells needed to complete spermatogenesis and to maintain accessory sex glands, secondary sex characteristics, and libido. Testosterone has a negative feedback effect on pituitary gonadotropins. Oxytocin and prostaglandins are important in the transport of sperm during ejaculation. Prostaglandins increase LH output and testosterone production and are the reason why sexual foreplay increases ejaculatory output and total number of sperm.

Testosterone is of little value in the treatment of infertility, except to increase libido for 2 to 3 days following administration of low doses. Prolonged use causes testicular degeneration and a negative feedback effect on LH release.

In copulation, the male responds to the female in estrus by biting and nuzzling her neck and licking her flanks and perineal region. The male mounts and clasps the female's hindquarters at the rear flank with his forelegs. After pelvic copulatory movement, intromission of the nonerect penis takes place, after which erection of the penis inside the vagina occurs. Ejaculation of the presperm and sperm-rich fractions of semen occurs during the most vigorous pelvic thrusting of the male, after which the male dismounts and, with the engorged penis still entrapped inside the vagina, lifts a hindleg over the rear quarters of the female and stands end to end with her in copulatory lock, or tie. During the tie, which may last from 5 to 60 minutes, the dog ejaculates the third and most voluminous fraction of semen, the prostatic fluid. Some male dogs rebreed within 2 hours of separation.

···········Feline Female

Puberty in the feline female occurs at 4 to 12 months of age. The reproductive life is 8 to 10 years. The feline female is seasonally polyestrous (January through September in the Northern Hemisphere, continuous if 14 hours of light are available daily). Ovulation is induced by coitus or simulated coitus. Estrus occurs every 4 to 30 days. For cellular characteristics of the vagina, see p. 484. Proestrus lasts 0 to 2 days, during which pheromones increase and a very slight mucoid discharge from the Bartholin glands may occur.

Estrus lasts 6 to 10 days in most queens (range = 2 to 12 days), and estrus length is not influenced by whether ovulation occurs. Following nonfertile induction of ovulation, the corpora lutea last 30 to 40 days, and the cycle averages 6 weeks. The feline female has a characteristic call, rubs the head against objects with affection, purrs, crouches with forelegs, elevates rear quarters and treads, and deflects tail laterally. Ovulation occurs 24 to 50 hours after copulation (sensory nerves stimulate the hypothalamus to release gonadotropin-releasing hormone, which acts on the anterior pituitary to release a surge of LH, causing ovulation). Sperm requires 24-hour capcitation in the uterus to be fertile, and fertilization may occur up to 48 hours after ovulation.

Fertilized ova are in the oviduct for 4 days. Implantation occurs 14 days after breeding, and an endotheliochorial zonary placenta forms. Gestation length is 58 to 70 days (usually 60 to 63 days).

Postestrus occurs if the queen is not induced to ovulate. This stage is 7 to 21 days long; the ova degenerate, and then the queen returns to estrus.

Anestrus lasts 1 to 6 months, depending on photoperiod; during anestrus the queen does not mate.

···········Feline Male

Puberty occurs at about 6 months (depending on age at the beginning of the breeding season). See p. 465 for data about artificial insemination and feline sperm. The tom has depressed sexual activity in the fall. He has rigid territorial and behavioral habits regarding the breeding ritual, and the feline male does much calling and fighting to retain his home territory.

The male approaches the female, makes chattering sounds, and rubs his face over her shoulder and body. Foreplay is limited; the tom grasps the queen's neck skin in his teeth and mounts.

REFERENCES

Concannon PW, Lein DH: Hormonal and clinical correlates of ovarian cycles, ovulation, pseudopregnancy, and pregnancy in dogs. *In* Kirk RW, ed: Current Veterinary Therapy X. Small Animal Practice. Philadelphia, WB Saunders, 1989.

Ettinger SJ, Feldman EC, eds: Textbook of Veterinary Internal Medicine, ed 4. Philadelphia, WB Saunders, 1995.

Feldman EC, Nelson RW: Canine and Feline Endocrinology and Reproduction, ed 2. Philadelphia, WB Saunders, 1996.

Finn ST, Wrigley RH: Ultrasonography and ultrasound-guided biopsy of the canine prostate. *In* Kirk RW, ed: Current Veterinary Therapy X. Small Animal Practice. Philadelphia, WB Saunders, 1989.

Johnson CA: Disorders of the vagina and uterus. *In* Nelson RW, Cuoto CG, eds: Essentials of Small Animal Internal Medicine. St Louis, Mosby–Year Book, 1992, pp 654–664.

Johnson SD, Romagnol SE, eds: Symposium on canine reproduction. Vet Clin North Am Small Anim Pract 21:1991.

Nicoletti P: Diagnosis and treatment of canine brucellosis. *In* Kirk RW, ed: Current Veterinary Therapy X. Small Animal Practice. Philadelphia, WB Saunders, 1989.

Nervous System

The animal is examined to ascertain the site and nature of the lesion responsible for signs of nervous system disease. In examining the animal with a neurologic disorder, three basic questions should be answered: (1) Where is the lesion in the nervous system? (2) What type of lesion is present (inflammation, degeneration, neoplasm, malformation, or injury)? (3) What causes the lesion?

Follow an outline in performing an examination of the nervous system. Examine the animal in quiet surroundings. The following equipment is helpful in performing a neurologic examination: reflex hammer, penlight, and hemostat.

..........SIGNALMENT AND HISTORY

The breed, sex and age of the animal should be noted; considered together with the chief complaint, they may help direct the line of questioning in the historical review. Certain breeds are predisposed to specific neurologic ailments, and the age of the animal may tend to reduce the possibility of certain neurologic diseases.

The history should include a summary of all past medical and surgical illnesses and the facts surrounding the present complaint. The line of questioning will be influenced by the chief complaint. However, general questions should include the dosage of and response to medications administered for the condition, the vaccination history, and the health status of littermates or other animals in the household.

..........Injury

1. When did it occur? Was it observed?
2. Describe the animal's initial condition.
3. How has the animal's condition changed since the accident?

..........Seizures

1. Describe completely. How do they start? How does the animal act during the seizure? Is the animal conscious? How long does the seizure last? How does the animal act during the recovery? Is the animal normal between seizures? What are the intervals between seizures? Is a period of abnormal behavior associated with the seizure?
2. List the age of the first seizure, date of the seizure(s), and total number of seizure(s).
3. What anticonvulsant medication has been used (include date of initiation, dosage, and response)?
4. Is there a past history of an injury?
5. When does the animal eat, and what does it eat?
6. Is there any source of intoxication, especially lead?
7. Has the animal been ill recently?

..........Weakness or Ataxia

1. Describe the first appearance of these signs. Was the onset sudden or gradual?
2. When did the signs begin? How have the signs changed since? Have the signs been progressively getting worse, or have they been intermittent?
3. Has the animal had periods of being normal since the first onset of the signs?
4. Have there been any seizures or periods of abnormal behavior or other signs of disturbed cerebral function?

............Puppy With Neurologic Signs

1. Were the signs present at birth or at least as soon as the pup could walk?
2. How have the signs changed since then?

............Neurologic Examination

The neurologic examination can be divided into five parts: mental attitude and behavior, gait, postural reactions, spinal nerve reflexes, and cranial nerve reflexes. In this description, an intact *reflex* requires the function of only the peripheral nerves being tested and the segments of the spinal cord or brain stem in which the afferent axon enters and the cell bodies and axons of the efferent neurons are located. A *reaction* depends on the same components as the reflex, plus the ascending pathways through the white matter of the spinal cord and brain stem to the cerebellum and sensorimotor cortex of the cerebrum and the descending pathways that return from the cerebrum by way of its internal capsule and the white matter of the brain stem and spinal cord. The lower motor neuron (LMN) has its cell body and dendritic zone in the ventral gray column of the spinal cord or specific cranial nerve nucleus in the brain stem. Its axon leaves the CNS and courses through peripheral nerves to its telodendron in the group of muscle fibers it innervates. The upper motor neurons (UMNs) have cell bodies and dendritic zones in collections of gray matter in the cerebrum (motor cerebral cortex) or brain stem (red nucleus, reticular nuclei). The axons of the UMNs descend in tracts through the white matter in the brain and spinal cord to end in telodendria in the vicinity of the LMN that they ultimately influence (Fig. 2–25).

The precise order in which the parts of a neurologic examination are performed varies with the preference of the examiner and the attitude of the patient. An initial assessment should be made of the patient's mental attitude and behavior. If the animal is resting quietly in a cage at the time of examination, the cranial nerve examination may be done first. If the animal is excited or apprehensive, it may be more convenient to perform the cranial nerve

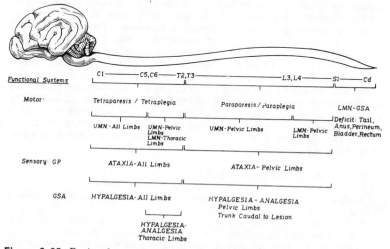

Figure 2–25. Regional neurologic signs in spinal cord disease. LMN, lower motor neuron; GSA, general somatic afferent; UMN, upper motor neuron.

examination after the animal has been handled during the examinations of gait, postural reactions, and reflexes.

............Mental Attitude and Behavior

An assessment should be made of the patient's mental attitude, sensorium, and behavior. The owner is usually the best judge of subtle changes in the patient's behavior and should be questioned about this. Is the animal bright, alert, and responsive initially and throughout the examination? The various terms that characterize alterations of this attitude and behavior are depression, lethargy, unresponsiveness, stupor, coma, anxiety, disorientation, hyperactivity, hysteria, propulsion, and aggression.

As a rule, these alterations in the animal's normal sensorium reflect disturbances in the diencephalon and telencephalon and often implicate some portion of the limbic system. It is especially important to evaluate these carefully in the recumbent animal. Cervical spinal cord disease that produces recumbency will not alter the animal's mental attitude, except that some animals may become frantic and hyperexcitable if they are unable to get up. The same degree of tetraplegia can occur with a brain stem lesion that severely alters the animal's responsiveness to its environment. However, cranial nerve abnormalities are generally noted with brain stem lesions.

............Gait

The gait should be examined in a place where the animal may be allowed to move freely, unleashed, and where the ground surface is not slippery. The floor of many examining rooms is too slippery for adequate evaluation of the animal's gait. In some patients with vertebral column injury with spinal cord contusion resulting in paresis and ataxia, moving the patient on a slippery floor may cause a fall, and further injury may result. A carpeted room is ideal.

The degree of functional deficit dictates the necessity for further examination of strength and coordination. A patient that is tetraplegic—unable to support its weight or move its limbs when the weight is borne on them—need not have further tests performed for the postural reactions. A grade 0 paraplegic patient need not be examined for postural reactions in the pelvic limbs, but the thoracic limbs should be examined carefully. Occasionally, a patient with progressive myelitis may present as paraplegic because of an extensive thoracolumbar spinal cord location of the lesion; the patient will also have an asymmetrical thoracic limb gait because of a less severe focus of the lesion in the cervical spinal cord. An early sign in dogs with ascening myelomalacia associated with an acute severe intervertebral disk extrusion may be a hesitant, stumbling, awkward gait in the thoracic limbs. The severity of advanced pelvic limb dysfunction is evaluated best by holding the animal suspended at the base of the tail and observing its gait. Pelvic limb function may be graded according to the following scheme:

5—Normal strength and coordination
4—Can stand to support: *minimal paraparesis and ataxia*
3—Can stand to support but frequently stumbles and falls: *mild paraparesis and ataxia*
2—Unable to stand to support; when assisted, moves limbs readily but stumbles and falls frequently: *moderate paraparesis and ataxia*
1—Unable to stand to support; slight movement when supported by the tail: *severe paraparesis*
0—Absence of purposeful movement: *paraplegia*

.... *Postural Reactions*

Following observation of the gait for strength and coordination, the postural reactions can be tested, especially to determine whether there are less obvious deficits in strength and coordination when the gait appears to be normal. Each of these reactions requires that all major components of the peripheral and central nervous systems be intact. They are not of localizing value by themselves.

Wheelbarrowing The thoracic limbs may be tested by supporting the animal under the abdomen so that the pelvic limbs are off the ground surface and forcing the animal to walk on its thoracic limbs. The normal animal walks with symmetric movements of both thoracic limbs and with the head extended in normal position. Animals with lesions of the peripheral nerves of the thoracic limbs, cervical spinal cord, or brain stem may have asymmetric movements, with stumbling or knuckling over on the dorsum of the paw of the affected limb. Hypermetria is occasionally observed. With more severe lesions in this area, there is a tendency to carry the head flexed with the nose close to and occasionally reaching the ground surface for support. Animals with neuromuscular disease affecting neck muscles will carry their neck partially flexed and have difficulty with normal extension. If no deficit is observed, extend the neck while the animal is wheelbarrowed. This sometimes reveals a mild deficit, a tendency to knuckle over on the dorsum of the paw, which was not observed previously. This may be helpful to confirm a cervical spinal cord lesion in Great Danes or Doberman pinschers that have a cervical vertebral malformation and show mild pelvic limb paresis and ataxia but no overt thoracic limb signs.

Hopping—Thoracic Limb While still supporting the pelvic limbs, hop the animal on one thoracic limb while holding the other off the ground surface so that the entire weight of the body is supported by the limb to be tested. Move the dog forward and to each side but especially laterally, and observe the strength and coordination of the limb. Repeat this on the other thoracic limb and compare the response. Asymmetry occurs with paresis or ataxia. Hypermetria may be seen with general proprioceptive or cerebellar deficits. This is an effective way of determining minor deficits when the gait appears to be normal, as occurs with contralateral cerebral sensorimotor cortex lesions. Animals with neuromuscular disease that can still move their limbs will usually struggle to hop, but will collapse when all the weight of the animal is borne on the limb being tested. If the weight is held up, the limb to be tested will often respond fairly well, indicating that proprioceptive function is not impaired.

Extensor Postural Thrust The same responses to tests can be obtained on the pelvic limbs. The extensor postural thrust reaction is performed by holding the animal off the ground surface by supporting it caudal to the scapulae, lowering it to the ground surface, and observing the animal extend its pelvic limbs to support its weight. Moving the animal forward and backward in this position test the symmetry of pelvic limb function, strength, and coordination.

Hopping—Pelvic Limb Continuing to support the animal by the thorax so that the thoracic limbs are not in contact with the ground surface, hold up one pelvic limb, and force the animal to hop laterally or forward on the supporting limb. Both pelvic limbs should be tested this way and the responses compared. It is important to compare the pelvic limb hopping responses with each other and not with the ipsilateral thoracic limb. Normally, the hopping response of the pelvic limb seems more stiff or hypertonic, with a slightly larger excursion than that of the thoracic limb.

Hemistanding and Hemiwalking The animal's ability to stand and walk with the thoracic and pelvic limbs on one side can be tested by holding the opposite thoracic and pelvic limbs off the ground surface and forcing the animal to walk forward or to the side. These reactions are referred to as the hemistanding and hemiwalking reactions. With a large dog or uncooperative patient that resists hopping, you may be able to evaluate the hopping responses by observing the responses of the limbs during hemiwalking.

An animal with a unilateral lesion of the sensorimotor cortex or internal capsule may have a normal gait but show deficits in its postural reactions on the side opposite the lesion. Attempts to hemiwalk on the contralateral side are delayed or exaggerated (hypermetric) and spastic, and stumbling may occur. With unilateral cervical spinal cord lesions, the limbs on the same side as the lesion show a deficiency in the gait and are poorly responsive to postural reaction testing, including the animal's inability to respond in the hemiwalking reaction.

Placing Other postural reactions that can be tested include placing with the thoracic limbs. The animal is supported off the ground surface and its thoracic limbs are brought to the edge of a table or similar surface so that the dorsal surface of the paws makes contact. This test should be performed on both thoracic limbs simultaneously and individually, with and without blindfolding the animal. Vision can compensate for the sense of position when the general proprioceptive system is abnormal, so tactile placing (blindfolded animal) is tested before visual placing.

Tonic Neck Reaction The tonic neck reaction involves extension of the head and neck so that the nose is directed dorsally. The normal patient responds by extension of all the joints of both thoracic limbs. An animal with disease of the general proprioceptive system in the cervical spinal nerves, cervical spinal cord, or medulla fails to extend its carpus or digits or both, and these joints passively flex so that the weight is borne on the dorsal surface of the paw. The same response may occur if an animal is paretic as a result of disease of the motor neurons that innervate the thoracic limb or in the white matter of the spinal cord that influences these motor neurons.

Proprioceptive Positioning Proprioceptive positioning tests this afferent system by determining the animal's ability to recognize when the paw has been flexed so that the weight is borne on its dorsal surface. The normal animal returns the paw to its usual position. In patients with severe paresis, this test may also be deficient.

............Spinal Nerve Reflexes

Spinal nerve evaluation includes assessment of muscle tone and size, spinal reflexes, and cutaneous sensation. Muscle tone and spinal reflexes are evaluated best when the animal is in lateral recumbency and as relaxed as possible. It is important to test muscle tone, tendon reflexes, and the flexor reflex to noxious stimuli, in that order, to maintain the cooperation of the animal.

Muscle Tone Muscle tone is evaluated by passive manipulation of the limbs individually. The degree of resistance is determined to be less than normal (hypotonic), normal, or more than normal (hypertonic). The last may be referred to as spasticity. The degree of spasticity varies from a mild increased resistance, to passive manipulation, to rigid extension.

Hypotonia usually occurs with LMN disease, whereas UMN disease may be characterized by hypertonia or spasticity. However, normal muscle tone without spasticity can occur in some animals with UMN disease. The functional integrity of the LMN is necessary to cause muscle cell contraction to maintain muscle tone. Functional integrity of the LMN is also necessary to maintain the normal health of the muscle cell it innervates. When denervated, these cells degenerate. The degeneration is observed clinically as neurogenic atrophy and can be detected electromyographically by the production of abnormal potentials in resting muscle. The UMN influences the activity of the LMN to produce voluntary motor activity and to maintain muscle tone for support of the body against gravity. Although the UMN includes both facilitatory and inhibitory functions on the activity of the LMN, when the UMN is diseased the result usually observed is a release of the LMN from inhibition and overactivity of the facilitory mechanism. This release is seen as hypertonia or spasticity.

Dogs that are tetraplegic should be held in a supporting position to observe the muscle tone in the limbs and any voluntary responses. Usually, dogs with cervical spinal cord lesions rostral to the brachial plexus have rigidly extended limbs, and the entire trunk and limbs feel stiff when the dog is held up and the limbs moved along the ground surface. The hypertonia may be severe enough to permit the animal to stand unsupported. Tetraplegic dogs with diffuse neuromuscular diseases such as polyradiculoneuritis are hypotonic or atonic and appear and feel limp when held in a supporting position. There is no reflex tension of the limb, and no support is elicited by placing the paws on the ground. Instead, the limbs buckle under the weight of the body.

Patellar Reflexes The most reliable tendon reflex is the patellar reflex. It is the only tendon reflex that is present in all normal animals. However, the reflex may normally be difficult to detect in older large-breed dogs. It is obtained by lightly tapping the patellar tendon with the animal in lateral recumbency and as relaxed as possible for proper evaluation. A pediatric neurologic hammer is the most useful instrument, but any hard object such as forceps handles can be used. The reflex can be elicited in all normal dogs and is mediated by the femoral nerve through the L4–6 spinal cord segments. The degree of normal response varies with the breed. Large breeds of dogs have a brisker reflex than the short-limbed breeds such as the dachshund. The response should be evaluated as absent (0), hyporeflexic (+1), normal (+2), hyperreflexic (+3), or clonic (+4). This reflex should be tested with the animal lying, on each side. An absent reflex or hyporeflexia occurs when there is disease of a portion of the reflex arc. Hyperreflexia or clonus is often present is UMN disease.

Biceps and Triceps Reflexes In the thoracic limb, the biceps and triceps reflexes can be elicited in many dogs that are relaxed and in lateral recumbency. Lightly tapping the tendon of insertion of the triceps proximal to the olecranon elicits a slight extension of the elbow. The reflex is mediated by the radial nerve through the C7 and C8 and the T1 and T2 spinal cord segments. The biceps reflex is elicited by placing a finger on the distal ends of the biceps and brachialis muscles at the level of the elbow. Tapping this finger with the hammer elicits a slight flexion of the elbow. The muscle contraction can be palpated in some instances when no movement of the joint is seen. The musculocutaneous nerve mediates this reflex through the C6–8 spinal cord segments. The normal animal has a mild reflex response to these stimuli. In a few normal animals, these reflexes are difficult to elicit. They are absent when there is disease of some portion of the reflex arc. They may be hyperactive in some animals with disease of the UMN.

Flexor Reflex—Pelvic Limb The flexor reflexes to noxious stimuli determine the integrity of the reflex arc as well as the pathway in the CNS that is concerned with the animal's response to noxious stimuli. The most reliable stimulus is pressure exerted on the base of the toenail with hemostats. Many normal animals do not respond to the stimulus of a pin. The pelvic limb is maintained perpendicular to the long axis of the pelvis by placing a hand on the anterior surface of the limb above the stifle when applying the noxious stimuli. The normal animal with UMN lesions will flex the limb at the stifle. The flexor reflex is mediated by the sciatic nerve through the L6 and L7 spinal cord segments and the S1 segment. A depressed or absent flexor indicates a lesion in one of these structures. Abnormality of the motor portion of the sciatic nerve distal to the pelvis causes paralysis, hypotonia, and atrophy of the flexors of the stifle, tarsus, and digits, as well as of the extensors of the hip, tarsus, and digits. There is no resistance to flexion or extension of the tarsus. In the animal walking with a sciatic nerve paralysis, the tarsus is lower on the affected side and the paw may be placed on its dorsal surface; however, the limb is able to support weight as long as the femoral nerve is intact.

Sensory branches of the peroneal nerves supply the dorsal surface of the paw. The plantar surface is supplied by tibial nerve sensory branches. The medial side of the paw is supplied by the saphenous nerve, a brach of the femoral nerve at the femoral triangle. The saphenous nerve enters the spinal cord through the L4–6 segments. A patient may have a contused sciatic nerve from a pelvic fracture and have no function of the muscles innervated by this nerve and analgesia of the lateral, dorsal, and plantar surfaces of the paw. However, the intact saphenous nerve provides sensation to the medial surface of the paw. If this area is stimulated, the animal will flex the hip with the intact innervation of the iliopsoas muscle, but the stifle, tarsus, and digits fail to flex. For this reason, both the medial and lateral surfaces of the paw should be tested for reflex responses as well as nociception.

Nociception Animals show signs of pain perception by a behavioral response (e.g., crying, biting), not a flexor reflex. The impulses generated by a noxious stimulus enter the spinal cord over the peripheral nerves and dorsal roots and are relayed to tracts in the lateral funiculi of the spinal cord bilaterally. These tracts ascend the spinal cord in the lateral funiculi and continue through the medulla, pons, and mesencephalon to specific nuclei in the thalamus for relay to the somatic sensory cerebral cortex. Pain may be evidenced when the impulses reach the thalamus or cerebrum.

Flexor Reflex—Thoracic Limb In the thoracic limb, the thoracodorsal, axillary, musculocutaneous, median, ulnar, and radial nerves are responsible for flexion of the shoulder, elbow, carpus, and digits when a noxious stimulus is applied to the paw. These nerves arise from the C6–T2 spinal cord segments. The specific sensory nerve stimulated depends on the location of the stimulus. The median and ulnar nerves innervate the skin of the palmar surface of the paw; the radial nerve supplies the dorsal surface. In the forearm, the radial nerve supplies the skin on the cranial and lateral surfaces. The ulnar nerve supplies the caudal surface, and the musculocutaneous nerve supplies the medial surface. Be aware of the amount of overlap of the cutaneous innervation by these nerves. The thoracic limb is maintained in a position similar to that described for the pelvic limb. Following a noxious stimulus, the normal animal and the animal with a UMN lesion will flex the limb at the elbow. A depressed or absent flexor reflex indicates a lesion in one of the structures that mediate the flexor reflex.

Crossed Extensor Reflex In animals with UMN disease and release of the LMN, a crossed extensor reflex may be elicited in the recumbent animal when the flexor reflex is stimulated. The crossed reflex occurs in the limb opposite the one being tested for a flexor reflex. To avoid voluntary extension of the contralateral limb as a response to a noxious stimulus, the flexor reflex first should be elicited with as mild a stimulus as is necessary and the opposite limb observed for extension. When elicited in an animal in lateral recumbency, this is an abnormal reflex, indicative of UMN disease.

Perineal Reflex The perineal reflex is elicited by stimulating the anus with a noxious stimulus and observing contraction of the anal sphincter and flexion of the tail. The reflex is mediated by branches of the sacral and caudal nerves through the sacral and caudal segments of the spinal cord.

Cutaneous Reflex The cutaneous reflex is the contraction of the cutaneous trunci in response to mild stimulation of the skin of the trunk. It can be elicited in normal animals from the thoracic and most of the lumbar region. The regional segmental spinal nerves contain the sensory neurons that are stimulated. The impulses are carried into the related spinal cord segments and then relayed through the white matter of the spinal cord cranially to the C6 spinal cord segment. Here synapse occurs on LMNs of the lateral thoracic nerve that innervate the cutaneous trunci. When the cutaneous response is present, it indicates the spinal cord white matter is intact from the level tested to the C8 spinal cord segment. This reflex may require multiple stimulation to elicit, and occasionally normal animals resist this stimulation; dehydrated animals and animals with advanced generalized muscle atrophy show no reflex.

.... Cranial Nerve Reflexes

The cranial nerve examination should be performed at the time when the animal is in the most cooperative attitude. The procedure for examining the cranial nerves is described here, with the specific cranial nerves being examined indicated in parentheses.

Observe the head for any evidence of a head tilt (vestibular, VIII), facial muscle asymmetry from weakness or contracture–hemifacial spasm (VII), or atrophy of the muscles of mastication (motor, V). Palpate these muscles for tone and atrophy. With one eye of the patient covered, menace the opposite eye with threatening gestures of the hand, being careful to avoid striking the patient or stimulating the hair with air currents (II through VII). Repeat this on the opposite side. If the response is absent, check the eyelids for ability to close (VII). Observe the symmetry of the pupils and their reaction to light in either eyeball (II through III). Observe the eyes for evidence of abnormal position, strabismus (III; IV; VI; vestibular, VIII), or abnormal nystagmus (vestibular, VIII). Move the head from side to side to generate normal vestibular nystagmus. This stimulates the vestibular nerve (VIII), and impulses pass through the vestibular nuclei (medulla) and medial longitudinal fasciculus (medulla-pons-midbrain) to abducent neurons in the medulla for abduction and oculomotor neurons in the midbrain for adduction. Test the corneal and palpebral reflexes (sensory, V through VII), ear movement (VII), and the position of the philtrum (VII). Examine the commissure of the lips for hypotonia that exposes mucosa and allows saliva to escape (VII). Check the skin sensation to blunt forceps from the corners of the eyelids (V) and the mucosa of the nasal septum (ophthalmic, V). If further evaluation is necessary, a pin can be used over the entire surface of the head. If evaluation is difficult and a deficit is suspected, the most sensitive area to test with a blunt object is the mucosa of the nasal septum inside each naris. Observe the jaws for normal closure (motor, V). Open the mouth and observe whether resistance is normal (motor, V). Observe the position of the tongue, its movements and size (atrophy), and pull on it to test its strength (XII). Check the gag reflex by probing the pharynx with a tongue depressor (IX, X).

Additional Tests—Visual (see p. 443)

Additional Tests—Vestibular Clinical signs associated with vestibular disease are summarized in Table 2–11. To examine the vestibular system (VIII), the head should be held laterally over each shoulder with the exposed eye covered except for the limbus. Observe the eye for the development of a positional nystagmus. Make a similar observation with the head and neck extended and both eyes covered with the lower eyelids except for the limbus at the superior portion of the eye. In the normal patient, no spontaneous nystagmus develops and the corneas remain in the center of the palpebral fissure. In patients with unilateral disease of the vestibular system, the eye on the affected side is depressed and does not elevate into the center of the fissure, and spontaneous nystagmus may be observed. The head should be moved from side to side, and the normal vestibular nystagmus elicited should be observed. In bilateral peripheral vestibular disease or severe lesions in the brain stem, this response may be absent. This lack of normal eye movement offers a poor prognosis in animals with intracranial injury. In unilateral vestibular lesions, the rapidity of the response may not be equal in both directions of head movement.

The presence of a spontaneous or positional nystagmus or a postrotatory

Table 2–11. Responses/Clinical Observations in Patients With Central vs. Peripheral Vestibular Disease

Peripheral Vestibular System Disease	Central Vestibular System Disease
Seldom roll	More tendency to roll
Nystagmus: quick phase always to the side away from the lesion	Nystagmus: quick phase may change directions with different head positions
Other signs: facial paresis, paralysis	Other signs
Horner's syndrome (cat, dog)	Ipsilateral hemiparesis, ataxia
	Slow postural reactions
	Depression
	Head tremor, hypermetria
	Dysphagia
	Medial strabismus
	Weak jaw, atrophy of masticatory muscles
	Facial hypalgesia

nystagmus that is markedly different on each side is evidence of disturbance of the vestibular system. With disturbance of the peripheral portion of this system (VIII), the abnormal spontaneous or positional nystagmus is either horizontal or rotatory, with the quick phase directed toward the side opposite the lesion. The postrotatory nystagmus developed after spinning the animal to the opposite side from the lesion is depressed when compared with the response observed on spinning the animal toward the side of the lesion. With extensive bilateral peripheral vestibular disease, the examiner may not be able to elicit nystagmus.

A horizontal, rotatory, or vertical spontaneous or positional nystagmus occurs with disturbance of the central portion of the vestibular system. In addition, with central vestibular lesions the direction of the nystagmus may vary with changes in the position of the head. A rapid pendular congenital nystagmus may occur in puppies with or without abnormalities of the visual system.

Vestibular system disease is characterized by loss of balance. Disease on one side produces ipsilateral head tilt, and the patient will lean, fall, or roll toward the side of the lesion. Strength and postural reactions are normal but may be difficult to elicit in severely affected animals. Abnormal nystagmus may occur and may be spontaneous or positional. Peripheral vestibular system lesions cause a jerk nystagmus directed away from the side of the lesion (quick phase).

The sense of smell (I) and hearing (cochlear, VIII) are difficult to evaluate unless the deficit is complete. Usually the owner's observations of the patient in its natural environment are more reliable for determination of these sensations.

...........Summary of Signs With Lesions at Specific Locations in the Spinal Cord

...........Lumbosacral: Fourth Lumbar to Fifth Caudal Segment

Complete malacia from fourth lumbar through fifth caudal segments:

Flaccid paraplegia: no support, gait, or movement of pelvic limbs and tail; normal thoracic limbs

No postural reactions in pelvic limbs
Areflexia: flexor, patellar, perineal reflexes
Atonia: soft muscles, no resistance to manipulation of pelvic limbs or tail
Neurogenic atrophy: in chronic lesions
Dilated anus
Analgesia from pelvic limbs, tail, and perineum

Partial malacia of gray and white matter between the fourth lumbar and fifth caudal segments:

Flaccid paraparesis and ataxia of pelvic limbs with normal thoracic limbs
Postural reactions of pelvic limbs attempted, but poorly accomplished
Hyporeflexia or areflexia: flexor and patellar reflexes
Hypotonia: normal or weak resistance to manipulation of pelvic limbs
Slight neurogenic atrophy: in chronic lesions
Normal or depressed nociception (hypalgesia) from pelvic limbs, tail, and perineum

2

............*Thoracolumbar: Third Thoracic to Third Lumbar Segment*

Complete malacia—focal site between third thoracic and third lumbar segments.

Spastic paraplegia: no voluntary support, gait, or movement of pelvic limbs; normal thoracic limbs. With acute lesions, the thoracic limbs may be spastic (Schiff-Sherrington syndrome). With cranial thoracic lesions, there may be more difficulty in standing up on the thoracic limbs from a recumbent position, and loss of trunk support may also be observed when the animal is walked on the thoracic limbs with the pelvic limbs supported by the tail. The trunk may sway to the side abnormally.
No postural reactions in pelvic limbs.
Reflexes normal or hyperactive: flexor and patellar.
Crossed extensor reflex may occur.
Muscle tone normal or hypertonic, no atrophy.
Analgesia from area caudal to the lesion.

Partial malacia—focal site between third thoracic and third lumbar segments.

Spastic paraparesis and ataxia of pelvic limbs with normal thoracic limbs.
All postural reactions poorly performed in pelvic limbs.
Reflexes normal or hyperactive: flexor and patellar.
Crossed extensor reflex may occur.
Muscle tone normal or hypertonic, no atrophy.
Nociception normal or depressed from area caudal to the lesion.
Note: Lesions confined to the white matter from L4–6 or L7 may produce the same signs.

............*Caudal Cervical: Fifth Cervical to Second Thoracic Segment*

Partial malacia of gray and white matter between fifth cervical and second thoracic segments:

Tetraparesis and ataxia of all four limbs, with the thoracic limb deficit sometimes worse than that of the pelvic limb, or tetraplegia, with the patient in lateral recumbency. Lesions confined to the white matter at this level usually cause more abnormality in the pelvic limbs than the thoracic limbs.

Thoracic limbs: hyporeflexic or areflexic; normal tone or hypotonic; neurogenic atrophy if a chronic lesion. Lesions confined to the white matter at this level cause hypertonia, hyperreflexia, and no atrophy.

Pelvic limbs: normal reflexes or hyperreflexia; normal tone or hypertonia; no atrophy.

Nociception: normal or depressed from all four limbs or depressed from thoracic limbs only.

All postural reactions poorly performed with the thoracic limb function sometimes worse than that of the pelvic lamb.

Miosis, protruded third eyelid, ptosis, and enophthalmos (T1–3 lesion).

Decreased-to-absent cutaneous reflex (C8).

............Cranial Cervical: First Cervical to Fifth Cervical Segment

Partial malacia—focal site between first and fifth cervical segments:

Spastic tetraplegia with patient in lateral recumbency: (1) no postural reactions present; (2) reflexes normal or hyperactive in all four limbs; (3) crossed extensor reflexes may occur; (4) muscle tone is usually hypertonic, occasionally normal; and (5) hypalgesia from area caudal to the lesion.

Spastic tetraparesis and ataxia of all four limbs. The deficit in the pelvic limbs is often worse than that in the thoracic limbs. Occasionally, the opposite is found:

1. Postural reactions are poorly performed.
2. Reflexes are normal or hyperactive.
3. Crossed extensor reflexes may occur.
4. Muscle tone is usually hypertonic, occasionally normal.
5. Nociception is normal or depressed from area caudal to the lesion.

Dogs with cervical spinal cord disease that have a significantly worse abnormality in the forelimbs than in the hindlimbs usually have two possible locations for lesions. Extensive lesions in the cervical intumescence with gray matter involvement cause hypotonic hyporeflexic throacic limbs and a more severe thoracic limb deficit. An extramedullary lesion that compresses the central region of any segment of the cervical spinal cord from a ventral midline site has also been observed with this disparity in limb abnormality. Most commonly these are midline intervertebral disk extrusions, less commonly atlantoaxial subluxations or neoplasms. The spinal cord is "tented" over the compressing mass, which apparently interferes more with the medially situated UMNs to the cervical intumescence.

............Micturition

Bladder dysfunction often accompanies severe spinal cord disease. Total LMN paralysis occurs with sacral spinal cord lesions. Severe or total focal thoracolumbar spinal cord lesions produce a UMN type of paralysis. Paralysis is less common with cervical spinal cord lesions unless the lesions is severe. With both LMN and UMN paralysis, retention of urine occurs. Overflow takes place with both but is more constant with LMN disease. Overflow is less frequent in UMN disease, because greater intraluminal pressure is required to overcome the tone in the striated urethral muscle. If the integrity of the bladder wall is retained, reflex urination may follow within a variable period of time. Reflex urination is more efficient in UMN disease, using the intact peripheral nerves and sacral spinal cord segments. In LMN disease, reflex urination must be mediated within the wall of the bladder and is very inefficient.

..........Summary of Signs With Lesions in Specific Segments of the Brain (Tables 2-12 and 2-13)

..........Medulla and Pons

Lesions in the medulla and pons result in spastic tetraparesis and ataxia of all four limbs or tetraplegia, ipsilateral spastic hemiparesis and ataxia (unilateral lesions), central vestibular signs, depression and irregular respirations and heartbeat, and hypalgesia of the trunk and limbs.

Signs of cranial nerve deficit are as follows: facial hypalgesia or analgesia (sensory, V); paresis or paralysis of masticatory muscles (motor, V); medial strabismus (VI); facial paresis or paralysis (VII); pharyngeal paresis (IX, X); tongue paresis (XII); and loss of balance, head tilt, and abnormal nystagmus (VIII).

..........Cerebellum

With diffuse lesions, the signs are symmetric ataxia with preservation of voluntary motor activity, dysmetric gait (hypermetria), truncal ataxia, head tremor, muscle hypertonia, occasional abnormal nystagmus, and bilateral menace deficit.

With unilateral lesions, the signs are ipsilateral. The body and the head tilt toward the side of the lesion or occasional away from the side of the lesion, and there may be ipsilateral menace deficit.

With severe rostral lesions, there may be opisthotonos and rigidly extended forelimbs, and the pelvic limbs are extended forward by hip flexion.

..........Midbrain (Mesencephalon)

With lesions in this area, the following signs occur: opisthotonus with rigid extension of all limbs (decerebration); spastic tetraparesis and ataxia of all four limbs; spastic hemiparesis if the lesion is unilateral (usually contralateral); depression; stupor (semicoma) or coma; and hypalgesia of the head, trunk, and limbs. Signs of cranial nerve deficit are ventrolateral strabismus (III) and mydriasis and nonreactive pupil (III). There is deviation of the eye in certain positions of the head, and the head and neck are flexed laterally, with the nose directed toward the shoulder with severe midline or unilateral lesions in the tegmentum. Visual deficits may be observed in acute lesions.

..........Thalamus and Hypothalamus (Diencephalon)

Bilateral lesions of the diencephalon produce the following signs: slows postural reactions bilaterally, mild ataxia, bilateral visual deficit with dilated unresponsive pupils (optic tracts), and bilateral hypalgesia.

Unilateral lesions are indicated by contralateral deficient postural reactions, contralateral visual deficit with normal pupils, contralateral hypalgesia (most noticeable in the head), and the adversive syndrome—propulsive circling and head and eye deviation, usually toward the side of the lesion.

With lesions that are either bilateral or unilateral, the manifestations are depression, stupor (semicoma) or coma, behavioral changes, seizures, and hypothalamohypophysical disorders of body temperature, glucose metabolism, appetite control, autonomic nervous system, water balance, gonadal function, and thyroid and adrenal function.

Text continued on page 346

Table 2–12. Evaluation of Cranial Nerves

Nerve	Sign of Dysfunction	Test/Responses
I Olfactory	Anosmia	Observe response to smell of food or some mild volatile oils
II Optic	Visual deficit, bumping objects	No menace response—failure to close eyelids or retract head when affected eye is menaced
	Unilateral disease	Light in affected eye—no pupillary response from either eye
	Mild mydriasis in affected eye (slight anisocoria) or none	Light in either eye—no pupillary constriction
	Bilateral disease	Examine with ophthalmoscope
III Oculomotor	Marked mydriasis bilaterally	Light in affected eye—only pupil of normal eye constricts
	Marked mydriasis	Light in normal eye—only pupil of normal eye constricts
	Severe anisocoria	Incomplete adduction of affected eye on moving head side to side
	Ventrolateral strabismus	Inability to elevate upper eyelid completely
	Ptosis	
IV Trochlear	Slight extorsion of eyeball, which may be visualized in the dog only by ophthalmoscopic examination of the position of the retinal veins	
V Trigeminal	Dropped jaw; unable to close mouth if bilateral disease	
	No motor deficit if unilateral disease	
	Atrophy of muscles of mastication	
	Hypalgesia or analgesia of face	Hypalgesia can be determined by patient's lack of response to touching nasal septum with forceps

Cranial Nerve	Deficit	Test/Sign
VI Abducent	Medial strabismus	Incomplete abduction of affected eye on moving head from side to side
VII Facial	Paresis/paralysis of facial muscles—inability to close palpebral fissure, drooped hypotonic lip with drooling of saliva, inability to move ear, but the ears will not droop in all patients (cats and some prick-eared dogs); incomplete dilation of naris on inspiration	
VIII Vestibulocochlear		
Cochlear	Deafness (unilateral is difficult to determine)	Lack of response to commands or any noise
Vestibular—Unilateral disease	Head tilt and ataxic toward side of lesion—lean, fall, circle toward side of lesion	Unequal response or postrotatory testing—spin away from side of lesion causes depressed response; extend neck and eye on affected side does not elevate completely (vestibular strabismus); hold head to side or dorsally and observe for positional nystagmus
	Abnormal resting or positional nystagmus with quick phase away from side of lesion	
Vestibular—Bilateral disease	Crouched gait, stumble to either side	Inability to generate nystagmus on moving head from side to side or spinning—no postrotatory response
	No abnormal nystagmus, wide excursions of head	
IX Glossopharyngeal	Dysphagia, gagging on eating	
X Vagus	Dysphagia, gagging on eating	
	Inspiratory dyspnea	
XI Accessory	None	
XII Hypoglossal	Atrophy of affected side of tongue	
	May deviate toward affected side on protrusion	

Table 2–13. Relationship of Clinical Signs to Anatomical Site of Lesion

Clinical Signs	Functional System	Anatomical Location
Inability to prehend	Masticatory and tongue muscles	Cranial nerves V, XII, pons-medulla
Dysphagia	Tongue, palate, pharynx, esophagus	Cranial nerves IX, X, XI, XII, medulla
Drooling	Facial paralysis, dysphagia	Cranial nerve VII, middle ear, medulla
		Cranial nerves IX, X, medulla
		Inner ear, medulla, cerebellum
Head tilt	Vestibular system	
Nystagmus	Vestibular system	
Loss of balance	Vestibular system	Medulla, cerebellum (inner ear)
Rolling	Vestibular system	Cranial nerves III, IV, VI, midbrain-medulla
Strabismus	Cranial nerves to extraocular muscles, vestibular system	Inner ear, medulla, cerebellum
Circling	Vestibular system	Frontal lobe, rostral thalamus
With loss of balance	Limbic system(?)	
Without loss of balance		
Head and eye deviation—turning to one side	Limbic system(?)	Frontal lobe, rostral thalamus

Clinical Sign	System	Location
Pacing, head-pressing	Limbic system(?)	Frontal lobe, rostral thalamus
Opisthotonos	UMN	Rostral cerebellum, midbrain
Blindness	Visual system	
	Dilated, unresponsive pupils	Eye, optic nerves
	Normal pupils	Visual cortex-cerebellum (midbrain)
Depression, semiconscious, coma	Ascending reticular activating system	Pons to thalamus-cerebral cortex
Seizures	Ascending reticular activating system	Cerebrum, thalamus-hypothalamus
Hyperesthesia, hyperactivity to external stimuli	Limbic system	Thalamus, cerebrum
Aggressive behavior, mania, hysteria, odontoprisis		Thalamus, cerebrum
Tremor		
Associated with movements of head and neck	Cerebellar system	Cerebellum
Associated with movements of head, trunk, and limbs	Multiple systems	Diffuse in CNS
Episodic, not associated with movements of head, trunk, and limbs		Thalamus, cerebrum
Bradycardia, hypothermia, hyperthermia	UMN for general visceral efferent system	Hypothalamus
Irregular, ataxic respirations	UMN for respiratory muscle LMN	Pons-medulla

From deLahunta A: Veterinary Neuroanatomy and Clinical Neurology, ed 2. Philadelphia, WB Saunders, 1983.
UMN, upper motor neuron; LMN, lower motor neuron; CNS, central nervous system.

.... *Cerebrum (Telencephalon)*

Lesions in this area are evidenced by changes in several ways. Changes in behavior or temperament include depression (lethargy, obtundation); stupor (semicoma); lack of recognition of owner or environment and bewilderment; loss of trained habits; and irritable, hysterical maniacal, or aggressive behavior. In propulsion, the animal often paces and circles in one direction and turns the head and eyes in one direction; this direction is usually toward a unilateral lesion, called the *adversive syndrome* (turn to). This may require a rostral thalamic involvement in the lesion. Seizures are partial (contralateral face or limbs or both) or generalized (grand mal, psychomotor). The gait is usually normal, but contralateral postural reactions are deficient. Bilateral lesions produce blindness. Unilateral lesions produce a contralateral visual deficit with normal pupil responses to light. Occasionally, contralateral facial hypalgesia occurs. Rarely, the hypalgesia is observed in the contralateral trunk and limbs. Acute diffuse lesions may produce bilateral miosis. Pseudobulbar paresis rarely may be observed on voluntary movement: contralateral lower facial paresis (lip and nose), pharyngeal paresis, and tongue paresis (see Tables 2–12 and 2–13).

REFERENCES

Berry WL: Episodic weakness in dogs. Compend Cont Educ Pract Vet 12:141–154, 1990.
deLahunta A: Veterinary Clinical Neuroanatomy, ed 2. Philadelphia, WB Saunders, 1986.
Ettinger SJ, Feldman EC, eds: Textbook of Veterinary Internal Medicine, ed 4. Philadelphia, WB Saunders, 1995.
Fenner WR: The neurologic evaluation of patients. *In* Ettinger SJ, ed: Textbook of Veterinary Internal Medicine. Philadelphia, WB Saunders, 1989, pp 549–577.
Meric SM: Canine meningitis. J Vet Intern Med 2:26–35, 1988.
Meric SM: The neurologic examination. *In* Nelson RW, Cuoto CG, eds: Essentials of Small Animal Internal Medicine. St Louis, Mosby–Year Book, 1992, pp 725–731.
Oliver LM: Handbook of Veterinary Neurology, ed 2. Philadelphia, WB Saunders, 1993.

Musculosketal System

.... ORTHOPEDIC EXAMINATION

Examination of the musculoskeletal system involves methods similar to those used in any other organ system by requiring the clinician to obtain a history, perform a physical examination, and order ancillary tests.

Consideration of the patient's body size, breed, age, lameness severity, onset, clinical course, and sometimes sex often provides important insights into the examination (Table 2–14). Certain body sizes and specific breeds are more at risk for particular orthopedic conditions. For example, large, rapidly growing dogs seem to be predisposed to conditions such as osteochondrosis dissecans of the shoulder, elbow, stifle, and tarsal joints and disorders of osteochondrosis in general. Hip dysplasias, fragmented coronoid processes, an ununited anconeal process, and bone tumors are further examples of syndromes seen in larger dogs, whereas small, miniature, and toy breeds are predisposed to conditions such as Legg-Calvé-Perthes disease and medial patella luxation.

Age can determine what conditions are considered likely for diagnosis on the examination. Immature dogs will have a certain differential diagnosis, while mature dogs, over 1 year old, will have others. For example, a grade II forelimb lameness of insidious onset and progressive course may indicate osteochondritis dissecans of the shoulder, whereas the clinician would not initially consider this condition in a mature dog of the same breed with the same history.

···········Lameness

The presenting complaint requiring an orthopedic examination is usually lameness, which can be acute or of chronic insidious onset. Acute onset of lameness is often characteristic of traumatic disorders and infections. Chronic insidious lameness is characteristic of degenerative abnormalities and immune-mediated arthropathies. Some lameness can present insidiously and with cyclic or shifting limb signs. Examples are panosteitis, infectious polyarthritis, and immune-mediated arthropathies or myopathies. Knowing the progression of clinical signs and whether there has been any response to medications provides the clinician with an understanding into diagnosis. For example, several immune-mediated lamenesses will not respond well to aspirin or other nonsteroidal anti-inflammatory drugs (NSAIDs); however, many of the degenerative arthropathies will respond to these medications. The course of the lameness can provide clues. For example, an animal exhibiting grade I lameness for a prolonged time due to medial patella luxation may acutely develop a grade III lameness. This often is the result of acute loss of stability provided by the cruciate ligament. The grade of lameness does not necessarily correspond with the severity of the orthpedic problem but the grade can sometimes give clues to the problem.

However, the clinician needs to be careful as these lameness grades can change during the course of a disease process. Dogs with cruciate syndrome may show grade I or II lameness during early stages of partial tearing and degeneration only to exhibit grade III or IV lameness when a major portion of the ligament acutely tears. Intermittent or episodic non–weight-bearing lameness may be noted in dogs having patellar instability or nerve root disease. The former becomes non–weight-bearing while running; the latter tends to lift the limb off the floor when standing (Table 2–15).

Often it must be determined whether the lameness is due to an orthopedic or neurologic problem. A cursory examination of the spinal column and assessment of the neurologic status of the affected limb should precede orthopedic examination of the extremity. However, one must be careful when performing the neurologic evaluation. Several common orthopedic problems, such as bilateral hip or stifle abnormalities, can appear as neurologic conditions. Animals with these problems can be reluctant to bear full weight on either limb. However, the clinician can be misled by a cursory assessment of the neurologic status when evaluating proprioceptive deficits using the knuckling test. This is because when performing the knuckling test the animal is reluctant to shift the weight to the contralateral limb to instantaneously correct the paw and continues to bear weight on the dorsum of the overturned digits. The following are guidelines that suggest neurologic lameness to help in the differentiation from orthopedic conditions:

- Limb appears weak, movement awkward or uncoordinated
- Segmental reflex abnormalities
- Sensory status abnormalities of paw
- Willing to bear significant weight on the overturned paw with the knuckling test
- Shuffling gaits or movements that are uncoordinated and allow the limb to cross over the midline into the path of the opposite limb
- Audible sound as the digits scuff the floor

···········Physical Examination

Sometimes the most difficult aspect of the orthopedic examination is determining which limb is lame, a problem with grade I lameness. As a guide the presence of a "head bob" is suggestive of lameness. The head and neck move

Table 2–14. History and Signalment

Condition	Size Predisposition Dog Small	Medium	Large	Giant	Cat	Breed	Sex	Lameness Grade	Age at Onset	Onset	Course
Hip dysplasia	+	2+	3+	3+	+	Several		II	I, M	Slow	Wax and wane, progressive, frequently bilateral
Cruciate syndrome	2+	2+	3+	2+	+	Rottweiler, Labrador, Newfoundland, Staffordshire terrier	♂c, ♀s	Any	M	Any	Wax and wane, progressive, frequently bilateral
Medial patella luxation	3+	2+	+	+	+	Toy breed	♀	I, II, III	I, M	Slow	Intermittent, progressive, frequently bilateral
Lateral patella luxation	+	+	2+	3+	+	Flat-coated retriever, Great Dane, Saint Bernard, Irish wolfhound		I, II, III	I, M	Slow	Intermittent, progressive, frequently bilateral
Bicipital tenosynovitis	+	+	2+	+				I, II	M	Slow	Intermittent, progressive, sometimes bilateral

Condition						Breed	Sex		Age	Onset	Clinical course
Mineralization of supraspinatus tendon	+	+	2 +			Rottweiler, Labrador		I, II	M	Slow	Intermittent, progressive, sometimes bilateral
Neoplasia	+	+	3 +	3 +				II, III	M	Slow	Progressive
Panosteitis	+	3 +	3 +	+	+	German shepherd	♂	II	I, M	Rapid	Variable, self-limiting, multiple limbs
Osteochondrosis	+	2 +	3 +	3 +		Rottweiler, Labrador, German shepherd, Great Dane	♂	II	I	Slow	Wax and wane, progressive, frequently bilateral
Legg-Calvé-Perthes disease	3 +					Terrier, toy breed		II	I	Slow	Progressive, sometimes bilateral
Fragmented coronoid process		+	3 +	2 +		Rottweiler, Labrador, golden retriever, German shepherd, Newfoundland, chow, Bernese mountain dog	♂	I, II	I, M	Slow	Wax and wane, progressive
Ununited anconeal process	2 +	3 +	+			German shepherd, basset, English bulldog	♂	II, III	I	Slow	Wax and wane progressive
Hypertrophic osteodystrophy		+	3 +	3 +				III	I	Rapid	Variable, self-limiting, multiple limbs, painful, anorectic, febrile

3 +, frequent; 2 +, sometimes; +, seldom; I, immature; M, mature; ♂c, male castrate; ♀s, female spayed; ♂, male; ♀, female.

Modified from Schrader SC, Prieur WD, Bruse S: Diagnosis: Historical, physical, and ancillary examinations. *In* Olmstead ML, ed: Small Animal Orthopedics. St Louis, Mosby–Year Book, 1995.

Table 2–15. Lameness Severity

Grade	Clinical Signs
I: Hardly perceptible lameness	Minor trauma
	Biceps brachii tenosynovitis or supraspinatus tendon calcification
	Traumatic injury of the iliopsoas muscle
	Hip dysplasia
	Early cruciate ligament disease
II: Noticeable weight-bearing lameness:	Degenerative joint disease
	Immune-mediated arthropathies
	Infraspinatus contracture
	Panosteitis
	Legg-Calvé-Perthes disease
	Fragmented coronoid process
	Ununited anconeal process
	Osteochondritis dissecans of shoulder, elbow, stifle, and tarsus
	Patella luxation
	Moderately early cruciate ligament disease
III: Severe lameness with only toe touching for balance	Hypertrophic osteodystrophy
	Infections
	Neoplasia
	Advanced patella luxation or cruciate ligament disease
IV: No weight-bearing; the limb is carried	Fracture
	Luxation
	Foreign body or laceration of paw
	Nerve root disease

Modified from Chambers JN: Lameness. *In* Lorenz MD, Cornelius LM, eds: Small Animal Medical Diagnosis, ed 2. Philadelphia, JB Lippincott, 1993.

upward as the problematic forelimb touches the floor, and downward when the affected rearlimb touches down. This action helps to reduce the load carried by the limb. The stride is shortened on the affected side; the animal will offload the abnormal limb more quickly than the normal one. Less time is spent on the abnormal limb. Audible clicks are sometimes heard in young dogs with hip dysplasia or in dogs that have a meniscus abnormality secondary to rupture of the cranial cruciate ligament.

..........Palpation and Manipulation

It is best to first examine the lame limb without sedation, if possible, to determine the source of discomfort or instability. The limb is palpated and manipulated from the toes proximally. The patient is turned and the procedure repeated on the other side as the contralateral limb can often serve as a normal control when bilateral conditions are not present. An equivocal asymmetric finding requires repeating the examination as many times as necessary to confirm or rule out its presence. Lastly, the animal is walked again, because a subtle lameness is often exacerbated by the manipulation. The following should be looked for when palpating, manipulating, and observing the orthopedic patient:

- Cardinal signs of inflammation (pain, swelling, heat, redness, and loss of function)

- Muscle atrophy, muscle tremors, the most severe atrophy localized to the muscle group primarily responsible for moving the painful part
- Laxity, effusion, crepitation, localized temperature increase, abnormal joint motion, and stability
- Range of motion of joint(s) different from contralateral side
- Normal to carrying 60% of weight on the fore limbs
- Body weight shifted to unaffected limb
- Digits of normal limb spread further apart than the digits of the affected limb
- Back arches dorsally as weight is shifted to fore- or hindlimbs
- Hindlimb stance wide-based and a bowlegged appearance when weight is shifted to the hindlimbs
- Nails of affected limb longer than those of the contralateral limb; nails that are excessively short when the limb is not lifted high enough to avoid scuffing
- Hairless areas over joints caused by constant licking or chewing
- Conformational difference among breeds: rottweiler, chow, and Akita tending to have a very straight or erect hindlimb stance; German shepherds assuming a more crouched posture

...........Specific Palpation

Often the goal of palpation is only to localize the specific site giving the animal discomfort or pain. Putting together the location of pain with the other known information will frequently lead to a diagnosis. For example, pain on palpation of the elbow joint in an immature German shepherd should lead the clinician to think of an ununited anconeal process rather than fragmentation of the medial coronoid process of the ulna. Fragmentation of the medial coronoid process is more frequently seen in retrievers, rottweilers, basset hounds, and Bernese moumtain dogs than in German shepherds. The following guidelines are kept in mind when palpating specific areas of the body:

- Digits need to be examined for lacerations, foreign bodies, ingrown nails, or burns, especially with grade III and IV lameness.
- Bite wounds of the limbs are the most common source of lameness in cats.
- In toy and miniature breeds, medial patella luxation results in a toe-in and bowlegged (genu varum) posture. Chronic cases are frequently complicated by rupture of the cranial cruciate ligament due to chronic instability of the stifle. This rupture may lead to an acute-onset presentation following a relatively chronic problem.
- Multiple subluxated joints are often associated with immune-mediated joint disease.
- Abnormal enlargements in diameter of long bones, especially in the metaphyseal regions, may indicate a developmental bone disease such as hypertrophic osteodystrophy or primary bone neoplasia.
- Palpation of the diaphyses of multiple long bones may produce pain in cases of neoplasia, fractures, infection, and panosteitis.
- Pain on palpation of the shoulder with peracute onset of lameness in a large athletic dog may be the result of bicipital tenosynovitis, mineralization of the supraspinatus tendon, or avulsion of the supraglenoid tubercle.
- Pain, lameness, fever, and anorexia are frequently associated with hypertrophic osteodystrophy in large rapidly growing breeds.
- Traumatic injury of the iliopsoas muscle may have a clinical presentation similar to hip dysplasia.

The cruciate syndrome in dogs can have a varied clinical presentation. Onset can be acute or chronically insidious. Any lameness grade is possible; however, grade II progressing to grade III lameness in middle-aged neutered obese dogs is very common. Palpation for the cranial drawer test can reveal obvious laxity, but subtle laxity is common with early or late disease. Early, the ligament is degenerating but mostly intact, while late, the ligament is severely degenerated and torn, but there is much fibrosis of the joint preventing gross laxity. Thus, frequently examination of the stifle joint for cruciate syndrome requires either sedation or general anesthesia to appreciate the subtleties. Palpation signs for cruciate ligament disease are a subtle or grossly positive cranial drawer test, increased internal rotation of the tibia on the femur, and medial joint thickening. When palpating for the cranial drawer, position the stifle in different flexion and extension angles while performing the maneuver. The normal joint will give an abrupt endpoint "thud" to the maneuver, as the ligament normally stretches. Minimal cranial translation of the tibia on the femur but with a soft "gushy" feel may indicate early degeneration and partial tearing or advanced degeneration and major tearing with fibrosis.

Clinical signs of hip dysplasia include lameness, gait abnormalities, reluctance to exercise, and pelvic limb muscle atrophy. Specific maneuvers, including Barlow's, Ortolani's, and Barden's signs, are useful to evaluate the degree of joint laxity, both when screening young puppies and in performing diagnostics in clinically lame dogs. None of the signs are definitive tests for hip dysplasia, but should be performed as sequential maneuvers in the examination. Pelvic radiography is mandatory to definitive diagnosis of hip dysplasia but should not be the first step in the examination, because other diagnoses or concurrent conditions may be missed.

···········Radiographs

Along with the history and physical examination, radiographs play an important part of the examination of the orthopedic patient. Mostly the two standard views, craniocaudal and lateromedial, are sufficient to define the problem. Proper technique is very important when obtaining radiographs, as it is easy to miss lesions when technique is less than adequate. Less frequently, oblique views or "stress views" are needed to help define the situation. Rarely, special imaging techniques such as tomography, bone scans, and arthrograms are needed. A common error made in veterinary medicine is to use the radiograph as a predictor of the severity of a problem and let it dictate clinical treatment or prognosis. For example, osteochondrosis dissecans of the shoulder joint in the dog may be demonstrated on the radiograph, but surgical exploration is not warranted unless lameness develops. It is difficult and often misleading to predict the severity of degenerative joint disease from radiographs alone; noncartilaginous changes, such as osteophytes, are what can be seen on radiographs. Conversely, inflammatory joint disease, when nonerosive, can be very severe and there will be minimal or no radiographic changes noted. The following are guidelines to be considered when using radiographs as part of the orthopedic examination.

- Radiograph the opposite limb whenever necessary to clarify suspected lesions.
- Consider stress views when suspecting collateral ligament damage to the stifle, elbow, carpus, and tarsus.
- Radiograph both shoulders when considering osteochondrosis dissecans, bicipital tenosynovitis, and mineralization of the supraspinatus tendon.
- Radiograph both elbows when considering elbow dysplasias.
- Radiograph both elbows for dysplasias when considering osteochondrosis of the shoulders and, likewise, both shoulders when diagnosing elbow dysplasias.
- Radiograph both stifles when considering cruciate ligament disease.

- Radiograph both hips when considering hip dysplasia or hip degeneration.
- Radiograph both hips when considering cruciate ligament disease.
- Radiograph hips, with or without mechanical aids, while viewing luxation or reduction angles with the animal positioned in dorsal recumbency. This can be used to help determine predisposition to hip dysplasia at a young age.

...........Other Diagnostic Aids

Besides radiographs, there are other diagnostic aids used with the orthopedic examination. Arthrocentesis and joint fluid analysis is a common diagnostic aid (Table 2–16). Other tests include arthroscopy, rheumatoid factor testing, antinuclear antibody testing, *Borrelia burgdorferi* testing, synovial membrane examinations, and other serologic tests and measurement of immune complexes.

REFERENCES

Chambers JN: Lameness. *In* Lorenz MD, Cornelius LM, eds: Small Animal Medical Diagnosis, ed 2. Philadelphia, JB Lippincott, 1993, p 389.
Schrader SC, Prieur WD, Bruse S: Diagnosis: Historical, physical, and ancillary examinations. *In* Olmstead ML, ed: Small Animal Orthopedics. St Louis, Mosby–Year Book, 1995, p 3.
Toombs JP, Widmer WR: Bone, joint, and periskeletal swelling or enlargement. *In* Lorenz MD, Cornelius LM, eds: Small Animal Medical Diagnosis, ed 2. Philadelphia, JB Lippincott, 1993, p 397.
Trotter EJ: Orthopedic examination. *In* Bistner BS, Ford RB, eds: Handbook of Veterinary Procedures and Emergency Treatment, ed 6. Philadelphia, WB Saunders, 1995, p 351.
Wilkins RJ; Joint serology. *In* Bojrab MJ, ed: Disease Mechanisms in Small Animal Surgery. Philadelphia, Lea & Febiger, 1993, p 705.

Respiratory System

When evaluating an animal with respiratory disease, it is important to (1) *observe* the animal while listening to the *history*; (2) examine the *whole animal*; and (3) *palpate, percuss*, and *auscultate* the thorax and neck. The completeness of the evaluation is tentative, depending on the animal's condition (Table 2–17).

...........OBSERVATION

Before the animal is disturbed, determine its respiratory rate and pattern. Normally, the dog breathes 10 to 30 times per minute (when not panting) and the cat breathes 20 to 60 times per minute. An increase in the respiratory rate (tachypnea) does not always mean that a respiratory disease is present. An increased respiratory rate may be caused by excitement, heat, exercise, pain, shock, or anemia. A decreased respiratory rate may result from narcotic poisoning or metabolic alkalosis. An animal may have dyspnea and respiratory disease with a normal respiratory rate. The pattern or rhythm of breathing can help categorize disease.

Labored breathing or dyspnea can be slow, deep, and deliberate, or it can be rapid and shallow. The dyspneic animal may assume a characteristic posture in a squatting position with abducted elbows. The dyspnea may be principally inspiratory, expiratory, or both. Inspiratory dyspnea is seen as difficulty in expanding the lungs with a relatively easy expiratory effort. Inspiratory dyspnea is observed most frequently in diseases that are restrictive. These diseases include those that restrict expansion of the lung because of disease of the pleura, chest wall, or neuromuscular apparatus or diseases with infiltrate

Text continued on page 358

Table 2–16. Joint Fluid Analysis

	Normal	Degenerative	Hemarthrosis	Rheumatoid	Lupus Erythematosus (LE)	Neoplastic	Aseptic	Septic
Color	None or straw-colored	Pale yellow	Red	Yellow to blood-tinged	Yellow to blood-tinged	Yellow to blood-tinged	Yellow to blood-tinged	Yellow to sanguineous
Turbidity	Clear	Clear to slight	Blood-tinged	Slight to moderate	Slight to moderate	Slight to moderate	Slight to moderate	Turbid to purulent
Viscosity	Normal	Normal	Reduced	Reduced	Reduced	Reduced	Reduced	Reduced
Mucin clot	Good	Good	Fair	Poor	Fair	Good	Fair	Poor
Red blood cells	Rare	Few	Many	Few to moderate	Few to moderate	Few to moderate	Few to moderate	Moderate
White blood cells	0.1–2.0×10^3 μL	Few	Moderate	Marked	Marked	Moderate	Moderate to marked	Marked
Neutrophils	1%–10%	Few	Moderate	Many	Many	Moderate	Moderate	Many
Lymphocytes	50%–60%	Moderate	Few	Few	Few to moderate	Few	Few to moderate	Few
Macrophages	Rare	Moderate	Few	Few	Few to moderate	Moderate	Moderate	Few

Synovial cells	Moderate	Moderate to many	Rare	Few	Few	Moderate	Few to moderate	Few
Synovial glucose–blood glucose ratio	0.8:1.0	0.8:1.0	1.0	0.5:0.8	0.5:0.8	0.5:0.8	0.5:0.8	<0.5
Other	Rare neutrophils and red blood cells unless blood contamination			Phagocytes	LE cells	Neoplastic cells		Toxic changes to cells, micro-organisms
Causes		Conformation, age, osteochondrosis	Trauma, bleeding disorder	Rheumatoid arthritis	Lupus	Synovial, periosteal bone, connective tissue	Trauma, local inflammation, immune-mediated, Lyme disease, viral, rickettsiael, mycoplasmas	Hematogenous, wounds

Modified from Wilkins RJ: Joint serology. In Bojrab MJ, ed: Disease Mechanisms in Small Animal Surgery. Philadelphia, Lea & Febiger, 1993.

Table 2-17. Approach to the Patient With Respiratory Distress

Emergency!	Potential Emergency	Nonemergency

1. Treat and observe
   Oxygen delivery choices
     Intubate
     Mask
     Cage
     Intranasal
     Intratracheal
   Mucous membrane color
     Cyanosis obvious
     Cyanosis not detected
   Obvious evidence of injury
   Apparent history—e.g. trauma
   Noises heard
     Stridor
     Wheezing
     Silent
   Respiratory pattern
     Open mouth
     Tachypneic
     Dyspneic
     Forced inspiration
     Forced expiration
     Weak or frantic
2. Auscultate, percuss, palpate
3. Differential diagnosis
   Upper airway:
     Brachycephalic syndrome
	1. Examine respiratory system and treat with oxygen by mask if tolerated
	2. Draw conclusions from examination and then treat accordingly
	             or
	3. If animal can tolerate radiographs, take them
	4. Differential diagnosis
	   All listed under Emergency; apply and add the following:
	     Lower airway
	       Aspiration pneumonia
	     Pleural disease
	       Pleural effusion
	       Cardiac
	       Hemorrhage
	       Pyothorax
	     Other
	       Neuromuscular weakness
	       Anemia
	5. Therapeutic choices as under Emergency
		1. Do complete examination
		2. Cases range from an acute problem that is not life-threatening to a chronic problem
		3. Other possible tests after history and physical examination:
		     Radiographs
		     Tracheobronchial washing
		     Bronchoscopy
		     Support laboratory data (e.g., ECG, CBC, titers)
		     Lung biopsy
		4. Differential diagnosis for dyspnea and coughing
		5. Therapy based on diagnosis

Laryngeal edema, paralysis, collapse, spasm
Obstruction (intraluminal or extraluminal)
Rupture of airway
Lower airway
  Asthma-like syndrome
  Acute pulmonary edema
  Pulmonary embolism
  Pulmonary hemorrhage and contusion
  Aspiration (e.g., drowning or near drowning)
Pleural disease
  Pneumothorax
  Diaphragmatic hernia
Other
  CNS injury or paralysis
  Shock
  Heat stroke
4. Possible choices of therapy in addition to oxygen and minimizing stress:
  Bronchodilators
  Thoracocentesis
  Corticosteroids
  Diuretics
  Tracheostomy
  Positive-pressure ventilation
  General anesthesia for therapeutic reasons (e.g., remove foreign body from trachea)
  Fluids or blood
5. Radiograph if possible or indicated to confirm diagnosis

ECG, electrocardiogram; CBC, complete blood count; CNS, central nervous system.

within the lung parenchyma that displace alveolar air. Restrictive diseases are characterized by a reduced vital capacity and a small resting lung volume without an increase in airway resistance relative to lung volume. Elastic recoil is increased, and air is exhaled rapidly. The lung's compliance is decreased. Examples of restrictive pulmonary disorders are pneumothorax, pleural effusions, or diffusely infiltrating diseases such as pneumonias or neoplasia. Inspiratory dyspnea is also observed with upper airway obstructions such as laryngeal paralysis.

Expiratory dyspnea is seen as difficulty in expelling air from the lungs. Normally, expiratory time is shorter than inspiratory time. Expiratory dyspnea is observed most frequently in obstructive lung disease. Airway obstruction due to increased resistance to air flow can be caused by conditions inside the lumen, in the bronchial wall, or in the surrounding bronchial region. A combination of these problems can exist in disease. An airway lumen may be compromised by bronchiectasis, severe pulmonary edema, or aspiration of fluid. Contraction of bronchial smooth muscle (which occurs in bronchial asthma), hypertrophy of mucous glands, or inflammation and edema of the airway wall can cause obstruction. Obstruction outside an airway can be caused by destruction of lung parenchyma that results in loss of radial traction and narrowing, as in emphysema. Narrowing can also be caused by peribronchial edema. With obstructive disease, air can usually get into the lungs, and lung volumes are normal or even elevated. With partial airway obstruction, inspiratory forces open the airway to allow air to enter the lung, but because of dynamic compression, expiratory forces can cause collapse of the airway. Dynamic compression is the narrowing of the airways that occurs during expiration due to increases in intrathoracic pressure and is a normal phenomenon that is exaggerated in situations of increased airway resistance and low lung volume. Inspiratory dyspnea and expiratory dyspnea may be observed together in various diseases, depending on the pulmonary changes present. Frequently, pulmonary edema is characterized by both types of dyspnea.

When a dog or cat is dyspneic, the respiratory pattern is one that makes the work of breathing easiest with the least expenditure of energy. With reduced compliance or stiff lungs due to parenchyma or pleural disease, an animal will tend to take small, rapid breaths, whereas an animal with airway obstruction will take deeper, slower breaths. These patterns reflect the altered forces (elastic, viscous resistance) that must be overcome in the breathing process. The cost of an increase in the work of breathing (oxygen consumed) will alter the ability of the animal to exercise.

Cyanosis is the appearance of a bluish tinge to the skin as a result of excess deoxyhemoglobin. For cyanosis to be observed readily, 5 g of deoxygenated hemoglobin must be present; therefore, marked hypoxemia may be present but not appreciated by observation of mucous membranes.

·············HISTORY

The cardinal signs of respiratory disease are cough, dyspnea, production of abnormal secretions, noisy breathing, sneezing, and change in the characteristics of the sounds the animal makes. Animals with pulmonary disease may not be presented with clinical signs that direct attention to the pulmonary system. Determine the presence or absence of:

1. *Nasal discharge.* The discharge may be unilateral or bilateral. Determine the character (bloody, yellow, clear) and duration (acute, chronic) of the discharge.
2. *Sneezing.* Note the frequency and accompanying discharge, if any.
3. *Coughing* (see p. 392). A *true cough* (sudden forced expulsion of air through a closed glottis) is characterized by the animal lowering its head and opening

its mouth during expiration. The cough itself may be moist and productive, or dry, nonproductive, and paroxysmal, and can be accentuated by collar pressure, exercise, or cold air. It should be noted whether the cough is productive or nonproductive. *Caution*: Most dogs swallow their coughed-up secretions, so the cough may appear to be nonproductive. Examine the coughed-up material for amount, color, consistency, cell content, foreign bodies, parasites, and so on. Hemoptysis is rare but many indicate tumor or *Paragonimus* or heartworm infestations.

4. *"Reverse sneeze or cough"*. This is characterized by the animal extending its head parallel to the ground and closing its mouth during inspiration. The episode commonly ends with the animal gagging, gulping, choking, or expectorating.

5. *Dyspnea*. Questions to the owner should help determine when the animal has difficulty (e.g., at rest, after exercise) and how severe the dyspnea is (e.g., open-mouth breathing, cyanosis).

6. *Noisy breathing*. Abnormal breathing sounds may be generated from the upper or lower airway. The owner should be questioned about the perceived origin of the abnormal sounds. In general, a noisy airway is an obstructed airway.

............HELPFUL ANATOMICAL LANDMARKS

Diaphragm The diaphragm attaches dorsocaudally at the 13th rib and is slanted forward to attach anteroventrally at the costal cartilage of the 8th, 9th, and 10th ribs. It bells forward as far as the 6th rib, a quarter of the way up from the sternum. In normal respiration, the diaphragm moves 1½ vertebral spaces forward and back.

Lungs Both lungs extend anterior to the first rib. The right lung consists of cranial, middle, caudal, and accessory lobes. A cardiac notch is situated low on the right hemithorax at ribs 4 and 5. The left lung consists of the cranial and caudal lobes. The cranial lobe has a cranial and a middle portion (Figs. 2–26 and 2–27).

Tracheal Bifurcation The bifurcation is situated dorsal to the cranial border of the heart at the fifth rib.

............PALPATION

Palpate bones of the maxillary and frontal sinus for any indication of fractures, swelling, or pain. Palpate the trachea for deformities and to induce coughing. Regional lymph nodes in the neck should be palpated. Palpate the thorax for rib or sternal deformities (e.g., pectus excavatum, masses). Gently compress the anterior thorax of cats to identify a large mediastinal mass.

............PERCUSSION

In addition to examination of the thoracic cavity, percussion of the maxillary bones and sinuses and frontal sinuses can be done, listening for changes in resonance.

............Methods

Place the middle finger of the left hand firmly on the chest and use it as a pleximeter. Rap the distal phalanx abruptly with the middle finger of the right hand. Three rules must be applied in percussion:

1. In defining boundaries, always move from the more resonant to the less resonant areas.

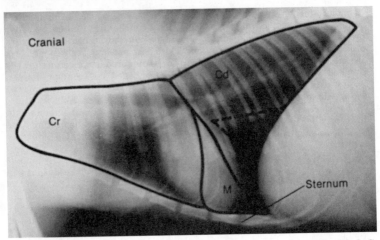

Figure 2–26. Lateral radiograph of a normal cat with lung lobes identified. Cr, right and left cranial lung lobes; M, right middle lung lobe; Cd, right and left caudal lung lobes.

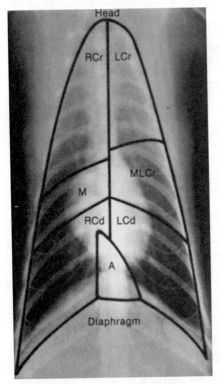

Figure 2–27. Dorsoventral radiograph of a normal cat with lung lobes identified. RCr, right cranial lung lobe; M, right middle lung lobe; RCd, right caudal lung lobe; A, accessory lung lobe; LCr, cranial portion of the left cranial lung lobe; MLCr, middle portion of the left cranial lung lobe; LCd, left caudal lung lobe.

2. The long axis of the pleximeter (finger) must be parallel to the boundary of the edges of the organ being percussed.

3. The progression of the line of percussion should be at right angles to the edge of the organ.

Application and interpretation of percussion are more difficult in small animals than in large animals. Differences in sound are slight, and it is helpful to percuss the throax systemically by tapping the ribs while a stethoscope is held firmly against the opposite chest wall. The percussion tones are thus greatly magnified by the instrument and differences are more obvious.

............Interpretation (see Table 2–6 on p. 309)

Chest radiographs are accurate in outlining anatomical structures, but changes in resonance offer additional helpful information.

Resonance is increased when the pleural cavity contains air and the lung is collapsed. In this case, the musical "bell sound" may also be heard. A coin is held flat aganist the chest wall and firmly tapped by a second coin. The observer listens to the transmitted sound through a stethoscope held against the opposite thoracic wall. Resonance may also be increased by emphysema (rare).

Resonance is decreased when the lung is more solid than usual, as with edema, pneumonia, or tumor; when the pleura is thickened; when the pleural cavity contains fluid; or when an abdominal viscus is displaced into the thoracic space.

............AUSCULTATION
............The Stethoscope

Some stethoscopes are better designed acoustically than others. The bell transmits low-pitched sounds, and the diaphragm transmits soft, high-pitched sounds best. For best results:

1. Be sure the stethoscope is seated firmly in the ear.
2. Perform the auscultation in a room as free of noise as possible.
3. Hold the stethoscope firmly against the chest.
4. Do not breathe on the tubing.
5. Avoid hair friction and muscle noises. Wetting the subject's hair is helpful.
6. Listen with the animal breathing quietly, if possible.
7. Close the mouth of a panting animal; stop the subject from shivering or trembling.
8. Stop cats from purring. Shake them gently, bring a dog into their view, or turn on a water faucet.
9. Concentrate on each part of the respiratory or cardiac cycle separately. Listen intently!

............Character of Respiratory Sounds

The terminology used in describing normal and abnormal lung sounds is still debated and still changing. Auscultation of the lung sounds is dependent not only on the actual intensity of the sounds but also on the reflection and transmission of the sounds of the stethoscope. Normal breath sounds are usually louder in the cat, kitten, and puppy than in the dog because the transmission of the sounds to the chest wall is greater. Previously, the sounds produced in the smaller airways were termed "vesicular" and the sounds generated in the larger airways were termed "bronchial," and a combination of these sounds was termed "bronchovesicular." The term "breath sounds" is probably more appropriate, although the other terms are still used. Increased breath sounds may be heard with increased ventilation, which may or may not reflect lung disease. Breath sounds may be decreased in intensity with conditions that decrease transmission, such as pleural effusion, pneumothorax, or chest wall thickness. With pleural fluid, the breath sounds are quiet ventrally but loud dorsally. With emphysema or complete airway obstruction, the lungs are too quiet.

Adventitial sounds are sounds that are added to the breath sounds. Crackles and wheezes are the terms used to describe these additional sounds. Crackles are discontinuous or interrupted sounds that sound like the crackling noise of a fire or the sound made when hair is rubbed between the fingers near the ear. Coarse or loud crackles are heard when the airways contain exudate or fluid. Fine crackles are heard when equalization of pressure occurs between airways following the reopening of collapsed airways. Late inspiratory crackles are heard in restrictive lung diseases such as pulmonary edema. With restrictive lung diseases, the lung volume is reduced and many airways are collapsed, and the opening of such airways produces crackles. Continuous, musical sounds that are high-pitched, sibilant, or squeaky are called wheezes. Wheezing can occur during inspiration (laryngeal paralysis) or expiration (obstructive bronchial disease). It is important to realize that the absence of abnormal lung sounds does not guarantee that the lungs are normal.

..........DIAGNOSTIC TESTS FOR ANIMALS WITH RESPIRATORY DISEASE

..........Nasal Disease

Animals with signs of nasal disease are evaluated by nasal radiography, rhinoscopy, and nasal biopsy. Computed tomography (CT) is helpful in difficult cases. Exploratory rhinotomy and turbinectomcy is considered if a diagnosis cannot be obtained less invasively. Tests for specific differential diagnosis include nasal exudate cytologic examination for cryptococcosis, cryptococcal antigen test (serum), aspergillus culture, and aspergillus antibody titers.

..........Laryngeal and Tracheal Disease

Lateral radiographs of the neck may be helpful in identifying metallic foreign bodies (e.g., sewing needles), masses, and tracheal collapse (neck films exposed during inspiration). Laryngoscopy is usually indicated. Laryngeal motion is observed under light anesthesia using a regimen that maintains laryngeal motion (e.g., minimal administration of a short-acting barbiturate or ketamine and diazepam). Following assessment of motion, deeper anesthesia is induced and the larynx, caudal nasopharynx, and proximal trachea are examined using a laryngoscope. When available, fiberoptic endoscopes are helpful. Grossly abnormal tissue is biopsied for histologic examination.

..........Pulmonary Disease

..........*Radiographic Study*

For evaluation of an animal with pulmonary disease, the most important initial diagnostic test is the thoracic radiograph. Two views, lateral and dorsoventral or ventrodorsal projections, are needed for best evaluation. Recognition of the different abnormal patterns (alveolar, vascular, interstitial, bronchial) and distribution (diffuse, focal, localized) and lung lobe involvement is vital for correct interpretation. Abnormalities commonly presented for emergency care for which the radiograph is paramount for correct diagnosis include pneumothorax, pleural effusions, diaphragmatic hernia, pulmonary edema, lower airway obstruction, lung contusions, and tracheal foreign body.

.... Tracheal Wash (see p. 499)

Cytologic and microbiologic evaluation of pulmonary specimens is extremely helpful for the diagnosis and management of the majority of animals with lung disease. Tracheal wash is minimally invasive and is recommended for most patients. Results are particularly helpful in animals with signs of airway or alveolar involvement. Further diagnostic testing or treatment is generally based on the combined results of history, physical examination, thoracic radiography, and tracheal wash evaluation.

.... Arterial Blood Gases (see p. 591)

Arterial blood gases can be measured at most laboratories and human hospitals, making them accessible to nearly all veterinarians. Blood gas measurement is useful for identifying pulmonary dysfunction, differentiating hypoventilation from ventilation-perfusion abnormalities, determining appropriate emergency management of animals in distress, and monitoring both short- and long-term response to therapy.

.... Bronchoscopy

Bronchoscopic examination of the airways is useful for the identification of structural abnormalities such as airway collapse, masses, foreign bodies, lung lobe torsions, parasitic nodules, and strictures. It also allows the collection of visually guided specimens from the airways or deep lung through bronchial brushings, bronchial and transbronchial biopsy, and bronchoalveolar lavage. Specimens can be collected for cytologic, histologic, or microbiologic examination. General anesthesia is required.

.... Transthoracic Lung Aspirates (see p. 499)

Mass lesions adjacent to the chest wall can readily be sampled by transthoracic lung aspiration. Specimens can also be obtained for cytologic analysis from animals with diffuse interstitial lung disease, if a diagnosis is not possible by less invasive means. Risks include pneumothorax, hemothorax, and pulmonary hemorrhage.

.... EXPLORATORY THORACOTOMY

This procedure should be carried out if required. A diagnosis can be confirmed, and in many cases (hernia, cyst, tumor, laceration of the lung, foreign body) therapy can be provided in one step.

.... Tests for Specific Diseases

Specific tests that may be considered in evaluating patients with lung disease include microfilarial examination, occult heartworm test, fecal examinations for pulmonary parasites, serology for infectious diseases (e.g., blastomycosis, histoplasmosis, toxoplasmosis), and angiography or nuclear scans for pulmonary thromboembolism.

.... PLEURAL DISEASE

.... Thoracocentesis

Cytologic evaluation of pleural fluid is indicated in all patients with effusion. The specimen should be collected prior to the administration of systemic therapy (e.g., antibiotics or steroids). Protein concentration, total nucleated cell count, differential cell count, and examination for abnormal cell morphology (degenerative or toxic changes, criteria of malignancy) and organisms are always performed. If infection is suspected, both aerobic and anaerobic cultures are indicated. If chylothorax is suspected, triglyceride and cholesterol concentrations are measured. Further diagnostic evaluation is based on the type of fluid obtained (see p. 768).

............Ultrasonography

Ultrasonography can be useful in evaluating the pleural cavity for masses. Effusion facilitates the examination, while aerated lung or air within the pleural cavity prevents the passage of sound.

REFERENCES

Aron DN, Crome DT: Upper airway obstruction: General principles and selected conditions in the dog and cat. Vet Clin North Am Small Anim Pract 15:891–918, 1985.

Bauer T, Thomas WP: Pulmonary diagnostic techniques. Vet Clin North Am Small Anim Pract 13:273, 1983.

Ettinger SJ, Feldman EC, eds: Textbook of Veterinary Internal Medicine, ed 4. Philadelphia, WB Saunders, 1995.

Hawkins EC: Respiratory disorders, part 2. In Nelson RW, Cuoto CG, eds: Essentials of Small Animal Internal Medicine. St Louis, Mosby–Year Book, 1992, pp 153–253.

King LG, Boothe DM: Bacterial Infections of the Respiratory Tract in Dogs and Cats. Trenton NJ, Veterinary Learning Systems, 1997.

Roudebush P, Ryan J: Breath sound terminology in the veterinary literature. J Am Vet Med Assoc 194:1415, 1989.

Skin

............THE SYSTEMATIC APPROACH TO DIAGNOSIS

If the veterinarian examines patients with skin disease in a cursory manner and attempts to make snap judgments, confusion and incorrect diagnoses will often result. In no other system of the body is a careful plan of examination and evaluation more important than in skin. Ideally, a thorough examination and appropriate diagnostic procedures should be accomplished the first time the patient is seen and before any masking treatments have been initiated. The points in Table 2–18 should be systematically considered and correlated for a rational, accurate dermatologic diagnosis.

............CLINICAL EXAMINATION

............Records

Recording historical facts, physical findings, and laboratory data in a systematic way is particularly important for patients with skin disease. Many dermatoses are chronic, and skin lesions are slow to change. For this reason, outline sketches of the patient enable the clinician to draw in the location and extent of lesions. One sketch is worth many words, and comparison of sketches made at different intervals graphically portrays changes in the lesions over time.

Figure 2–28 illustrates a satisfactory record form for noting physical and laboratory findings for dermatology cases. The special form enables one to circle pertinent descriptive terms, saves time, and ensures that no important

Table 2–18. Steps to a Dermatologic Diagnosis

1. Clinical examination: Record age, sex, breed, and general medical and dermatologic history. The inquiry should determine the chief complaint and data about the original lesion's location, appearance, onset, and rate of progression. Also determine the presence and degree of pruritus, contagion to other animals or people, and possible seasonal incidence. Relationship to diet and environmental factors and response to previous medications are also important.
2. Physical examination:
   a. Determine the distribution pattern and regional location of affected areas.
   b. Closely examine the skin to identify primary and secondary lesions. Evaluate alopecias or hair abnormalities.
   c. Observe the configurations of specific skin lesions and their relationship to each other; certain patterns are diagnostically significant.
3. Diagnostic and laboratory aids: Diagnostic aids such as skin scrapings, Wood's light examination, impression smears, and fungal or bacterial cultures should be done routinely. Biopsies, hormonal assays, chemistry panels, hemograms, immunologic and other special tests are also performed when indicated by clinical findings.
4. Correlation of the data: Make a list of differential diagnoses.
5. Narrowing the list of differential diagnoses: Plan additional tests, observations of therapeutic trials, etc., to narrow the list and provide a definitive diagnosis.

Modified from Muller GH, Kirk RW, Scott DW: Small Animal Dermatology, ed 4. Philadelphia, WB Saunders, 1989.

information is omitted. This form details only dermatologic data and should be used as a supplement to the general history and physical examination record. A special dermatologic history form is also useful, especially for allergic and chronic cases (Fig. 2–29). This form should be filled out by the client.

History

The clinician should obtain a complete medical history in all cases. Some dermatologists prefer to examine the skin quickly at first, so that pertinent questions can be emphasized in taking the history and inappropriate items can be omitted. However, it is vital to use a systematic, detailed method of examination and history taking so that important information is not overlooked.

Age

Some dermatologic disorders are age-related, so age is important in the dermatology history. For example, demodicosis usually begins in young dogs before sexual maturity. Allergies tend to appear in more mature individuals, probably because repeated exposure to the antigen must occur before clinical signs develop. Hormonal disorders tend to occur in animals between 6 and 10 years of age, and most neoplasms develop in mature to older patients.

Sex

The sex of the patient obviously limits the incidence of certain problems, but it is especially important in sex hormone imbalances. Perianal adenomas are seen almost exclusively in male dogs. One should determine whether the
Text continued on page 370

DERMATOLOGY EXAMINATION

DISTRIBUTION OF LESIONS

Weight ____

Ventral

Dorsal

PRIMARY LESIONS (Check)

Macule ____	Patch ____	Purpura ____	Wheal ____
Papule ____	Nodule ____	Plaque ____	Tumor ____
Pustule ____	Vesicle ____	Bullae ____	Cyst ____
Abscess ____			

SECONDARY LESIONS (Check)

Scale ____	Crust ____	Alopecia ____	Erythema ____
Erosion ____	Ulcer ____	Fissure ____	Scar ____
Excoriation ____	Collarettes ____		Nikolsky ____
Hyperpigmentation ____	Hypopigmentation ____		Callus ____
Hyperkeratosis ____	Lichenification ____		Comedone ____
Sinus ____	Hyperhidrosis ____		Necrosis ____

SKIN CHANGES (Check)

Normal ____	Thick ____	Thin ____	Fragile ____
Hypotonic ____	Hyperextensible ____	Increased Laxity ____	

OTHER FINDINGS

Pinal-Pedal Reflex ____

Lymph Nodes ____

366

HAIRCOAT CHANGES (Check)

Alopecia _____   Hypotrichosis _____   Hypertrichosis _____
Dry Coat _____   Brittle Coat _____   Oily Coat _____
Easy Epilation _____   1°Hairs _____   2°Hairs _____   Both _____
Hair Casts _____   Color Associated Hair Loss _____

CONFIGURATION OF LESIONS (Check)

Linear _____   Follicular _____   Grouped _____
Annular _____   Other _____

PRURITUS (Check)

Seasonal _____   Nonseasonal _____   Lesional _____
Face _____   Ears _____   Feet/Legs _____   Rump _____
Axillae _____   Abdomen _____   Other _____

CUTANEOUS PAIN (Check)

Absent _____   Mild _____   Moderate _____   Severe _____

PARASITES (Check)

Fleas _____   Flea Dirt _____   Lice _____   Ticks _____
Ear Mites _____   Other _____

*Can have either dog or cat outline here

Ears L _____
     R _____

Oral _____
Anogenital _____
Footpads _____
Nails _____
Other _____

LABORATORY

Scrape _____
Scotch Tape _____
Fungal Cult _____
Wood's Light _____
Hair Exam _____
ID Hist _____   Flea 15 _____   Flea 24 _____
Cytology _____
1. _____
2. _____
3. _____
4. _____

DIAGNOSIS/DIFFERENTIAL

_____
_____
_____

Figure 2-28. Dermatology examination sheet.

2

When was the problem first noted? _____ Day _____ Month _____ Year

Where on the body did the problem begin? _____

Is the problem: _____ Year Round _____ Seasonal _____ Unknown

If seasonal, in which season(s) is it worse? _____ Spring _____ Summer _____ Fall _____ Winter

If nonseasonal, is it worse in any season? _____

Does the animal itch (scratch, chew, lick, rub)? _____ Yes _____ No

Is the itching: _____ Mild _____ Moderate _____ Severe _____ Constant _____ Periodic

Where does the animal itch? Check those areas which are itchy.

Face: _____	Abdomen: _____	Lower Back: _____
Ears: _____	Front Feet/Legs: _____	All Over: _____
Arm Pits: _____	Back Feet/Legs: _____	

What medications have been used?

Drug	How Much	How Often	Did It Help?

Do parents, littermates, other animals in the house or other animals in the area have a similar problem? _____ Yes _____ No

On the reverse side, please provide any information which you feel is important.

DERMATOLOGY HISTORY

Chief Complaint:

_____ Itching   _____ Sores

_____ Hair loss   _____ Ear Disease

_____ Other _____

Aside from the skin problem is the animal healthy?

_____ Yes   _____ No

(Please Specify) _____

_____

_____

_____

_____

_____

Figure 2–29. Dermatology history sheet (to be completed by owner).

patient is sexually intact and, if so, whether the skin problem bears any relationship to the estrous cycle.

·········· Breed

Breed predilection determines the incidence of some skin disorders. For example, seborrhea is common in cocker spaniels; acanthosis nigricans usually occurs in dachshunds; adult-onset hyposomatotropism occurs in Pomeranians, keeshonds, and chows; dermatomyositis is found in Shetland sheepdogs and collies; zinc-responsive dermatosis occurs in Siberian huskies and Alaskan malamutes; and many of the wire-coated terrier breeds (Scotties, Cairns, Sealyhams, West Highland whites, Irish terriers, and Welsh terriers) seem to be particularly predisposed to allergic skin disease.

In a study of dogs in northern California conducted at the University of California at Davis, elevated risk for the development of skin diseases was found for 31 breeds, including Doberman pinscher, Irish setter, Dalmatian, dachshund, golden retriever, various terrier breeds, Shar Pei, chow, and Akita. In the same study, decreased risk for skin disease was found for dogs of mixed breeding and for 12 pure breeds, including Saint Bernard, standard poodle, beagle, basset hound, German short-haired pointer, Afghan hound, and Australian shepherd.

·········· Owner's Complaint

The owner's complaint or chief cause of concern is often the major sign used in compiling a differential diagnosis. The clinician who can draw out a complete history in an unbiased form has a valuable skill. It is important that the questions presented to the client do not suggest answers or tend to shut off discussion. A friendly "Let's help this patient together" attitude often stimulates the client to reveal more information.

Next, the following information should be obtained from the owner's history sheet (see Fig. 2–29): date of onset, original locations of the lesions, description of the initial lesions, tendency to progression or regressions, factors affecting the course, and previous treatment (home, proprietary, or pet shop remedies used, as well as veterinary treatment).

·········· PHYSICAL EXAMINATION

In dermatology, the clinician can observe the pathologic lesions directly and need not rely on radiologic shadows or referred sounds to determine abnormality, as skin lesions are clearly visible. By careful, systematic inspection alone, the diagnosis of many dermatoses becomes apparent.

The examination should be performed with good lighting. Normal daylight without glare is best, but any artificial light of adequate candlepower is sufficient if it produces bright, uniform lighting. The lamp should be adjustable to illuminate all body areas. A combination loupe and light provides magnification of the field as well as good illumination.

Before concentration on the individual lesions begins, the entire animal should always be observed from a distance of several feet for a general impression of abnormalities and to observe distribution patterns.

Does the animal appear to be in good health? Is it fat or thin, unkempt or well-groomed? Is the problem generalized or localized? What is the distribution of the lesions? Are they bilaterally symmetric or unilaterally irregular?

In order that some of these questions can be answered, the patient must be examined more closely. The dorsal aspect of the body should be inspected by viewing it from the rear, as elevated hairs are more obvious from that angle.

Then the lateral surfaces should be observed carefully. Next, the clinician should turn the patient over for a careful examination of the ventral region.

···········Close Examination of the Skin

After an impression is obtained from a distance, the skin should be examined more closely. Palpation now becomes important too. What is the texture of the hair? Is it coarse or fine, dry or oily, and does it epilate easily? A change in the amount of hair present is often a dramatic finding. Alopecia is a complete lack of hair in areas where hair is normally present. Hypotrichosis implies a partial alopecia that may be developmental, hormonal, neoplastic, inflammatory, or idiopathic. Hypertrichosis is excess hair and, although very rare in animals, is usually hormonal or developmental in nature.

The texture, elasticity, and thickness of the skin should be determined and impressions of heat or coolness recorded. It is important to examine every inch of skin and mucous membranes. It is easier to find important skin lesions in some breeds than in others, depending on the thickness of the coat. There is a variation in density of an individual's coat in different body areas. Lesions can be discerned more easily in sparsely haired regions. However, the clinician must part or clip the hair in many areas to observe and palpate lesions that are partially covered. It is useful to clip hair over an area of abnormal skin with a surgical blade (such as No. 40 Oster) to expose the area for identification of lesions. The clipped area is then cleansed with alcohol. Lesions previously hidden by hair and debris can now be clearly seen and interpreted. It is as if a "window" appears giving a new view of the skin disease. When abnormalities are discovered, it is important to establish their general distribution as well as their configuration within an area. Are they single, multiple, discrete, diffuse, grouped, or confluent? With sharp observation, linear or annular configuration of the lesions may be noted.

Two special techniques for close examination of the skin are noteworthy:

1. *Diascopy* is a technique that involves pressing a clear piece of plastic or glass over an erythematous lesion. If the lesion blanches on pressure, the reddish color is due to vascular engorgement. If the lesion does not blanch, there is hemorrhage into the skin (petechiae or ecchymoses).
2. *Nikolsky's sign* is elicited by applying pressure on a vesicle or pustule or at the edge of an ulcer or erosion or even on normal skin. The result is positive when the outer layer of the skin is easily rubbed off or pushed away. This indicates poor cellular cohesion, as found in the pemphigus complex, pemphigoid, and toxic epidermal necrolysis.

At this point one should focus on individual lesions and examine them minutely with good light and a hand lens or a head loupe with four- to six-power magnification.

···········Lesional Changes

The evolution of lesions should be determined from the history or by finding different stages of lesions on the same patient. Papules often develop into vesicles and pustules, which may rupture to leave erosions or ulcers with epidermal collarettes and finally crusts. An understanding of these processes helps in the diagnostic process. As lesions develop in special patterns, they also involute in characteristic ways. Acute lesions often appear suddenly and disappear quickly and completely. Chronic lesions may leave diagnostically important pigmentation or scars that persist for months or permanently (i.e., chronic generalized demodicosis and juvenile cellulitis, respectively) (Table 2–19).

Table 2–19. Classification of Skin Lesions

Primary Lesions (Lesions of First Diagnostic Importance)

Macule—patch	Pustule	Tumor—neoplasm	
Papule—plaque	Nodule	Vesicle—bulla	Wheal

Secondary Lesions (Evolutionary or Complicating Lesions of Secondary Diagnostic Importance)

Scale—epidermal collarette	Comedo	Pigmentary abnormalities
Crust	Fissure	(hyperpigmentation or
Scar	Excoriation	hypopigmentation)
Erosion—ulcer	Lichenification	Hyperkeratosis—callus

From Muller GH, Kirk RW, Scott DW: Small Animal Dermatology, ed 4. Philadelphia, WB Saunders, 1989, p 104.

..........Morphology of Skin Lesions

Morphology of skin lesions is the essential feature of dermatologic diagnosis and sometimes is the *only* guide if laboratory procedures yield no useful information. The clinician must learn to recognize primary and secondary lesions.* A primary lesion is one that develops spontaneously as a direct reflection of underlying disease. Secondary lesions evolve from primary lesions or are artifacts induced by the patient or by external factors such as trauma or medications (see Table 2–20). Careful inspection of the diseased skin will frequently reveal a primary lesion suggestive of a specific dermatosis. In many cases, however, the significant lesion must be differentiated from the mass of secondary debris. The ability to discover a characteristic lesion and understand its significance is the first step toward mastering dermatologic diagnosis. Variations are common, since early as well as advanced stages exist in most skin diseases. In addition, the appearance of skin lesions may change with medication, self-inflicted trauma, and secondary infection.

Most skin diseases, however, are characterized by a single type of lesion. This primary lesion varies slightly from its initial appearance to its full development. Later, through regression, degeneration, or traumatization, it changes in appearance and in its new, altered form becomes a secondary lesion.

..........Cutaneous Manifestations of Systemic Disease

Cutaneous changes that accompany internal disease may result from simultaneous involvement of skin and internal organs with identical pathologic mechanisms (multicentric disease); direct extension of an internal disease process to the skin; immunologic manifestations of a deficient or hyperactive immune system; hormonal deficiency or excess; or metabolic derangements. These cutaneous changes may be obvious or subtle, mild or extensive, or incidental or specific. When the cutaneous change has a high correlation to a specific internal disease process, the lesions are referred to as a marker of internal disease (Table 2–21). Clinicians must examine the patient with dermatologic disease while considering internal pathologic factors.

Internal disease should be suspected in patients with dermatologic disorders when the following conditions are seen:

---

*Illustrations and definitions of these lesions are presented in Muller GH, Kirk RW, Scott DW: Small Animal Dermatology, ed 4. Philadelphia, WB Saunders, 1989, pp 105–122.

Table 2–20. Systemic Diseases With Cutaneous Lesions

Disease	Skin Lesions or Signs
Atopy	Pruritus
Castration-responsive dermatosis	Alopecia
Cold agglutinin disease	Erytherma, purpura, necrosis, ulceration
Diabetes mellitus	Atrophy, ulceration, pyoderma, seborrhea
Dirofilariasis	Erythema, alopecia, pruritus, nodules
Erythema multiforme	Macules, papules, vesicles, wheals
Feline leukemia virus infection	Pyoderma, seborrhea, poor healing, cutaneous horns on footpads
Hepatocutaneous syndrome	Mucocutaneous crusts and ulcers, footpad hyperkeratosis and ulcers
Hyperadrenocorticism	Alopecia, hyperpigmentation, calcinosis cutis, pyoderma, seborrhea, phlebectasias, thin and hypotonic skin
Hypothyroidism	Alopecia, hypothermia, seborrhea, pyoderma, hyperpigmentation, myxedema, galactorrhea
Leishmaniasis	Erythema, nodules, ulceration, exfoliative dermatitis
Male feminizing syndrome	Alopecia, seborrhea, hyperpigmentation, gynecomastia, galactorrhea
Mycoses, deep	Nodules, ulceration, fistulas
Mycosis fungoides	Erythroderma, plaques, nodules, ulceration
Ovarian imbalances	Alopecia, hyperpigmentation, seborrhea
Pemphigus	Purulent exudate, crusting, vesiculation, ulceration/erosion
Pituitary dwarfism	Alopecia, cutaneous degeneration, hyperpigmentation
Sertoli cell tumor	Alopecia, gynecomastia, hyperpigmentation
Systemic lupus erythematosus	Pyoderma, seborrhea, ulceration, pruritus, erythema
Thallium toxicosis	Alopecia, erytherma, ulceration
Toxic epidermal necrolysis	Ulceration, blisters, pain
Tuberculosis	Nodules, ulceration, fistulas

From Muller GH, Kirk RW, Scott DW: Small Animal Dermatology, ed 4. Philadelphia, WB Saunders, 1989, p 100.

Table 2–21. Examples of Cutaneous Markers of Internal Disease

Cutaneous Lesion/Disease	Systemic Disease
Nodular dermatofibrosis	Renal cystadenocarcinoma Uterine leiomyosarcoma
"Alabama" rot (cutaneous ulcerations) in greyhounds	Renal vasculopathy
Superficial necrolytic dermatitis (hepatocutaneous syndrome)	Glucagonoma (diabetes mellitus) Hepatic disease
Xanthomas	Hyperlipidemia syndromes (cat)
Calcinosis cutis	Hyperadrenocorticism

1. Dermatologic disease concurrent with systemic illness, such as fever, depression, or clinical signs consistent with a particular organ system (e.g., diarrhea, lameness)
2. Bizarre or atypical dermatoses
3. Chronic recurring dermatoses, including pyoderma, scaling, and so forth
4. Dermatoses in unexpected patients (e.g., age, breed, sex)
5. Dermatologic signs following illness or drug administration

..........Distribution Patterns of Skin Lesions

A dramatic change becomes apparent when a skin disorder affects an animal whose body is covered with a dense hair coat. Even the most casual observer is aware of the loss or hair in certain areas. The alopecic pattern, which is often sharply demarcated, assumes a new meaning when it is accurately interpreted. When alopecia and other hair changes are evaluated according to their distribution pattern over the entire body, significant diagnostic clues appear. Comparatively speaking, only on the human scalp is alopecia as striking and meaningful.

In animals, the primary or secondary skin lesions are often hidden under the hair coat; in fact, it requires painstaking observation to see them. In short-coated animals, if you stand behind the animal and use both hands to roll the skin into a horizontal fold, it is possible to see between the erected hair shafts to the skin surface. By rolling the fold backward, you can see progressively new areas of skin surface and get "an impression" of the distribution of lesions. Only when the animal is clipped can the distribution pattern of such lesions be seen with ease and accuracy. Consequently, in animals there are two distinctly different patterns that aid in diagnosis: (1) the changes in external hair coat and (2) the definition and distribution of primary and secondary skin lesions. These two factors do not necessarily have a reciprocal relationship. In addition, it is important to recognize whether the lesions present a symmetric distribution on either side of the midline or an asymmetric distribution.

..........Different Stages

As a skin disease progresses from its earliest appearance to its final fully developed state, the pattern necessarily changes. A small patch or alopecia can enlarge into almost total hair loss in some cases. Obviously, if all intermediate stages of such a disease were drawn diagrammatically, the result would be more confusing than helpful. Therefore, it is necessary to select for each skin disorder the single distribution pattern that is of greatest diagnostic value. Different stages of each disease exist, and the total impact of the diagram should be interpreted with that fact always in mind. In addition, note that the distribution pattern represents alopecia or changes of the skin surface or both.

..........Regional Diagnosis

When a dermatosis is confined to a specific region, several diagnoses are often possible. Table 2–22 lists areas or parts of the body and the skin diseases that are commonly localized or especially severe in those areas. This table should be useful in suggesting several differential diagnosis.

..........DIAGNOSTIC AND LABORATORY PROCEDURES

Diagnostic tests and laboratory procedures are valuable aids in almost every dermatologic case. Most tests are simple, quick, and inexpensive to perform. Some tests should be done "routinely," because many dermatoses are, in fact,

Text continued on page 379

Table 2–22. Regional Diagnosis

Area	Disease
Head	Atopy
	Demodicosis
	Dermatophytosis
	Facial fold dermatitis
	Feline food allergy
	Feline leprosy
	Juvenile cellulitis
	Otic vascular necrosis
	Pemphigus erythematosus
	Pemphigus foliaceus
	Scabies, feline
	Sporotrichosis
	Sterile pyogranuloma syndrome
	Systemic lupus erythematosus
	Vasculitis
	Zinc-responsive dermatosis
Ear	Alopecia, pattern
	Atopy
	Ceruminal gland tumor
	Cold agglutinin disease
	Demodicosis
	Fly dermatitis
	Frostbite
	Melanoderma and alopecia of Yorkshire terriers
	Otitis externa
	Bacterial
	Candidiasis
	Ceruminosis
	Demodicosis
	Malassezia (yeast)
	Otodectes cynotis
	Trombiculidiasis
	Scabies, canine and feline
	Seborrhea, marginal (pinna)
	Solar dermatitis, feline
	Sterile eosinophilic pinnal folliculitis
Eyelid	Chalazion
	Demodicosis
	Dermatophytosis
	Distichiasis
	Entropion
	Folliculitis, bacterial
	Hordeolum
	Seborrheic blepharitis
	Trichiasis

Table continued on following page

Table 2–22. Regional Diagnosis *Continued*

Area	Disease
Nasal area	Contact dermatitis (plastic, rubber) Demodicosis Dermatophytosis Discoid lupus erythematosus Facial fold dermatitis Folliculitis, bacterial Nasodigital hyperkeratosis Pemphigus erythematosus Pemphigus foliaceus Sporotrichosis Squamous cell carcinoma Sterile pyogranuloma syndrome Vitiligo-like lesions Vogt-Koyanagi-Harada–like syndrome (uvea-dermatologic syndrome)
Lip	Acne, canine and feline Candidiasis Contact dermatitis (plastic, rubber) Demodicosis Indolent ulcer, feline Juvenile cellulitis Lip fold dermatitis Oral papillomatosis, canine Vitiligo-like lesions Vogt-Koyanagi-Harada–like syndrome
Oral cavity (mucosal lesions)	Bullous pemphigoid Candidiasis Discoid lupus erythematosus Eosinophilic granuloma, canine and feline Eosinophilic plaque, feline Erosions, chemical Erosions, viral, feline Fibrosarcoma Fusospirochetal stomatitis Gingival hypertrophy Indolent ulcer, feline Malignant melanoma Marginal gingivitis, ulcerative, dental Mycosis fungoides Oral papillomatosis Pemphigus vulgaris Plasma cell stomatitis, feline Squamous cell carcinoma Systemic lupus erythematosus Thallium toxicosis Vegetative glossitis (foreign body)

Table 2–22. Regional Diagnosis *Continued*

Area	Disease
Mucocutaneous margins	Bullous pemphigoid Candidiasis Erythema multiforme Hepatocutaneous syndrome Mycosis fungoides Pemphigus vulgaris Systemic lupus erythematosus Thallium toxicosis Toxic epidermal necrolysis
Chin	Acne, canine and feline Demodicosis Juvenile cellulitis Eosinophilic granuloma, feline Furunculosis, bacterial
Neck	Contact dermatitis (collars) Dermoid sinus Flea bite hypersensitivity, feline Flea collar dermatitis
Lower chest	Contact dermatitis Fibrovascular papilloma Sternal callus
Axilla	Acanthosis nigricans Atopy Bullous pemphigoid Contact dermatitis Pemphigus vulgaris
Back	Atopy Calcinosis cutis Cheyletiellosis Comedo syndrome, schnauzers Flea bite hypersensitivity Folliculitis, bacterial Food hypersensitivity Hypothyroidism Pediculosis Psychogenic dermatitis/alopecia, feline
Trunk	Demodicosis, generalized Eosinophilic plaque, feline Folliculitis, bacterial Hyperadrenocorticism Hyposomatotropism Hypothyroidism Male feminizing syndrome Ovarian imbalance Panniculitis, sterile Sebaceous adenitis Sertoli cell tumor Sterile eosinophilic pustulosis Subcorneal pustular dermatosis Vitamin A–responsive dermatosis

2

Table continued on following page

Table 2–22. Regional Diagnosis *Continued*

Area	Disease
Abdomen	Bullous pemphigoid
	Calcinosis cutis
	Contact dermatitis (ventral abdomen)
	Eosinophilic plaque, feline
	Feline symmetric alopecia
	Folliculitis, bacterial
	Hookworm dermatitis
	Hyperadrenocorticism
	Impetigo
	Mycobacteriosis, atypical, feline
	Panniculitis, sterile, feline
	Pelodera dermatitis
	Psychogenic dermatitis/alopecia, feline
	Subcorneal pustular dermatitis
	Trombiculidiasis
Flanks	Bullous pemphigoid
	Folliculitis, bacterial
	Hyposomatotropism
	Mechanical irritation (flank suckers)
	Ovarian imbalance
Tail	Acute moist dermatitis
	Cold agglutinin disease
	Cryoglobulinemia
	Feline symmetric alopecia
	Flea bite hypersensitivity
	Frostbite
	Hyperplasia of tail gland, stud tail
	Mechanical irritation (tail suckers)
	Psychogenic dermatitis/alopecia, feline
	Tip-of-tail trauma
Anus	Anal sac dermatitis
	Anal sac disease
	Bullous pemphigoid
	Perianal adenoma
	Perianal fistulas
	Perianal gland hyperplasia
Legs	Acral lick dermatitis
	Calcinosis circumscripta
	Contact dermatitis
	Decubital ulcers
	Demodicosis
	Elbow callus
	Elbow callus pyoderma
	Hygroma
	Eosinophilic granuloma, feline
	Feline leprosy
	Lymphangitis, bacterial, fungal
	Lymphedema
	Pelodera dermatitis
	Scabies, canine

Table 2–22. Regional Diagnosis *Continued*

Area	Disease
Feet	Acral mutilation
	Atopy
	Collagen disease of German shepherd footpads
	Contact dermatitis
	Demodicosis
	Dermatophytosis
	Digital hyperkeratosis of Irish terriers
	Digital pad hyperkeratosis
	Food hypersensitivity
	Hepatocutaneous syndrome
	Hookworm dermatitis
	Interdigital foreign bodies (foxtails, thorns)
	Leishmaniasis
	Pelodera dermatitis
	Pemphigus foliaceus
	Pododermatitis
	Plasma cell, feline
	Traumatic
	Sterile pyogranuloma syndrome
	Trombiculidiasis
	Tyrosinemia
	Zinc-responsive dermatosis
Nails	Hyperthyroidism, feline
	Leishmaniasis
	Onychomadesis
	Onychogryphosis
	Bullous pemphigoid
	Pemphigus vulgaris
	Oncychomycosis
	Onychorrhexis
	Paronychia
	Arteriovenous shunt
	Bacterial
	Feline leukemia
	Trauma
	Systemic lupus erythematosus
	Traumatic injury

From Muller GH, Kirk RW, Scott DW: Small Animal Dermatology, ed 4. Philadelphia, WB Saunders, 1989, pp 124–126.

complex problems with more than one cause. It would be embarrassing to miss a case of demodectic mange or dermatomycosis because a simple test was not run to check for a secondary problem in what superficially looked like a single primary disease.

Detailed discussions of dermatologic tests are presented in Section 4, p. 492.

REFERENCES

Ihrke PJ: Pruritus. *In* Ettinger SJ, Feldman EC, eds: Textbook of Veterinary Internal Medicine, ed 4. Philadelphia, WB Saunders, 1995, pp 214–219.

Scott DW, Miller WH, Griffin CE: Muller and Kirk's Small Animal Dermatology, ed 5. Philadelphia, WB Saunders, 1995.

...........Urinary Tract

Attempt to answer the following questions when completing the history, physical examination, and laboratory evaluation of the patient with suspected urinary tract disease:

1. Is urinary tract disease present?
2. Does the disease involve the upper (kidneys and ureters) or lower (bladder and urethra) urinary tract?
3. What is the current status of the patient's renal function?
4. Can the disease be treated?
5. What is the prognosis?
6. What nonurinary complicating factors are present (e.g., dehydration, infection)?

...........HISTORY

Take a complete history, including signalment (age, breed, sex), presenting complaint, husbandry, and review of body systems. The history of the presenting complaint should include information about onset (acute or gradual), progression (improving, unchanging, or worsening), and response to previous therapy. Information about husbandry includes the animal's immediate environment (indoor or outdoor); use (pet, breeding, show, or working animal); geographic origin and travel history; exposure to other animals; vaccination status; diet; and information about previous trauma, illness, or surgery. A brief review of body systems may be obtained by determining the presence or absence of the following abnormalities: lethargy, anorexia, vomiting, diarrhea, coughing, sneezing, exercise intolerance, polyuria, polydipsia, weight loss, lameness, pruritus, alopecia, and exposure to drugs or toxins.

Questions related to the urinary tract include those about changes in water intake and the frequency or volume of urination. The owner should be questioned about pollakiuria, dysuria, or hematuria. Care must be taken to distinguish dysuria and pollakiuria from polyuria and to differentiate polyuria from urinary incontinence (see p. 441). The distinction between pollakiuria and polyuria is very important because polyuria may be a sign of upper urinary disease, whereas pollakiuria and dysuria usually are indicative of lower urinary tract disease. Occasionally, an owner will complain that the dog is incontinent because it is urinating in the house when in reality the dog is polyuric but is not allowed outdoors frequently enough. Nocturia may be an early sign of polyuria but also can occur as a result of dysuria. Normal urine output ranges from 20 to 45 mL/kg/day in dogs and cats.

Information about the initiation of urination and diameter of the urine stream may be helpful because animals with partial obstruction may experience difficulty initiating urination or may have an abnormal urine stream. If hematuria is present, question the owner about its timing. Blood at the beginning of urination may indicate a disease process in the urethra or genital tract. Blood at the end of urination or throughout urination may signify a problem in either the bladder or upper urinary tract (kidneys or ureters).

Polydipsia usually is more easily detected by the owner than polyuria. Water intake should not exceed 90 mL/kg/day in dogs and 45 mL/kg/day in cats. It is helpful to describe amounts in quantitative terms familiar to the owner, such as cups (approximately 250 mL per cup) or quarts (approximately 1 L/q). Question the owner about exposure about exposure of the animal to nephrotoxins such as ethylene glycol in antifreeze (especially during fall and spring), aminoglycosides, amphotericin B, thiacetarsamide, and NSAIDs. Also, determine whether the animal has received any drugs that could cause polydipsia and polyuria, such as corticosteroids or diuretics.

..........PHYSICAL EXAMINATION

Perform a complete physical examination, including funduscopic and rectal examinations. Pay careful attention to evaluation of hydration from skin turgor, position of the eyes in the orbits, moistness of mucous membranes, pulse rate and character, capillary refill time, and heart rate. The minimal amount of dehydration detectable clinically is approximately 5% of body weight; 15% dehydration is the maximal amount compatible with life. Skin elasticity and subcutaneous fat affect the reliability of skin turgor in the assessment of hydration. Obese animals may be dehydrated yet demonstrate normal skin turgor, whereas emaciated animals may have abnormal skin turgor yet not be dehydrated. Changes in weight can be used to monitor changes in hydration on an acute basis, since 1 L of fluid is equal to 1 kg of body weight. Evaluate the animal for the presence of ascites or subcutaneous edema, which may occur in patients with nephrotic syndrome.

2

..........Oral Cavity

Examine the oral cavity for ulcers, which may occur in the presence of uremia, especially in dogs. Tongue-tip necrosis occasionally occurs in uremic dogs because of fibrinoid necrosis of vessels in the tongue. Examine the mucous membranes for pallor suggestive of anemia. Vascular injection may be observed in the sclera and soft palate of some uremic dogs. Examine the fundus for evidence of systemic hypertension, which can complicate renal disease: retinal edema, retinal detachment, retinal hemorrhage, and vascular tortuosity. Young growing animals with renal failure may develop marked fibrous osteodystrophy characterized by enlargement and deformity of the maxilla and mandible, but this is uncommon in older dogs with renal failure.

..........Abdomen

Perform abdominal palpation. Both kidneys can be palpated in most cats and the left kidney can be palpated in up to 20% of dogs. Evaluate the kidneys for size, shape, consistency, pain, and location. Unless empty, the bladder can be palpated in most dogs and cats. Note the degree of bladder distention, the presence or absence of pain, and thickness of the bladder wall. Evaluate the bladder for intramural (e.g., tumors) or intraluminal (e.g., stones, clots) masses. In the absence of obstruction, a distended bladder in a dehydrated animal suggests abnormal renal function or administration of drugs that impair urinary concentrating ability (e.g., corticosteroids, diuretics).

..........Pelvic Examination and Genitalia

Palpate the prostate gland (males) and pelvic urethra (males and females) by rectal examination. The perianal and sublumbar areas should be palpated carefully during rectal examination to determine the presence of tumors. Evaluate the prostate gland for size, symmetry, pain, and location. Exteriorize and examine the penis and palpate the testes for symmetry, consistency, masses, or pain. In the female dog, perform a vaginal examination to evaluate for abnormal discharge, masses, and the status of the urethral orifice.

..........LABORATORY EVALUATION (see also p. 772)

The following tests or procedures may be useful in evaluation of animals with suspected urinary tract disease:

1. Daily water intake and urine output over several days

2. Routine urinalysis including urine sediment examination (the sample should be collected before administration of parenteral fluids to avoid confusion in interpretation of the urine specific gravity value)
3. Complete blood count (CBC)
4. Blood urea nitrogen (BUN) and serum creatinine concentrations
5. Serum cholesterol, albumin, and total protein concentrations
6. Serum sodium, potassium, chloride, calcium, and phosphorous concentrations
7. Total carbon dioxide content or blood gas analysis
8. Urine culture and sensitivity
9. Arterial blood pressure determination
10. Plain abdominal radiography
11. Excretory urography
12. Contrast cystography and urethrography
13. Abdominal ultrasonography
14. Endogenous or exogenous creatinine clearance
15. Urine protein excretion in 24 hours
16. Urine protein–urine creatinine ratio
17. Fractional excretion of sodium, potassium, chloride, and phosphorous
18. Urine-plasma osmolality ratio
19. Water deprivation test
20. Exogenous vasopressin test
21. Phenolsulfonphthalein half-life
22. Sodium sulfanilate half-life
23. Ammonium chloride challenge test
24. Renal biopsy
25. Cystometrogram, urethral pressure profile, and electromyography
26. Cystoscopy

REFERENCES

Grauer GF: Clinical manifestations of urinary disorders. *In* Nelson RW, Cuoto CG, eds: Essentials of Small Animal Internal Medicine. St Louis, Mosby–Year Book, 1992, pp 449–465.

Kruger JM: Clinical evaluation of cats with lower urinary tract disease. J Am Vet Med Assoc 199:211–216, 1991.

Lorenz MD, Cornelius LM: Small Animal Medical Diagnosis, ed 2. Philadelphia, JB Lippincott, 1991.

Osborne CA, Finco DR, eds: Canine and Feline Nephrology and Urology. Baltimore, Williams & Wilkins, 1995.

Section 3

··

CLINICAL SIGNS

3

· ·

Abdominal Enlargement and Ascites

............DEFINITION

Ascites, an abnormal accumulation of fluid in the peritoneal cavity, can result from a variety of inflammatory, infectious, metabolic, degenerative, and neoplastic disorders. Ascites is best confirmed by abdominal radiographs or ultrasound examination and abdominocentesis. Abdominal enlargement can be physiologic (in a postprandial puppy or kitten) or may be the result of metabolic or neoplastic disorders not associated with fluid accumulation.

............ASSOCIATED SIGNS

Clinical signs associated with abdominal enlargement are common. Once characterized, the associated signs can provide critical information relevant to the underlying diagnosis. The history may include increased water consumption and urination, diarrhea, vomiting, increased or decreased appetite, pain, apparent or real weight gain, and loss of muscle mass.

On physical examination, verify the abdominal enlargement to determine whether or not the enlargement is caused by fluid accumulation. Examine the patient for the presence of a heart murmur and palpable arrhythmia. If fluid is not present, determine the presence or absence of a mass within the abdominal cavity. When fluid is present, analyze the fluid character biochemically and cytologically (see p. 768).

............DIFFERENTIAL DIAGNOSIS (see Table 3–1)
............DIAGNOSTIC PLANS

1. Physical examination, to establish or rule out cardiopulmonary disease. Evaluate skin and hair coat for signs supporting endocrine disease. Assess abdominal enlargement by palpation and auscultation (see p. 280).
2. Abdominal radiograph and ultrasound, to confirm the presence of fluid, fat, or organomegaly.
3. If fluid *is* present, abdominocentesis, fluid analysis, and, if available, abdominal ultrasound. A laboratory database also is recommended (see pp. 651 and 718).

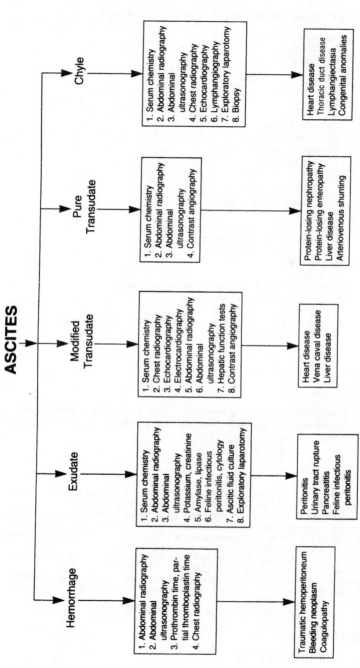

Figure 3–1. Diagnostic workup of patients with ascites. (From King L, Gelens H: Ascites. Compend Contin Educ 14:1063, 1992.)

Table 3–1. Differential Diagnosis of Abdominal Enlargement

Physiololgic Enlargement
Postprandial
Pregnancy

Without Fluid Accumulation
Organomegaly
Neoplasia
Obstipation
Gastric dilation
Hyperadrenocorticism
Ruptured prepubic tendon
Bladder distention
Pneumoperitoneum

With Fluid Accumulation
High protein: >2.5 g/dL
  Hepatic failure
  Right-sided congestive heart failure
  Inflammatory-infectious (e.g., FIP)
  Chemical/drug peritonitis
  Trauma
  Neoplasia
  Hepatic vein thrombosis or vascular anomaly
  Chyloabdomen
Low protein: <2.5 g/dL
  Hypoproteinemia (renal, hepatic, or gastrointestinal cause)
  Portal hypertension subsequent to primary liver disease
  Neoplasia

FIP, feline infectious peritonitis.

4. If fluid *is not* present, contrast radiography of the bowel (barium series), dexamethasone suppression test, abdominal laparotomy, or, if available, abdominal ultrasound (see p. 526).

REFERENCES

Bunch SE: Abdominal effusion. *In* Ford RB, ed: Clinical Signs and Diagnosis in Small Animal Practice. New York, Churchill Livingstone, 1988, pp 521–540.

Center SA: Chronic hepatitis, cirrhosis, breed-specific hepatopathies, copper storage hepatopathy, suppurative hepatitis, granulomatous hepatitis, and idiopathic hepatic fibrosis. *In* Guilford WG, Center SA, Strombeck DR, eds: Strombeck's Small Animal Gastroenterology, ed 3. Philadelphia, WB Saunders, 1996, pp 705–765.

Cornelius LM: Abdominal distention. *In* Lorenz MD, Cornelius LM, eds: Small Animal Medical Diagnosis. Philadelphia, JB Lippincott, 1987, pp 73–77.

Ettinger SJ, Barrett KA. Ascites, peritonitis, and other causes of abdominal distention. *In* Ettinger SJ, Feldman EC, eds: Textbook of Veterinary Internal Medicine, ed 4. Philadelphia, WB Saunders, 1995, pp 66–71.

King L, Gelens H: Ascites. Compend Contin Educ Pract Vet 14: 1063, 1992.

Aggression

·········· DEFINITION

Aggression in either the dog or cat is a behavior that leads to the destruction or injury of an animal or person. Furthermore, aggression can be categorized as offensive or defensive. Specific knowledge of the pattern and type of aggression is critical if effective intervention is to be accomplished. To meet the criteria of this definition, it is assumed that organic causes of aggression (e.g., pain or intracranial mass) have been ruled out.

············ASSOCIATED SIGNS

Although rare, aggression may be the result of organic disease, particularly disorders affecting the brain. In these patients, the onset of aggressive behavior is usually acute and may be associated with other neurologic signs suggesting cerebral dysfunction (e.g, seizures and circling). However, animals with pain may also manifest aggressive behavior, an apparent secondary response to discomfort. Animals with unilateral or bilateral blindness or deafness may bite or manifest aggressive behavior when approached and touched from the blind, or deaf, side. This behavior is probably the result of the animal's being startled and is far less likely to be representative of abnormal behavior.

············DIFFERENTIAL DIAGNOSIS (see Tables 3–2 and 3–3)

············DIAGNOSTIC PLANS

An accurate diagnosis and informed prognosis are essential to effective intervention. The most effective plan for diagnosis and therapy may be for the clinician to make the owners aware of the clinical signs of aggression, alert them to the usual sequelae of early patterns, and direct them to a behavior specialist. Administration of a psychotropic drug as empiric therapy for aggression is *not* recommended prior to determining a possible cause and attempting to modify behavior through training.

Table 3–2. Aggressive Behavior in the Dog: Differential Diagnosis According to Origin

Pathophysiologically Based Aggressive Behavior
Rabies
Intracranial neoplasia
Cerebral hypoxia
Seizure activity
Neuroendocrine disturbances
Species-Typical Aggressive Behavior*
Dominance aggression
Possessive aggression
Protective aggression
Predatory aggression
Fear-induced aggression
Intermale and interfemale aggression
Pain-induced, punishment-induced, and irritable aggression
Maternal aggression
Redirected aggression

*These behavior patterns are not pathologic states. They are typical patterns of the species and are, therefore, normal. Familiarity with normal, species-typical aggressive patterns of the dog enables differentiation of species-typical patterns from pathophysiologically based aggression. Like many animal behavior problems, their species-typicality does not lessen their disruptiveness or danger.

From Young MS: Aggressive behavior. *In* Ford RB, (ed): Clinical Signs and Diagnosis in Small Animal Practice. New York, Churchill Livingstone, 1988, p 137.

Table 3–3. Aggressive Behavior in the Cat: Differential Diagnosis According to Origin

Pathophysiologically Based Aggressive Behavior
Rabies
Intracranial neoplasia and lesions
*Species-Typical Aggressive Behavior**
Intermale aggression
Predatory aggression
Play aggression
Territorital aggression
Fear-induced aggression
Pain-induced aggression
Maternal aggression
Redirected aggression

*These behavior patterns are not pathologic states. They are typical patterns of the species and are, therefore, normal. Familiarity with normal, species-typical aggressive patterns of the cat enables differentiation of species-typical patterns from pathophysiologically based aggression. Like many animal behavior problems, their species-typicality does not lessen their disruptiveness or danger.

From Young MS: Aggressive behavior. *In* Ford RB, ed: Clinical Signs and Diagnosis in Small Animal Practice. New York, Churchill Livingstone, 1988, p 137.

REFERENCES

Beebe AD, Overall K: Feline behavioral disorders. *In* Morgan RV, ed: Handbook of Small Animal Practice, ed 3. Philadelphia, WB Saunders, 1997, pp 1206–1211.
Houpt KA, Reisner IR: Behavioral disorders. *In* Ettinger SJ, Feldman EC, eds: Textbook of Veterinary Internal Medicine, ed 4. Philadelphia, WB Saunders, 1995, pp 179–187.
Overall KL: Canine behavioral disorders. *In* Morgan RV, ed: Handbook of Small Animal Practice, ed 3. Philadelphia, WB Saunders, 1997, pp 1193–1195.

Alopecia (see Hair Loss, p. 412)

Ataxia, Incoordination

··········**DEFINITION**

Ataxia is defined as the loss of coordination *without* spasticity, paresis, or involuntary movement. In practice, however, it is possible for ataxia to be accompanied by additional neurologic signs. Ataxia is the result of disorders of the conscious or unconscious proprioceptive system, disorders of the cerebellum, or disorders of the vestibular system.

··········**ASSOCIATED SIGNS**

In the spectrum of disorders causing ataxia, lesions of the vestibular system predominate. However, vestibular signs may result from other brain disorders and spinal cord syndromes. Associated signs include head tilt, nystagmus, circling, and hemiparesis. Patients with cerebellar lesions typically have symmetric signs: hypermetria, abnormally long range of movement (goose-stepping gait); hypometria, abnormally short range of movement; or tremor, particularly of the head.

...........DIFFERENTIAL DIAGNOSIS (see Table 3–4)
...........DIAGNOSTIC PLANS

1. Physical examination, with particular attention to the external ear and tympanic membrane (see p. 320).
2. Neurologic examination, to include assessment of the cranial nerves with the intent of localizing the lesion (see p. 330).
3. Laboratory database, to rule out metabolic causes (see p. 718).
4. Skull radiographs, to include the tympanic bullae.
5. Spinal tap and an examination of cerebrospinal fluid (CSF) (see p. 516).
6. Special diagnostics, depending on availability (e.g., electroencephalogram [EEG] and computed tomography [CT].

REFERENCES

Oliver JE, Lorenz MD, Kornegay JN: Handbook of Veterinary Neurology, ed 3. Philadelphia, WB Saunders, 1997.
Shores A: Ataxia, paresis and paralysis. In Ettinger SJ, Feldman EC, eds: Textbook of Veterinary Internal Medicine, ed 4. Philadelphia, WB Saunders, 1995, pp 145–149.

Table 3–4. Differential Diagnosis of Ataxia

Congenital (Signs Present Before 3 Months of Age)
Reported in Siamese and Burmese cats and several dog breeds. Multiple congenital disorders are present with multiple neurologic signs, including ataxia. Bilateral congenital vestibular disorders have been observed in Doberman pinschers, beagles, and Akitas (see p. 824).

Inflammatory
Otitis interna, as an extension of otitis externa and media
Neuritis of the eighth cranial nerve
Infections

Toxic
Drug-induced aminoglycoside therapy

Nutritional
Thiamine deficiency (cat only—rare)

Metabolic
CNS signs secondary to other diseases (e.g., hepatic, renal)

Traumatic-Vascular
Head trauma with concussive injury to the cerebellum and brain stem

Neoplastic
Any tumor

Degenerative
Storage diseases
Demyelinating diseases
Neuropathies
Cerebellar abiotrophy

Idiopathic (Particularly Common Cause of Vestibular Signs)
Feline vestibular syndrome
Geriatric canine vestibular syndrome
Acute labyrinthitis

Selcer B: Radiographic imaging in canine lumbosacral disease. Vet Med Rep 1:282, 1989.
Simpson ST: Ataxia, head tilt, nystagmus, circling, and hemiparesis. *In* Ford RB, ed: Clinical Signs and Diagnosis in Small Animal Practice. New York, Churchill Livingstone, 1988, pp 257–267.

Blindness

(See Vision Loss, p. 443)

Coma

............DEFINITION

Coma refers to a state of complete reversible or irreversible unconsciousness that can result from neurologic as well as non-neurologic disease. Coma can be a consequence of diffuse or multifocal lesions of the cerebrum or a lesion affecting the rostral brain stem and ascending reticular activating system. A variety of organic central nervous system (CNS) disease leading to metabolic or toxic encephalopathy can also produce coma. In addition to a thorough neurologic examination, a cardiac examination and comprehensive laboratory profile are justified in the initial assessment of the comatose patient.

............ASSOCIATED SIGNS

Despite the fact that the comatose patient is unconscious, a complete neuro-ophthalmologic examination should be completed. Altered pupil size and pupillary light responses usually indicate brain stem disease. Emergency cardiac assessment of the unconscious patient justifies an electrocardiogram (ECG) and thoracic radiographs. Laboratory assessment of the comatose patient includes hepatic enzymes and, when feasible, hepatic function, electrolytes, and glucose level.

............DIFFERENTIAL DIAGNOSIS (see Table 3–5)

............DIAGNOSTIC PLANS

1. Assessment of vital signs, to evaluate airway, breathing, and circulation (pulse, heartbeat, and ECG). Take thoracic radiographs if indicated. If cerebral edema is suspected, administer ventilation support, hyperosmotic agents (e.g., mannitol 20%, 1 to 2 g/kg of body weight q6h IV), and glucocorticoids (see p. 152).
2. Neurologic examination, directed toward evaluation of brain stem function, including motor function, pupillary light response, and eye movement.
3. Comprehensive laboratory profile, to include hematologic data, biochemical profile, and urinalysis (Table 3–6) (see pp. 651 and 718).
4. Special diagnostic tests as appropriate:
   a. Metabolic coma. Serum ammonia, bile acids, glucose, blood and urine lead levels (see pp. 734 and 772).
   b. Neurologic coma. Spinal tap CT, EEG (see p. 516).

REFERENCES

Oliver JE, Lorenz MD, Kornegay JN: Handbook of Veterinary Neurology, ed 3. Philadelphia, WB Saunders, 1997.
Shell L: Altered States of consciousness: Coma and stupor. *In* Ettinger SJ, Feldman EC, eds: Textbook of Veterinary Internal Medicine, ed 4. Philadelphia, WB Saunders, 1995, pp 149–152.

Table 3–5. Differential Diagnosis of Coma

	Neurogenic	**Non-Neurogenic**
Acute, nonprogressive	Intracranial hemorrhage Brain malformations	— —

Acute, progressive	Metastatic lesions
	Epidural, subdural
	  hemorrhage
	Meningoencephalitis
	Cerebral edema
		Hypoglycemia
		Diabetic coma
		Heat stroke
		Hepatic/uremic
		  encephalopathy
		Infectious
		Hypoxia
		Thiamine deficiency (cat)
		Heavy metal and drug
		  toxicity
		Carbon monoxide
		  poisoning

Chronic, progressive	Hemorrhage (rare) Storage diseases Hydrocephalus Encephalitis	Heavy metal toxicity

Table 3–6. Types of Abnormalities Causing Coma

Primary Brain Disease
Space-occupying lesions (neoplasm, hemorrhage, abscess)
Injury (concussion, epidural or subdural hematoma, cerebral edema, brain
  stem contusion)
Infarction (diffuse cerebral or brain stem lesion)
Infection (viral, mycotic)
Degenerative disease (lipodystrophy, terminal)
Hydrocephalus

Secondary Encephalopathy
Renal disease (uremia, acidosis)
Liver disease (hypoglycemia, hyperammonemia)
Pancreatic disease (beta cell neoplasm hypoglycemia, diabetes mellitus
  hyperglycemia, ketoacidosis)
Myocardial disease (ischemic anoxia)
Pulmonary disease (anoxic anoxia, acidosis)
Nutritional deficiency (thiamine)
Anemia (carbon monoxide poisoning, hemorrhage)
Endocrine disease (hypoadrenocorticoidism, hypothyroidism)
Postictal depression
Exogenous toxicity (hexachlorophene, cyanide, barbiturates, ethylene glycol,
  benzene hexachloride, carbon tetrachloride, lead salts, kerosene,
  nitrobenzene, turpentine, arsenic, zinc, phosphide)

Abnormal Osmotic States
Hyperosmolar states: hyperglycemia, diabetes mellitus, hypernatremia,
  diarrhea, diabetes insipidus, severe water loss
Hypo-osmolar states, such as water intoxication

Shores A, Simpson ST: Coma and stupor. *In* Ford RB, ed: Clinical Signs and Diagnosis in Small Animal Practice. New York, Churchill Livingstone, 1988, pp 269–281.

Constipation, Obstipation, Dyschezia

............DEFINITION

Infrequent or difficult passage of feces characterizes *constipation; obstipation* is intractable constipation resulting in fecal impaction through the rectum and possibly the colon. In both dogs and cats, either state is most likely to be acquired. *Dyschezia*, the act of straining to defecate or painful defecation, is the likely manifestation of constipation or obstipation and typically represents the reason for which a constipated dog or cat is presented (see Dyschezia, p. 403).

There is no strict definition of bowel regularity; therefore, there is no "normal" number of daily or weekly bowel movements, deviations from which constitute constipation. Practically, constipation can be considered to exist when a significant delay in frequency of passing formed stools has been noted or when the stool is observed to be of unusually hard or dry consistency. Constipation is categorized under one of the following headings:

- Neurogenic
- Mechanical (physical)
- Muscular (smooth muscle)
- Iatrogenic (drug-induced)

The owner who perceives a pet as straining to defecate may, in fact, be observing a pet that is straining to urinate. This is particularly true among cats with disorders of the lower urinary tract; e.g., feline urologic syndrome (FUS). In the context of this discussion, dyschezia is discussed only insofar as it is associated with constipation and obstipation. See Algorithm, p. 394.

............ASSOCIATED SIGNS

Animals with neurogenic causes of constipation may have significant perianal or rectal pain associated with focal lesions. Other patients may present with nonpainful neurologic disease or long-term complications stemming from previous pelvic or spinal trauma.

Mechanical causes are either extraluminal or intraluminal. Abdominal and rectal palpation is indicated in both male and female dogs and cats. Narrow or blood-tinged feces may signal the presence of an intraluminal lesion, whereas in patients with extraluminal lesions, associated clinical signs may not be manifested.

Muscular causes are the least common and are generally the result of extreme metabolic aberrations. Idiopathic colonic atony is reported, but constipation may also result from severe catabolic states. Laboratory evidence of endocrine disease and electrolyte abnormalities should be assessed (see p. 630).

............DIFFERENTIAL DIAGNOSIS (see Table 3–7)

............DIAGNOSTIC PLANS (see Fig. 3–2)

REFERENCES

Ford RB: Constipation and dyschezia. *In* Ford RB, ed: Clinical Signs and Diagnosis in Small Animal Practice. New York, Churchill Livingstone, 1988, pp 491– 503.

DeNovo RC: Constipation, tenesmus, dyschezia and fecal in continence. *In* Ettinger SJ, Feldman EC, eds: Textbook of Veterinary Internal Medicine, ed 4. Philadelphia, WB Saunders, 1995, pp 115–123.

Table 3–7. Differential Diagnosis of Constipation

Neurogenic Causes	*Muscular Causes*
Cortical (pain-induced)	Colonic atony
Perianal neoplasia	Severe malnutrition and cachexia
Anal sac disease	Hypothyroidism
Perianal fistulas	Hypercalcemia
Myiasis	Hyperkalemia
CNS disease	Hyperparathyroidism
Spinal trauma	Segmental dilation subsequent to
Spinal neoplasia	surgery
Degenerative myelopathy	
Peripheral nerve disease (e.g.,	*Drug-Induced Causes*
complication following pelvic trauma)	Anesthetics
	Anticholinergics (e.g., atropine)
Mechanical Causes	Anticonvulsants
Extraluminal	Barium sulfate
Prostate (neoplasia or hyperplasia)	Diuretics
Large intra-abdominal tumors	Prolonged laxative therapy
Pregnancy (?)	Monoamine oxidase inhibitors
Pelvic fracture	Heavy metal toxicity (e.g., lead)
Intraluminal	
Rectal stricture (e.g., adenocarcinoma)	*Behavioral*
Colonic stricture	Soiled or odiferous litter
Granulomas (e.g., histoplasmosis)	No litter available
Benign colorectal tumors	
Fecalith	
Rectal-colonic prolapse	
Intussusception	

3

Salisbury KS: Feline megacolon. Vet Med Rep 3:131, 1991.
Welches CD, Scavelli TD, Aronsohn M, et al: Perineal hernia in the cat: A retrospective study of 40 cases. J Am Anim Hosp Assoc 28:431, 1992.
Wheaton LG: Common questions about megacolon management. Vet Med Rep 3:161, 1991.

Cough

·········· DEFINITION

A *cough* is the sudden, forceful expiratory response to irritating stimuli (e.g., secretions) situated in the tracheobronchial tree. Cough is the most frequent clinical problem, followed by dyspnea and hemoptysis, that is referable to the lower respiratory tract. At presentation, cough should be characterized as "acute" (duration <2 weeks) or "chronic" (duration ≥2 weeks). It should be noted that attempting to define cough as productive or nonproductive can be difficult in animals and, furthermore, seems to have little value in the overall diagnostic plan.

·········· ASSOCIATED SIGNS

Although cough is a principal sign of lower respiratory tract disease, particularly lower airway (tracheal and bronchial) disease, it may also occur in animals with nonpulmonary disease, particularly cardiac and intrathoracic diseases. Associated signs, therefore, may include a wide spectrum of findings; there may also be no associated signs. Particular attention should be given to determining the character of the cough: it can be paroxysmal and severe, which usually indicates the need for immediate intervention, or mild but persistent.

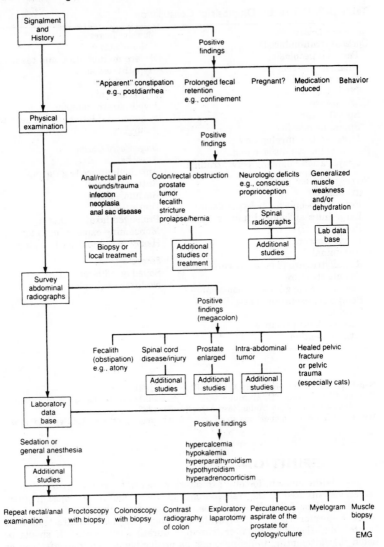

Figure 3–2. Clinical algorithm for constipation in the dog or cat. EMG, electromyogram. (From Ford RB, ed: Clinical Signs and Diagnosis in Small Animal Practice. New York, Churchill Livingstone, 1988.)

Animals in need of immediate attention are those with cough associated with syncope, dyspnea, or hemoptysis. *Orthopnea*, the inability to breathe without assuming a particular (usually upright) position, is a serious sign that suggests compromised respiratory function and also warrants immediate attention. Nasal discharge, tachypnea, and hyperpnea are less commonly associated with cough.

Cough can be misinterpreted as vomiting, particularly in dogs with tracheobronchitis. Coughing episodes in affected dogs typically terminate in the expectoration of tracheal secretions. The white, foamy phlegm expelled as the dog retches may appear to the untrained eye as vomitus.

............DIFFERENTIAL DIAGNOSIS (see Table 3–8)

............DIAGNOSTIC PLANS

1. A thorough history and physical examination, to focus on known breed and age predispositions. Physical examination is particularly valuable in determining the extent of respiratory tract involvement and characterizing the type of cough present, particularly when the cough can be elicited.
2. Careful thoracic auscultation, to determine the presence or absence of murmur or abnormal lung or airway sounds (see p. 282).
3. Thoracic radiographs, using lateral and ventrodorsal projections. These are critical, particularly when the patient has associated signs compatible with respiratory distress. Oxygen should be available to the dyspneic patient throughout the radiographic procedure. Patients with suspected tracheal collapse should be radiographed twice in the lateral position to assess changes in the intrathoracic tracheal and bronchial diameters between inspiration (open) and expiration (closed). Patients suspected of having neoplasia should undergo left and right lateral thoracic projections in addition to the ventrodorsal projection.
4. A laboratory profile, to include hematologic studies, biochemistry panel,

3

Table 3–8. Differential Diagnosis of Cough

Primary Respiratory Tract Disease	*Pulmonary Vascular Disease*
Airway diseases	Pulmonary edema (multiple
Tonsillitis and pharyngitis	causes)
Tonsillar neoplasm	Pulmonary hypertension, esp.
Pharyngeal polyp (cat)	heartworm disease
Laryngeal cyst	
Laryngeal neoplasm	*Pulmonary Parenchymal Disease*
Laryngeal paralysis	Bacterial pneumonia
Tracheobronchitis and tracheitis	Systemic mycoses (e.g.,
Tracheal hypoplasia	histoplasmosis)
Segmental tracheal stenosis	Pulmonary neoplasia
Tracheal collapse—acquired and	Pulmonary abscess
congenital	Protozoan pneumonia (e.g., feline
Tracheal neoplasia	toxoplasmosis)
Tracheal osteochondral dysplasia	Viral pneumonia
Foreign body	Allergic pneumonitis (e.g., feline
Bronchiectasis	asthma)
Bronchial collapse	Metabolic and endocrine (e.g.,
Immotile cilia syndrome	hyperadrenocorticism)
Aspiration	
Respiratory parasites (e.g.,	*Cardiovascular Diseases*
Capillaria aerophila in cats;	Left heart disease
Filaroides osleri in dogs)	Left heart failure (cardiogenic
	pulmonary edema)
	Intrathoracic Disease
	Mediastinal abscess
	Mediastinal neoplasia

fecal flotation, urinalysis, heartworm test, and the feline leukemia virus/feline immunodeficiency virus (FeLV/FIV) test in the cat (see pp. 676 and 680).
5. Special diagnostics:
   a. Primary respiratory disease: transtracheal aspiration, bronchial lavage, bronchoscopy, contrast bronchography, fluoroscopy, and radionuclide assessment of mucociliary transport (see p. 521).
   b. Primary pulmonary disease: fine-needle lung aspiration, arterial blood gases, fungal serology, nuclear studies (perfusion-ventilation), lung biopsy.
   c. Primary cardiac disease: ECG, echocardiogram (M-mode and two-dimensional), and nonselective angiography (see p. 311).

REFERENCES

Ettinger SJ, Barrett KA: Coughing. In Ettinger SJ, Feldman EC, eds: Textbook of Veterinary Internal Medicine, ed 4. Philadelphia, WB Saunders, 1995, pp 57–61.
Ford RB, Roudebush P: Chronic cough. In Ford RB, ed: Clinical Signs and Diagnosis in Small Animal Practice. New York, Churchill Livingstone, 1988, pp 203–219.

Cyanosis

..........DEFINITION

Cyanosis is the bluish discoloration of the skin and mucous membranes resulting from excessive concentration (>5 g/dL) of reduced hemoglobin in the blood. In dogs and cats, cyanosis may develop acutely in hypoxic states or may be chronic. Although cyanosis can develop during hypoxia, the terms are not synonymous.

The increased concentration of reduced hemoglobin in blood is the result of either an increase in the quantity of venous blood in the cutaneous tissues (passive venous congestion) or a decrease in oxygen saturation in capillary blood. It is the absolute, rather than the relative, amount of reduced hemoglobin that actually causes the cyanosis to develop. If the concentration of hemoglobin is also reduced, the absolute concentration of *reduced* hemoglobin is also decreased. Therefore, even in severe anemia, cyanosis is not evident. On the other hand, patients with an elevated red blood cell (RBC) mass, or polycythemia, tend to be cyanotic at higher levels of arterial oxygen saturation than patients with a normal RBC mass. Cyanosis also occurs when functional abnormalities of hemoglobin (e.g., methemoglobinemia [dark-brown blood], sulfhemoglobinemia) exist. In the dog and cat, disorders affecting the oxygen-carrying capacity of hemoglobin are usually drug- or chemical-induced. As little as 1.5 g/dL of methemoglobin or 0.5 g/dL of sulfhemoglobin will produce cyanosis.

..........ASSOCIATED SIGNS

Cyanosis can result from disorders affecting the cardiovascular system, ventilation, or oxygen-carrying capacity of RBCs. Several cardiovascular diseases, particularly those that compromise cardiac output or are associated with right-to-left vascular shunts, predispose to cyanosis. Therefore, animals with both acquired and congenital cardiac disease are susceptible. Associated signs include cough, respiratory distress, and syncope. The most common congenital heart defects associated with right-to-left shunts are (1) pulmonary valve stenosis as seen in tetralogy of Fallot, stenosis, and ventricular septal defect, (VSD); and (2) pulmonary hypertension as seen in patent ductus arteriosus (PDA) and VSD.

Respiratory disorders affecting ventilation predispose to cyanosis. Severe infiltrative lung disease (e.g., neoplasia, pulmonary edema, or generalized pneumonia) can produce cyanosis associated with increased respiratory effort.

Animals that do present with cyanosis not associated with clinical signs other than increased respiratory rate may have abnormal hemoglobin levels which, if present in sufficient concentration, will cause cyanosis. Associated signs include methemoglobinuria and methemoglobinemia.

Central cyanosis is defined as compromised oxygen saturation or abnormal hemoglobin; *peripheral cyanosis* is compromised blood flow.

⋯⋯⋯⋯ DIFFERENTIAL DIAGNOSIS
⋯⋯⋯⋯ DIAGNOSTIC PLANS

1. Provide 100% oxygen, particularly in patients with respiratory distress. Reassess color of the mucous membranes at 2- or 3-minute intervals. Auscultate the heart and lungs (see pp. 282 and 610).
2. Thoracic radiographs. Oxygen should be available at all times.
3. Hematologic studies, with particular emphasis on RBC morphology (Heinz bodies in the cat and hematocrit values), biochemical profile, and urinalysis (see pp. 662 and 772).
4. Special diagnostics: arterial blood gases (with and without 100% oxygen), ECG, echocardiogram, and nonselective angiogram (see p. 282).

REFERENCE

Jacobs G: Cyanosis. *In* Ettinger SJ, Feldman EC, eds: Textbook of Veterinary Internal Medicine, ed 4. Philadelphia, WB Saunders, 1995, pp 192–197.

Deafness, Hearing Loss

⋯⋯⋯⋯ DEFINITION

Loss of hearing, either partial or complete, in one or both ears does occur in both dogs and cats but is particularly difficult to confirm. Partial loss of hearing occurs most commonly in older animals but is rarely confirmed. Deafness is generally first detected by astute owners who observe diminished or absent responses to noise in an animal with no previous history of hearing difficulty.

Deafness can result from abnormalities at any one of several levels from the ear to the brain. *Peripheral deafness* is categorized as either *conduction deafness*, involving abnormalities of the transduction apparatus (external ear canal, tympanic membrane, auditory ossicles in the middle ear), or *nerve deafness*, involving the hearing receptors in the cochlea or the auditory branch of the eighth cranial nerve. *Congenital deafness* is usually nerve deafness and is the result of abnormal development of the spiral organ or auditory receptors. CNS hearing loss is uncommon, since auditory pathways in the brain are multisynaptic.

⋯⋯⋯⋯ ASSOCIATED SIGNS

Although rare, invasive lesions or panencephalitis could conceivably cause central hearing loss. However, the associated neurologic signs would be extensive and hearing loss becomes a secondary or insignificant clinial issue.

Animals with peripheral hearing loss due to acquired unilateral lesions may manifest a variety of signs referable to the vestibular apparatus, particularly head tilt and, less often, circling. Pain or increased sensitivity may be associated with invasive lesions affecting hearing in either ear. Physical evidence of otitis externa is readily detected during routine examinations. Severe swelling associated with a chronic inflammation, a ruptured or damaged tympanic membrane, and infections of the middle ear may effectively decrease hearing acuity. Hypothyroidism may also be associated with degeneration of the cochlea and subsequent decrease in hearing acuity. The clinical history is important and should include any prior exposure to drugs known to be toxic to the cochlear nerve and organ of Corti (e.g., aminoglycosides).

Congenital (hereditary) deafness is associated with a white or merle hair coat in both dogs and cats. In dogs, the highest incidence is in the Dalmatian. However, several breeds are reported to be affected.

............DIFFERENTIAL DIAGNOSIS (see Table 3–9)

............DIAGNOSTIC PLANS

1. Assessment of response to noise while the animal is relaxed or asleep.
2. Thorough physical examination, particularly of the external ear canal and tympanic membrane.
3. Neurologic examination.
4. Assessment of thyroid hormone levels (see p. 639).
5. Radiography of the head, with particular emphasis on the tympanic bullae, for evidence of otitis media.
6. Electrophysiologic studies, including electroencephalography, tympanometry, and auditory evoked potentials (BAER test).

REFERENCES

Knowles K: Deafness. *In* Morgan RV, ed: Handbook of Small Animal Practice, ed 3. Philadelphia, WB Saunders, 1997, pp 1104–1108.
Lorenz MD, Cornelius LM: Small Animal Medical Diagnosis, ed 2. Philadelphia, JB Lippincott, 1991.
Strain GM: Congenital deafness in dogs and cats. Comp Contin Educ Pract Vet 13:245–253, 1991.

Table 3–9. Differential Diagnosis of Deafness

Acquired Hearing Loss
Degenerative causes
  Neurogenic deafness in the geriatric dog and cat
  Subsequent to chronic inflammatory disease (?)
Metabolic (endocrine) causes
  Hypothyroidism
Neoplastic causes
  Invasive tumors of the pharynx and retropharyngeal tissue
Infectious-inflammatory causes
  Otitis externa and media
  Canine distemper virus infection
  Protothecosis (in the dog)
Toxic
  Aminoglycoside antimicrobials, especially gentamicin, streptomycin, and neomycin
Traumatic
Idiopathic

Congenital Hearing Loss—Breed Predisposition
White, blue-eyed cats (may be unilateral or bilateral)
Several breeds affected, particularly those with a white or merle hair coat

Decreased Urine Production: Oliguria and Anuria

...........DEFINITION

Reduced amount of urine production and output in relation to fluid intake defines *oliguria*. Affected patients are said to be oliguric. Patients in which urine production ceases have *anuria*, or are considered to be anuric. In contrast to polyuric states, neither oliguria nor anuria is likely to be the primary problem for which a dog or cat is presented to a veterinarian. The metabolic consequences of decreased urine production are severe and generally represent significant compromises in renal blood flow or in the functional status of a critical nephron mass. If this condition is sustained, the patient will die.

The daily urine volume at which oliguria begin is a function of solute load and renal concentrating ability. In general, oliguria exists when daily urine production is reduced by 75% or more. Production of 0.5 to 1.0 mL/kg/hr of urine is indicative of adequate renal perfusion in the dog. Anuria begins or terminates with oliguria; therefore, early detection and treatment of the underlying cause are critical to the overall prognosis.

...........ASSOCIATED SIGNS

The problem(s) for which an oliguric or anuric patient is presented will likely be related to the metabolic consequences of compromised renal function. Uremia, characterized by vomiting, hematemesis, diarrhea, lethargy, or anorexia, predominates. Any one or a combination of signs may at the time of initial examination. Some patients may present in a comatose or semiconscious state, in which case it is essential that renal function and urinary output be established immediately (see p. 772).

Since acute renal failure (ARF) is the principal differential diagnosis in oliguria and anuria, once it has been established the clinician must obtain a thorough clinical history and laboratory profile, including urinalysis if possible, in an attempt to determine the cause of renal failure and to institute corrective therapy.

...........DIFFERENTIAL DIAGNOSIS (see Table 3–10)
...........DIAGNOSTIC PLANS

1. Initiation of fluid therapy and placement of an indwelling urinary catheter, to establish the rate of urine production (see p. 585).
2. History, to address any possible exposure to toxins, particularly antifreeze, as well as recent drug treatment.
3. Radiographs of the abdomen. These may reveal enlarged kidneys, thereby supporting a diagnosis of ARF. Do not rule out the diagnosis of ARF if kidney size appears normal. Ultrasound imaging of kidneys is also helpful in establishing diagnosis.
4. Complete blood count (CBC). The biochemical profile should include electrolytes as well as blood urea nitrogen (BUN) and creatinine levels. Urinalysis (must include urine specific gravity) with microscopic examination of sediment for evidence of crystalluria, RBCs, white blood cells (WBCs), and casts is essential even if only a small volume of urine can be obtained.
5. Blood gases, to assess for metabolic acidosis, which may be severe in ARF (see p. 591).
6. Urine protein-creatinine ratio, to assess proteinuria (see p. 781).
7. If possible, determinations of serum osmolality and serum osmole gap.
8. Special diagnostics: intravenous pyelogram (IVP), renal biopsy, and determinations of lead and other heavy metals in the blood as indicated.

Table 3–10. Differential Diagnosis of Acute Renal Failure

Inflammatory-Infectious Causes
Leptospirosis
Pyelonephritis
Immune complex glomerulonephritis
   Systemic lupus erythematosus
   Heartworm disease
   Pyometra
   Endocarditis
   Feline leukemia virus infection
Viral
   Canine distemper virus infection
   Infectious canine hepatitis infection (rare)
   Canine herpesvirus infection (rare)

Primary Renal Causes (Nephroses)
Hypoperfusion (ischemia)
Extreme dehydration
Hemorrhage
Trauma
Sepsis
Surgery
Thromboembolic diseases

Nephrotoxins
Heavy metals (lead, arsenic, thallium, mercury)
Carbon tetrachloride
Ethylene glycol (antifreeze)
Aminoglycoside antibacterials (amikacin, gentamicin)
Antibiotics (cephaloridine, amphotericin B)
Hypercalcemia
Anesthetics (fluoride metabolites of methoxyflurane)

REFERENCES

Brown SA, Grauer GF: Acute renal failure. *In* Morgan RV, ed: Handbook of Small Animal Practice. Philadelphia, WB Saunders, 1997, pp 508–512.
Chew DJ, DiBartola SP: Renal failure. *In* Fenner WR, ed: Quick Reference to Veterinary Medicine, ed 2. Philadelphia, JB Lippincott, 1991, pp 216–238.
Osborne C, Finco D: Canine and Feline Nephrology and Urology. Baltimore, Williams & Wilkins, 1997.

Diarrhea, Acute

···········DEFINITION

The term *diarrhea* not only denotes the pattern of defecation characterized by passage of unformed stool but also applies to an increase in the frequency of defecation and in the volume of stool whether or not stool has form. Establish whether the diarrhea is acute or chronic. *Acute diarrhea* can be defined as a sudden change in bowel pattern, characterized as increased fluidity, frequency, or volume, that is sustained for 1 to 2 weeks despite empiric or supportive therapy (see also Diarrhea, Chronic).

Fundamentally, diarrhea occurs when the amount of water and other intestinal contents reaching the colon exceeds the ability of the colon to store the feces and adequately remove the excess water. *Osmotic diarrhea* is common in small animal pratice and occurs as the osmotic gradient in the bowel favors the movement of water into the gut lumen over that of absorption. Disorders of digestion and absorption readily generate such an intraluminal osmotic gradient. In simple osmotic diarrhea, clinical signs should resolve when the patient is fasted and the osmotic gradient equilibrates. Diarrhea may also result from *abnormal gut permeability*. In health, fluid constantly moves from the vascular system into the gut lumen and is reabsorbed. Normally, the net effect favors absorption, yet the volume of fluid exchange per day is very large. Disease affecting this fluid homeostasis, depending on the region of the bowel affected, have the ability to alter the consistency of the stool. Inflammatory lesions of the intestine alter mucosal permeability and promote exudation into the gut lumen.

 Secretory diarrhea results from the effect of various substances (e.g., enterotoxins, gut hormones) that act as secretagogues. The gut is stimulated to secrete fluids without concurrent changes in permeability, absorptive capacity, motility, or osmotic gradients. *Abnormal bowel motility* may occur in several primary disorders of the gastrointestinal (GI) tract, but it appears unlikely that abnormal motility is a primary cause of diarrhea. Normally, peristaltic contractions move chyme aborally, whereas segmental activity retards the movement of chyme, thereby performing the important functions of mixing intestinal contents and maximizing contact with the brush border enzyme systems. As segmental contractions are diminished, intestinal contents flow freely through the flaccid gut.

 In the patient with acute diarrhea, it is conceivable that only one of these mechanisms is involved. However, the longer the underlying cause of the diarrhea persists, the more likely that homeostatic and compensatory mechanisms will be overwhelmed. The pathogenesis of the patient's diarrhea is then related to a combination of events.

············ASSOCIATED SIGNS

Acute diarrhea is a common presenting sign for which a multitude of diagnostic possibilities exist. The list of associated signs can be, in the clinical setting, extensive. Among the most common signs encountered in an animal presented for acute diarrhea are vomiting, dehydration, slight weight loss, and hematochezia. Abdominal pain, halitosis, flatulence, and borborygmus are other gut-associated signs. However, not all patients with acute diarrhea have primary intestinal disease, such as those with renal or hepatic failure or hypoadrenocorticism. Therefore, icterus, oral ulcers, muscle weakness, and so on, may also be encountered. Fever, anorexia, and lethargy may also accompany acute diarrhea in the dog and cat.

············DIFFERENTIAL DIAGNOSIS
············DIAGNOSTIC PLANS

1. Thorough history and physical examination, including abdominal palpation. Establish possible exposure to infectious agents and associated signs.
2. Intravenous fluids, which may be a critical part of the early evaluation in severely dehydrated patients.
3. Laboratory profile, to include routine hematology valves, biochemistry profile (to include amylase or lipase and sodium and potassium), urinalysis, examination of feces (direct and flotation). Perform several examinations before ruling out parasitic disease. Cats should be tested for both FeLV and FIV. Dogs should be tested for parvovirus antigen in stool.
4. Abdominal radiographs.
5. Special diagnostic tests as indicated: duodenoscopy and mucosal biopsy;

stool culture for viruses or bacteria; serologic studies for rickettsial, viral, and fungal disease; and abdominal laparotomy (see p. 16).

REFERENCES

Guilford BG, Center SA, Strombeck DR, Williams DA, Myer DJ, eds: Strombeck's Small Animal Gastroenterology, ed 3. Philadelphia, WB Saunders, 1996.
Jergens AE: Diarrhea. *In* Ettinger SJ, Feldman EC, eds: Textbook of Veterinary Internal Medicine, ed 4. Philadelphia, WB Saunders, 1995, pp 111–114.
Lorenz MD, Cornelius LM: Small Animal Medical Diagnosis, ed 2. Philadelphia, JB Lippincott, 1991.
Pidgeon GL: Acute onset diarrhea. *In* Ford RB, ed: Clinical Signs and Diagnosis in Small Animal Practice. New York, Churchill Livingstone, 1988, pp 437–451.

Diarrhea, Chronic

·········· DEFINITION

Chronic diarrhea can be defined as a persistent or gradual change in bowel pattern, characterized as increased fluidity, frequency, or volume of stool, that is sustained for more than 2 weeks despite empiric or supportive therapy (see also Diarrhea, Acute). In the clinical setting, the clinical history and associated signs can be used to further characterize chronic diarrhea as *large bowel* or *small bowel*.

·········· ASSOCIATED SIGNS

Clinical differentiation of small bowel and large bowel diarrhea is fundamentally important for the diagnosis and treatment of chronic diarrhea (Table 3–11).

Less specific signs associated with chronic diarrheal diseases include dehy-

Table 3–11. Clinical Differentiation of Diarrhea of the Small Bowel and Large Bowel Types

Clinical Signs	Small Bowel	Large Bowel
Fecal volume	Markedly increased daily output (large quantity of bulky or watery feces with each defecation)	Normal or slightly increased daily output (small quantities with each defecation)
Frequency of defecation	Normal or slightly increased	Very frequent: 4–10 times/day
Urgency of tenesmus	Rare	Common
Mucus in feces	Rare	Common
Blood in feces	Dark black (digested)	Red (fresh)
Steatorrhea (malassimilation)	May be present	Absent
Weight loss and emaciation	Usual	Rare
Flatulence	May be present	Absent
Vomiting	Occasional	Occasional

From Sherding RG: Chronic diarrhea. *In* Ford RB, ed: Clinical Signs and Diagnosis in Small Animal Practice. New York, Churchill Livingstone, 1988, p 466.

dration, poor-quality hair coat, and fever. On abdominal palpation, discrete masses, thickened bowel loops, pain, or gas may occasionally be detected. Edema, ascites, and pleural effusion in patients with chronic diarrhea suggest substantial protein losses through the bowel. The patient with pallor should be assessed for intestinal bleeding, as well as an anemia of chronic inflammatory disease (see p. 656).

Hematologic signs of most significance include eosinophilia (allergic or inflammatory) and lymphopenia (lymphangiectasia). Hypoproteinemia is associated with extreme malnutrition, protein-losing enteropathies, and enteric blood loss. Hyperglobulinemia is associated with basenji enteropathy.

··········DIFFERENTIAL DIAGNOSIS (see Table 3–12)
··········DIAGNOSTIC PLANS

1. Clinical history and physical examination findings, to classify the diarrhea as small bowel or large bowel. Routine patient screening should include hematologic studies, biochemical profile, fecal flotation and direct examination, and urinalysis (see pp. 761 and 772).
2. Diagnosis of intestinal parasites. Perform a visual examination of the feces and anus for proglottids, a zinc sulfate flotation test for *Giardia* and *Coccidia* cysts, a saline suspension for protozoan trophozoites, and a sedimentation or Baermann determination for *Strongyloides* larvae. Adult whipworms can be seen in the colon on colonscopy (see p. 521).
3. Additional fecal studies. Beyond routine fecal flotation and direct examination, several other fecal tests are indicated, including microscopic examinations for fat (Sudan preparation), starch (iodine preparation), and cytologic staining (Gram stain and Wright's stain) to assess for presence of leukocytes and infectious agents. Malassimilation can be assessed through quantitative fecal fat analysis and fecal weight (daily output), although in clinical practice these tests are seldom performed. Several special biochemical and physical tests can also be carried out on feces: fecal water content, nitrogen content (for azotorrhea and malassimilation), electrolytes, pH, osmolality, fecal occult blood, and cultures for both fungi and bacteria.
4. Tests of absorptive and digestive function, such as trypsin-like immunoreactivity (TLI), serum folate, and vitamin B_{12} assay (see p. 764).
5. GI radiography and ultrasonography.
6. GI endoscopy (gastroscopy, duodenoscopy, and colonoscopy), with biopsy of intestinal mucosa. Duodenal intubation and aspiration can be performed to obtain specimens for cytologic examination and culture.
7. Exploratory laparotomy and intestinal biopsy.
8. Response to empiric treatment: Enzyme replacement or treatment of occult parasite infections.

REFERENCES

Burrows CF: Canine colitis. Compend Contin Educ Pract Vet 14:1347, 1992.
Jacobs G: Lymphocytic plasmacytic enteritis in 24 dogs. J Vet Intern Med 4:45, 1990.
Jergens AE: Diarrhea. *In* Ettinger SJ, Feldman EC, eds: Textbook of Veterinary Internal Medicine, ed 4. Philadelphia, WB Saunders, 1995, pp 111–114.
Leib MS: Inflammatory bowel disease. Semin Vet Med 7:1992.
Sherding RG: Chronic diarrhea. *In* Ford RB, ed: Clinical Signs and Diagnosis in Small Animal Practice. New York, Churchill Livingstone, 1988, pp 453–489.

Dyschezia

··········DEFINITION

Dyschezia refers to painful or difficult evacuation of feces from the rectum. In the clinical setting, dyschezia may be a difficult problem to ascertain unless

Table 3–12. Diagnosis of Specific Chronic Diarrheal Disorders

Diarrhea	Diagnostic Test/Procedure
Small Bowel Type	
Exocrine, pancreatic insufficiency	Serum trypsin-like immunoreactivity (TLI)
Chronic inflammatory small bowel disease	
Eosinophilic enteritis	Eosinophilia, biopsy
Lymphocytic-plasmacytic enteritis	Biopsy
	Serum protein electrophoresis
Immunoproliferative enteropathy of basenjis	Radiography, biopsy
Granulomatous enteritis	
Lymphangiectasia	Lymphopenia, biopsy
Villous atrophy	
Gluten enteropathy	Response to gluten-free diet
Idiopathic	Biopsy
Histoplasmosis	Serology, cytology, biopsy
Lymphosarcoma	Biopsy
Bacterial overgrowth syndrome	Culture intestinal aspirate, folate, response to antibiotics
Giardiasis	Fecal examinations, response to parasiticides
Lactase deficiency	Response to lactose-free diet
Large Bowel Type	
Chronic colitis	Colonoscopy, colon biopsy
Idiopathic	
Histiocytic	
Eosinophilic	
Abrasive colitis	Dietary history, inspection of feces
Whipworm colitis	Fecal flotation, colonoscopy, response to fenbendazole
Protozoan colitis	Saline fecal smears
Amebiasis	
Balantidiasis	
Trichomoniasis	
Histoplasma colitis	Fecal cytology, colon biopsy, serology, culture
Salmonella colitis	Culture
Campylobacter colitis	Culture
Prototothecal colitis	Colon biopsy
Rectocolonic polyps	Digital palpation, barium enema
Colonic adenocarcinoma	Colonscopy, barium enema, possibly abdominal ultrasound
Colonic lymphosarcoma	Barium enema, colonoscopy
Functional diarrhea (irritable colon)	History, diagnostic workup excludes all other diseases

the owner is particularly astute and is able to distinguish effort to urinate (see Dysuria) from effort to defecate in cats and female dogs. Therefore, a concerted effort on the part of the clinician is usually necessary to differentiate disorders affecting the urinary outflow tract and micturition from disorders affecting defecation.

The most likely cause for any animal to present with dyschezia is rectal or perianal pain. The origin of the pain may be mucosal, mucocutaneous (anal), or extraluminal lesions. Rectal strictures are uncommon but may contribute to constipation and associated dyschezia. Strictures typically develop subsequent to neoplasia or deep, nonpenetrating injury to the rectum. Although uncommon, dyschezia may also occur subsequent to lesions in the lumbar spinal cord or sacrum.

···········ASSOCIATED SIGNS

The most common response to dyschezia is constipation, although many owners do not recognize this as a primary problem. Not uncommonly, the pain associated with rectal lesions is intense during attempts to defecate. The animal may cry or turn abruptly and lick the anus in response to the pain. Dogs may circle while assuming the position to defecate. Cats are more likely to make many attempts at defecation or may manifest inappropriate defecation in locations outside of the litter box. Unless attempting defecation, the animal is likely not to manifest pain at all.

Physical examination should include digital examinaation of the rectum and inspection of the perineum and each anal sac for evidence of lesions. It is **3** important to consider shaving the perineum to assess the integrity of the skin for evidence of lesions, particularly neoplasia.

···········DIFFERENTIAL DIAGNOSIS (see Table 3–13)
···········DIAGNOSTIC PLANS

1. History and physical examination, to determine the ability of the patient to urinate vs. defecate. Physical examination must include:
   a. Rectal temperature, as a means of detecting source of pain.

Table 3–13. Differential Diagnosis of Dyschezia

Constipation (see Table 3–7)
Idiopathic Ulcerative and Inflammatory Lesions   Colon (colitis)   Rectum (proctitis)   Anal sacs (determined at surgery)
Neoplasia   Mucosa (e.g., carcinoma)   Intestinal wall (e.g., carcinoma, sarcoma)   Extramural (intra-abdominal prostate)   Anal glands   Perineum (particularly skin/mucocutaneous tissues)
Direct Rectal Injury   With stricture formation   Without stricture formation (e.g., linear foreign body)
Perineal Hernia

    b. Rectal examination, expressing both anal glands and assessing the character of the discharge (sedation may be required).

    c. Evaluation of the perianal skin (shaving the perineum is recommended).

2. Fecal examination for occult blood.
3. Abdominal radiographs, to assess prostate size (in male dogs only), intra-abdominal masses, and presence of fecalith formation.
4. Colonoscopy or proctoscopy, with rigid or flexible endoscope and biopsy of any obvious lesions. Recovered tissues should be examined cytologically and by histopathology. Anesthesia is rarely required for this procedure unless the integrity of the rectal mucosa is substantially compromised or pain is significant.
5. Rarely, exploratory laparotomy, to further elucidate the nature of abnormal intra-abdominal findings.

REFERENCES

DeNovo RC: Constipation, tenesmus, dyschezia, and fecal incontinence. *In* Ettinger SJ, Feldman EC, eds: Textbook of Veterinary Internal Medicine, ed 4. Philadelphia, WB Saunders, 1995, pp 115–122.

Dennis JS, Kruger JM, Mullaney TA: Lymphocytic plasmacytic colitis in cats: 14 cases. J Am Vet Med Assoc 202:313, 1993.

Dysphagia

............DEFINITION

Dysphagia refers to painful or difficult swallowing. Clinically, dysphagic animals characteristically are presented for making frequent forced attempts to swallow with or without regurgitation. Signs are most apparent immediately following prehension of food or water.

    Swallowing is a complex reflex requiring coordination of multiple muscular and neurologic reactions involving the tongue, palate, pharynx, larynx, esophagus, and gastroesophageal junction. The swallowing reflex is coordinated by cranial nerves V, VII, IX, X, and XI; therefore, neurologic lesions affecting nuclei in the brain stem and reticular formation can alter normal swallowing.

    Dysphagia may occur as a result of disorders affecting any one of the three swallowing phases:

1. Oropharyngeal.
2. Esophageal.
3. Gastroesophageal.

    Both morphologic as well as functional lesions affecting the oropharynx, esophagus, stomach, and brain or brain stem may result in dysphagia.

    Functional or motility disorders that affect swallowing include spasticity, incoordination, or failure of muscular contractions, and they result from neurologic disorders, disorders of neuromuscular transmission, or primary muscle disease. Such disorders may be either congenital or acquired. Disorders affecting the oropharyngeal phase of swallowing are responsible for causing pronounced dysphagia, whereas disorders affecting the esophageal and gastroesophageal phases of swallowing are associated with regurgitation.

............ASSOCIATED SIGNS

Dysphagia is observed in young animals, particularly in association with congenital esophageal motility disorders and as an acquired condition in older animals. This is more common as a presenting sign in dogs than in cats. There is no sex predisposition.

Prehension of food in animals presented for dysphagia is characteristically normal. Hypersalivation may occasionally be reported, particularly in animals with nasal discharge associated with regurgitation.

Regurgitation is an inconsistent sign associated with dysphagia that does not necessarily correlate with the severity of the underlying disorder. Generally, regurgitation is a consequence of abnormalities of the esophageal and gastroesophageal phases of swallowing. Although most dysphagic patients have a normal to increased appetite (polyphagia), anorexia, weight loss, and coughing may be associated with severe or chronic obstructive esophageal disease or esophageal ulceration.

···········DIFFERENTIAL DIAGNOSIS (see Table 3–14)
···········DIAGNOSTIC PLANS

1. Observation of the patient's attempt to swallow food and water.
2. Hematologic studies, a biochemistry profile, and urinalysis. Findings are usually of little diagnostic value but are important in assessing overall patient status. A fecal flotation test for parasite ova can be diagnostic for *Spirocerca lupi*.
3. Special laboratory tests, including antinuclear antibody (ANA) titer and lupus erythematosus (LE) cell results, to assess for the presence of immune-mediated disease. Serum thyroxine (T_4) and thyroid-stimulating hormone (TSH) tests are indicated to rule out peripheral neuropathy due to primary hypothyroidism (see p. 639).
4. Noncontrast thoracic *and* cervical radiographs.
5. Positive contrast esophogram, both thoracic and cervical.
6. Esophagoscopy, which may be therapeutic if esophageal foreign body can be retrieved. Esophageal endoscopy is not a reliable means for diagnosing megaesophagus (see p. 521).

3

Table 3–14. Differential Diagnosis of Dysphagia

Cardiovascular
Megaesophagus secondary to congenital persistent fourth aortic arch

Lymphatic and Immune
Mandibular, retropharyngeal, and less commonly bronchial lymphadenopathy associated with lymphosarcoma, thymic neoplasia in FeLV-positive cats, and systemic mycoses (histoplasmosis or blastomycosis)
Epidermolysis bullosa–induced esophagitis (rare)

Gastrointestinal
Esophageal obstruction due to foreign body, parasitic granuloma (*Spirocerca lupi*), stricture, esophageal neoplasia
Cricopharyngeal achalasia (young dogs)
Megaesophagus secondary to pyloric obstruction in cats
Esophageal diverticula
Traumatic esophageal rupture
Reflux esophagitis
Feline herpesvirus–induced esophagitis (rare)

Neurologic
Congenital and acquired megaesophagus
Myasthenia gravis in dogs
Rabies virus infection

FeLV, feline leukemia virus.

7. Fluoroscopic evaluation of esophageal motility.
8. Visual examination of the oropharynx in the anesthetized patient. (Findings are of low diagnostic value).

REFERENCES

Guilford WG, Strombeck DR: Diseases of Swallowing. *In* Gilford WG, Center SA, Strombeck DR, et al, eds: Strombeck's Small Animal Gastroenterology, ed 3. Philadelphia, WB Saunders, 1996, pp 211–238.
Jergens AE: Diseases of the esophagus. *In* Morgan RV, ed: Handbook of Small Animal Practice, ed 3. Philadelphia, WB Saunders, 1996, pp 323–333.

Dysuria

............DEFINITION

Dysuria, characterized by painful or difficult urination, is a relatively common presenting sign in both dogs and cats. Until the patient has been thoroughly evaluated, dysuria should be regarded as an urgent situation worthy of immediate attention. Owner observations are not entirely reliable in describing dysuria. Therefore, physical examination is usually necessary to differentiate attempts to defecate from attempts to urinate and to distinguish between incontinence and dysuria.

Dysuria generally results from disorders of the lower urinary tract (bladder or urethra) or genital tract (prostate or vagina), or both, that induce an impediment to urinary outflow resulting in abnormal micturition or inappropriate urination. However, a variety of neurologic lesions, particularly lesions in the caudal lumbar spine and sacrum affecting either parasympathetic or sympathetic innervation to the lower urinary tract, can result in dysuria. Neurologic dysurias are among the most difficult to characterize and to treat.

............ASSOCIATED SIGNS

Clinical signs associated with dysuria can often be localized to the point of the primary lesion in the lower genitourinary tract. Dysuria is commonly associated with discolored urine (particularly hematuria), pyuria, or both, subsequent to mucosal inflammation and infection. Certain causes of urinary incontinence may also result in dysuria. The owner may also report frequent attempts at urination by the animal.

Distinguish between two additional clinical signs associated with dysuria: *polyuria* (increased volume) vs. *pollakiuria* (increased frequency). Patients with dysuria may also manifest *strangury*, defined as a slow, painful discharge of urine caused by spasm of the bladder and urethra. In male dogs, dysuria caused by an enlarged prostate may also be associated with constipation.

............DIFFERENTIAL DIAGNOSIS (see Table 3–15)

............DIAGNOSTIC PLANS

1. Preliminary measures. The initial diagnostic plan depends on confirmation of dysuria at presentation and whether, on abdominal palpation, the urinary bladder is empty or distended (Fig. 3–3).
2. Routine hematology and biochemical profile (see pp. 651 and 718).
3. Urinalysis, with specific attention to color, specific gravity, protein, glucose, occult blood, and microscopic evaluation of urine sediment (see p. 772).
4. Radiography of the abdomen, including the lower urinary tract. Follow nondiagnostic studies with contrast radiography of the lower urinary tract

Table 3–15. Differential Diagnosis of Dysuria

Infectious and Inflammatory Causes	*Congenital* (continued)
Bacterial cystitis	Urethra
Urethritis	Transitional cell carcinoma
Prostatitis/benign prostatic	Transmissible venereal tumor
hyperplasia (male dog)	Vagina and penis
Vaginitis	Transmissible venereal tumor
Feline urologic syndrome	Fibroma
	Sarcoma
Cystic and Urethral Calculi	Carcinoma
Neoplasia	*Trauma*
Urinary bladder	Ruptured bladder
Transitional cell carcinoma	Urethral laceration (bite wound,
Rhabdomyoma or fibrosarcoma	calculus)
Prostatic carcinoma	Urethral stricture
Congenital	*Neurologic Causes*
Ectopic ureters (esp. female)	Reflex dyssynergia
Various vaginal malformations	Vesicular-urethral asynchronization

(contrast urethrography, contrast cystography, and double-contrast cystography).

REFERENCES

Guilford WG, Center SA, Strombeck DR, Williams DA, Myer DJ, eds: Strombeck's Small Animal Gastroenterology, ed 3. Philadelphia, WB Saunders, 1996.

Lorenz MD, Cornelius LM: Small Animal Medical Diagnosis, ed. 2. Philadelphia, JB Lippincott, 1991.

Lulich JP, Osborne CA: Diseases of the urinary bladder. In Morgan RV, ed: Handbook of Small Animal Practice. ed 3. Philadelphia, WB Saunders, 1996, pp 531–543.

Wolf AM: Hematuria and dysuria. In Ford RB, ed: Clinical Signs and Diagnosis in Small Animal Practice. New York, Churchill Livingstone, 1988, pp 541–563.

Edema, Peripheral

··········DEFINITION

Edema is the abnormal accumulation in the volume of fluid within a defined tissue space. Peripheral edema refers to a pathologic increase in the fluid volume of the interstitium of soft tissue. Generally, the distribution pattern of peripheral edema can be characterized as generalized, regional, or focal.

Physiologically, the distinction bewteen normal and abnormal increases in interstitial fluid volumes is difficult to establish clinically. Moderate to severe increases (30%) in interstitial fluid volume are evident on visual examination of the patient as a result of the physical changes in the tissue caused by the fluid. Any increase in the interstitial fluid volume identified by any means (e.g., histopathology, physical examination) constitutes peripheral edema.

Albumin is the smallest plasma protein and is the primary source of plasma colloidal oncotic pressure. Edema may become clinically evident as the serum albumin concentration falls below 2 g/dL. However, other factors are also involved in the formation of edema, such as decreased plasma volume and increased extracellular space associated with decreased renal excretion of sodium.

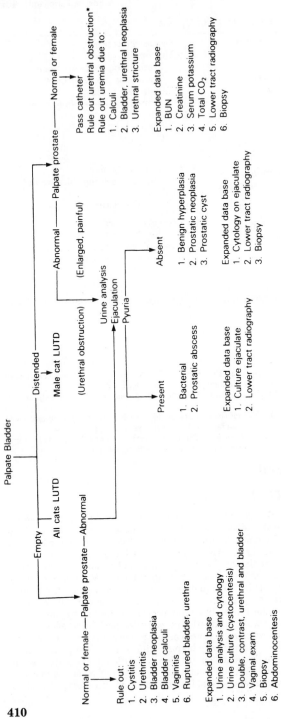

Figure 3–3. Algorithm for the differential diagnosis of dysuria. LUTD, lower urinary tract disease; BUN, blood urea nitrogen. (From Lorenz MD, Cornelius LM, eds: Small Animal Medical Diagnosis Philadelphia, JB Lippincott, 1987.)

* If no obstruction exists, pursue bladder detrusor or neurologic dysfunction.

...........ASSOCIATED SIGNS

Patients that are presented with peripheral edema may manifest other signs. Evidence of chronic inflammatory disease, vasculitis, cardiac disease, allergy, or trauma (including burns) should be considered. Patients with peripheral edema may also have primary protein-losing (renal or GI) disorders. These patients may be presented with increased water consumption or urination or diarrhea and weight loss. Severe hepatic disease may result in diminished synthesis of albumin, thereby contributing to the formation of edema.

...........DIFFERENTIAL DIAGNOSIS (see Table 3–16)
...........DIAGNOSTIC PLANS

1. History and physical examination, to focus on cardiac, hepatic, GI, and urinary system disease. Particular attention is given to the presence of jugular vein distention or pulsations, tachycardia, and ascites.
2. Clinical pathology.
   a. Routine hematology.
   b. Biochemical profile, including electrolytes, total protein, and albumin.
   c. Urinalysis (see p. 772).
   d. Urine protein-creatinine ratio.
3. Special laboratory testing, as indicated:

Table 3–16. Differential Diagnosis of Edema

Increased Capillary Hydrostatic Pressure
Functional or structural obstruction to blood flow
  Congestive heart failure
  Venous obstruction
  Compression of a vessel by a mass lesion
Arteriovenous fistula

Decreased Capillary Oncotic Pressure (Hypoalbuminemia)
Protein-losing enteropathies
Protein-losing nephropathies
Decreased hepatic synthesis
Decreased dietary intake (protein malnutrition)
Chronic hemorrhage
Exudative lesion with large surface (e.g., burns, peritonitis)

Permeability
Chronic inflammatory disease
Vasculitis
Vascular trauma
Toxins
Infections
Neurogenic, physical, or other vasoactive stimuli

Decreased Lymphatic Drainage (Lymphedema)
Congenital (primary) lymphedema—an autosomal dominant
  trait primarily affecting the hindlimbs by 3–6 mo of age
Acquired (secondary) lymphedema (focal or regional)
Infectious, granulomatous, neoplastic, traumatic injury, or
  compression of lymphatics

Increased Interstitial Gel Matrix
Myxedema (hypothyroidism)—rare

a. Bile acids.
b. Quantitative urinary clearance studies (see p. 780).
c. Serology—viral or rickettsial infections.
d. ANA titer, LE cell preparation, and rheumatoid factor assay (see p. 703).
4. Central venous pressure (CVP) (see p. 519).
5. Radiography:
   a. Thorax. Look for evidence of pericardial effusion, pleural effusion, or cardiac disease.
   b. Abdomen. Look for liver or mass lesions in particular, and peritonitis.
   c. Abdominal ultrasound.
6. Contrast radiography. Angiograms or lymphangiograms are indicated to confirm an obstructive lesion or the presence of an arteriovenous fistula.
7. Serologic studies, particularly for ehrlichiosis and Rocky Mountain spotted fever.
8. Edema fluid analysis. Collect by direct insertion of a 22-gauge needle into edematous tissue. A sample is collected into plain and edetic acid (EDTA)–containing tubes. Fluid is analyzed for color, consistency, and turbidity as well as protein and cellularity.
9. Postcapillary venous pressure and oxygen saturation, to confirm proximal obstruction to venous drainage or an arteriovenous fistula. (Normal postcapillary venous pressure = 13 ± 4 mm Hg).
10. Cytology and histopathology. Studies are particularly useful in evaluating mass lesions associated with edematous tissue. Indirect fluorescent antibody (IFA) staining of affected tissue may facilitate detection of immune-mediated disorders.

REFERENCES

Bright JM: Peripheral edema. *In* Ettinger SJ, Feldman EC, eds: Textbook of Veterinary Internal Medicine, ed 4. Philadelphia, WB Saunders, 1995, pp 100–103.
Fossum TW, Millet MW: Lymphedema: Etiopathogenesis. J Vet Intern Med 6:283, 1992.
Olivier NB: Peripheral edema. *In* Ford RB, ed: Clinical Signs and Diagnosis in Small Animal Practice. New York, Churchill Livingstone, 1988, pp 123–134.

Edema, Pulmonary

(See Respiratory Distress or Difficulty [Dyspnea], p. 431).

Hair Loss

·········· DEFINITION

Hair loss, also called *alopecia*, refers to loss or absence of hair in any amounts and any distribution that is the result of one or a combination of disorders affecting the integrity of the hair coat. Therefore, physiologic loss of hair (e.g., normal shedding or hereditary hair loss, e.g., in the Rex cat breed) is excluded from this definition. In clinical practice, hair loss, with and without pruritus, is among the most common reasons a cat, and particularly a dog, is presented. In most cases, the loss of hair is secondary to some underlying disorder rather than being a primary event. The distribution of hair loss is important in that it can be characteristic of the underlying etiology.

Alopecia can be classified on the basis of distribution as (1) diffuse, (2) regional, (3) multifocal, and (4) focal. The causes for hair loss are varied and often complex. Abnormalities of follicular structure may be inherited, ranging from complete absence of hair follicles to selective absence of follicles that produce hair of a specific color. Inflammatory skin diseases that incorporate the hair follicle may disrupt hair growth and maintenance. Bacterial folliculitis, demodectic mange, and follicular hyperkeratosis are examples.

Disorders disrupting the normal follicular cycles can interrupt hair growth without loss or injury to the hair follicle. The cycle are as follows:

- Anagen (growth phase)
- Catagen (transitional phase)
- Telogen (resting phase)

··········ASSOCIATED SIGNS

The complex pathogenesis of alopecia supports a multitude of associated clinical signs in any animal presented for hair loss. Pruritus is an important associated sign if present. Allergic, inflammatory, and parasitic skin diseases are likely to cause pruritus. Secondary traumatic excoriation of the skin may further provoke cutaneous injury, thereby intensifying the pruritus. Alopecia caused by endocrine, genetic, and metabolic factors is less likely to be associated with pruritus, although pruritus may become a factor if the exposed skin becomes particularly dry or sunburned. Immune-mediated diseases leading to alopecia are variably pruritic, depending on the distribution and type of skin injury. Nutritional alopecia is rarely confirmed but can be a source of dermatitis and associated pruritus.

Alopecia without pruritus may be associated with dramatic physical signs resulting from endocrine or metabolic disorders. Dermatologic signs include thickened skin, hyperpigmentation, and dry and brittle hair coat (hypothyroidism). On the other hand, skin may appear thin and lack elasticity (canine Cushing's syndrome, Sertoli cell tumor). Gynecomastia, skin softness, calcinosis cutis, and pigmented macules are other dermatologic signs associated with alopecia.

··········DIFFERENTIAL DIAGNOSIS (see Table 3–17)
··········DIAGNOSTIC PLANS

1. Thorough history and physical examination, to determine the nature and extent of primary and secondary skin lesions. Distribution, pattern of alopecia, and associated cutaneous lesions should be characterized. Use the physical examination to determine whether or not evidence of systemic disease is present. Time of onset or the seasonal nature of alopecia may be significant, particularly when accompanied by pruritus.
2. Examination (macroscopic and microscopic) of affected and nonaffected hair.
3. Skin scraping (multiple), fungal cultures, and bacterial cultures (particularly of pustules).
   a. Fine-needle aspiration of discrete intracutaneous masses.

Table 3–17. Differential Diagnosis of Genetic Disorders Causing Alopecia

Hairless breeds (e.g., African sand dog, Abyssinian dog, Chinese crested dog, xoloitzcuintli, Turkish naked dog; sphinx cat, Rex cat [seasonal alopecia])
Ectodermal and follicular dysplasias (e.g., miniature poodles)
Hypotrichosis
Black hair follicular dysplasia
Color-mutant alopecia
Pattern baldness
Feline alopecia universalis
Demodicosis

   b. Skin biopsy, to include normal and affected skin (see p. 496).
4. Laboratory database, to include hematology, biochemical profile, urinalysis, and fecal flotation. In addition, cats should be tested for FeLV and FIV.
5. Special diagnostics:
   a. Allergic skin disease: Intradermal antigen inoculation, radioallergosorbent test (RAST) (IgE).
   b. Endocrine alopecia: T_4 before and after TSH stimulation, adrenocorticotropic hormone (ACTH) stimulation, dexamethasone suppression, serum testosterone (see p. 630).
6. Elimination testing.
7. Environmental allergen or irritant.
8. Food allergy elimination diet.

REFERENCES

Foil CS: Pruritus. *In* Ford RB, ed: Clinical Signs and Diagnosis in Small Animal Practice. New York, Churchill Livingstone, 1988, pp 605–630.
Noxon JO: Alopecia. *In* Ettinger SJ, and Feldman EC, eds: Textbook of Veterinary Internal Medicine, ed 4. Philadelphia, WB Saunders, 1995, pp 211–214.
Scott DW, Miller WH Jr, Griffin CE: Acquired alopecias. *In* Muller and Kirk's Small Animal Dermatology, ed 5. Philadelphia, WB Saunders.
Scheidt V: Alopecia. *In* Ford RB, ed: Clinical Signs and Diagnosis in Small Animal Practice. New York, Churchill Livingstone, 1988, pp 577–604.

Hematemesis (see also Vomiting, p. 447)

..........DEFINITION

Hematemesis, the vomiting of blood, is an uncommon presentation in the dog and is particularly rare in the cat. Although the presence of blood in the vomitus is, by strict definition, hematemesis, repeated episodes of vomiting in which the vomitus is composed of large blood clots, frank, uncoagulated blood, or the so-called coffee-ground appearance of blood denatured by gastric acid represents a serious clinical finding.

..........ASSOCIATED SIGNS

Hematemesis does not localize the diagnosis to the stomach or GI tract. Since a variety of metabolic and coagulation disorders may result in severe hematemesis, a wide spectrum of physical signs may also be present in affected animals. In addition, blood emanating from the upper respiratory tract may be swallowed and, subsequently, vomited, giving the appearance that bleeding is from the stomach.

Anorexia and vomiting are the most common associated, but nonspecific, signs. Weight loss, weakness, dark stool (melena), dehydration, and inactivity are other related signs having low diagnostic yield. Severe anemia can result from sustained gastric hemorrhage and, if acute, may justify exploratory laparotomy to identify the source of the bleeding.

Increased water consumption and urination may suggest underlying renal or hepatic disease. Intracutaneous or subcutaneous tumors, specifically mast cell tumors, can be associated with severe gastric ulceration and bleeding. Ulcerative lesions in the mouth may indicate recent ingestion of caustic or toxic compounds. The frenulum in the mouth should always be examined to rule out linear foreign bodies.

Table 3–18. Differential Diagnosis of Hematemesis

Primary Gastric Disorders	Systemic Metabolic Disorders
Gastritis	Acute pancreatitis
Infectious (e.g., parvovirus)	Adrenocortical insufficiency
Toxic	(Addison's disease)
Bile reflux–bilious vomiting syndrome	Toxins (e.g., lead, ethylene glycol)
Foreign body	Hepatic failure
Gastric ulcers	Renal failure
Drug-induced (e.g., aspirin)	Neoplasia
Idiopathic	
Metabolic (e.g., renal failure)	
Neoplastic	

············ **DIFFERENTIAL DIAGNOSES** (see Table 3–18)

············ **DIAGNOSTIC PLANS**

1. Comprehensive history. This is critical and should focus on:
   a. Recent medications administered, both prescription and nonprescription.
   b. Known and potential exposure to toxic or poisonous substances.
   c. Duration of the primary and associated signs.
   d. Physical appearance of the vomitus.
   e. Physical status of other pets in the family, if applicable.
2. Laboratory profile, including, as a minimum, hematologic values, particularly in anemic patients; biochemistry findings; urinalysis; and fecal flotation. Emphasis should be placed on renal, adrenal, and hepatic function (see pp. 651, 718).
3. Testing of feces for the presence of parvovirus antigen.
4. Activated coagulation time (ACT). A coagulation panel, including partial thromboplastin time (PTT), prothrombin time (PT), fibrin degradation products (FDPs), fibrinogen, and total platelet count, is indicated as appropriate (see p. 687).
5. Fine-needle aspiration of any intracutaneous or subcutaneous tumors.
6. Abdominal and thoracic radiographs; abdominal ultrasound.
7. Gastroscopy and esophagoscopy.
8. Exploratory laparotomy and gastrotomy.

Note: In patients with severe hematemesis, surgery may be indicated prior to obtaining results from the laboratory profile.

REFERENCE

Magne ML, Twedt DC: Vomiting. *In* Ford RB, ed: Clinical Signs and Diagnosis in Small Animal Practice. New York, Churchill Livingstone, 1988, pp 425–435.

Hematuria, Hemoglobinuria, Myoglobinuria

············ **DEFINITION**

To most owners, the appearance of small blood clots in recently voided urine, blood-tinged urine, or brown or red urine denotes urinary tract bleeding. The presence of blood in the urine, whether gross or occult, denotes *hematuria* and is most often indicative of upper or lower urinary tract bleeding, although

Table 3–19. Causes of Hematuria in Dogs and Cats Classified by Anatomical Site of Origin

Site	Diseases
Kidney	Pyelonephritis
	Glomerulopathy
	Neoplasia
	Calculi
	Renal cysts
	Infarction
	Trauma
	Benign renal bleeding
	Hematuria of Welsh corgis
	Dioctophyma renale infection
	Microfilaria of *Dirofilaria immitis*
	Chronic passive congestion
Bladder, ureter, urethra	Infection
	Calculi
	Inflammation—LUTD
	Neoplasia
	Trauma
	Capillaria plica infection
	Cyclophosphamide
Any site	Coagulation disorders
	Heatstroke, DIC
Extraurinary causes (genital tract or spurious hematuria)	Prostate
	Neoplasia
	Infection
	Hypertrophy
	Uterus
	Estrus
	Subinvolution
	Infection
	Neoplasia
	Vagina
	TVT
	Trauma
	Penis
	TVT
	Trauma

From Lorenz MD, Cornelius LM, eds: Small Animal Medical Diagnosis. Philadelphia, JB Lippincott, 1987, p 333.

DIC, disseminated intravascular coagulation; TVT, transmissible venereal tumor; LUTD, lower urinary tract disease.

systemic coagulopathies and reproductive tract disorders may also cause hematuria. The presence of hemoglobin in urine *(hemoglobinuria)* is not necessarily a reflection of urinary tract disease. Systemic disorders, (e.g., those leading to intravascular hemolysis) can be associated with significant hemoglobinuria in the presence of a normal urinary system.

Distinguishing hemoglobinuria from hematuria is an important diagnostic consideration. Conventional urine test strips (dipsticks) do not differentiate between the two; therefore, microscopic examination of urine sediment for the presence of significant numbers of RBCs is critical.

Myoglobinuria is characterized by brown to dark-red urine, the absence of RBCs in the urine sediment, and a positive test for occult blood. Bilirubinuria can also cause dark-brown to dark-orange urine but alone will not produce a positive test for occult blood. Myoglobinuria is a serious sign and denotes generalized muscle disease.

...........ASSOCIATED SIGNS

Hematuria associated with the urinary tract may not be associated with any other clinical signs. In patients with significant bleeding of renal origin, evidence of systemic illness may be present but is unlikely to localize the source of hematuria. Hematuria originating from the bladder is more likely to be associated with clinical signs, particularly pollakiuria and dysuria. Reproductive tract disorders (e.g., prostatitis and vaginitis) can also cause significant hematuria. Patients with hematuria or hemoglobinuria should be examined carefully for evidence of systemic bleeding, coagulopathies, and neoplasia.

...........DIFFERENTIAL DIAGNOSIS (see Tables 3–19 and 3–20)
...........DIAGNOSTIC PLANS

1. Thorough history and physical examination, with emphasis on examination of the genitalia, palpation of the prostate, and caudal abdominal palpation.
2. If practical, assessment of urethral patency and the patient's ability to urinate. Attempt to pass a urethral catheter if significant dysuria and evidence of lower urinary tract obstructions are present (see p. 486).
3. Complete urinalysis. Using a fresh sample, include assessment of gross appearance, specific gravity, biochemical reagent strips (dipsticks), and microscopic examination of urine sediment. Ideally, two samples should be

Table 3–20. Differential Diagnosis of Hemoglobinuria

Intravascular Destruction of Red Blood Cells
Immune-mediated hemolytic anemia
Transfusion hemolysis
Sepsis
Red blood cell parasites (e.g., *Babesia* spp.)
Chemical-induced
    Phenothiazine
    Acetominophen
    Methylene blue
    Copper
Hypo-osmolality

Extravascular Destruction of Red Blood Cells
Red blood cell parasites (e.g., *Hemobartonella* spp.)
Immune-mediated hemolytic anemia
Pyruvate kinase deficiency (basenji and beagle)
Congenital porphyria (cats)
Hereditary stomatocytosis (malamute)
Microangiopathic disease (e.g., hepatic cirrhosis, hemangiosarcoma)

Lysis of Red Blood Cells in Urine
Hematuria combined with very dilute urine
Hematuria in stored urine

collected: a voided urine sample followed by a urine sample collected by cystocentesis (see p. 490).

4. Culture and sensitivity, if bacteria are present (see p. 466).
5. Routine laboratory profile, to include hematology and biochemistry panel (see pp. 651 and 718).
6. Coagulation profile, if hemoglobinuria is present.
7. Abdominal radiographs, for evidence of calculi, prostatic enlargement, and soft tissue masses.
8. Contrast radiography of the upper and lower urinary tracts.
9. Ultrasound examination of the prostate, urinary bladder, and kidneys.
10. Exploratory laparotomy.

REFERENCES

Lulich JP, Osborne A: Diseaes of the urinary bladder. *In* Morgan RV, ed: Handbook of Small Animal Practice, ed 3. Philadelphia, WB Saunders, 1997, pp 531–543.
Moreau PM, Lees GE: Incontinence, enuresis, nocturia, and dysuria. *In* Ettinger SJ, Feldman EC, eds: Textbook of Veterinary Internal Medicine, ed 4. Philadelphia, WB Saunders, 1995, pp 164–169.
Wolf AM: Hematuria and dysuria. *In* Ford RB, ed: Clinical Signs and Diagnosis in Small Animal Practice. New York, Churchill Livingstone, 1988, pp 541–563.

Hemoptysis

...........DEFINITION

Hemoptysis is the expectoration, during cough, of blood. Seldom is the volume of blood loss sufficient to cause anemia; however, once confirmed, hemoptysis is a severe clinical finding indicative of bleeding into or from the lower airways. Hemoptysis can be attributed to direct injury of the pulmonary, or, less commonly, the tracheobronchial blood vessels; pulmonary hypertension; or coagulopathy. Although an uncommon presenting sign, hemoptysis is more prevalent in dogs than in cats.

Since vomiting can be mistaken by the owner for coughing, it becomes essential to differentiate between hemoptysis and hematemesis during the initial examination. Hemoptysis is regarded as an emergency presentation.

...........ASSOCIATED SIGNS

The most common, and least significant, sign associated with hemoptysis is *melena,* or dark-red or black discoloration of stool, that occurs subsequent to swallowing expectorated blood. More serious associated signs include coughing, hyperpnea, orthopnea, and cyanosis. Apparent episodic weakness and collapse may also be reported.

...........DIFFERENTIAL DIAGNOSIS (see Table 3–21)

...........DIAGNOSTIC PLANS

1. Thorough history and physical examination. In addition, an attempt should be made to determine that the sign for which the patient was presented is, in fact, expectoration of blood during coughing and not bloody vomitus.
2. Routine laboratory profile, to assess the patient's overall health status. Emphasis should be placed on the fecal examination and heartworm tests. Multiple attempts to locate parasite ova in the stool should be made, since lung parasites may be few in number and ova shed intermittently.
3. Thoracic radiographs.

Table 3–21. Differential Diagnosis of Hemoptysis

Cardiovascular Hemoptysis
Thromboembolic disease
   Heartworm disease (in the dog and cat)
   Hyperadrenocorticism
   Cardiomyopathy
   Renal amyloidosis (in the dog)
   Idiopathic
Acute pulmonary edema
Arteriovenous fistula

Parasitic Hemoptysis
Lung flukes (e.g., *Paragonimus* spp.)
Lungworms (e.g., *Aelurostrongylus* spp.)

Inflammation-Induced Hemoptysis
Chronic bronchitis
Pneumonia
Mycotic lung infection
Lung abscess

Neoplasia
Either primary or metastatic

Miscellaneous
Coagulation disorder
Direct injury or trauma
Transtracheal aspirate

4. Coagulation profile, particularly in those animals with significant bleeding from other sites (see p. 687).
5. Transtracheal aspiration with cytologic studies or bacterial culture and sensitivity (see p. 499) tests, or both.
6. Special procedures, including ultrasonography of the lung, particularly when discrete masses are seen on radiographs; echocardiography; blood gas analysis; bronchoscopy; bronchography; and angiography.
7. Radionuclide scans. Although of limited availability, they may be able to detect areas of pulmonary embolization.

REFERENCES

Armstrong PJ: Hemoptysis. *In* Ford RB, ed: Clinical Signs and Diagnosis. New York, Churchill Livingstone, 1988, pp 239–256.
Hawkins EC: Clinical manifestations of lower respiratory tract disorders. *In* Nelson RW, Couto CG, eds: Essentials of Small Animal Internal Medicine. St Louis, Mosby–Year Book, 1992, pp 180–184.

Hemorrhage
(See Spontaneous Bleeding, p. 437)

Icterus (Jaundice)

............DEFINITION

Yellow discoloration of tissue caused by an increased concentration of bilirubin is termed *icterus,* or *jaundice*, and is indicative of underlying hepatocellular disease or intravascular hemolytic disease. Hyperbilirubinemia is required for icterus to develop but may not occur concurrently with icterus.

In practice, icterus is an uncommon presenting complaint, since the dense hair coat of cats and dogs precludes early detection of bile pigment in skin. Icteric tissues are most evident in the sclera and in the oral, vaginal, and preputial mucous membranes, particularly in anemic patients. Icterus can occur subsequent to the accumulation of either unconjugated (lipid-soluble) or conjugated (water-soluble) bilirubin in the blood.

Icterus can originate at any of three levels:

1. Prehepatic (hemolytic disease).
2. Hepatic (hepatocellular disease).
3. Posthepatic (obstructive or reduced bile flow).

Unconjugated hyperbilirubinemia results from rapid hemolysis (a common cause in the dog and cat), ineffective erythropoiesis, impaired hepatic uptake of conjugated bilirubin, or impaired conjugation. Conjugated (water-soluble) hyperbilirubinemia is generally the result of disorders intrinsic to the liver that affect bilirubin transport. Cholestatic disease is associated with reduced bile flow and can be characterized by significant bile acidemia and icterus.

............ASSOCIATED SIGNS

Icterus can be detected in a dog or cat without overt clinical signs; however, RBC values and hepatic function should be assessed. Prehepatic icterus is characteristically associated with rapid-onset anemia and with generalized weakness, lassitude or acute collapse (caval syndrome), and bright-orange urine. Pallor can be difficult to assess in patients with marked icterus. Hepatic icterus and posthepatic icterus are generally associated with lethargy and decreased appetite and are therefore difficult to distinguish clinically. Depending on the type of hepatic injury or the level of obstruction, episodic vomiting or diarrhea, weight loss, abdominal distention, polyuria or polydipsia, peripheral edema associated with hypoproteinemia, and prolonged bleeding (uncommon) may be reported.

............DIFFERENTIAL DIAGNOSIS (see Table 3–22)
............DIAGNOSTIC PLANS

1. Thorough history. This should focus on current and previous drug therapy, including heartworm preventative, as well as duration of illness and associated signs. Physical examination confirms the presence of icterus but is unlikely to reveal the underlying cause. Abdominal palpation may reveal hepatomegaly, a discrete mass, or the presence of fluid.

   Note: In obviously anemic patients, when practical, transfusion should be avoided until laboratory test results have been interpreted.
2. Laboratory evaluation of the icteric patient. This is essential and should initially include a CBC, biochemistry panel (to include total and direct bilirubin), fecal analysis, urinalysis, heartworm test (in dogs), serum electrophoresis (in cats), and a test for FeLV antigen and FIV antibody.
3. Anemic patient: Coombs' test; ANA titer; peripheral blood smear for the presence of parasites; blood cultures, particularly if the patient is febrile; and IFA test on bone marrow for FeLV antigen (in cats) (see p. 680).
4. Nonanemic patient: Abdominal radiographs, abdominocentesis with fluid analysis and cytologic study, fine-needle aspiration of liver, plasma ammo-

Table 3–22. Differential Diagnosis of Icterus

Prehepatic (Hemolytic)
Immune-mediated hemolytic anemia (Coombs'-positive anemia)
Heartworm disease, especially postcaval syndrome
Hemolytic septicemia
Transfusion-induced hemolysis

Hepatic (Hepatocellular)
Cholangitis/cholangiohepatitis
Chronic active liver disease
Copper storage disease (Bedlington terriers and Doberman pinschers)
Drug-induced/vaccine-induced
    Thiacetarsamide—sporadic occurrence
    Imidazole anthelmintics—sporadic occurrence
    Anticonvulsants, especially primidone
    Acetaminophen/methylene blue (in cats)
Hepatic fibrosis
Septicemia
    Gram-negative bacteremia
    Leptospirosis
Viral
    Canine viral hepatitis
    Feline leukemia
    Feline infectious hepatitis
Neoplasia, primary or metastatic

Posthepatic (Obstructive)
Cholangitis/cholangiohepatitis
Hepatic fibrosis
Neoplasia
Acute pancreatitis
Extrahepatic neoplasm (by compression)
Bile duct trauma
Ruptured gallbladder (usually traumatic)
Cholelithiasis

nia, bile acids, serum amylase, and lipase if not included in the biochemistry panel.
5. Special diagnostic tests. Coagulation profile, followed by liver biopsy (percutaneous or at laparotomy) or exploratory celiotomy with biopsy (see pp. 16 and 687).
6. Abdominal ultrasound, CT, and perfusion scintigraphy (special facilities required).

REFERENCES

Anderson J, Washabau RJ: Icterus. Compend Contin Educ Pract Vet 14:1045, 1992.
Dimski DS: Jaundice. *In* Ettinger SJ, Feldman EC, eds: Textbook of Veterinary Internal Medicine, ed 4. Philadelphia, WB Saunders, 1995, pp 205–208.
Meyer DJ: Jaundice. *In* Ford RB, ed: Clinical Signs and Diagnosis. New York, Churchill Livingstone, 1988, pp 505–519.

Jaundice

(See Icterus, p. 419)

Joint Swelling

(See also Lameness, p. 346)

............DEFINITION

Joint swelling, or enlargement, refers to any abnormal increase in size, either visible or palpable, or any joint that is *not* directly caused by a proliferation of tissue. In practice, joint swelling is the primary presenting sign only occasionally. Pain and associated lameness are more likely causes for presentation, whereas actual enlargement of a joint is detected during physical examination. However, there is not necessarily an association between joint swelling and pain.

Joint swelling, or effusion, occurs subsequent to injury to the synovial membrane in which there is not only an increase in volume of synovial fluid produced, but quantitative biochemical and cellular changes as well. Most joint swelling is attributed to inflammation of the synovial membrane, or synovitis. Abnormal synovial fluid accumulation (effusion) may be classified as serous, fibrinous, purulent, septic, or hemorrhagic (see Table 3–23).

............ASSOCIATED SIGNS

Although lameness is the most common clinical sign associated with joint swelling, it is not consistently present. Joint swelling may also be associated

---

Table 3–23. Arthropathies in the Dog

Noninflammatory
Degenerative joint disease (osteoarthritis, osteoarthrosis)
  Primary
  Secondary
    As a sequel to acquired or congenital defects of the joints and supporting
      structures
Traumatic
Neoplastic involvement
Drug-induced

Inflammatory
Infectious
  Bacterial
  Mycoplasmal
  Fungal
  Protozoal
  Rickettsial (neurophilic erlichiosis, Rocky Mountain spotted fever)
  Spirochetal (Lyme disease)
Noninfectious
  Immunologic
    Erosive (deforming)
      Rheumatoid arthritis
    Nonerosive (nondeforming)
      Systemic lupus erythematosus
      Arthritis resulting from chronic infectious disease
      Idiopathic nonerosive arthritis
      Drug reactions (sulfadiazine reaction)
  Nonimmunologic
    Crystal-induced arthritis (gout, pseudogout)
    Chronic hemarthrosis (coagulation defects, congenital or acquired)

with, or mistaken for, hyperplasia, metaplasia, or neoplasia of the synovium, joint capsule, articular cartilage, or periarticular bone. Hemorrhagic joint effusion (hemarthrosis) may be associated with coagulopathy and spontaneous bleeding from the respiratory, *GI*, or urinary tract. Subluxation or fracture of a carpus, tarsus, or stifle may also be associated with detectable joint swelling. Arthritis associated with systemic disease (e.g., infectious or immune-mediated) can also be accompanied by significant joint swelling.

··········DIAGNOSTIC PLANS

1. History. The history generally focuses on associated signs rather than primary joint swelling and should address duration, exposure to ticks, known injury, and evidence of spontaneous bleeding. Physical examination establishes the presence of joint swelling and the number of joints involved. Evidence of inflammation, crepitus, joint laxity, abnormal range of motion, a drawer sign, luxations, or fractures should be determined.
2. Radiography of the affected joint(s).
3. Synovial fluid analysis, including biochemical, cytologic, and culture findings (see p. 770).
4. Coagulation profile in the presence of hemarthrosis (see p. 687).
5. Immune function testing: ANA titer, rheumatoid factor, and LE cell preparation (see p. 703).
6. Contrast arthrography.
7. Joint capsule–synovial membrane biopsy.
8. Periarticular bone biopsy.
9. Surgical exploration of the affected joint.

REFERENCES

Feldman DG: Joint effusion. *In* Ettinger SJ, Feldman EC, eds: Textbook of Veterinary Internal Medicine, ed 4. Philadelphia, WB Saunders, 1995, pp 113–136.
Milton J: Canine arthritis. Vet Med Rep 2:64, 1990.
Roush JK: Diseases of joints and ligaments. *In* Morgan RV, ed: Handbook of Small Animal Practice, ed 3. Philadelphia, WB Saunders, 1997, pp 813–829.

Lymphadenopathy—Lymph Node Enlargement

··········DEFINITION

Any change in the size or consistency of a lymph node or group of lymph nodes denotes *lymphadenopathy*. For purposes of this discussion, lymphadenopathy refers to those lymph nodes that are larger than expected with or without commensurate changes in consistency. Involved nodes may be unusually soft, firm, or painful, suggestive of inflammation; whereas enlarged, firm, nonpainful lymph nodes are suggestive of neoplasia. Lymphadenopathy is usually not a presenting problem, with the possible exception of generalized enlargements of all superficial lymph nodes.

Lymph nodes become enlarged as a result of inflammation (pyogenic or granulomatous), reactive lymphoid hyperplasia, or neoplasia (primary or neoplastic). In pyogenic inflammation, neutrophils dilate and engorge the sinuses, whereas in granulomatous inflammation an infiltrate or macrophages is present (e.g., systemic mycoses). Reactive lymphoid hyperplasia is associated with an increase in the number of germinal centers within the lymph node and an infiltrate of plasma cells. In neoplastic lymph nodes, tumor cells may invade the sinuses (metastatic), gradually destroying the normal node architecture, or the architecture of the lymph node is entirely replaced by malignant lymphocytes (lymphosarsoma); i.e., histologically, the sinuses are obliterated and germinal centers cannot be found.

...........ASSOCIATED SIGNS

Characterize the consistency and number of affected nodes as well as their location (i.e., generalized or regional). Lymph node pain is an inconsistent finding usually associated with inflammatory disease rather than neoplasia. Associated signs are likely to be regional, as is the lymph node enlargement (i.e., tissue injury or infection). Patients with generalized lymphadenopathy may not have associated signs, or there may be nonspecific signs, including weight loss, fever, decreased appetite, and lassitude as a result of systemic illness.

...........DIAGNOSTIC PLANS

1. History and physical examination, to determine the duration and type of associated signs, if any, and the duration of lymph node enlargement, if known.
2. Laboratory profile, with emphasis on CBC, including platelet count; biochemistry panel, and urinalysis.
3. Specific tests for infectious diseases, as indicated (e.g., FeLV antigen and FIV antibody).
4. Thoracic and abdominal radiographs, as indicated.
5. Fine-needle aspiration of affected lymph node(s) (see p. 496).
6. Serum protein electrophoresis (see p. 703).
7. Bone marrow aspirate (see p. 666).
8. Lymph node biopsy and, if indicated, culture (see p. 496).

REFERENCES

Barton CL: Lymphadenopathy. *In* Ford RB, ed: Clinical Signs and Diagnosis in Small Animals. New York, Churchill Livingstone, 1988, pp 171–187.

McCaw D: Lumps, bumps, masses, and lymphadenopathy. *In* Ettinger SJ, Feldman EC, eds: Textbook of Veterinary Internal Medicine, ed 4. Philadelphia, WB Saunders, 1995, pp 219–223.

Vail DM: Diseases of lymph nodes and lymphatics. *In* Morgan RV, ed: Handbook of Small Animal Practice ed 3. Philadelphia, WB Saunders, 1997, pp 719–729.

Painful Defecation

(See Dyschezia, p. 403)

Polyuria, Polydipsia

...........DEFINITION

In practice, *polyuria* (PU) and *polydipsia* (PD) are loosely interpreted to mean an increase in urination and water consumption, respectively. The fact that polyuria is an abnormal increase in urine production, usually of low specific gravity, is seldom confirmed in practice. Likewise, although polydipsia is an abnormal or absolute increase in water consumption usually associated with increased thirst, water intake is seldom quantitated. Use of the terms polyuria and polydipsia is usually justified when a client presents a dog or cat for subjective increases in urination frequency and water intake as the primary problem. When clear evidence of increased urination and increased thirst is not present, actual documentation of 24-hour urinary output and water intake may be necessary.

Polydipsia is a compensatory sign that develops subsequent to polyuria. Primary polydipsia with compensatory polyuria is uncommon.

The pathophysiology behind polyuria is complex in that several renal and nonrenal mechanisms can be involved. Diseases affecting proximal tubules (e.g., primary renal failure, renal glycosuria) or those causing high solute loads overwhelming proximal tubule absorptive capacity (e.g., diabetes mellitus) cause osmotic diuresis. Water conservation is also affected at the level of the loop of Henle (e.g., primary renal disease, diuretics) and in the distal tubules and collecting ducts. Disorders of the distal tubule and collecting duct are frequently responsible for polyuria, including diabetes insipidus, pyometra, hyperadrenocorticism, liver failure, and hypercalcemia.

Polyuria does result in subsequent failure of the sodium chloride pump in the loop of Henle, leading to significant decreases in the renal medullary osmotic gradient. Liver failure resulting in urea depletion and prolonged polyuria can cause medullary washout.

Primary polydipsia subsequent to increased thirst can cause secondary polyuria but is an uncommon clinical finding. Compulsive water drinking (pseudopsychogenic polydipsia) is probably the most important type of primary polydipsia, although the underlying cause is not known. Hypothalamic lesions, hypercalcemia, and increased levels of plasma renin are less common causes of primary polydipsia.

·········· ASSOCIATED SIGNS

3

Signs associated with PU or PD are varied and dependent on the underlying disease. Generalized signs include weakness, decreased appetite, weight loss, diarrhea, and fever. Polyphagia with weight loss occurs in animals with diabetes mellitus and in cats with hyperthyroidism. Paraneoplastic syndromes, particularly hypercalcemia, may develop in conjunction with PU or PD. A comprehensive physical examination and a laboratory assessment are justified in all patients presented with PU or PD as the primary complaint.

·········· DIFFERENTIAL DIAGNOSIS (see Table 3–24)
·········· DIAGNOSTIC PLANS

1. History and physical examination, to facilitate verification of the problem in addition to determining the duration of the problem and associated signs. Of particular importance is knowledge of the recent administration of medication.
2. Laboratory database. The primary focus of the diagnostic plan is interpreting results from a laboratory database, including a CBC, biochemistry profile, urinalysis, fecal culture, heartworm test (in dogs), FeLV and FIV tests (in cats), and urine culture.
3. Collecting urine and measuring water intake over a 24-hour period, to document the problem, if necessary.
4. Abdominal radiographs, if indicated.
5. Special diagnostic tests, if indicated, on the basis of results from a laboratory database:
   a. Water deprivation and modified-water deprivation tests (contraindicated in the presence of azotemia, dehydration, or hypercalcemia).
   b. Antidiuretic hormone (ADH, vasopressin) response test.
   c. Glucose tolerance test.
   d. ACTH stimulation or dexamethasone suppression.
   e. Serum T_4.

Table 3–24. Differential Diagnosis of Polyuria and Polydipsia

Polyuria of Renal Origin
Renal failure
   Glomerulonephritis
   Tubular dysfunction
   Renal medullary dysfunction
Postobstructive diuresis (e.g., feline urologic syndrome)
Diabetes insipidus (nephrogenic)
Hypercalcemic nephropathy
Fanconi's syndrome
Medullary washout

Polyuria of Nonrenal Causes
Diabetes insipidus (neurogenic)
Diabetes mellitus
Hyperadrenocorticism
Liver disease (nonspecific)
Pyometra
Pseudopsychogenic polydipsia

Drug-Induced Polyuria
Glucocorticoids (esp. in dogs)
Mannitol, IV
Dextrose, concentrations >50 mg/dL (5.0%)
Alcohol
Diuretic therapy (e.g., furosemide)
Phenytoin
Vitamin D intoxication

   f. Liver function studies, e.g., serum ammonia, bile acids.
   g. Abdominal ultrasound.
   h. Tissue biopsy (e.g., renal and hepatic).
   i. Exploratory laparotomy.

These can be evaluated in diagnosis using the algorithm of polyuria (Fig. 3–4).

REFERENCES

Allen TA, Wilke WL: Polyuria and polydipsia. *In* Ford RB, ed: Clinical Signs and Diagnosis in Small Animals. New York, Churchill Livingstone, 1988, pp 55–73.

Feldman EC, Nelson RW: Canine and Feline Endocrinology, ed 2. Philadelphia, WB Saunders, 1996.

Meric SM: Polyuria and Polydipsia. *In* Ettinger SJ, Feldman EC, eds: Textbook of Veterinary Internal Medicine. Philalelphia, WB Saunders, 1995, pp 159–164.

Nichols R: Polyuria and polydipsia. Probl Vet Med 2:610, 1990.

Pruritus (Itching)

(See also Hair Loss, p. 412)

···········DEFINITION

In veterinary medicine, *pruritus* is the term used to describe abnormally frequent scratching or biting that results from an unpleasant, sometimes intense, epidermal stimulation.

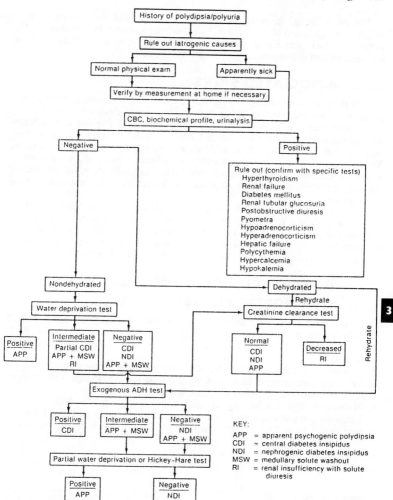

Figure 3–4. Clinical approach to the patient with polydipsia and polyuria. CBC, complete blood count; ADH, antidiuretic hormone. (From Fenner WR: Quick Reference to Veterinary Medicine, ed 2. Philadelphia, JB Lippincott, 1991, p 110.)

Histamine, endopeptidases, and other polypeptides liberated from skin cells serve as mediators of pruritus. Histamine is the primary mediator of itch associated with wheal-and-flare reaction. Histamine-mediated itching cannot be completely inhibited by either H_1- or H_2-receptor antagonists (blockers). Other polypeptides (such as bradykinin), β-endorphin, and neuropeptides, such as substance P, can induce itching when applied directly to skin. The close association between itching and inflammation of the skin is attributed to the fact that many of the endogenous mediators and potentiators are released in situ during inflammatory events.

Itching, although a protective response, can become more harmful than helpful. As a feature of dermatitis, itch mediators cannot be removed by the patient. In fact, scratching and biting eventually serve to promote more inflammation and subsequently perpetuate the itching.

..........ASSOCIATED SIGNS

Skin lesions are commonly associated with pruritus; however, it becomes important to characterize the lesion and to distinguish those that are primary from those that are secondary to scratching or biting. Papules and pustules are characteristic primary lesions that may ultimately develop into secondary lesions, such as crusts, ulcers, scale in collarettes, and pigmented macules. Vesicles and bullae, plaques, and urticaria (wheals) can also occur as primary skin lesions. Linear crusts, irregular ulceration, lichenification, diffuse scaling and pigmentation, and patchy alopecia are characteristic lesions that develop secondary to excoriation.

Pruritus can also occur without primary lesions (i.e., "essential" pruritus). This type of itching is a manifestation of systemic disease, although mediation may be central or cutaneous. Causes include atopy, dry skin, and neurogenic and psychogenic disorders. A spectrum of renal, hepatic, hematopoietic, allergic, and endocrine diseases are associated with essential pruritus.

..........DIFFERENTIAL DIAGNOSIS (see Table 3–25)
..........DIAGNOSTIC PLANS

1. History and physical examination, to characterize the skin lesion and its distribution, to determine whether or not the condition appears to be contagious, and to determine whether or not systemic disease is present (see p. 364).
2. Laboratory database, if evidence of systemic disease is present.
3. Skin and coat examination. Perform multiple skin scrapings, and examine skin and hair coat with Wood's light (see p. 492).
4. Microbiologic testing for bacteria and dermatophytes (see p. 466).
5. Immunologic testing, to include intradermal skin testing and direct fluorescent antibody testing of skin (both normal and affected) biopsy specimens (see p. 364).
6. Skin biopsy with dermatohistopathology (see p. 492).
7. Provocative exposure to selected environmental agents, diet, and drugs.

REFERENCES

Foil CS: Pruritus. *In* Ford RB, ed: Clinical Signs and Diagnosis in Small Animals. New York, Churchill Livingstone, 1988, pp 605–630.
Ihrke PJ: Pruritus. *In* Ettinger SJ, Feldman EC, eds: Textbook of Veterinary Internal Medicine, ed 4. Philadelphia, WB Saunders, 1995, pp 214–219.
Scott DW, Miller WH Jr, Griffin CE: Muller and Kirk's Small Animal Dematology, ed 5. Philadelphia, WB Saunders, 1995.
White S: Clinical approach to the pruritic dog: Advances and basics. J Am Anim Hosp Assoc 24:489, 1991.

Rectal and Anal Pain

(See Dyschezia, p. 403)

Regurgitation

(See also Dysphagia and Vomiting, pp. 406 and 447)

Table 3–25. Differential Diagnosis of Pruritus

Pustular Dermatitis
Infectious
　Puppy pyoderma
　Folliculitis and furunculosis
Immune-mediated
　Pemphigus foliaceus
　Vesicle-forming disorders (e.g., drug eruption)
　Linear IgA γ dermatosis
Idiopathic
　Puppy strangles
　Subcorneal pustular dermatosis

Vesicular/Bullous Eruption
Bullous dermatoses
Systemic lupus erythematosus (SLE)
Toxic epidermal necrolysis
Drug eruption
Acute contact dermatitis

Plaque Formation
Infectious dermatitis
Immune-mediated dermatitis
Neoplasia (e.g., mast cell tumor)

Papular Eruption (Dog)
Infectious
　Folliculitis (bacterial, fungal, demodectic)
　Parasitic (*Sarcoptes*, *Cheyletiella*, lice, fleas)
　Vasculitis (Rocky Mountain spotted fever)
Immune
　Allergy
　Autoimmune (pemphigus foliaceus, SLE)
Idiopathic

Papular Eruption (Cat)
Infectious (bacterial folliculitis)
Dermatophytosis
Parasitic (otodectic and notoedric mange, *Cheyletiella*, lice)
Immune-mediated (hypersensitivity to food)
Idiopathic miliary dermatitis

Ulcerative Dermatitis
SLE
Leukocytoclastic vasculitis
Erythema multiforme
Toxic epidermal necrolysis
Mycosis fungoides
Epidermolysis bullosa complex
Dermatomyositis
Acute contact dermatitis
Vogt-Koyanagi-Harada syndrome

...........DEFINITION

Rabies vaccination status should be assessed before examining any case of difficult swallowing or regurgitation in the dog and cat. The term *regurgitation* implies retrograde esophageal transport of ingesta subsequent to a mechanical, neurogenic, or myogenic swallowing disorder. Both regurgitation and vomiting imply a backward flowing of ingesta through the esophagus; however, regurgitation is a relatively effortless act in contrast to the retching and abdominal pressure characteristic of vomiting. Regurgitation localizes the problem to the esophagus.

The pathophysiology of esophageal function is addressed and referenced in the article on dysphagia (see p. 406). Both acquired (e.g., foreign body) and congenital (e.g., familial megaesophagus) forms and esophageal disease can lead to regurgitation. Many esophageal problems remain undiagnosed if regurgitation is not present.

...........ASSOCIATED SIGNS

Physical signs recognized by owners of dogs or cats with regurgitation include dysphagia characterized by difficulty swallowing food, frequent attempts to swallow food, and hypersalivation. Belching may also be reported subsequent to the entrapment of air in the esophagus. Inappetence and weight loss subsequently develop. Esophageal dilatation may be observed at the level of the lower cervical esophagus or thoracic inlet.

Owners may report expulsion of blood-tinged saliva subsequent to esophageal mucosal injury. Paroxysms of coughing and retching, particularly when eating, may be present along with difficult breathing in animals with significant pneumonia. Nasal discharge may consist of mucoid to mucopurulent exudates or of food and liquid recently consumed.

Rarely, affected animals present with swollen joints, lameness, and severe weakness associated with hypertrophic osteodystrophy subsequent to an intrathoracic lesion. Atypical signs include inspiratory dyspnea, regurgitation unrelated to eating, and recurrent gastric bloating associated with aerophagia.

...........DIFFERENTIAL DIAGNOSIS (see Table 3–26)
...........DIAGNOSTIC PLANS

1. History and physical examination, to characterize the nature of the problem, to distinguish between vomiting and regurgitation, and to establish the character of the regurgitated material.
2. Laboratory database, to assess patient status, particularly if secondary complications are present.
3. Survey thoracic and cervical radiography, to assess presence of megaesophagus, radiopaque intraesophageal lesion, or both.
4. Contrast esophagram, to confirm any interference with normal bolus transport at the point of obstruction, changes in mucosal integrity or luminal displacement, and the presence of extraluminal gas. (Oral suspension of barium sulfate is recommended over other contrast materials.)
   Note: Contrast medium retention in the esophagus is the hallmark of a motor disorder and often localizes the site of dysmotility.
5. Endoscopy and, as indicated, biopsy, to determine the cause of megaesophagus rather than to diagnose megaesophagus. In some instances, especially foreign body obstruction, endoscopy may be therapeutic.
6. Special procedures, to include contrast esophagram during fluoroscopy, CT, and exploratory laparotomy.

Table 3–26. Differential Diagnosis of Regurgitation

Functional Megaesophagus*
Primary (or congenital)
Secondary (or acquired)
  Foreign body
  Esophageal stricture
  Esophageal diverticula
  Neurogenic (e.g., myasthenia gravis, rabies)
  Myopathy, smooth muscle
  Extraesophageal compressive lesion (e.g.,
  neoplasia)
  Vascular anomaly

Esophagitis
Gastric reflux
Neoplastic

Restrictive Lesion Without Megaesophagus
Foreign body obstruction
Intrathoracic mass
Vascular ring anomaly
Esophageal stricture

---

*The most prevalent cause.

3

REFERENCES

Guilford WG, Strombeck DR: Diseases of swallowing. *In* Guilford WG, Center SA, Strombeck DR, et al, eds: Strombeck's Small Animal Gastroenterology, ed 3. Philadelphia, WB Saunders, 1996, pp 211–238.

Jergens AE: Diseases of the esophagus. *In* Morgan RV, ed: Handbook of Small Animal Practice, ed 3. Philadelphia, WB Saunders, 1996, pp 323–333.

Watrous BJ: Dysphagia and regurgitation. *In* Ford RB, ed: Clinical Signs and Diagnosis in Small Animals. New York, Churchill Livingstone, 1988, pp 389–423.

Respiratory Distress or Difficulty (Dyspnea)

·········· DEFINITION

For purposes of this discussion, respiratory distress or difficulty refers to pathologic breathlessness (true *dyspnea*) ascribed to the unpleasant, distressful sensation of labored breathing most commonly associated with cardiac or pulmonary disease. What actually *is* and *is not* true breathlessness in veterinary medicine is difficult to define in clinical practice. Serious respiratory distress associated with substantive respiratory compromise may appear, to the owner at least, as only a minor problem. Physical examination and patient assessment are critical to the recognition and interpretation of this clinical sign.

Respiratory distress may result from (1) the need for oxygen, (2) metabolic aberrations leading to acidosis (a compensatory mechanism), (3) high environmental temperatures (heat stroke), (4) CNS disease, (5) disorders affecting motor innervation to the muscles of respiration, and (6) pain. In any event, once confirmed, diagnostic evaluation of the patient presented in respiratory distress should not be delayed.

·········· ASSOCIATED SIGNS

The most common respiratory signs that characterize distress or dyspnea include (1) tachypnea (increased respiratory rate), (2) hyperpnea (increased respiratory rate and depth), (3) orthopnea, and (4) cough. In obstructive upper airway diseases, stridor and stertorous breathing may be present on the initial examination.

Fluid accumulation in the thoracic cavity may be accompanied by ascites and hepatomegaly. Physical evidence of hyperadrenocorticism supports thrombolic pulmonary disease. Cyanosis, pallor, evidence of physical trauma, shock, and coma are serious signs often associated with respiratory distress.

............DIFFERENTIAL DIAGNOSIS (see Table 3–27)

............DIAGNOSTIC PLANS

1. Physical examination. This is justified even before a comprehensive history is completed. Patient stabilization, as required, must be accomplished (see p. 353).
2. History. Historical information relevant to duration, progression, and exposure to noxious substances or trauma is indicated. Knowledge of all current medications, including heartworm preventative, is established.
3. Laboratory profile, to include a CBC, biochemistry panel, urinalysis, heartworm test (in dogs), and FeLV and FIV tests (in cats). Cytologic, bacteriologic, and biochemical assessments of body cavity effusions are indicated.
4. Thoracic and cervical radiographs. Presence of a heart murmur, cardiac arrhythmia, or both, should be further evaluated by electrocardiography and echocardiography (see p. 282).
5. Examination of the upper respiratory tract *in the anesthetized patient* and endoscopy when signs of tracheal and bronchial disease exist.

REFERENCES

Hawkins EC: Emergency management of respiratory distress. *In* Nelson RW, Couto CG, eds: Essentials of Small Animal Internal Medicine. St Louis, Mosby–Year Book, 1992, pp 245–246.
Hribernik T: Respiratory distress or difficulty. *In* Ford RB, ed: Clinical Signs and Diagnosis in Small Animals. New York, Churchill Livingstone, 1988, pp 221–238.

Seizures (Epilepsy, Convulsions, Ictus)

............DEFINITION

The terms *seizure, convulsion, epilepsy, epileptic attack,* and *fit* all describe a clinical sign that is characterized by involuntary contraction of a series of voluntary muscles. Seizures result from disorders of the brain that cause spontaneous depolarizations and excitation of cerebral neurons. As a presenting problem, seizures are much more common in the dog than in the cat. Such disorders may originate from extracranial causes, metabolic or toxic diseases, and intracranial causes (e.g., organic brain disease). When seizures occur in the absence of detectable organic or metabolic CNS abnormalities, the seizures are described as *idiopathic*. Idiopathic epilepsy is the most common type of seizure reported in companion animal species.

A distinction is made between *partial seizures* (also called *focal seizures*) and *generalized seizures*. Three classes of partial seizure are recognized:

1. Partial motor seizures (the most common type of seizure in animals).
2. Psychomotor seizures.
3. Sensory seizures.

Partial seizures are caused by a cortical lesion or focus that periodically disrupts cerebral function. Generalized motor seizures represent a widespread

Table 3-27. Causes of Dyspnea in Dogs and Cats

Upper Airway	Lower Airway	Restrictive	Miscellaneous
Stenotic nares	Bronchial diseases	Pneumothorax	Anemia
Rhinitis/sinusitis	COPD	Pleural effusion	Methemoglobinemia
Laryngeal diseases	Allergic bronchitis (asthma,	Right heart failure	Compensation for metabolic
Necrotic laryngitis	PIE)	Neoplasia	acidosis
Edema	Lungworms	Hypoalbuminemia	Heatstroke
Paralysis of vocal folds	Pneumonia	Hemothorax	Damage to respiratory center
Everted saccules	Pulmonary edema	Chylothorax	Head trauma
Laryngeal collapse	Left heart failure	Pyothorax	Encephalitis
Intraluminal tracheal or	Hypoalbuminemia	Feline infectious peritonitis	Neoplasia
bronchial foreign body or	Others	Pericardial effusion	Neuromuscular weakness
mass	Pulmonary thromboembolism	Diaphragmatic hernia	Polyradiculoneuritis
Extraluminal tracheal or	Heartworm disease	Intrathoracic neoplastic mass	(coonhound paralysis)
bronchial obstruction	Hyperadrenocorticism	Thoracic wall trauma	Diaphragmatic paralysis
Mediastinal mass	Others	Flail chest	Others
Tracheal or bronchial collapse	Pulmonary contusions (trauma)	Extreme obesity	Pain
Hilar lymphadenopathy	Pulmonary fibrosis	Severe hepatomegaly	Fractured ribs or vertebrae
	Pulmonary granulomatosis	Marked ascites	Pleuritis
	Deep mycosis	Large intra-abdominal mass	Others
		Severe gastric distention	Paraquat poisoning
		(gastric volvulus)	

COPD, chronic obstructive pulmonary disease; PIE, pulmonary infiltrates with eosinophils.
From Lorenz MD, Cornelius LM, eds: Small Animal Medical Diagnosis. Philadelphia, JB Lippincott, 1987, p 216.

disorder not referable to any single anatomical or functional system. Clinical manifestations suggest widespread activation of the brain.

Seizures may be repeated frequently in groups of two or three, or they may occur singly. If a series of seizures occurs and the patient fails to regain consciousness during the interictal period, the term *status epilepticus* applies. In contrast to a single seizure, status epilepticus is a serious, life-threatening condition that justifies emergency intervention.

............ASSOCIATED SIGNS

Generalized motor seizures are the most prevalent type of seizure encountered in veterinary medicine. Most cases are diagnosed as idiopathic epilepsy on the basis that organic causes of seizure activity cannot be identified. The interictal period in animals with a history of generalized motor seizures is characteristically described by owners as normal. The immediate postictal period, regardless of the cause of the seizure activity, is often associated with transient disorientation, blindness, stumbling, polydipsia, or polyphagia.

The spectrum of possible clinical signs associated with seizure activity is extensive. Before a diagnosis of idiopathic epilepsy is reached, it is important that the patient be evaluated for cardiovascular disease, trauma, toxicity, infectious disease, parasites, neoplasia, and metabolic disorders, particularly those affecting the kidney, liver, and endocrine pancreas.

............Age of Animal

Seizures in young animals (<1 year old) are commonly caused by developmental abnormalities, hydrocephalus, lissencephaly, encephalitis (infectious), lead poisoning, severe intestinal parasitism, portacaval shunt abnormalities, and juvenile hypoglycemia. Idiopathic epilepsy usually begins when animals are 1 to 3 years of age. Animals over 5 years of age are more likely to have CNS tumors or hypoglycemia from insulin-secreting beta cell pancreatic neoplasms.

............Breed Predisposition

Some basic knowledge about breed predisposition to seizure disorders may be helpful in establishing a diagnosis. Idiopathic epilepsy has been seen in numerous dog breeds, particularly German shepherds, Belgian Tervurens, keeshonds, Saint Bernards, standard and miniature poodles, beagles, Irish setters, cocker spaniels, Alaskan malamutes, Siberian huskies, and Labrador and golden retrievers. Juvenile hypoglycemia is most prevalent in toy breeds. Hydrocephalus is common in the toy and brachycephalic breeds. Neoplastic diseases are common in brachycephalic breeds over 5 years of age.

Concerning disorders of CNS metabolism, leukodystrophy is most common in Cairn and West Highland whites; lipodystrophy in German shorthaired pointers and English setters; lissencephaly in the Lhasa apso; and portacaval shunts and hyperlipoproteinemia in miniature schnauzers. A unique, usually fatal, encephalitis occurs in pugs.

............Environment

Exposure to infectious agents or other sick animals may be important, as is exposure to sources of intoxicants, such as lead in paints, linoleum, tar, batteries, or roofing material; hexachlorophene soap; ethylene glycol (antifreeze); metaldehyde snail bait; and various other insecticides, including chlorinated hydrocarbons, organophosphates, and rodenticides. Dogs and cats on the same premises with swine may be exposed to *Herpesvirus suis* (pseudorabies, or

Auzjesky's disease). A high protein diet exacerbates hepatic encephalopathy. Thiamine deficiency may result from some fish diets or from cooking the food.

··········DIFFERENTIAL DIAGNOSIS (see Table 3-28)
··········DIAGNOSTIC PLANS

1. History, to take into consideration breed predisposition, environmental exposures, past medical illnesses, and medication. Because most seizures are of short duration and the physical (tonic-clonic) manifestations of a seizure are so dramatic, requesting the owner to describe the type and duration of seizure may elicit unreliable information.
2. Thorough physical examination, to include careful neurologic examination, with particular attention to cranial nerves, funduscopic examination, and cardiac auscultation (see p. 330).
3. Laboratory database, essential to rule out metabolic causes. In addition to a CBC, biochemistry profile, urinalysis, and fecal culture, any or all of the following tests are indicated: serum ammonia, bile acids, serum insulin in hypoglycemic patients, blood lead test, and serial blood cultures.
4. Survey radiographs of the skull. These are rarely helpful, as intracranial neoplasms are not detectable.
5. Electrocardiogram or echocardiogram, if indicated.
6. Serologic studies for canine distemper, rabies, feline infectious peritonitis (FIP), FeLV, FIV, toxoplasmosis, and systemic (deep) mycoses.

Table 3–28. Causes of Seizures in Symptomatic Epilepsy

Intracranial	Extracranial
Congenital	Intoxication
Hydrocephalus	Lead
Lissencephaly	Organophosphates
Other malformations	Chlorinated hydrocarbons
Storage diseases	Strychnine
Vascular anomaly	Drugs
Traumatic	Garbage
Immediate	Metabolic
Post trauma	Hypoglycemia
Inflammatory	Hypocalcemia
Distemper	Hyperkalemia
Rabies	Acid-base
Feline infectious peritonitis	Hepatic encephalopathy
Feline leukemia virus	Uremia
Toxoplasmosis	Hyperlipoproteinemia
Mycosis	Nutritional
Bacteria	Thiamine
Reticulosis	Parasites?
Parasites	Hypoxia
Neoplasia	Cardiovascular disease
Primary	Respiratory disease
Metastatic	Birth
Vascular—cerebrovascular accident	Anesthetic accident
	Hyperthermia

From Russo ME: Seizures. *In* Ford RB, ed: Clinical Signs and Diagnosis in Small Animal Practice. New York, Churchill Livingstone, 1988, p 290.

7. CSF analysis, including biochemistries, antibody titers, and cytologic parameters (see p. 891).
8. EEG. Although limited in availability, the EEG may be useful in detecting inflammatory brain disease and congenital intracranial abnormalities (e.g., hydrocephalus).
9. Contrast studies, requiring special equipment or facilities: radioisotope brain scan, cerebral angiography, pneumoencephalography, and CT scan.

REFERENCES

Chrisman CL: Seizures. *In* Ettinger SJ, Feldman EC, eds: Textbook of Veterinary Internal Medicine, ed 4. Philadelphia, WB Saunders, 1995, pp 152–157.
Meric SM: Seizures. *In* Nelson RW, Couto CG, eds: Essentials of Small Animal Internal Medicine. St Louis, Mosby–Year Book, 1992, pp 752–763.
Podell M: Seizures and sleep disorders. *In* Morgan RV, ed: Handbook of Small Animal Practice, ed 3. Philadelphia, WB Saunders, 1997, pp 220–229.

Sneezing and Nasal Discharge

..........DEFINITION

Sneezing is a protective reflex described as a sudden, involuntary, and forceful, even violent, expulsion of air from the upper respiratory tract. Sneezing is easily recognized by clients. Although sneezing is a physiologic response to irritating stimuli, increased frequency and paroxysmal sneezing episodes are readily recognized as abnormal. Like sneezing, a nasal discharge, regardless of its consistency, is a clinical sign that is accurately interpreted by the client and reliably described to the clinician.

Sneezing is the outward manifestation of nasal passage irritation by extraneous (foreign material) or endogenous (antigen-antibody interaction) agents. Afferent impulses travel via the fifth cranial nerve to the medulla, where the initial reflex is triggered. Chronic nasal discharge is a clinical sign that localizes a disorder to the upper respiratory passages, particularly the nasal cavity and frontal sinuses.

..........ASSOCIATED SIGNS

Important associated signs suggesting systemic involvement include facial asymmetry (neoplasia or fungal infection), atrophy of the masseter and temporal muscles, difficulty prehending or masticating food, conjunctivitis, and ocular discharge. *Epistaxis*, which is distinguished from blood-tinged nasal discharge, is an important associated sign that further supports intranasal disease or coagulopathy. Cleft palate is a common cause of nasal discharge in neonates. Erosion and depigmentation of the planum nasale is often associated with nasal aspergillosis in dogs, whereas cats with nasal cryptococosis may have a detectable granuloma at the rostral aspect of the nose. Occasionally, cough is associated with purulent nasal discharges and sneezing.

..........DIFFERENTIAL DIAGNOSIS (see Table 3–29)
..........DIAGNOSTIC PLANS (see Fig. 3–5)

REFERENCES

Ford RB: Sneezing and nasal discharge. *In* Ford RB, ed: Clinical Signs and Diagnosis in Small Animal Practice, New York, Churchill Livingstone, 1988, pp 189–202.
Hawkins EC: Disorders of the nasal cavity. *In* Nelson RW, Couto CG, eds: Essentials of Small Animal Internal Medicine. St Louis, Mosby–Year Book, 1992, pp 163–171.

Table 3–29. Differential Diagnosis of Nasal Discharge

Intranasal Causes
Serous nasal discharge
    Acute viral upper respiratory infection (feline)
    Feline chlamydiosis
    Intranasal parasites
    Oronasal fistula (canine tooth)
    Rhinosporidiosis (canine, rare)
Purulent Nasal Discharge
    Viral upper respiratory infection with secondary bacterial infection
      (dog and cat)
    Mycotic nasal disease
    Foreign body rhinitis
    Traumatic rhinitis or sinusitis
    Cleft palate
    Neoplasia (several types possible)
    Nasopharyngeal polyps (feline, rare)
    Benign nasal polyps (canine, rare)
    Oronasal fistula
Mucoid to Mucopurulent Nasal Discharge
    Mycotic nasal disease (e.g., aspergillosis, cryptococcosis, blastomycosis)
    Neoplasia (especially adenocarcinoma)
Epistaxis
    Acute nasal trauma
    Oronasal fistula

Extranasal Causes
Purulent Nasal Discharge
    Bacterial pneumonia
    Megaesophagus with aspiration pneumonia, congenital or acquired
    Achalasia with nasal reflux of food
    Acquired esophageal stricture
Epistaxis
    von Willebrand's disease (most common canine coagulopathy)
    Factor VIII deficiency (classic hemophilia)
    Other inherited factor deficiencies
    Thrombocytopenia (infectious or immune-mediated)
    Disseminated intravascular coagulation
    Hyperviscosity syndrome

Modified from Ford RB: Sneezing and nasal discharge. *In* Ford RB, ed: Clinical Signs and Diagnosis in Small Animal Practice. New York, Churchill Livingstone, 1988, pp 189–202.

Mckiernan BC: Diseases of the nasal and nasopharyngeal cavities and paranasal sinuses. *In* Morgan RV, ed: Handbook of Small Animal Practice. Philadelphia, WB Saunders, 1995, pp 138–147.

Spontaneous Bleeding

##·········· DEFINITION

Spontaneous or prolonged bleeding is an abnormal condition resulting from a failure of the hemostatic mechanism. It results from deficiencies in platelet numbers or function, in the extrinsic or intrinsic coagulation cascades, or in vascular integrity (see also p. 687).

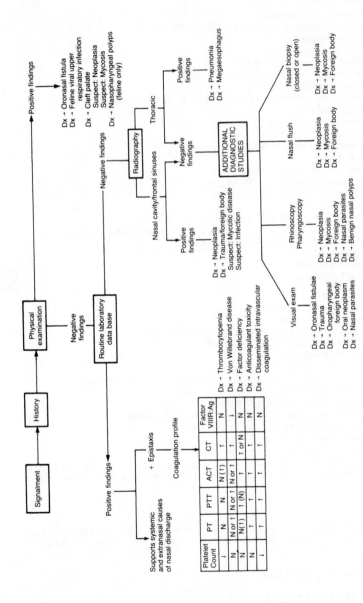

Figure 3–5. See legend on opposite page

The hemostatic response is a complex defense system that fulfills three basic functions:

1. Ensures that blood is confined to the vascular system of the normal animal (vascular integrity).
2. Causes the arrest of bleeding at sites of vascular injury.
3. Maintains the patency of the vascular network.

These functions are accomplished through complex interactions between blood platelets, the blood vessel wall, and a variety of plasma enzyme systems. Disorders affecting these interactions can result in spontaneous or prolonged bleeding.

The *primary phase* of hemostasis occurs with platelet aggregation and the formation of the relatively unstable platelet plug. The *secondary phase* of hemostasis, essential to complete hemostasis, reinforces the platelet plug with fibrin. Secondary hemostasis depends on adequate plasma concentration of procoagulant proteins and on their proper interaction. Coagulation can be initiated through an intrinsic pathway, which involves components normally found within the vasculature and which is activated by contact with a foreign surface. The extrinsic pathway is an alternative mechanism through which clotting is initiated.

Secondary hemostasis is regulated by inhibitory products that limit the extent of enzymatic reaction and prevent their dissemination: antithrombin III, a potent inhibitor of kallikrein; factors IXa, XIa, XIIa, and Xa; and thrombin. The fibrinolytic system, another plasma protein–enzyme system, serves to remove the hemostatic plug once its function has been served.

··········ASSOCIATED SIGNS

Bleeding disorders are most apparent when bleeding develops spontaneously from one or more body orifices and is prolonged. Bleeding into the skin or mucous membranes (e.g., petechiation) may not be immediately apparent to even the most observant owner. Excessive or prolonged bleeding into soft tissues (hematoma) or joints (hemarthrosis) may be seen as physical enlargement of the affected tissues with pain and lameness.

There may be a history of recurrent minor bleeding episodes in some animals. The severity of clinical signs is dependent upon such factors as type of defect, degree of clotting factor activity, and individual variation. Moderately to severely affected animals are typically young at the time of presentation. Prolonged bleeding subsequent to elective surgical procedures may be the first sign of a bleeding disorder.

··········DIFFERENTIAL DIAGNOSIS (see Table 3–30)
··········DIAGNOSTIC PLANS

1. History. Age (inherited vs. acquired), sex (sex-linked vs. autosomal), and breed (inherited vs. acquired) of the bleeding patient must be carefully

---

Figure 3–5. Clinical algorithm for the patient presented for sneezing, nasal discharge, or both. ACT, activated clotting time; PT, prothrombin time; PTT, partial thromboplastin time; CT, clotting time; Factor VIIIR:Ag, factor VIII–related antigen; ↓, decreased (numbers); ↑, prolonged (time); N, normal; N (↑), usually normal, occasionally prolonged; ↑ (N), usually prolonged, occasionally normal. (From Ford RB: Sneezing and nasal discharge. *In* Ford RB, ed: Clinical Signs and Diagnosis in Small Animal Practice. New York, Churchill Livingstone, 1988.)

Table 3–30. Differential Diagnosis of Spontaneous Bleeding

Hereditary Disorders—Factor Deficiencies
Hypoprothrombinemia (factor II)—boxers
Hypoproconvertinemia (factor VII)—beagles, malamutes
Hemophilia A (factor VIII)—most dog breeds and cats
Hemophilia B (factor IX)—several dog breeds and British short-hair cats
von Willebrand's disease (vWD factor)—most dog breeds
Stuart factor deficiency (factor X)—cocker spaniels
Plasma thromboplastin antecedent (PTA) deficiency (factor XI)—springer
    spaniels, Great Pyrenees, Kerry blue terriers
Hageman factor deficiency (factor XII)—cats

Hereditary Platelet Disorders
Thrombocytopenia
Platelet dysfunction
    Thrombasthenia (Glanzmann's disease)*
    Thrombopathia (e.g., osteogenesis imperfecta, Ehlers-Danlos syndrome)*

Acquired Clotting Factor Disorders
Primary hyperfibrinolysis
Disseminated intravascular coagulation (DIC)
Chemical- or drug-induced
    Vitamin K deficiency
    Rodenticide ingestion
    Prolonged enteric antimicrobial therapy*
Circulating anticoagulants
    Heparin
    Warfarin
    Warfarin-like chemical (e.g., diphacinone)
    Plasma expander therapy*
    Antifactor antibody*
Liver disease
    DIC
    Vitamin K deficiency
    Decreased factor synthesis subsequent to severe liver disease*

Acquired Platelet Disorders
Thrombocytopenia (relatively common)
    Decreased or ineffective thrombopoiesis*
    Immunologic destruction: immune-mediated, infectious, drug-induced
    Consumption: DIC, vasculitis
    Sequestration: splenomegaly subsequent to neoplasia*
    Dilutional: IV fluid administration*
Platelet dysfunction
    Secondary to underlying disease: renal failure and uremia, hepatic failure,
        polycythemia*
    Drug-induced: aspirin, phenylbutazone, estrogen, phenothiazines, plasma
        expanders*

*These occur rarely.

considered. Bleeding disorders in related animals should also be considered.
A detailed history of recent or current drug administration and vaccination
is critical.
2. Physical examination. This may be normal. However, evidence of melena,
   hematuria, epistaxis, and hematoma or hemarthrosis should be pursued.

The skin and mucous membranes should be inspected for evidence of pete-chiae or ecchymoses.

3. Routine laboratory database, indicated in all bleeding patients to assess for the presence of underlying contributory diseases, as well as the possible consequences of bleeding within major organs.

4. Antibody titers for ehrlichiosis and Rocky Mountain spotted fever (see p. 700).

5. Coagulation screening tests (see p. 687):
   a. Peripheral blood smear (for the presence of platelets).
   b. Cuticle bleeding time.
   c. Platelet count.
   d. Assessment of clot retraction.
   e. PT.
   f. Activated partial thromboplastin time (APTT).
   g. Thrombin clotting time.
   h. Fibrinogen.
   i. FDPs.
   j. Clot lysis.

6. Specialized laboratory tests (special facilities required):
   a. Specific factor activity assays.
   b. Platelet function studies (adhesion, aggregation, secretion).
   c. Antiplatelet antibody.
   d. Antithrombin III.
   e. Kallikrein.
   f. Electron microscopic assessment of platelets.

3

REFERENCES

Boudreaux MK: Platelet and coagulative disorders. *In* Morgan RV, ed: Handbook of Small Animal Practice. Philadelphia, WB Saunders, 1997, pp 698–717.

Dhupa N, Littman MG: Epistaxis. Compend Contin Educ Pract Vet 14:1033, 1992.

Johnstone IB: Spontaneous or prolonged bleeding. *In* Ford RB, ed: Clinical Signs and Diagnosis in Small Animal Practice. New York, Churchill Livingstone, 1988, pp 103–116.

Urinary Incontinence

···········DEFINITION

Urinary incontinence referes to the lack of normal ability to prevent discharge of urine from the body. Urinary incontinence is suspected when an animal that previously exhibited normal control of urination begins passing urine at times or in places that are inappropriate. Determining whether or not the presenting complaint of inappropriate urinary behavior is involuntary can be a formidable task in a dog or cat. Distinguishing between voluntary and involuntary urination is fundamental to the diagnostic plan.

The normal micturition reflex is a result of the complex interaction of the autonomic and somatic nervous systems. Normal control of micturition can be divided into a series of nervous pathways.

1. Sensory neurons have stretch receptors in the bladder wall that relay information through ascending spinal cord tracts to the brain stem and somesthetic cortex of the frontoparietal lobes. This pathway is the basis for the perception of a full bladder.

2. Frontoparietal motor cortex projects to the brain stem reticular formation centers for micturition that are responsible for storage and evacuation of urine.

3. From these centers, reticulospinal tracts descend the spinal cord to influence

gray matter centers responsible for the storage or evacuation of urine. For evacuation, the visceral efferent neurons in the sacral segments that innervate the detrusor muscle via the pelvic nerves are facilitated. The somatic efferent neurons in the sacral segments that innervate the striate urethralis muscle via the pudendal nerve are inhibited. Facilitation of these pudendal somatic neurons prevents urination.

Urinary incontinence is the physical manifestation of any one of several disorders affecting voluntary urine retention in the bladder. Neurologic lesions involving either upper motor or lower motor neuron segments of the micturition reflex arc result in urinary incontinence. A paralytic bladder usually results in bladder overdistention and urine dribbling. Urine can be easily expressed by manual compression of the bladder in affected patients. A "cord bladder" is caused by a lesion between the brain and the spinal reflex center of micturition. There is usually temporary bladder paralysis followed by involuntary reflex micturition subsequent to manual compression.

Non-neurogenic urinary incontinence may be due to anatomical or functional disorders (e.g., ectopic ureters) affecting the storage phase of micturition. Hormone-responsive incontinence is also a common form of non-neurogenic urinary incontinence. In these patients, the detrusor reflex is normal and the animal exhibits normal urination behavior in addition to urine dribbling.

A number of disorders of micturition are associated with excessive outlet resistance (e.g., urethral calculi, neoplasia) during voiding. Bladder overdistention and urine dribbling are frequently accompanied by dysuria and hematuria.

............ASSOCIATED SIGNS

Evidence of urine or blood-tinged urine on the hair coat around the genitalia or on the patient's sleeping surface is frequently the first sign of a micturition disorder recognized by owners. Patients with neurogenic urinary incompetence may show evidence of spinal cord disease with conscious proprioceptive deficits in the hindlimbs, foot drag, and abrasions on the dorsal aspect of the hindfeet. However, lesions involving the cerebral cortex and cerebellum may also be associated with incontinence, as can behavioral disorders.

Obvious straining to urinate, particularly if associated with an enlarged abdomen, may indicate obstructive disease. Affected patients may be uremic, manifesting characteristic signs of lethargy, anorexia, and vomiting.

............DIFFERENTIAL DIAGNOSIS (see Table 3–31)
............DIAGNOSTIC PLANS

1. History and physical examination. The size of the urinary bladder must also be determined.
2. Neurologic examination. A thorough neurologic examination should be performed in an attempt to establish or rule out a neurogenic cause. Particular emphasis is given to the spinal cord and sacral nerve roots. The bulbourethral and perineal reflexes should be assessed (see p. 330).
3. Catheterization of urinary bladder, to determine residual urine (normal = 0.2 to 0.4 mL/kg in the dog and cat). Urine collected is submitted for urinalysis and, as indicated, for culture and sensitivity (see p. 486).
4. Laboratory database, to evaluate patient health status.
5. Survey radiographs of the caudal abdomen and spinal cord.
6. Contrast studies, as needed, including, pneumocystogram (only in the absence of hematuria), contrast urethrogram, and excretory urogram (also called intravenous pyelogram).
7. Cystometrogram. Special equipment is required.

Table 3–31. Differential Diagnosis of Urinary Incontinence

Neurogenic
Cerebral lesions
Cerebellar lesions
Brain stem lesions
Spinal cord lesions
Spinal nerve root lesions

Non-neurogenic without Distended Bladder
Ectopic ureter(s)
Patent urachus
Hormone-responsive incontinence
Urethral incompetence
Neoplasia
Reduced bladder capacity
Cystitis

Non-neurogenic with Distended Bladder
Urethral obstruction, calculi, or neoplasia
Detrusor-urethral dyssynergia
Overflow incontinence (associated with polyuric states)

REFERENCES

Grauer GF: Disorders of micturition. *In* Nelson RW, Couto CG, eds: Essentials of Small Animal Internal Medicine. St Louis, Mosby–Year Book, 1992, pp 517–524.
Lane IF: Disorders of Micturition. *In* Morgan RV, ed. Handbook of Small Animal Practice, ed 3, Philadelphia, WB Saunders, 1997, pp 545–557.
Moreau PM, Lee GE: Incontinence, enuresis, nocturia, and dysuria. *In* Ettinger SJ, Feldman EC, eds: Textbook of Veterinary Internal Medicine, ed 4. Philadelphia, WB Saunders, 1995, pp 164–169.

Vision Loss

············DEFINITION

Blindness is the inability to perceive visual stimuli. Because decreased visual function in animals is evidenced only by a change in behavior, the ability of pet owners to detect vision loss depends on their awareness of changes in the animal's awareness of and interaction with its surroundings. Visual deficits, such as partial vision loss or unilateral blindness, are unlikely to be detected by an owner because of the animal's ability to compensate.

Blindness can occur in any of four ways:

1. Lesions causing opacification of clear ocular media (e.g., cornea, aqueous humor, or lens).
2. Failure of the retina to process visual images.
3. Failure of neurologic transmission.
4. Failure in the final image processing (i.e., cortical blindness).

············DIFFERENTIAL DIAGNOSIS

When an animal is presented with acute visual loss, the owner is usually describing a bilateral ocular disease problem or the possibility of a CNS problem. Acute unilateral visual loss problems are not often recognized except by the very astute animal owner or observer. For the veterinarian, initial assessment of the animal with acute visual loss depends initially on confirming that the ocular media are clear and allow light to pass from the anterior ocular segment and reach the photoreceptor cells (rods and cones) in the posterior ocular segment. A strong, focal light source such as a 3.5-V halogen-illuminated Finoff transilluminator (Welch-Allyn Co., Skaneateles, N.Y.) should be used to evaluate the ocular media. Such conditions as acute bilateral uveitis, severe corneal edema, bilateral acute keratitis, rapidly developing metabolic cataracts, or acute cyclitis with vitreous involvement may alter the ocular media to interfere with light transmission. Both direct and indirect pupillary responses should be evaluated while evaluating the anterior ocular media. Once it has been determined that light can reach the posterior ocular segment, a fundus evaluation should be done. *Fundic abnormalities associated with acute visual loss* may include acute chorioretinitis, often with exudative retinal detachments; acute choroidal hemorrhages, often associated with abnormal blood pressure in chronic renal disease; and acute optic neuritis.

Acute visual loss in the dog *without accompanying fundic lesions* that can be seen on ophthalmoscopic examination may be associated with a retrobulbar optic neuritis or with the syndrome of sudden acquired retinal degeneration in the dog (SARDS). SARDS is poorly understood. The syndrome appears to involve middle-aged to old female dogs and there is a breed predilection for the dachshund. The visual loss may first start as a nyctalopia and progress over a period of weeks to complete visual loss. In some cases the visual loss is generalized and acute. Associated systemic signs of polydipsia, polyuria, polyphagia, obesity, and hepatomegaly may be present. Laboratory profiles may show abnormal differentials in the WBC count, elevated liver enzymes, an abnormal response to ACTH stimulation testing, or an abnormal response to low-dose dexamethasone suppression testing. The fundus may appear absolutely normal or early signs of retinal thinning and atrophy may be evident. Differential diagnosis with an optic neuritis are based on electroretinography (ERG) testing in which the ERG response is flat in SARDS but the ERG response is normal in optic neuritis. The cause of SARDS is unknown.

Acute visual loss in the dog associated with tumors of the CNS, particularly CNS tumors that involve the optic chiasm, are infrequently reported in the dog. In humans, tumors of the pituitary gland may be associated with a bitemporal hemianopsia. The pituitary gland of the dog is directed caudoventrally and the diaphragmatic sella is incomplete in the dog, allowing pituitary tumors to grow dorsocaudally. Thus, pituitary tumors must become macroadenomas before invading and involving midbrain structures and the optic chiasm region. It is not uncommon for macroadenomas to be nonfunctional; thus, the affected animal may not develop any clinical metabolic abnormalities. Papilledema is rarely observed with brain tumors in dogs. Although pituitary macroadenomas that produce chiasmal compression and visual loss are rare in dogs, the differential diagnosis must still be considered.

The availability at large teaching centers of CT has provided the ability to diagnose tumors of the hypophysis that may be associated with acute visual loss. Additionally, the use of the same technique has made visualization of the adrenal glands and the ability to diagnose bilateral adrenal gland hyperplasia easier. Pituitary macroadenomas are larger than 1 cm in diameter. In evaluating the possible role of the pituitary gland in producing endocrine abnormalities, the following techniques of patient evaluation may be of value:

1. Careful evaluation of the patient, including history of possible endocrine imbalance; careful examination of the skeleton and skin; evaluation of the eyes, including a complete fundus evaluation; possible role of ERG in distinguishing causes of acute visual loss problems.
2. Evaluate systemic hormonal levels.
3. Visualize the pituitary with CT scans.

Optic neuritis may present as an acute visual loss problem. There may or may not be observable ophthalmoscopic changes of the optic nerve. Ophthalmoscopic abnormalities are characterized by edema of the disk, hemorrhages in and around the disk, edema, and inflammation of the surrounding retinal tissue. Acute optic neuritis often persists as a retrobulbar lesion without any ophthalmoscopically observable lesions. Pupils are widely dilated and nonresponsive or poorly responsive to light. In suspected acute optic neuritis a complete physical examination, including a neurologic evaluation, peripheral blood count, and CSF analysis, should be performed, if possible. The presence of pleiocytosis and increased protein content in the CSF is of significance. It may be difficult to specifically diagnose the cause of acute optic neuritis. Granulomatous meningoencephalitis (reticulosis) of the CNS can result in optic nerve inflammation. Granulomatous meningoencephalitis is a specific entity of the canine CNS characterized by a proliferation and accumulation of mesenchymal cells around the blood vessels of the CNS. These reactive cells may also invade the parenchyma of the CNS. Histologically, the cellular accumulation is predominantly macrophages, lymphocytes, and plasma cells. The condition may be focal or diffuse or involve the uveal tract and the optic nerves of the eyes. Treatment involves the early use of immunosuppressive doses of corticosteroids.

■ HEMORRHAGE IN THE VITREOUS CAVITY OR RETINA

Chorioretinitis

Hypertensive retinopathy

Acute cyclitis

Retinal detachment

Trauma hyperviscosity syndrome

Coagulation factor disorders or platelet disorders

Persistent hyperplastic primary vitreous/Persistent hyperplastic hyaloid vasculature

---

■ INTRAOCULAR HEMORRHAGE

Coagulation factor disorders or platelet disorders

Trauma

Secondary to acute anterior uveitis and cyclitis

Retinal detachment

Intraocular neoplasia

Persistent hyperplastic primary vitreous/Persistent hyperplastic hyaloid vasculature

---

··········DIAGNOSTIC AND TREATMENT PLANS
(see Fig. 3–6)

1. Evaluate pupillary light responses and vision by evaluating the animal's vision in an obstacle course and in altered light conditions.
2. Perform an ophthalmic examination to evaluate the clarity of the ocular media and the ability of light to reach the photoreceptor cells. Evaluate the posterior ocular segment by performing an ophthalmoscopic examination.
3. Evaluate the general physical condition of the animal including a basic neurologic examination:

Fundic
reflection ──→

↓

1. Absent

A. Acute anterior
   uveitis, cyclitis with
   cells, flare, blood in
   anterior chamber

B. Acute edema of
   cornea as in
   uveitis, lens luxation
   Acute glaucoma

C. Opacity of lens
   cataract

D. Vitreous opacity,
   blood, inflammation,
   asteroid hyalosis

Present
↓

2. Normal

Lesions of lateral
geniculate
nucleus
Optic radiations or
occipital cortex
   Trauma
   Necrosis
   Hydrocephalus
   Toxicity
   Infection
   Mass
   Degeneration
   Biochemical

3. Miotic

A. Acute uveitis

B. CNS disorders

4. Mydriatic with no
   fundus abnormalities

A. SARDS

B. Acute retrobulbar optic
   neuritis

5. Mydriatic with fundus
   lesions

A. Acute optic neuritis

B. Atrophy of optic nerve
   Chronic glaucoma

C. Retinal disease
   Hypertensive retinopathy
   Retinal detachment
   which may be secondary
   to congenital defect,
   inflammation,
   hemorrhage, trauma

Figure 3–6. An algorithm for sudden acquired blindness. SARDS, syndrome of sudden acquired retinal degeneration in the dog.

a. If acute retinal or vitreal hemorrhage is present, determine if the bleeding involves only the eyes or if there is evidence of bleeding elsewhere in the body (see p. 687). Determine if blood pressure is normal (see p. 75) and if there is evidence of chronic renal disease, hyperadrenocorticism, or hyperthyroidism.

b. If active chorioretinitis with or without exudative retinal detachment is present, determine if the inflammation appears granulomatous; if it does, consider systemic fungal infections and consider performing a vitreal or subretinal aspiration and cytologic examination to look for fungal agents. If inflammation is not granulomatous, perform a complete physical examination, CBC, and chemistry panel, and look for evidence of other systemic inflammatory diseases.

c. If acute visual loss is *unaccompanied* by any fundus abnormalities, perform a complete physical examination, including a basic neurologic evaluation (see p. 330); if acute retrobulbar optic neuritis is suspected, a CBC and CSF examination (see p. 519) should be considered; an ERG may be indicated to distinguish between SARDS and acute optic neuritis.

REFERENCES

Bistner S: Recent Developments in Comparative Ophthalmology. Compend Contin Educ Pract Vet 10:1304–1318, 1992.
McLaughlin SA, Hamilton HL: Acute vision loss. In Ettinger SJ, Feldman, EC, eds: Textbook of Veterinary Internal Medicine, ed 4. Philadelphia, WB Saunders, 1995, pp 208–210.
Nasisse MP: Vision loss. In Ford RB, ed: Clinical Signs and Diagnosis in Small Animals. New York, Churchill Livingstone, 1988, pp 673–721.

Vomiting

·········· DEFINITION

The forceful ejection of food or fluid through the mouth from the stomach and, occasionally, the proximal duodenum describes *vomiting*. The term applies to those animals with overt evidence of effort associated with the expulsion of food and is characterized by vigorous abdominal pressing, arched back, gagging or retching, and hypersalivation. *Projectile vomiting* is the term used to describe the violent ejection of stomach contents without nausea or retching. *Regurgitation*, on the other hand, denotes expulsion of food or fluid from the esophagus and is a considerably more passive act than in vomiting.

Cough-induced gagging associated with tracheitis or tracheobronchitis is often accompanied by the expulsion of mucus from the respiratory tract and can be a forceful act. As such, productive coughs may appear to the owner to be vomiting.

Vomiting is a complex reflex that entails coordination of the GI tract, musculoskeletal system, and nervous system. Although the CNS vomiting center initiates vomiting, it must first be stimulated. Even when vomiting is drug-induced, stimulation of the vomiting center is accomplished subsequent to stimulation of a medullary chemoreceptor trigger zone that forwards impulses to the vomiting center. Emetic impulses can be mediated by many sensory nerves. Therefore, intense pain (especially abdominal); nervous (psychogenic) stimuli; disagreeable odors, tastes, and smells; sensations from the labyrinth and pharyngeal areas; various toxins and drugs; and, presumably, the retention of metabolic waste products all may lead to vomiting. Numerous receptors for vomiting are located in the abdominal viscera, especially the duodenum. Afferent nerve fibers are found in the vagal and sympathetic nerves.

Vomiting can be quite debilitating. When excessive, it causes severe extra-

Table 3–32. Differential Diagnosis of Vomiting

Infectious Causes
Feline panleukopenia virus infection
Canine parvovirus infection
Canine coronavirus infection
Infectious canine hepatitis
Leptospirosis
Bacterial enteritis
Parasitic enteritis
Heartworm disease (cats)

Inflammatory
Pyometra
Prostatitis
Peritonitis
Acute pancreatitis
Gastritis and enteritis
Gastric ulcers

Obstructive Causes
Intestinal foreign body
Gastrointestinal neoplasia
Gastric dilation–volvulus syndrome
Pyloric stenosis
Trichobezoar (hairballs)
Diaphragmatic hernia

Metabolic Causes
Renal failure (uremia)
Hepatic disease
Diabetic ketoacidosis
Hypoadrenocorticism (Addison's disease)
Hypokalemia, regardless of cause
Hyperthyroidism (cats)

Chemical Causes
Heavy metals, pesticides, solvents
Digitalis, salicylates, mebendazole, penicillamine, chloramphenicol,
  morphine, antineoplastic drugs, others

Idiopathic/Miscellaneous Causes
Psychogenic, vestibular (car sickness)
Overconsumption of food, especially puppies
Various CNS diseases
Bilious vomiting syndrome
Autonomic epilepsy
Constipation/obstipation
Ileus, paralytic

---

cellular fluid deficits, particularly of sodium, potassium, and chloride ions and water. Loss of mainly gastric contents results in loss of hydrogen ions, a high serum bicarbonate concentration, and metabolic alkalosis. Vomited material from the proximal intestinal tract contains high concentrations of bicarbonate.

Clinically, vomiting should be addressed as a problem that originates from the GI tract (primary causes) or from causes outside the GI tract; i.e., metabolic causes (secondary).

···········ASSOCIATED SIGNS

Depending on the underlying cause, vomiting may be associated with a number of significant clinical signs. Primary causes of vomiting are generally associated with other GI signs, such as diarrhea, abdominal pain, obvious foreign bodies (e.g., a linear foreign body entrapped proximally under the tongue), ingestion of known irritant materials or drugs, hematochezia, or palpable abdominal tumors. Animals with metabolic or secondary causes of vomiting may appear lethargic, anorectic, and weak, particularly when the vomiting episodes have been sustained for several days. In some animals, polyuria or polydipsia, anuria, icterus, cough, and anemia are present.

···········DIFFERENTIAL DIAGNOSIS (see Table 3–32)
···········DIAGNOSTIC PLANS

1. Verification that the patient is vomiting, not gagging or retching subsequent to tracheal disease. Determine duration, precipitating causes, and current drug therapy. Assess associated signs.
2. Laboratory database, fundamental to the diagnostic plan. It must include CBC, biochemistry profile, urinalysis, and fecal flotation. Cats should also be tested for heartworm disease, FeLV, FIV, and hyperthyroidism. Perform serologic studies, as needed, to rule out systemic infections (e.g., systemic mycoses).
3. Radiographs of the thorax and abdomen; abdominal ultrasound.
4. Contrast radiographic studies of the stomach and small bowel (e.g., barium series).
5. Exploratory laparotomy, depending on patient condition.
6. Special diagnostic procedures: endoscopy, GI biopsy, double-contrast studies of the stomach and small bowel, and gastric motility studies (fluoroscopy).

REFERENCES

Guilford WG, Center SA, Strombeck DR, et al: Strombeck's Small Animal Gastroenterology, ed 2. Philadelphia, WB Saunders, 1996.
Tams TR: Vomiting, regurgitation, and dysphagia. *In* Ettinger SJ, Feldman EC, eds: Textbook of Veterinary Internal Medicine, ed 4. Philadelphia, WB Saunders, 1995, pp 103–111.
Willard M: Clinical manifestations of gastrointestinal disorders. *In* Nelson RW, Couto CG, eds: Essentials of Small Animal Internal Medicine, ed 2. St Louis, Mosby–Year Book, 1998, pp 346–369.

Section 4

···

CLINICAL
PROCEDURES

4

●●●

ROUTINE DIAGNOSTIC PROCEDURES

Abdominal Paracentesis

(See also Diagnostic Peritoneal Lavage, p. 18)

Abdominal paracentesis refers to the surgical puncture of the abdominal cavity for the purpose of removing fluids. Always weigh the animal before and after removing abdominal fluid. Any subsequent gain in weight indicates a reaccumulation of abdominal fluid. Place the animal in left lateral recumbency and restrain it in this position (Fig. 4–1). Clip and surgically prepare a 1- to 3-in. square between the bladder and the umbilicus just lateral to the midline. If the bladder is distended, empty it before paracentesis is performed. Infiltrate the paracentesis site with lidocaine (Xylocaine) 0.5%, using a 22- to 24-gauge needle. In most cases, local anesthesia is not necessary. Abdominal puncture can be made with an 18- to 20-gauge needle. When the abdominal puncture has been made, the animal should be allowed to rest quietly to facilitate drainage of the fluid. Some clinicians recommend tapping while the patient is in a standing position in the hope of obtaining more complete drainage. Changing the patient's position after the tapping may cause laceration of the abdominal contents. Aspiration may be easier if a specially adapted needle with multiple holes drilled in the shaft is used because it is less likely to become plugged with omentum. Ideally, four quadrants of the abdomen should be tapped. Single needle taps are not as accurate as instilling a lavage fluid (warmed lactated Ringer's solution) into the abdomen and examining the lavage fluid (see p. 18). Measure the amount of fluid obtained, and examine the fluid to determine whether it is an exudate or a transudate (see p. 768). Cytologic examination and culture may also be performed. Rather than drain the abdominal fluid completely, it may be better to spare protein loss and mobilize the fluids with diuretics. Paracentesis can also be performed by using a sterile intravenous catheter to enter the abdomen (Fig. 4–2). When performing paracentesis, ultrasonographic guidance can prove very valuable in placing the needle into the compartmental space desired and in avoiding complications. The major complications in abdominal paracentesis are perforated hollow viscus, laceration of abdominal organs, and iatrogenic peritonitis.

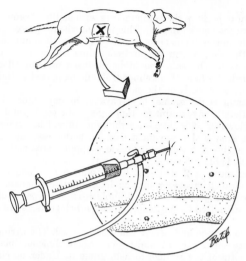

Figure 4–1. A 3-in. square to the right of the midline between the bladder and umbilicus has been clipped and surgically prepared. Paracentesis is performed using a needle and three-way valve to facilitate fluid collection. An improved technique is to use an extension tube from the needle hub to the three-way valve. This allows manipulation of the valve and syringe without disturbing the needle and may reduce possible trauma.

REFERENCES

Meyer DJ, Harvey J: Veterinary Laboratory Medicine, ed 2. Philadelphia, WB Saunders, 1998.
Paddelford RR, Harvey RC: Critical care techniques. Vet Clin North Am Small Anim Pract 19:1079–1094, 1989.

4

Blood Collection

Venipuncture of the dog or cat may be accomplished by using the cephalic, jugular, femoral, or recurrent tarsal veins. In large dogs, the cephalic vein is preferred. In cats and smaller dogs, the jugular vein is frequently used. A peripheral blood sample can be obtained by deep clipping of a toenail, but this method is often undesirable.

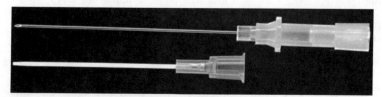

Figure 4–2. JELCO IV catheter (reference #4059) 20 gauge, 1¾ in. (Courtesy of Johnson & Johnson Medical, Arlington, TX.)

It is essential to perform the venipuncture with as little trauma as possible so as to preserve the vein's integrity. This is vital when repeated taps must be performed. With show animals or for aesthetic reasons, it is undesirable to clip the hair over the site, but in long-haired animals, careful clipping aids in identifying the vein. The skin should be cleansed and an effective topical antiseptic applied. The hair (if not clipped) should be parted so that the sterile needle can be placed directly on the skin.

Proper restraint of the animal is of paramount importance for successful venipuncture. Details of restraint for tapping specific veins are discussed in a later section. However, it is necessary that the animal be comfortable while restrained. The area of the vein must be held motionless, the skin stretched firmly to help anchor the vein, and pressure applied proximal to the site of puncture to occlude blood flow.

In most instances, a 2- to 5-mL blood sample is adequate for routine hematology, clinical chemistry, or enzyme determinations. In small dogs and in cats, jugular vein samples are collected (Table 4–1). The types of blood samples that should be submitted for particular clinicopathologic tests are discussed on p. 859.

A dry, sterile syringe and needle can also be used. The syringe should be held lightly between the thumb and fingers. Some clinicians place the index finger near the tip of the syringe to help guide it. Under no circumstances, however, should the finger touch the needle.*

In most cases, it is best to penetrate the skin just lateral to the vein. The needle is further advanced to puncture the vein from the side. Blood usually enters the syringe spontaneously but can be encouraged to enter by applying gentle suction. Some clinicians maintain continuous suction in the syringe (after the skin and fascia have been punctured) while probing for the vein so that penetration of the vein is indicated by the appearance of blood. Inadequate flow into the syringe may be caused by too much suction, which collapses the vein; partial occlusion of the needle; circulatory failure; hematoma formation; or piercing the vein wall without entering the lumen. Occasionally, the tip of the needle becomes snagged in the opposite wall of the vein. Slight retraction and rotation of the needle correct the problem. The flow of blood is often

....

*Becton Dickinson and Co., Sparks, MD.

Table 4–1. Evacuated Tubes for Blood Samples

Color of Rubber Stopper	Anticoagulant	Purpose
Red	None	Electrolytes Enzymes Serologic studies
Lavender	EDTA	Blood cell counts
Blue	Citrate	Prothrombin time Partial thromboplastin time
Gray	NaF	Blood sugar
Green	Heparin	Serologic studies Blood gases
Yellow	ACD AD PBS	Acid-citric-dextrose* Acid-dextrose* Physiologic saline

*All tubes for blood storage are sterile.
EDTA, ethylenediaminetetraacetic acid; PBS, phosphate-buffered saline.

improved by alternating occlusion and release of the vein combined with slight passive motion of the leg drained by the vein. The complications of venipuncture include minor hemorrhage, subcutaneous hematoma formation, vascular trauma, and thrombophlebitis.

The use of a Vacutainer has simplified obtaining blood samples from small animals, especially when larger veins are tapped to collect blood. Do not use large-volume Vacutainer containers in small veins because the wall of the vein will collapse and samples will not be obtained. To ensure that the proper anticoagulant-blood ratio is obtained, all tubes with anticoagulants should be filled until the vacuum is exhausted.

............HANDLING BLOOD SAMPLES (see p. 859)

Use syringe and needle or evacuated blood collection tubes when handling blood samples. All equipment must be chemically clean and *dry*.

Hemolysis is avoided by using clean, dry equipment and avoiding trauma to the red blood cells (RBCs). Trauma to RBCs is often the result of application of excessive or fluctuating suction during the aspiration procedure, excessive force in expelling blood from the syringe to the container, or excessive agitation of blood after collection.

Hemolysis may interfere with the following tests:

1. *Serum lipase*. With 0.5 g of hemoglobin per deciliter, 50% inhibition occurs.
2. *Serum bilirubin*. Large negative errors in the presence of hemoglobin may be due to the conversion of hemoglobin to methemoglobin by nitrous acid in the test and not in the control.
3. *Urea nitrogen*. Falsely elevated by the color in the protein-free filtrate.
4. *Inorganic phosphate*. Increases rapidly in hemolyzed serum because RBCs contain a high concentration of inorganic phosphate esters, which are hydrolyzed by serum phosphatases.
5. *Serum potassium*. In dogs and cats hemolysis has no noticeable effect on serum potassium concentration.
6. *Alkaline phosphates*. Increased.
7. *Total protein*. May be spuriously raised by hemoglobinemia.
8. *Transaminase*. Hemolysis has less influence on dog serum than on serum of human origin because of the variation in the ratio of transaminases between RBCs and serum.
9. *Lactic (acid) dehydrogenase* (LDH). The ratio between RBCs and serum may vary from 160:1 in humans to 1.38:1 in the dog.
10. *Blood pH*. Decreased slightly by hemolysis.
11. *Calcium concentration*. Artifactually raised by hemolysis.
12. *Creatinine concentration*. Artifactually raised by hemolysis.
13. *Chloride*. Decreased by hemolysis.
14. *Prothrombin*. Hemolysis has a negligible effect on prothrombin by the one-stage technique, but it causes interference with prothrombin consumption tests.

An effort should be made to fast the animal 12 hours prior to the collection of blood specimens to avoid postprandial lipemia. Lipemia, attributed to metabolic disorders as well as recent meals, is a common cause of factitious test results. Total protein, albumin, glucose, calcium, phosphorus, and bilirubin are examples of tests that can be markedly affected by lipemia. The clinician should become familiar with the testing procedures performed by the clinical laboratory handling the blood specimens to become aware of the tests that are affected by lipemia as well as hemolysis and various anticoagulants.

............Blood for Hematology

Ethylenediaminetetraacetic acid (EDTA) is the anticoagulant of choice for hematology. Heparin is especially to be avoided if blood films are to be made from blood mixed with anticoagulant. Heparin is acceptable for most routine procedures using blood plasma. It should be remembered that the anticoagulant effect of heparin is transitory. Specimens may clot after 1 to 3 days.

Blood films should be made immediately after blood collection. Cell morphology deteriorates progressively after collection. Although blood films made immediately after addition of blood to EDTA are acceptable, a better practice is to make films from blood remaining in the blood collection needle because this blood has not been exposed to anticoagulant. *Blood exposed to heparin should never be used for making blood films.*

Incorrect proportions of blood to anticoagulant may result in water shifts between plasma and RBCs. Such shifts may alter the packed cell volume (PCV), especially when small volumes of blood are added to tubes prepared with sufficient anticoagulant for much larger volumes of blood.

Erroneous laboratory results may also be obtained when small volumes of blood are placed in a relatively large container; these errors are due to evaporation of plasma water and adherence of cells to the surface of the container.

Liquid blood mixed with anticoagulant should be refrigerated after collection if there is to be a delay in making the laboratory determinations. White blood cell (WBC) and RBC counts, PCV, and hemoglobin level can be measured up to 24 hours after blood collection. Platelet counts, however, should be done within 1 hour after collection of blood. Dried, unfixed blood films can be stained satisfactorily with most conventional stains 24 to 48 hours or even longer after being made. If a considerable delay before staining is unavoidable, blood films should be fixed by immersion in absolute methanol for at least 5 minutes. Such fixed films are stable indefinitely. Unfixed blood films must never be placed in a refrigerator because condensation forming after removal from the refrigerator will ruin the film. Care should be taken to leave unfixed blood films face down on a countertop or in a closed box. Special stains, such as peroxidase, may require fresh blood films.

............Blood for Clinical Chemistry Procedures
(see also p. 878)

Most clinical chemistry procedures are done with serum. The serum is obtained by collecting blood without any anticoagulant and allowing the blood to clot in a clean, dry tube. Serum should be separated from cells within 45 minutes of venipuncture. Special vacuum tube vials are available (Corvac vials*) that produce a strong barrier between the clot and the serum so that it is not necessary to draw off the serum into a separate vial. Clotting of the blood and retraction of the clot occur best and maximum yields of serum are obtained at room temperature or at body temperature. Refrigeration of the specimen impairs clot retraction. When the blood is firmly clotted, free the clot from the walls of the container by "rimming" with an applicator stick or tapping sharply on the outside of the tube. After the clot is freed, allow clot retraction to occur; then centrifuge and draw off the clear supernatant serum using a pipette and suction bulb. Serum yield is usually approximately one third of the whole blood volume.

Many clinical chemistry procedures can be done on plasma as well as serum. The advantage of using plasma is that separation of cells can be accomplished immediately without waiting for clot formation and retraction. The disadvan-

*Corvac vials, Corning Glass, Corning, NY.

tage of plasma is the presence of the anticoagulant, which interferes with many chemistry procedures. Plasma is often somewhat less clear than serum, which may be an additional disadvantage. Plasma and serum are virtually identical in chemical composition except that plasma has fibrinogen and the anticoagulant. For many chemical procedures in which plasma or whole blood is to be used, heparin is the anticoagulant of choice. Heparinized blood is the only acceptable specimen for pH and blood gas studies. Although blood containing EDTA is acceptable for certain chemical procedures, it cannot be used for determinations of plasma electrolytes because it both contributes electrolytes to and sequesters them from the specimen. In addition, EDTA can interfere with alkaline phosphatase levels, decrease the carbon dioxide–combining power of blood, and elevate blood nonprotein nitrogen.

Serum or plasma should be separated and removed from the cells as soon as possible after blood is collected because many constituents of plasma exist in a higher concentration in the blood cells. With time, these substances leak into the plasma and cause spurious elevations of the plasma values obtained. Magnesium, potassium, phosphorus, and transaminase are examples of constituents for which this may be a serious problem. Under no circumstances should whole blood be sent through the mail; serum derived from such specimens is usually visibly hemolyzed and the results are often inaccurate. The serum should be separated and transferred to a clean, dry tube for shipment.

Whole blood collected in Gas-Lyte syringes (Marquest Medical Products) can be used to measure sodium, potassium, and ionized calcium. The syringe contains dry (reduced) heparin product, which eliminates the dilution effects caused by liquid heparin products. Specimen stability is: for blood gases, 60 minutes on ice; for ionized Ca and Na, 60 minutes on ice; for K, 20 minutes.

REFERENCES

Lumsden JH, Jacobs RM: Clinical chemistry. Vet Clin North Am Small Anim Pract 19:875, 1989.

Meyer DJ, Harvey JW: Veterinary Laboratory Medicine, ed 2. Philadelphia, WB Saunders, 1998.

Raskin R, Meyer DJ: Update on Clinical Pathology. Vet Clin North Am Small Anim Pract 26: 1996.

·········· VENIPUNCTURE OF DOGS

To restrain a dog for venipuncture of the cephalic vein, place the dog on the table in sternal recumbency. If the right vein is to be tapped, the assistant stands on the left side of the dog, places his left arm under the dog's chin to immobilize the head and neck, and reaches across and grasps the right foreleg just distal to the elbow joint (Fig. 4–3). The thumb rotates the vein laterally while the hand immobilizes the leg in slight extension. It is important to keep the dog pressed down on the table if a struggle ensues. The person making the venipuncture grasps the leg at the metacarpals and begins the skin puncture at the medial side of the vein slightly above the carpus.

For a recurrent tarsal vein tap, restrain the dog in lateral recumbency. The assistant holds the under foreleg and presses the dog's neck to the table with the forearm. Hold the upper rear leg above the knee joint and in extension. The vein is not easily visualized in some animals unless the hair is clipped. The vein is also very mobile subcutaneously, which may cause difficulty in inserting the needle.

The jugular vein is easily visualized in short-coated, long-necked breeds. If the dog has a heavy coat, it is probably better to clip the hair. Positioning is most important to make the vein pop out into view, especially for puppies and

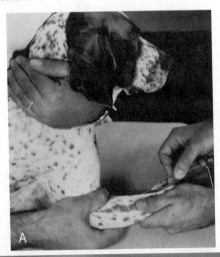

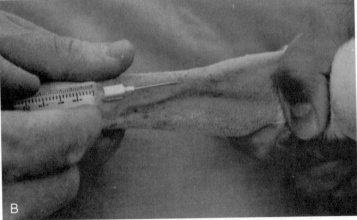

Figure 4–3. A, Cephalic venipuncture in right foreleg. A restraining arm is placed under the dog's chin, his neck and chest are held close to the assistant's body, and the cephalic vein is rolled laterally by thumb pressure. Proper restraint to prevent struggling is important. (The person doing venipuncture should hold the leg in the region of the metacarpals and should start the venipuncture just proximal to the carpus.) B, Medial view of technique for cephalic venipuncture.

kittens less than 1 week old. Small breeds or puppies, with their feet hanging free, are held by an assistant who places the right arm under the dog's chest and holds the dog at his side. The right hand grasps one or both of the dog's forelegs below the elbows. The assistant's left hand is used to lift the dog's chin up and back, thus extending the neck. If the dog's head is rotated slightly, the veins will be seen more easily. The person making the tap places the left thumb in the jugular furrow at the thoracic inlet. The right hand manipulates the Vacutainer or syringe to make the venipuncture. Larger dogs are restrained in sternal recumbency on a table, with their necks in extreme dorsal extension (Fig. 4–4).

··········VENIPUNCTURE OF CATS

Jugular puncture in the cat or kitten is accomplished in a manner that is basically similar to that used for dogs (Fig. 4–5). However, a cat bag or a blanket or heavy towel is more efficient in restraining the cat and protecting the operator.

Puncture of the femoral vein of a cat is an effective way to obtain blood or to give medications. Because of its loose subcutaneous support, however, this vein is very mobile and, after puncture, almost always develops a hematoma. The quiet or depressed cat can be held gently on its side, the medial surface of the thigh clipped of hair, and the venipuncture made with minimal restraint. Most normal active cats can be managed as follows:

1. Grasp the loose skin of the anterior neck close to the ears with the right hand.
2. Lay the cat on its right side on a blanket-padded table (so that the cat's front paws can grasp the blanket with its claws).
3. Use the left hand to hold and firmly control the left rear leg, and extend the cat so that its spine rests along the handler's right forearm.

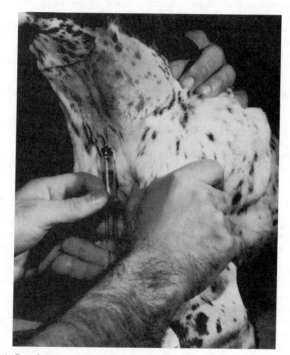

Figure 4–4. Jugular puncture in the dog. The hair on the neck has been clipped, and the skin has been prepared with alcohol. The head and neck are extended, and the thumb is placed in the jugular furrow to distend the vein. A Vacutainer is being used to collect blood.

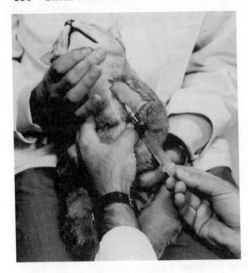

Figure 4–5. Jugular puncture in the cat. The cat is positioned comfortably on the restrainer's lap, and the head and neck are extended to make the jugular vein protrude.

4. Use the edge of the left palm to press down on the medial surface of the cat's right thigh, thus compressing the femoral vein.
5. The person drawing the blood holds and extends the cat's right hindleg. The refractory animal requires more stringent measures. We prefer to roll the cat in a blanket and to pull out one hindleg.
6. The medial aspect is clipped, and the tap is performed as described previously.

Small amounts of blood can be collected easily from the marginal ear vein. Pluck hair from an area of skin about 0.5 in. in diameter at the medial dorsal edge of the ear over the vein. Wipe the skin with alcohol, and apply pressure at the base of the ear to make the blood well up in large droplets on the skin following venipuncture. Incise the vein with a lancet or No. 11 Bard-Parker blade. Blood can be aspirated from the surface of the skin directly into a pipette. Hemorrhage stops quickly with gentle finger pressure. The whole procedure is quite painless and rarely upsets the animal.

·········· COLLECTING AN ARTERIAL BLOOD SAMPLE

The femoral artery is of sufficient size in the dog and the cat to collect arterial blood. These samples are used for blood gas content and acid-base status although venous samples may also be used (see p. 591). Hair must be clipped from over the femoral artery and the skin prepared with povidone-iodine (Betadine) and alcohol. Stretch the skin between the thumb and forefinger of one hand. Palpate the artery. Use a 22-gauge needle with the bevel of the needle up. Use a 3-mL syringe rinsed with 0.25 mL of heparin. Aspirate the sample. Immediately apply pressure over the artery with a sterile piece of cotton and maintain pressure for 3 to 5 minutes. Submit the sample on ice with the needle end sealed with a rubber stopper.

REFERENCE

Crow S, Walshaw S: Manual of Clinical Procedures in the Dog, Cat, and Rabbit, ed 2. Philadelphia, Lippincott-Raven, 1997.

Collection and Evaluation of Semen

Semen is collected for examination for breeding soundness, for investigation of infertility or prostatic disease, and for artificial insemination.

...........CANINE SEMEN COLLECTION

............Equipment

............Sterile

Sterile rubber cone (artificial vagina) connected to a semen collection tube
Glass, polytef (Teflon), or plastic test tubes
Saline solution, 0.9%
Sterile aqueous lubricant

............Nonsterile

Microscope slides and coverslips (warmed)
A quick Romanowsky's stain, buffered formalin
Hemocytometer—counting chamber and 1:100 WBC dilutor pipette or Unopette
Microscope with oil immersion objective ($\times 1000$) and light
Muzzle gauze

............Collecting Semen

The following procedures should be carried out when collecting semen:
1. Take the male and an estrous teaser bitch (if available) to a quiet room where there will be no distractions and where there is good traction (rubber mats or rug) for mounting by the male.
2. Hold the female, and allow the male to "flirt" for several minutes. If the female is in heat, a brief period of foreplay with both dogs unrestricted is beneficial.
3. If necessary, have assistants restrain the muzzled female and control the male by a collar and leash. Bring the male up to the rear end of the female, and allow him to either mount her or keep his nose in the region of her perineal area.
4. Attach the artificial vagina (AV) to the semen collection tube, and apply a scant amount of lubricant to the opening of the AV.
5. If mounting occurs, allow the male to grasp the bitch and start to thrust his pelvis in an attempt to copulate. Gently, from the side of the sheath, grasp the penis by the prepuce and move the prepuce back over the engorged bulbus glandis; while applying the AV to the shaft of the penis, apply pressure with the thumb and forefinger proximal to the exposed glandis. This can usually be done with one motion as the male is thrusting. If the male is shy and not interested, massage the penis slightly in the prepuce or in the AV to cause erection. When erection of the bulbus is felt, reflect the prepuce posteriorly to free the bulbus. Apply pressure with the thumb and forefinger behind the bulbus, circling the shaft of the penis. After completion of the most rapid pelvic thrusting and ejaculation of the sperm-rich fractions of semen (1 to 3 mL), the penis should be twisted 180 degrees backward in a horizontal plane, between the hindlegs, so that the penis remains in the same plane as in the forward position with the thumb and forefinger still applying pressure around the circumference of the penis proximal to the

bulbus. The penis cannot be twisted unless the prepuce is reflected posterior or proximal to the bulbus glandis. Twisting the penis in this position simulates a natural "tie" and allows the person collecting the semen to better visualize the collection (AVs are widely available now and are much preferred because they simulate the natural pressure of the vagina). The first drops of ejaculate may be discarded, especially if any urine is present. The sperm-rich fraction should be collected separately. A clear ejaculate is prostatic fluid, which may be collected separately for examination.

6. After semen collection, the penis is placed in the forward position, the prepuce is straightened out to avoid paraphimosis, and the female is removed from the room. Allow the stud to lick the erect penis and lose the erection. The stud should be checked for evidence of paraphimosis before he is released or caged.

7. The ejaculate consists of three fractions:
   a. Urethral secretion (usually clear fluid)—0.1 to 2 mL within 50 seconds, pH 6.3. If evidence of urine is present, discard this fraction and do not add it to the sperm-rich fraction. In most ejaculates collected from dogs, the first and second semen fractions are collected together.
   b. Sperm-containing secretion (milky opaque fluid)—0.5 to 3 mL within 1 to 2 minutes, pH 6.1.
   c. Prostatic secretion (usually clear fluid)—2 to 20 mL within 30 minutes, pH 6.5. The total specimen is 0.3 to 20 mL, pH 6.4.

8. Because the first and third fractions are clear, water-like material and the second fraction is milky-opaque, the clinician can separate them by changing collecting tubes as each fraction is ejaculated. It is best to collect only enough prostatic fluid to rinse the sperm fraction into the test tube. Too much prostatic fluid may be detrimental to the longevity of sperm in storage. Collecting individual fractions may be important in determining the site of an inflammatory reaction, but for artificial insemination only the sperm-rich, low-volume ejaculate is needed for insemination, dilution, or freezing.

9. The male is returned to his cage. The female is retained until the semen is examined, if insemination is to be performed.

..........Evaluation of Semen

The evaluation of semen should include the following procedures:

1. Immediately after semen collection, slowly invert the tube several times to mix the semen gently.

2. Determine motility. Place 1 drop of semen on a warmed microscope slide. Cover the slide with a coverslip, and observe the specimen under low power for progressive motility. There will be no "waves," but general vigorous forward motion should be evident. If the sample is too concentrated for individual sperm to be found, mix 1 drop of semen with 1 drop of saline at body temperature on a warmed microscope slide. Using high power, count 10 different groups of 10 sperm, observing the numbers of motile and nonmotile sperm. Total motility for a suitable sample should be 80% or greater. Motility less than 60% is not satisfactory.

3. Determine the number of sperm in the total ejaculate. Sperm concentration may be determined in a hemocytometer with a 1:100 blood cell dilutor kit (Unopette), and concentration is then multiplied by volume to determine sperm numbers per ejaculate. Remember that more dilute samples will be obtained when prostatic fluid is collected, but total sperm numbers in the ejaculate will be only marginally influenced by dilution with prostatic fluid. Total sperm per ejaculate should exceed 300 million in a normal male and may approach 2 billion in large dogs. A minimum number of 200 million sperm per insemination is needed on average for conception.

4. Determine morphology. Make a smear of a drop of semen like a blood smear and allow it to air-dry. Then stain with Diff-Quik stain; dip the slide into the fixative and solutions 1 and 2 for 2 to 3 minutes each. Then count 100 sperm at ×1000 magnification, noting normal and abnormal sperm. If there is any question about abnormality, 500 sperm cells should be examined.

Normal canine sperm are 63 nm long; the heads are 7 nm long. The percentage of abnormal sperm should be less than 20%. Differential abnormality is important, and the following abnormalities should not be exceeded in any sperm count: abnormality of the head, 10% to 12%; midpiece abnormalities, 3% to 4%; tail abnormalities, 3% to 4%; and retained protoplasmic droplets, 3% to 4%. Abnormalities that should be counted and recorded are shown in Figure 4–6. It is important to note the presence and location of distal or proximal protoplasmic droplets, which may indicate cell immaturity.

Defects of the cells within the testes are generally more serious than defects that occur in the sperm during epididymal transport or after ejaculation (such as fractured heads, retained protoplasmic droplets, or bent tails). Usually, a biopsy should not be done on material from testes unless the testes are azoospermic. Damage produced after the sperm have left the testes may indicate epididymal disease or may be the result of cold, trauma, or osmotic or urinary contamination. When abnormalities are found, it is wise to obtain two or three semen samples within a few days for baseline evaluation and then repeat the studies in 4 to 6 weeks to determine whether there is a healing or regressing trend. There are usually 64 days from the date of sperm formation to the date of ejaculation—54 days in the testes and 10 days in transport and maturation in the epididymis.

Normal male dogs can be used at stud once every other day indefinitely or once every day for 7 to 9 days, after which sperm numbers in the ejaculate will decline but not to less than the numbers needed to achieve conception.

············INSEMINATING THE BITCH
············Equipment

Dry, warm, sterile 5- or 10-mL syringes
Rubber adapter tubing, 0.75 in. long
A 6- to 9-in. plastic or polypropylene inseminating pipette
A sterile examination glove
Alcohol
Cotton

Do not use lubricating materials.

············Procedure

The procedure for insemination includes the following steps:

1. Determine the correct time to inseminate by test-teasing with a male, by cytologic examination of vaginal smears, or by vaginoscopic examination to determine the day when vaginal folds change from round to angular. Breed the day after the bitch first stands staunchly to accept service and "flags" her tail or during cytologic indications of estrus (complete cornification of vaginal epithelial cells) but before WBCs reappear in the smears. Breed at 48-hour intervals until the female goes out of heat or for three or four inseminations.
2. If the vulva is soiled, clean it thoroughly with alcohol swabs.
3. Gently aspirate semen through the inseminating pipette into the warm syringe.

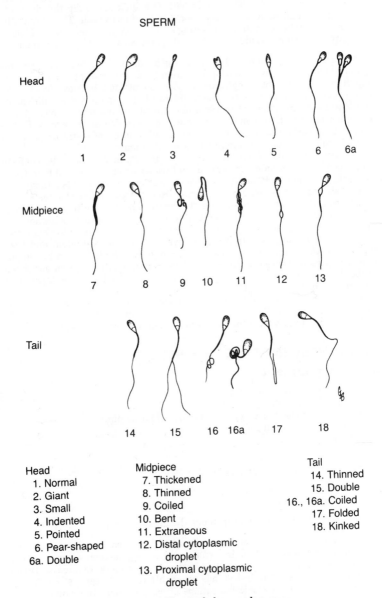

Figure 4–6. Chart of abnormal sperm.

4. Using a gloved left index finger (not lubricated) as a guide, insert the pipette through the vulva and dorsally into the vagina and forward to the cervix. Elevate the bitch's rear quarters to a 45-degree angle by having an assistant pick up the bitch by holding the hock region so that no pressure is applied to the ventral abdomen and uterus. Eject the semen gently and slowly. A bubble of air should be ejected to push all the semen through the pipette. Deposit the semen in the anterior vagina.

5. Remove the pipette, and hold the bitch in an elevated position for 5 minutes. During this time, the finger encased in a sterile glove should be used to "feather" the ceiling of the vagina to stimulate constrictor activity. This may be important to simulate a "tie" and transport semen into the uterus.

6. Lower the bitch to the normal position, and immediately walk her for 5 minutes so that she does not sit down or jump up on a person and allow semen to run back out of the vagina.

7. For best conception, inseminate undiluted fresh semen immediately.

8. It is best to use refrigerated extended semen within 24 to 48 hours if possible. However, refrigerated semen has been kept viable for up to 9 days with proper care.

Skim milk has been used as an economical and adequate extender. Milk is heated to 92° to 94°C for 10 minutes, cooled, and skimmed at room temperature. To each milliliter, add 1000 units of crystalline penicillin. If *Pseudomonas* spp. affect the semen, polymyxin B may be added at 200 units/mL of extender. Semen is diluted with extender at a semen-extender ratio of 1:1 to 1:4. Seager extends canine semen for freezing with a diluent containing 11% lactose, 4% glycerin, and 20% egg yolk. The 1:4 diluted semen is refrigerated; then 0.05-mL portions are pipetted into depressions in a block of dry ice and held for 8 minutes to freeze. The frozen pellets are stored in liquid nitrogen. Frozen semen can be thawed in buffered saline at 30° to 37°C. Good semen may be stored in liquid nitrogen for many years without significant loss of motility. Conception is best when large numbers of thawed motile sperm are deposited in the cervix or uterine cavity. Conception is poor when thawed semen is placed in the anterior vagina, as done in artificial breeding with raw semen.

··········FELINE SEMEN COLLECTION AND INSEMINATION

4

Semen can be collected by means of electroejaculation while the tom is anesthetized. For semen collection with an AV, the tom must be trained for several weeks and not all males will ejaculate even then; thus, the AV method is not generally used except in larger catteries. Teaser queens can be produced by injecting spayed females with 0.25 mg of estradiol cyclopentylpropionate (ECP), or normal queens in heat can be used. An AV can be made by cutting off the bulb end of a 2-mL rubber bulb pipette and inserting a 3-mm × 44-mm test tube into the cut end. The apparatus is placed into a 60-mL plastic bottle filled with warm water (52°C). The rolled end of the rubber pipette is stretched over the rim of the bottle. The opening of the pipette ("vagina") is sparingly lubricated with sterile aqueous lubricant. A teaser queen is placed in a quiet cage with the tom. As the male mounts the queen and develops an erection, the AV is placed over the penis. The ejaculation takes 1 to 4 minutes, the semen volume is 0.05 mL (range = 0.03 to 0.3 mL), and the semen contains 50 million to 100 million sperm. Motility is normally 80% to 90%, and pH is 7.4. There should be less than 10% abnormal sperm. The semen can be diluted for insemination to contain 10 million sperm in 0.1 mL of saline; then each 0.1 mL is an adequate insemination volume. With such small samples, microequipment is essential to avoid losing semen by surface absorption. Toms can undergo this collection procedure three times weekly and maintain excellent semen quality and libido.

Queens can be detected in estrus by stroking their backs and necks daily and noting the arching of the back and the extended and treading action of the rear feet when they are in receptive heat. Estrus is verified by examination of vaginal smears, which show epithelial cell cornification with pyknotic nuclei. Insemination is carried out with a 0.25-mL syringe and a bulb-tipped 9-cm spinal needle. Ovulation is induced by intramuscular (IM) injection of 25 μg of gonadotropin-releasing hormone or 250 IU of human chorionic gonadotropin. If insemination is repeated 24 hours later, the conception rate improves from 60% to 75%.

REFERENCES

Bartlett DJ: Studies on dog semen. I. Morphologic characteristics. II. Biochemical characteristics. J Reprod Fertil 3:174, 1962.

Feldman EC, Nelson RW: Canine and Feline Endocrinology and Reproduction, ed 2. Philadelphia, WB Saunders, 1996.

Freshman JL, Amann RP, Bowen RA: Clinical evaluation of infertility in dogs. Compend Contin Educ Pract Vet 10:443–460, 1988.

Johnston SD: Diagnostic and therapeutic approach to infertility in the bitch. J Am Vet Med Assoc 176:1335–1338, 1980.

Johnston SD, Larsen RE, Olson PNS: Canine Theriogenology. Hastings, NE, American Society for Theriogenology, 1982.

Larsen RE: Breeding soundness examination of the male dog. *In* Kirk RW, ed: Current Veterinary Therapy VIII: Small Animal Practice. Philadelphia, WB Saunders, 1983, p. 956–959.

Seager SWJ: Successful pregnancies utilizing frozen dog semen. Artif Insem Dig 17:6, 1969.

Wright PJ, Parry BW: Cytology of the canine reproductive system. Vet Clin North Am Small Anim Pract 19:851–874, 1989.

Bacterial Cultures

..........PRINCIPLES OF COLLECTION

Collect a representative sample of bacteria and examine the material promptly.

1. Collect specimens from areas where organisms are most likely to be found, such as the edge of a spreading skin lesion, from incised pustules, or from contaminated cavities.
2. Collect specimens prior to the use of antibiotics, when possible.
3. Avoid accidental contamination of the specimen.
4. Label all specimens clearly and carefully.
5. Inoculate culture material into appropriate media *promptly.*

..........ROUTINE PROCEDURE FOR A BACTERIOLOGIC CULTURE

..........Routine Smear

Prepare a smear by collecting material on a sterile cotton swab and rolling the material onto a clear glass slide. Heat-fix and stain the slide with Diff-Quik stain or Gram stain. Fluids should be centrifuged, and the sediment should be examined and used for cultures.

............Routine Culture

Inoculate material for culture on blood agar plates or in cystine lactose–electrolyte-deficient (CLED) medium as an acceptable alternative. CLED medium stimulates growth, detects lactose fermentation, and prevents spreading of *Proteus*. CLED serves as a basis for the isolation of most aerobic microorganisms. Selective media may be necessary for the isolation and identification of specific microorganisms. Biopsy material may be ground in sterile sand and placed in sterile broth.

............Multiple-Media Plates

Multiple-media plates have been developed commercially to facilitate direct antibiotic sensitivity and tentative identification of common pathogenic bacteria. These prepackaged, relatively inexpensive plates help the small laboratory identify pathogenic bacteria by their characteristic behavior on selective media. Some companies have different kits for different suspected infections. In general, kits are most useful for evaluating conjunctivitis, otitis, pyoderma, wound infections, uterine or anterior vaginal infections, fresh necropsy material, and urinary infections. Multiple-media plates are not recommended for culturing areas that have a large population of normal microbial organisms (such as the respiratory tract, throat, and vulva), for fecal samples, or for blood cultures to determine bacteremia (see Table 4–2).

............SPECIFIC CULTURE AND SMEAR METHODS
............Blood Culture

Bacteria can enter the blood from extravascular sites by way of the lymphatic circulation. Direct entry of bacteria into the bloodstream can be observed in the presence of endocarditis, suppurative phlebitis, infected IV catheters, dialysis cannulas, osteomyelitis, and so forth. Bacteremias can be transient, intermittent, or continuous. Transient bacteremia is produced by manipulation of an abscess, dental procedures, urethral catheterization, or surgery on contaminated areas. Intermittent bacteremia is associated with undetected and undrained abscesses. Most dogs with bacteremia, especially gram-negative bacteremia, are febrile and have an abnormal peripheral blood picture with an increased WBC count, increased number of band and segmented neutrophils, increased number of monocytes, and lymphopenia. An exception to this is osteomyelitis, in which dogs with bacteremia associated with staphylococci have basically normal hemograms. Large-breed male dogs with valvular insufficiency, congestive heart failure, or thromboembolism should be suspects for infectious endocarditis. The mitral valve is most often involved, followed by the aortic, tricuspid, and pulmonary valve.

The material for culture must be collected under aseptic conditions. Clip and surgically prepare the skin over the cephalic, recurrent tarsal, or jugular vein. Blood for culture should not be drawn through an indwelling IV or intra-arterial catheter. Use a Becton Dickinson blood culture bottle,*† which can be used for both aerobic and anaerobic blood cultures. Add 10 mL of blood to the enriched culture medium. Immediately after collection, mix the contents of bottles or tubes to prevent clotting.

Blood for cultures should be taken 1 hour before temperature spikes if intermittent fevers are present (see Table 4–3). Three separate blood culture specimens should be taken over a 24-hour-period. With a 1:10 dilution of blood

4

---

*Becton Dickinson and Co., Sparks, MD; Remel, Inc., Lenexa, KS.
†Bactec and Bactec Plus aerobic medium, Becton Dickinson and Co., Sparks, MD.

Table 4–2. Common Bacterial Culture Results

Site	Commensals	Pathogens
External ear canal		
Dog	Malassezia, Clostridium, Staphylococcus (a few), Bacillus (a few); never Streptococcus, Pseudomonas, or Proteus	Many Staphylococcus and Malassezia together; Pseudomonas, Proteus, Streptococcus, Escherichia coli
Cat	Not documented	Staphylococcus aureus, β-hemolytic streptococcis, Pasteurella, Pseudomonas, Proteus, E. coli, Malassezia
Skin		
Dog	Micrococcus, Clostridium, diphtheroids, Staphylococcus epidermidis, Corynebacterium, Malassezia	S. aureus (coagulase positive), Proteus, Pseudomonas, E. coli
Cat	Micrococcus, Streptococcus, S. aureus (?), S. epidermidis	S. aureus, Pasteurella multocida, Bacteroides, Fusobacterium, hemolytic streptococci
Conjunctiva	Staphylococcus, Streptococcus, Bacillus, Corynebacterium, diphtheroids, Neisseria, Pseudomonas	S. aureus, Bacillus, Pseudomonas, E. coli, Aspergillus
Vagina	Staphylococcus, Streptococcus, Enterococcus, Corynebacterium, E. coli, Haemophilus, Pseudomonas, Peptostreptococcus, Bacteroides	Brucella canis; pure culture of organism (esp. E. coli, Staphylococcus, Pseudomonas) when accompanied by tissue reaction at vaginal cytology
Urine	<1000* organisms/mL; presence of several organisms suggests contamination	More than 100,000* organisms/mL and often pure culture. E. coli, enterobacteria, Klebsiella, Proteus, Pseudomonas aeruginosa, Pasteurella multocida, Staphylococcus, Streptococcus

*Absolute numbers of bacteria depend on the collection technique (see p. 472).

Table 4-3. Recommendations for Blood Culture

Patient's Clinical Status	No. of Cultures	Period Within Which Cultures Are Collected	Interval Between Cultures	Timing of Culture
Fever of unknown origin	3	24 hr	At least 1 hr	Preferably before predicted temperature spike
Subacute bacterial endocarditis	2–3	24 hr	At least 1 hr	Unimportant
Overwhelming acute sepsis	3	30 min–1 hr	15 min	At least two cultures before antibiotics are administered
Subacute sepsis	3	24 hr	At least 1 hr	Before temperature spike, if possible
Patient currently receiving antibiotics	3–6	48–72 hr	12–24 hr	Before temperature spike, if possible

From Dow SW, Jones RL: Bacteremia: Pathogenesis and diagnosis. Compend Contin Educ Pract Vet 11:438, 1989.

in broth, antibiotics that may have been administered systemically are usually diluted to noninhibitory concentrations. The addition of sodium polyanethole-sulfonate (SPS) to commercial culture media inactivates aminoglycosides present in clinical concentrations.

Other media that may be used as selective agents include MacConkey (MC) agar, brain-heart infusion agar, mannitol salt agar, Streptosel agar, urea agar, blood agar, and eosin–methylene blue (EMB) agar. Special techniques make it possible to determine total bacteria counts and whether an organism is coagulase-positive or -negative.

...........Anaerobic Culture

Because anaerobes may be present in significant numbers in positive cultures from blood, abscesses, wounds, and urine, it may be advisable to make these special examinations. Anaerobes are present in the normal flora in fecal, throat, and bronchial swabs, so the anaerobic culture of these samples may be difficult to evaluate.

Specimens for anaerobic examination should be protected from air, held at room temperature, and inoculated in culture media as soon as possible. They should not be used with transport or enrichment media but should be inoculated directly from the specimen. Specimens for anaerobic culture can be placed in modified Cary-Blair transport medium, the Vacutainer Anaerobic Specimen Collector,* or the BBL Port-A-Cul Transport System.* Specimens can be held for short periods in sterile, carbon dioxide–filled, tightly stoppered tubes or bottles. The sample should be inoculated onto prereduced anaerobically sterilized medium under oxygen-free gas. Specimens can be inoculated deep into thioglycolate medium for transfer and subculture.

With anaerobic organisms, it is especially important to make a smear and a Gram stain and to record all morphotypes present and the relative numbers of each (see Table 4–4).

...........Urine Culture

Urine, as it is secreted by the kidneys, is sterile unless the kidney is infected. Most urinary tract infections are ascending infections by organisms introduced through the urethra. The most common sites of infection in female animals are the urethra and urinary bladder. Chronic prostatitis is common in male dogs and is often associated with relapsing urinary tract infections (UTIs).

*Becton Dickinson and Co., Sparks, MD.

Table 4–4. Signs Indicative of Anaerobic Infections in the Dog and Cat

Fight wounds (claw and bite wounds)
Foul-smelling discharges
Presence of gas in tissues or discharges
Necrotic tissues
Septic pleuritis and peritonitis
Fractures associated with trauma to soft tissues
Aspiration pneumonias
Infections following surgery on gastrointestinal tract or septic processes such as pyometra
Granulomas
Actinomycotic sulfur granules in pus
Infections near or on mucous membranes
Nonresponse to gentamicin or other aminoglycosides

Urine specimens can be collected by catheterization, by collecting a clean voided midstream sample, or by cystocentesis (Table 4–5) (see p. 486). Cystocentesis is the preferred method for qualitative and quantitative bacterial culture. To calibrate bacterial counts in urinary cultures, use a standard platinum milk dilution loop calibrated to deliver 0.001 mL of urine to one half of a blood agar plate. The initial loop of urine is streaked onto the plate. One hundred colonies or more signifies a bacterial count in the original specimen greater than or equal to 10^5/mL. The number of bacteria that is significant varies with the method of collection. With cystocentesis, a bacterial count greater than 10^3/mL of urine is significant; with catheterization, greater than 10^5/mL is significant. An MC agar plat can be used in addition to a blood agar plate.

Cystocentesis samples collected from animals that have received antimicrobial therapy should have 5 mL of urine centrifuged at 2500 rpm for 5 minutes, and the sediment should be streaked onto blood agar and MC agar.

MC agar and EMB agar are selective and differential media that are used to identify urinary tract organisms. MC agar prevents early growth of *Proteus*, inhibits growth of gram-positive bacteria, and allows separation of gram-negative bacteria in lactose-positive and lactose-negative subgroups.

Several commercial methods for urinary culture are available for screening urine for bacterial infection. Microstix* has proved 92% accurate in detecting bacteriuria of greater than 10^5/mL. If urine is collected by cystocentesis, significant bacteriuria may not be observed. Samples positive by Microstix should be recultured using calibrated loop or pour plate techniques.

Catheterization with aseptic technique or antepubic cystocentesis (see p. 491) should be used to collect urine for culture. Specimens of urine should be refrigerated within a few minutes after collection if culture is not done immediately. Bacterial culture of the specimen should be carried out within 2 hours of collection. Becton Dickinson† supplies a Vacutainer urine transport kit for urine culture. The Vacutainer tube can hold 5 mL of urine, which can be taken from a midstream catch or cystocentesis. The collection tube has a bacteriostatic fluid that preserves unrefrigerated urine specimens for up to 24 hours for culture.

·········· Prostatic Cultures

Inflammation or bacterial infection of the prostate may result in a nidus of infection that can cause recurrent UTI in male dogs. An effective way to evaluate the prostate for bacterial infection is to examine the prostatic fraction of the male ejaculate; if separation proves to be too difficult, the whole ejaculate specimen can be used for culture. To better interpret the results of the prostatic culture, obtain urethral cultures prior to the ejaculate sample.

·········· Culture of Urethral Specimens from the Male Dog

Wipe the end of the penis with 1:1000 Zephiran swab. Use a Calgi‡ urethral swab, and insert the swab 5 cm into the urethra. Place the swab in enrichment broth (brain-heart infusion or thioglycolate) by cutting the end of the swab off with sterile scissors. Refrigerate the broth and send it to the laboratory. Make subcultures with 0.1-mL loops of broth onto blood agar, MC agar, and mycoplasma medium.

···

*Ames Co., Elkhart, IN
†Becton Dickenson, Sparks, MD.
‡Spectrum Diagnostics, Glenwood, IL.

Table 4–5. Interpretation of Quantitative Urine Cultures in Dogs and Cats*

Collection Method	Colony-Forming Units/mL Urine					
	Significant		Suspicious		Contaminant	
	Dogs	Cats	Dogs	Cats	Dogs	Cats
Cystocentesis	≥1000	≥1000	100–1000	100–1000	≤100	≤100
Catheterization	≥10,000	≥1000	1000–10,000	100–1000	≤1000	≤100
Voluntary voiding	≥100,000†	≥10,000	10,000–90,000	1000–10,000	≤10,000	≤1000
Manual compression	≥100,000†	≥10,000	10,000–90,000	1000–10,000	≤10,000	≤1000

*The data represent generalities. On occasion, bacterial urinary tract infections may result in colony counts of 10,000/mL or more in some dogs (i.e., false-negative results).

†*Caution:* Because contamination of midstream samples may result in colony counts of 10,000/mL or more in some dogs (i.e., false-positive results), they should not be used for routine diagnostic culture of urine from dogs.

From Osborne CA, Finco DR: Canine and Feline Nephrology and Urology. Baltimore, Williams & Wilkins, 1995.

...........Culture of Prostatic Ejaculate

Collect the ejaculate fraction into a sterile side-mouth container (such as a 12-mL sterile plastic syringe container). Make subcultures with 0.1 mL of ejaculate onto differential media as for urethral swabs.

The prostatic ejaculate culture shows significant bacterial infection if the number of bacteria in the prostatic culture is greater than 2 logs of growth compared with the bacteria in the urethral culture.

...........Laboratory Diagnosis of Bacterial Diarrhea

Acute infectious diarrhea can be caused by bacteria, viruses, and protozoa (see p. 760). The major bacteria in feces are non–spore-forming anaerobic bacilli, but gram-negative facultative anaerobic bacteria such as *Escherichia coli* and other members of the Enterobacteriaceae family are usually present.

The clinical picture in acute infectious diarrhea is frequent loose stools containing pus or blood, abdominal pain, and fever. Damage to the intestinal tract may be produced by an enterotoxin, as with *Staphylococcus aureus* or *Escherichia coli*, or by invasion of the mucosa of the small intestine and colon. The most common bacterial pathogens of the intestinal tract in small animals are *E. coli*, *Salmonella* spp., and *Campylobacter jejuni*.

■ INDICATIONS FOR BACTERIAL CULTURES IN DIARRHEA

Acute onset of bloody diarrhea in association with exposure to contaminated food, garbage, after kenneling, after attendance at a dog show, after contact with an animal with infectious disease

■ Evidence of sepsis on clinicopathology, or evidence on fecal examination of large number of fecal neutrophils, and large populations of bacteria

■ Evidence of young, elderly, or infirm persons in the environment of the affected animal

---

Stool specimens can be collected in screw-cap glass or plastic containers or waxed cardboard containers with leakproof covers. If feces are not available, a rectal swab can be obtained using a Culturette.* A small amount of stool can be prepared on a slide and stained with Löffler's alkaline methylene blue stain for pus cells, and another slide can be prepared with Gram stain.

...........Submission Samples for *Chlamydia psittaci*

The importance of *Chlamydia* as the cause of a variety of common diseases in animals and birds is now firmly established. *C. psittaci* is the causative agent of psittacosis, enzootic abortion of ewes, bovine encephalomyelitis, feline pneumonitis, and ovine polyarthritis. The public health risk and the marked economic losses associated with this agent necessitate rapid and sensitive diagnostic procedures.

...........Laboratory Techniques
...........Direct Smears

Cell scrapings taken from conjunctiva during the phase of inflammation (first 10 to 14 days) and stained with Giemsa stain may show typical intracytoplas-

---

*Culturette Culture Collection System, Marion Scientific Laboratories, Kansas City, MO.

mic inclusions of initial and elementary bodies accompanied by a polymorpho-nuclear inflammatory cellular reaction.

............Isolation and Identification

For isolation, columnar epithelial cells (not exudate) should be obtained. Calcium alginate (not wooden) swabs should be used. Swabs should be placed directly into liquid-holding medium on wet ice. The most commonly used transport medium is 2-SP, composed of 0.2M sucrose and 0.02M phosphate (pH = 7.2) with added antibiotics. This can be supplied by the laboratory that is doing the isolations.

Monolayers of McCoy and HeLa cells are best for isolation of *Chlamydia*. Egg (yolk sac) inoculation of embryonated eggs has been abandoned. Chlamydial inclusions are detected by fluorescent antibody techniques.

............Puncture Fluids

Aspirate material using aseptic technique (see p. 496). Centrifuge the aspirated material at high speed, and stain a smear of the sediment with Gram stain. Culture the sediment on blood agar, in thioglycolate medium, on Sabouraud dextrose agar, or on one of the multiple-media plates. Also consider anaerobic cultures.

............Wounds and Ulcers

In dealing with an abscess (except those of the eye), clip and clean the abscess site. Aspirate material from the abscess into a sterile syringe and culture in blood agar and thioglycolate broth or on one of the multiple-media plates. In open wounds, use a sterile cotton swab and obtain fresh exudate from the deeper portion of the lesion. Also consider anaerobic cultures.

............Throat Cultures

It is very difficult to obtain a good representative sample from the throat without contamination from the mouth. Pass a sterile cotton swab over the tonsillar area and posterior pharyngeal walls. In some animals, this may have to be done under a short-acting general anesthetic. Place the swab onto blood agar colistin nalidixic acid (CNA) blood agar for gram-positive bacteria and MC agar for gram-negative bacteria. Because of the abundant normal flora, multiple bacteria will usually grow and evaluation of pathogenicity will be difficult.

............Spinal Fluid

If the spinal fluid is cloudy, make a direct smear and stain with Gram and Giemsa stains. If the fluid is fairly clear, centrifuge for 10 minutes, make a smear, and stain the sediment with Gram stain. Make cultures of the sediment on blood agar, in thioglycolate medium, or on one of the multiple-media plates, and on Sabouraud dextrose agar.

............Ear Cultures

Collect material on sterile cotton swabs, make a smear, and stain it with Gram stain. Place the swab on blood agar or CNA blood agar and EMB agar. Look for star-shaped colonies (yeasts) after 48 hours on EMB agar.

............Eye Cultures

Use a sterile cotton swab moistened with sterile saline or broth, and pass it over the conjunctiva of the inferior fornix of each eye. Use one half of a blood agar plate and one half of a mannitol plate for each eye. Material should also be placed into thioglycolate medium. Alternatively, use one of the commercial multiple-media plates. Make two conjunctival scrapings and stain one with Gram stain and the other with Giemsa stain.

............Skin Cultures

Cultures made from the surface of the epidermis or open ulcers are of little significance because they usually grow a mixture of nonpathogenic organisms. A culture made from the deep tissue of a biopsy specimen may be helpful in the diagnosis of a bacterial, atypical mycobacterial, or subcutaneous mycotic infection. Diagnostic isolates may be obtained from cultures of tissue sections from ulcers, fistulas, abscesses, enlarged nodes, or granulomatous lesions. Smears and cultures made from exudates of deep fistulas and node aspirates may be useful in some cases.

Intact pustules are satisfactory lesions for making smears and cultures. After the skin surface has been carefully sterilized, the pustule's fluid content may be gently aspirated with a sterile needle and syringe for inoculation into appropriate media; alternatively, the pustule roof may be opened and a culture taken (by swab) from the fluid inside. In all these procedures, the utmost care must be taken to prevent contamination from tissues outside the area of primary involvement.

When any fluid material or tissue is cultured, it is always desirable to use a portion of the sample to make stained smears. Stained smears often provide immediate clues to the diagnosis (organisms present [yeast, bacteria, or fungi] and indications as to the host response [cell types, phagocytosis, or eosinophils]. Examine the slides for the presence of bacteria and for cell morphology.

REFERENCES

Barsanti JA, Prasse KW, Crowell WA, et al: Evaluation of various techniques for diagnosis of chronic bacterial prostatitis in the dog. J Am Vet Med Assoc 183:219–224, 1983.

Calvert C, Greene CE: Bacteremia in dogs: Diagnosis, treatment and prognosis. Compend Contin Educ Pract Vet 8:179–186, 1986.

Calvert CA, Greene CE, Hardie E: Cardiovascular infections in dogs: Epizootiology, clinical manifestations, and prognosis. J Am Vet Med Assoc 187:612, 1985.

Dow S: Diagnosis of bacteremia in critically ill dogs and cats: *In* Bonagura J, ed: Current Veterinary Therapy XII. Small Animal Practice. Philadelphia, WB Saunders, 1995.

Dow SW, Curtis CR, Jones RL, et al: Bacterial culture of blood from critically ill dogs and cats: 100 cases (1985–1987). J Am Vet Med Assoc 195:113–117, 1989.

Greene CE: Infectious Diseases of the Dog and Cat, ed 2. Philadelphia, WB Saunders, 1998.

Hardie EM, Rawlings CA, Calvert CA: Severe sepsis in selected small animal surgical patients. J Am Anim Hosp Assoc 22:33–41, 1986.

Hirsh DC, Indiveri MC, Jang S, et al: Changes in prevalence and susceptibility of obligate anaerobes in clinical veterinary practice. J Am Vet Med Assoc 186:1086–1089, 1985.

Osborne C: Three steps to effective management of bacterial urinary tract infections: Compend Contin Educ Pract Vet 17:1233–1248, 1995.

Osborne CA, Finco DR: Canine and Feline Nephrology and Urology. Baltimore, Williams & Wilkins, 1997.

Scott DW, Miller WH Jr, Griffin CE: Muller and Kirk's Small Animal Dermatology, ed 5. Philadelphia, WB Saunders, 1997.

4

Fungal Cultures

...........PRINCIPLES OF COLLECTION

Positive cultures depend on proper selection of the culture site, proper collection of specimens, and appropriate use of selective media. Cultures are made from hair, skin, nails, and biopsy tissues.

...........Hair

If the hair is grossly dirty, it should be cleaned with soap and water; if not, wash it carefully with alcohol. Allow the hair to dry thoroughly. Select a site at the edge of an active lesion, and look for broken or stubby hairs. Use a forceps (curved Kelly or mosquito hemostats), and epilate hair from these areas by pulling parallel to the direction of the hair growth. It is important to get the hair root and not break off the hair shaft. Pluck many hairs and implant (push) the roots of the hair into the selected agar. The hair shaft should then be gently laid down to contact the surface of the medium. Hairs for inoculation can often be selected by choosing those that fluoresce with a Wood's light.

It is desirable to examine some of the plucked hairs with a potassium hydroxide (KOH) or wet-mount preparation for spores, hyphae, and so on. Specimens should never be taken from areas that have been treated within 1 week.

If samples are to be sent to a laboratory, the dry hair can be placed in a clean, tightly sealed envelope and mailed.

...........Skin

Dermatophyte or yeast infections may affect glabrous skin. If necessary, cleanse culture sites with *alcohol gauze swabs* (cotton will leave excess fibers) and allow to dry. Using a fine scalpel blade, collect superficial scrapings of scales, crusts, and epidermal debris at the periphery of typical lesions. Dermatophytes live in a dry state for several weeks, but yeast infections should be cultured immediately or placed in transport medium to prevent drying.

...........Nails

Although hard keratin fungal infections are rare in animals, diseased nails should be avulsed, scraped, or ground into fine pieces for collection in a sterile Petri dish. Pieces can be examined directly for arthrospores or hyphae and placed on appropriate media for culture.

...........Tissue Biopsy

Tissue core or excision samples can be sliced and the newly exposed surface used for impression smears or inoculation of medium. Samples also may be chopped or ground and placed in medium. Small amounts should be placed in sterile saline or broth for referral to an appropriate laboratory for further processing.

...........Dermatophyte Media

Sabouraud dextrose agar has been used traditionally in veterinary mycology for isolation of fungi; however, other media are available with bacterial and fungal inhibitors, such as dermatophyte test medium (DTM), potato dextrose agar, and rice grain medium. Mycosel and mycobiotic agar are formulations of

Sabouraud dextrose agar with cycloheximide and chloramphenicol added to inhibit fungal and bacterial contaminants. If a medium with cycloheximide is used, fungi sensitive to it will not be isolated. Organisms sensitive to cycloheximide include *Cryptococcus neoformans,* many members of the Zygomycota, some *Candida* spp., *Aspergillus* spp., *Pseudoallescheria boydii*, and many agents of phaeohyphomycosis. DTM is essentially a Sabouraud dextrose agar containing cycloheximide, gentamicin, and chlortetracycline as antifungal and antibacterial agents. The pH indicator phenol red has been added. Dermatophytes use protein in the medium first, and alkaline metabolites turn the medium red. When the protein is exhausted, the dermatophytes use carbohydrates and give off acid metabolites, and the medium's color returns to yellow. Most other fungi use carbohydrate first and protein later, so they too may produce a red change in DTM, but only after a prolonged incubation (10 to 14 days or more). Consequently, DTM cultures should be examined daily for the first 10 days. Fungi such as *Blastomyces dermatitidis, Sporothrix schenckii, Histoplasma capsulatum, Coccidioides immitis, P. boydii,* some *Aspergillus* spp., and others may cause a red change in DTM, so microscopic examination is essential to avoid an erroneous presumptive diagnosis. Because DTM may (1) depress development of conidia, (2) mask colony pigmentation, and (3) inhibit some pathogens, fungi recovered on DTM should be transferred to plain Sabouraud dextrose agar for identification.

Potato dextrose agar is useful for promoting sporulation and observing pigmentation. On potato dextrose agar, *Microsporum canis* has a lemon-yellow pigment, whereas *Microsporum audouinii* has a salmon- or peach-colored pigment. Rice agar medium promotes conidia formation in some dermatophytes, especially *M. canis* strains, which produce no conidia on Sabouraud dextrose agar.

Skin scrapings, nails, and hair should be inoculated onto Sabouraud dextrose agar, DTM, mycosel, or mycobiotic agar. Cultures should be incubated at 30°C with 30% humidity. A pan of water in the incubator will usually provide enough humidity. Cultures should be checked every 2 to 3 days for fungal growth. Cultures on DTM may be incubated for 10 to 14 days, but cultures on Sabouraud dextrose agar should be allowed 30 days to develop.

Practitioners can usually identify dermatophytes in cultures in their hospital laboratories.

Diagnosis should depend on characteristic gross identification of cultures and careful inspection of elements from those cultures using slide preparations and slide cultures for microscopic examination. Table 4–6 and Figure 4–7 may be helpful guides. The reference by Scott et al. is helpful.

Cultures of fungi other than dermatophytes should probably be made by commercial or institutional laboratories with appropriate equipment and special expertise.

REFERENCES

Attleberger MH: Practical diagnostic procedures for mycotic diseases. *In* Kirk RW, ed: Current Veterinary Therapy VII: Small Animal Practice. Philadelphia, WB Saunders, 1983, p 1157.

Dow. S: Diagnosis of bacteremia in critically ill dogs and cats. *In* Bonagura J, ed: Current Veterinary Therapy XII. Small Animal Practice. Philadelphia, WB Saunders, 1995, p 137.

Dow SW, Curtis CR, Jones RL, et al: Bacterial culture of blood from critically ill dogs and cats: 100 cases (1985–1987). J Am Vet Med Assoc 195:113–117, 1989.

Greene CE: Infectious Diseases of the Dog and Cat, ed 2. Philadelphia, WB Saunders, 1998.

Table 4–6. Serologic Tests in Systemic Fungal Disease

	Agar Gel Immunodiffusion (AGID)	Complement Fixation (CF)	Counterimmuno-electrophoresis (CIE)	Latex Agglutination (LA)	Passive Hemagglutination (PHA)
Aspergillosis* No good test for invasive aspergillosis except histology	Used for noninvasive aspergillosis; most widely used test; Aspergillus fumigatus, Aspergillus flavus, Aspergillus niger				
Blastomyces dermatitidis† Confirm by demonstrating organisms in tissues	Preferred test in the dog	(Replaced by AGID)			
Coccidioidomycosis Reaction to coccidioidin, which is mycelial-arthrospore antigen; confirm by demonstrating organisms in tissues	Available (TP test); detects IgM precipitins	Available; fourfold rise in CF titer is confirmatory; CF titer 1:16 or more suggestive of disseminated infection			Detects positive circulating IgM antibody during wk 2–3 of illness; never performed on CSF

Cryptococcus Testing for cryptococcal polysaccharide capsular antigen			Available	Highest sensitivity LA test; can be used on CSF; titers ≥1:8 are diagnostic§	Available
Histoplasmosis‡ Elevated titers may not be evident in fulminant disseminated disease; radioimmunoassay (RIA) test also becoming available; titers greater than 1:16 are significant	Available but regarded to be unreusable; simpler than CF	Most available; serologic test to antibodies to yeast phase; serum reaction 1:32 or greater or fourfold increase in titer. False negatives are common	Available	Available: simpler than CF but is neither sensitive nor specific	False positives in LA test, 50%

CDC, Centers for Disease Control and Prevention; TP, tube precipitin.

*Aspergillosis—false-negative results occur. Cross-reaction with antibodies to *Penicillium* sp. is common.

†AGID is test of choice in *Blastomyces* infection because this test does not cross-react with aspergillosis or other systemic fungal agents—the sensitivity is 91% to 94%.

‡Histoplasmosis—the serologic diagnosis is unreliable and used only to establish presumptive diagnosis.

§An ELISA (enzyme-linked immunosorbent assay) with polyclonal antibody capture and monoclonal detection is available as an alternative test.

4

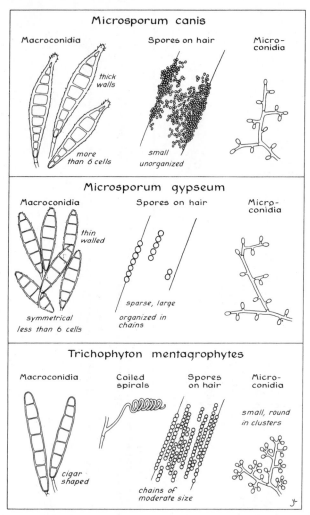

Figure 4–7. Characteristic microscopic morphologies of pathogenic fungi causing dermatophytosis. The conidia and spirals are microscopic structures. The hair shafts are much larger. (From Muller GH, Kirk RM, Scott DW: Small Animal Dermatology, ed 4. Philadelphia, WB Saunders, 1989, p 140.)

Scott DW, Miller WH Jr, Griffin CE: Muller and Kirk's Small Animal Dermatology, ed 5. Philadelphia, WB Saunders, 1997.

Examination of the Vagina

Vaginal examination is indicated for collection of material from the mucosal wall for culture and exfoliative cytology and for vaginoscopic examination of vaginal and cervical mucosa.

···········EQUIPMENT

The following equipment is necessary for examination of the canine vagina:

Sterile vaginal speculum (e.g., adjustable-spreading, stainless steel, or disposable plastic; cylindrical; glass, plastic, stainless steel, nylon)
Sterile otoscope heads of variable size for small dogs
Sterile protected culture swabs (Tiegland type or other)
Sterile culture swabs (Culturettes)
Amies transport medium with charcoal
Viral transport media
Glass slides and coverslips
Sterile proctoscope (Welch Allyn, human pediatric type) or other endoscope, flexible or rigid
Sterile offset biopsy punch

···········TECHNIQUE

Examination of the vagina for culture and cytology or vaginoscopic examination can be done with the aid of an assistant to restrain the bitch on an examination table (or on the floor for large breeds). Bitches that can be restrained for other minor examinations (ears, teeth, toenails, anal sacs, and blood samples) easily tolerate vaginal examinations. Those that need further restraint may require tranquilization or administration of a short-acting barbiturate anesthetic.

If the vulva appears clean, no preparation prior to examination is needed. If the vulva is soiled or vulvar hair is matted or soiled, the hair should be trimmed and the area washed with a germicidal or surgical scrub such as povidone-iodine (Betadine, Purdue Frederick, Norwalk, CT) or a general grooming and bath should be done 24 hours prior to examination. If prior preparation is not possible and cultures must be obtained, remove any matted hair and use cotton wetted with rubbing alcohol to remove visible soiling. Water and germicidal soap will usually not control surface contamination by *Pseudomonas* and *Proteus* spp., which frequently contaminate culture swabs. Bitches with long hair should have the leg hair pinned to one side with clips and the tail bandaged before examination.

A deep vaginal culture should be obtained before other vaginal examination causes contamination. A sterile, warm vaginal speculum without lubricating gel is passed into the posterior vagina while an assistant spreads the lips of the vulva open. The speculum is guided into the vagina by placing the speculum into the vulva just at the dorsal commissure of the vulvar lips and applying pressure up and out against the commissure. The speculum is directed dorsally toward the rectum until resistance is met and is then directed horizontally into the cranial vagina. This procedure bypasses the clitoral fossa, urethral opening, and pelvic arch and causes minimal pain. Lubricating jelly is not used because it contaminates the swabs for culture and cytology.

A guarded culture swab (swab covered by a protective plastic pipette) is taken from its individual sterile bag and passed inside the vaginal speculum to the anterior vagina or cervical area. The swab is then exposed from the protective plastic tubing and rotated against the mucosa. The swab is retracted into the protective plastic tubing and carefully removed from the vagina. The protected swab may then be placed back in its original sterile bag until it is either processed for culture (30 minutes) or placed in Amies transport medium with charcoal. Amies transport medium with refrigerator packs and a styrofoam-insulated mailing box will retain fastidious organisms for 72 to 96 hours. Bacterial, *Mycoplasma,* and *Ureaplasma* cultures should be processed for potential infectious agents. Viral transport medium can be used for a separate sterile swab if viral agents such as the genital form of canine herpesvirus are suspected.

Immediately after the swabbing for culture, while the vaginal speculum is still in place, a clean or sterile swab moistened with sterile physiologic saline solution is advanced carefully into the anterior vagina to make a smear for cytology. Vaginal epithelial cells are gently scraped from the ceiling of the vagina at or cranial to the region of the external urethral orifice. Samples should not be collected from the region of the clitoral fossa, which is lined by stratified squamous epithelium at all stages of the estrous cycle. Gently rub the swab on the vaginal mucosa. Remove the swab and roll it smoothly onto two or three clean glass slides. The smears may be fixed immediately in 95% alcohol, sprayed with a commercial fixative or hair spray, or left to dry in air.

A drop of new methylene blue (NMB) stain placed on a coverslip and inverted on the smear can be used to examine a wet-mount preparation immediately. This stain is not permanent and precipitates when it dries, and NMB-stained smears cannot be used for comparison with other smears made later in the cycle. A better and quick method that provides a permanent record is the use of the Diff-Quik or Leukostat stain. Giemsa stain, toluidine blue, Wright's stain, Shorr's stain, or phase-contrast microscopy can also be used. The smear should be examined for stage of estrous cycle and evidence of active inflammation. These findings should be compared with culture results and vaginoscopic findings to interpret evidence for an active genital tract infection, a carrier state of a potential infectious agent, or a possible contaminant at culture. A diagnostic laboratory with the ability to isolate specific infectious agents should indicate the number of organisms (few, moderate, many, or heavy) and report whether the isolates are pure or mixed and their significance.

⋯⋯⋯⋯EXAMINATION

The vagina of the bitch is long, and the mucosa forms longitudinal folds. The clitoris is in a well-developed fossa in the floor of the vestibule. We have found that the vagina can be completely visualized with a small sterile proctoscope or fiberscope. Lubricate the warmed, sterile instrument, and pass it to the region of the cervix. Examine first without insufflation for true color and vaginal fluids or discharge. When insufflation is performed while the vulva is compressed around the sterile proctoscope, the vagina balloons and its entire wall can be viewed completely as the instrument is withdrawn.

The normal canine vagina has a uniform light-pink color and longitudinal folds. During proestrus and estrus, the folds become more prominent and cross-striations give the surface a cobblestone appearance. This cobblestone appearance remains smooth when estrogen levels are high but quickly becomes angular (worn cobblestone appearance) when estrogen levels drop during the luteinizing hormone (LH) peak (ovulation), and progesterone levels increase. This change can be used to indicate ovulation and the ideal time for breeding. The hyperemia causes the vagina to appear reddish and congested. The pressure of air insufflation balances the mucosa. The canine vulva has a large cranial dorsal median fold that may obscure the cervix. In fact, ridges near the dorsal fold may give a false impression that this fold is the cervix. During estrogen stimulation, the cervix may be open and uterine blood may be escaping. In the management of dystocia, the vaginoscope can be used to detect puppies in the birth canal and to diagnose malpositions and aid in the correction of these conditions.

During the endoscopic examination, small tumors or polyps can be removed or large masses can be sampled with the biopsy punch. Ulcers or erosions can be cauterized, and foreign bodies can be removed.

A complete vaginal examination must include careful palpation of the vaginal wall and pelvic canal. This palpation is accomplished by digital examination through the vulva (using a sterile glove) and is assisted by palpation through the posterior abdominal wall. Incomplete hymen rings, vaginal fibrous stenotic rings, or pelvic malformation can be diagnosed. A digital rectal examination may be needed for vaginal masses or pelvic deformities.

············CHARACTERISTICS OF THE CANINE VAGINA DURING THE ESTROUS CYCLE (see Fig. 4–8)

The canine reproductive cycle begins at the age of 6 to 12 months and repeats at intervals of 4 to 12 months. In the average bitch, ovulation occurs spontaneously 1 to 3 days after the onset of estrus; in normal bitches ovulation may occur between 3 days before and 11 days after the onset of estrus. Sperm live in the uterus of the estrous bitch up to 11 days, and the ovum lives up to 5 days after ovulation. The fertilized ovum takes 4 to 10 days to reach the uterus, and implantation takes place 18 to 20 days after ovulation. The gestation

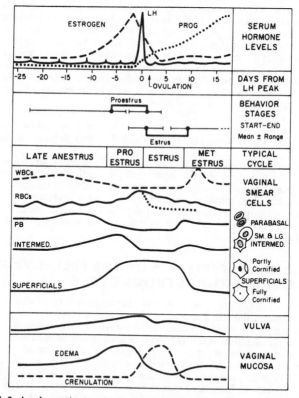

Figure 4–8. A schematic summary of temporal relationships among periovulatory endocrine events, behavioral and vulval changes, and changes in vaginal exfoliate cytology associated with proestrus and estrus periods in the bitch. LH, luteinizing hormone; PROG, progesterone; WBCs, white blood cells; RBCs, red blood cells. (From Kirk RW, ed: Current Veterinary Therapy X: Small Animal Practice. Philadelphia, WB Saunders, 1989, p 1272.)

period from the first breeding is 57 to 72 days and from the LH peak is 64 to 66 days.

Anestrus Anestrus is characterized by dryness of the mucosa and a thin vaginal wall with stratified squamous epithelial cells a few cells to several layers thick but without cornification. Noncornified epithelial cells and WBCs are present in a ratio of 1:5 in the vaginal smear. The WBCs are polymorphonuclear. The noncornified epithelial cells are 15 to 51 nm in diameter and have round free edges, granular cytoplasm, and large nuclei with distinct chromatin granules. The period of anestrus is 2 to 3 months or longer in some breeds.

Proestrus In proestrus, the vaginal wall is thicker than in anestrus and the mucosa shows prominent cornified squamous epithelium (20 to 30 cells thick) with rete pegs. The longitudinal and transverse vaginal folds are thick, smooth, and round. The vaginal wall becomes impervious to WBCs, but there is extravasation of RBCs to the surface epithelium. The RBCs are discharged. Vaginal smears show predominantly RBCs and noncornified epithelial cells, which become cornified as proestrus progresses. WBCs are present but their numbers decrease as estrus approaches. Debris and bacteria are abundant for 7 to 10 days.

Estrus The vagina is thick with longitudinal and transverse folds that become angular as estrogen levels decrease and progesterone levels increase. There is abundant fluid, often tinged with blood. Noncornified epithelial cells and WBCs are absent. Cornified epithelial cells, which are polyhedral and contain pyknotic nuclei or no nucleus, are predominant; their presence seems to be related to the appearance of flirting by the bitch and acceptance of the stud. WBCs reappear about 36 to 96 hours after ovulation. Bacteria and debris are absent during estrus, but they are seen again in the smears after ovulation when WBCs reappear 7 to 10 days later.

Diestrus The number of WBCs increases rapidly, the number of cornified epithelial cells decreases, and the number of noncornified epithelial cells increases. After 5 to 7 days, the number of WBCs may decrease to 10 to 30 per field.

Following parturition, much cellular debris, WBCs, RBCs, and a few epithelial cells are present for several days, until placental sloughing is complete. The presence of masses of degenerate WBCs (and bacteria) indicates metritis or endometritis. The continued presence of blood-tinged fluids containing abundant RBCs, a few noncornified epithelial cells, and occasional WBCs (nontoxic) plus necrotic cells for months post partum is evidence of subinvolution of placental sites.

.... CHARACTERISTICS OF THE FELINE VAGINA DURING THE ESTROUS CYCLE

Most of the characteristics just discussed that apply to bitches also pertain to queens. However, the small size of the feline vagina precludes palpation and early vaginoscopy. A sterile, warm, small-animal otoscope speculum enables fairly good visualization of the vaginal mucosa and can be used with a small, 4-mm-diameter sterile swab* to obtain smears for culture procedures. Use of the speculum is easiest following parturition or during estrus.

Vaginal cells for cytologic examination can be obtained with a moistened 3-mm cotton swab (Calgiswab) inserted 2 cm into the vagina. In some cases, flushing the vagina with sterile saline injected and aspirated with a clean glass eyedropper is more successful. Use of an eyedropper may trigger ovulation, as it simulates coitus.

....

*Calgiswab Type IV, Inolex Divison, American Can Co., Glenwood, IL.

Unlike the bitch, the queen shows no diapedesis of RBCs during proestrus or throughout the estrous cycle.

Cytologic examination of feline vaginal smears reveals the following.

Anestrus or Prepuberty Scarce debris; numerous small round epithelial cells with a high nuclear-cytoplasmic ratio, frequently in groups (seasonal—from September to January in the Northern Hemisphere).

Proestrus Increased debris; fewer but larger nucleated epithelial cells with a low nuclear-cytoplasmic ratio (0 to 2 days).

Estrus Markedly less debris; numerous large polyhedral cornified cells with curled edges and small dark pyknotic nuclei or loss of nuclei (6 to 8 days) following coitus or induced ovulation.

Early Diestrus Hazy, ragged-edged cornified cells; zero to numerous WBCs with numerous bacteria and increased debris.

Late Diestrus Increasing numbers of small basophilic cells with WBCs still present (total period of metestrus, 7 to 21 days). If ovulation does not occur, the smear will return to an anestrous stage with few to no WBCs.

The feline estrous cycle is continuous every 14 to 36 days if 12 to 14 hours of light is present daily. Ovulation is induced 24 to 30 hours post coitus. Sperm require 2 to 24 hours for capacitation in the uterus. Implantation occurs 13 to 14 days post coitus.

REFERENCES

Concannon PW: Clinical and endocrine correlates of canine ovarian cycles and pregnancy. *In* Kirk RW, ed: Current Veterinary Therapy IX: Small Animal Practice. Philadelphia, WB Saunders, 1986, pp 1214–1224.

Feldman EC, Nelson RW: Canine and Feline Endocrinology and Reproduction, ed 2. Philadelphia, WB Saunders, 1996.

Van Camp SD, Estill CT: Manipulating the canine estrous cycle. Vet Med Rep 2:4, 1990.

Laboratory Diagnosis of Viral Infections

The following procedures and materials should be used for diagnosing viral infections:

1. Swabs. Specific types of swabs with carrier media are available for viral culture: Culturette and Calgiswab.
2. Media. Several types of media have been used for the transport of viral specimens: modified Stuart, modified Hanks, Leibovitz-Emory, all with added serum.
3. For short-term transit (≤5 days), specimens for viral isolation should be held at 4°C rather than frozen.
4. Submit blood serum samples for possible antibody response (especially paired serum samples) with tissues or tissue fluids for viral isolation.
5. Fluorescent antibody technique. Four types of specimens can be used for immunofluorescence diagnosis: frozen sections, impression smears, lesion scrapings, and resuspended cells in centrifuged sediment.
6. Electron microscopy (EM). EM techniques are applicable in situations in which viral infections produce titers of virus in the specimen of 10^6 to 10^7/mL. Specimens such as feces, vesicle fluid, brain tissue, urine, or serum can be negatively stained for EM.
7. ELISA assays for detection of FELV, CPV, FIV.
8. Applied molecular diagnostics
   a. Immunoblotting
   b. PCR

REFERENCES

Greene CE: Infectious Diseases of the Dog and Cat, ed 2. Philadelphia, WB Saunders, 1998.
Hoskins JD, Loar AS: Feline infectious diseases. Vet Clin North Am Small Anim Pract 23:1993.

Urine Collection

Urine can be removed from the bladder by one of four methods: (1) natural micturition, (2) manual compression of the urinary bladder, (3) catheterization, or (4) cystocentesis.

For routine urinalysis, collection of urine by natural micturition is often very satisfactory. The major disadvantage is the contamination of the sample with cells, bacteria, and other debris located in the genital tract. The first portion of the stream should be discarded because it contains the most contamination and debris.

Manual compression of the bladder may be used in collecting urine samples from dogs and cats. Excessive digital pressure should not be used; if moderate digital pressure does not induce micturition, the technique should be discontinued. The technique can be difficult to use in male dogs and male cats.

Urinary catheters are hollow tubes made of rubber, plastic, nylon, latex, or metal and are designed to serve four purposes:

1. To relieve urinary retention
2. To test for residual urine
3. To obtain urine directly from the bladder for diagnostic purposes
4. To perform bladder lavage and instillations

The size of catheters (diameter) is usually calibrated in the French (F) scale; each French unit is equivalent to roughly 0.33 mm. The openings adjacent to the catheter tips are called "eyes." Human urethral catheters are routinely used in male and female dogs; 4F- to 10F-catheters are satisfactory for most dogs (Table 4–7). Catheters should be individually packaged and sterilized by autoclaving or ethylene oxide gas.

............CATHETERIZATION OF THE MALE DOG

Equipment needed to catheterize a male dog includes a sterile catheter (4F to 10F, 18 in. long, with one end adapted to fit a syringe), sterile lubricating jelly, povidine-iodine soap or benzalkonium chloride, sterile rubber gloves or a sterile hemostat, a 20-mL sterile syringe, and an appropriate receptacle for the collection of urine.

Proper catheterization of the male dog requires two people. Place the dog in lateral recumbency on either side. Pull the rear leg that is on top forward, and then flex it (Fig. 4–9). Alternatively, long-legged dogs can be catheterized easily in a standing position.

Next, retract the sheath of the penis and cleanse the glans penis with a solution of povidone-iodine 1%, triclosan (Septisol), benzalkonium chloride, or bichloride of mercury solution diluted 1:1000. The distal 2 to 3 cm of the appropriate-size catheter is lubricated with sterile lubricating jelly. The catheter is never entirely removed from its container while it is being passed because the container enables one to hold the catheter without contaminating it. The catheter may be passed with sterile gloved hands or by using a sterile hemostat to grasp the catheter and pass it into the urethra. Alternatively, cut a 2-in. "butterfly" section from the end of the thin plastic catheter container. This

Table 4–7. Recommended Urethral Catheter Sizes for Routine Use in Dogs and Cats

Animal	Urethral Catheter Type	Size (French Units*)
Cat	Flexible vinyl, red rubber, or Tom Cat catheter (polyethylene)	3.5
Male dog (≤25 lb)	Flexible vinyl, red rubber, or polyethylene	3.5 or 5
Male dog (≥25 lb)	Flexible vinyl, red rubber, or polyethylene	8
Male dog (>75 lb)	Flexible vinyl, red rubber, or polyethylene	10 or 12
Female dog (≤10 lb)	Flexible vinyl, red rubber, metal, or polyethylene	5
Female dog (10–50 lb)	Flexible vinyl, red rubber, metal, or polyethylene	8
Female dog (>50 lb)	Flexible vinyl, red rubber, metal, or polyethylene	10, 12, or 14

*The diameter of urinary catheters is measured on the French (F) scale. One French unit equals roughly 0.33 mm.

From Crow S, Walshaw S: Manual of Clinical Procedures in the Dog, Cat, and Rabbit, ed 2. Philadelphia, Lippincott-Raven, 1997.

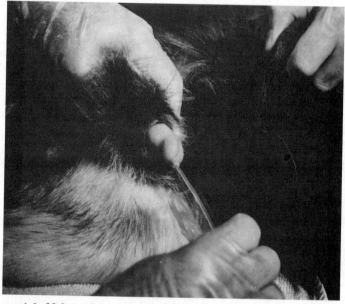

Figure 4–9. Male canine urethral catheterization. The subject is in lateral recumbency with the upper hindleg pulled forward (to the right) and held by an assistant. The penile sheath is retracted, and the glans penis is cleaned. A sterile catheter is protected in its covering until it enters the urethra.

section can be used as a cover for the sterile catheter, and the cover can be used by the clinician to grasp and advance the catheter without using gloves.

If the catheter cannot be passed into the bladder, the tip of the catheter may be caught in a mucosal fold of the urethra or there may be a stricture or block in the urethra. In small breeds of dogs, the size of the groove in the os penis may limit the size of the catheter that can be passed. Difficulty may also be experienced in passing the catheter through the urethra where the urethra curves around the ischial arch. Occasionally, a catheter of small diameter may kink and bend on being passed into the urethra. When the catheter cannot be passed on the first try, the size of the catheter should be reevaluated and the catheter gently rotated while being passed a second time. The catheter should never be forced through the urethral orifice.

Effective catheterization is indicated by the flow of urine at the end of the catheter, and a sterile 20-mL syringe is used to aspirate the urine from the bladder. Walk the dog immediately following catheterization to encourage urination.

............CATHETERIZATION OF THE FEMALE DOG

Equipment needed to catheterize a female dog includes flexible human ureteral or urethral catheters identical to those used in the male dog. Sterile metal or plastic female catheters can also be used; however, they tend to traumatize the urethra. The following materials should also be on hand: a Brinkerhoff's speculum or small nasal speculum, a 20-mL sterile syringe, lidocaine 0.5%, sterile K-Y jelly, a focal source of light, appropriate receptacles for urine collection, and 5 mL of povidone-iodine solution.

Strict asepsis should be used. Cleanse the vulva with a solution of povidone-iodine, triclosan, benzalkonium chloride, or bichloride of mercury diluted 1:1000. Instillation of lidocaine 0.5% into the vaginal vault helps to relieve the discomfort of catheterization. The external urethral orifice is 3 to 5 cm cranial to the ventral commissure of the vulva. In many instances, the female dog may be catheterized in the standing position by passing the female catheter into the vaginal vault, despite the fact that the urethral tubercle is not directly visualized.

In the spayed female in whom "blind catheterization" may be difficult, the use of Brinkerhoff's speculum or a nasal speculum with a light source will help to visualize the urethral tubercle on the floor of the vagina (Figs. 4–10 and 4–11). In difficult catheterizations, it may be helpful to place the animal in dorsal recumbency and pull the hindlegs forward. Insertion of a speculum into the vagina almost always permits visualization of the urethral tubercle and facilitates passage of the catheter. Be careful not to pass the catheter into the fossa of the clitoris because this is a blind passage.

............INDWELLING URETHRAL CATHETER

For continuous urine drainage, a closed collection system should be used to help prevent UTI. A soft urethral or Foley catheter can be used, and polyvinyl chloride (PVC) tubing should be connected to the catheter and to the collection bottle outside the cage. The collection bottle should be below the level of the animal's urinary bladder. An Elizabethan collar should be placed on the animal to prevent chewing on the catheter. Apply antibacterial ointment to the urethral orifice. Despite care of the catheter, UTI still may develop with an indwelling catheter. The animal should be observed for development of fever, discomfort, pyuria, or other evidence of UTI. Cultures should be made with catheter material if UTI develops.

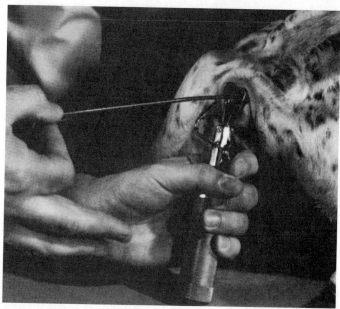

Figure 4–10. Female canine catheterization. Subject is standing or is placed in sternal recumbency. A sterile, lighted, nasal speculum is used to visualize the urethral opening, and a catheter is passed. An otoscope cone may also be used effectively.

REFERENCES

Barsanti JA, Blue J, Edmunds J: Urinary tract infection due to indwelling bladder catheters in dogs and cats. J Am Vet Med Assoc 187:384, 1985.
Crow S, Walshaw S: Manual of Clinical Procedures in the Dog, Cat, and Rabbit, ed 2. Philadelphia, Lippincott-Raven, 1997.
Osborne CA, Finco DR: Canine and Feline Nephrology and Urology. Baltimore, Williams & Wilkins, 1995.
Stone EA, Barsanti JA: Urologic Surgery of the Dog and Cat. Philadelphia, Lea & Febiger, 1992.

4

·········· CATHETERIZATION OF CATS

Catheterization of the male cat may require sedation or the use of dissociative anesthesia. Very ill cats or uremic cats can usually be catheterized with systemic sedation, although the use of a topical anesthetic such as proparacaine HCl flushed into the urethral orifice may minimize discomfort. When the cat is anesthetized, place it on its back and pull the hindlegs forward. Draw the penis from the sheath and gently pull the penis backward. Pass a sterile, flexible plastic or polyethylene (PE 60 to 90) catheter or 3- to 5-in., 3.5F urethral catheter* into the urethral orifice and gently into the bladder, keeping the catheter parallel to the vertebral column of the cat. The catheter should never be forced through the urethra. The presence of concretions within the urethral lumen may require the injection of 3 to 5 mL of sterile water, saline,

*Monojet, Sherwood Manufacturing Co., St. Louis, MO.

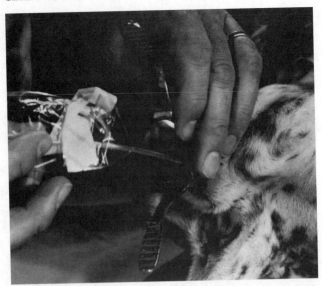

Figure 4–11. Female canine catheterization. The subject is in dorsal recumbency with the hindlegs pulled forward and held by an assistant. A Brinkerhoff speculum is helpful in visualizing the urethral opening. A sterile plastic catheter is being passed.

or Walpole's solution* to flush out the concretions so that the catheter can be passed (Fig. 4–12) (see also p. 122).

Catheterization of female cats can be accomplished with the use of a plastic, blunt-ended Tom Cat catheter. The vaginal vault is first anesthetized by instilling lidocaine 0.5% Cleanse the lips of the vulva with an appropriate antiseptic and then grasp and pull them caudally. Insert the Tom Cat catheter along the floor of the vagina, and gently guide the tip into the urethral orifice. The procedure is usually accomplished without difficulty, even though the urethral orifice is not visualized.

..........CYSTOCENTESIS

Diagnostic cystocentesis involves insertion of a needle through the abdominal wall and bladder wall to obtain urine samples for urinalysis or bacterial culture. The technique prevents contamination of urine by urethra, genital tract, or skin, and reduces the risk of iatrogenic production of a UTI. Cystocentesis may also be needed to decompress a severely overdistended bladder temporarily in an animal with urethral obstruction. In these cases, it should be performed only if urethral catheterization is impossible.

..........Equipment

Equipment required for cystocentesis includes a 22-gauge, 0.5- to 3.0-in.needle and a 5- to 10-mL syringe (depending on the size of the animal).

....

*Acetic acid 0.2 M—57 mL; sodium acetate 0.2 M—43 mL; use Millipore filtration and sterilization; otherwise the solution will grow molds.

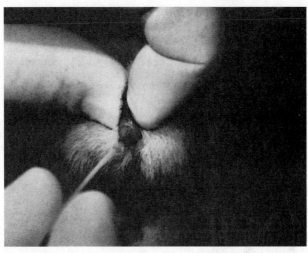

Figure 4–12. Catheterization of a male cat. With the cat on his back and the hindlegs pulled forward, the penis is withdrawn from its sheath and held. A sterile catheter is passed into the urethra, keeping the catheter parallel to the vertebral column of the cat.

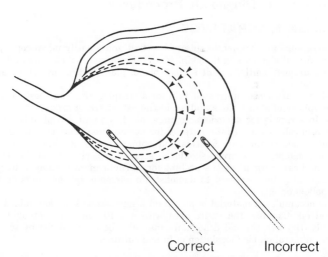

Correct   Incorrect

Figure 4–13. Schematic drawing illustrating correct and incorrect sites of insertion of a needle into the bladder for the purpose of evacuating urine. The needle should be inserted a short distance cranial to the junction of the bladder with the urethra rather than at the vertex of the bladder. This will permit removal of urine and decompression of the bladder without need for reinsertion of the needle into the bladder lumen. (From Osborne CA, Johnston GR, Shenk MP: Cystocentesis: Indications, contraindications, technique, and complications. Minn Vet 17:13, 1977.)

............Procedure

Clip and surgically prepare the skin over the cystocentesis site on the ventral abdomen. Cystocentesis is performed by placing the needle in the ventral abdominal wall slightly (3 to 5 cm) cranial to the junction of the bladder with the urethra. Insert the needle at a 45-degree angle (see Fig. 4–13). The bladder must contain a sufficient volume of urine to permit palpation through the abdominal wall prior to cystocentesis. One hand is used to hold the bladder steady within the peritoneal cavity while the other guides the needle.

Although this procedure is relatively safe, the bladder must have a reasonable volume of urine, the tap should not be made without identifying and immobilizing the bladder, and there must be adequate cooperation or sedation of the patient.

REFERENCES

Osborne CA, Finco DR: Canine and Feline Nephrology and Urology. Baltimore, Williams & Wilkins, 1995.
Stone EA, Barstanti JA: Urologic Surgery of the Dog and Cat. Philadelphia, Lea & Febiger, 1992.

....
SPECIAL DIAGNOSTIC PROCEDURES

Dermatologic Diagnostic Procedures

............SKIN SCRAPINGS

Skin scrapings are frequently obtained to find and identify microscopic parasites or fungal elements in the skin. Material required includes mineral oil in a small dropper bottle, a dull scalpel blade, glass slides, coverslips, and a microscope.

Select undisturbed, untreated skin for a scraping site. It is best to scrape the periphery of skin lesions and avoid the excoriated or traumatized center areas. In scraping for demodectic mange, pinch a small fold of affected skin firmly and collect the surface material for examination. This procedure forces the mites out of the hair follicles and onto or near the skin surface. For sarcoptic mange, large areas should be scraped. Select sites on the elbows, hocks, and ear margins when searching for sarcoptic mange. Many or frequent scrapings may be necessary to demonstrate sarcoptic mange mites or their fecal pellets or eggs.

The accumulated material is placed on a microscope slide and mixed with mineral oil. Examine the entire area with a ×10 objective thoroughly and carefully. Dry keratin and dead hairs may also be accumulated by scraping without mineral oil for inoculation of fungal cultures.

............WOOD'S LIGHT EVALUATION

Ultraviolet light filtered through nickel oxide produces a beam called *Wood's light*. If an animal is taken into a dark room and its hair and skin are exposed to a Wood's light, fluorescence may show for several reasons. Hair shafts affected by some species of *Microsporum* fungi fluoresce a bright yellow-green (like the color of a fluorescing watchface). However, iodide medications, petroleum, soap, dyes, and even keratin may produce purple-, blue-, or yellow-colored fluorescence. The positive fungal fluorescence is a valuable aid in selecting affected hairs for culture inoculation. Remember, a negative fluorescence does not preclude a possible diagnosis of fungal infection. There are both false negatives and false positives.

............ACETATE (SCOTCH) TAPE PREPARATION

This is one of the simplest diagnostic procedures. Bend clear (not frosted) acetate tape into a loop around the fingers with the sticky side facing out. Part the animal's hair coat, and press the tape firmly onto the skin and hair. The sticky tape picks up all loose particles it touches. Cut the loop of tape and place the strip of tape, sticky side down, on a clean microscope slide. Use a low-power microscope to look through the tape at the collected particles. This technique is excellent for trapping and identifying biting and sucking lice, *Otodectes* and *Cheyletiella* mites, flea dirt and larvae, fly larvae, or dandruff scales.

Acetate tape also is useful for studying hair abnormalities. Use a strong hemostat to securely clamp and quickly avulse a group of 10 to 20 hair shafts. The pointed distal ends can be pressed onto sticky acetate tape (lined up like pickets in a fence), and the hair shafts can be cut off in the middle with a scissors. The butt ends with the hair roots are likewise pressed onto another piece of tape. The tape holding the hair is then pressed onto a microscope slide to allow low-power examination of the hairs through the clear tape. The tips of the hairs will be well oriented and controlled; thus, it is easy to evaluate whether they are split, broken, or bitten off and whether the hair roots are in the anagen or telogen growth stage.

............BACTERIAL CULTURE (see p. 466), FUNGAL CULTURE (see p. 476)

............DIRECT (IMPRESSION) SMEAR

This simple, direct, and inexpensive technique may yield significant information within a short time. Cytologic examination can be made of material obtained from pustules, vesicles, or the raw, ulcerated, or cut surfaces of a lesion. To make the smear, press a clean microscope slide firmly against a raw or ulcerated lesion to transfer cellular material to the slide. Exudates may be collected by sterile swab or aspirated into a sterile syringe. Roll the swab gently across the slide, or place a drop of fluid from the syringe onto the slide and carefully spread the fluid in a uniform film. Material from a block of tissue can be transferred to the slide by gently pressing the tissue onto the slide in several locations. Use various stains for different conditions.

Rapid stains such as NMB or Diff-Quik are useful and convenient for office procedures, but even Wright's and Gram stains for evaluation of bacterial infections are easy to use. The presence of many bacteria, especially mixed types, may mean only surface contamination, whereas single types of bacteria, abundant polymorphonuclear WBCs, and especially phagocytosis support the diagnosis of infection and the host's response to it. A *few* acantholytic cells (loose epidermal cells) in the smear may be compatible with infectious processes, but large numbers, or "rafts," of acantholytic cells are highly suggestive of pemphigus and imply the need for more complex tests for positive diagnosis.

Large numbers of eosinophils are sometimes found in stained smears. Contrary to popular opinion, they usually do not mean allergy. They are most commonly seen with furunculosis and may be associated with the eosinophilic granulomas, eosinophilic plaques, sterile eosinophilic pustulosis, pemphigus complex, and ectoparasites. Yeasts (usually *Malassezia,* rarely *Candida*) are commonly found as budding cells in masses of wax and debris from ear smears.

Tumor cells may be recognized in some impression or aspiration samples where Giemsa is a preferred stain. Although special expertise is needed, cases of mastocytoma, histiocytoma, and lymphoma are most easily recognized. Formalin-fixed tissues for histologic diagnosis should always be prepared in tumor evaluations.

............SKIN BIOPSY

Histologic examination of diseased skin can serve as a means for diagnosis of cutaneous lesions. The etiologic agent is often found in both acute and chronic skin infections.

Punch biopsy of the skin is a quick and accurate means of removing a small sample of diseased skin for histopathologic examination. Select a site that is well developed but not traumatized or excoriated. The sample should include little or no normal tissue. If the lesion (pustule, vesicle) can be identified early in its development and if the biopsy sample is taken only from the lesion, one may obtain a superior specimen. It is best not to take too large a sample that contains much normal skin; by mistake, the technician might take a section that misses the lesion. Proper selection of the biopsy site is crucial to accurate diagnosis. The hair should be carefully clipped from the lesion. The skin should be lightly blotted with 70% alcohol. Avoid superficial trauma while cleaning the skin. A small subcutaneous bleb should be made with 2.0% lidocaine to deaden the area. Special equipment needed for the biopsy includes a 4- to 6-mm biopsy punch and 10% formalin solution. After the area has been anesthetized with lidocaine, press and rotate the biopsy punch through the skin until the subcutaneous tissue is penetrated. Remove the biopsy specimen by "spearing" the subcutaneous fat with a fine needle. Do not grasp the specimen with a forceps. Blot the specimen gently between two paper towels. Spread the tissue out gently (like a pancake), place the specimen epidermal side up on a piece of cardboard or tongue depressor, press the specimen gently to cause adhesion, and drop the specimen into the formalin fixative. The skin defect may be closed with one or two simple interrupted sutures. If deep subcutaneous tissue or large biopsy samples are needed, a punch biopsy is inadequate. Use a small (No. 15) scalpel blade to obtain an appropriate sample. In all cases in which skin biopsies are made, *multiple* samples should be taken to increase the odds that at least one will have diagnostic lesions. Specimens submitted to laboratories should be accompanied by extensive, detailed clinical information, including a differential diagnosis. Skin biopsies are routinely stained with hematoxylin-eosin (H&E); however, periodic acid–Schiff (PAS), Gomori's methenamine silver (GMS), and Verhoeff's stains are used for special problems.

............SKIN ALLERGY TESTS

The intradermal skin test can be used as a means of identifying specific allergens capable of inducing immediate hypersensitivities in dogs and cats. The test will not routinely give positive reactions for delayed hypersensitivities such as those from allergic contact dermatitis. Also, the test has not proved accurate for food-induced allergic dermatitis. Other diagnostic methods such as provocative exposure or patch testing must be used to identify the allergen causing food allergy or contact dermatitis.

Test antigens are purchased in concentrations of 1000 or 1500 protein nitrogen units (PNU)/mL. Aqueous antigens are ordered from a manufacturer of veterinary antigens. The following antigen groups are suggested for routine testing.

·········· Seasonal Allergens

(The contents of the list will vary according to locale; for helpful suggestions contact a local physician allergist.) Seasonal allergens include trees, flowers, grasses, weeds, and fleas.

·········· Nonseasonal Allergens

Nonseasonal allergens include molds and individual allergens such as house dust,* animal dander, feathers,* tobacco, newsprint, wool, and kapok.

Control agents include a *negative control* (diluent or buffered saline) and a *positive control* (histamine phosphate).

A negative diluent control and a positive histamine phosphate control are used. Two weeks prior to testing, the animal should be taken off all corticosteroids, antihistamines, and tranquilizers; 1 to 2 months or longer may be necessary if a long-acting steroid has been given. If there is doubt, a test with histamine can be made to demonstrate the animal's reactivity. The animal should not be tranquilized for the procedure, but it can be given xylazine (Rompun), diazepam (Valium), or ketamine, or can be anesthetized with short-acting barbiturates, if necessary. If the animal is firmly restrained on its side on a comfortable pad and its head covered with a towel to obscure its vision, it will usually lie quietly after a few moments. Gently clip the hair from the lateral thorax, and do not prepare the skin. Make intradermal injections of 0.05 mL of each antigen and each control. Use a 25- to 27-gauge 0.375-in. needle attached to a 1-mL disposable syringe. Space the injections about 2 cm apart, and mark each with a felt pen. The reactions are recorded in terms of centimeters and are read at intervals of 15 minutes after injection in dogs and every 5 to 15 minutes in cats, whose reactions are more difficult to read. Flea and staphylococcal injections are also read at 24 hours. A positive reaction looks more like the histamine reaction than the saline reaction. The histamine control should be diluted 1:10 with saline (1:100,000 histamine phosphate) before injection. This dilution will give a good 4+ reaction (a wheal 10 to 15 mm in diameter) in most dogs and is necessary to show that the patient is capable of responding to histamine.

A positive reaction indicates that the patient is hypersensitive to the test antigen or to a similar antigen. A negative reaction could mean any of the following: (1) the patient was not sensitive to the antigens used, (2) the antigen used was not present in sufficient quantity to give a positive reaction (combination antigens), (3) the patient is allergic but does not possess sufficient reagin antibody to give a positive skin test reaction, (4) an improper technique was used, or (5) inhibitory effects of other medications interfered.

One should always remember that a negative skin test does not mean that the patient is not allergic. Positive reactions can be false, too (e.g., house dust, some molds, some danders); therefore, the test reactions should correlate with the history if one expects to achieve good results from hyposensitization.

The National Pollen Calendar is helpful in correlating history and reactions with allergens. It is available in the third edition of this book or from manufacturers of allergy test kits.

Allergy skin testing is expensive and requires dedication, interest, and experience with many cases to make it a useful diagnostic method. If the clinician is not interested in allergic states and does not see many allergy cases, he or she should refer the cases to someone who is more familiar with them.

··

*House dust and feathers produce significant reactions in many normal dogs, so they might need to be diluted further.

REFERENCES

Baker E: Small Animal Allergy. Philadelphia, Lea & Febiger, 1990.
Reedy LM, Miller WH Jr, Willemse T: Allergic Skin Diseases of Dogs and Cats, ed 2. Philadelphia, WB Saunders, 1989.
Scott DW, Miller WH Jr, Griffin CE: Muller and Kirk's Small Animal Dermatology, ed 5. Philadelphia, WB Saunders, 1997.

Biopsy Techniques

............GENERAL CONSIDERATIONS

Numerous biopsy techniques are available, and the selection of the appropriate technique is based on the tissue to be examined, the condition of the patient, and the skill of the examiner.

Excisional Biopsy This technique refers to the surgical removal of the entire lesion and histologic examination. Excisional biopsy is most frequently used for skin lesions (see Skin Biopsies, p. 494) cases in which an entire organ may have to be removed (such as an eye or an internal organ that has developed a tumor).

Incisional Biopsy This technique refers to the surgical removal of a *portion* of a lesion. A representative area of the lesion should be chosen for biopsy. Include lesion margins, if possible.

Needle Aspiration In this form of biopsy, a variety of needles and a syringe are used to remove a small amount of tissue from the body.

............Needles

Various types of needles are available for biopsy. The selection of type, gauge, and length of needle should be based on the site of the biopsy and the characteristics of the tissues to be examined. *Thick-walled needles* with a stylet are needed for collection of material from bone and sclerotic tissue. On the other hand, *fine-needle aspiration* can be used in soft tissues. A 25-gauge needle and 12-mL syringe can be used.

The length of the needle is dependent on the location of the tissue. The *Menghini needle* is a coring and aspirating biopsy needle. It has an extremely thin wall and a 45-degree convex cutting edge. The needle is available in diameters of 1.0, 1.2, and 1.4 mm and lengths of 3.5 and 7.0 cm. Although only a small number of cells can be obtained, the danger of trauma to tissues with resultant postbiopsy complications is greatly reduced. Needles are available that will remove a small core of tissue by a cutting action. When the overall architecture of a tissue is important in making a diagnosis, a *punch (core) biopsy* is preferable to a needle biopsy.

............Touch Imprints and Scrapings

Touch imprint is the term used when an incised tissue mass has been cut to reveal a fresh surface and the mass is gently blotted onto glass slides imprinting cells. *Scrapings* are the result of scraping the surface of a lesion with a scalpel blade or "spatula"-type blade to obtain exfoliated cells for examination.

............NEEDLE BIOPSY

In this technique, a core or plug of tissue is removed by the cutting action of the biopsy instrument. Both cells and the supporting architecture of the tissue are removed. Needles available for punch biopsies include (1) the Franklin-modified Vim-Silverman needle, which has an outside 14-gauge cannula and an inner stylet and cutting prongs; and (2) the Tru-Cut disposable biopsy needle (see Fig. 4–14).

··········Characteristics of Cellular Malignancy

1. Enlargement of nucleus—nuclei larger than 10 nm
2. Decreased nuclear-cytoplasmic ratio
3. Multinucleation because of abnormal mitosis
4. Abnormal or frequent mitosis
5. Variations in size and shape of nuclei
6. Increase in size and number of nucleoli
7. Increased basophilia of cellular cytoplasm—increased RNA content
8. Anisokaryosis or pleomorphism
9. Multinucleated giant cells

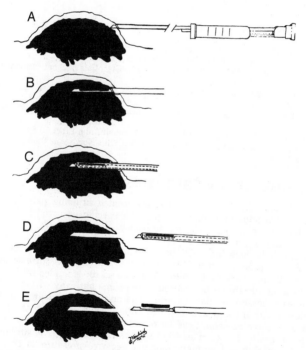

Figure 4–14. Mechanism of action of Tru-Cut biopsy needle for typical nodular biopsy. A small skin incision is made with a No. 11 blade to allow insertion of the instrument. A, With the instrument closed, the outer capsule is penetrated. B, The outer cannula is fixed in place, and the inner cannula with specimen notch is thrust into the tumor. Tissue then fills the notch. C, The inner cannula is now fixed while the outer cannula is moved forward to cut off the biopsy specimen. D, The entire instrument is removed. E, The inner cannula is pushed ahead to expose tissue in the specimen notch. (From Withrow SJ, Lowes N: Biopsy techniques in small animal oncology. J Am Anim Hosp Assoc 14:899–902, 1981.)

............LYMPH NODE ASPIRATION

Lymph node aspiration is used (1) in generalized lymphadenopathy, (2) in focal lymphadenopathy of unknown cause, and (3) in suspected instances of tumor metastases. Surgically prepare the skin over the node from which a biopsy specimen is to be taken. With one hand, localize and immobilize the lymph node; with the other hand, guide the aspiration biopsy needle into the affected node. Affix a syringe onto the needle, and advance the needle into the lymph node. When the needle is in position in the node, gradually draw negative pressure on the syringe. Cellular material within the needle is ejected onto clean glass slides. Lymph node aspirates must be handled gently. To make slides, place two slides together and pull the slides apart to avoid shearing the cells. Do not compress or force slides together.

Lymph node biopsy specimens can be obtained by excisional or punch (core) techniques, if desired.

REFERENCES

Barr F: Percutaneous biopsy of abdominal organs under ultrasound guidance. J Small Anim Pract 36:105–113, 1995.
Burkhard MJ, Meyer DJ: Invasive cytology of internal organs: Cytology of the thorax and abdomen. Vet Clin of North Am Small Anim Pract 26:1203, 1996.
Couto GC: Oncology. In Nelson RW, Couto GC, eds: Essentials of Small Animal Internal Medicine. St Louis, Mosby–Year Book, 1992.
Cowell R: Diagnostic Cytology of the Dog and Cat. St. Louis, Mosby–Year Book, 1998.
Ehrhart N: Principles of tumor biopsy. Clin Tech Small Anim Pract 13:1998.
Meyer D, Harvey J: Veterinary Laboratory Medicine, ed 2. Philadelphia, WB Saunders, 1998.
Mills JN: Lymph node cytology. Vet Clin North Am Small Anim Pract 19:697–717, 1989.
Wellman ML: Cytologic diagnosis of neoplasia. Vet Clin North Am Small Anim Pract 20:919–938, 1990.

............FINE-NEEDLE BIOPSIES

Potential lesions or abnormal tissues are located utilizing palpation, radiographs, or ultrasound imaging techniques.The specific areas to be biopsied and the needle path is determined and the biopsy site is surgically prepared. The type of sedation or anesthesia is dependent on the temperament of the animal and the site to be biopsied. A 22-gauge needle without stylet is attached to a 12-mL syringe prefilled with 5 mL of air via a flexible 84-cm extension set. Needle length may vary from 1.0 to 3.5 in. The needle is guided into the proper site and the needle tip is then moved in the same pathway within the site 10 to 12 times to loosen cellular material. The needle is withdrawn rapidly and the material within the needle expelled onto glass slides using the air in the syringe. This same procedure can be repeated with a new needle to obtain an additional three to five samples from alternative sites. This technique allows samples to be obtained without applying negative pressure to the syringe, which may damage cells.

Ultrasound-guided needle aspirations from abdominal tissues is a safe technique, especially when obtaining samples from smaller animals. Automatic-trigger needles such as Cook or Temno biopsy needles (14- to 18-gauge) can be used. The risks associated with fine-needle aspiration include: rupture of an encapsulated inflammatory process, dissemination of an infectious agent, seeding of neoplastic cells in the needle tract, and hemorrhage. All specimens obtained by fine-needle aspiration should be placed in a vial containing EDTA to prevent clot formation. Both direct and sedimentation specimens should be prepared.

REFERENCES

Menard M, Papgeorges M: Fine needle biopsies: How to increase diagnostic yield. Compend Contin Educ Pract Vet 19:738, 1997.

Menard M, Papgeorges M: Ultrasound-guided liver fine needle biopsies in cats: Results of 307 cases. Vet Pathol 33:570, 1996.

Meyer D, Harvey J: Veterinary Laboratory Medicine, ed 2. Philadelphia, WB Saunders, 1998.

··········FINE-NEEDLE ASPIRATION OF LUNG

Percutaneous aspiration needle biopsy and punch (core) biopsy can be helpful in establishing a diagnosis in conditions such as (1) chronic inflammatory disease of the lung—e.g., granulomatous lung disease caused by mycotic organisms; (2) chronic inflammatory disease; (3) metastases to the lung; and (4) primary lung tumors. The biopsy may provide enough diagnostic information to preclude performing an exploratory thoracotomy. Lung biopsy is contraindicated in animals with hemorrhagic disease or thoracic disease that produces forceful breathing and coughing.

The biopsy site is clipped and surgically prepared. The skin, subcutaneous tissue, muscle, and parietal pleura are infiltrated with 1% to 2% lidocaine.

In diffuse parenchymal lung disease, it is recommended that biopsy material be taken from the diaphragmatic lobes. The dorsal portions of the seventh to ninth intercostal spaces are preferred for percutaneous biopsies. In diffuse lesions, biopsy material should be taken from the right lung.

Fewer complications occur with a percutaneous aspiration biopsy than with a punch biopsy; however, a lung aspirate will yield only cells, fluid, and small pieces of tissue. A 20-gauge, 1.5-in. disposable needle (such as a Yale spinal needle) with stylet can be used for thoracic aspiration biopsy. The stylet is left in the needle until the lung substance has been entered. The stylet is then quickly removed, a gloved finger is placed over the needle opening to prevent air from entering the thoracic cavity, and a 10- to 20-mL syringe is placed on the needle. Suction and a back-and-forth movement of the needle are used to aspirate the lung material.

Contraindications to fine-needle aspiration are bleeding diathesis and coagulopathy, uncontrolled coughing, pulmonary hypertension, pulmonary cysts, and bullous emphysema.

4

··········TRANSTRACHEAL ASPIRATION

Transtracheal aspiration is a safe and clinically useful method for obtaining material for cytologic and bacteriologic examination from the lower respiratory tract of medium-sized to large dogs without invading the oval cavity. The technique can be performed on the unanesthetized animal, although some sedation may be necessary in fractious animals. In small dogs and cats, tracheal aspirates are collected by passing the catheter through sterile tracheal tubes. Light levels of anesthesia are used to accommodate coughing, as well as tracheal intubation.

Place the animal in sternal recumbency, and elevate and extend the head. Clip the area around the larynx, and surgically prepare the skin. The cricothyroid membrane is located by moving the finger cranially along the trachea until the large ventral ridge of the cricoid cartilage is felt. Use a 16-gauge, 0.5-in. IV catheter to collect material through the trachea (Fig. 4–15). Puncture the cricothyroid membrane with the 16-gauge needle, and pass the catheter into the trachea until it reaches the distal trachea or main stem bronchus. (Alternatively, in large dogs, the catheter can be inserted between the tracheal rings at the junction of the middle third and distal third of the cervical trachea.)

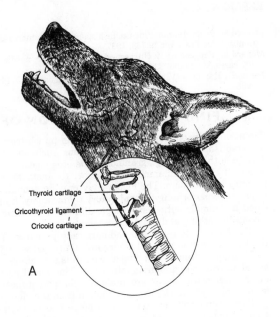

Thyroid cartilage

Cricothyroid ligament

Cricoid cartilage

A

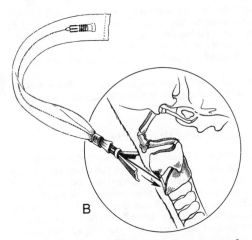

B

Figure 4–15. A, Diagrammatic representation of anatomical structures involved with transtracheal aspiration technique. The best landmark for percutaneous puncture is the cricothyroid ligament of the larynx, although the tracheal lumen can also be entered between cervical tracheal rings. B, The needle is advanced and directed slightly caudad until the trachea is entered. Once the needle is positioned within the tracheal lumen, the catheter is advanced through the needle and down the trachea. (From Kirk RW: Current Veterinary Therapy VIII: Small Animal Practice. Philadelphia, WB Saunders, 1983, p 223.)

Withdraw the needle, and leave the catheter in place. Attach a 12-mL syringe containing sterile saline solution to the catheter. Expel 1 to 2 mL of saline from the syringe. When the animal coughs, aspirate the syringe to collect cells and mucus for bacteriologic and cytologic examination. When material has been collected, remove the catheter and bandage the animal's neck. Material present in the syringe is cultured in blood agar and in thioglycollate medium. Prepare material from aspiration for cytologic examination. Large plugs of mucus are pressed between two clean glass slides, and thin smears are stained with either Wright's or Giemsa stain.

Complications of transtracheal aspiration biopsy include catheter trauma to the lower airway or needle trauma to the larynx, resulting in bleeding, subcutaneous emphysema, pneumomediastinum, pneumothorax, or airway obstruction.

REFERENCES

Bauer T, Thomas WP: Pulmonary diagnostic techniques. Vet Clin North Am Small Anim Pract 13:273, 1983.
Cowell RL, Tyler RD: Diagnostic Cytology of the Dog and Cat. Goleta, CA. American Veterinary Publications, 1989.
Roudebush P, Green R, Diglio KM: Percutaneous fine-needle aspiration of the lung in disseminated pulmonary disease. J Am Anim Hosp Assoc 17:109, 1981.

·········· BRONCHOALVEOLAR LAVAGE (see p. 499)
·········· LIVER BIOPSY

The diagnosis of liver disease can be made on the basis of clinical signs coupled with clinicopathologic results obtained by performing a "liver profile." The development of a more specific diagnosis and prognosis in liver disease may be greatly aided by information obtained in a liver biopsy. Percutaneous liver biopsies are of much greater value in generalized liver disease such as cirrhosis, generalized acute hepatic necrosis, or amyloidosis than in focal hepatic disease. The major indications for performing a liver biopsy are (1) to explain an abnormal liver profile, (2) to define reasons for abnormal liver size, (3) to identify a possible liver tumor, (4) to obtain a prognosis and rational approach to management, and (5) to identify the cause of ascites.

There are numerous procedures for obtaining liver tissue; however, needle biopsy of the liver, when performed properly, can be very helpful. Careful physical and clinicopathologic examination should precede a liver biopsy. Abnormalities in normal hemostatic mechanisms should be detected and corrected prior to needle biopsy of the liver. Contraindications to hepatic biopsy are (1) possible hemorrhage associated with coagulation abnormality, (2) suspicion of hepatic abscess or cyst, and (3) extrahepatic biliary obstruction.

·········· Equipment

Equipment necessary for liver biopsy includes the following:

    Local anesthetic
    Franklin-modified Vim-Silverman or similar biopsy needle
    Cutdown tray (sterile)
    Suitable fixative for tissue specimen

·········· Technique

Percutaneous needle biopsy of the liver can be performed with the patient under effective sedation and local anesthesia, but general anesthesia is recommended in most cases. Biopsy sites in the liver can best be selected when needle biopsy techniques are used in conjunction with laparoscopy or ultrasound techniques. Blind percutaneous needle biopsies of the liver are easily performed when the liver is enlarged and easily palpated. If the liver is not palpable, blind percutaneous transabdominal and transthoracic liver biopsies should be performed only by experienced clinicians.

A modified percutaneous liver biopsy can be performed by the following method. Prior to biopsy, the animal should be fasted and any ascitic fluid should be removed. The animal is placed in dorsal recumbency, and a local block is placed in the midline of the skin and abdomen at the caudoventral aspect of the left hepatic lobe. The incision into the peritoneal cavity should be large enough to accommodate the gloved index finger. Make a separate skin puncture site in the abdominal wall to accommodate the biopsy needle. Use the index finger to manually fix the left hepatic lobe (or other desired hepatic lobe) against the diaphragm or other adjacent structures, and insert the outer cannula and stylet through the abdominal wall in the isolated hepatic lobe. Remove the stylet, and rapidly insert the cutting prongs. If properly placed, the cutting prongs should not go through the entire hepatic lobe. Advance the outer cannula over the blades of the cutting prongs, thus entrapping the hepatic tissue material within the cutting prongs. Remove the biopsy needle. Using a wooden applicator stick, very carefully place the biopsy specimen into fixative. Biopsy samples can be used to prepare slides for cytologic examination, and the biopsy needle may be cultured. Close the abdominal incision in the routine manner.

Another liver biopsy technique uses the Tru-Cut biopsy needle.* Place the dog in dorsal recumbency. Clip a 5-cm² area over the triangle formed by the xiphoid cartilage and left costal arch, and prepare the area as for aseptic surgery. Make a small paramedian incision large enough to accommodate a sterile otoscope head 7 mm in diameter. Use a halogen-illuminated otoscope head to visualize the liver. A Tru-Cut biopsy needle is passed through the otoscope cone to obtain a biopsy specimen of the liver.

REFERENCES

Bunch SE, Polak DM, Hornbuckle WE: A modified laparoscopic approach for liver biopsy in dogs. J Am Vet Med Assoc 187:1032, 1985.

Guilford WG, Center SA, Strombeck DR, et al: Strombeck's Small Animal Gastroenterology, ed 3. Philadelphia, WB Saunders, 1996.

Kerwin S: Hepatic aspiration and biopsy techniques. Vet Clin North Am Small Anim Pract 25:275, 1995.

Kristensen AT, Klausner J, Weiss D, et al: Liver cytology in cases of canine and feline hepatic disease. Compend Contin Educ Pract Vet 12:797–808, 1990.

Selcer B, Cornelius LM: Percutaneous liver biopsy. Vet Med Rep 1:412, 1989.

············ PERCUTANEOUS RENAL BIOPSY

Renal biopsies can be valuable in confirming or eliminating a diagnosis of renal disease that is based on history, physical examination, and radiographic and laboratory data. In addition, biopsy may be a way of arriving at a prognosis in generalized renal disease and a better means of evaluating the type of treatment to be instituted. When performing renal biopsy, ultrasonographic guidance can prove very valuable in placing the needle into the tissue desired and in avoiding complications.

*Travenol Laboratories, Deerfield, IL.

.... Equipment

Equipment necessary for percutaneous renal biopsy includes the following:

A Franklin-Silverman biopsy needle
Sharp, pointed tissue scissors and scalpel
Thumb forceps
Hemostats
Needle holder, skin suture, sponges
Local anesthetic; surgical preparation tray; small drape; formalin 10% for fixation of specimen

.... Precautions in Renal Biopsy

Prior to renal biopsy the animal should have a baseline evaluation of coagulation (see p. 687) including an activated coagulation time (ACT), platelet count, and bleeding time. Biopsies should be obtained from the renal cortex. Fluids should be administered to patients prior to and after biopsy.

■ CONTRAINDICATIONS TO RENAL BIOPSIES

Coagulation abnormalities
A single functional kidney
Marked hydronephrosis
Markedly contracted kidneys
Large cysts
Acute pyelonephritis

.... Technique

Many patients with generalized renal disease are critically ill and debilitated, and general anesthesia is contraindicated. In these cases, a neuroleptanalgesic agent may be used for sedation. If the animal is a good anesthetic risk and renal function will permit it, a general anesthetic can be used.

Surgically prepare the area over the kidney from which the biopsy specimen is to be obtained. Infiltrate the skin and paralumbar muscles caudal to the last rib just below the ventral border of the lumbar muscles with a local anesthetic. Make a paralumbar incision large enough for the index finger in this site over the caudal pole of the kidney. Dissect muscle and fascia until the peritoneum is reached, and enter the peritoneal cavity. With the sterile, gloved index finger, examine the posterior pole and remaining portions of the kidney. Make a small stab incision in the skin just anterior to paralumbar entry into the peritoneal cavity, and insert the biopsy needle into the peritoneal cavity (Fig. 4–16). Guide the needle toward the posterior pole of the kidney with the index finger. Hold the kidney so that it is immobilized against the body wall and, placing the long axis of the biopsy needle away from the renal pelvis, insert the needle just through the renal capsule. Replace the stylet in the needle with the cutting prongs, and rapidly thrust the cutting prongs into the renal cortical tissue. Keeping the cutting prongs in the same position, move the outer cannula down over the blades, rotating the cannula. Remove the cutting prongs and outer cannula, and place the biopsy specimen in fixative. Close the surgical wound, ensuring that excessive hemorrhage is not present.

Alternatively, a Tru-Cut biopsy needle can be used to perform the kidney biopsy. Figure 4–14 illustrates the use of this biopsy needle.

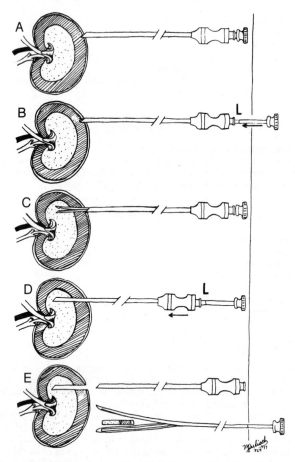

Figure 4–16. Mechanism of action of Franklin-Silverman biopsy needle. A, Outer cannula with stylet in place should just penetrate the capsule. B, The outer cannula is held in place and the stylet is removed. Cutting prongs are introduced until the prongs just contact the organ or up to the line marked on the shaft of the cutting prongs (L). C, The outer cannula is fixed in place while cutting prongs are thrust rapidly into tissue. D, The cutting prongs are now held fixed while the outer cannula is gently rotated back and forth over the prongs until the line on the shaft of the prongs can be seen. E, Both the cannula and prongs are removed together. The prongs are then removed from the cannula, and the biopsy specimen is gently removed. (From Withrow SJ, Lowes N: Biopsy techniques in small animal oncology. J Am Anim Hosp Assoc 14:899–902, 1981.)

In dogs, renal biopsy can be performed under ultrasound guidance using probes with channels for biopsy needle insertion.

............Fixation and Preparation of Biopsy Material

The choice and concentration of the fixative to be used depend on the type of tissue specimen. In general, when a piece of tissue has been removed for biopsy by excision, the specimen should be no more than 0.5 to 1.0 cm thick and a 10:1 ratio of fixative volume to tissue volume should be used.

Various types of fixatives are available for processing tissue biopsies:

1. *Neutral buffered 10% formalin solution.* For routine examination of tissues by light microscopy. The amount of formalin used should be 10 times that of the tissue present. Fix for at least 18 hours.
2. *Bouin's solution.* For fixation of testicular, endocrine, and intestinal mucosal tissue. Fix in Bouin's solution for not more than 24 hours. Bouin's solution is a combination of picric acid, formalin, and glacial acetic acid.
3. *Zenker's acetic acid solution.* Tends to preserve nuclear structures very well. This solution, which is very good for fixation of eyes, is a combination of mercuric chloride and potassium dichromate. Zenker's solution does not remain stable in acetic acid, and 5 mL of acetic acid must be added to 95 mL of Zenker's solution just prior to use.
4. *Freezing.* For frozen sections.
5. *Glutaraldehyde.* Used for tissues to be prepared for electron microscopy.

Special techniques are required to prepare fluids that have a low cellular count:

1. Centrifugation of the specimen at 1500 to 2000 rpm for 10 minutes can allow concentration of cellular material.
2. Special filters such as the Millipore filter (five-pore size) or the nucleopore filter can be used to isolate cells.
3. Fluids can be fixed in 40% ethyl alcohol combined with 18% neutral buffered formalin if special stains are required, and the cells can be isolated on filters.

4

REFERENCES

Burkhard MJ, Meyer DJ: Invasive cytology of internal organs: Cytology of the thorax and abdomen. Vet Clin North Am Small Anim Pract 6:103, 1996.
Osborne CA, Finco DR: Canine and Feline Nephrology and Urology. Baltimore, Williams & Wilkins, 1995.
Stone E: Biopsy: Principles, technical considerations, and pitfalls. Vet Clin North Am Small Anim Pract 25:33, 1995.
Tvedten H: Cytology of neoplastic and inflammatory masses. *In* Willard MD, Tvedten H, Turnwald GH, eds: Small Animal Clinical Diagnosis by Laboratory Methods. Philadelphia, WB Saunders, 1990, pp 327–348.

............PROSTATE BIOPSY (see also p. 380)

A transperineal approach can be used for prostatic biopsy. General anesthesia or neuroleptanalgesia is required to perform this technique. The perineal area is surgically prepared, and a 0.5-cm skin incision is made 2 to 4 cm lateral to the anus on the side of the prostate from which the biopsy specimen is to be obtained. A Tru-Cut disposable biopsy needle is used. The prostate gland should be manually pushed toward the pelvic brim by placing pressure on the abdominal viscera. This can best be done with the dog in lateral recumbency. The clinician should wear sterile gloves. Palpate the prostate per rectum with one hand. Hold the biopsy needle with the other hand, and insert the needle through the tissue lateral to the anus and medial to the tuber ischii. Direct the needle anteriorly, parallel to the rectum, until the prostate is reached.

Prostatic biopsy may also be performed transabdominally or via exploratory laparotomy.

REFERENCES

Barsanti JA: Canine prostatic disease. *In* Ettinger SJ, Feldman EC, eds: Textbook of Veterinary Internal Medicine, 4th ed. Philadelphia, WB Saunders, 1995, pp 1162–1185.
Osborne CA, Finco DR: Canine and Feline Nephrology and Urology. Baltimore, Williams & Wilkins, 1995.
Stone EA, Barsanti JA: Urologic Surgery of the Dog and Cat. Philadelphia, Lea & Febiger, 1992.

............NASAL BIOPSY

Nasal Specimen Collection (see Fig. 4–17):

Advance a 3.5F catheter into the nares to the desired position. Attach a syringe filled with 10 to 20 mL of sterile saline. Inject the saline slowly, moving the catheter in and out. Collect the effluent in a sterile receptor for culture and cytologic examination. If a mass is identified in the nares, a 10F polyethylene

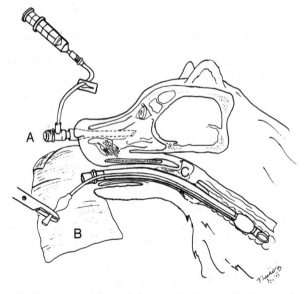

Figure 4–17. Illustration of nasal flush technique. Stiff plastic tubing (A) is measured to a length corresponding to the distance from the external nares to the medial canthus of the eye. Gauze sponges are placed on the table near the nares (B) and behind the soft palate (C) to trap dislodged tissue. Intermittent positive and negative pressure is applied with saline via the syringe while the catheter is pushed in and out of the turbinates to cut or dislodge cores of tissue. (From Withrow SJ, Lowes N: Biopsy techniques in small animal oncology. J Am Anim Hosp Assoc 14:889, 1981.)

catheter that has been cut sharply at a beveled angle is passed into the nares to a depth that corresponds to the location of the mass. Use a syringe filled with sterile saline and collect pieces of the tissue mass as well as effluent for cytologic examination.

REFERENCES

Crow S, Walshaw S: Manual of Clinical Procedures in the Dog, Cat, and Rabbit, ed 2. Philadelphia, Lippincott-Raven, 1997.
Withrow SJ, Susaneck SJ, Macy DW, et al: Aspiration and punch biopsy technique for nasal tumors. J Am Anim Hosp Assoc 21:551–554, 1985.

Pharyngostomy

This technique allows placement of a gastroesophageal tube for the repeated oral alimentation required in a wide variety of disease conditions. Pharyngostomy obviates the necessity of repeated passage of a stomach tube and is well tolerated by most animals.

...........EQUIPMENT

Equipment for pharyngostomy includes:

Standard surgical pack and suture material.
Plastic or rubber feeding tube. The tube length should be from canine teeth to anterior or midthoracic esophagus. The tube should be of the end-hole type as opposed to the side-hole type. Use a 10F to 12F catheter for cats and dogs under 10 kg, 16F to 20F for larger dogs.

...........TECHNIQUE

A short-acting anesthetic can be used in animals that are good surgical risks. A neuroleptanalgesic agent with local anesthesia or local anesthesia alone can be used in debilitated patients.

4

1. Prepare the ventrolateral portion of the neck from the thyroid cartilage to the cranial border of the mandibular ramus. The tube can be placed in the right or left pharynx (Fig. 4–18).
2. Feel the epihyoid bone, and put the gloved finger above the epiglottis. Palpate the lateral wall of the pharynx caudodorsal to the hyoid apparatus.
3. Make an incision in the skin directly over this area. Using a curved Kelly forceps, bluntly dissect a tunnel toward the finger in the oral cavity. Place the tube into the esophagus. Use blunt dissection through the skin, and use a hemostat to place the pharyngostomy tube into the esophagus. By having the tube enter the esophagus in the posterior pharynx *above* the epiglottis, respiratory difficulties and gagging are avoided. The end of the tube should terminate in the midthoracic or caudal esophagus to prevent reflux esophagitis and ulceration. Occlusion of the jugular vein permits visualization of the external maxillary and linguofacial veins.
4. Palpate the ventral border of the digastric muscle. The hypoglossal nerve and lingual artery are caudal to the pharyngostomy site. The incision is caudal to the digastric muscle and parallel to the facial branch of the linguofacial vein. A safety pin may be laced through the lumen of the tube to maintain its position, or a friction suture of 2-0 or 0 silk can be used to keep the tube in place. The tube should be capped when not in use (see p. 537 for nutrients that can be administered via pharyngostomy tube).

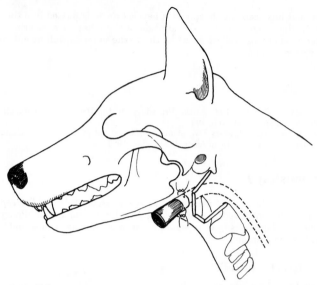

Figure 4–18. Tube in position within the pharynx and esophagus. (From Bojrab MJ, ed: Current Techniques in Small Animal Surgery, ed 2. Philadelphia, Lea & Febiger, 1983, p 103.)

5. Clean the incision in the skin and the entrance site of the tube daily with soap and water. Povidone-iodine ointment is applied to help prevent infection. The wound is allowed to heal by second intention when the tube is removed.

A pharyngostomy incision has also been used to place an endotracheal tube when surgery is necessary to treat oral or pharyngeal lesions and mandibular or maxillary fractures.

REFERENCE

Armstrong PJ, Hand MS, Frederick GS: Enteral nutrition by tube. Vet Clin North Am Small Anim Pract 20:237–275, 1990.

Percutaneous Gastrostomy Tube Placement

Percutaneous gastrostomy tubes are routinely used to administer nutrients and medications orally (PO) over days or weeks to cats and dogs who cannot have nutrients administered by mouth or who will not eat (e.g., because of feline hepatic lipidosis, oropharyngeal neoplasms, maxillary or mandibular fractures, oral reconstructive surgery, esophageal masses or foreign bodies, severe pharyngitis). The percutaneous gastrostomy tube is placed so that it extends through the skin and left cranial abdominal wall of the abdomen into the body of the stomach.

·········**PREPARATION OF THE CATHETER**

1. Use the French-Pezzar mushroom-tipped catheter.
2. Cut off 1.5 cm of the open(distal) end of the catheter with scissors.
3. Cut 3-mm holes on either side of the 1.5-cm piece (outer flange).
4. Cut the distal end of the catheter to form a sharp bevel point.
5. Measure the length of the tube from the mushroom tip to 2 cm below the bevel.

·········**PREPARATION OF THE STOMACH TUBE PLACEMENT DEVICE**

1. Use a smooth-ended vinyl stomach tube.
2. Measure the length of the tube needed to reach the stomach by laying the tube along the animal's side with the rounded end 1 to 2 cm caudal to the last rib.
3. Mark the tube with an indelible marker or adhesive tape at the tip of the muzzle and cut off excess tube.
4. Put the tube in the freezer for 30 minutes prior to beginning the procedure to stiffen the tube.

·········**PLACEMENT OF PERCUTANEOUS GASTROTOMY TUBE**

1. Clip and surgically prepare the skin over the left abdominal wall.
2. Place the mouth speculum between the right canine teeth.
3. Place the stomach tube in the esophagus to the level of the cardia.
4. Rotate the tube counterclockwise while carefully advancing it through the cardia.
5. Turn the tube back clockwise and advance the tube until it can be visualized through the abdominal wall 1 to 2 cm caudal to the last rib (Fig. 4–19).

4

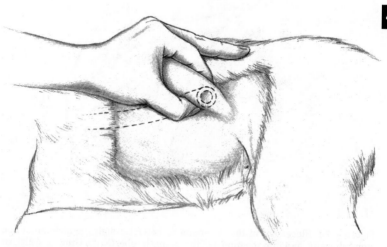

Figure 4–19. Locating the end of the rigid stomach tube at the left lateral abdominal wall. (From Crow S, Walshaw S: Manual of Clinical Procedures in the Dog, Cat, and Rabbit, ed 2. Philadelphia, Lippincott-Raven, 1997, p 183.)

6. Rotate the tube so that the tip lies against the stomach and abdominal wall one-third the distance between the epaxial muscles and the ventral midline.

7. Make a 2- to 3-mm skin incision directly over the lumen of the stomach tube.

8. Use a Sovereign catheter (over the needle) and puncture the abdominal and stomach walls, placing the catheter inside the lumen of the stomach tube. Remove the needle (Fig. 4–20).

9. Thread a long rigid suture through the catheter and advance it through the stomach tube until the end is observed at the mouth end of the tube (Fig. 4–21).

10. Carefully remove the plastic catheter from the stomach tube opening and place a hemostat clamp at the end of the suture material.

11. Remove the stomach tube over the oral end of the stiff introduction suture line.

12. Attach the open, beveled end of the French-Pezzar catheter stomach tube to a plastic Sovereign catheter using a mattress suture (Fig. 4–22).

13. Force the tip of the rubber stomach tube into the large end of the Sovereign catheter.

14. Advance the catheter-tube through the mouth and esophagus into the stomach by placing traction on the abdominal end of the introduction line.

15. The catheter will emerge through the skin incision followed by the rubber tube. Grasp the tube with forceps and pull it through the incision opening (Fig. 4–23A).

16. Remove the catheter by cutting it off 2 cm below the beveled tip. Pull the rubber tube through the abdominal wall until slight resistance is felt (Fig. 4–23B).

17. Slide the outer flange over the end of the tube down to the skin level (Fig. 4–24).

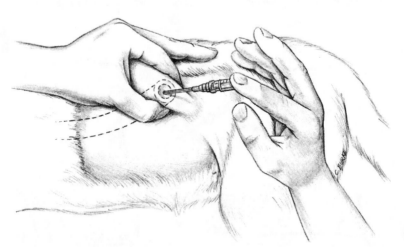

Figure 4–20. Placement of the Sovereign catheter through the abdominal and stomach walls, and into the lumen of the stomach tube. (From Crow S, Walshaw S: Manual of Clinical Procedures in the Dog, Cat, and Rabbit, ed 2. Philadelphia, Lippincott-Raven, 1997, p 184.)

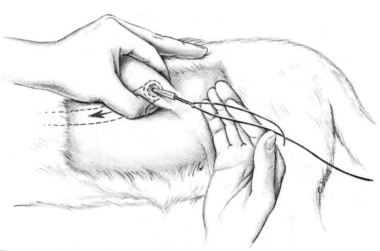

Figure 4–21. Threading the introduction line retrograde through the Sovereign catheter and stomach tube. (From Crow S, Walshaw S: Manual of Clinical Procedures in the Dog, Cat, and Rabbit, ed 2. Philadelphia, Lippincott-Raven, 1997, p 185.)

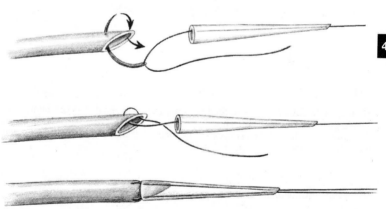

Figure 4–22. Suturing the introduction line to the beveled end of the gastrostomy catheter. (From Crow S, Walshaw S: Manual of Clinical Procedures in the Dog, Cat, and Rabbit, ed 2. Philadelphia, Lippincott-Raven, 1997, p 186.)

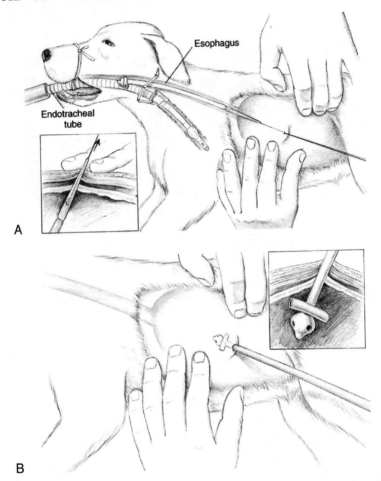

Figure 4–23. Catheter-tube assembly being pulled through (A) the mouth and esophagus and (B) the stomach and abdominal walls. (From Crow S, Walshaw S: Manual of Clinical Procedures in the Dog, Cat, and Rabbit, ed 2. Philadelphia, Lippincott-Raven, 1997, p 186.)

18. Apply antimicrobial ointment and a sterile gauze sponge over the skin incision.
19. Bandage the gastrostomy tube in place (Fig. 4–25).

REFERENCES

Armstrong PJ, Hardie EM: Percutaneous endoscopic gastrotomy—a retrospective study of 54 clinical cases in dogs and cats. J Vet Intern Med 4:202–206, 1990.
Crow S, Walshaw S: Manual of Clinical Procedures in the Dog, Cat, and Rabbit, ed 2. Philadelphia, Lippincott-Raven, 1997.

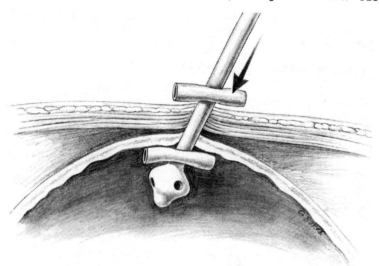

Figure 4–24. Diagram showing the inner and outer flanges in place against stomach mucosa and skin, respectively. (From Crow S, Walshaw S: Manual of Clinical Procedures in the Dog, Cat, and Rabbit, ed 2. Philadelphia, Lippincott-Raven, 1997, p 187.)

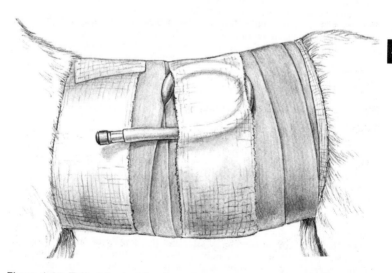

Figure 4–25. Full abdominal bandage showing the plugged end of the gastrostomy tube emerging dorsally. (From Crow S, Walshaw S: Manual of Clinical Procedures in the Dog, Cat, and Rabbit, ed 2. Philadelphia, Lippincott-Raven, 1997, p 188.)

Crowe DT, Downs MO: Pharyngostomy complications in dogs and cats and recommended technical modifications: Experimental and clinical investigations. J Am Anim Hosp Assoc 22:493, 1986.

Bone Marrow Aspiration

Collection of bone marrow may prove valuable in diseases of the blood in which examination of the peripheral blood reveals abnormal cells or cell counts. Conditions such as leukopenia, thrombocytopenia, nonregenerative anemias, agranulocytosis, pancytopenia, and leukemias may be present because of pathologic changes within the bone marrow.

Bone marrow in the young animal is very cellular and exists in the flat bones (sternum, ribs, pelvic bones, and vertebrae) and in the long bones (humerus and femur).

As the animal ages, the cellular content of the marrow decreases, especially in the long bones. In older animals, bone marrow cells still exist in the flat bones; however, in conditions of stress in which new blood cells must be produced in large numbers, primitive cells in the bone marrow of the long bones again become active.

Interpretation of the bone marrow smear may be limited by:

1. The technique used to obtain a bone marrow specimen. Technique is important because contamination with peripheral blood should be avoided.
2. The specialized knowledge necessary to interpret bone marrow cells.

............BONE MARROW COLLECTION (DOG)

The biopsy techniques that may be used in the examination of bone marrow are aspiration, core, and incisional biopsy. The most frequently used technique is aspiration biopsy. When aspiration biopsy fails to produce bone marrow cells (as in advanced myelofibrosis, neoplasia, or marrow aplasia), a core biopsy of bone marrow is indicated. Bone marrow aspiration needles may be a 16-gauge Rosenthal needle or Illinois needle for medium-sized dogs; an 18-gauge Rosenthal needle for small dogs and cats; or a Jamshidi bone marrow biopsy needle, 12-gauge for most adult dogs and 14-gauge for small dogs and cats.

............Equipment

All equipment should be sterile. Equipment necessary for bone marrow collection includes the following:

Rubber gloves
Lidocaine 0.5%
Skin disinfectant
Clear glass slides
One 12-mL syringe
One scalpel
Sponges

The selection of needles for aspiration biopsy of bone marrow is based on the biopsy site, the depth of the biopsy site, and the density of cortical bone. For bone marrow aspiration, the modified disposable Illinois sternal-iliac bone marrow aspiration needle works well. For a core biopsy of bone marrow, the Jamshidi bone marrow biopsy-aspiration needle (pediatric, 3.5-in., 13-gauge) can be used.

The iliac crest is the site for marrow aspiration in dogs. The head of the humerus is an alternative site. A short-acting anesthetic may occasionally be needed, but tranquilization together with local anesthesia is usually sufficient. Place the animal in lateral recumbency, and clip the hair over the area of the iliac crest. Surgically prepare the site. To aspirate marrow, have the needle enter the widest part of the iliac crest and stop the needle just after penetration of the bone. Remove the stylet, place a 12-mL syringe on the needle, and aspirate 0.2 mL of marrow.

Contamination of the bone marrow with peripheral blood results if (1) the marrow is not aspirated immediately after the needle enters the marrow cavity, or (2) too much negative pressure is placed on the syringe, thus rupturing small sinusoids in the bone marrow.

Marrow can also be obtained from the proximal end of the femur via the trochanteric fossa. Make a small skin incision over the trochanteric fossa just medial to the summit of the trochanter major. The bone marrow aspiration needle is inserted medial to the trochanter major, and the long axis of the needle is placed parallel to the long axis of the femur. Using firm pressure and an alternating rotary motion, insert the bone marrow needle 0.5 in. into the femoral canal. Remove the stylet from the needle, and aspirate with a 12- or 20-mL syringe (Fig. 4–26). It is important for accurate bone marrow interpretation that smears contain marrow particles. The marrow particles appear as small white grains. A "squash" preparation of the marrow particles can be made using two glass slides. Smears are air-dried. Liquid bone marrow clots rapidly and should be collected into vials containing EDTA.

···········BONE MARROW COLLECTION (CAT)

Accessible sites for bone marrow sampling in the cat are the iliac crest and the proximal end of the femur via the trochanteric fossa. The latter is generally the more useful site. The techniques just described for the dog can be used; however, caution is advised against using vigorous restraint with a severely anemic cat, as such restraint may precipitate severe cyanosis, apnea, and cardiac arrest. Adequate sedation with supplemental oxygen administration and local anesthesia usually suffices.

4

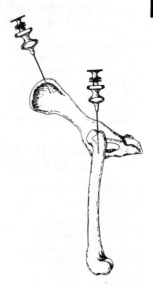

Figure 4–26. Diagram of the ilium and femur, illustrating the sites for bone marrow biopsy. The angle of the needle is variable for the ilial site. The needle may approach a more vertical position in larger bones, in which case the needle is started more caudally on the wing of the ilium. (From Bojrab MJ, ed: Current Techniques in Small Animal Surgery, ed 2. Philadelphia, Lea & Febiger, 1983, p 492.)

Smears of bone marrow should be made immediately after aspiration of material. Extrinsic thromboplastin present in bone marrow tissue will cause the marrow to clot within 30 seconds. In addition, small pieces of marrow can be fixed in formalin for histologic preparation. Staining with NMB, Wright's, May-Grünwald, or Giemsa stain may be used. A peroxidase stain may be helpful in differentiating granulocytic elements from lymphocytes.

Another method is to aspirate the bone marrow into a syringe containing 1 to 2 mL of 4% EDTA solution. The aspirate is expelled into a sterile Petri dish, and the firm marrow particles can be picked out and prepared on glass slides for staining.

REFERENCES

Crow S, Walshaw S: Manual of Clinical Procedures in the Dog, Cat, and Rabbit, ed 2. Philadelphia, Lippincott-Raven, 1997.

Grindem CB: Bone marrow biopsy and evaluation. Vet Clin North Am Small Anim Pract 19:669–696, 1989.

Jacobs RM, Valli VEO: Bone marrow biopsies: Principles and perspectives of interpretation. Semin Vet Med Surg 3:176, 1988.

Meyer D, Harvey J: Veterinary Laboratory Medicine, ed 2. Philadelphia, WB Saunders, 1998.

O'Keefe D: Bone marrow biopsy: Indications and techniques. In Kirk RW, ed: Current Veterinary Therapy XI. Small Animal Practice. Philadelphia, WB Saunders, 1991, p 488.

Cerebrospinal Fluid Collection

In the dog, the preferred site for obtaining cerebrospinal fluid (CSF) is the cerebellomedullary cistern (cisterna magna) at the atlanto-occipital articulation.

..........CONTRAINDICATIONS TO CSF FLUID COLLECTION

1. Congenital abnormalities involving malformations of the foramen magnum, or suspected neural malformations in the region of the cisterna magna
2. Fractures, dislocations, or subluxations of the occipital region of the skull or rostral cervical region, resulting in distortion of the brain stem, medulla, or cervical cord
3. Suspected brain herniation
4. Infection of soft tissue overlying the puncture site

..........COMPLICATIONS OF CSF FLUID COLLECTION

1. No CSF fluid obtained
2. Herniation of the brain
3. Contamination of the CSF fluid with blood
4. Pithing of the medulla or the rostral spinal cord
5. Infection of the CNS
6. Respiratory or cardiac arrest
7. Vestibular dysfunction
8. Paresis or paralysis

............EQUIPMENT

Sterile test tubes
A 20- to 22-gauge, 1.5- to 3.5-in. spinal needle with a short bevel and stylet
Spinal fluid manometer for pressure readings
Three-way stopcock
Two sterile 5-mL syringes
Sterile sponges

............TECHNIQUES

In order to perform an adequate cisternal puncture and not injure the animal, a short-acting general anesthetic is required. Place the animal in either ventral or lateral recumbency. Clip and surgically prepare the area of skin from the external occipital protuberance to the wings of the atlas. The dog should be positioned in left lateral recumbency for right-handed personnel and in right lateral recumbency for left-handed personnel. Position the animal with the prepared area at the edge of the table. The head should be flexed ventrally and maintained at a right angle to the long axis of the neck. Flexion of the neck will serve to separate the occipital bone from the atlas.

To find the site of entrance for the needle into the cistern, draw an imaginary line across the neck from the prominent cranial lateral portion of the wings of the atlas. At a point where this line bisects an imaginary line drawn craniocaudally from the external occipital protuberance, pass the needle inward at a right angle to the dorsal line of the neck (Fig. 4–27). As the needle is advanced,

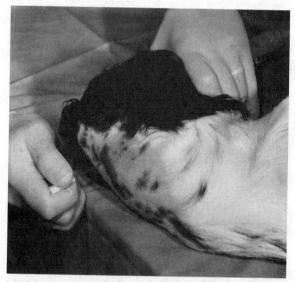

Figure 4–27. Collection of cerebrospinal fluid. The dog is in left lateral recumbency. The area from the external occipital protuberance to the wings of the atlas has been clipped and surgically prepared. The head is flexed ventrally. The needle is inserted at the junction of a line that bisects the cranial wings of the atlas and the external occipital protuberance. One person should hold the dog's head carefully and firmly in a flexed position while a second person makes the tap.

the stylet is removed periodically to see whether CSF appears in the hub. During this procedure, the hub of the needle must be held tightly to prevent any movement of the needle. Occasionally, resistance is felt just before the needle passes through the dura, but this cannot be depended on; therefore, remove the stylet frequently to avoid injury to the spinal cord. If bone is felt with the tip of the needle, the needle can be walked caudally or cranially to the atlanto-occipital space. Occasionally, blood without CSF is obtained as a result of puncture of a branch of the vertebral venous plexus. Obtain another clean sterile needle and repeat the procedure. This repetition should not contaminate the CSF with blood. Any fresh blood that appears in the CSF may be associated with rupture of small blood vessels during the tap or may be part of the disease process.

When the cisternal space is entered and fluid is seen at the needle hub (Fig. 4–28), allow 2 mL of CSF to flow passively into a sterile vial. The initial CSF examination should include inspection for color and turbidity, total cell count, differential cell count, and protein determination. Further tests such as glucose levels, creatine kinase (CK) levels, and cultures may be indicated, depending on the clinical situation.

All animals on which a cisternal tap was performed should be closely observed for the next 5 to 7 days for signs of adverse effects such as infection.

See p. 891 for normal CSF values.

REFERENCES

Bailey CS, Higgins RJ: Characteristics of cerebrospinal fluid associated with canine granulomatous meningoencephalomyelitis: A retrospective study. J Am Vet Med Assoc 188:418, 1986.
Bailey CS, Higgins RJ: Characteristics of cisternal cerebrospinal fluid associated with

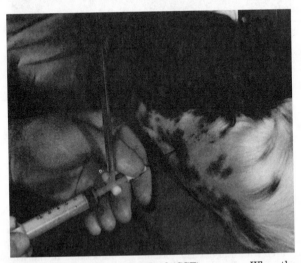

Figure 4–28. Recording cerebrospinal fluid (CSF) pressure. When the cisternal space is entered and fluid is seen at the needle hub, the spinal fluid pressure manometer is attached and the opening and closing CSF pressure is recorded. If CSF pressures are recorded, extreme care must be taken to avoid trauma to the spinal cord with the needle.

primary brain tumors in the dog: A retrospective study. J Am Vet Med Assoc 188:414, 1986.

Meyer D, Harvey J: Veterinary Laboratory Medicine, ed 2. Philadelphia, WB Saunders 1998.

Oliver J, Lorenz M, Kornegay J: Handbook of Veterinary Neurology, ed 3. Philadelphia, WB Saunders, 1997.

Measurement of Central Venous Pressure (Dog)

Central venous pressure (CVP) is the blood pressure within the intrathoracic portions of the cranial or caudal vena cava. Measurement of CVP in the dog provides an excellent index for determining circulation efficiency. The CVP is controlled by interaction of the circulating blood volume, cardiac pumping action, and alterations in the vascular bed. The CVP is not a measure of blood volume but an indication of the ability of the heart to accept and pump blood brought to it. The CVP reflects the interaction of the heart, vascular tone, and circulatory blood volume. When the heart action and vascular tone remain constant, CVP reflects blood volume. When blood volume and vascular tone are constant, CVP reflects heart action. When blood volume and heart action are constant, CVP can be used to measure vascular tone.

In addition, the placement of a jugular catheter can be helpful in long-term fluid management and in parenteral alimentation of critically ill animals (see p. 585).

··········· INDICATIONS

Measurement of CVP is indicated (1) in acute circulatory failure that has not responded to initial treatment; (2) in administration of large volumes of blood or fluids, as may occur in acute shock; (3) as part of the monitoring procedure in poor-risk surgical patients; and (4) in abnormal urine production for which fluids are being administered.

··········· EQUIPMENT

The following equipment is necessary for CVP measurement:

4

One Intracath needle, 17- or 18-gauge
One metric rule, 80 cm long
One three-way stopcock
One bottle of isotonic sodium chloride 500 mL, and IV tubing
One extra piece of tubing, 3 ft long, or a Becton Dickinson or Batten disposable CVP set

··········· PROCEDURE

For CVP measurement, a catheter must be placed in the external jugular vein so that the catheter is in direct fluid continuity with the right atrium.

Place the animal in lateral recumbency, and clip the hair over the jugular vein. Surgically prepare the skin in the clipped area.

Make a percutaneous puncture of the jugular vein with the Intracath catheter needle, and advance the tip to approximately the third intercostal space (tip of the catheter at the right atrium). Fasten the catheter securely to the neck of the patient by passing adhesive tape around the neck and the hub of the catheter needle so that the hub of the needle comes to lie at the base of the ear. Connect a three-way stopcock to the catheter. Connect an IV setup of isotonic sodium chloride to one end of the stopcock, and to the other end of the stopcock attach a piece of IV tubing, which should be taped vertically to a pole or a piece of doweling (Fig. 4–29). The metric rule is placed so that the 0 level is aligned with the midpoint of the trachea at the thoracic inlet, and the rule is taped to the vertical pole.

To fill the CVP manometer, turn the three-way stopcock so that fluid will flow from the bottle of saline into the manometer and will exceed the 15-cm mark. Next, turn the stopcock so that a column of fluid exists from the superior vena cava to the manometer. The fluid in the manometer will fall until it reflects the level of the CVP.

It is desirable to allow fluid to flow frequently through the catheter so that the catheter tip does not become plugged with a blood clot. Periodic flushing with heparinized saline will help maintain the patency of the catheter. This setup allows easy administration of fluids and medication IV to the patient and collection of blood, if necessary.

There is no absolute value for a normal CVP. The CVP for the normal dog is -1 to $+5$ cm H_2O. Elevations of $+5$ to $+10$ are borderline; however, values above 10 cm H_2O may indicate an abnormally expanded blood volume, and those above 15 cm H_2O may indicate congestive heart failure. It is the trend of the CVP that should be monitored and correlated with the regimen of treat-

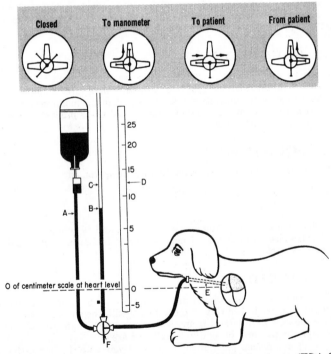

Figure 4–29. Central venous manometer. A, Standard intravenous (IV) infusion tube. B, Central venous pressure level. C, Thirty-inch IV extension tube. D, Centimeter scale. E, Plastic tube in great veins in thorax or right atrium via jugular vein. F, Three-way stopcock set in measuring position (open from manometer to catheter). *Note*: This procedure should be performed with the dog in right lateral recumbency. (From Sattler FP: Shock. *In* Kirk RW, ed: Current Veterinary Therapy III. Philadelphia, WB Saunders, 1968.)

ment. One must be constantly aware of the interrelationship between blood volume, cardiovascular function, and vascular tone. If the CVP is at levels of 10 to 15 cm H_2O, the pulmonary venous pressure is approaching 20 to 22 mm Hg and additional IV fluids should not be administered.

REFERENCES

Haskins SC: Monitoring the critically ill patient. Vet Clin North Am Small Anim Pract 19:1059–1078, 1989.

Wingfield WE: Veterinary Emergency Medicine Secrets. Philadelphia, Hanley & Belfus, 1997.

ENDOSCOPY PROCEDURES

Laryngoscopy and Tracheobronchoscopy

Laryngoscopy and tracheobronchoscopy may be of value in the diagnosis of upper airway obstructions such as eversion of the lateral ventricles, collapsed arytenoid cartilages, hyperplasia of the vocal cords, presence of nodules on the vocal cords, overly long soft palate, and traumatic injuries to the neck. Lesions of the trachea and main stem bronchi, such as collapsed trachea, mediastinal tumors, hilar lymph node enlargement, parasitic nodules *(Filaroides osleri)*, and foreign body aspiration, may also be diagnosed. In addition, tracheobronchoscopy is a valuable technique that permits culturing and cytologic examination of material from bronchi involved in chronic respiratory disease. Upper airway obstruction that is not responsive to conservative therapy is an indication for more extensive diagnostic procedures, such as bronchoscopy.

REFERENCES

4

Amis TC, McKiernan BC: Systematic identification of endobronchial anatomy during bronchoscopy in the dog. Am J Vet Res 47:2649–2657, 1986.

Hawkins E: Bronchoalveolar lavage in the cat. *In* Proceedings of the American College of Veterinary Internal Medicine, 1988, pp 94–96.

Roudebush P: Laryngoscopy. Vet Clin North Am Small Anim Pract 20:1291–1296, 1990.

Roudebush P: Tracheobronchoscopy. Vet Clin North Am Small Anim Pract 20:1297–1314, 1990.

Venker-Van Haagen AJ, Vroom WM, Heijn A, et al: Bronchoscopy in small animal clinics: An analysis of the results of 228 bronchoscopies. J Am Anim Hosp Assoc 21:521–526, 1985.

Gastrointestinal Endoscopy

Flexible fiberoptic endoscopy is a noninvasive, atraumatic means of visualizing the mucosal surfaces of the esophagus, stomach, and colon. Flexible endoscopes are available from several companies at a wide range of prices. The state-of-the-art endoscopy today is video endoscopy.

To minimize the risk of injury to the animal and to reduce the possibility of damage to the endoscope, place animals undergoing endoscopic examination under general anesthesia after routine preanesthetic preparation. A fast of 12 to 24 hours is recommended for most patients undergoing upper gastrointestinal (GI) endoscopy. However, for patients with indications of delayed gastric emptying, a longer fast (24 to 48 hours) may be needed to empty the stomach completely. In preparation for colonoscopy, a 24- to 48-hour fast is recommended. A high warm-water enema is given the evening before and again 2 to 4 hours before the procedure. Such enemas should be given until the return is clear.

.... ESOPHAGOSCOPY

The clinical signs indicating esophageal disease and a potential benefit of esophagoscopy include repeated regurgitation, excessive drooling, ballooning of the esophagus, anorexia or dysphagia, and recurrent pneumonia. Esophagoscopy allows visualization of the mucosal lining of the esophagus and makes it possible to detect inflammation, ulcerations, dilations, diverticula, strictures, foreign bodies, tumors, and parasite infestations.

.... GASTROSCOPY

Endoscopic examination of the mucosal aspect of the stomach is indicated when the clinical signs or physical findings suggest the presence of gastric disease or when there is a need for confirmation or clarification of radiographic findings. In most cases, persistent vomiting is the chief complaint. Other clinical signs suggestive of serious gastric disease include hematemesis, melena, weight loss, anemia, and abdominal pain. Gastroscopy allows visualization of the mucosal lining of the stomach and enables detection of inflammation, ulceration, foreign bodies, and tumors. In most dogs and cats the endoscope can be passed into the proximal duodenum (first 6 in.).

.... COLONOSCOPY

The primary indication for colonoscopy is the presence of signs of large bowel disease, which typically include tenesmus and the passage of small, frequent stools containing fresh blood or excess mucus (see p. 402). Endoscopic examination of the colon allows direct visualization of the effects of mucosal inflammation, ulceration, mucosal polyps, malignant neoplasia, and strictures. Histologic examination of mucosal biopsy material will confirm the diagnosis of colonic disease.

REFERENCES

Brearley M, Cooper J, Sullivan M: A Color Atlas of Small Animal Endoscopy. St Louis, Mosby–Year Book, 1991.

Guilford WG, Center SA, Strombeck DR, et al: Stombeck's Small Animal Gastroenterology, ed 3. Philadelphia, WB Saunders, 1996.

Jones BD: Canine and Feline Gastroenterology. Philadelphia, WB Saunders, 1986.

Jones BD: Endoscopy of the lower gastrointestinal tract. Vet Clin North Am Small Anim Pract 20:1229–1242, 1990.

■ ENDOSCOPIC DIAGNOSTIC FINDINGS

Esophagus

Esophagitis
Reflux esophagitis
Esophageal stricture
Foreign body
Diverticula
Vascular ring anomaly
Hiatal hernia
Neoplasia

Stomach

Gastritis
Antral pyloric mucosal hypertrophy or erosion
Ulcer
Foreign body
Parasites *(Physaloptera, Ollulanus, Ascaris)*
Phycomycosis
Hiatal hernia
Polyp
Neoplasia

Duodenum

Inflammatory bowel disease
Lymphangiectasia
Ulcer
Foreign body
Giardiasis
Parasites
Bacterial overgrowth
Neoplasia

Colon

Colitis
Regional granulomatous colitis
Parasites (*Trichuria*, protozoa)
Strictures
Intussusception
Cecal inversion
Histoplasmosis
Polyp
Neoplasia
Foreign body

From Twedt DC. Perspectives on gastrointestinal endoscopy. Vet Clin North Am Small Anim Pract 23:481, 1993.

Jones B: Incorporating endoscopy in veterinary practice. Compend Contin Educ Pract Vet 20:307–313, 1998.

Tams TR: Handbook of Small Animal Gastroenterology. Philadelphia, WB Saunders, 1996.

Tams TR: Small Animal Endoscopy. St Louis, Mosby–Year Book, 1990.

Twedt DC: Perspectives on gastrointestinal endoscopy. Vet Clin North Am Small Anim Pract 23:481, 1993.

Proctoscopy

Protoscopy, the technique of examining the descending colon, rectum, and anus, is a valuable procedure. The technique is helpful in the definitive diagnosis of lower bowel lesions, such as granulomatous colitis, foreign bodies, tumors, lacerations, and other mucosal abnormalities.

.... TECHNIQUE

For the colonic mucosa to be visualized, the large bowel must be empty. This can be accomplished by withholding food for 24 hours and performing a colonic irrigation the evening before and again 2 hours before the examination. The material used for the enema must be nonirritating and nonoily. Mildly hypertonic saline solutions such as Fleet enemas work well if given 2 hours before examination so that gas and fluid can be passed completely. However, Fleet enemas should not be used in cats or small dogs.

If the general physical condition of the animal is poor and withholding food is not possible, feeding a low residue diet for 12 to 18 hours preceding proctoscopy can be helpful. This diet could consist of cooked eggs, small amounts of cooked beef or chicken, and small amounts of carbohydrate, such as a slice of toast or one-fourth to one-half cup of moist kibble. Maintain good hydration. If all food is contraindicated, oral electrolyte solutions such as Gatorade or Resorb (Bristol) can be used to maintain hydration without moving solids through the intestinal tract.

Give the animal a short-acting anesthetic and place it on a tilted table in lateral recumbency with the hindquarters elevated. Perform a digital examination of the rectum and pelvic cavity to ensure that there are no strictures, polyps, or other obstructions. Lubricate the proctoscope thoroughly with water-soluble jelly, and pass it gently through the anal sphincter. Press it forward slowly and carefully with a spiral motion. If any resistance is encountered, stop the motion, remove the obturator, and inspect the bowel to determine the cause of the resistance. If possible, replace the obturator and continue forward motion until the instrument is passed its full length. Withdraw the obturator, and observe the mucosa.

The major portion of the examination is conducted as the instrument is withdrawn. To view the colonic and rectal walls completely, it is necessary to move the anterior end of the proctoscope around the circumference of a small circle as the proctoscope is withdrawn. Occasional insufflation with the inflating bulb is helpful in smoothing out folds of tissue. Repeated instrumentation may produce petechiae and minor hemorrhages that are not pathologic.

For examination of the terminal rectum and anus, the Hirshman anoscope provides adequate, convenient visualization.

Newer techniques for visualizing the upper and lower GI tract are being used in dogs. The flexible fiberoptic endoscope enables one to visualize and photograph the esophagus, colon, and stomach. One is able not only to visualize lesions of the GI tract directly but also to assess motility and biopsy lesions and to remove foreign bodies.

REFERENCE

Guilford WG, Center SA, Strombeck DR, et al: Strombeck's Small Animal Gastroenterology, ed 3. Philadelphia, WB Saunders, 1996.

Laparoscopy

Laparoscopy is a procedure for visual examination of the peritoneal cavity and its contents after the establishment of pneumoperitoneum. The Needlescope* is a small fiberoptic laparoscope, 1.7 or 2.2 mm in diameter. It requires a bright light source but, because of its small size, can be readily inserted into the abdomen.

Abdominal insufflation and laparoscopy require either general anesthesia, neuroleptanalgesia with local anesthesia, or rarely (in the critically ill animal), regional local anesthesia alone. The depth and type of anesthesia or analgesia depend on the condition of the patient and the skill and experience of the examiner.

Prior to laparoscopy, a cleansing enema should be performed. The laparoscopy site is surgically prepared.

To insufflate the abdomen, use a Verees pneumoperitoneum needle. The needle is placed 3 to 4 cm below the umbilicus, along the linea alba. Saline 10 mL is injected through the needle, and aspiration is attempted to ensure that a blood vessel or hollow viscus has not been penetrated. The intra-abdominal pressure created should not be greater than 20 mm Hg. Any ascitic fluid that is present must be removed and examined (see p. 768).

Air is injected into the peritoneal cavity through an in-line filter with the Verees needle. Insufflation should be slow, and vital signs should be monitored. Following effective insufflation, the needle is removed, a small skin incision is made over the needle entry point, and the larger trocar and cannula are inserted at a 30-degree angle to the animal's longitudinal plane. Extreme care should be taken when placing the trocar into the abdomen. The endoscope (Needlescope) is moved cephalad along the abdominal wall while good insufflation is maintained. Rotate the animal into different positions to enable visualization of various internal organs. Biopsy specimens can be obtained through the Needlescope or through a separate incision while observing through the Needlescope. When endoscopic inspection has been completed, the Needlescope is removed, the insufflated air is allowed to escape, and skin sutures are placed.

Indications for laparoscopy include biopsy, visual diagnosis, follow-up examinations, and research needs.

Contraindications to laparoscopy include peritonitis, hernias, coagulation defects, obesity, abdominal adhesions, and inexperience of the clinician.

REFERENCES

Guilford WG, Center SA, Strombeck DR, et al: Strombeck's Small Animal Gastroenterology, ed 3. Philadelphia, WB Saunders, 1996.
Jones BD: Laparoscopy. Vet Clin North Am Small Anim Pract 20:1243–1263, 1990.

---

*Dyonics, Inc., Andover, MA.

....

SPECIAL TECHNIQUES OF RADIOGRAPHIC EXAMINATION

Gastrointestinal Studies

Contrast agents available for GI studies include barium suspension preparations or Micropaque*; and water-soluble agents (Gastrografin,† which is 60% meglumine and 10% sodium diatrizoate). Water-soluble agents are used if bowel perforation is suspected. Undiluted water-soluble agents are very hypertonic and should be diluted at a ratio of one part Gastrografin to two parts water.

............PROCEDURES

No single procedure is appropriate for all GI cases. The clinician needs to select procedures based on the location of the lesion based on clinical examination and endoscopy.

............Barium Swallow

Barium swallows and esophagograms necessitate that the animal be fasted for 12 hours prior to radiography. Remove all leashes from around the animal's neck, and obtain survey radiographs of the thorax. In esophageal contrast studies, barium suspension contrast medium 2 to 5 mL/kg body weight should be administered. Barium is contraindicated if a perforation of the esophagus is suspected. When the esophagus has been coated with radiopaque material, lateral, ventrodorsal (VD), and right VD oblique thoracic radiographs should be taken to visualize the esophagus. Animals with megaesophagus should *never* be placed back in their cage with an esophagus full of barium because the risk of aspiration is significant.

For barium swallows, the barium should be thick and pasty (like marshmallow fluff). Position the patient and cassette, and have the radiographic technique set up. Give a tablespoonful of barium orally. Make the exposure when the animal takes its second swallow after the barium has been given.

For esophageal studies and barium swallows, sedation with acepromazine 0.1 mg/kg and buprenorphine 0.015 mg/kg will produce no adverse alteration in GI motility. For cats, ketamine 10 mg and midazolam 0.2 mg/kg (combined) can be administered IM.

To achieve the maximum information from a GI study, the following preliminary steps are necessary:

1. Ensure that the hair of the animal is free from dirt, paint, and foreign material. Bathe the animal if necessary.
2. Withhold food for 18 to 24 hours.
3. If the colon is filled with feces, administer a bisacodyl suppository (Dulcolax‡, 5 mg) 30 minutes prior to the radiographic procedure or administer a Fleet enema, which leaves no abnormal residual gas patterns in the bowel. In dogs, a Fleet enema should be given 3 hours prior to the start of the GI

....

*Picker Corp., Cleveland, OH.
†E.R. Squibb & Sons, Princeton, NJ.
‡Boehringer Ltd., Burlington, Ont., Canada.

series. Fleet enemas should not be given to cats; they should receive only a mild soap and warm-water enema (see p. 584).

At the start of an upper GI series, obtain survey radiographs of the abdomen and establish a technique. A barium sulfate (micropulverized) preparation can be administered by stomach tube, or the animal can be induced to swallow the fluids. Flavored prepared barium suspensions are available. Dosage levels vary, but for barium suspensions approximately 10 mL/kg is usually given. When using organic iodide liquid preparations, administer 0.5 mL/kg by stomach tube. Obtain lateral and dorsoventral (DV) radiographs of the abdomen immediately following administration of the barium and at 30-minute, 1-hour, and 2-hour intervals. Water-soluble contrast material passes through the GI tract in approximately 30 to 90 minutes. Barium suspensions take 60 to 180 minutes to traverse the intestine. The colon is usually filled with barium 6 hours after oral administration, and may contain barium for 2 to 3 days following administration.

Contrast studies of the upper GI tract are frequently used in cases of nonresponsive vomiting, refractory diarrhea, hematemesis, suspected enteric foreign bodies, suspected neoplasms and obstructions, and for confirmation of displaced intestinal organs, as may be seen in diaphragmatic hernias.

Barium contrast radiography is contraindicated if perforation of the stomach or upper GI tract is suspected. In these cases, water-soluble contrast media such as the oral diatrizoates are used, because leakage into the abdomen will produce no foreign body granuloma. In addition, barium sulfate should not be administered when an obstruction of the lower bowel may be present. In these cases, barium may only contribute to the obstipation.

If chemical restraint is needed for GI studies, the following tranquilizers can be used: acetylpromazine maleate (Acepromazine*), triflupromazine hydrochloride (Vetame†), and ketamine hydrochloride (Vetalar,‡ for cats only).

The following radiographic views are recommended following administration of radiographic contrast material:

1. Survey radiographs of abdomen
   a. Views: VD and right lateral recumbency.
   b. Objectives: Evaluate for preparation of the patient, interpretation of disease, and reference point for contrast study.
2. Immediately following administration of contrast material—5 minutes
   a. Views: VD, right lateral recumbency, and left lateral recumbency. The right lateral view shows the pylorus of the stomach filled with barium, and the left lateral view shows the cardia and fundic portion filled with barium.
   b. Objective: Evaluate the distended stomach and initial gastric emptying.
3. Twenty to 30 minutes following administration of contrast material
   a. Views: VD and right lateral recumbency.
   b. Objective: Evaluate the stomach, pyloric function, and duodenum.
4. Sixty minutes following administration of contrast material
   a. Views: VD and right lateral recumbency.
   b. Objective: Evaluate the small intestine.
5. Two hours following administration of contrast material
   a. Views: VD and right lateral recumbency.
   b. Objective: Evaluate the passage of contrast material into the colon and complete emptying of the stomach; contrast material should be in the terminal portion of the small intestine.

*Ayerst Laboratories, New York, NY.
†E.R. Squibb & Sons, Princeton, NJ.
‡Parke-Davis, Detroit, MI.

The passage of contrast material through the normal GI tract is variable; however, the following guidelines have been suggested:

1. Contrast material is in the duodenum within 15 minutes in most patients. Excitement can delay this time to 20 to 25 minutes.
2. Contrast material reaches the jejunum within 30 minutes and is within the jejunum and ileum at 60 minutes.
3. Contrast material reaches the ileocecal junction in approximately 90 to 120 minutes.
4. At 3 to 5 hours after administration, contrast material has cleared the upper GI tract and is within the ileum and the large intestine.

Diatrizoate compounds are hypertonic and irritating to the bowel wall.

In evaluation of GI contrast studies, the following criteria may be considered: (1) the size of the intestinal mass, (2) the contour of the mucosal surface, (3) thickness of the bowel wall, (4) flexibility and motility of the bowel wall, (5) position of the small intestine, (6) continuity of the opaque column, and (7) transit time.

The upper GI tract is further examined with the technique of gastrography and upper GI contrast radiography.

In gastrography, the stomach is distended with either negative contrast material (air) or positive contrast material and is visualized radiographically. The animal should be fasted for 12 to 24 hours, and a technique of abdominal radiography should be established. To perform negative contrast gastrography, administer air at 5 to 10 mL/kg body weight via a stomach tube or 30 to 90 mL of a highly carbonated beverage by stomach tube.

In double contrast gastrography, the stomach is coated with barium sulfate suspension and then negative contrast material (air) is liberated into the stomach. Radiographs are taken in the VD, dorsovental (DV), and right and left lateral positions.

..........Barium Enema

Suspected clinical conditions for which barium enemas are indicated in the dog include ileocolic intussusception and cecal inversion, mechanical and functional large bowel obstruction, invasive lesions of the large bowel, a mass outside the large bowel compressing the bowel, and inflammation of the lower intestinal tract. Barium sulfate enemas are contraindicated in suspected obstruction of the colon and rupture or perforation of the colon.

The following procedures should be followed when giving barium enemas:

1. For the 24 hours preceding radiographs, maintain the animal on a liquid diet only, preferably water or broth.
2. During the 18 to 24 hours before the radiographs, administer a mild high colonic enema or give a saline laxative PO.
3. Do not give any irritating enemas within 12 hours of the scheduled radiographic examination; however, isotonic saline solution or plain water enemas should be administered prior to the examination to ensure that the bowel is clear.
4. Obtain survey radiographs of the abdomen, and examine the colon to ensure that this portion of the bowel is clear.
5. Do not force barium into the colon under pressure. Do not elevate the enema bag more than 18 in. above the animal.
6. Do not perform a proctoscopic examination on the same day that the barium enema is given.

Cuffed rectal catheters (Bardex Cuffed Rectal Catheters, 24F to 38F, and the Bardex Cuffed Pediatric Rectal Catheter, 18F*) can be used in dogs. For very small dogs and cats, smaller catheters are used. A plastic catheter adapter and a three-way stopcock are needed.

Various barium sulfate preparations can be used; however, the final concentration should be 15% to 20% w/v. A commercially available barium enema kit is helpful.†

To perform a barium enema effectively, sedate or anesthetize the animal. Place the cuffed rectal catheter so that the inflated bulb is cranial to the anal sphincter. Place the animal in right lateral recumbency and fill the colon with contrast material at a dose of 20 to 30 mL/kg body weight. Take the radiographs after infusion of a two-thirds dose of barium. If the colon is not filled, infuse more contrast agent. Obtain radiographs in the VD and lateral positions, and determine whether the colon is adequately distended. Remove as much of the contrast material as possible from the colon, and repeat the radiographs. Then insert air at 2 mL/kg into the colon, and repeat the radiographs. Deflate the cuff on the catheter, and remove the catheter from the rectum. Throughout the procedure of filling the colon with contrast material or air, care should be taken not to overdistend the colon, which may lead to rupture.

In carrying out a barium enema, look for the following radiographic lesions: (1) irregularity of the barium-mucosal interface; (2) spasm, stricture, or occlusion of the bowel lumen; (3) filling defects; (4) outpouching of the bowel wall due to diverticulum or perforation; and (5) displacement of the bowel.

REFERENCES

Burk RL, Ackerman N: Small Animal Radiology and Ultrasonography: A Diagnostic Atlas and Text, ed 2. Philadelphia, WB Saunders, 1996.

Dennis R: Barium meal techniques in dogs and cats. Practice 14:237–249, 1992.

Morgan JP: Techniques in Veterinary Radiography, ed 5. Ames, Iowa State University Press, 1993.

Thrall DE: Textbook of Veterinary Diagnostic Radiology, ed 3. Philadelphia, WB Saunders, 1997.

Excretory Urography

IV administration of organic iodinated compounds in high concentrations permits visualization in four phases: (1) the arteriogram, (2) the nephrogram, (3) the pyelogram, and (4) the cystogram. The arterial phase demonstrates renal blood flow; the nephrogram demonstrates the accumulation of contrast agent in the renal tubules and is used to evaluate renal parenchyma; the pyelogram phase evaluates the urinary collecting system, including the ureters; and the cystogram reveals the collection of contrast agent in the urinary bladder. Excretory urography does not result in any quantitative information about renal function and is not a substitute for renal function tests. The degree of visualization of contrast material within the renal excretory system depends on the concentration of iodine in the contrast medium, the technique of excretory urography performed, the state of hydration of the patient, renal blood flow, and the functional capacity of the kidneys.

*Bard Hospital Division, C.R. Bard, Inc., Murray Hill, NJ.
†Available from E-Z-EM Corporation, Inc., Westbury, NY.

............TECHNIQUE

The following steps should be used in carrying out excretory urography:

1. Fast the animal for 12 to 18 hours.
2. Administer a high colonic enema or give a saline laxative PO 12 to 18 hours prior to radiography.
3. Ensure that the animal's hair is free of dirt and debris.
4. Try to limit the animal's fluid intake in the 12 hours preceding radiography.
5. Empty the animal's bladder immediately before taking radiographs.
6. Take survey radiographs before administering contrast media.

............Low-Volume, Rapid Infusion Without Compression

The contrast medium most commonly used is a diatrizoate or iothalamate compound. Administer rapidly 850 mg/kg of an iodine compound IV. Obtain a VD radiograph at 10 seconds post injection, and repeat VD and lateral radiographs 1, 3, 5, 15, 20, and 40 minutes following injection. This method is the current standard technique. If the patient's blood urea nitrogen (BUN) level is greater than or equal to 50 mg/dL or the creatinine level is above 4 mg/dL, the dose rate should be doubled.

Lesions that can be detected by using IV urography are renal mass lesions—neoplasia; renal cysts; renal and ureteral traumatic lesions; pyelonephritis; hydroureter; hydronephrosis; renal agenesis; hypoplasia; pelvic and ureteral obstructions (calculi, blood clots); renal parasites; ectopic ureter; and duplication of the collecting system.

............Retrograde Contrast Urethrography

Retrograde urethrography is a diagnostic tool that can be used to localize diseases of the lower urinary tract of dogs and cats. Conditions such as urethral neoplasms, strictures, trauma, calculi, or other anomalies can be revealed by this method.

The technique involves the injection of an aqueous iodine contrast medium into the urethra through a ureteral or balloon-tipped catheter. The radiopaque contrast material is mixed to a three- to fivefold dilution with sterile lubricating jelly to increase the viscosity of the medium. A dilution of 1:3 contrast medium with sterile distilled water or saline can also be used. Before retrograde contrast urethography is performed, a cleansing enema should be given. Sedation or anesthesia may be necessary. Five to 10 mL of contrast medium should be injected. Near the end of the injection, while the urethra is still under pressure, a lateral radiograph is obtained.

If the urinary bladder is to be distended with contrast material or air, remove urine from the bladder. In the male dog, position the catheter so that the tip of the catheter is distal to the os penis. Inject lidocaine 1 to 2 mL into the urethral lumen to anesthetize the urethra adjacent to the balloon-tipped catheter. Extreme care should be taken in the amount of fluid placed in the bladder if the urethra is occluded by a balloon catheter. Overdistention of the bladder results in hematuria, pyuria, urinary bladder rupture, and mild to severe bladder inflammation. Palpate the bladder carefully during distention, and note the backpressure on the syringe used in filling the bladder.

Retrograde contrast urethrography is a definite aid in defining the extent of urethral damage (stricture) or in demonstrating urethral calculi in male cats. In male cats, a 4F balloon catheter or a 3.5F Tom Cat open-ended urethral catheter* should be used. The catheter should be inserted 1.5 cm into the penile urethra. If the urethra is patent, 2 to 3 mL of contrast material will enable visualization of the urethra, but increased amounts of contrast material (2 to 3 mL/lb) injected into the bladder are needed for maximum distention of the preprostatic urethra. A voiding positive contrast urethrogram is necessary to visualize the distal (penile) urethra. Apply external pressure to the bladder (using a wooden spoon or other external compression device), and radiograph the distal urethra.

·········· CYSTOGRAPHY—RADIOGRAPHIC VISUALIZATION OF THE BLADDER

There are three procedures that can be used to visualize the urinary bladder: positive contrast cystography, negative contrast (pneumo-) cystography, and double contrast cystography.

■ INDICATIONS FOR CYSTOGRAPHY

Persistent hematuria (pneumocystography is contraindicated)
Strangury
Pyuria
Crystalluria
Proteinuria
Dysuria
Persistent or recurrent UTI

Pneumocystography

The following steps should be followed in pneumocystographic examination:

1. Fast the animal for 18 to 24 hours preceding radiography.
2. Administer a high colonic enema, or give saline laxative PO 12 to 18 hours prior to taking radiographs. Administer a mild, warm-water enema 2 to 3 hours before the radiographs are to be taken.
3. Ensure that the animal's hair is clean.
4. Take survey radiographs of the bladder, and then empty the bladder of urine. The entire urinary tract—kidneys through urethra—should be included in the radiographs. Avoid the use of metal female catheters because they may cause traumatic injury to the bladder wall.
5. Using a syringe and a three-way valve, inject 4 to 10 mL/kg of carbon dioxide or nitrous oxide. Air can be used but an increased risk of air emboli is incurred. Palpate the bladder while filling it with air to avoid overdistention or rupture. Inject air until there is pressure on the syringe barrel or leakage of air around the catheter. Any air that escapes during the procedure should be replaced.
6. Take lateral and VD views of the abdomen.

Pneumocystography is not an innocuous procedure; fatal venous air emboli have occurred in dogs and cats. This complication is seen most commonly in cases of severe hematuria. Positive contrast cystography is preferred over pneumocystography in such cases if a soluble gas is not available. Inject air slowly. If possible, use a gas that is readily soluble in blood (such as carbon

··

*Monoject, Sherwood Medical Co., St. Louis, MO.

dioxide or nitrous oxide) for bladder insufflation. Place the animal in left lateral recumbency.

Positive Contrast Cystography

This technique involves injection of radiographic contrast material into the bladder and may be used for the following indications:

············CLINICAL

1. Frequent urination
2. Intermittent or chronic hematuria or small volumes of voided urine
3. Hematuria that is seen throughout or in the later stages of voiding
4. Dysuria
5. Persistent posttraumatic hematuria

············RADIOGRAPHIC

1. Areas of increased or decreased density associated with the urinary bladder
2. Nonvisualization of the urinary bladder after trauma
3. Evaluation of abnormal caudal abdominal masses and structures adjacent to the urinary bladder
4. Evaluation of abnormal bladder shape or location

The same principles of preparation apply as in performing a pneumocystogram. Use a urethral catheter with a three-way valve or a small Foley catheter with an inflatable cuff. Organic iodides are the contrast material of choice and should be used in 5% to 10% concentrations.

Double contrast cystography can also be performed. Catheterize the urinary bladder, and remove all urine. Inject a small volume (2 to 5 mL) of an aqueous organic iodine contrast medium into the bladder. Roll the animal over in an attempt to coat the bladder with contrast material. Then distend the bladder with air in the same manner as for pneumocystography.

Some of the routine lesions diagnosed with the aid of cystography are calculi (Table 4–8); neoplasia; cystitis, if proliferative changes are present; muscle hypertrophy; diverticula; duplications; adhesions, especially uterine stump; persistent urachus; ruptures; and atonic bladder.

Table 4–8. Radiopacity of Cystic Calculi on Plain Abdominal Radiographs

Calculus Composition	Density
Calcium oxalate	Radiopaque
Calcium carbonate	Radiopaque
Triple phosphate	Radiopaque—small calculi may be nonradiopaque
Cystine	Variable density—may have radiopaque stippling
Uric acid and urates	Nonradiopaque
Xanthine	Nonradiopaque
Matrix concretions	Nonradiopaque

From Park RD: Radiology of the urinary bladder and urethra. In O'Brien TR, ed: Radiographic Diagnosis of Abdominal Disorders in the Dog and Cat. Philadelphia, WB Saunders, 1978.

REFERENCES

Burk RL, Ackerman N: Small Animal Radiology and Ultrasonography: A Diagnostic Atlas and Text, ed 2. Philadelphia, WB Saunders, 1996.

Leveille R, Atiola M: Retrograde vaginocystography: A contrast study for evaluation of bitches with urinary incontinence. Compend Contin Educ Pract Vet 13:934, 1991.

Osborne CA, Finco DR: Canine and Feline Nephrology and Urology. Baltimore, Williams & Wilkins, 1995.

Pugh CR, Rhodes HW, Biery D: Contrast studies of the urogenital system. Vet Clin North Am Small Anim Pract 23:281, 1993.

Thrall DE: Textbook of Veterinary Diagnostic Radiology, ed 3. Philadelphia, WB Saunders, 1997.

Myelography

Myelography is the study of the spinal cord and vertebral canal made possible by the use of contrast media in the subarachnoid space. Ideally, the contrast material should be relatively nontoxic and absorbable, should provide good contrast, and should be evenly distributed throughout the subarachnoid space. Indications for myelography are progressive neurologic disease in which survey radiographs have failed to reveal substantive findings.

The nonionic water-soluble agents are currently preferred for myelography. The agents are iopamidol,* iohexol,† and ioxaglate.‡ These agents are stable in solution and much more convenient than metrizamide. These agents have low toxicity and low epileptogenic activity, are inert to nervous tissue, have no long-term side effects, and are resorbed and excreted rapidly from the CSF. They can be injected into the subarachnoid space at the cerebellomedullary cistern or at the caudal lumbar spine at a dose level of 0.22 mL/kg. Five minutes after cisternal injection, if there is no obstruction, the cervical and thoracic cord segments are outlined, and after 10 to 15 minutes the entire cord is outlined.

Patients undergoing myelography can be pretreated with diazepam at a dose of 0.25 mL/kg, not to exceed 10 mL in larger patients. It has a short biologic half-life of 30 to 45 minutes and may be better used after myelography if seizures do occur.

·········· TECHNIQUE

Myelographic examination involves the following procedures:

1. The animal is fasted for 18 to 24 hours preceding myelography if the procedure is elective.
2. Anesthetize the animal with a short-acting agent, and maintain the animal on the gas anesthetic of choice. Maintain an IV catheter and good hydration through fluid support.
3. Clip and surgically prepare the skin over the cisterna magna or in the lumbosacral area, depending on where one wishes to enter the spinal canal. When fluoroscopic visualization is available, myelograms can be done for all animals from a lumbar subarachnoid tap. Lumbar puncture can be made between L1 and L6 or between L4 and L5. A short-bevel spinal needle should be used (1.5-in. 22-gauge needle for dogs under 20 lb, and a 2.5-in., 22-gauge needle for larger dogs). The average dose for any of the four agents

*E.R. Squibb & Sons, Princeton, NJ.
†Omnipaque, Winthrop Laboratories, New York, NY.
‡Hexabrix, Mallinckrodt, Inc., St. Louis, MO.

is 0.22 mL/kg. More is needed per kilogram for small dogs and less per kilogram for large dogs (for cisterna magna puncture, see p. 517).

4. Inject the contrast medium through a flexible extension tube attached to the needle. The recommended dose of iohexol 300 mg/mL is for cervical myelogram (lumbar tap), 0.45 mL/kg; for cervical tap, 0.30 mL/kg; for thoracolumbar myelogram (lumbar tap), 0.30 mL/kg; for thoracolumbar myelogram (cervical tap), 0.30 mL/kg; and for cervicothoracolumbar myelogram (cervical or lumbar), 0.45 mL/kg.

REFERENCES

Burk RL, Ackerman N: Small Animal Radiology and Ultrasonography: A Diagnostic Atlas and Text, ed 2. Philadelphia, WB Saunders, 1996.

Roberts R, Selcer B: Myelography and epidurography. Vet Clin North Am Small Anim Pract 23:307, 1993.

Sande RD: Radiography, myelography, computed tomography and magnetic resonance imaging of the spine. Vet Clin North Am Small Anim Pract 22:811, 1992.

Thrall DE: Textbook of Veterinary Diagnostic Radiology. ed 3. Philadelphia, WB Saunders, 1997.

Nonselective Angiocardiography (see p. 311)

Cholecystography

Use of this technique depends on the ability of selected radiopaque compounds to be removed from the blood and excreted via active transport by hepatocytes. Contrast agents for cholecystography can be administered either PO or IV. PO cholecystographic examination requires that the contrast agent (1) enter the small bowel, (2) be absorbed and enter the portal circulation, and (3) be excreted into the bile and concentrated in the gallbladder. IV cholecystography eliminates some of the variables within the digestive tract and may be a more reliable technique in dogs and cats.

Following the administration of a selected contrast agent to produce cholecystography, DV and standing lateral projections for radiography are indicated at time intervals appropriate for the contrast material used.

Ultrasound

A very complete discussion of ultrasonography is presented in the text by Nyland and Mattoon. Certain important definitions and concepts are discussed here for the benefit of the student and technician.

Ultrasound is characterized by sound waves with a frequency higher than the upper range of human hearing, approximately 20,000 cps (20 kHz). Sound frequencies in the range of 2 to 10 Mhz are commonly used in performing diagnostic examinations. Selection of a transducer head results in selecting the ultrasound frequency that will enable the clinical investigator to perform examination of certain types of tissues: small dogs (<10 kg) and cats can be examined with a 7.5- or 10-Mhz transducer; medium-sized dogs require frequencies of 5.0 Mhz; large-breed dogs may require a 3.0-Mhz or lower frequency transducer. Multiple transducers are frequently used in the same examination to evaluate different organ tissues in the same animal.

Ultrasound imaging is based on the pulse-echo principle. There are three modes of echo display:

1. A-mode (amplitude mode) is the least frequently used but has been used in ophthalmic evaluations.
2. B-mode (brightness mode) displays the returning echoes as dots whose brightness or gray scale is used to determine tissue density and depth of tissue.
3. M-mode (motion or time-motion mode) is used for echocardiography along with B-mode evaluation of the heart. The echo tracings produced with M-mode are useful for precise cardiac chamber and wall measurements and quantitative evaluation of valve or wall motion with time.

Real time refers to the ability to see motion on the displayed ultrasound image. Real-time B-mode scanners display a moving gray-scale image of cross-sectional anatomy. Ultrasound is a technique that images anatomy in any desired tomographic plane. To interpret the ultrasound image, knowledge of three-dimensional anatomy is very helpful. Normal parenchymal organs and body tissues are visualized as various shades of gray. Blood or fluid that does not contain cells or debris is black on ultrasound.

REFERENCES

Barr F: Percutaneous biopsy of abdominal organs under ultrasound guidance. J Small Anim Pract 36:105–113, 1995.
Barthez P, Nyland T, Feldman E: Ultrasonography of the adrenal glands in the dog, cat, and ferret. Vet Clin North Am Small Anim Pract 28:869, 1998.
Feeney DA, Fletcher TF, Hardy RM: Atlas of Correlative Imaging. Anatomy of the Normal Dog: Ultrasound and Computed Tomography. Philadelphia, WB Saunders, 1991.
Green RW, ed: Small Animal Ultrasound. Philadelphia, Lippincott-Raven, 1996.
Nyland T, Mattoon J: Veterinary Diagnostic Ultrasound. Philadelphia, WB Saunders, 1995.
Nyland T, Mattoon J, Wisner E: Ultrasound-Guided Biopsy. In Nyland T, Mattoon J: Veterinary Diagnostic Ultrasound. W.B. Saunders, Philadelphia, 1995.
Penninck D, ed: Ultrasonography. Vet Clin North Am Small Anim Pract; 28 (No.4):1998.
Penninck D, Finn-Boder, S: Updates in interventional ultrasonography. Vet Clin North Am Small Anim Pract 28:1017, 1998.

4

THERAPEUTIC PROCEDURES AND TECHNIQUES

Administration of Medications

··········ORAL ADMINISTRATION OF CAPSULES AND TABLETS

··········Dogs

Probably the easiest method of administering pills is to hide them in food. Toss several chunks of unbaited cheese, meat, or some favorite food to the dog, and then give one that includes the pill. For anorectic dogs or when pills must be given without food, medications should be given quickly and decisively so that the "pilling" is accomplished before the animal realizes what has happened. With fairly large, placid dogs, hold the tablet between the tips of the second and third fingers of the right hand. Slip the thumb of the left hand through the interdental space, and press up on the hard palate. Use the thumb of the right hand to press down on the space behind the mandibular incisors (Fig.

4–30). Push the pill deep into the pharynx, withdraw the hand quickly, and close the animal's mouth. Often a brusque tap under the chin startles the dog and facilitates its swallowing. When the animal licks its nose, you can be confident that it has swallowed.

Dogs that offer more resistance can be induced to open their mouths by compressing their upper lips against their teeth. As they open their mouth, roll their lips medially so that if they attempt to close their mouth, they will pinch their own lips.

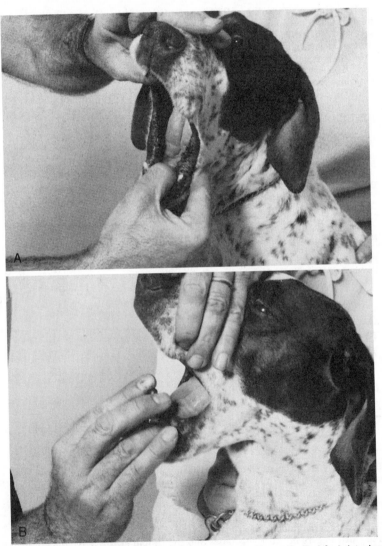

Figure 4–30. A, Placement of thumbs for opening dog's mouth. B, Administering capsule to dog. The capsule should be placed deeply into the pharynx.

Dogs that struggle and slash with their teeth are the most difficult, especially if they are aggressive toward the medicator. They can often be medicated by placing the tablet over the base of the tongue with a 6-in. curved Kelly hemostat or special pill forceps. Cubes of canned food or dried meat can often be "pushed down" a placid but anorectic patient by using the thumb as a lever. The fingers are kept out of the mouth, but the thumb is inserted behind the last molar of the open mouth and pushes the bolus down.

............Cats

Two methods of pilling are useful in cats. In both methods, the cat's head is elevated and tipped back. Use the left hand to hold the head from behind with the index finger at one commissure of the mouth and the thumb at the other. Use the index finger of the right hand to open the mouth by pressing down on the incisor teeth. Hold the mouth open by compressing inward with the fingers at the angle of the jaw. A tablet can be dropped deep in the pharynx and the mouth closed quickly. The cat is tapped under the jaw or on the tip of the nose to facilitate swallowing. Licking of the nose signals success. An alternative method is similar except a "pilling syringe" is used to deliver the oral capsule.

............ORAL ADMINISTRATION OF LIQUIDS
............Without the Stomach Tube

Small amounts of liquid medicine can be given successfully to dogs and cats by pulling the commissure of the lip out to form a pocket. The patient's head should be held level so that the medication will not ooze into the larynx. Spoons are ineffective because they measure fluids inaccurately and materials spill easily. A plastic hypodermic syringe makes a convenient, easy-to-use measuring device. The medicine is deposited in the "cheek pouch" and encouraged to flow between the teeth by tilting the head slightly. Patience and gentleness are needed for success.

............With the Stomach Tube

Stomach tubes can be passed through the nostrils (nasogastric), but the small lumen limits the types of solutions that can be administered. Nasogastric intubation can be done with a variety of tube sizes (Table 4–9). Newer polyurethane types,* when coated with a lidocaine lubricating jelly, are nonirritating and may be left in place with the tip at the level of the caudal esophagus. When placing the nasogastric tube, instill 4 to 5 drops of 0.5% proparacaine HCl in the nostril of the cat or 0.5 to 1.0 mL of 2% lidocaine HCl in the nostril of the dog. Elevate the head, and direct the tube dorsomedially to the alar fold. After the tip has been inserted 1 to 2 cm into the nostril, direct the tube ventrally down the esophagus. If the turbinates block the passage of the tube, reinsert the tube. The position of the tube can be checked by injecting 1 mL of sterile saline. If the animal coughs, reinsert the tube, because the trachea has been intubated. Nasogastric tubes can be left in place by securing them with a butterfly bandage that is taped and sutured to the external nares and using a collar or bucket to prevent the animal from removing the tube. Always flush the tube with sterile saline after having infused fluids or food. Orogastric tubes are simpler and more functional. Little restraint is needed to pass a stomach tube in a placid or depressed dog or cat.

Gavage in puppies and kittens can be effected by passing a soft rubber

*Dobbhoff Enteral Feeding Tube or Entriflex Feeding Tubes, Bioresearch Medical Products, Somerville, NJ.

Table 4–9. Tubes for Nasogastric and Nasoenteral Feeding

Composition	Sizes (F × cm length)	Tip Weight	Name	Manufacturer
Polyvinyl chloride*	5 × 16	No	Infant feeding tube	National Catheter Co.
	5 × 42	No		
	8 × 42	No		
	3.5 × 12	No		
	5 × 16, 5 × 36	No		Argyle, division of Sherwood Medical
	8 × 16, 8 × 42	No		
	10 × 42	No		
Polyurethane	5 × 20, 5 × 36	No	Indwell	
	8 × 42			
	6 × 31	No	Entron	Biosearch Medical Products
	8 × 36, 8 × 43	Yes	Entriflex	
Silicone	5 × 15, 8 × 15	No	Nutrifeed	American Pharmaseal
	6 × 42, 8 × 42	Yes		Ivac Corp.
	6 × 36, 7.3 × 36, 7.3 × 42	Yes	Keofeed	

*Will harden if left in stomach for more than 2 weeks.

From Lewis LD, Morris ML Jr, Hand MS: Small Animal Clinical Nutrition, ed 3. Topeka, KS, Mark Morris Associates, 1987.

urethral catheter as an orogastric tube. A 12F catheter is of an adequate diameter to pass freely, but it is too large to enter the larynx of infant animals up to 14 days of age. Mark the tube with tape or a ballpoint pen at a point equal to the distance from the tip of the nose to the last rib. The tube is merely pushed into the pharynx and down the esophagus to the caudal thoracic level (into the stomach). A syringe can be attached to the flared end, and medication is injected slowly.

Larger puppies and adult dogs tolerate intubation with little fuss, although they may have to be placed on a table and restrained. In some animals, the finger can be used to hold the jaws slightly apart. In most animals, a wooden spacer block or a partially used roll of adhesive tape is inserted behind the canine teeth to keep the mouth open. Pass the tube through a central hole in the tape or block. A 22F urinary catheter, 30 in. long, is an ideal tube. The catheter is attached to a funnel, bulb, or syringe which delivers the medication. In most cases, the tip of the tube should be wetted or lubricated with catheter jelly and then gently pushed into the pharynx.

When the dog swallows, advance the catheter down the esophagus to the level of the eighth or ninth rib. It is advisable to measure this distance on the tube first and mark it with a ballpoint pen or a piece of tape. It is almost impossible to pass the tube into the trachea in a conscious dog with its head held in a normal position. Always palpate the neck, however, to be certain that the tube can be located in the esophagus.

Cats usually offer more resistance to oral intubation than do dogs. The cat can be restrained in a bag or cat stocks or by rolling it in a blanket. The cat can be held in a vertical position by an assistant. The operator then grasps the cat's head, as for pilling, and quickly passes the prelubricated tube 6 to 10 in. down the esophagus. A 12F to 16F soft rubber catheter, 16 in. long, makes a suitable tube, and the plastic adapter on the end for attaching a syringe makes medication easy to administer (Table 4–10).

For most cats, a block of soft wood should be used as speculum to prevent severe damage to or severing of the stomach tube. Drill a vertical hole in each

Table 4–10. Maximum Feeding Volume for Cats and Dogs

	Body Weight (kg)	Volume (mL/kg)
Cats	0.5–1.0	70
	1.0–1.5	50
	1.5–4.0	40
	4.0–6.0	25
Dogs	All	80

Modified from Lewis LD, Morris ML Jr, Hand MS: Small Animal Clinical Nutrition, ed 3. Topeka, KS, Mark Morris Associates, 1987.

end of the block (wooden dowel) so that the upper and lower canine teeth can pass through. A horizontal hole in the center allows the tube to pass through. Force the cat to bite down on the block and close the jaws while intubation proceeds. Appetite stimulants can be used to promote the animal's eating (Table 4–11).

REFERENCES

Abood S, Buffington CA: Improved nasogastric intubation technique for administration of nutritional support to dogs. J Am Vet Med Assoc 199:577, 1991.

Abood S, Dimski D, Buffington T, et al: Enteral nutrition. In DiBartola S, ed: Fluid Therapy in Small Animal Practice. Philadelphia, WB Saunders, 1992.

Armstrong PJ, Hand MS, Frederick GS: Enteral nutrition by tube. Vet Clin North Am Small Anim Pract 20:237, 1990.

Crowe DT: Enteral nutrition for critically ill or injured patients, part 1. Compend Contin Educ Pract Vet 8:603, 1986.

Crowe DT: Enteral nutrition for critically ill or injured patients, part 2. Compend Contin Educ Pract Vet 8(10):719, 1986.

Crowe DT: Enteral nutrition for critically ill or injured patients, part 3. Topeka KS, Mark Morris Associates, 1987.

4

Table 4–11. Appetite-Stimulating Drugs for Cats Only

Drug*	Recommended Dose	How Supplied
Diazepam (Valium)†	1–2 mg PO or 0.5 mg IV	2-mg tablets or 5 mg/mL injectable solution
Oxazepam (Serax)†	0.3–0.4 mg/kg PO	15-mg five-sided tablets
Flurazepam (Dalmane)†	0.1–0.2 mg/kg PO	15-mg capsules
Chlordiazepoxide (Librium)†	1.25–2.5 mg PO	5-mg capsules
Cyanocobalamin (vitamin B_{12} injectable)	1000 µg SC	1000-µg/mL injectable solution
Boldenone undecylenate (Equipoise)	5 mg IM or SC	50-mg/mL injectable solution

*None of these drugs are consistently effective. Only trial-and-error usage will determine whether a particular drug will be effective in any given cat.

†If sedation occurs, reduce the dosage.

Adapted from Norsworthy GD: Providing nutritional support for anorectic cats. Vet Med 86:589, 1991.

Marks S: The principles and practical application of enteral nutrition. Vet Clin North Am Small Anim Pract 28:677, 1998.

...........TOPICAL MEDICATIONS

...........Ocular

There are numerous ways to apply medication to the eyes, including the use of drops, ointments, subconjunctival injections, and subpalpebral lavage. The route and frequency of medication depend on the disease being treated.

If more than 2 drops of aqueous material are administered, the fluid will wash out of the conjunctival sac and be wasted. Most drops should be applied every 2 hours (or less) to maintain effect. Ointments should be applied sparingly, and their effect may last a maximum of 4 to 6 hours.

Drops should be placed on the inner canthus without touching the eye with the dropper. Ointment (0.125-in.-long strip) should be placed on the upper sclera or lower palpebral border so that as the lids close they form a film across the cornea.

...........Otic

Powders and aqueous solutions are generally contraindicated in the external ear canal. Thin films of ointments or propylene glycol solutions may be effective vehicles. A few drops generally suffice, and the ear should be massaged gently after instillation to spread the medication over the lining of the ear canal.

...........Nasal

Isotonic aqueous drops are used and should be applied without touching the dropper to the nose. Oily drops are not advised, because they may damage the nasal mucosa or may be inhaled and produce a lipid pneumonia.

...........Dermatologic

There are several objectives that should be considered when treating dermatologic disorders: (1) eradication of causative agents; (2) alleviation of symptoms, such as reduction of inflammation; (3) cleansing and debridement; (4) protection; (5) restoration of hydration; and (6) reduction of scaling and callus. Many different forms of skin medications are available, but the vehicle in which they are applied is an extremely critical factor. In all cases, topical medications should be applied to a clean skin surface in a very thin film, because only the medication in contact with the skin is effective. In most cases, clipping hair from an affected area enhances the effect of medication.

...........Vehicles

The following is a list of vehicles in which skin medications are made available:

1. *Lotions* are suspensions of powder in water or alcohol. They are used for acute, eczematous lesions. Because they are less easily absorbed than creams and ointments, lotions need to be applied two to six times a day.
2. *Pastes* are mixtures of 20% to 50% powder in ointment. In general, they are thick, heavy, and difficult to use.
3. *Creams* are oil droplets dispersed in a continuous phase of water. Creams permit excellent percutaneous absorption of ingredients.
4. *Ointments* are water droplets dispersed in a continuous phase of oil. They are very good for dry, scaly eruptions.

5. *Propylene glycol* is a stable vehicle and spreads well. It allo̶̶ neous absorption of added agents.
6. *Adherent dressings* are bases that dry quickly and stick to the le̶
7. *Shampoos* are usually detergents designed to cleanse the skin. If s̶ are left in contact with the skin for a time, added medications may specific antibacterial, antifungal, or antiparasitic effects.

..........PARENTERAL ADMINISTRATION
..........Preparing the Skin

Before medications are aspirated from multiple-dose vials, carefully wipe the rubber diaphragm stopper with the same antiseptic used on the skin. This basic rule should be observed with all medication vials, even with modified live virus vaccines.

It would be admirable to prepare the skin surgically before making needle punctures to administer medications. Because such preparation is not practical, we should carefully part the hair and apply a good skin antiseptic such as benzalkonium chloride (Zephiran) in 70% alcohol. Place the needle directly on the prepared area, and thrust the needle through the skin.

Although the use of antiseptics on the vial and skin is not highly effective, the procedure removes gross contamination and projects an image of professionalism.

..........Subcutaneous Injections

The dog and cat have loose alveolar tissue and can easily accommodate large volumes of material in this subcutaneous (SC) space. Infection may be introduced inadvertently or vessels may rupture, causing hematomas. The dorsal neck should not be used for injections because accidents are more difficult to handle in this location and the skin of the dorsal neck is very thick. The dorsal back from the shoulders to the rump makes an ideal site for SC injection. Pick up a fold of skin in this region, prepare it with antiseptic, and pinch. Pinch the area a second time while making the injection. The patient rarely feels the injection. Gentle massage of the area after the injection is completed facilitates spreading and absorption of the medication. Only isotonic, buffered, or nonirritating material should be given SC.

..........Intramuscular Injections

Because the tightly packed muscular tissue cannot expand and accommodate large volumes of injectables without trauma, medications given by this route should be small in volume. These medications are often depot materials that are poorly soluble, and some may be mildly irritating. IM injections should never be given in the neck because of the fibrous sheaths there and the complications that may occur. We also believe that injections in the hamstring muscles may cause severe pain, lameness, and occasionally peroneal paralysis due to local nerve involvement. Unless the animal is extremely thin, give injections into the lumbodorsal muscles on either side of the dorsal processes of the vertebral column.

After proper preparation of the skin, insert the needle through the skin at a slight angle (if the animal is thin) or at the perpendicular (if the animal is obese). When any medication is injected by a route other than the IV one, it is *imperative* to retract the plunger of the syringe before injecting to be certain that a vein was not entered by mistake. This is especially crucial with oil suspension, microcrystalline suspension, or potent dose medications.

...jections

n Techniques and Equipment

rs and gauges depends on (1) species and size, and
(2) length of time that the catheter will be in place;
e delivered, its viscosity, and the rapidity of flow

and related equipment are available:

Catheter* with stylet, available in various sizes (see
Fig. .uge and 14-gauge catheters are used commonly; the
larger sizes are best.
2. Argyle Medicut Intravenous Cannula.†
3. Sovereign Indwelling Catheter,† available in 14-, 18-, and 20-gauge sizes—
i.e., an over-the-needle catheter fitting over 16-, 20-, or 22-gauge, 2-in.
needles. These catheters are a good size for placing in the cephalic vein.
4. The Abbocath T Catheter‡ works well in both dogs and cats.
5. The Vasculon TM Catheter System§ is an effective cephalic vein catheter in
small animals.
6. The Becton Dickenson injection cap is useful for intermittent closure of
catheters, which also allows injections.

..........Preparation of Catheterization Sites

Contamination and infection at the catheterization site are common complications of indwelling catheters and cannulas. Aseptic preparation of the site is,
therefore, of paramount importance. In emergency situations it may be necessary to perform catheterization under less than ideal circumstances and without time for adequate aseptic preparation. When the animal's condition is
stabilized, the catheter should be removed and placed properly elsewhere.

The hair is clipped or shaved over a wide area to facilitate disinfection of
the skin surface. The skin surface is scrubbed with a detergent solution for 1
to 2 minutes. The detergent is then removed with an iodine or alcohol solution,
and the skin is sprayed with an iodine-based solution. If it is necessary to
maintain the aseptic conditions of the procedure, sterile gloves should be worn
and the field should be draped with sterile towels or a fenestrated drape.

When the catheter is placed, it should be fixed in position. The catheter
should not be allowed to move in and out of the skin, as this will predispose to
mechanical vessel trauma and the introduction of bacteria. When the puncture
site is a large flat surface such as the medial femoral area or neck, apply a tag
of tape to the catheter at a point close to the puncture site and then suture the

....

*Bard Hospital Division of C.R. Bard, Inc., Murray Hill, NJ.
†Sherwood Medical Industries, St. Louis, MO.
‡Abbott Laboratories, North Chicago, IL.
§Pioneer Viggo, Inc., Beaverton, OR.

Table 4–12. Guidelines for Catheter Gauge

	Cephalic or Tarsal Vein (Catheter Gauge)	Jugular (Catheter Gauge)
Cat or small dog	20–24	18–22
Medium-sized dog	19–23	18–20
Large dog	17–20	14–18

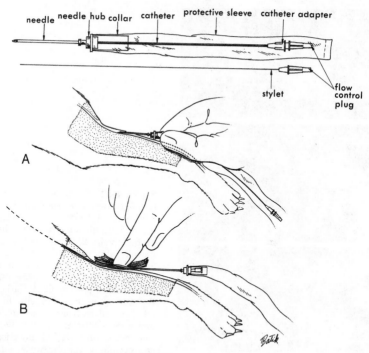

Figure 4–31. A, Percutaneous needle puncture of cephalic vein. The needle should be inserted close to the carpus. The catheter is advanced through the needle into the vein. B, After the catheter is placed in the vein, the needle is withdrawn, pressure is applied over the veinpuncture site, the catheter is taped in place, and the needle guard is placed around the needle.

tape to the skin. When the puncture site is on a circular appendage, the catheter may be taped in place (Fig. 4–32A). Pass the adhesive tape around the entire circumference of the catheter, and then tape the catheter to the appendage. Additional tape may be applied to isolate the injection site from the underlying skin and to secure the catheter cap. An antibiotic-antifungal ointment should be placed at the puncture site and wrapped occlusively if the catheter is to remain in place for more than a few hours.

···········Percutaneous Jugular Vein Catheter Insertion
(see Fig. 4–32)

The immobilization procedure for the jugular vein is particularly important because of the tendency of the vein to roll in the loose subcutaneous tissues of the neck. The vein is occluded by digital pressure in the thoracic inlet so that the skin and underlying tissues are retracted toward the body. The head is extended to provide traction on the upper portion of the vein. All of this positioning is accomplished by a second person.

A catheter-inside-the-needle system is easy to maintain sterile, but the needle leaves a larger hole in the vessel than is filled by the remaining catheter, and early postcatheterization hemorrhage may be a problem. The position of

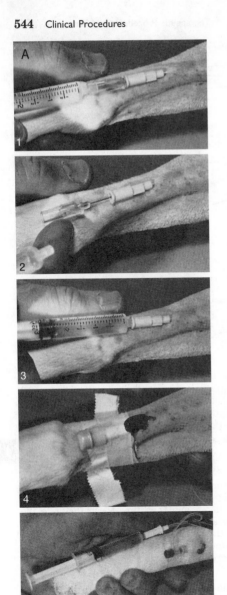

Figure 4–32. Placement and fixation of catheters. A, Cephalic vein placement: 1, Syringe with catheter and needle inserted into the cephalic vein. 2, Needle being removed from inside the catheter. 3, Heparin and saline solution is injected to flush the catheter and check proper placement. 4, Catheter and skin insertion site has been coated with povidone-iodine ointment. Catheter hub has Becton Dickenson Luer Lok injection cap occluding the entrance, and the tape is wrapped around the hub and leg for fixation. Note tape is folded back on tag ends for easy removal. 5, Extension set with "T" is attached to the catheter.

the vessel is located with one hand, and the needle is inserted subcutaneously with the other hand. The needle is placed directly over the jugular vein and below the palpating index finger. The needle is advanced steeply at first to secure the superficial wall of the vessel and then more parallel to the vein to allow insertion of the needle into the lumen without penetrating the deep wall of the vessel. The position of the needle within the vein is ascertained by

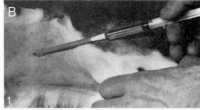

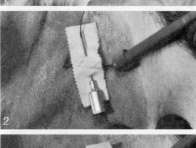

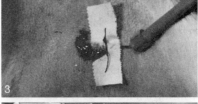

Figure 4–32 *Continued.* B, Jugular vein placement: 1, Syringe with catheter and needle is inserted into the jugular vein. 2, The catheter is slightly withdrawn and secured with two pieces of tape. Needle penetrates the tape and skin so the suture can be used to secure the catheter to the skin (a suture needle could also be used for this technique). 3, Suture is tied and povidone-iodine ointment is applied at the catheter-skin juction. 4, Knit bandage wrap is used to secure and protect the catheter. Note extension set with "T" attached for versatility of injections.

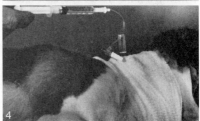

4

feeling the needle "pop" through the vessel wall and seeing the reflux of blood into the catheter. If, after the initial plunge, the needle is not in the vessel lumen, withdraw the needle slowly. It is a common occurrence for the needle to penetrate the deep wall of the vein. Constant traction on the syringe plunger will aspirate blood into the catheter if the needle passes back through the vessel lumen during withdrawal.

When it has been ascertained that the needle is within the lumen, gently thread the catheter into the vein without moving the vein or the needle. The catheter is inserted to its full length. If the catheter cannot be fully advanced, consider that (1) the tip of the needle may not have been entirely within the vessel lumen, (2) the vessel and needle may have moved with respect to one another during the initial threading process, (3) the catheter may be caught at the thoracic flexure (change the position of the head), or (4) the catheter may be caught in one of the tributaries to the front legs (change the position of the front leg). Care should be exercised when withdrawing the catheter through the needle. The catheter can catch on the needle bevel and be cut off, resulting in catheter embolization.

When the catheter has been inserted to the desired length, the needle is removed from the skin and the needle guard is placed. Air is aspirated from the catheter, which is then flushed with heparinized saline. If blood cannot be aspirated from the catheter, consider that (1) the catheter may be kinked or compressed by the needle guard, (2) the catheter tip may be against a vessel wall (withdraw the catheter slightly), (3) the catheter may be clotted (if the clot cannot be aspirated, remove the catheter), or (4) the catheter may not be in the vein.

············Surgical Approach to Jugular Vein Catheterization

Make a skin incision over or next to the jugular vein. The normal jugular vein is very superficial and usually rises with venous occlusion. Location of the jugular vein following repeated unsuccessful attempts at percutaneous catheterization is more difficult because of the resultant hematoma. The vein is always located in the middle of the hematoma, and there is a temptation to skirt the hematoma with the dissection procedure. The vein can be identified during blunt dissection by the appearance of an off-white longitudinal structure against the dark background of the hematoma.

Isolate the vein and suspend it by two sutures. Visually introduce the needle into the lumen of the vein, and take care not to penetrate the deep wall of the vessel. Insert the catheter and relax the proximal suture to allow passage of the catheter. Remove both stay sutures (the vein is not tied), and close the incision in a routine manner.

············Percutaneous Dorsal Metatarsal Artery Catheterization

The tarsus is taped in an extended position, and the skin is prepared with antiseptic solution. The vessel is palpated as it courses across the anteromedial surface of the metatarsus. The artery is palpated with one or two fingers of one hand. A relief incision is made completely through the skin with the beveled edge of an 18-gauge hypodermic needle without entering the artery. A thin-wall catheter-outside-the-needle system is positioned subcutaneously on top of the artery (bevel up). The needle tip and the artery are simultaneously palpated with the finger(s) of the opposite hand, and the catheter is inserted into the artery. Insert the catheter steeply at first so that the tip of the needle just penetrates the superficial wall of the artery, and then advance the catheter flat against the skin surface and parallel with the longitudinal axis of the artery so that the bevel of the needle and the end of the catheter lie entirely within the lumen of the artery without penetrating the deep wall. The presence of the needle tip within the lumen can be verified by the reflux of blood into the hub of the needle. At this point, neither vessel nor needle should be moved while the catheter is gently rotated into the artery to its full length. The needle is then rapidly removed and replaced with a three-way stopcock or an infusion plug, and the catheter is flushed with heparinized saline and taped in place. Catheter flushing is poorly tolerated by awake patients and should be done with care.

············Percutaneous Femoral Artery Catheterization

The leg is taped in a caudally extended position, and the skin is prepared with antiseptic solutions. The vessel is palpated as it courses distally on the medial surface of the leg and anterior to the pectineus muscle. A small relief hole is made in the skin over the palpated artery with an 18-gauge hypodermic needle. A long, 5- to 6-in. catheter-outside-the-needle system is utilized. The catheter is inserted through the relief hole so that the needle tip rests in the subcutaneous tissue between the artery and the palpating index finger. The needle is advanced steeply at first to secure the superficial wall of the vessel, and then more parallel to allow catheter insertion into the lumen without penetration of the deep wall of the vessel. When the needle and catheter tip are within the vessel lumen, as ascertained by feel and by the spontaneous reflux of blood into the syringe, the catheter is inserted. The needle is removed and quickly replaced by a catheter cap. The catheter is flushed with heparinized saline and sutured to the skin via a tag of tape.

Excessive movement between the skin and the vessel puncture sites will cause dislodgement of short catheters; therefore, long catheters must be used. Long catheters are available only in large sizes, 16-gauge or larger; therefore, percutaneous catheterization of small femoral arteries is difficult or impossible. Excessive movement will also cause subcutaneous kinking of indwelling catheters. Hematoma formation following catheter removal may be a problem.

Surgical Cutdown for Femoral Artery Catheterization

Following appropriate aseptic skin preparation, a 4- to 5-cm skin incision is made over the femoral artery. The caudal edge of the sartorius muscle is found by blunt dissection and then reflected anteriorly to expose the underlying femoral artery, vein, and nerve. Taking care to avoid tearing any vessel branches, gently isolate 2 to 3 cm of the femoral artery from the surrounding fascia. The vessel is elevated by two stay sutures that have been passed under the artery, and a long catheter-outside-the-needle system is inserted into the lumen of the artery without penetrating the deep wall. The catheter is gently inserted into the vessel, the needle removed, and the catheter capped and flushed. The incision is closed and the catheter affixed to the skin via a tape tag.

Maintenance of Indwelling Catheters

Indwelling catheters should be redressed and inspected every 1 to 2 days. Discard all soiled bandage material. Clean the puncture site with antiseptic solutions and fresh antibiotic-antifungal ointment, and reapply the occlusive wrap. Inspect the skin puncture site and the vessel at each redressing. There is normally a very small ring of inflammation at the puncture site. Excess inflammation, diffuse tissue swelling, expulsion of exudate from the puncture site upon palpation, and tenderness or pain upon palpation are signs of untoward effects of the indwelling catheter. Phlebitis may be caused by mechanical, chemical, or infectious irritation of the vein. Phlebitis is recognized as warm, erythematous skin overlying a tender, indurated vessel. Purulent thrombophlebitis is heralded by all of the signs of simple phlebitis plus free exudate, which may drain exteriorly with or without palpation or may drain internally and result in a severe septicemia. Thrombotic occlusion of the vessel is recognized by severe hardening ("ropiness") of the vessel. Thrombotic occlusion is associated with inability to infuse fluids by gravity and may result in severe subcutaneous fluid accumulation if the fluids are administered with a pump. Occult infection of the IV site may occur in the absence of local inflammatory, thrombotic, or exudative signs. Unexplained fever and leukocytosis may be the only early signs. The diagnosis may be confirmed by obtaining a culture of material from the catheter tip.

The catheter should be removed if there is evidence of cellulitis, phlebitis, thrombosis, purulent thrombophlebitis, or catheter-associated bacteremia or septicemia; if the catheter ceases to function properly because of thrombosis or catheter occlusion by a clot or kink; after 3 days, if there is another location to which it can be moved; if the patient begins to lick or chew at the bandages; and when it is no longer necessary.

Catheter patency may be maintained by continuous fluid infusion, by intermittent flushing with heparinized saline (1000 units/250 to 500 mL t.i.d. or q.i.d.), by filling the catheter with pure heparin (1000 units/mL once daily), or by filling the catheter with low-molecular-weight dextran once daily.

Infusion fluids and administration tubing must be sterile. Connections should not be disconnected unless it is absolutely necessary and then must be disconnected aseptically. All injection caps should be cleaned well with an antiseptic solution prior to needle insertion. The fluid bottles and all administration tubing should be changed every 1 to 2 days. Tubing should be changed after blood or colloid infusion. The primary catheter or infusion line should not be used for the collection of blood samples except in emergencies. The fluid bottle should be clearly marked if any drug or concentrate has been added to the bottle. In-line filters are not necessary for infection control for routine fluid administration.

............Intradermal Injections

Intracutaneous (or intradermal) injections are used for testing purposes. The skin should be prepared by carefully clipping the hair with a No. 40 clipper blade. If the skin surface is dirty, it can be gently cleaned with a moist towel. Scrubbing and disinfection are contraindicated because they may produce iatrogenic trauma and inflammation, which interfere with the test. Stretch the skin by lifting a fold, and use a 25- to 27-gauge intradermal needle attached to a 1-mL tuberculin syringe. The point of the needle, bevel up, is inserted in a forward lifting motion as if to pick up the skin with the needle tip. The needle is advanced as the syringe is pushed (levered) downward until the bevel is completely within the skin. A bleb of 0.05 to 0.10 mL of fluid is injected. If the procedure is done correctly, the small bleb will appear translucent.

............Intraosseous Injections

Intraosseous infusion of blood, fluids, or medications is useful whenever rapid, direct access to the circulatory system is required and peripheral or central access is impossible or too time-consuming. This technique can be set up rapidly (3 minutes), is certain, and is especially useful for unusually small patients, especially kittens and puppies.

Intraosseous infusion is particularly indicated in shock or circulatory collapse syndromes, edematous states, severe burns, and obesity, and when peripheral veins are thrombosed. This method is contraindicated in birds (whose bones contain air), for infusion into fractured bones, or in cases of sepsis, as osteomyelitis may develop.

Substances injected into the bone marrow reach the general circulation at about the same rate as those injected directly into peripheral veins. Blood and blood components and solutions of colloids, crystalloids, electrolytes, drugs, and nutrients can be given—even in large volumes.

...........Technique

The two easiest and most desirable sites for marrow access are (1) the flat medial side of the proximal tibia but distal to the tibial tuberosity and the proximal growth plate, and (2) the trochanteric fossa of the proximal femur.

1. Prepare the skin site aseptically, and inject 1% lidocaine into the skin and periosteum.
2. Stabilize the leg, and make a small stab incision through the skin. Needles of 18- to 20-gauge are preferred and can be ordinary hypodermic needles (short bevel desired) or special stylet needle sets, such as a spinal needle or

an Illinois bone marrow needle.* A needle with a stylet is preferred so that the needle is not occluded with cortical bone or marrow during introduction.

3. Point the needle slightly distally and rotate with firm pressure until it enters the near cortex. A properly seated needle will feel stable and firm. Use a 10-mL syringe to aspirate marrow, fat, and bony debris. Prefill the needle prior to administering fluids.
4. Attach a regular fluid infusion set, and start fluids. The rate should not exceed 11 mL/min by gravity or 24 mL/min with pressure up to 300 mm Hg. Gravity flow through a single catheter may be adequate for patients up to 16 lb. For larger animals, multiple catheters in separate bones or pressurized flow, or both, may be needed for rapid infusions.
5. Encase the needle hub in a butterfly tape, and suture the tape in place. Place antibiotic ointment around the skin incision, and protect and immobilize the whole apparatus with a bulky bandage wrap.
6. Manage intraosseous catheters in the same way as IV catheters. Flush the catheter every 6 hours with heparinized saline, and place the catheter in a new bone every 72 hours. The same bone can be reused at another location if 25 to 36 hours is allowed for occlusion and healing of the original site.

···········Complications

Infection is the primary concern. Fat embolism and damage to the growth plates are other concerns. Extravasation of fluid from the bone marrow into the subcutaneous tissue may occur if the needle punctures both cortices or if more than one hole is made in the cortex. In such cases, remove the needle and select another bone.

REFERENCES

Crow S, Walshaw S: Manual of Clinical Procedures in the Dog, Cat, and Rabbit, ed 2. Philadelphia, Lippincott-Raven, 1997.
Hansen BD: Technical aspects of fluid therapy. *In* DiBartola S, ed: Fluid Therapy in Small Animal Practice. Philadelphia, WB Saunders, 1993.
Otto CM, Kaufman GM, Crowe DT: Intraosseous infusion of fluids and therapeutics. Compend Contin Educ Pract Vet 11:421–430, 1989.
Wingfield WE: Veterinary Emergency Medicine Secrets. Philadelphia, Hanley & Belfus, 1997.

4

Bandaging and Splinting Techniques

···········GENERAL INDICATIONS

In general, bandages and splints are applied to either open or closed wounds. They serve several functions:

1. Exert pressure to obliterate dead space, reduce edema, and minimize hemorrhage
2. Prevent pressure on wounds
3. Pack a wound
4. Absorb exudate and debride a wound
5. Protect a wound from environmental bacteria
6. Protect the environment from wound blood, exudate, and bacteria
7. Immobilize a wound and support underlying osseous structures

*Allegiance Health Care Corp., McGraw Park, IL.

8. Make the patient comfortable
9. Serve as a vehicle for antiseptics and antibiotics
10. Serve as an indicator of wound secretions
11. Provide an aesthetic appearance

............MATERIALS

There are three component layers of bandage. When pressure relief or immobilization are necessary, splint material is also needed.

1. Contact (primary) layer
2. Intermediate (secondary) layer
3. Outer (tertiary) layer

The materials and methods for bandaging depend on the stage of healing, the need for pressure and immobilization, or the need to prevent pressure. There are six types of wounds for which bandaging is required:

1. Open contaminated and infected wounds
2. Open wound in repair stage of healing
3. Closed wound
4. Wound in need of pressure bandage
5. Wound in need of pressure relief
6. Wound in need of immobilization

............Open Contaminated and Infected Wounds

............Wounds with Loose Necrotic Tissue, Foreign Matter, and Copious Quantities of Exudate

............Materials Needed

1. Contact layer
   a. Wide-mesh gauze sponges with no cotton filling
      i. Dry (wounds with low viscosity exudate)
      ii. Wet (wounds with viscous exudate)
         (a) Physiologic saline balanced electrolyte solution
         (b) Antiseptic solution (i.e., 0.05% chlorhexidine solution—1:40 dilution of chlorhexidine diactate or gluconate in water)
      iii. Dry with topical medication (see Acute Superficial Tissue Injuries, VII. Open Wounds, B. Topical Medications)
   b. Foam sponge—dry, wet, or with topical medication (see Acute Superficial Tissue Injuries, VII. Open Wounds, B. Topical Medications)
   c. Calcium alginate
   d. Acemannan freeze-dried gel
2. Intermediate layer—thick absorbent wrapping material
3. Outer layer—porous adhesive tape

............How to Bandage

1. The contact layer is placed over the wound.
2. The intermediate layer is wrapped over the contact layer.
3. Tape strips are placed over the intermediate layer with overlap of tape strips.

············Complications and Disadvantages

1. Dry wide-mesh gauze sponges
   a. After wound fluid has been absorbed and evaporated and the bandage is dry again, it is painful to remove the adherent contact layer from the wound.
   b. Tissues may desiccate if left in contact with the dry bandage too long.
   c. Any reparative tissue in the wound may be damaged when the bandage is removed.
2. Wet wide-mesh gauze sponges
   a. Bacteria may flourish in the wet environment.
   b. Tissues may become macerated.
   c. If fluid reaches the outer layer, bacteria may move centrally toward the wound.
   d. After fluids have evaporated from the bandage and the bandage becomes dry, it is painful to remove the adherent contact layer from the wound.
   e. Any reparative tissue in the wound may be damaged when the contact layer is removed.
3. Foam sponge
   a. As the wound becomes smaller by contraction and epithelialization with less fluid production, the sponge may adhere to the wound edges.
4. Calcium alginate
   a. With insufficient wound fluid to convert the calcium alginate to a gel, a calcium alginate eschar forms which is difficult to remove.

············Result of Bandaging

1. Dry wide-mesh gauze sponges
   a. When the bandage is removed after it is dry, necrotic tissue and debris that adhere to the contact layer are removed with it.
2. Wet wide-mesh gauze sponges
   a. The wetting agent dilutes viscous exudate and enhances its absorption.
   b. When the bandage is removed after it is dry, necrotic tissue and debris that adhered to the contact layer are removed with it.
3. Foam sponge
   a. Large amounts of exudate are absorbed.
   b. When used to deliver liquid medication, infection may be controlled and wound healing enhanced.
4. Dry wide-mesh gauze sponge or foam sponge with topical medication (see Acute Superficial Tissue Injuries, VII. Open Wounds, B. Topical Medications)
   a. Bacterial control (antibiotic/antibacterial agents)
   b. Healing stimulation (hydrophilic agent and hydrogel wound dressing)
   c. Enzymatic debridement (enzymatic agent)
5. Calcium alginate
   a. Large amounts of exudate are absorbed.
   b. Enhanced granulation tissue formation.
   c. Mechanical hemostasis of capillary hemorrhage.
   d. Bacteria entrapped in the gel are removed when the gel is lavaged from the wound.
6. Acemannan freeze-dried gel
   a. Large amounts of exudate are absorbed.
   b. The gel is delivered to the wound to enhance healing.

············Open Wound in the Repair Stage of Healing
············*Early Stage of Repair*

The *early* stage of repair is characterized by new granulation tissue, some exudate, and no epithelialization. An early nonadherent bandage is required.

············Materials Needed

1. Contact layer
   a. Wide-mesh, petrolatum-impregnated gauze (commercial or prepared by autoclaving gauze sponges with petrolatum)
   b. Wide-mesh gauze sponges lightly coated with nitrofurazone dressing or petrolatum-based antibiotic ointment
   c. Foam sponge
   d. Hydrogel dressing
   e. Hydrocolloid dressing
2. Intermediate layer. Absorbent wrapping material
3. Outer layer. Porous adhesive tape

············How to Bandage

1. The contact layer is placed over the wound.
2. The intermediate layer is wrapped over the contact layer.
3. Tape strips are placed over the intermediate layer with overlap of the tape strips.

············Complications and Disadvantages

1. Wide-mesh, petrolatum-impregnated gauze
   a. Rapidly growing granulation tissue may grow into mesh openings of the petrolatum-impregnated gauzes between bandage changes. Hemorrhaging may occur at the time of bandage removal.
   b. Impregnated gauzes prepared by autoclaving petrolatum and gauzes together may have their interstices occluded if too much petrolatum is used in preparation or as gauzes from the lower part of the gauze stack are used.
   c. Petrolatum gauzes used after epithelialization has started will slow epithelialization.
2. Foam sponge
   a. The absorbent foam dressing may remain adhered to the wound edge when the dressing is changed as the wound gets smaller by contracting and epithelialization and produces less fluid.
3. Hydrogel dressing
   a. May tend to cause exuberant granulation tissue
   b. May cause tissue maceration
4. Hydrocolloid dressing
   a. Hydrocolloid gel is tenacious and hard to remove from skin.
   b. May cause tissue maceration.
   c. Causes reduced wound contraction.

············Result of Bandaging

1. Wide-mesh, petrolatum-impregnated gauze
   a. The wide-mesh openings of the gauze allow the more viscous exudate that may be present in the early reparative wound healing stage to move on into the intermediate layer.
2. Wide-mesh gauze lightly coated with nitrofurazone dressing or petrolatum-based antibiotic ointment
   a. Gauzes coated with nitrofurazone or petrolatum-based antibiotic provide a nonadherent bandage that has some antibacterial properties along with allowance for exudate absorption.

3. Foam sponge
   a. The absorbent foam dressing absorbs considerable exudate and yet maintains a moist wound environment without a gel left in the wound.
   b. Requires less frequent change.
4. Hydrogel dressing.
   a. Enhances epithelialization
   b. Requires less frequent bandage change and allows wound visualization
   c. Relieves pain
5. Hydrocolloid dressing
   a. Enhances epithelialization
   b. Requires less frequent bandage change
   c. Relieves pain

............Late State of Repair

The wound is characterized by granulation tissue, serosanguineous drainage, and epithelialization. A late nonadherent bandage is needed.

............Materials Needed

1. Contact layer
   a. Commercially available nonadherent dressing
   b. Wide-mesh gauze sponges lightly coated with nitrofurazone dressing
   c. Foam sponge
   d. Hydrogel dressing
   e. Hydrocolloid dressing
2. Intermediate layer. Absorbent wrapping material
3. Outer layer. Porous adhesive tape

............How to Bandage

1. The contact layer is placed over the wound.
2. The intermediate layer is wrapped over the contact layer.
3. Tape strips are placed over the intermediate layer with overlap of the tape strips.

4

............Complications and Disadvantages

1. Commercially available nonadherent dressing
   a. Exudate that is still viscous will not be absorbed well.
2. Foam sponge
   a. As the wound becomes smaller by contraction and epithelialization with less fluid production, the sponge may adhere to the wound edges.
3. Hydrogel dressing
   a. May tend to cause exuberant granulation tissue
   b. May cause tissue maceration
4. Hydrocolloid dressing
   a. Hydrocolloid gel is tenacious and hard to remove from skin.
   b. May cause tissue maceration.
   c. Causes reduced wound contraction.

............Result of Bandaging

1. Commercially available nonadherent dressing
   a. Excess serosanguineous fluid is absorbed by the contact layer and transported to the intermediate layer while some fluid is retained by the contact layer to enhance epithelialization.

2. Foam sponge
   a. The absorbent foam sponge maintains a moist environment over the wound without leaving a gel over the wound.
   b. Requires less frequent change.
3. Hydrogel dressing
   a. Enhances epithelialization
   b. Requires less frequent bandage change and allows wound visualization
   c. Relieves pain
4. Hydrocolloid dressing
   a. Enhances epithelialization
   b. Requires less frequent bandage change
   c. Relieves pain

.... Closed Wound
.... Wound With No Drainage

Closed-wound bandages are required.

.... Materials Needed

1. Contact layer. Commercially available nonadherent dressing
2. Intermediate layer. Absorbent wrapping material
3. Outer layer. Porous adhesive tape

.... How to Bandage

1. The contact layer is placed over the wound.
2. The intermediate layer is wrapped over the contact layer.
3. Tape strips are placed over the intermediate layer with overlap of the tape strips.

.... Complications and Disadvantages

1. There should be no major inherent complications with this type of bandage.

.... Result of Bandaging

1. The small amount of material that drains from the wound is absorbed by the nonadherent dressing pad. The pad does not adhere to the wound to cause discomfort.
2. The function of the intermediate layer is more protective than absorptive.

.... Wound With Drainage

There is considerable drainage via a drain tube.

.... Materials Needed

1. Contact layer. Commercially available nonadherent dressing and several layers of absorbent wide-mesh gauze over the distal drain end
2. Intermediate layer. Thick, absorbent wrapping material
3. Outer layer. Porous adhesive tape

.... How to Bandage

1. The contact layer is placed over the suture line, and several layers of absorbent wide-mesh gauze are placed over the distal end of the drain.

2. The intermediate layer is wrapped over the contact layer.
3. Tape strips are placed over the intermediate layer with overlap of the tape strips.

···········Complications and Disadvantages

1. If insufficient padding is placed over the end of the drain on a heavily draining wound, the drainage fluid may reach the outer bandage layer.

···········Result of Bandaging

1. When the bandage is removed, the surgeon can note the amount and nature of the fluid that drains from the wound by observing the gauzes placed over the end of the drain and can determine when the drain should be removed.

···········Wounds in Need of Pressure Bandage
···········*Minor Hemorrhage*
···········Materials Needed

1. Contact layer. Commercially available nonadherent dressing
2. Intermediate layer. Thick, absorbent wrapping material
3. Outer layer. Elastic adhesive tape (Vet Wrap, 3M, St. Paul, Minn.)

···········How to Bandage

1. The contact layer is placed over the wound.
2. The intermediate layer is wrapped over the contact layer.
3. The elastic adhesive tape is *carefully* wrapped over the intermediate layer with overlap of wraps. (The pressure bandage should not be left on for long periods of time.)
4. When applied to a limb, the third and fourth digits should be left exposed just enough that they can be monitored for sensation and circulation several times a day.

4

···········Complications and Disadvantages

1. Pressure bandages that are placed too tightly or left on too long may interfere with nerve function and circulation and result in sloughing of tissue.
2. Wound drainage may be reduced, which encourages infection.

···········Result of Bandaging

1. Hemorrhage is controlled.

···········Edema

There are areas of edema, especially passive edema.

···········Materials Needed

1. Contact layer. In accordance with the type of wound present
2. Intermediate layer. Thick, absorbent wrapping material
3. Outer layer. Elastic adhesive tape

.... How to Bandage

1. The contact layer is placed over the wound.
2. The intermediate layer is wrapped over the contact layer, usually in an amount greater than when used for minor hemorrhage control.
3. The elastic adhesive tape is *carefully* wrapped over the intermediate layer with overlap of wraps.
4. When applied to a limb, the third and fourth digits should be left exposed just enough that they can be monitored for sensation and circulation several times daily.
5. If the bandage is on a limb, the patient should be positioned with that limb uppermost.

.... Complications and Disadvantages

1. Pressure bandages that are placed too tightly or left on too long may interfere with nerve function and circulation and result in sloughing of tissue.
2. Wound drainage may be reduced, which encourages infection.

.... Result of Bandaging

1. Edema is controlled.

.... *Initial Fracture Immobilization*

.... Materials Needed

1. Contact layer. In accordance with the type of wound present, if any
2. Intermediate layer. Thick, absorbent wrapping material
3. Outer layer. Elastic adhesive tape

.... How to Bandage

1. The contact layer, if needed, is placed over the wound.
2. The intermediate layer is wrapped over the contact layer, usually in an amount thicker than when used for minor hemorrhage control.
3. The elastic adhesive tape is *carefully* wrapped over the intermediate layer with overlap of wraps.
4. When applied to a limb, the third and fourth digits should be left exposed just enough that they can be monitored for sensation and circulation several times a day.

.... Complications and Disadvantages

1. Pressure bandages that are placed too tightly or left on too long may interfere with nerve function and circulation and result in sloughing of tissue.
2. Wound drainage may be reduced, which encourages infection, when the bandage is used with a compound fracture.

.... Result of Bandaging

1. Fracture immobilization

.... *Exuberant Granulation Tissue*

.... Materials Needed

1. Contact layer. Commercially available nonadherent dressing
2. Intermediate layer. Thick, absorbent wrapping material
3. Outer layer. Elastic adhesive tape

·········· How to Bandage

1. The contact layer is placed over the wound. A topical wound medication containing a corticosteroid may also be placed on the wound to help control exuberant growth of granulation tissue.
2. The intermediate layer is wrapped over the contact layer.
3. The elastic adhesive tape is *carefully* wrapped over the intermediate layer with overlap of wraps.
4. When applied to a limb, the third and fourth digits should be left exposed just enough that they can be monitored for sensation and circulation several times daily.

·········· Complications and Disadvantages

1. Pressure bandages that are placed too tightly or left on too long may interfere with nerve function and circulation and result in sloughing of tissue.
2. Wound drainage may be reduced, which encourages infection.

·········· Result of Bandaging

1. Excess granulation tissue is reduced.

·········· *Obliteration of Dead Space*
·········· Materials Needed

1. Contact layer. Commercially available nonadherent dressing
2. Intermediate layer. Absorbent wrapping material
3. Outer layer. Elastic adhesive tape

·········· How to Bandage

1. The contact layer is placed over the suture line, and several layers of absorbent wide-mesh gauze are placed over the distal end of any drain that might be in place to also help obliterate dead space.
2. The intermediate layer is wrapped over the contact layer.
3. The elastic adhesive tape is *carefully* wrapped over the intermediate layer with overlap of wraps.

4

·········· Complications and Disadvantages

1. Pressure bandages to obliterate dead space are usually used on the trunk where there is sufficient tissue to allow dead space. If used on the thoracic area, tight bandages could result in restricted respiratory function.

·········· Result of Bandaging

1. The dead space is obliterated.

·········· **Wounds in Need of Pressure Relief**

Wounds typified by decubitus ulcers, pressure bandage or cast ulcers, or impending ulcer areas, and surgical repair sites of ulcers can be managed in four ways:

1. Modified doughnut bandage
2. Doughnut-shaped bandage

3. Pipe insulation bandage
4. Splints

............*Modified Doughnut Bandage*

............Materials Needed

1. Cast padding material
2. Thick wrapping material
3. Porous adhesive tape

............How to Bandage (Fig. 4–33)

1. This type of bandage is used over bony prominences on the limbs when there are early signs of pressure over these areas, (i.e., hyperemia) to help prevent further pressure injury.
2. Several layers of cast padding are folded together, making a 3-in. × 3-in. pad (Fig. 4–33A).
3. The pad is folded on itself and a slit is cut in its center; the slit is formed into a hole (Fig. 4–33B and C).
4. The hole in the pad is placed over the bony prominence (Fig. 4–33D).
5. The wrapping material is wrapped over the pad.
6. Tape strips are placed over the wrapping material with overlap of the tape strips.

............Complications and Disadvantages

1. The pad becomes compressed after two or three bandage changes and must be replaced.

............Result of Bandaging

1. Pressure is relieved over the bony prominence, the hyperemia disappears, and further skin breakdown is prevented.

............*Doughnut-Shaped Bandage*

............Materials Needed

1. Hand towel rolled and taped in a doughnut shape
2. Porous adhesive tape

............How to Bandage (see Fig. 4–34)

1. This type of bandage should be used over bony prominences on the distal limbs, (e.g., over the lateral malleolus). It is used if more padding is indicated than would be provided by a modified doughnut bandage.
2. The hand towel is rolled tightly, and tape is wrapped around the roll.
3. The towel is formed into a doughnut shape of the proper size to fit around the ulcer or surgical repair site and then cut to the proper length.
4. The ends of the towel are taped together to form the doughnut bandage.
5. The doughnut bandage is centered over the wound or impending ulcer and taped to the surrounding skin with strips of adhesive tape so that it will not slip (see Fig. 4–34).
6. The wound can be treated as indicated through the hole in the bandage.

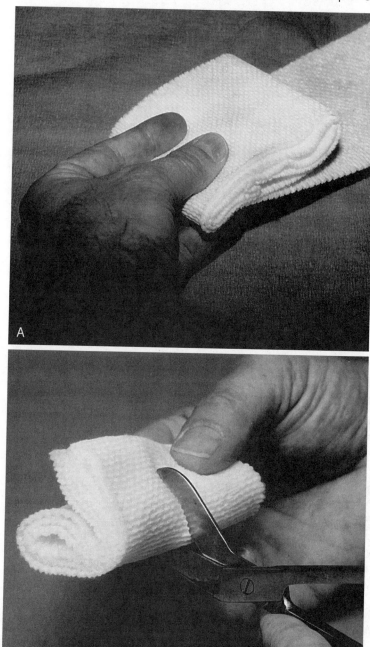

Figure 4–33. Modified doughnut bandage. A, Several layers of cast padding are folded together. B, The pad is folded on itself and a slit is cut in its center.

Illustration continued on following page

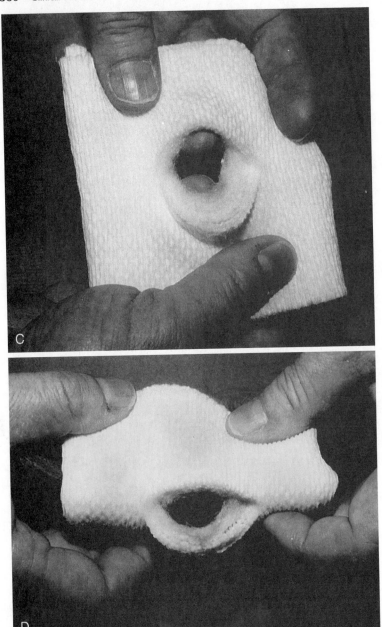

Figure 4–33 *Continued.* C, The slit is formed into a hole. D, The hole is placed over the bony prominence. (From Swaim SF, Henderson RA: Small Animal Wound Management, ed 2. Media, PA, Williams & Wilkins, 1997.)

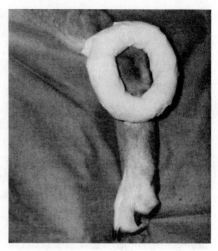

Figure 4–34. The doughnut-shaped bandage is taped with the hole over an area of impending decubital ulcer formation. (From Swaim SF, Henderson RA: Small Animal Wound Management, ed 2. Media, PA, Williams & Wilkins, 1997.)

·········· Complications and Disadvantages

1. If not securely taped, the doughnut bandage may not stay in the proper position.
2. Tape applied directly to the skin to hold the bandage in place may cause some irritation of the skin.
3. Doughnut-type bandages may be difficult to apply to some areas on some dogs, e.g., to the hock on a dachshund.

·········· Result of Bandaging

1. Prevention of pressure over the ulcer or a surgical repair site enables the wound to heal.

·········· *Elbow Loop Splint*

·········· Materials Needed

1. Thick wrapping material
2. Aluminum splint rod
3. Porous adhesive tape

·········· How to Bandage (Fig. 4–35)

1. This splint is used to prevent pressure over the olecranon in the presence of an impending ulcer, a pressure ulcer, or an ulcer repair site.
2. Cut an appropriate length of aluminum splint rod and bend it into a basic rectangular loop. Tape the ends of the rod together.
3. Bend the loop at its center to conform to the natural cranial radial-humeral curvature.
4. Bend the loop at its ends to conform to the cranial curvature of the radial-humeral area.
5. Pad the ends of the loop (Fig. 4–35A).

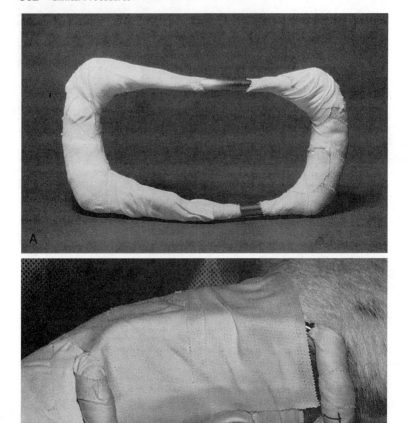

Figure 4–35. Elbow loop splint. A, The ends of an aluminum rectangular-shaped splint are padded. B, The splint is placed over the cranial surface of the radial-humeral joint over a bandage and taped in place. (From Swaim SF, Henderson RA: Small Animal Wound Management, ed 2. Media, PA, Williams & Wilkins, 1997.)

6. Wrap the radial-humeral area with thick wrapping material; do not place extreme pressure over the olecranon.
7. Place the elbow loop splint over the cranial surface of the bandage with the bend in the center of the loop at the level of the radial-humeral joint (Fig. 4–35B).
8. Tape strips are placed over the elbow loop splint and wrapping material with overlap of the tape strips.

···········Complications and Disadvantages

1. If there is insufficient curvature at the ends of the loop to conform to the curvature of the humerus and radius, the loop may tend to twist out of position.

···········Result of Bandaging

1. The elbow loop splint prevents elbow flexion, forces the dog into lateral recumbency, and thus keeps pressure off the olecranon area.
2. If the dog does get into sternal recumbency, the splint helps keep the olecranon off the resting surface to prevent pressure.

···········*Prefabricated, Padded, Fiberglass Elbow Splint*

···········Materials Needed

1. Thick wrapping material
2. Prefabricated, padded, fiberglass splint material (C-splint, Johnson & Johnson Orthopaedics, Raynham, MA.)
3. Porous adhesive tape

···········How to Bandage (Fig. 4–36)

1. This splint is an alternative means of preventing pressure over the olecranon in the presence of an impending ulcer, a pressure ulcer, or an ulcer repair site.
2. Wrap the radial-humeral area with the thick wrapping material, without placing extreme pressure over the olecranon.
3. Place the prefabricated, padded, fiberglass splint material in warm water for about 1 minute and knead it.
4. Wring the splint material out and place it on the cranial aspect of the forelimb, extending from the midhumeral area to the metacarpal area (Fig. 4–36A).
5. The splint material is molded to the front of the extended limb and held in position until it hardens.
6. The limb is then wrapped again with the thick wrapping material (Fig. 4–36B).
7. Tape strips are placed over the wrapping material with overlap of the tape strips.

···········Complications and Disadvantages

1. On obese dogs with a short length of humerus, it may be difficult to get a secure fit of the splint in the midhumeral area.

···········Result of Bandaging

1. The splint prevents elbow flexion, forces the dog into lateral recumbency, and thus keeps pressure off of the olecranon area.
2. If the dog does get into sternal recumbency, the splint helps prevent elbow flexion to keep the olecranon off the resting surface to prevent pressure.

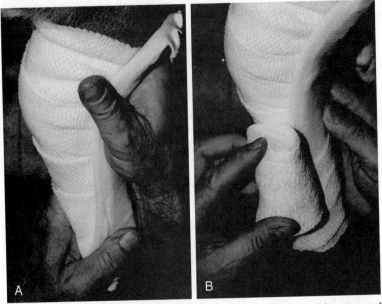

Figure 4–36. Prefabricated, padded, fiberglass elbow splint. A, After removal from warm water, the splint is molded to the cranial surface of the bandage-wrapped forelimb, extending from the midhumeral to the metacarpal area. B, The splint is wrapped in place with bandage wrap followed by tape wraps.

··········Pipe Insulation Bandage

··········Materials Needed

1. Pipe insulation of appropriate length and diameter
2. Cast padding
3. Thick wrapping material
4. Short aluminum splint rod loop
5. Porous adhesive tape

··········How to Bandage (Fig. 4–37)

This bandage is an alternative means of preventing pressure over the olecranon in the presence of an impending ulcer, a pressure ulcer, or an ulcer repair site. It is indicated when more pressure relief is necessary.

1. Dogs with a long length of humerus
   a. Two or three pieces of foam rubber pipe insulation of the proper diameter and length are split lengthwise.
   b. A hole large enough to go around the ulcer or surgical repair site is cut in the center of each piece of split foam rubber (Fig. 4–37A). The pieces are stacked and taped together.
   c. The cranial surface of the radial-humeral joint is *well* padded with cast padding material, and the foam rubber pad is placed with the hole over the olecranon (Fig. 4–37B).
   d. A short segment of aluminum splint rod material can be bent into a

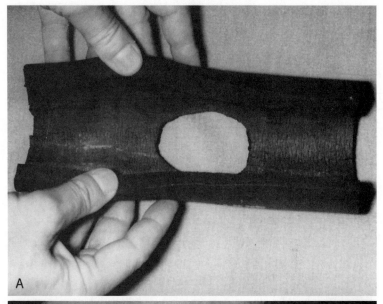

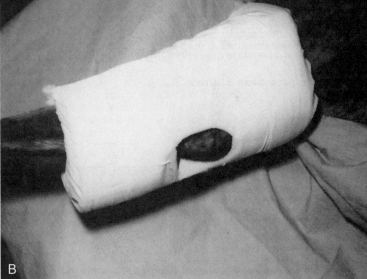

Figure 4–37. Pipe insulation pressure relief bandage. A, A piece of foam rubber pipe insulation is split lengthwise with a hole to accommodate the olecranon area. B, The cranial surface of the radial-humeral joint is well padded with cast padding; the foam rubber pad is placed with the hole over the olecranon area and is taped in place. (From Swaim SF, Henderson RA: Small Animal Wound Management, ed 2. Media, PA, Williams & Wilkins, 1997.)

loop and included in the cranial surface of the bandage (see Elbow Loop Splint).

   e. The cast padding and foam rubber padding are taped in place with strips of adhesive tape.

   f. The wound may be treated as indicated through the hole.

2. Dog with a short humerus length or obesity (spica-type bandage)

   a. Thick wrapping material and adhesive tape are used to place a circumferential body bandage just behind the forelimbs.

   b. A strip of 2-in. adhesive tape is placed from the dorsal body bandage area onto the cranial surface of the forelimb.

   c. See steps 1a–e above.

   d. The strip of adhesive tape that was placed from the body bandage onto the cranial surface of the forelimb is twisted and placed back onto the elbow and onto the body bandage. This forms a "stirrup" to hold the elbow bandage up.

   e. The wound may be treated as indicated through the hole.

............Complications and Disadvantages

1. On a very large dog or an active dog, the bandage may be difficult to keep in place.

2. On a obese dog with a short humerus length, more bandage material is needed for the spica-type bandage.

............Result of Bandaging

1. Prevention of pressure over the olecranon enhances wound healing. Inclusion of a short aluminum splint rod loop in the cranial surface of the bandage helps prevent elbow flexion. Thus, the dog cannot attain sternal recumbency and pressure over the olecranon is averted.

............*Extended Side Splints*

............Materials Needed

1. Rolled cast padding
2. Porous adhesive tape
3. Padded aluminum splint (4 in. × 18 in.)

............How to Bandage (Fig. 4–38)

1. These splints are indicated to relieve pressure over the ischiatic tuberosities in the presence of an impending ulcer, a pressure ulcer, or an ulcer repair site.

2. The rolled padding material is used to place a body bandage on the dog that extends from the axillary regions to the folds of the flanks.

3. Porous adhesive material is placed over the padding material.

4. A padded aluminum splint is placed along each side of the dog so that each splint extends beyond the ischiatic tuberosity approximately 3 to 4 in.

5. Porous adhesive tape is paced around the trunk to affix the splints to the body bandage (see Fig. 4–38).

............Complications and Disadvantages

1. The bandage and splints may require adjustment to maintain proper position of the splints to prevent the dog from attaining a sitting position and placing pressure over the ischiatic tuberosity.

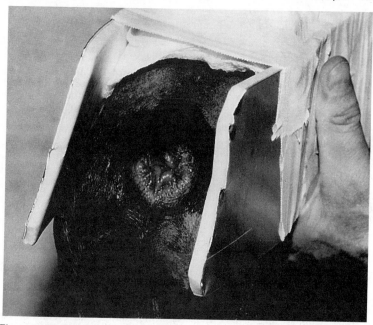

Figure 4–38. Padded aluminum side splints are taped along each side of the dog over a body bandage. Each splint extends approximately 3 to 4 in. beyond each ischiatic tuberosity. (From Swaim SF, Hanson RR, Coates JR: Pressure wounds in animals. Compend Contin Educ Pract Vet 18:203, 1996.)

············ Results of Bandaging

1. The extended splints keep the dog from attaining a sitting position and placing pressure over the ischiatic tuberosity causing decubital ulcers.

············ **Wounds in Need of Immobilization (Immobilizing Bandage)**

An immobilizing bandage is needed for wounds with underlying orthopedic damage (see also p. 100).

············ *External Pin Splints*

············ Materials Needed

1. Contact layer. In accordance with the type of wound present (see p. 257)
2. Intermediate layer. In accordance with the type of wound present (see p. 257)
3. Outer layer. Porous adhesive tape or elastic adhesive tape

············ How to Bandage (Fig. 4–39)

1. These splints are indicated when there are fractures or luxations associated with open wounds.

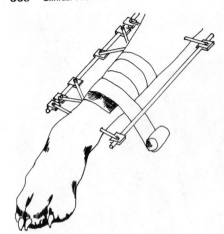

Figure 4–39. An external pin splint is applied proximal and distal to a fracture site with a bandage being applied to the wound. (From Swaim SF, Henderson RA: Small Animal Wound Management, ed 2. Media, PA, Williams & Wilkins, 1997.)

2. An external pin splint is placed on the limb with pins in the bone above and below the wound or fracture site.
3. The contact layer is placed over the wound.
4. The intermediate layer is wrapped over the contact layer.
5. Tape strips are placed over the intermediate layer with overlap of the tape strips.

............Complications and Disadvantages

1. It may be difficult to bandage under the bars of the pin splint in such a way that the bandage is in proper contact with the wound.

............Result of Bandaging

1. The external pin splint provides good immobilization of the fracture site for healing, while the wound is treated as an open wound.

............*Metal or Plastic Splints*

............Materials Needed

1. Contact layer. In accordance with the type of wound present (see p. 257)
2. Intermediate layer. In accordance with the type of wound present (see p. 257)
3. Outer layer. Porous adhesive tape or elastic adhesive tape

............How to Bandage

1. These splints are indicated when there are fractures or luxations associated with open wounds.
2. The contact layer is placed over the wound.
3. The intermediate layer is wrapped over the contact layer with sufficient thickness to fit snugly into the metal or plastic splint.
4. A metal or plastic splint is placed over the intermediate layer.
5. Strips of adhesive tape are placed over the splint to hold it in place.

########### Complications and Disadvantages

1. Removal of the splint for bandage changes may cause movement of the fracture site, and further orthopedic surgery may be necessary after soft tissues have healed.

########### Result of Bandaging

1. The fracture may heal, and the fibrosis of scar tissue from healing overlying soft tissues may add stability to the fracture site.

########### *Cup Splints*

########### Materials Needed

1. Contact layer. In accordance with the type of wound present (see p. 257)
2. Intermediate layer. In accordance with the type of wound present
3. Outer layer. Porous adhesive tape
4. Paw cup portion of a metal limb splint

########### How to Bandage

1. This splint is indicated when bandaging pad wounds.
2. The contact layer is placed over the wound.
3. The intermediate layer is wrapped over the contact layer sufficiently to provide a *well*-padded bandage especially on large dogs.
4. The paw cup portion cut from a metal limb splint is placed on the palmar or plantar surface of the paw or bandage.
5. Strips of adhesive tape are placed over the splint and intermediate layer.

########### Complications and Disadvantages

1. On very large or active dogs, the splint may not be sufficient to prevent spreading of the pad wound when the dog places weight on the paw.

4

########### Result of Bandaging

1. The cup splint helps absorb and distribute pressure so weight bearing does not result in spreading of the pad wound edges to inhibit healing.

########### *Clamshell Splints*

########### Materials Needed

1. Contact layer. In accordance with the type of wound present
2. Intermediate layer. In accordance with the type of wound present
3. Outer layer. Porous adhesive tape
4. Two metal limb splints

########### How to Bandage (Fig. 4–40)

1. These splints are indicated when bandaging pad wounds and it is necessary to alleviate as much pressure as possible.
2. The contact layer is placed over the wound.
3. The intermediate layer is wrapped over the contact layer sufficiently to provide a *well*-padded bandage, especially on large dogs.
4. Strips of adhesive tape are placed over the intermediate layer.

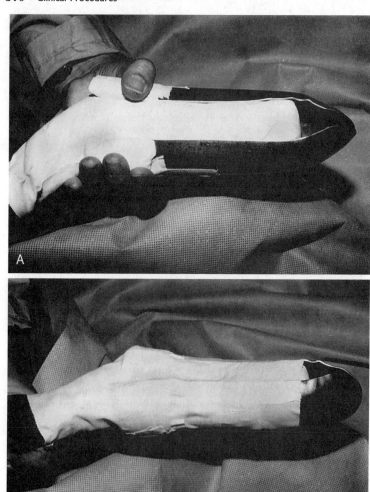

Figure 4-40. Clamshell splints. A, Metal limb splints are placed on the dorsal and palmar or plantar surface of a paw bandage with the concave surfaces of the paw cups facing each other and extending beyond the bandage about 1 in. B, The splints are taped in place with circumferential wraps of adhesive tape.

5. Two metal limb splints are cut to the appropriate length and the proximal (cut) ends are padded.
6. One splint is placed on the dorsal surface of the bandage and one on the palmar or plantar surface of the bandage so that the concave surface of the paw cups face each other and extend about 1 in. beyond the end of the bandage (Fig. 4-40A).

7. The splints are taped in place with circumferential wraps of adhesive tape (Fig. 4–40B).

···········Complications and Disadvantages

1. A large or active dog will in time gradually push the end of the paw bandage toward the end of the splints.

···········Results of Bandaging

1. The splints put the paw in a vertical position and when weight is borne, it is on the splints and not directly on the pads. Thus, pads heal faster.

REFERENCE

Swaim SF, Henderson RA: Small Animal Wound Management, ed 2. Media. PA, Williams & Wilkins, 1997.

Blood Component Therapy

Blood component therapy is the mainstay of the initial management of hematologic emergencies. It involves the specific replacement of component deficits. Blood components provide temporary support of the critically ill patient until the underlying disease process is controlled. The separation of blood into its cellular and plasma components:

- Allows for more specific replacement of the animal's deficits
- Decreases the risk of transfusion reactions
- Allows for more efficient use of donor blood

■ APPROACH TO BLOOD COMPONENT THERAPY

4

Red Blood Cell Support Necessary

- Packed cell volume (PCV) drops rapidly to less than 20% in the dog and less than 12% to 15% in the cat.

- Greater than 30% of blood volume is lost (approximately 30 mL/kg in the dog, 20 mL/kg in the cat).

- Blood loss is associated with collapse.

- Ongoing hemorrhage is present.

- Poor response to shock therapy.

Platelet Support Necessary

- Life-threatening bleeding from thrombocytopenia or thrombocytopathia is present.

- Surgery is necessary in the animal with thrombocytopenia or thrombocytopathia.

Plasma Necessary

- Life-threatening hemorrhage associated with decreased coagulation factor activity.

Box continued on following page

■ APPROACH TO BLOOD COMPONENT THERAPY *(Continued)*

■ Surgery is necessary in an animal with decreased coagulation factor activity.

■ Severe hypoproteinemia is present.

■ As colloid replacement in hypovolemic shock.

··········· CONSIDERATIONS IN BLOOD COMPONENT THERAPY

Prior Transfusion History or Sensitization of the Animal Has the animal received any blood components prior to the present admission? Was crossmatching done prior to administration if RBCs were given? What donors were used? Were the donors random or typed? Did the patient exhibit any signs of transfusion reaction during the past administration? Is it a female intended for breeding (in which case crossmatching and typing is optimal prior to any further administration of RBCs)?

Does the Animal Need Component Administration? Type of loss and replacement needed is determined by clinical signs, continuing fluid losses, and clinicopathologic findings.

Precautions—Crossmatching A crossmatch should be performed in both dogs and cats prior to any RBC administration if at all possible. A crossmatch is done to decrease the risk of a hemolytic transfusion reaction (rapid destruction of donor RBCs) in a sensitized animal. Even if crossmatching is done prior to transfusion, transfusion reactions can still occur. The crossmatch does not check for the presence of incompatible WBCs or platelet antigens, which are the main source of many immediate transfusion reactions. Dogs that are transfused for the first time (nonsensitized) can have a compatible crossmatch, despite differing blood types, because they often do not have naturally occurring isoantibody. Even if type-specific blood components are used for the transfusion, crossmatching is still advised.

In dogs, if neither crossmatching nor typing is available, or it is an emergency situation with no time for crossmatching, universal donor blood (DEA 1.1, 1.2, and 7 negative) should be given. There is no universal feline blood donor.

Transfusion Reaction Prophylaxis Diphenhydramine 0.5 mg/kg IM or IV 15 minutes prior to component therapy may help to minimize transfusion reactions.

Preparation of Component All components except platelet-rich plasma (PRP): warm in a 37°C water bath, incubator, or use fluid warmer directly on administration lines. Do not heat any component above 40°C to avoid hemolysis and destruction of coagulation factors. With packed RBCs (PRBCs) add warm (maximum 37°C) sodium chloride 20 to 100 mL depending on the unit size and the animal's volume status. In the hypovolemic patient, add 150 to 250 mL. Cryoprecipitate: resuspend cryoprecipitate 1:1 in 0.9% NaCl and mix prior to administration.

Simultaneous Fluid Administration (Same Catheter) Avoid any calcium-containing or hypotonic fluid solutions. Calcium may activate the clotting system and simultaneous administration of hypotonic solutions can cause hemolysis. Normal saline (0.9%) is the optimal choice.

··········· SPECIFIC CONSIDERATIONS FOR BLOOD COMPONENT THERAPY

Transfusion of RBC Components (Tables 4–13 through 4–16). The amount of blood components needed to achieve a specific increment in packed

Table 4–13. Indications for Blood Component Therapy

Component	Indications
Fresh whole blood (FWB) (rarely needed)	1. Coagulopathy with active bleeding (e.g., ITP, DIC) 2. Massive acute hemorrhage 3. No stored blood available
Stored whole blood (SWB)	1. Massive acute → ongoing hemorrhage 2. Shock due to blood loss, unresponsive to conventional fluid therapy 3. Unavailability of equipment to prepare components
Packed red blood cells (PRBCs)	Anemia 1. Nonregenerative 2. Autoimmune hemolytic anemia 3. Correction of anemia prior to surgery 4. Blood loss—acute or chronic hemorrhage

Platelet-rich plasma (PRP)	1. Thrombocytopenia
	    With active life-threatening bleeding (ITP)
	    Prior to surgery (ITP)
	2. Platelet function abnormality
	    Congenital (e.g., thrombasthenia—basset hounds)
	    Acquired (NSAIDs, other drugs)

Fresh frozen plasma (FFP)	1. Factor depletion associated with active bleeding
	    Congenital (von Willebrand's disease, hemophilia A, hemophilia B)
	    Acquired (warfarin toxicity, DIC)
	2. Acute hypoproteinemia (e.g., severe burns)
	3. Chronic hypoproteinemia (hepatic, renal, intestinal losses)
	    Prior to surgery

Plasma (include stable clotting factors)	1. Acute plasma loss 2. Acute hypoproteinemia 3. Chronic hypoproteinemia (see FFP 3) 4. Colostrum replacement—neonates 5. Hemophilia B and selected clotting factor deficiencies

Cryoprecipitate (CP) (concentration of factor VIII, von Willebrand's factor, and fibrinogen, 10×)	1. Congenital factor deficiencies (routine or prior to surgery) von Willebrand's disease
	    Hemophilia A
	    Hypofibrinogenemia
	2. Acquired factor deficiencies

ITP, immune-mediated thrombocytopenia; DIC, disseminated intravascular coagulation, NSAIDs, nonsteroidal antiinflammatory drugs.

cell volume (PCV) depends on whether PRBCs or whole blood is administered. Because the PCV of PRBC units is high (usually around 80% for greyhound units), a smaller volume is needed to achieve the same increase in hematocrit as if whole blood were given. In general, 10 mL/kg of PRBCs or 20 mL/kg of whole blood will increase the PCV 10 points. If the animal is hypovolemic and whole blood is given, fluid is redistributed into the extravascular compartment during the first 24 hours after the transfusion, resulting in a secondary rise in

Table 4–14. Blood Component Dose and Administration Rates

Component	Dose	Administration Rate	
Whole blood	20 mL/kg, will ↑ PCV 10%	Normovolemia Max 22 mL/ kg/24 hr	Hypovolemia Max 22 mL/kg/ hr
PRBCs	10 mL/kg, will ↑ PCV 10%		*Critically ill patients:* (e.g., cardiac failure, renal failure) 3–4 mL/kg/hr
Fresh frozen plasma Plasma	10 mL/kg body weight (repeat 2–3/day for 3–5 days or until bleeding stops) → monitor ACT, APTT, PT before and 1 hr after transfusion	4–10 mL/min or use rates as for whole blood (infuse within 3–6 hr)	
Cryoprecipitate (CP)	*General:* 1 unit/10 kg/12 hr or until bleeding stops *Hemophilia A:* 12–20 units of factor VIII/kg—1 unit of CP contains approximately 125 units of factor VIII	4–10 mL/min or use rates as for whole blood (infuse within 3–6 hr)	
Platelet-rich plasma (PRP)	1 unit/10 kg (1 unit of PRP will ↑ platelet count 1 hr after transfusion by ≈10,000/μL)	2 mL/min Check platelet count before and 1 hr after transfusion	

PRBCs, packed red blood cells; PCV, packed cell volume; ACT, activated clotting time; APTT, activated partial thromboplastin time; PT, prothrombin time.

PCV 24 hours after transfusion in addition to the initial rise 1 hour after transfusion caused by the RBCs.

Use of Fresh Frozen Plasma The volume of plasma transfused will depend upon individual patient need. This generally should not exceed 6 to 10 mL/kg of body weight once or twice daily or not more than 22 mL/kg during a 24-hour period for normovolemic animals. Following thawing, plasma is administered with the aid of a standard drip-type administration set. The average rate of administration for normovolemic animals should not exceed 22 mL/kg/hr. In acute-need situations, plasma may be delivered at rates up to 4 to 6 mL/min. For cardiac or other compromised animals who may have circulatory problems, rates should not exceed 5 mL/kg/hr. Plasma should not be mixed with or used in the same IV administration lines as lactated Ringer's

Table 4–15. Storage of Blood Components

Component	Anticoagulant	Shelf Life	Comments
WB	Heparin, 625 IU/ 50 mL WB	37 days, 4°C	No preservation, coagulation factor inhibition
	ACD, 10 mL/60 mL WB	24 hr, 4°C	ACD rarely used
	CPDA-1 1 mL/7 mL WB	21 days, 4°C	Will maintain 75% PTV*
	AS-1*	35 days, 4°C	
PRBCs	CPDA-1	20 days, 4°C	Will maintain 75% PTV*
	AS-1*	37 days, 4°C	
Platelet-rich plasma	CPDA-1	3–5 days, 23°C 2 hr, 4°C	Needs constant agitation
Fresh frozen plasma	CPDA-1	1 yr, −30°C 3 mo, −18°C	Frozen <6 hr after collection of blood; all coagulation factors present
Plasma/ cryopoor plasma	CPDA-1	4 yr, −30°C 35 days, 4°C	Does not contain factors V and VIII
Cryoprecipitate	CPDA-1	1 yr, −30°C	High concentration of factor VIII, vWF, and fibrinogen

WB, whole blood; PRBC, packed red blood cells; ACD, acid-citrate-dextrose; PTV, post-transfusion viability (FDA standard); CPDA-1, citrate acid-dextrose-adenine; vWF, von Willebrand's factor; AS, additive solution.

*Fenwal Laboratories, Baxter, Deerfield, IL.

solution or any other solution containing divalent cations. The safest fluid to mix with plasma is 0.9% NaCl. In cases of significant bleeding, as may occur with rodenticide toxicity, fresh frozen plasma may be administered in one or two doses at 6 to 10 mL/kg over a 24-hour period along with vitamin K_1 (see also p. 184). *A general guideline for plasma therapy is that 1 mL of plasma contains approximately 1 unit of coagulation factor activity.*

Use of Plasma Cryoprecipitate (Concentrated Fresh Frozen Plasma) Indicated in severe forms of von Willebrand's disease (von Willebrand's factor levels below 1% or 2%), and hemophilia A (factor VIII deficiency). It is available through commercial services such as Hemopet.*

Use of Fresh Platelet-Rich Plasma Indicated in significant bleeding or risk of bleeding in animals with severe chronic thrombocytopenia, as in oncology patients on chemotherapy. Animals with immune-mediated thrombocytopenia are not good candidates for this therapy, as platelets may be rapidly destroyed. Animals with immune-mediated thrombocytopenia should be managed by immunomodulating techniques (see also p. 695) and the administration of fresh frozen plasma.

....

*Canine and feline blood products, including whole blood and plasma, are commercially available from Animal Blood Bank, Dixon, CA, and Eastern Veterinary Blood Bank, Annapolis, MD.

Table 4-16. Complications and Adverse Reactions Associated With Blood Component Therapy

Type	Cause	Clinical Symptoms	Action Required
Nonimmune Immediate			
Circulatory overload	Excess volume administration Patient with cardiovascular disease	Coughing, dyspnea, vomiting, signs of pulmonary edema and congestive heart failure	Slow transfusion rate or stop transfusion; administer diuretic (furosemide)
Sepsis	Bacterial growth in blood component	Pyrexia, chills, nausea, vomiting, diarrhea, shock	Stop transfusion, Gram-stain blood, culture blood, antibiotic therapy
Coagulopathy	Massive transfusion → dilution of coagulation factors	Bleeding	Monitor hemostasis Factor replacement (FFP)
Air embolism	Air infused during administration	Pain, cough, dyspnea	Place patient on left side
Pulmonary microembolism	Debris (platelets and fibrin)	Cough, dyspnea	Stop transfusion Use 40-μm filter in critically ill patients
Hypocalcemia	Citrate intoxication in massive transfusion (>1 blood volume/24 hr)	Pyrexia Tremors, restlessness, vomiting, arrythmias	Slow transfusion Administer Ca gluconate
Hypothermia	Administration of cold components	Chills, hypothermia	Warm component prior to transfusion Heating pad
Acidosis	↓ pH in stored RBC component (massive transfusion)	↓ TCO_2	HCO_3^- replacement
Nonimmune Delayed			
Disease transmission	Contaminated component	Depending on disease	Check donors, therapy depending on disease

576

Immune Immediate

Hemolysis	Incompatible blood	Pyrexia, nausea, chills, vomiting, hypotension, anorexia, shock, hemoglobinemia, hemoglobinuria	Stop transfusion; administer dexamethasone 4 mg/kg IV; shock therapy if necessary; administer diuretic (furosemide); monitor urine output; monitor ACT (risk of DIC); heparin, therapy
Acute hypersensitivity	Type I—foreign protein reaction	Pruritus, urticaria, bronchospasm, anaphylaxis	Stop transfusion; administer antihistamine, corticosteroids, and epinephrine if severe reaction
Leukocyte/platelet reactivation	Antigens	Pyrexia, chills, dyspnea, pulmonary edema, tachycardia	Stop transfusion. Usually self-limiting. Administer dexamethasone, furosemide, and aminophylline if ARDS develops

Immune Delayed

Hemolysis	Incompatible RBCs Product of isoantibody	Anemia, icterus, anorexia, bilirubinemia, bilirubinuria	Coombs' test (becomes positive), self-limiting. Future transfusions: crossmatch and type
Purpura	Product/presence of platelets isoantibody	Petechiae, ecchymoses (anemia)	Usually self-limiting. PRP if bleeding is severe

FFP, fresh frozen platelets; RBCs, red blood cells; ACT, activated clotting time; DIC, disseminated intravascular coagulation; ARDS, acute respiratory distress syndrome; PRP, platelet-rich plasma; TCO_2, Total CO_2 (reflect HCO_3^-).

4

577

............BLOOD TRANSFUSIONS

Great advances have been made in the field of veterinary transfusion medicine. Today, qualified laboratories are making blood components for animals commercially available (see p. 580). This type of therapy in a wide variety of hemostatic disorders is a proven form of therapeutic management. Despite this, veterinarians are still faced with emergency and lifesaving situations where whole blood is still administered. The availability of commercial corporations that will type animal blood donors will assist the practitioner in making this type of blood component administration more effective and less dangerous. Because veterinarians must still administer whole blood transfusions in selected cases, the following information is presented.

............Cats

Blood transfusions for cats are usually administered for medical reasons, and repeated small doses of fresh whole blood are desirable. Cats have an AB blood group system. *Cats possess naturally occurring alloantibodies against the blood type antigen they lack. Cats do not need to be sensitized by previous transfusions and incompatibility reactions can develop with the first transfusion.* Studies conducted in the United States indicate that fewer than 1% of cats have type B blood. Certain lines of purebred cats have a higher incidence of type B blood than found in the domestic short-hair and long-hair cat. Cats with type B usually have anti-A (natural alloantibodies of the IgM class) in their serum and will hemolyze RBCs of type A when their anti-A titers are as low as 1:64. Cats with type A blood have a low incidence of anti-B antibody, with titers rarely exceeding 1:2.

If type A or type B blood is transfused into a matched recipient, the RBC half-life will be 33 days. If type B blood is transfused into a type A cat, the RBC half-life will be 2.3 days with a mild systemic reaction. If type A blood is transfused into a type B cat, the RBC half-life will be 1.4 hours and a moderate to severe reaction will occur. If cats are to be kept as in-hospital blood donors, their blood can be typed*; *type A donors are preferred. Eastern Veterinary Blood Bank, Annapolis, MD, provides feline type A and type B blood.*

............Equipment

The following equipment is necessary for feline blood transfusions:

Ketamine
150-mL citrate-phosphate-dextrose (CPD) blood collection bag or heparin 2 units/mL whole blood or CPD 0.14-mL solution per milliliter of whole blood
One scalp vein infusion set
Adhesive tape, 1 in. wide
Blanket
Clear plastic bag
Oxygen tank
Flowmeter

............Technique

For feline donors sedation is always necessary. Ketamine (11 mg/kg) alone or a ketamine combination (ketamine 6 mg/kg; midzolam [Versed] 0.1 mg/kg; atro-

....

*Blood can be typed by Stormont Laboratories, Woodland, CA; Eastern Veterinary Blood Bank, Annapolis, MD; Animal Blood Bank, Dixon, CA; and Hemopet, Irvine, CA.

pine 0.04 mg/kg) can be given IM. The blood can be stored in acid-citrate-dextrose (ACD) or CPD solution 150-ml donor packs. Donor cats should be healthy, vigorous, and free of blood disorders. A 40-mL donation from these animals can be repeated safely every 3 weeks. *Feline donors should receive replacement fluids if more that 50 mL are removed.* All donor cats should be checked for feline leukemia virus (FeLV) and feline immunodeficiency virus (FIV). Cat blood should not be stored. Administration of fresh blood is preferable.

···········Administering Blood

Cats needing blood are usually extremely depressed, toxic, or anoxic and require blood to correct anemia or for other medical reasons. Struggling or violent exertion may cause these patients to collapse and die. Therefore, extreme gentleness and care are mandatory in handling and restraint. Critically anemic cats should be cradled gently on a towel or blanket. Although it admittedly does little to improve oxygenation of anemic cats, some clinicians advocate placing the cat's head in a clear plastic bag into which oxygen is being infused at 4 to 6 L/min.

Blood can be administered IV by way of the jugular, cephalic, or femoral vein, using a 22- to 24-gauge scalp vein infusion set. Intramedullary infusion is possible through the femur by way of the intratrochanteric fossa. However, intramedullary infusion may be impractical and presents dangers of intramedullary infection. Intraperitoneal infusion can be done safely with good utilization of RBCs. About 45% of the infused RBCs are in the circulation within 24 hours, and 65% are in the circulation within 48 hours.

The average 2- to 3-kg cat can accept 30 to 40 mL of blood injected IV over a period of 30 minutes (give filtered blood 5 to 10 mL/kg/hr). Small, repeated injections are safer and more desirable than a large, single injection. Single intraperitoneal injections (40 mL) are safe.

Transfusion reactions are rare in cats but, when they occur, can be life-threatening. Prodromal signs of a transfusion reaction are pawing at the face, tachypnea, restlessness, fever, urticaria, and vomiting. If these signs are noted, stop administration of blood; start administration of warmed lactated Ringer's solution at three times basal administration levels, and administer hydrocortisone 50 mg IV (see also p. 32).

The following formula can be used to estimate the volume of blood needed for transfusion in the cat:

$$\text{Anticoagulated blood volume (mL)} = \text{body weight (kg)} \times 70 \times \frac{\text{PCV desired} - \text{PCV of recipient}}{\text{PCV of donor in anticoagulant}}$$

···········Dogs

The blood group system of the dog has been worked out. The ideal blood donor should be (DEA-1) A-negative and (DEA-7) Tr-negative, healthy, and 1 to 6 years of age; should weigh 20 kg (44 lb) or more; and should not have been transfused. The greyhound is the breed of choice as a blood donor (i.e., has high PCV, easily accessible veins, low frequency of DEA-1 and DEA-7). Donor dogs can be bled at a rate of 10 to 20 mL/kg every 3 weeks. Greyhounds heavier than 60 lb work well as donor dogs. Dogs used for donors should be healthy (free of heartworm, *Brucella canis*, *Ehrlichia canis*, *Rickettsia riskettsii*, *Trypanosoma cruzi*, *Babesia*, and *Borrelia burgdorferi*). There is a high endemic prevalence of *Babesia* spp. in the racing greyhound industry (estimated to be as high as 30% to 50% in greyhound kennels in Florida, Arizona, and Colorado).

In clinical practice, few transfusion reactions are observed, because about 40% of the random dog population is A-negative and multiple transfusions are usually not required. When dogs are to be kept as blood donors, their blood can be typed by a commercial laboratory.*

...........Blood Donor Programs

The following canine blood banks will ship blood components overnight:

Animal Blood Bank, Dixon, CA.
Eastern Veterinary Blood Bank, Annapolis, MD.
Hemopet, Irvine, CA.

...........Equipment

The following equipment is necessary for canine blood transfusions:

Oxymorphone 0.1 to 0.2 mg/kg or ketamine 6 mg/kg plus diazepam 0.2 mg/kg combination
Blood donor kit, preferably a CPD-containing blood pack (Fenwal-Baxter) or an SMB (storage medium for blood) anticoagulant
Blood recipient kit containing a 5-mL syringe with saline and an IV catheter
Sterile IV cutdown kit containing a scalpel, thumb forceps, needle holder, sharp-pointed scissors, two pairs of mosquito forceps, curved needle, plain catgut, fine silk, and sponges

...........Collecting Blood

Blood may be drawn from a donor dog aseptically via the jugular vein or femoral artery or by left ventricular puncture. When repeated withdrawals of blood are to be made from a donor dog, the jugular vein should be used. The way in which blood is removed, preserved, and stored determines its viability. Blood is routinely collected in plastic bags containing CPD solution and allowed to flow through the solution while the bag is gently agitated. When the bag is filled, the tubing should be clamped without allowing air to enter (CPDA-1 anticoagulant 1 mL/7 mL blood).

Recent experiments have demonstrated the advantage of collecting canine blood in a solution consisting of ascorbate phosphate, citric acid, sodium citrate, sodium phosphate, and dextrose. With this solution, viability remained above 70% for 6 weeks when blood was kept at 4°C. Oxygenated blood so collected can be stored under refrigeration at 4°C. In general, do not use stored whole blood more than 3 weeks old. Plasma can be harvested from blood and frozen for later use. The donor dog should be healthy, parasite-free, vaccinated for the usual diseases. A mature, thin, 22-kg (48-lb) animal makes an ideal donor.

Component storage of blood is the most efficient way to use whole blood or blood products for treatment of bleeding patients. Component storage involves separating and freezing the plasma from fresh units of whole blood. The remainder can be stored as packed cells at 4°C for up to 6 weeks for blood collected in CPD or SMB and 3 to 4 weeks in ACD. The clotting factors in plasma are preserved by freezing, and the PRBCs are available for immediate use. A blood bank centrifuge is required to separate cellular components effectively. If a centrifuge is not available, the RBCs can be allowed to settle by gravity overnight at 4°C and the supernatant plasma is removed. Plasma stored at −40° to −70°C will last for up to 1 year. At a household freezer temperature of −20°C, plasma will last for 2 to 4 months.

---

*Stormont Laboratories, Woodland, CA.

...........Administering Blood (Dog)

In dogs, blood is invariably given IV. The cephalic vein is commonly used, but the jugular vein is routinely used when an IV catheter is placed in the animal. The recipient set should be filled so that blood in the drip chamber covers the filter (normal 170-μm filter). With small amounts of blood (50 mL) or critically ill patients, use the 40-μm filter. Avoid latex filters for platelet and cryoprecipitate administration. Blood can be administered at variable rates, but the routine figure of 4 to 5 mL/min is often used. Normovolemic animals can receive blood at 22 mL/kg/day. Dogs in heart failure should be infused at no more than 4 mL/kg/hr. Volume is given as needed. To calculate the approximate volume of blood needed to raise hematocrit levels, the following formula can be used for the dog:

Anticoagulated blood volume (mL) =

$$\text{body weight (kg)} \times 90 \times \frac{\text{PCV desired} - \text{PCV of recipient}}{\text{PCV of donor in anticoagulant}}$$

An alternative formula that can be utilized is:

$$2.2 \times \text{recipient weight (kg)} \times 30 \text{ (dog)} \times \frac{\text{PCV desired} - \text{PCV of recipient}}{\text{PCV of donor in anticoagulant}}$$

Surgical emergencies and shock may require several times this volume within a short period (see p. 32). If greater than 25% of the blood volume is lost, supplement with colloids as fluid replacement (see p. 585). One volume of RBCs achieves the same increase in plasma as two to three volumes of plasma.

If the blood type of the patient is unknown and CEA-1 or CEA-2 (type A-negative blood) is not available, any dog blood can be given to patients in acute need if they have not had previous transfusions. If mismatched blood is given, however, the patient will become sensitized and after 9 days, destruction of the donated RBCs will begin. In addition, any subsequent mismatched transfusions may cause an immediate reaction (usually mild) and rapid destruction of the donated cells.

The clinical signs of *blood transfusion reaction* are seen only when type A blood is given to a non–type A recipient that has previously been sensitized. Incompatible blood transfusions to breeding females can result in isoimmunization and in hemolytic disease in puppies. The A-negative bitch transfused with A-positive blood who produces a litter from an A-positive stud can have puppies with neonatal isoerythrolysis.

...........Transfusion Reactions

Immunologic and metabolic abnormalities may develop during the course of a transfusion. There are a number of types of transfusion reactions:

1. Acute immunologic reaction: e.g., if type A RBCs are transfused into a type B cat, acute hemolysis develops and may result in disseminated intravascular coagulation (DIC), acute renal failure, and shock. Milder reactions may produce urticaria and noncardiogenic pulmonary edema.
2. Delayed immunologic reaction.
3. Acute nonimmunologic transfusion reaction: This results from abnormal blood products accumulating, e.g., hyperkalemia following transfusion because of lysis of blood cells, embolism associated with blood clots, circulatory overload, infections secondary to transfusions.

............How to Prevent Transfusion Reactions

1. Correct selection of blood donor types.
2. Appropriate crossmatching.
3. Strict aseptic technique.
4. Administer blood through a filtration set.
5. Monitor patient during the transfusion procedure—temperature, respirating, heart rate.

The signs of an acute immunologic transfusion reaction are usually seen within 1 hour of the time of the beginning of the transfusion. Hemoglobinemia and hemoglobinuria result. Fever, emesis, incontinence of urine, tremors, hives, and transient prostration may be observed. If a transfusion reaction is observed, (1) discontinue the transfusion if it is still in progress; (2) institute immediate infusion of crystalloids to maintain blood pressure and urine output; (2) give soluble corticosteroids IV; (3) measure coagulation parameters and institute therapy for DIC if indicated; (4) ensure complete rest; (5) give oxygen, if necessary; and (6) if blood is necessary, crossmatch blood of donor with that of recipient. Crossmatching is important when repeated transfusions are to be performed (see p. 49).

REFERENCES

Authement J: Blood transfusion therapy. *In* DiBartola S, ed: Fluid Therapy in Small Animal Practice. Philadelphia, WB Saunders, 1992.

Callan MB, Oakley D, Shofer F, et al: Canine red blood cell transfusion practice. Am Anim Hosp Assoc 32:303, 1996.

Cotter SM: Comparative transfusion medicine. Adv Vet Sci Comp Med 36:1991.

Giger U, Buchler J: Transfusion of type A and type B blood to cats. J Am Vet Med Assoc 198:411, 1991.

Giger U: Feline transfusion medicine. *In* Hohenhaus AE, Kay WJ, Brown NO, eds: Problems in Veterinary Medicine. Philadelphia, JB Lippincott, 1992, pp 600–611.

Giger U, Gelens CJ, Callan MB, et al: An acute hemolytic transfusion reaction caused by dog erythrocyte antigen 1.1 incompatibility in a previously sensitized dog. J Am Vet Med Assoc 206:1358, 1995.

Griot-Went ME, Giger U: Feline transfusion medicine: Blood types and their importance. Vet Clin North Am Small Anim Pract 5:1305–1322, 1995.

Hohenhaus A: Transfusion reactions: Prevention and Management. *In* Proceedings of 14th Annual Forum of the American College of Internal Veterinary Medicine, San Antonio, Texas, 1996, p. 26

Hohenhaus AE, ed: Transfusion medicine. Probl Vet Med 4:1992.

Kerl ME, Hohenhaus AE: Packed red blood cell transfusions in dogs: 131 cases. J Am Vet Med Assoc 202:1495–1499, 1993.

Kirby R: Transfusion therapy in emergency and critical care medicine. Vet Clin North Am Small Anim Pract 25:1365–1386, 1995.

Kristensen AT, Feldman BF: General principles of small animal blood component administration. Vet Clin North Am Small Anim Pract 25:1365–1386, 1995.

Norsworthy GD: Clinical aspects of feline blood transfusions. Compend Contin Educ Pract Vet 14:469, 1992.

Wingfield WE: Veterinary Emergency Medicine Secrets. Philadelphia, Hanley & Belfus, 1997.

Endotracheal Intubation

In selecting an appropriate-size endotracheal tube, consider the size of the animal and select the tube with the largest diameter that can be introduced without force (Table 4–17).

It is better to use high-volume, low-pressure cuffs on endotracheal tubes.

Table 4–17. Recommended Sizes for Endotracheal Tubes

	Body Weight (kg)	Magill Size	French Size	Internal Diameter (mm)
Dogs	2	2	22	6
	4	4–5	26–28	8
	6	6–7	28–30	9
	9	8	32	10
	12	9–10	34–36	11–12
	14	9–10	34–36	11–12
	16	10–11	36–38	11–12
	18–20	11–12	38–44	12
Cats	1	00	13	4
	2	0	16	5
	4	1	20	5

Overinflation of tracheal cuffs can lead to tracheal ulceration, tracheitis, hemorrhage, tracheomalacia, fibrosis, and stenosis. Occlusion of high-volume, low-pressure cuffs can be achieved at 25 mm Hg or less.

Always check the cuff of a cuffed tube to ensure that there are no leaks and that the cuff is working properly prior to intubation. The selected endotracheal tube should be lubricated with material such as K-Y jelly. The animal to be intubated should be given a short-acting anesthetic or be under the influence of an analgesic-tranquilizer combination. Intubation in the dog and cat may cause an increase in sympathetic activity or vagal stimulation and result in cardiac arrhythmias. Atropine or glycopyrrolate may be given to canine and feline patients to avoid certain arrhythmias that are often associated with induction of anesthesia and intubation. One of these agents should always be given when narcotic analgesics or xylazine is used or when ocular surgery is being performed.

Caution in the use of atropine is warranted, and the animal's cardiovascular function should be monitored during surgery. Atropine will (1) increase anatomical dead space in the pulmonary compartment by 50% to 100%; (2) remove vagal control over the myocardium and increase the heart rate, thus increasing oxygen demand and irritability of damaged myocardial tissue; and (3) change the nature of bronchial secretions so that they become more tenacious.

Atropine *should not* be given to animals with heart rates over 140 bpm or to dogs receiving xylazine for cystometry. Glycopyrrolate may have some distinct advantages over atropine.

··········· TECHNIQUE

Direct visualization of the larynx is the best method for intubating dogs and cats. A laryngoscope should be used for intubation. The blades are detachable from rechargeable handles. MacIntosh, Miller, or Bizarri-Guiffrida blades work well in animals. Small blades (pediatric) are needed in cats and small dogs. Place the animal in lateral, sternal, or dorsal recumbency, according to preference. Hold the laryngoscope in the left hand, and open the animal's mouth with the right hand. In large dogs or animals under light anesthesia, the use of a mouth gag may be helpful. Pull the tongue forward with the right hand, being careful not to lacerate the ventral aspect of the tongue on the lower incisor teeth. In large dogs, it may be helpful to hold the tongue between the small and ring fingers to prevent it from moving excessively. Place the tip of the laryngoscope blade at the base of the tongue at the glossoepiglottic fold. Press the tip of the blade ventrally to move the epiglottis and expose the glottis. In some dogs, especially those that are brachycephalic, it may be necessary to put the laryngoscope tip directly on the epiglottis. Holding the endotracheal tube in the right hand, insert the endotracheal tube. A piece of aluminum wire temporarily placed inside a very flexible plastic tube will provide enough rigidity to make intubation simpler. Place the tube between the vocal folds, using a slight rotating motion rather than try to push the tube through. Never try to force too large a tube into position. If partial closure of the glottis or laryngeal spasm occurs during attempted intubation, deepen the level of anesthesia, administer a muscle relaxant such as succinylcholine, or apply to the larynx a local anesthetic such as 2% lidocaine as a spray or on a soaked cotton swab.

The cuff of a cuffed endotracheal tube should be at a level just beyond the larynx. Overinflation of the cuff may lead to a pressure necrosis of tracheal epithelium.

In cats induced with thiamylal sodium, intubation may be difficult because of laryngospasm. It is easier to intubate cats if ketamine is administered as a preanesthetic at a dosage of 6 to 8 mg/kg. A Warne neonatal endotracheal tube has proved to be very easy to use in the cat. The tube is noncuffed. The tube should be coated with 4% lidocaine jelly prior to being placed in the trachea.

REFERENCES

Muir W, Hubbell J, Skarda R, et al: Handbook of Veterinary Anesthesia, ed 2. St Louis, Mosby–Year Book, 1995.
Short CE: Principles and Practice of Veterinary Anesthesia. Baltimore, Williams & Wilkins, 1987.

Enema

It is best if two people give an enema to a dog. The patient should stand in an outdoor exercise run or in a bathtub. One person restrains the dog by holding its head and collar; the second person holds the dog's tail and gives the enema.

If the contents of the rectum and colon are soft, irrigation once or twice with relatively small volumes of tepid soapy water usually is effective. However, if the stool is hard and inspissated, the procedure may be difficult. In these instances, administer dioctyl sodium sulfosuccinate PO the day before the enema to help soften the dry stool. Adding the same liquid to the enema solution (especially if the solution is to be partially retained) will also act to hydrate the stool.

We recommend a tepid solution of water and Ivory soap for routine irrigation. The amount varies with the size of the dog. Place the solution in an enema can suspended 4 to 5 ft above the dog's back, and use a soft rubber tube to infuse the rectum. Move the tube back and forth, and, as the feces are expelled, advance the tube forward into the rectum. Avoid trapping the fluid in the rectum or using a fast flow because reverse peristalsis may occur and cause vomiting. If these precautions are followed, the can may be refilled for irrigation several times if needed. Occasionally, a gloved finger or a closed sponge forceps or clamshell forceps can be inserted into the rectum to break up hard feces. *Do not work on these difficult cases more than 20 minutes at one time.* The stress can be acute, and it is better to allow time for the solution to soften the feces and try again several hours later. If impactions are severe, anesthesia may be needed for some procedures. Resolution of severe impactions may take several sessions over several days.

Phosphate enemas are *contraindicated* in cats and small dogs but are used by some clinicians for rapid, easy enemas in large, healthy dogs.

Cat enemas require special conditions. Usually the cat is best handled under ketamine sedation and placed on a special work table. Be gentle and use small amounts of solution under low pressure and flow. Feces from a constipated cat have a particularly disagreeable odor. Always wear gloves when giving an enema.

REFERENCES

Burrows CF: Constipation. *In* Kirk RW, ed: Current Veterinary Therapy IX. Small Animal Practice. Philadelphia, WB Saunders, 1986, pp 904–908.

Guilford WE, Center SA, Strombeck DR, et al: Strombeck's Small Animal Gastroenterology, ed 3. Philadelphia, WB Saunders, 1996.

Fluid Therapy

...........GENERAL PRINCIPLES

1. Three major body fluid compartments should be considered when designing a fluid therapy plan: intravascular, interstitial, and intracellular.
2. These three compartments are separated by semipermeable membranes that are freely permeable to water. The distribution of water across each of these membranes is determined by the osmotic gradient on each side of the membrane. The volume of water within each compartment is determined by the total number of osmotic particles within the respective compartment.
3. Sodium and its related anions (predominantly Cl^- and HCO_3^-) are primarily responsible for the osmotic attraction and retention of water in the extracellular fluid compartments (intravascular and interstitial). The endothelial membrane is freely permeable to these small electrolytes. Sodium is excluded from cells by Na^+, K^+-ATPase (adenosinetriphosphatase) in the cell membrane.
4. Large colloidal particles (albumin and globulins), to which the endothelial membrane is not readily permeable, are responsible for the osmotic attraction and retention of water in the intravascular compartment (oncotic pressure).
5. Naturally occurring fluid losses can be divided into four categories:
   a. Whole blood loss.
   b. Fluids lost through vomiting, diarrhea, diuresis, and third-space losses. Fluids lost have an electrolyte composition similar to that of extracellular fluid.
   c. Fluids lost as exudates, transudates, and some types of diarrhea. Fluids lost have an electrolyte composition similar to that of extracellular fluid but are higher in protein.
   d. Pure water loss (evaporation from the respiratory tract and skin). Fluids lost are derived proportionately from all three fluid compartments.
6. Some patients are presented with fluid and electrolyte disturbances that represent combinations of the above categories.
7. The clinical signs of an intravascular volume deficit are those associated with the normal compensatory response to hypovolemia: tachycardia and vasoconstriction (pale mucous membranes, prolonged capillary refill time, cool appendages), oliguria, high urine specific gravity. Pulse quality and

Table 4–18. Laboratory Reference Values for Dogs and Cats

	Dog	Cat
Blood volume (mL/kg)	80–90	50–55
Packed cell volume (%)	37–55	25–45
Hemoglobin (g/dL)	14–18	9–16
Total plasma protein (g/dL)	6.0–8.0	6.0–8.0
Heart rate (bpm)	70–140	110–140
Mean arterial pressure (mm Hg)	90–110	100–150
Cardiac output (mL/kg/min)	100–200	120
Central venous pressure (cm H_2O)	0–10	0–5
Respiratory rate (breaths/min)	10–30	24–42
Sodium (mEq/L)	140–150	150–160
Osmolality (mOsm/kg)	290–310	300–320
Potassium (mEq/L)	3.5–5.5	3.5–5.5
Bicarbonate (mEq/L)	18–26	18–23
Chloride (mEq/L)	105–115	115–125
Arterial pH	7.34–7.45	7.31–7.44
Arterial P_{CO_2} (mm Hg)	31–42	28–36
Arterial P_{O_2} (mm Hg)	85–105	100–115
Base deficit (mEq/L)	0 – – 4	–1 – –8
Core temperature (°C)	37–40	37–40

amplitude and central venous and arterial blood pressures usually are low. Hypovolemia of varying magnitude is expected in all categories of fluid loss.

8. An interstitial fluid deficit causes decreased skin turgor (i.e., tendency of the skin to retain its position after it has been lifted into a fold). An interstitial fluid deficit is expected in all categories of fluid loss except whole blood loss. A patient with decreased skin turgor is said to be dehydrated. A dehydrated patient is, by definition, hypovolemic, because the electrolyte composition of interstitial fluid is virtually identical to that of the intravascular compartment and the two are in equilibrium.

9. The diagnosis of an intracellular water deficit is based more on the presence of hypernatremia or hyperosmolality than on clinical signs. An intracellular water deficit is expected when free water loss (normal insensible and urinary losses and most fluids lost by vomiting, diarrhea, or diuresis contain free water) is not matched by free water intake.

10. The above considerations allow assessment of the volume of the fluid compartments. Also important in the development of a fluid therapy plan is the assessment of the concentrations of the important electrolytes in these fluid compartments (Table 4–18). The fluid therapy plan should accommodate alterations in these concentrations as well.

..........NORMAL VALUES AND INTERPRETATION OF ABNORMAL VALUES

..........History

Animals with a history of excessive fluid losses or inadequate fluid intake are expected to be volume deficient even if they do not exhibit signs of hypovolemia or dehydration.

..........Vasomotor Tone

Animals should have pink mucous membranes and a capillary refill time of about 1 second. Pale mucous membranes and a prolonged capillary refill time indicate vasoconstriction and, with a history of fluid loss, suggest hypovolemia. Pale mucous membranes also could be due to anemia. Vasoconstriction, while supporting blood pressure, diminishes peripheral (visceral) organ perfusion and, if prolonged, may contribute to organ failure. If vasoconstriction is thought to be due to hypovolemia, fluids should be administered in quantities sufficient to relieve the vasoconstriction.

·······Skin Turgor

The skin should return rapidly to its normal resting position after it has been lifted into a fold. If the skin tone returns slowly, the animal is said to be 5% dehydrated. If the skin stands in a fold, the animal is said to be 12% dehydrated. Intermediate skin pliability is estimated between 5% and 12% (e.g., dorsal, cervical, or lumbar region).

Skin turgor should be tested at the same location with the animal in the same position (e.g., standing or lateral recumbency) by the same person each time to minimize error. Skin turgor also is reduced by emaciation. Skin turgor should not be used as a guide to fluid therapy in emaciated patients; instead, administer fluids until other signs of dehydration are corrected (e.g., dry mucous membranes, vasoconstriction, decreased central venous pressure, oliguria). Obesity obscures decreases in skin turgor due to dehydration. Animals vary greatly in skin turgor response to dehydration; an animal may be very dehydrated and exhibit little or no decrease in skin turgor.

·······Packed Cell Volume

PCV is an indicator of the number of RBCs in the active circulation and consequently is an indicator of the oxygen-carrying capacity of the blood. PCVs below 20% in acute anemia, and 15% in chronic anemia may be associated with inadequate oxygen delivery to the tissues, especially in patients with debilitating systemic disease. RBCs should be administered to maintain the PCV above these levels.

·······Colloid Oncotic Pressure

Albumin is responsible for 65% and globulin for 15% of intravascular oncotic pressure. Albumin concentrations below 1.5 g/dL and total protein concentrations below 3.5 g/dL may be associated with inadequate fluid retention in the intravascular compartment. Plasma or artificial colloids (dextran 70 or hetastarch) should be administered to maintain total plasma protein above 3.5 g/dL.

·······Arterial Blood Pressure (see also p. 75)

Mean arterial pressures below 60 mm Hg and systolic blood pressures below 80 mm Hg may be associated with inadequate perfusion of the brain and heart. Blood pressure can be measured indirectly by Doppler blood flow (systolic) or oscillometric techniques or can be measured directly by arterial catheterization. Weak, thready pulses are more a measure of stroke volume than of blood pressure, although thready pulses and hypotension often occur together. Rapid blood volume expansion is the treatment of choice for hypovolemic hypotension.

·······Potassium (see also p. 720)

The ratio of intracellular to extracellular potassium concentration determines the resting membrane potential. Hyperkalemia (Table 4–19) decreases the resting potential, making the cell more susceptible to depolarization. Hyperka-

Table 4–19. Causes of Hyperkalemia

Pseudohyperkalemia
  Thrombocytosis
  Hemolysis
Increased intake
  Unlikely to cause hyperkalemia in presence of normal renal function unless
    iatrogenic (e.g., continuous infusion of potassium-containing fluids at an
    excessively rapid rate)
Translocation (ICF → ECF)
  Acute metabolic acidosis (e.g., HCl, NH_4Cl)
  Insulin deficiency (e.g., diabetic ketoacidosis)
  Acute tumor lysis syndrome
  Reperfusion of extremities after aortic thromboembolism in cats with
    cardiomyopathy
  Hyperkalemic periodic paralysis (one case report in a pit bull)
  Drugs
    Nonspecific β-blockers (e.g., propranolol)*
Decreased urinary excretion
  Urethral obstruction
  Ruptured bladder
  Anuric or oliguric renal failure
  Hypoadrenocorticism
  Selected gastrointestinal disease (e.g., trichuriasis, salmonellosis, perforated
    duodenal ulcer)
  Chylothorax with repeated pleural fluid drainage
  Hyporeninemic hypoaldosteronism
  Drugs
    ACE inhibitors (e.g., captopril, enalapril)*
    Potassium-sparing diuretics (e.g., spironolactone, amiloride, triamterene)*
    Prostaglandin inhibitors*
    Heparin*

ICF, intracellular fluid; ECF, extracellular fluid; ACE, angiotensin-converting enzyme.
*Only likely to cause hyperkalemia in conjunction with other contributing factors (e.g., decreased renal function, concurrent administration of potassium supplements.)
From DiBartola SP: Fluid Therapy in Small Animal Practice. Philadelphia, WB Saunders, 1992, p 108.

lemia usually is associated with characteristic changes in the electrocardiogram (ECG) (tall, tented T waves; small P waves; prolonged P–R intervals; widened QRS complexes) and may be associated with bradycardia, ventricular fibrillation, or asystole.

Hypokalemia (Table 4–20) increases the resting potential, hyperpolarizing the cell. Hypokalemia may be associated with U waves and ventricular arrhythmias, but the ECG changes are not as characteristic as they are with hyperkalemia.

Measured potassium concentrations below 3.0 or above 7.0 mEq/L require intervention. Inorganic metabolic acidosis increases plasma potassium concentration because potassium is redistributed from intracellular to extracellular fluid.

·····Bicarbonate

Hydrogen ion concentration has an important influence on the structure and function of proteins in cells. The metabolic contribution to acid–base balance

Table 4-20. Causes of Hypokalemia

Decreased intake
  Alone, unlikely to cause hypokalemia unless diet is aberrant
  Administration of potassium-free fluids (e.g., 0.9% NaCl, D5W)
Translocation (ECF → ICF)
  Alkalemia
  Insulin/glucose-containing fluids
  Catecholamines
  Hypothermia?
  Hypokalemic periodic paralysis (Burmese cats)
Increased loss
  Gastrointestinal (FE_K <6%)
  Vomiting of stomach contents
  Diarrhea
  Urinary (FE_K > 6%)
    Chronic renal failure in cats
    Diet-induced hypokalemic nephropathy in cats
    Distal (type I) RTA
    Proximal (type II) RTA after $NaHCO_3$ treatment
    Postobstructive diuresis
    Dialysis
    Mineralocorticoid excess
    Hyperadrenocorticism
    Primary hyperaldosteronism (adenoma, hyperplasia)
Drugs
  Loop diuretics (e.g., furosemide, ethacrynic acid)
  Thiazide diuretics (e.g., chlorothiazide, hydrochlorothiazide)
  Amphotericin B
  Penicillins

D5W, 5% dextrose in water; ECF, extracellular fluid; ICF, intracellular fluid; FE_K, excreted fraction of filtered potassium; RTA, renal tubular acidosis.
From DiBartola SP: Fluid Therapy in Small Animal Practice. Philadelphia, WB Saunders, 1992, p 99.

4

(Tables 4–21 and 4–22) can be estimated by measuring total carbon dioxide concentration or by measuring pH and partial pressure of carbon dioxide (PCO_2) and calculating bicarbonate or base deficit values. Acidemia is severe enough to warrant therapy if the bicarbonate concentration is below 12 mEq/L, if the base deficit is below −10 mEq/L, or if the pH is below 7.2.

...........Sodium and the Anion Gap

The volume of extracellular fluid is determined by total body sodium content, whereas the osmolality and sodium concentration of extracellular fluid are determined by water balance. Serum sodium concentration is an indication of the amount of sodium relative to the amount of water in extracellular fluid and provides no direct information about total body sodium content. Patients with hyponatremia or hypernatremia may have decreased, normal, or increased total body sodium content. An increased serum sodium concentration (see Table 4–23) implies hyperosmolality, whereas a decreased serum sodium concentration (see Table 4–24) usually, but not always, implies hypoosmolality. The severity of the clinical signs of hyponatremia and hypernatremia are related more to the rapidity of onset than to the magnitude of the associated plasma hypo- or hyperosmolality. Neurologic signs (e.g., disorientation, ataxia, sei-

Table 4–21. Causes of Metabolic Acidosis

Increased Anion Gap (Normochloremic)
Ethylene glycol intoxication
Salicylate intoxication
Other rare intoxications (e.g., paraldehyde, methanol)
Diabetic ketoacidosis*
Uremic acidosis†
Lactic acidosis

Normal Anion Gap (Hyperchloremic)
Diarrhea
Renal tubular acidosis
Carbonic anhydrase inhibitors (e.g., acetazolamide)
Ammonium chloride
Cationic amino acids (e.g., lysine, arginine, histidine)
Posthypocapnic metabolic acidosis
Dilutional acidosis (e.g., rapid administration of 0.9% saline)
Hypoadrenocorticism‡

---

*Patients with diabetic ketoacidosis may have some component of hyperchloremic metabolic acidosis in conjunction with increased anion gap acidosis.
†The metabolic acidosis early in renal failure may be hyperchloremic and later convert to increased anion gap acidosis.
‡Patients with hypoadrenocorticism typically present with uncorrected hypochloremia due to impaired water excretion (dilutional effect) and absence of aldosterone. Factors that may mask hyperchloremia include lactic acidosis and chronic vomiting.
From DiBartola SP: Fluid Therapy in Small Animal Practice. Philadelphia, WB Saunders, 1992, p 218.

---

zures, coma) may occur at serum sodium concentrations below 120 or above 170 mEq/L in dogs.

Therapy of hyponatremia with hypertonic saline or of hypernatremia with free water solutions (e.g., D5W) such that rapid changes occur in the extracellular sodium concentration may cause intracellular dehydration or edema, respectively, even though the actual measured sodium concentration has not been restored to normal. Therefore, it is essential to restore sodium concentrations to normal slowly, over the course of 48 to 72 hours. Treatment with 0.9% NaCl (for hyponatremia) or 0.45% NaCl (for hypernatremia) is recommended initially.

··········Osmolality (see also p. 772)

Osmolality is measured by freezing point depression or vapor pressure osmometry and may be calculated as $2([Na^+]+[K^+])+BUN/2.8 + glucose/18$, where

Table 4–22. Causes of Metabolic Alkalosis

Vomiting of stomach contents
Diuretic therapy (e.g., loop diuretics, thiazides)
Post hypercapnia
Primary hyperaldosteronism (rare)
Hyperadrenocorticism
Oral administration of sodium bicarbonate or other organic anions
  (e.g., lactate, citrate, gluconate, acetate)

From DiBartola SP: Fluid Therapy in Small Animal Practice. Philadelphia, WB Saunders, 1992, p 249.

Table 4–23. Causes of Hypernatremia

Pure Water Deficit
  Primary hypodipsia (e.g., miniature schnauzers)
  Diabetes insipidus
    Central
    Nephrogenic
  High environmental temperature
  Fever
  Inadequate access to water

Hypotonic Fluid Loss
  Extrarenal
    Gastrointestinal
      Vomiting
      Diarrhea
      Small intestinal obstruction
    Third-space loss
      Peritonitis
      Pancreatitis
    Cutaneous
      Burns
  Renal
    Appropriate
      Osmotic diuresis
        Diabetes mellitus
        Mannitol
      Chemical diuretics
    Inappropriate
      Chronic renal failure
      Nonoliguric acute renal failure
      Postobstructive diuresis

Impermeate Solute Gain
  Salt poisoning
  Hypertonic fluid administration
    Hypertonic saline
    Sodium bicarbonate
    Hyperalimentation fluid
    Sodium phosphate enema
  Hyperaldosteronism
  Hyperadrenocorticism

From DiBartola SP: Fluid Therapy in Small Animal Practice. Philadelphia, WB Saunders, 1992, p 64.

sodium and potassium are measured in milliequivalents and BUN and glucose in milligrams per deciliter. Osmolalities below 260 mOsm/kg or above 360 mOsm/kg are serious enough to warrant therapy.

The difference between the measured osmolality and the calculated osmolality (the osmolal gap) should be about 10 mOsm/kg. A value greater than 20 mOsm/kg suggests the presence of an unmeasured osmole (e.g., ethylene glycol metabolites).

···········BASICS OF ACID-BASE PHYSIOLOGY

Normal pH in dogs and cats ranges between 7.30 and 7.45. Blood pH is maintained by three major mechanisms: (1) buffer systems, (2) respiratory

Table 4–24. Causes of Hyponatremia

With normal plasma osmolality
  Hyperlipemia
  Hyperproteineima
With high plasma osmolality
  Hyperglycemia
  Mannitol infusion
With low plasma osmolality
      and
  Hypervolemia
    Severe liver disease
    Congestive heart failure
    Nephrotic syndrome
    Advanced renal failure
      and
  Normovolemia
    Psychogenic polydipsia
    Syndrome of inappropriate antidiuretic hormone secretion
    Antidiuretic drugs
    Myxedema coma of hypothyroidism
    Hypotonic fluid infusion
      and
  Hypovolemia
    Gastrointestinal loss
      Vomiting
      Diarrhea
    Third-space loss
      Pancreatitis
      Peritonitis
      Uroabdomen
      Chylothorax with repeated pleural fluid drainage
    Cutaneous loss
      Burns
  Hypoadrenocorticism
  Diuretic administration
  Salt-losing nephritis

From DiBartola SP: Fluid Therapy in Small Animal Practice. Philadelphia, WB Saunders, 1992, p 73.

mechanisms that alter P_{CO_2}, and (3) metabolic (i.e., renal) mechanisms that alter HCO_3^- (Table 4–25).

Hyperventilation decreases blood P_{CO_2}, producing alkalosis of respiratory origin. Hypoventilation increases P_{CO_2}, producing acidosis of respiratory origin. The normal canine P_{CO_2} in arterial blood (Pa_{CO_2}) is 31 to 42 mm Hg. In cats, the normal Pa_{CO_2} is 28 to 36 mm Hg. Venous P_{CO_2} values are 33 to 50 mm Hg in dogs and 33 to 45 mm Hg in cats. The metabolic influence on pH can be examined by looking at bicarbonate concentration. Venous and arterial blood bicarbonate concentrations in normal dogs are 18 to 26 mEq/L. In cats, the normal concentrations are 17 to 23 mEq/L.

To interpret the acid–base status of an animal:

1. Consider the patient's blood pH. If the pH is outside of the normal range, an acid–base disturbance is present. If the pH is within the normal range, an acid–base disturbance may or may not be present. If the patient is

Table 4–25. Acid–Base Values in Acute Uncompensated Disturbances

Disturbance	pH	P_{CO_2}	HCO_3^-	$\dfrac{HCO_3^-}{(0.03 \times P_{CO_2})}$
Metabolic acidosis	↓	—	↓	<20
Respiratory acidosis	↓	↑	—	<20
Metabolic alkalosis	↑	—	↑	>20
Respiratory alkalosis	↑	↓	↓	>20

acidemic and the plasma HCO_3^- concentration is decreased, *metabolic acidosis* is present. If the patient is acidemic and P_{CO_2} is increased, *respiratory acidosis* is present. If the patient is alkalemic and plasma the HCO_3^- concentration is increased, *metabolic alkalosis* is present. If the patient is alkalemic and P_{CO_2} is decreased, *respiratory alkalosis* is present.

2. Calculate the expected compensatory response in the opposing component of the system (e.g., respiratory alkalosis as compensation for metabolic acidosis, metabolic alkalosis as compensation for respiratory acidosis) using the rules of thumb listed in Table 4–26. These rules of thumb were established using arterial blood gas results from normal dogs and should not be used for cats until further information is available about the normal compensatory responses of cats. If the patient's secondary or adaptive response in the compensating component of the system falls within the expected range, a *simple* acid–base disturbance is likely present. If the adaptive response falls outside of the expected range, a *mixed* disorder is present.

3. Attempt to determine whether the acid–base disturbance(s) is (are) compatible with the patient's history and clinical findings. The original interpretation of the blood gas data must be questioned if the acid–base disturbance does not fit the patient's history, clinical findings, and other laboratory data.

The most desirable method of assessing the acid–base status of an animal is with a blood gas analyzer. Arterial samples are preferred over venous sam-

4

Table 4–26. Renal and Respiratory Compensations to Primary Acid–Base Disorders in Dogs

Disorder	Primary Change	Compensatory Response
Metabolic acidosis	↓ $[HCO_3^-]$	0.7-mm Hg decrement in P_{CO_2} for each 1-mEq/L decrement in $[HCO_3^-]$
Metabolic alkalosis	↑ $[HCO_3^-]$	0.7-mm Hg increment in P_{CO_2} for each 1-mEq/L increment in $[HCO_3^-]$
Acute respiratory acidosis	↑ P_{CO_2}	1.5-mEq/L increment in $[HCO_3^-]$ for each 10-mm Hg increment in P_{CO_2}
Chronic respiratory acidosis	↑ P_{CO_2}	3.5-mEq/L increment in $[HCO_3^-]$ for each 10-mm Hg increment in P_{CO_2}
Acute respiratory alkalosis	↓ P_{CO_2}	2.5-mEq/L decrement in $[HCO_3^-$ for each 10-mm Hg decrement in P_{CO_2}
Chronic respiratory alkalosis	↓ P_{CO_2}	5.5-mEq/L decrement in $[HCO_3^-]$ for each 10-mm Hg decrement in P_{CO_2}

From DiBartola SP: Fluid Therapy in Small Animal Practice. Philadelphia, WB Saunders, 1992, p 207.

ples, and heparin is used as an anticoagulant. Arterial samples are sometimes difficult to obtain, and venous samples often are used. Capillary blood can be collected from the ear or a clipped nail and is satisfactory, provided that capillary blood is free-flowing. Obtain blood samples in plastic syringes, and insert the needles into a rubber stopper. Blood samples can be stored for only 15 minutes at room temperature without significant changes in values. Storage in an ice-water bath allows extending the time in which analysis will be reasonably accurate for up to 4 hours.

The acid–base status of an animal can also be evaluated by using a commercial kit* to measure the total carbon dioxide and an expanded pH meter to measure blood pH. This type of testing has the advantage of being more economical and practical. The total CO_2 test measures the *amount* of carbon dioxide released when HCO_3^- in the serum is mixed with a strong acid. This test is an estimate of plasma HCO_3^- concentration when the sample is handled aerobically and includes both HCO_3^- and dissolved carbon dioxide ($0.03 \times P_{CO_2}$) when the sample is handled anaerobically.

............Anion Gap

Sodium is balanced electrically predominantly by the anions Cl^- and HCO_3^-, and the difference between these concentrations, $[Na^+] - ([Cl^-] + [HCO_3^-])$, has been called the anion gap (AG). When the AG exceeds 25, the clinician should suspect an accumulation of unmeasured anions (lactate, keto acid anions, phosphate, sulfate, ethylene glycol metabolites, salicylate).

An AG of 12 to 25 mEq/L is normal for dogs and cats. Abnormalities of the AG may be helpful in determining the cause of metabolic acidosis (Fig. 4–41).

............*Important Causes of Increased Anion Gap*

1. Diabetic ketoacidosis
2. Lactic acidosis
3. Certain intoxications (e.g., ethylene glycol, salicylate)
4. Uremia (e.g., phosphates, sulfates)

............*Important Causes of Decreased Anion Gap*

1. IgG myeloma
2. Hypoalbuminemia
3. Dilution of plasma proteins by infusion of a crystalloid solution
4. Potassium bromide therapy for refractory epilepsy (i.e., bromide measured as chloride)
5. Pseudohyponatremia

Changes in the serum concentrations of unmeasured cations (e.g., calcium, magnesium) great enough to have substantial effects on the AG would likely be incompatible with life.

............*Metabolic Acidosis and Anion Gap*

Metabolic acidosis associated with a **normal AG** (hyperchloremic metabolic acidosis):

*Harleco CO_2 Apparatus Set, Harleco Division, American Hospital Supply Corp., Philadelphia, PA.

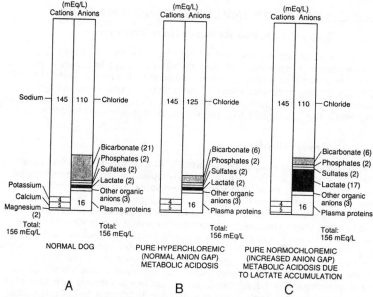

Figure 4–41. Theoretical examples of electrolyte distribution in (A) normal canine plasma, (B) a dog with pure hyperchloremic (normal anion gap) metabolic acidosis, and (C) a dog with normochloremic (increased anion gap) metabolic acidosis due to lactate accumulation (i.e., lactic acidosis). (Adapted from Toto RD: Metabolic acid–base disorders. *In* Kokko JP, Tannen RL, eds: Fluids and Electrolytes, ed 2. Philadelphia, WB Saunders, 1990, p 324.)

1. Diarrhea
2. Renal tubular acidosis
3. Early renal failure
4. Carbonic anhydrase inhibitors (e.g., acetazolamide)
5. Ammonium chloride
6. Cationic amino acids (e.g., lysine, arginine)
7. Posthypocapnic metabolic acidosis
8. Dilutional acidosis (e.g., rapid administration of 0.9% saline)
9. Some patients with diabetic ketoacidosis (i.e., efficient urinary excretion of ketones with renal retention of chloride)
10. Some cases of hypoadrenocorticism (uncorrected serum chloride concentration is low but when corrected for increased plasma water content, serum chloride concentration is normal or may be increased)

Metabolic acidosis associated with an **increased AG** (normochloremic metabolic acidosis):

1. Ethylene glycol intoxication
2. Salicylate intoxication
3. Other rare intoxications (e.g., paraldehyde, methanol)
4. Diabetic ketoacidosis
5. Uremic acidosis
6. Lactic acidosis

.............STEPS FOR IMPLEMENTING THERAPY
............Blood Volume Restoration Therapy

When evaluating an animal, first address its blood volume needs. If a dehydrated patient is hypovolemic or vasoconstricted, therapy to restore intravascular volume should be instituted and continued until the patient is out of danger. Life-threatening metabolic acidosis, hyperkalemia, hypoxemia, and hypoventilation also should be dealt with at this time. Oxygen therapy for hypoxemia and ventilation therapy for hypoventilation are not discussed in this section.

............Crystalloids

Begin intravascular volume replacement with a replacement solution such as lactated Ringer's solution, which has a composition similar to extracellular fluid (Table 4–27). These solutions are economical and readily available, and can be administered safely in large volumes to animals that do not have preexisting pulmonary edema, cerebral edema, or congestive heart failure without causing major changes in the concentrations of serum electrolytes. Measurement of central venous pressure can be helpful in guiding fluid therapy. Crystalloid solutions such as 0.9% NaCl or Ringer's solution do not contain organic anions that can be metabolized to bicarbonate. Consequently, they dilute extracellular bicarbonate, and cause dilutional acidosis when given in large quantities. Crystalloid solutions that are low in sodium, such as maintenance solutions (see Table 4–27) or D5W, are distributed to the intracellular fluid compartment and may cause detrimental CNS edema before adequate intravascular volume is restored.

Crystalloid fluids may have to be administered in quantities of 50 to 90 mL/kg or more to achieve adequate intravascular volume replacement. The cat has a smaller blood volume than the dog (see Table 4–18) and should receive proportionately less fluids. The specific endpoint of fluid administration is determined by monitoring the patient until the signs or measurements that indicated hypovolemia have normalized.

Crystalloid solutions are relatively ineffective intravascular volume expanders. After redistribution to the interstitial space (30 minutes), only one third of the infused volume remains in the vascular compartment. Thus, 2.5 to 3.0 times as much crystalloid solution must be given (as compared with a colloid solution) to effectively restore intravascular volume.

Early in the course of crystalloid fluid therapy, the PCV and total protein concentration should be measured. Administration of large volumes of crystalloid fluids may cause excessive hemodilution, especially in patients with preexisting anemia or hypoproteinemia.

............Whole Blood (see also p. 46)

If the PCV is below 20% or is likely to be reduced below 20% with crystalloid fluid therapy, PRBCs or whole blood should be administered as part of the fluid therapy program. Blood can be anticoagulated with ACD or CPD. Use CPD-A$_1$ if blood is to be stored; RBCs will be 70% viable for up to 4 weeks. After 4 weeks the plasma can be separated and stored frozen for up to 1 year; the RBCs should be discarded.

Canine Blood Approximately 15% of random first-time canine blood transfusions should be associated with a transfusion reaction due to naturally occurring alloantibodies. In practice, the frequency appears to be much lower, presumably because most reactions are subclinical. The frequency of clinical transfusion reactions will increase with repeated random transfusions. Even if donor blood is typed, in vitro crossmatching is recommended (see p. 49) before transfusion if the recipient has received a previous transfusion. Crossmatching is desirable even for first-time transfusions. Dogs kept as blood donors should be typed to be sure they are DEA-1.1-negative and DEA-1.2-negative.

Feline Blood Only two RBC antigens, A and B, have been identified in the domestic cat. In the United States, almost all domestic short-hair and long-hair cats are type A. Approximately 20% of purebred cats (e.g., Abyssinian, Persian) have type B blood. Type B cats have strong natural isoagglutinins against type A RBCs that can result in serious transfusion reactions. Consequently, pretransfusion crossmatching is recommended.

The amount of blood to be administered is calculated as 10 to 40 mL/kg (in the dog) or 5 to 20 mL/kg (in the cat); these ranges represent small to large transfusions. A dose of 22 mL/kg of whole blood or 10 mL/kg of PRBCs is expected to increase the PCV by approximately 10%. The post-transfusion PCV should be measured to determine whether the desired elevation has been achieved.

Infused blood should be filtered. Blood should be administered slowly (5 to 10 mL/kg/hr) so that reactions can be detected early and the infusion stopped, if necessary. Immunologic transfusion reactions may be manifested by restlessness, acute collapse, hypotension, dyspnea, urticaria, hemoglobinemia, hemoglobinuria, or fever. If any of these signs develop during a blood transfusion, the transfusion should be stopped immediately and the patient treated with glucocorticoids or antihistamines as necessary.

Autotransfusion of whole blood should be considered if the animal is bleeding excessively into the pleural or peritoneal cavity and an exogenous source of whole blood is not readily available. Blood for autotransfusion should be gently aspirated, anticoagulated, and filtered.

·········· Colloid Therapy

If the total protein concentration is below 3.5 g/dL or is likely to be reduced below this value with crystalloid therapy, plasma or a plasma substitute (e.g., dextran, hetastarch) should be administered as part of the fluid therapy regimen. Colloids are more effective intravascular volume expanders than are crystalloids and should be considered when the patient does not respond appropriately to crystalloid fluid infusion or when edema develops prior to adequate intravascular volume replacement. Colloids, although more expensive than crystalloids, promote better tissue perfusion at lower infusion volumes and equivalent colloid oncotic pressures and mean blood pressures.

Plasma may be separated from whole blood by centrifugation or gravity. Plasma infusion will result in an increase in plasma volume equivalent to approximately 50% of the infused volume.

Dextran 70 is a high-molecular-weight polysaccharide with a half-life of about 12 to 24 hours and a refractometric index of 4.6 g/dL. Dextran 70 will increase blood volume by 60% to 75% of the infused volume. Particles with molecular weights below 50,000 are rapidly excreted by the kidneys; larger particles are metabolized slowly by the liver. Overly rapid administration of dextran 70 may be associated with hemorrhagic diathesis. Approximately 5 to 10 mL/kg/hr is the proper dosage. Any hemorrhagic diathesis that does occur should subside within a few hours after cessation of the dextran infusion. The total daily dosage should not exceed 40 mL/kg/day.

Hetastarch (hydroxyethyl starch) has a molecular weight higher than 100,000 and a half-life of about 24 to 36 hours. Hetastarch will increase blood volume by about 50% of the infused volume. Like dextran, hetastarch can cause coagulopathy when infused too rapidly or in too large a volume. Hetastarch can be administered in volumes up to 30 mL/kg/day.

Table 4-27. Electrolyte Composition of Commercially Available Fluids

Solution	Glucose (g/L)	Na$^+$ (mEq/L)	Cl$^-$ (mEq/L)	K$^+$ (mEq/L)	Ca^{+2} (mEq/L)	Mg^{+2} (mEq/L)	Buffer (mEq/L)	Other Solute	Osmolarity (mOsm/L)	Calories (kcal/L)	pH
Solution Formulated to Replace a Water Deficit											
5% dextrose	50	0	0	0	0	0	0		252	170	4.0
Maintenance Solutions											
2.5% dextrose in 0.45% NaCl	25	77	77	0	0	0	0		280	85	4.0
2.5% dextrose in half-strength lactated Ringer's	25	65.5	55	2	1.5	0	14(L)		263	89	5.0
0.45% NaCl	0	77	77	0	0	0	0		154	0	5.0
Ionosol-T	50	40	40	35	0	0	20(L)		387	170	4.7
Normosol-M in 5% dextrose	50	40	40	13	0	3	16(A)		364	175	5.2
Plasma-Lyte 56	0	40	40	13	0	3	16(A)		112	5	5.5
Plasma-Lyte M in 5% dextrose	50	40	40	16	5	3	12(A) 12(L)		380	178	5.0
Replacement Solutions											
2.5% dextrose in lactated Ringer's	25	130	109	4	3	0	28(L)		398	94	5.0
5% dextrose in lactated Ringer's	50	130	109	4	3	0	28(L)		524	179	5.0
5% dextrose in 0.9% NaCl	50	154	154	0	0	0	0		560	170	4.0
0.9% NaCl	0	154	154	0	0	0	0		308	0	5.0
Ringer's	0	147.5	156	4	4.5	0	0		310	0	6.0
Lactated Ringer's	0	130	109	4	3	0	28(L)		272	9	6.5
Multisol-R	0	140	98	5	0	0	27(A) 23(G)		293	15	6.4

Normosol-R	0	140	98	5	0	3	27(A) 23(G)		296	15	6.4
Plasma-Lyte R	0	140	103	10	5	3	47(A) 8(L)		316	17	5.5
Plasma-Lyte 148	0	140	98	5	0	3	27(A) 23(G)		296	15	5.5
Normal Plasma Composition											
Dog	1	146	110	4.5	5	2.5	21(B)		300	—	7.36
Cat	1	156	120	4.5	4.5	2.0	19(B)		310	—	7.34
Special Solutions and Additives											
10% dextrose	100	0	0	0	0	0	0		505	340	4.0
20% mannitol	200(M)	0	0	0	0	0	0		1098	0	—
5% NaHCO$_3^-$	0	595	0	0	0	0	595(B)		1190	0	8.0
8.4% NaHCO$_3^-$	0	1000	0	0	0	0	1000(B)		2000	0	8.0
10% CaCl$_2$	0	0	2720	0	1360	0	0		4080	0	—
10% calcium gluconate	0	0	0	0	460	0	920(G)		1380	0	—
15% KCl	0	0	2000	2000	0	0	0		4000	0	—
50% dextrose	500	0	0	0	0	0	0		2780	1700	4.2
Colloids											
6% dextran 70 in 0.9% NaCl	0	154	154	0	0	0	0	D70 60 g	308	0	5.0
10% dextran 40 in 0.9% NaCl	50	154	154	0	0	0	0	D40 100 g	308	0	5.0
10% dextran 40 in 5% dextrose	00	0	0	0	0	0	0	D40 100 g	308	0	4.5
Hypertonic Saline Solutions											
3% NaCl	0	513	0	0	0	0	0		1026	0	5.0
5% NaCl	0	856	856	0	0	0	0		1712	0	5.0

A, acetate; B, bicarbonate; D40, dextran 40; D70, dextran 70; G, gluconate; L, lactate; M, mannitol.

.... *Alkalinization Therapy*

Animals with markedly reduced blood volume may suffer severe metabolic acidosis secondary to poor tissue perfusion. Treatment of metabolic acidosis is aimed at correction of the underlying disease process. Bicarbonate therapy may be indicated to support the pH of the patient until the underlying disease process can be stabilized. Bicarbonate therapy should always be conservative, with regard to both total dose and rate of administration, and frequently can be avoided. Bicarbonate should be administered if the blood pH is below 7.1 to 7.2 or if the bicarbonate concentration is below 12 mEq/L.

The dose of bicarbonate to administer can be determined in either of the following ways:

1. Multiply the base deficit $\times$ 0.3 $\times$ body weight in kilograms, where 0.3 $\times$ body weight (kg) is an estimate of the extracellular fluid volume and the early redistributive fluid space of the administered bicarbonate.
2. Use 1 to 2 mEq/kg of body weight (for moderate or severe degrees of acidosis, respectively).

Sufficient bicarbonate should be administered to restore the pH to at least 7.2 or the bicarbonate concentration to 10 mEq/L or more.

Potential complications of bicarbonate therapy include volume overload due to administered sodium, tetany from decreased serum ionized calcium concentration due to increased binding of calcium to plasma proteins, decreased oxygen delivery to tissues due to increased affinity of hemoglobin for oxygen, paradoxical CNS acidosis as hyperventilation abates and carbon dioxide diffuses into CSF, late development of alkalosis as metabolism of organic anions (e.g., ketoanions, lactate) replenishes body bicarbonate stores, and hypokalemia as potassium ions enter and hydrogen ions exit intracellular fluid in response to alkalinization of extracellular fluid.

.... *Therapy for Hyperkalemia*

Life-threatening hyperkalemia (see Table 4–19), indicated by severe ECG disturbances, should be treated. Calcium (2 to 10 ml of a 10% solution of calcium gluconate administered slowly IV with ECG monitoring) antagonizes the effect of hyperkalemia on the heart. The effects of calcium are short-lived (<1 hour), lasting only until the calcium is redistributed into its storage compartments. Glucose works by stimulating endogenous insulin release and moving potassium into cells. Its effects begin within an hour and last a few hours. Glucose-containing fluids (5% or 10% dextrose) or 50% dextrose (1 to 2 mL/kg) can be used for this purpose. Unless the patient is diabetic, administration of insulin with glucose usually is unnecessary and may cause hypoglycemia. Some clinicians do use insulin (0.55 to 1.1 units/kg regular insulin added to parenteral fluids) with glucose (2 g dextrose per unit insulin added). Sodium bicarbonate also works by moving K+ into cells as H+ ions leave cells to titrate administered bicarbonate in the extracellular fluid. Bicarbonate begins to work within an hour and its effects last a few hours. The usual dose is 1 to 2 mEq/kg IV and it can be repeated if necessary.

.... **Total Body Water and Electrolyte Restoration Therapy** (see Table 4–28)

When life-threatening hypovolemia has been corrected or is not present, the remaining fluid and electrolyte abnormalities can be managed. Three categories should be considered when developing a fluid therapy plan.

1. *The deficit.* How much and what type of fluid will be needed to restore the patient to normal?
2. *The maintenance.* How much and what type of fluid will be needed to accommodate the normal daily losses?
3. *The ongoing losses.* How much and what type of fluid will be needed to accommodate contemporary or ongoing losses (e.g., vomiting, diarrhea, polyuria)?

............Deficit Volume

An animal may be determined qualitatively to be dehydrated by clinical signs (e.g., reduced skin turgor, dry mucous membranes, oliguria, hemoconcentration, peripheral vasoconstriction). These signs do not, however, provide a quantitative estimate of the volume of fluids that should be administered. An acute change in body weight can be used as a quantitative guide to the volume of the deficit. Lean body mass normally is not lost or gained rapidly enough to produce major acute changes in body weight. Large volumes of fluid can accumulate in the intestinal lumen, in body cavities (e.g., peritoneal or pleural space), or in traumatized tissues and reduce effective extracellular fluid volume without changing body weight (so-called third-space loss). Changes in skin turgor often are the only quantitative indications of the magnitude of the existing deficit. If skin turgor is thought to be misleading because of obesity or emaciation, fluids should be administered until the qualitative signs are normalized.

Table 4–28. Outline of the Very Simple Fluid Therapy Planning Guide

1. Calculate a quantitative estimate of the deficit volume.
2. Start with lactated Ringer's or an equivalent replacement solution.
3. Supplement or do not supplement potassium.
4. Decide whether, and how much, bicarbonate to supplement.
5. Decide whether the sodium aberrations are severe enough to warrant switching from lactated Ringer's to one-half lactated Ringer's and one-half 5% dextrose in water or to saline plus sodium bicarbonate.
6. Calculate the maintenance volume requirement,* and administer as the predetermined maintenance solution.
7. Estimate or measure the abnormal ongoing losses as they occur, and replace as lactated Ringer's solution with or without potassium supplementation.
8. Round up and combine fluid volumes from all categories, and establish a convenient and practical plan for the order in which the fluids will be administered.
9. Divide the total volume of fluids to be administered by the number of hours available to determine the hourly infusion rate. If a route other than the intravenous route is to be used, decide on volumes and treatment intervals.
10. Distribute the additives to the individual fluid bottles as prescribed.
11. Calculate the rate of potassium infusion to ascertain that it abides by the rules of potassium therapy.
12. Monitor the patient during the day to make sure that all is going according to plan.

*See Maintenance (Normal Ongoing Losses), p. 604.

.... *Deficit Repair Fluid*

Lactated Ringer's solution or a similar replacement solution approximating extracellular fluid in composition usually (see Table 4–27) is a good choice for restoration of deficit volume. This replacement fluid should be administered without alteration when the dehydration is known to be due to accumulation of fluid within the intestinal lumen, peritoneal or pleural cavities, or traumatized tissues, or when the nature of the fluid loss is not known or cannot be estimated, or when electrolyte concentrations cannot be measured. The adequacy of the deficit repair solution to meet the needs of the patient may be improved by addressing the potassium, bicarbonate, chloride, and sodium needs of the patient.

.... Potassium Concentration

Abnormalities in potassium concentration, particularly hypokalemia, are common:

1. Some fluids that are lost (e.g., GI secretions) contain potassium in concentrations in excess of the normal extracellular fluid concentration.
2. To maintain extracellular fluid volume, the kidneys must reabsorb sodium by all available mechanisms. If there is a deficit of chloride (e.g., vomiting of stomach contents), the kidneys must reabsorb less sodium with chloride and more sodium in exchange for hydrogen and potassium ions. The latter two mechanisms contribute to perpetuation of the metabolic alkalosis and development of potassium depletion.
3. Many critically ill patients are anorectic and thus have no dietary replacement of lost potassium. Potassium balance is most easily evaluated by measuring serum potassium concentration. Nonorganic acidoses (but not organic acidoses) will increase and alkalosis will tend to decrease serum potassium concentration, but the extent of this change is very variable.

Increased potassium intake, translocation of potassium from intracellular to extracellular fluid, and decreased urinary excretion of potassium are the settings in which hyperkalemia develops. Increased intake is likely to be contributory only during excessive infusion of potassium-rich fluids or in the face of impaired renal excretion. Translocation of potassium from cells to extracellular fluid may occur with acute mineral acidosis, insulin deficiency, and acute tumor lysis syndrome. The most common disorders associated with decreased urinary excretion of potassium are urethral obstruction, ruptured bladder, anuric or oliguric renal failure, and hypoadrenocorticism. In these patients, a potassium-free fluid, such as 0.9% NaCl, is preferable to lactated Ringer's solution. The small amount of potassium in lactated Ringer's solution, however, should not be a major concern, and these solutions could be administered to all patients except those with life-threatening hyperkalemia, as long as effective therapy is instituted for hyperkalemia.

Decreased intake, translocation of potassium from extracellular to intracellular fluid, and increased GI or urinary loss of potassium may cause hypokalemia. Often, hypokalemia results from a combination of chronic anorexia, loss of muscle mass, and ongoing urinary or GI losses. Decreased intake may aggravate existing hypokalemia, but alone is unlikely to cause hypokalemia in dogs and cats. Hypokalemia commonly occurs during administration of potassium-free fluids, especially those containing glucose. Translocation of potassium from extracellular to intracellular fluid may occur with acute alkalosis or insulin-mediated glucose uptake by cells. Excessive GI (e.g., vomiting, diarrhea) and urinary (e.g., polyuric renal failure, postobstructive diuresis, loop diuretics) losses of potassium are common causes of hypokalemia in dogs and cats (see

Table 4–20). If the plasma potassium concentration is known, potassium may be added accordingly to the deficit repair solution (Table 4–29). If the potassium concentration is not measured, estimate the magnitude of the hypokalemia, based on the type and severity of the underlying disease processes. Mild hypokalemia might be expected if the fluid loss has been via vomiting, diarrhea, or diuresis but the animal has been eating. Moderate hypokalemia might be expected if the animal has not been eating, and has experienced abnormal GI or renal losses. Severe hypokalemia might be expected if the anorexia has been of long duration, if the abnormal GI or renal losses have been severe and of long duration, or if the animal is a ketoacidotic diabetic (the measured serum potassium concentration may not be very low, but total body potassium stores are very low and insulin and glucose therapy will cause intracellular redistribution of potassium and result in severe hypokalemia). If the potassium depletion is judged to be mild, moderate, or severe, add potassium at 20 to 40 mEq/L to the deficit repair solution.

More aggressive potassium supplementation should be accompanied by regular ECG monitoring for the electrical changes associated with iatrogenic hyperkalemia (tall, spiked T waves; small P waves; prolonged P–R intervals; bradycardia; widened QRS complexes; and prolonged Q–T intervals). Diseases such as hypoadrenocorticism can be difficult to diagnose before the first fluid therapy plan is implemented, and such patients may be hyperkalemic without any overt signs and will be intolerant of potassium loading. Potassium should not be administered at rates greater than 0.5 mEq/kg/hr.

············ Bicarbonate Concentration

Volume restoration alone results in self-correction of mild to moderate metabolic acidosis in many patients. Patients with moderate to severe metabolic acidosis (see Table 4–21) may benefit from bicarbonate therapy.

There are two types of vomiting: that in which the fluids come predominantly from the stomach and that in which fluids come from the stomach and the duodenum (after reflux of the fluids into the stomach). An animal that vomits as a result of pyloric obstruction is expected to be alkalotic. The bicarbonate concentration of the fluids lost by the "duodenal vomiter" is high compared with that in normal extracellular fluid because pancreatic secretions have very high bicarbonate concentrations. Consequently, the duodenal vomiter is expected to be acidotic. Duodenal vomiting is the more common of the two types and can be verified by observing green (bile) or yellow (gastric) coloration in the vomitus. Lactated Ringer's solution is a good deficit repair solution for

Table 4–29. Guidelines for Routine Intravenous Supplementation of Potassium in Dogs and Cats*

Serum Potassium Concentration (mEq/L)	mEq KCl to Add to 250 mL Fluid	mEq KCl to Add to 1 L Fluid	Maximal Fluid Infusion Rate (mL/kg/hr)
<2.0	20	80	6
2.1–2.5	15	60	8
2.6–3.0	10	40	12
3.1–3.5	7	28	18
3.6–5.0	5	20	25

*Do not exceed 0.5 mEq/kg/hr.

the duodenal vomiter. Normal saline, by virtue of its high chloride content (154 mEq/L), is indicated when the patient is a "gastric vomiter."

The metabolic contribution to acid–base balance is identified by measuring the total carbon dioxide content or calculating the bicarbonate concentration from pH and P_{CO_2} measurements. If these measurements are not available, one must estimate the acid–base disturbance from the severity of the underlying disturbance.

Mild, moderate, or severe acidemia is expected if the underlying disease is mild, moderate, or severe, and is known to be associated with acidemia: hypovolemic or traumatic shock, septic shock, ketoacidotic diabetes mellitus, or oliguric or anuric renal failure.

If measurements have provided a quantitative base deficit value, the amount of bicarbonate to add to the deficit repair solution is given by the equation: base deficit $\times$ 0.3 $\times$ kg of body weight. If the metabolic acidosis is estimated to be mild, moderate, or severe, add sodium bicarbonate at 1, 3, or 5 mEq/kg of body weight, respectively, to the deficit repair solution. The acidotic diabetic may not require much bicarbonate, because metabolism of the keto acids will have an alkalinizing effect.

.... Sodium Concentration

In the absence of a serum sodium concentration, an animal is expected to be hypernatremic if it has suffered an exogenous fluid loss and has not been drinking water, and is expected to be hyponatremic if water consumption has continued in the presence of the fluid loss.

In almost all circumstances, volume restoration will allow the animal to restore its own sodium balance. If the hypernatremia persists after repair of dehydration, subsequent fluids should contain a lower sodium concentration (e.g., 0.45% NaCl in 2.5% dextrose). If hyponatremia persists after repair of the dehydration, subsequent fluids should be changed to 0.9% NaCl (sodium 154 mEq/L).

.... *Maintenance (Normal Ongoing Losses)*

The volume of fluids required to replace the normal ongoing losses can be determined from predictive charts (Tables 4–30 and 4–31). if a chart is not available, the maintenance volume is assumed to be 40 to 60 mL/kg/day (higher values per kilogram for smaller dogs and cats and lower values per kilogram for larger dogs and cats).

The nature of the fluids used for maintenance is distinctly different from that of fluids used to replace extracellular volume deficits. The average concentration of normal urine and insensible losses is 40 to 50 mEq/L, and the potassium concentration is 15 to 20 mEq/L. Administration of a replacement solution to an animal for its maintenance requirements predisposes to hypernatremia (most animals are able to eliminate the excess sodium) and hypokalemia.

Lactated Ringer's solution or equivalent replacement solutions are poor maintenance solutions because they predispose to hypernatremia and hypokalemia. In one version of a homemade maintenance solution, a replacement solution is supplemented with potassium (15 to 20 mEq/L) to accommodate the potassium losses that normally occur. A further modification is dilution of the replacement solution with one to two parts of D5W per one part of replacement solution. The easiest approach is to use commercial maintenance solutions.

Maintenance solutions, likewise, should not be used to replace extracellular volume deficits because they may cause hyponatremia and hyperkalemia when administered in large volumes. If a patient is receiving a maintenance solution

Table 4–30. Approximate Daily Energy and Water Requirements of Dogs Based on Body Weight*

Body Weight (kg)	Total Energy (kcal) or Water (mL)		
	Per Day	Per Kilogram	Per Hour
1	132	132	5.5
2	222	111	9.5
3	301	100	12.5
4	373	93	15.5
5	441	88	18.5
6	506	84	21
7	568	81	23.5
8	628	78	26
9	686	76	28.5
10	742	74	31
11	797	72	33
12	851	71	35.5
13	904	70	37.5
14	955	68	40
15	1006	67	42
16	1056	66	44
17	1105	65	46
18	1154	64	48
19	1201	63	50
20	1248	62	52
21	1295	62	54
22	1341	61	56
23	1386	60	58
24	1431	60	59.5
25	1476	59	61.5
26	1520	58	63.5
27	1564	58	65
28	1607	57	67
29	1650	57	68.5
30	1692	56	70.5
35	1899	54	79
40	2100	52	87.5
45	2293	51	95.5
50	2482	50	103.5
55	2666	48	111
60	2846	47	118.5
70	3195	46	133
80	3531	44	147
90	3857	43	161
100	4174	42	174

*132 kcal/kg$^{0.75}$.

From Nutritional Requirements of the Dog, National Research Council, Bethesda, MD, 1985.

Table 4–31. Approximate Daily Energy and Water Requirements of Cats Based on Body Weight*

Body Weight (kg)	Total Energy (kcal) or Water (mL)		
	Per Day	Per Kilogram	Per Hour
1.0	80.0	80	3
1.5	108.4	72	5
2.0	134.5	67	6
2.5	159.1	64	7
3.0	182.4	61	8
3.5	204.7	58	9
4.0	226.3	57	9
4.5	247.2	55	10
5.0	267.5	53	11

*80 kcal/kg$^{0.75}$.
From Nutritional Requirements of the Cat, National Research Council, Bethesda, MD, 1987.

and is noted to be dehydrated or hypotensive, a replacement solution should be administered.

..........Abnormal Ongoing Losses

Ongoing losses that occur via transudation into one of the major body cavities, into the tissues, or through burn wounds are similar in composition to extracellular fluid and should be replaced with lactated Ringer's solution or an equivalent replacement solution. Ongoing losses that occur via vomiting, diarrhea, or diuresis should be replaced with lactated Ringer's solution or an equivalent solution that has been supplemented with potassium (10 to 30 mEq/L). One exception is the patient that has been chronically vomiting stomach contents, a situation in which 0.9% NaCl supplemented with potassium (10 to 30 mEq/L) is recommended.

When the fluid therapy plan is being developed, it is not known how much fluid the animal will lose over the day. One can leave this category blank initially and then, as losses occur during the day, add equivalent volumes of the appropriate fluid to the fluid therapy regimen. Alternatively, if the patient has a disease that is known to be associated with severe ongoing fluid losses (e.g., parvovirus gastroenteritis), one can fill in an estimated volume initially and then adjust upward or downward as the day progresses.

..........IMPLEMENTING THE FLUID THERAPY PLAN

The fluid therapy prescription is the best guess as to the requirements of the patient. It is important to try and enact a fluid therapy regimen that is as close as possible to the prescription; however, considering the inherent inaccuracies in the assumptions used to construct the prescription, it is not imperative to administer exactly what has been prescribed. There are many acceptable ways to administer the prescribed fluids. One way is to mix all of the fluids and additives from each category into one large bottle and administer them throughout the day. Another way is to administer the fluids simultaneously, in parallel, throughout the day in one administration line. A third way is to administer the fluids in series. Administer the prescribed fluids in a manner that is convenient for your practice situation.

1. To determine the rate of IV infusion of the fluids and additives, take the total volume of the fluids that have been prescribed and divide the total volume by the total number of hours in the day that are available for safe administration of the fluids. There should be no need to front-load the deficit repair fluid volume as long as the intravascular volume has been stabilized previously.
2. Administer the fluids over as many hours as possible to allow the patient as much time as possible to redistribute and fully utilize the administered fluids and electrolytes. With faster administration, a diuresis will occur and more of the fluids will be excreted in urine. Fluids should not be administered continuously IV when the patient cannot be observed periodically to ascertain if the fluids are continuing to run at an appropriate rate and that the administration line has not become disconnected. If the available time is limited (i.e., less than 12 hours) or if extra time is needed for safe administration of the fluids, an alternative plan (e.g., administering some of the required fluids SC) is indicated.
3. IV administration of fluids is the preferred route because the fluid is rapidly dispersed and immediately available to the patient. IV administration may be inconvenient in some practice settings. The prescribed fluid can be administered SC in several divided doses. The SC route is usually well tolerated by patients, and therapy often is efficacious. However, the SC route is slower in onset than the IV route, is less efficacious than the IV route because some patients (especially those that are severely dehydrated and vasoconstricted) do not absorb the fluids well or at all, and it carries a slight risk of infection. Fluids can be administered PO or via stomach tube, in several divided doses, as long as the GI tract is functional. Fluids also can be administered intraperitoneally. The intraperitoneal route is characterized by the same advantages and disadvantages as the SC route, but in addition there is a danger of injury or perforation of an abdominal organ. Fluids can also be administered via the intramedullary route. Intramedullary administration is more difficult than SC or intraperitoneal administration, but is associated with much more rapid and reliable systemic uptake. The intramedullary route may be useful when venous access is difficult (e.g., a severely dehydrated kitten or puppy).
4. Fluids may be administered through central or peripheral veins. Indwelling catheters must be introduced and maintained aseptically. All fluids and administration sets must be sterile. Fluids with osmolalities below 600 mOsm/L can be safely administered via a peripheral vein. Fluids with osmolalities above 700 mOsm/L should be administered via a large central vein, because hyperosmolar fluids may cause thrombophlebitis if administered via small peripheral veins.
5. It is difficult to control the infusion rate when fluids are administered by gravity. This problem is eliminated by use of an infusion pump.

............RATES OF ADMINISTRATION
............Establishing Rates of Flow

Differences among IV infusion sets:

- Cutter—20 drops/mL
- Abbott and McGaw—15 drops/mL
- McGaw—15 drops/mL
- Travenol—10 drops/mL

To calculate drops per minute:

$$\frac{\text{Fluid volume to be infused (mL)}}{\text{No. of hours available (hr)}} = \text{mL/hr}$$

For adult drip sets:

Cutter: $\text{mL/hr} \div 3 = \text{drops/min}$
Abbott and McGaw: $\text{mL/hr} \div 4 = \text{drops/min}$
Travenol: $\text{mL/hr} \div 6 = \text{drops/min}$

Most pediatric drip sets deliver 60 drops/mL ($\text{mL/hr} = \text{drops/min}$). Fluid orders should be written so that the volume to be administered is recorded as mL/day, mL/hr, and drops/min. This will allow personnel to detect major calculation errors more easily. The clinician should not assume that the animal has received the volume of fluid ordered, and the volume actually received should be noted in the record by nursing personnel. All additives should be clearly listed on the bottle; adhesive labels for this purpose are available. A strip of adhesive tape can be attached to the bottle and marked appropriately to provide a quick visual estimate of the volume of fluid received.

REFERENCES

Chew DJ, Kohn CW, DiBartola SP: Disorders of fluid balance and fluid therapy. *In* Fenner WR, ed: Quick Reference to Veterinary Medicine, ed 2. Philadelphia, JB Lippincott, 1991, pp 561–585.
Crowe DT: Autotransfusion in the trauma patient. Vet Clin North Am Small Anim Pract, 10:581–597, 1981.
de Morais HSA, Chew DJ: Use and interpretation of serum and urine electrolytes. Semin Vet Med Surg (Small Anim) 7:262–274, 1992.
DiBartola SP: Fluid Therapy in Small Animal Practice. Philadelphia, WB Saunders, 1992, p 720.
Haskins SC: A simple fluid therapy planning guide. Semin Vet Med Surg (Small Anim) 3:227–236, 1988.
Ilkiw JE, Rose RJ, Martin ICA: A comparison of simultaneously collected arterial, mixed venous, jugular venous, and cephalic venous blood samples is assessment of blood gas and acid base status in the dog. J Vet Intern Med 5:294–298, 1991.
Mathews KA: The various types of parenteral fluids and their indications. Vet Clin North Am Small Anim Pract 28:483, 1998.
Otto CM, McCall-Kauffman G, Crowe DT: Intraosseus infusion of fluids and therapeutics. Compend Contin Educ Pract Vet 11:421–430, 1989.
Phillips S, Polzin D: Clinical disorders of potassium homeostasis: Hyperkalemia and hypokalemia. Vet Clin North Am Small Anim Pract 28:545, 1998.
Schaer M.: Advances in fluid and electrolyte disorders. Vet Clin North Am Small Anim Pract 28:1998.
Schaer M, ed: Fluid and electrolyte disorders. *In* Vet Clin North Am Small Anim Pract 203–385, 1989.
Smiley LE: The use of hetastarch for plasma expansion. Probl Vet Med 4:652, 1992.
Willard MD: Disorders of potassium homeostasis. Vet Clin North Am Small Anim Pract 19:241–263, 1989.
Wingfield WE: Veterinary Emergency Medicine Secrets. Philadelphia, Hanley & Belfus, 1997.

Nebulization Therapy

Inhalation therapy is most useful for humidifying air in the respiratory tract and moistening the mucous membranes. Drying causes irritation, which in turn causes swelling, bronchial gland hypertrophy, goblet cell proliferation, and loss of ciliary epithelium. Respiratory secretions become thick and tenacious, and efficient bronchial drainage is impaired.

·········· OBJECTIVES

The aims of aerosol therapy are:

1. Humidification of bronchial mucous membranes
2. Deposition of minuscule amounts of potent drugs in smaller airways to obtain optimal topical therapeutic effects with minimal systemic side effects (e.g., bronchodilators)
3. Deposition of moderate amounts of potent agents or agents that are only effective topically (e.g., antibiotics and mucolytics)
4. Deposition of relatively large quantities of bland substances that promote bronchial drainage with minimal irritation (e.g., saline, propylene glycol, glycerine, detergents)

Nebulization therapy is used (1) in combination with oxygen therapy; (2) in tracheostomy care; (3) in acute respiratory diseases such as tracheobronchitis, bronchiolitis, upper respiratory disease of cats, pneumonia, and postoperative atelectasis and pneumonia; and (4) in chronic respiratory diseases such as chronic bronchitis, bronchopneumonia, collapsed trachea with secondary tracheobronchitis, emphysema, and bronchiectasis.

·········· PRINCIPLES OF ACTION

Large water particles (10 to 60 μm) in the high-velocity air flow of the nose and throat settle on the mucosa of the larynx, nose, and throat. Particles smaller than 10 μm (2 to 10 μm) are deposited in the bronchi, but only the smallest particles reach the bronchioles. Ultrasonic aerosol generators are the most effective machines for nebulization. Their mists can be directed into a cage or a face mask. If nebulization is used with an endotracheal or tracheostomy tube, inspired gases should be warmed to body temperature.

Dense mist from an unheated jet nebulizer contains only slightly more water than is needed to humidify air with temperature increasing from 22° to 37°C. Evaporation of the aerosol solution can be prevented by stabilization, i.e., by heating it to 35°C or by reducing the vapor pressure by adding 10% propylene glycol. Because distilled water and hypertonic solutions are irritating to the mucosa, only isotonic or half-strength isotonic saline should be used.

Although continuous, low-level humidification of the oxygen tent atmosphere is necessary, periodic medication by aerosol spray is permissible. High levels of water can be introduced several times daily for 10 to 15 minutes per treatment, or drugs can be added to the solution during these times. Many drugs have been used; isoproterenol, epinephrine, and phenylephrine are some of the drugs that may cause bronchodilation and decreased airway resistance.

It is important to differentiate obstruction of the bronchi due to pulmonary edema from that due to bronchial secretions. In both cases, the patient cannot ventilate because of fluids or semifluid liquids in the bronchi. In pulmonary edema, the fluid turns to a frothy, bubbly material that produces a rattling in the throat. Patients suffering from pulmonary edema should be treated with antifoaming substances such as 12% alcohol in water, given by nebulization. If used to treat tenacious exudates, these agents increase viscosity and thus the obstruction.

Thick, inflammatory exudates, on the other hand, must be thinned by detergent materials that liquefy bronchial secretions. However, these agents increase frothing and, indirectly, anoxia if used in pulmonary edema.

In pulmonary edema, antifoaming agents (12% alcohol) should be used. In bronchial exudates (thick), detergents (liquefying agents such as acetylcysteine) should be used.

Heated aerosol units (vaporizers) produce large water droplets that do not penetrate small bronchioles and may overheat the patient. These units should not be used for intensive therapy.

·········· DRUGS

Drugs that can be applied by nebulizer include:

1. Bronchodilators: always use bronchodilators when administering drugs that may be irritating and constricting.
   a. Bronkosol (isoetharine HCl 1% and phenylephrine 0.25%)—0.5 to 1.0 mL in 2 to 3 mL of saline t.i.d.
2. Antibiotics: poorly absorbed from the respiratory mucosa. Systemic administration of most antibiotics produces adequate pulmonary concentration for antibacterial effect. For *Bordetella* spp. that are located at the tips of bronchial cilia, topical contact via nebulization may be useful.
   a. Kanamycin—250 mg in 5 mL saline b.i.d.
   b. Gentamicin—50 mg in 5 mL saline b.i.d.
   c. Polymyxin B—333,000 IU in 5 mL saline b.i.d.
3. Bland solutions: use in large volume for prolonged mist effect.
   a. Saline—5 to 200 mL as needed
   b. Glycerine—5% in saline
   c. Detergents (see below)
   d. Propylene glycol—10% to 20% solution in saline
4. Detergents and mucolytics: these compounds are irritating and are not recommended by most authors.
5. Antifoaming agents.
   a. Ethyl alcohol—70% solution 5 to 10 mL b.i.d.

REFERENCE

Haskins SC: Management of pulmonary disease in the critical patient. *In* Zaslow IM, ed: Veterinary Trauma and Critical Care. Philadelphia, Lea & Febiger, 1984, pp 339–384.

Oxygen Therapy

·········· TISSUE OXYGENATION

The basic indication for oxygen therapy is inadequate tissue oxygenation (hypoxia).

The partial pressure of oxygen (PO_2) is a convenient figure to use in following oxygen utilization. Inspired air has a PO_2 of 150 mm Hg. As the inspired air is mixed with air in the alveolus, the PO_2 drops to 100 mm Hg. Arterial blood saturated with oxygen has a PO_2 of 95 mm Hg, and when tissues have been supplied, the PO_2 of venous blood is about 40 mm Hg. Tissue levels of oxygen are normally approximately 35 mm Hg.

Oxygen is transported in the blood in combination with hemoglobin and in physical solution in the plasma. If an adequate amount of hemoglobin is normally saturated with oxygen while the animal is breathing room air, breathing high concentrations of oxygen will only slightly increase the amount of oxygen carried by hemoglobin. However, moderate increases in dissolved plasma oxygen will be obtained. On the other hand, if inadequate hemoglobin saturation is obtained by breathing normal air, breathing high concentrations of oxygen may markedly raise hemoglobin saturation and improve tissue oxygen tensions. The additional oxygen in physical solution would be helpful, too.

············MONITORING PULMONARY FUNCTION

1. Observe the physical signs of the animal; rate (8 to 25 breaths per minute); rhythm.
   a. Hypoventilation—lower than normal alveolar minute volume
   b. Cheyne-Stokes breathing—cyclic hyperventilation and hypoventilation associated with acidosis and alterations in medullary center response
   c. Biot's breathing—hypoventilation with periods of apnea, indicating severe medullary disease
   d. Tachypnea—rapid breathing without any comment on the volume of air moved
2. Auscultate the thorax (see p. 353)
3. Evaluate mucous membranes – capillary perfusion.
4. Radiograph the chest if the procedure will not decompensate (overly stress) the animal.
5. Obtain some idea of ventilation volume—normal values are 10 to 20 mL/kg for tidal volume, 150 to 250 mL/kg for minute volume, and 8 to 20 breaths per minute. Ventilometers are valuable when placed on the expiratory end of the breathing circuit.
6. Measure arterial blood gases, if possible (see p. 591)

············HYPOXIA
············Signs

Measurement of arterial blood gases and pH is the only reliable means of measuring hypoxia. The clinical signs of hyperpnea, dyspnea, tachycardia, and cyanosis may be dominant features in some patients, but these signs are nonspecific and unreliable.

············Types
············Hypoxic Hypoxia

Alterations of respiratory function may lead to a lowered partial pressure of arterial oxygen (PaO_2), which in turn may be caused by the following:

1. *Alveolar hypoventilation,* which is the result of depressed respirations of increased resistance to chest movements. Hypercapnia is present. With a normal lung, adequate ventilation with air should help to correct the problem. In acute pneumothorax caused by leakage of air into the pleural cavity from ruptured lung or bronchi (see p. 242), additional administration of air or oxygen under positive airway pressure will further increase the tension pneumothorax and kill the animal. In this case, air must be effectively removed from the pleural space.
2. An *arteriovenous shunt* within the heart or lungs due to a congenital defect or to perfusion of a section of lung that is not ventilated (consolidated or atelectatic segment). If the rest of the lung is hyperventilated, hypercapnia will not develop. Correction of the shunt is necessary, and oxygen inhalation is only partially helpful.
3. A *diffusion defect* in which the alveolar membrane is altered by fibrosis, emphysema, or thromboembolic disease. Hypercapnia usually is not present because carbon dioxide can diffuse 20 times as fast as oxygen. Inhalation of oxygen may be helpful.

4. *Uneven blood flow and ventilation* throughout the lung may be caused by many pulmonary diseases and is probably the most common cause of hypoxia. Hypercapnia may or may not be present. Hyperventilation with air and oxygen inhalation are helpful.

Reduced oxygen-carrying capacity of the blood may be due to a low or abnormal hemoglobin level. Therapy must increase the amount of active hemoglobin.

............Circulatory Hypoxia

Inadequate perfusion of tissues may be due to shock, low cardiac output, or vascular obstruction. Tissues do not live on oxygen alone, so improved circulation is imperative.

............Histotoxic Hypoxia

Toxic tissue cells may be unable to use oxygen. Inhalation of oxygen is of no value.

............METHEMOGLOBINEMIA

Methemoglobinemia refers to methemoglobin content in blood above 1.5% of total hemoglobin. Methemoglobinemia is suspected when arterial blood with normal or increased Po_2 is dark-colored. Significant methemoglobinemia has been associated with clinical cases of benzocaine, acetaminophen, and phenazopyridine toxicities in cats and dogs. These oxidants can also produce Heinz body hemolytic anemias.

............INDICATIONS FOR OXYGEN THERAPY

1. In veterinary medicine, oxygen therapy is indicated in acute cases of respiratory insufficiency (hypoxic hypoxia) leading to a low Pao_2. Oxygen therapy, for economic and practical considerations, is rarely indicated for any chronic condition.
2. Altered ventilation-perfusion relationships are often indications for oxygen therapy. However, measures designed to treat infection, reduce airway obstruction, or improve the mechanics of breathing may reduce the need for oxygen.
3. Circulatory failures such as shock and reduced cardiac output cause hypoxia because of poor perfusion. Giving oxygen is an ancillary treatment, subordinate to the measures directed at the primary cause. However, oxygen therapy may be the critical factor in raising tissue oxygen levels above hypoxic levels.
4. In anemic hypoxia, blood transfusions are needed and oxygen therapy is helpful only if the hemoglobin is abnormal (carboxyhemoglobin).
5. In histotoxic hypoxia oxygen is unlikely to be beneficial but it should be administered.
6. When possible, arterial blood gas analysis should be used to assess the need for oxygen therapy. Analysis should include Po_2, Pco_2, and blood pH.

............NORMAL VALUES

Po_2: 85 to 95 mm Hg (arterial); 40 to 60 mm Hg (venous)
Pco_2: 29 to 36 mm Hg (arterial); 29 to 42 mm Hg (venous)
Blood base excess: ±2.5 mEq/L
Plasma bicarbonate: 17 to 24 mEq/L
Blood pH: 7.31 to 7.42

···········ADMINISTERING OXYGEN

The goal of oxygen therapy is to increase the amount of oxygen carried in the blood by raising the PaO_2 to normal in hypoxic hypoxia and by increasing the PaO_2 above normal in circulatory and anemic hypoxia.

The requirements of an oxygen tent environment include the following:

1. Usually, 30% to 40% oxygen is more than adequate to treat cases of hypoxia correctable by oxygen therapy. (Higher concentrations may be needed in severe circulatory failure.) Initially, high flow rates of 10 L/min are required to wash out residual nitrogen in the cage. A maintenance flow of 5 L/min is usually sufficient.
2. Adequate humidification (often 40% to 60%) is absolutely essential.
3. Maintenance of carbon dioxide at less than 1.5% is necessary. Oxygen tents equipped with carbon dioxide absorbers can maintain carbon dioxide levels at 0.7%.
4. Control of environmental temperature at 65° to 70°F is necessary in almost all cases.

Methods of oxygen administration include face mask, tracheal catheter, nasal catheter, oxygen tent, endotracheal tube, and intermittent positive-pressure breathing (IPPB) respirator. Obviously, endotracheal intubation and IPPB can be used only in the anesthetized or comatose animal. Tight-fitting masks are usually resented by the animal, and its struggling causes further hypoxia.

Supplemental oxygen may be administered via a catheter (8F) placed either through the cricothyroid ligament or between the tracheal rings. Either of these techniques overcomes the occasional lack of cooperation by the patient with nasal catheters. This method has proved especially useful for administration of supplemental oxygen to dogs too large for the oxygen cages. A large, sterile, pliable male urinary catheter is utilized. Humidified oxygen at a flow rate of 10 mL/kg/min should achieve an oxygen concentration that maintains 97% hemoglobin saturation.

A small 5F to 8F soft rubber nasal catheter may also be used effectively to deliver oxygen to small animals. The catheter should have multiple side holes. Instill 2% lidocaine into the nose of the dog and proparacaine HCl into the nose of the cat. Insert a lubricated, soft, red rubber catheter to a level of the midnasal region by placing it in the ventral nasal meatus. The catheter is sutured in place into the external nares with 2-0 or 3-0 silk suture. The catheter is extended up the face between the eyes and over the head and is sutured into the skin to maintain its position. An Elizabethan collar is useful. Administer oxygen by nebulizing the flow through a bottle of warmed saline. Oxygen flow rates should be 50 to 200 mL/min/kg to bring the oxygen concentrations to 40% or greater. The catheter may also be placed in the nasopharyngeal area in an attempt to deliver oxygen at higher rates to the animal or to deliver some form of continuous airway positive pressure (CAPP). Difficulties with this technique include aerophagia, gastric dilation, and irritation and gagging.

For controlled positive-pressure ventilation, either orotracheal intubation or tracheostomy is indicated. Awake animals will not tolerate orotracheal intubation. The technique is used in comatose, anesthetized, or heavily sedated (with neuroleptanalgesic) animals. Neuromuscular blocking agents are *not* recommended for any but the briefest of positive-pressure procedures.

In orotracheal intubation (see p. 582), high-volume, low-pressure endotracheal cuffs are used and the time limit for maintaining intubation depends on the condition of the patient and the degree of chemical restraint required. Prolonged tracheal intubation necessitates a tracheostomy (see p. 623).

Oxygen tent equipment to provide these conditions is rarely found in veterinary hospitals. The best equipment includes a mechanical, thermostatically controlled compressor cooling unit, a circulatory fan, nebulizers or humidifiers to moisten the air, and a carbon dioxide absorber. The ice-chest oxygen diffusion tents are *very poor* for long-term maintenance therapy in hypoxemic animals. Small incubator isolettes have been used with good success in cats and puppies.

The animal should be maintained in the tent continuously, not on an intermittent basis. Animals with chronic respiratory disease or hypoxemia from other causes such as depressant drugs or cerebral trauma have become adjusted to a high carbon dioxide level and rely on the chemoreceptor reflex to maintain respiration. Administration of high levels of oxygen may depress the "hypoxic drive" and result in a lowered respiratory rate, apnea, and increased hypoxia. Therefore, animals with chronic hypoxia should be observed closely for respiratory depression when oxygen therapy is administered.

REFERENCES

Drobatz K, Hackner S, Powell S; Oxygen Supplementation. *In* Bonagura J, ed: Current Veterinary Therapy XII. Small Animal Practice. Philadelphia, WB Saunders, 1995, p. 175.

Fitzpatrick RK, Crowe DT: Nasal oxygen administration in dogs and cats: Experimental and clinical investigations. J Am Anim Hosp Assoc 22:293–300, 1986.

Hendricks J: Pulse oximetry *In* Bonagura J, ed: Current Veterinary Therapy XII. Small Animal Practice. Philadelphia, WB Saunders, 1995, p. 117.

Mann FA, Wagner-Mann C, Allert JA, et al: Comparison of intranasal and intratracheal oxygen administration in healthy, awake dogs. Am J Vet Res 53(5):856, 1992.

Peritoneal Dialysis

The peritoneum serves as a passive, semipermeable barrier to the diffusion of plasma water and peritoneal fluid. The movement of solutes from plasma water to dialysis solution is thought to result from diffusion or solvent drag effects of bulk flow, or both. The fluid instilled into the peritoneum is called the dialysate.

Factors that alter peritoneal clearance are blood flow to the peritoneum and changes in peritoneal membrane permeability. Peritoneal clearance can be increased by (1) increasing the dialysate exchange volume, (2) decreasing the time dialysate fluid stays in the peritoneal cavity, (3) increasing the temperature of the dialysate fluid to body temperature, or (4) adding glucose in hypertonic concentration to the dialysis fluid. Commercial dialysis solutions made for human patients can be used in dogs, but the sodium and chloride concentrations are low for dogs. Additional sodium and chloride ions should be added to commercially available solutions. Commercially available dialysate solutions may contain 1.5% or 4.25% glucose. A dextrose solution containing 1.5 g/dL is moderately hypertonic to normal plasma (350 mOsm/L), whereas a solution containing 4.25 g/dL (490 mOsm/L) can be used to produce negative fluid balance in overhydrated animals.

The major use of peritoneal dialysis in dogs is to treat and maintain patients with acute oliguric renal failure until they compensate for renal damage.

Technique for Continuous Ambulatory Peritoneal Dialysis In performing peritoneal dialysis, place the animal in left lateral recumbency. Clip and surgically prepare a site midway between the umbilicus and pelvis. Empty the bladder if it is filled. Using local anesthetic (e.g., 2% lidocaine), infiltrate the skin and abdominal musculature just lateral to the midline and a few centimeters posterior to the umbilicus. Commercial peritoneal dialysis sets*

....

*Stylocath and Inpersol Peritoneal Catheter (with stylet), Abbott Laboratories, North Chicago, IL; Diacath, Travenol Laboratories, Inc., Deerfield, IL.

are available, or Silastic tubing* of 0.025-in. inside diameter (ID) with multiple fenestrations can be used. When the catheter is placed, suture it to the skin and bandage the abdomen and catheter. Inject enough warm (38° to 39°C) dialysate fluid to distend the abdomen mildly (200 to 2000 mL). Lactated Ringer's solution with added glucose (to 2%) is a satisfactory lavage fluid, but Peridial, 1.5%, and Inpersol 1.5% are balanced more correctly. After 1 hour, drain the abdomen of solution. Remove the dialysate by siphoning it back into the original sterile container. During the first dialysis period, some fluid will be absorbed; thus, the entire volume that was placed in the peritoneal cavity will not be collected. In patients with severe renal failure, peritoneal dialysis may have to be repeated three to five times a day. For each liter of dialysate, add 1000 units of heparin to prevent fibrin from plugging the catheter. Commercial human peritoneal dialysis sets may function for a short period of time in the dog but then become blocked with tissue and fibrin.

The surgically implanted column disc catheter for peritoneal dialysis has recently been discontinued. An alternative catheter, namely the fluted-T peritoneal catheter† has proved successful in the dog. The catheter is made of silicone with two Dacron cuffs. The junction of the catheter is to be placed against the parietal peritoneum and oriented in a cranial-to-caudal plane. In this type of dialysis technique, called continuous ambulatory peritoneal dialysis (CAPD), Dianeal 137 with 1.5% dextrose‡ is used. The dialysis solution is available in 250-mL, 500-mL, 1-L, and 2-L bags. For each liter of dialysate, add 1000 units of heparin to prevent fibrin from plugging the catheter. Instill a sufficient volume of warmed dialysate solution to distend the abdomen mildly (40 mL dialysate per kilogram). Peritoneal dialysis must be done under aseptic conditions. A mask and gloves must be worn. As the fluid flows rapidly from the Silastic bag into the peritoneum, roll up the bag; when the bag is empty, tape it to the body wall. Dialysate solution is allowed to remain in the peritoneal cavity for 45 to 50 minutes. Record the volume of solution instilled and remove from the abdomen during each exchange. When dialysis fluid is to be collected, unroll the bag; gravity permits collection of dialysate. As the patient improves, the frequency of dialysis may be decreased to three or four times per day and the dwell time for the fluid in the abdomen may be increased to 4 to 6 or even 8 to 12 hours.

··········· COMPLICATIONS

There is always a danger of peritonitis resulting from peritoneal dialysis. Daily peritoneal infusion of ampicillin 1 g/2L of dialysate may be used to prevent bacterial contamination of the dialysis catheter and peritoneal cavity. Peritoneal infection is indicated by the presence of turbid drainage fluid with WBC counts exceeding 100 to 200/mm^3. Gram staining and culture and sensitivity tests should be done on the fluid. Blood culture media should be inoculated with dialysate fluid, and culture plates should be inoculated to identify gram-positive and coliform organisms.

If peritonitis is suspected, antimicrobial therapy should be begun by adding tobramycin 16 mg/2L of dialysate and of cephalothin sodium 250 mg/2L of dialysate per exchange. Systemic cephalexin should be used at 20 mg/kg b.i.d.

*Silastic brand medical grade tubing, Dow Corning Corp., Midland, MI.
†Ash Advantage Peritoneal Catheter, Medigroup, Aurora, IL.
‡Dianeal–Viaflex–Transfer Set Tubing, Travenol Laboratories, Inc., Deerfield, IL.

Other antibiotics that may be added to dialysate fluid, depending on bacterial sensitivity results, are penicillin G 50,000 units/L, ampicillin 50 mg/L, cloxacillin 100 mg/L, ticarcillin 100 mg/L, vancomycin 30 mg/L, amikacin 50 mg/L, clindamycin 50 mg/L, or trimethoprim-sulfadiazine 5 to 25 mg/L. Additional complications that can occur are intraabdominal trauma or perforation during catheter placement, electrolyte imbalances and excessive protein loss, and cardiovascular or respiratory complications resulting from too rapid fluid injections.

REFERENCES

Chew D, DiBartola S, Crisp S: Peritoneal dialysis. *In* DiBartola S, ed: Fluid Therapy in Small Animal Practice. Philadelphia, WB Saunders, 1992.

Cowgill LD: Application of peritoneal dialysis and hemodialysis in the mangement of renal failure. *In* Osborne CA, ed: Canine and Feline Nephrology and Urology. Philadelphia, Lea & Febiger, 1995.

Crisp MS, Chew DJ, DiBartola SR, et al: Peritoneal dialysis in dogs and cats. J Am Vet Med Assoc 195:1262, 1989.

Dyzban L, Labato M, Ross L: Peritoneal dialysis. *In* Bonagura J, ed: Kirk's Current Veterinary Therapy 13. Philadelphia, WB Saunders, 2000.

Physical Therapy

Most physiotherapeutic modalities have a stimulating effect, and their action is directed toward the musculoskeletal system or the skin.

............HYDROTHERAPY

Water baths or soaks are among the easiest and most versatile modes of physical therapy in small animal practice. Wet packs, water soaks, or whirlpool baths can be helpful in adding moisture to (hydrating) or removing moisture from (dehydrating) the skin. Cyclic repetitions of moistening and drying the skin many times a day serve to dehydrate (similar to the chapped lips and hands seen in humans). Constant moisture hydrates and even macerates the skin.

Whirlpool baths are the most efficient and popular means of applying hydrotherapy and, often, antiseptic medication to the skin. Whirlpool baths combine moist heat, gentle massage, and the solvent properties of water, with or without the mechanical impact of water from a whirlpool, to remove dirt, pus, and necrotic debris. Dry or scaly skin is softened and moisturized. Whirlpools may increase edema and are contraindicated in acute traumatic and inflammatory conditions or in cases of impaired sensation or circulation (unless treated with extreme caution). Whirlpools are particularly beneficial for skin infections, chronic dryness, open or infected wounds, skin grafts, adhesions, arthritis, postsurgical fractures, amputations, muscle spasms, and stiff joints. This modality is especially useful for cleaning and stimulating the skin of patients who are predisposed to decubital ulcers.

The patient should be placed in an appropriate water bath at a temperature of 39° to 42°C (102° to 108°F). A low-suds detergent or antiseptic solution (povidone-iodine, chlorine, chlorhexidine) can be added for cleansing or germicidal effects. Allow the water turbine to circulate the water around and against the affected parts for 10 to 15 minutes once or twice daily. Support and reassure the animal during treatment, and never leave an animal unattended. Following therapy, ensure that the tub and turbine are thoroughly cleaned and sanitized.

Commercial whirlpool baths or Jacuzzi-type agitators are a good investment for a busy practice. A less expensive alternative is a variable-temperature bath with agitation provided by a pressure hose.

............HEAT
............Effects

The effects of heat in physical therapy include the following:

1. Hyperemia and dilation of cutaneous vessels
2. Increase in pulse, blood pressure, and pulmonary ventilation
3. Increased metabolite transfer across capillary membranes
4. General muscle relaxation
5. Sedative and analgesic effect
6. Improved extensibility of connective tissue

In the presence of trauma, swelling, and edema, circulation may be impeded and the application of heat may cause necrosis. Cold is more beneficial in the early acute stages of inflammation and edema.

............Superficial Heat

Infrared radiation is produced by long-wave generators that glow red and produce heat that penetrates only 1 to 2 mm. Short-wave generators produce invisible light; their heat penetrates 10 to 12 mm and reaches blood-carrying layers of tissue, where the heat is dispersed by the circulation. Because of their penetration, short waves do not produce a burning sensation; however, one should check the skin meticulously during therapy to ensure that it is not overheated. A warm sensation is normal. If the skin feels hot to the touch, the heat is too intense. Short-wave therapy is contraindicated in acute trauma and inflammation. Superficial heat is beneficial for subacute and chronic problems, skin infections, and abscesses. Treat for 15 to 20 minutes once or twice daily.

Hot packs or wet towels can be used to apply mild, gentle heat. The indications are the same as for infrared heat, but additional precautions are needed. Hot packs may spread contagious skin disease, and the weight of the packs in an insensitive area is more likely to cause burns or tissue damage. This modality has the advantage of providing moist heat, which is particularly beneficial for chronic soft tissue problems such as arthritis, myositis, and contractures. Hot packs should be applied for 10 to 15 minutes several times a day. Check the skin under the packs frequently during therapy.

Whirlpool baths combine moist heat, gentle massage, and the solvent properties of water to remove dirt, pus, and necrotic debris. The moist heat is especially indicated for extensive involvement of musculoskeletal disorders. Warm-water baths can be repeated two to three times daily for 10 to 15 minutes and can often be followed with a gentle massage and passive flexion and extension exercises to improve range-of-motion and soft-tissue flexibility.

............Deep Heat

Short-wave diathermy transmits physical energy deep into tissues; because the body tissues resist the flow of high-frequency current (27 million cps [Hz]), heat is produced. In dissipating heat, there marked vascular dilation, sedation, analgesia, and relief of muscle spasm. However, edema may increase. Absolute contraindications are the presence of imbedded metal implants, ischemia, malignancy, and pregnancy. No water can be in the field, and splints and bandages must be removed. This therapy can result in electrical shock to both the patient and technician, so all cables, electrodes, and other equipment must be in excellent condition. Safety cannot be overemphasized. Each unit should be calibrated and adjusted individually to produce only a sensation of warmth. Treatment daily is applied for 15 to 20 minutes.

Microwave techniques produce about the same effects as diathermy except that more localized heating occurs (one side of a joint may be treated at a time). Microwaves are more readily absorbed by water, so great care must be used around the eye or in the presence of edema to ensure that the effects are not excessive.

Ultrasound produces the deepest heat. Ultrasound produces mechanical vibrations (1 million/second) in the elastic media of the body. Ultrasonic waves are reflected from boundaries between different types of tissues. The vibrations produce a micromassage that accelerates fluid absorption by increasing permeability. Ultrasonic therapy can be dangerous if the intensity or application is concentrated too long in a small area. Burn or tissue destruction may result. Ultrasonic therapy is contraindicated in neoplasms, the eye, heart, spine, and brain; near growing bony epiphyses; and in acute infections. Otherwise, its beneficial effects are similar to those of other forms of deep heat. Ultrasound is particularly indicated for softening scar tissue and reducing the pain of neuromas and degenerative joint disease. It can be used over and around metal implants.

Ultrasonic waves are applied via a transducer and using coupling media such as water or contact gels. The transducer is moved constantly over a small area (usually 6 to 8 sq in., depending on the size of the transducer). It is best to shave the skin before therapy to enhance contact (or use a water bath).

The dose varies with each patient. Most ultrasonic generators have an output of 700,000 to 1 million Hz at intensities of 0.1 to 1.0 W/cm^2. It is best to use the lowest intensity possible. The maximum dose should be 1.0 W/cm^2 for 5 minutes of application to the affected tissues. This application can be repeated once daily for 5 days and then every other day for five treatments. Then it should not be repeated for at least 1 month. Do not use ultrasonic therapy in acute injuries, inflammations, or infections.

For cervical intervertebral disease, use 0.3 W/cm^2 for 3 minutes daily for 5 days and then every other day for five treatments.

For arthritis, bursitis, and myositis, use 0.2 W/cm^2 for 3 minutes for joints of the extremities. Repeat two times weekly.

............COLD

Cold can be applied by blowing cold air on the skin, by evaporation of volatile liquids from the skin, or by direct contact of the cooling substance with the skin surface.

............Effects

The effects of cold in physical therapy include:

1. Decreased tissue temperature
2. Decreased blood flow, vasoconstriction
3. Decreased tendency to edema
4. Decreased delivery of nutrients, phagocytes
5. Decreased phagocytic action
6. Transient vasoconstriction followed by vasodilation and increased blood flow (brief cold applications)

Cold reduces extravasation of blood and fluid into tissues after trauma, reduces pain and spasticity, and is indicated in acute traumatic and inflammatory conditions.

Overtreatment with cold may produce maceration and frostbite. Prolonged cold produces a vascular response with stasis of blood, occlusion of vessels, and tissue anoxia and necrosis.

Cold packs over a damp towel applied to the affected area and covered with a folded dry towel to prevent rapid warming can be used for 15 to 20 minutes. Treatment is repeated several times daily. It is important to keep the rest of the patient's body warm, dry, and comfortable during treatment. Cold treatments are often more effective when alternated with heat treatments (immersion bath or moist warm packs). The combined treatment is most effective when heat for 3 to 4 minutes is alternated with 1 to 2 minutes of cold. This regimen can be repeated for 15 to 20 minutes and should always end with the hot phase.

Cold immersion baths for one or several extremities may be useful. The temperature should be 15.5° to 21°C (60° to 70°F) and can be decreased by adding ice or cold water. Continue treatment until the muscles are relaxed or the animal cannot tolerate the cold, usually 2 to 5 minutes. Modification of this technique can be used for heat stroke, but one must be careful not to overchill such patients.

············ELECTRICITY

Medical galvanism is the physiologic use of direct current. This treatment will produce the same effects as heat except that it has no tendency to produce edema. The treatment is beneficial for acute, subacute, or chronic traumatic and inflammatory problems, i.e., arthritis, decubital sores, neuralgia, tenosynovitis, or postfracture repair. Electricity should not be used near the brain, heart, or neoplasms.

Low-intensity therapy (0.5 to 1.0 mA/sq in. of electrode) is desirable. Electrodes should be wet and held in firm contact with the skin. No metal should be in or near the area being treated. Halfway through the treatment, the intensity of current should be reduced to zero, the polarity reversed, and the intensity returned to starting levels.

Electrical stimulation of partially or wholly innervated muscle is possible with alternating current. Intact or denervated muscle will contract when stimulated with interrupted pulses of direct current. These kinds of stimulation improve circulation and nutrition of the muscle, promote venous return, remove lymph, relax spasm, reduce edema, and assist in muscle reeducation. Muscle atrophy and weakness can be retarded or controlled. Each muscle or group of muscles can be stimulated 10 to 20 times for one procedure, depending on the condition. Avoid overtreatment.

············MASSAGE

Massage is the use of the hands and fingers to manipulate soft tissues. Massage is usually used in combination with heat, cold, or whirlpool treatments. Massage improves circulation, reduces edema, loosens and stretches fibrotic or contracted tissue, and has a soothing or sedative effect. Massage should not be used in acute, inflammatory, traumatic, and painful lesions or with tumors, hemorrhages, and perhaps contagious conditions. Massage is indicated for tight or contracted tendons, ligaments, or muscles; chronic traumatic or inflammatory problems; and subacute or chronic edema.

In performing massage, keep the strokes in the direction of venous flow. Firm, rapid pressure tends to be stimulating, whereas slow, light strokes are soothing. Some type of lubricating powder or oil can be used to reduce friction.

The massage can be stroking, kneading, or applied with friction. Stroking and kneading assist circulation, whereas friction and kneading tend to loosen adhesions and scars and to stretch tissues. Massage should last 15 or 20 minutes and can be repeated several times daily if desired.

............EXERCISE

Therapeutic exercise should strengthen musculoskeletal function, improve range-of-motion flexibility, improve endurance or coordination, and increase cardiovascular and respiratory capabilities. Exercise should never be forced but should be kept within safe tolerance of the patient's cardiac and respiratory capacity. Active exercise (such as walking, running, or swimming) is most desirable, because endurance and strength increase with repetition. Passive exercise is useful when paralysis or traumatic injuries preclude active exercise.

Movements should never be forced, but stabilization of parts and controlled pressure should be used to activate only the structures of concern. When attempting to increase range of motion, use smooth, controlled pressure to move the joint slightly beyond its limited range; hold the stretch for a count of five, and slowly release the traction. Several repetitions can be performed two or three times daily. Gradual improvement can be expected within several weeks.

REFERENCES

Moore M, Rasmussen J: Physical therapy in small animals, part I. Anim Health Tech 2:199–211, 1981.
Moore M, Rasmussen J: Physical therapy in small animals, part II. Anim Health Tech 2:242–250, 1981.

Thoracentesis and Pericardiocentesis

Thoracentesis refers to the aspiration of fluid or air from the thoracic cavity. The procedure may be performed for diagnostic or therapeutic purposes. It may be impossible to remove all of the fluid or air that is present; however, either of the two should be removed as much as possible. If repeated withdrawal of air or fluid from the chest is contemplated, a chest tube is safer. Clip and surgically prepare the thoracic wall from the 5th to the 11th intercostal space. If fluid or air is present on only one side of the thoracic cavity (a rarity in dogs and cats), only that side should be aspirated. If fluid is to be aspirated, infiltrate lidocaine, 0.5%, into a spot low in the seventh intercostal space using a 1-in., 22- to 24-gauge needle. (Use of local anesthesia is not always necessary.) Then fit a 20- to 22-gauge needle to extension tubing, which in turn is fitted to a two-way stopcock and then to a 20-mL sterile syringe. Insert the needle into the thoracic cavity until the tip is just through the pleura but does not lacerate the lung. Any fluid aspirated should be saved and analyzed to determine whether it is a transudate or an exudate. A safer and better way to remove quantities of fluid from the thoracic or pericardial cavity is to use the IV Intrafusor system (see Fig. 4–2).* Needles in this system are available in 14- and 15-gauge, with a radiopaque, through-the-needle catheter attached. The catheter can be passed through the needle in the appropriate cavity, the needle removed, and a three-way valve used to remove fluid or air.

In dogs that require repeated aspirations of air or fluid from the chest, the

....

*Sorenson Research Co., Salt Lake City, UT.

suprapubic Cystocath* drainage system works well. Prepare the ches
over the 6th to 11th intercostal spaces by clipping and surgical prepar
Starting at the 11th rib, make a small incision in the skin and slide the sp
trocar-cannula to the middle of the dorsal eighth intercostal space (Fig. 4–
This can be done easily by drawing the skin cranially until the incision is o\
the eighth intercostal space. (When the skin is later released to return to 1
original location, a subcutaneous tunnel is formed.) Push the trocar into th
chest cavity, leave the cannula in place, and clamp the cannula after removing
the trocar. Place the silicone catheter in the chest cavity, attach a three-way
valve and a syringe, and aspirate air. Tape the cannula and catheter to the
chest wall.

■ SIZE OF THE DOG AND APPROPRIATE CHEST CATHETER SIZE

<7 kg—14F to 16F.
7 to 15 kg—18F to 22F.
16 to 30 kg—22F to 28F.
>30 kg—28F to 36F.

Cytologic examination may be performed, and cultures of this fluid may be
made. Thoracentesis in pneumothorax is carried out in the same manner
as aspiration of fluid; however, because air rises in the thoracic cavity, the
thoracentesis puncture should be made high up in the seventh intercostal
space.

....

*Silastic Cystocath Suprapubic Drainage System, Dow Corning Corp., Midland, MI. This
system can be reused after cleaning and gas autoclaving.

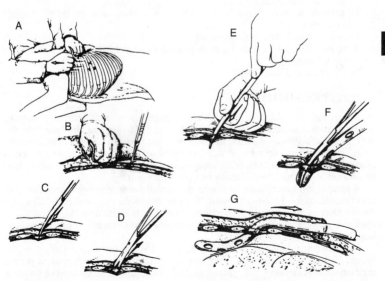

Figure 4–42. Placement of thoracostomy tube (see text for description of the
technique). (From Crowe DT: The Surgical Laboratory. Athens, College of Veterinary Medicine, University of Georgia, 1986.)

Pericardiocentesis is the surgical puncture of the pericardium for the purpose of aspirating effusions. Sedate the animal with morphine or a neuroleptanalgesic agent (sedation is not always necessary). Surgically prepare both sides of the thorax. Place the animal in lateral recumbency. Infiltrate the muscles of the fourth intercostal space at a level with the junction of the ventral and middle thirds of the thorax with lidocaine 1%, using a 22-gauge needle. Use a Venocath (16-gauge needle) or an Intrafusor system; place a three-way stopcock on the syringe adapter end of the Venocath. Have an assistant place a 30-mL syringe on the three-way stopcock, and maintain negative pressure on the syringe as the chest is entered. Carefully advance the 16-gauge Intracath needle into the fourth intercostal space, advancing toward the heart, while maintaining negative pressure in the syringe. When fluid enters the syringe, the needle may be drawing fluid from the thoracic cavity. Advance the needle until resistance of the pericardium is felt and a sudden release indicates that the pericardial sac has been entered. If the needle is advanced too far (into the myocardium), ventricular premature contractions (VPCs) will be seen on the ECG monitor. Thread the Intracath polyethylene tubing through the 16-gauge needle so that the end of the tubing lies securely within the pericardial sac, and remove the needle from the intrathoracic space. Continue aspirating fluid. This technique should prevent trauma to the myocardium. The ECG monitoring during pericardiocentesis will also warn of trauma to the myocardium. All aspirated fluid should be examined as described on p. 768.

Tracheotomy and Tracheostomy

............INDICATIONS

Tracheotomy is indicated in the following situations:

To relieve upper respiratory tract obstructions

To facilitate removal of respiratory secretions

To decrease the dead air space

To provide a route for inhalant anesthesia when oral or facial surgery is complex

To reduce resistance to respiration

To reduce the risk of closed glottis pressure (cough) following pulmonary or cranial surgery

To facilitate artificial respiration

............TECHNIQUE

In an emergency situation in which asphyxiation is imminent, any cutting instrument will suffice in making a tracheotomy. Moistening the hair over the ventral neck facilitates midline incision over the trachea. The first few tracheal rings (between the second and third or third and fourth) are incised to allow placement of any firm tube (e.g., ballpoint pen barrel), or the knife blade may be rotated 90 degrees to maintain the tracheal opening.

A specialized instrument has been developed for emergency tracheotomy or cricothyroidotomy. This instrument is a percutaneous special-slotted 13-gauge needle that is passed into the trachea through the cricothyroid ligament. A special tracheostomy tube* is guided through the split needle into the tracheal lumen (Fig. 4–43).

In less demanding circumstances, aseptic surgical technique should be followed. Make an exact midline skin incision just caudal to the larynx to permit incision and retraction of the paired sternohyoid muscles, exposing the trachea.

....

*Available from Pertrach, Inc., Long Beach, CA.

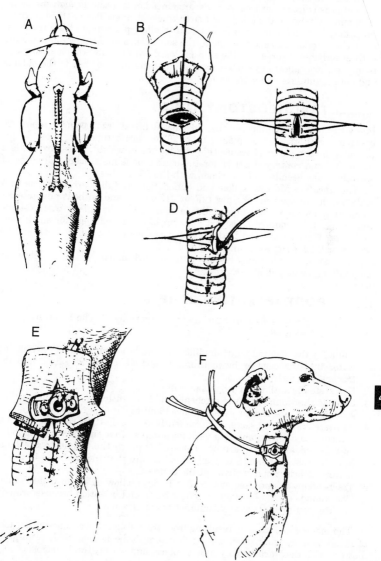

Figure 4–43. Tracheostomy technique (see text for description). (From Aron DN, Crowe DT: Upper airway obstruction. Vet Clin North Am Small Anim Pract 15:897, 1985.)

4

Then elevate and immobilize the trachea by passing 0.25-in. umbilical tape around it as traction sutures. A transverse incision is made through the annular ligament between the third and fourth tracheal rings. Two or three tracheal rings may be incised or partially resected to allow placement of the tracheostomy tube. Following tube placement, the soft tissues are *loosely* approximated with absorbable sutures and the skin is closed with nonabsorbable sutures. It is important to allow any air escaping around the tube to vent to the outside and *not* accumulate under the skin.

...........TRACHEOSTOMY TUBES

Many of the shortcomings of the old curved metal tracheostomy tubes are overcome with the newer plastic tubes. The plastic tubes are often better tolerated by the patient because they are lighter in weight, more flexible, less irritating, and contoured better for the canine or feline trachea. Crusting of secretions has been less of a problem with the PVC tubes.

The uncuffed Morrant-Baker and cuffed Bassett tubes are available in a wide variety of sizes for the dog (2F to 21F), with and without adapters for connection to respirators or anesthesia machines. The infant tracheostomy tubes (Great Ormond St. Hospital pattern) have proved ideal for small dogs and cats. We also use the Portex* cuffed tracheostomy tubes that have an obturator that permits cleaning of the tube.

Tracheostomy tubes may become plugged with mucus, blood, or debris, or may fall out or be pulled out.

...........POSTOPERATIVE CARE

Postoperative care is as important as the surgery itself. The following procedures should be used:

1. Humidify the inspired air. Humidification can be accomplished by nebulizing water into the cage or by instilling 1 to 3 mL of sterile saline into the trachea at hourly intervals.
2. Use systemic antibiotics prophylactically.
3. Cleanse the wound and the tracheal tube frequently. By using the traction sutures, the tube can easily be removed and replaced.
4. Aspirate respiratory secretions frequently. A soft urethral catheter (12F.) is attached to a T-tube and to a vacuum pump so that suction can be applied or released at will. This tube is passed through the wound to the large bronchi. Instillation of 3 to 5 ml of saline into the trachea helps to loosen mucous debris. Then suction out the debris.
5. Tracheotomy wounds heal within 7 to 10 days following removal of the tube. The wounds should be allowed to heal by second intention because primary closure may predispose to subcutaneous emphysema.

The major complications resulting from tracheostomy are coughing because of intubation, gagging when the tracheostomy tube is aspirated, respiratory distress with the tracheostomy tube in place, and tracheal wall necrosis.

REFERENCES

Fingland, R: Temporary tracheostomy. *In* Bonagura J, ed: Current Veterinary Therapy XII. Small Animal Practice, Philadelphia, WB Saunders, 1995 p. 179.

*Portex Blue Line Tracheostomy Unit, Wilmington, MA.

Hedlund C: Tracheostomies in the management of canine and feline upper respiratory disease. Vet Clin North Am Small Anim Pract 24:873, 1994.

Muir W, Hubbell J, Skarda R, et al: Handbook of Veterinary Anesthesia, ed 2. St Louis, Mosby–Year Book, 1995.

Paddleford RR, Harvey RC: Critical care surgical techniques. Vet Clin North Am Small Anim Pract 19:1082, 1989.

Wingfield WE: Veterinary Emergency Medicine Secrets. Philadelphia, Hanley & Belfus, 1997.

Urohydropropulsion

Urohydropropulsion is a therapeutic procedure for removal of foreign material, namely, uroliths, from the urethra of the male dog. The animal is placed in lateral recumbency and the prepuce retracted and the penis exposed as for urethral catherization. Sterile technique is used to pass an appropriately sized (see also p. 487) flexible catheter which is advanced to the point of obstruction. Attach a syringe containing 60 mL of sterile saline to the catheter. Place your lubricated, gloved finger in the rectum and occlude the lumen of the pelvic

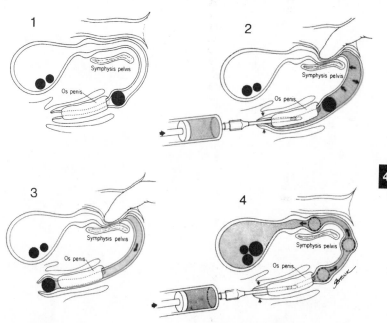

Figure 4–44. Removal of urethrolith in a male dog by urohydropropulsion: 1, Urethrolith originating from the urinary bladder has lodged behind the os penis. 2, Dilation of the urethral lumen is achieved by injecting fluid with pressure. Digital pressure applied to the external urethral orifice and the pelvic urethra has created a closed system. 3, Sudden release of digital pressure at the external urethral orifice and subsequent movement of fluid and urethroliths toward the external urethral orifice. 4, Sudden release of digital pressure at the pelvic urethra and subsequent movement of fluid and urethrolith toward the urinary bladder. (From Osborne CA, Finco DR: Canine and Feline Nephrology and Urology. Baltimore, Williams & Wilkins, 1995.)

urethra using the thumb and index finger. Inject saline rapidly to dilate the urethra and then suddenly release pressure on the proximal urethra allowing small stones to pass the os penis and eject from the urethra. Large stones may not be able to pass through the os penis and surgery would then be indicated.

REFERENCE

Osborne CA, Finco DR: Canine and Feline Nephrology and Urology. Baltimore, Williams & Wilkins, 1995.

Section 5

INTERPRETATION OF LABORATORY TESTS

In this section, the interpretation of results of laboratory tests that vary from normal is discussed. This section provides information about the possible causes of these variations and touches on points of differential diagnosis. However, the discussion is *not* a complete evaluation of the differential merits of each test.

The information discussed here is not intended to give specific directions for performing laboratory tests. For such directions, the reader should consult standard texts on clinical pathology.

5

CEREBROSPINAL FLUID

Analysis of cerebrospinal fluid (CSF) is a valuable aid in establishing a diagnosis in neurologic disease. Changes in CSF depend mainly on the location and extent of the lesion.

In the dog and cat, CSF is collected by puncture of the cerebellomedullary cistern (see p. 516). Slowly remove 2 mL of CSF for examination. A maximum of 1 mL/5 kg body weight can be removed.

............GROSS APPEARANCE

............Color

Normal CSF is clear and colorless. A pinkish or reddish color usually indicates hemorrhage, which may be caused by the spinal tap itself or may be due to CNS disease. The supernatant will be clear following centrifugation if the hemorrhage was caused by the tapping procedure. A yellow, or xanthochromic, color of the spinal fluid indicates previous hemorrhage from injury or cerebrovascular accident or progressive brain disease (such as inflammation or neoplasia). Mild CSF contamination with blood will not alter white blood cell (WBC) or protein determinations. Leukocytosis of 10,000/cm³ in the CSF indicates gross blood contamination, and the tap should be repeated. In some cases of previous hemorrhage, centrifuging the CSF will reveal the supernatant to be yellow and the sediment to be red or brown. In other cases, a clot forms, resulting in few loose cells. A gray or green color may indicate suppuration.

............Turbidity

A cloudy CSF usually indicates the presence of a high cell count (pleocytosis). Neutrophils are found in bacterial meningitis, immune-mediated meningitis, bacterial encephalitis, abscess, and hemorrhage. Increased numbers of mononuclear cells are found in the CSF in viral encephalitis, fungal infections, postvaccinal reactions, uremia, and chronic and toxic conditions. A greatly elevated CSF WBC count may not indicate a guarded prognosis. In steroid-responsive meningoencephalomyelitis (SRM), the WBC count may return to normal and clinical signs abate with the administration of systemic corticosteroids. In SRM the neutrophils are intact and nondegenerative and no bacteria are observed. A high percentage of degenerative neutrophils in the CSF may be indicative of a bacterial infection.

Cytologic examination should be done within 30 minutes after obtaining the sample; otherwise, cell disintegration will take place. The normal cell count is fewer than six cells per microliter for the dog but could be less for the cat.

............Coagulation

Normal CSF does not coagulate. Increased fibrinogen, found in inflammation such as acute suppurative meningitis, produces coagulation.

............PROTEIN

The main protein in normal CSF is albumin. Increases in the total protein levels in disease usually reflect increases in the globulin levels. If blood is present in the CSF, the globulin levels will also be high. Protein examination may be qualitative or quantitative. The Pandy test used for qualitative determination of proteins measures only globulins. Quantitative protein determinations are more critical and measure lower levels of protein, including both albumins and globulins. Normally, the protein level is less than 25 mg/dL.

............BACTERIOLOGIC EXAMINATION

If the CSF is turbid, it should be cultured and a Gram stain or new methylene blue (NMB) stain should be made. Gram stain and NMB stain will also show cryptococci; NMB will also show the capsule. Culture the CSF on blood agar, in thioglycolate culture medium, or in Sabouraud dextrose agar, depending on the findings in the direct smear. If the fluid is not turbid, centrifuge it before staining and culturing the sediment. India ink can be used to see the capsule of the cryptococcal organisms in a smear.

··········CREATINE KINASE

Elevated creatine kinase (CK) levels in serum (see p. 725) usually indicate muscle disease, and elevated CK levels in the CSF are usually independent of the serum concentration. Elevated CK levels in CSF are of little value in differential diagnosis but may indicate a guarded to poor prognosis.

REFERENCES

Bagley R: Intracranial pressure in dogs and cats. Compend Contin Educ Pract Vet 18:605, 1996.
Bailey CS, Higgins RJ: Characteristics of cisternal cerebrospinal fluid associated with primary brain tumors in dogs. J Am Vet Med Assoc 188:414–417, 1986.
Bailey CS, Higgins RJ: Characteristics of cerebrospinal fluid associated with canine granulomatous meningoencephalomyelitis. J Am Vet Med Assoc 188:418–421, 1986.
Chrisman CL: Cerebrospinal fluid analysis. Vet Clin North Am Small Anim Pract 22:781, 1992.
Christopher MM, Perman V, Hardy RM: Reassessment of cytologic values in canine cerebrospinal fluid by use of cytocentrifugation. J Am Vet Med Assoc 192:1726–1729, 1988.
DeLahunta A: Veterinary Neuroanatomy and Clinical Neurology, ed 2. Philadelphia, WB Saunders, 1983.
Kline KL, Joseph RJ, Averill DR: Feline infectious peritonitis with neurologic involvement: Clinical and pathological findings in 24 cats. J Am Anim Hosp Assoc 30:345–350, 1994.
Meric SM: Canine meningitis. J Vet Intern Med 2:26–35, 1988.
Meyer D, Harvey J: Veterinary Laboratory Medicine, ed 2. Philadelphia, WB Saunders, 1998.
Oliver JE, Lorenz M, Kornegay J: Handbook of Veterinary Neurology, ed 3. Philadelphia, WB Saunders, 1997.
Thomson CE, Kornegay JN, Stevens JB: Analysis of cerebrospinal fluid from the cerebellomedullary and lumbar cisterns of dogs with focal neurologic disease: 145 cases (1985–1987). J Am Vet Med Assoc 196:1841–1844, 1990.
Tipold A: Diagnosis of inflammatory and infectious disease of the central nervous system in dogs: A retrospective study. J Vet Intern Med 9:304–314, 1995.
Tipold A, Jaggy A: Steroid responsive meningitis-arteritis in dogs: Long term study of 32 cases. J Small Anim Pract 35:311–316, 1994.

ENDOCRINE FUNCTION

··········HANDLING AND SHIPPING GUIDELINES—ENDOCRINE ASSAYS

5

Clot activator present in serum separator tubes may adversely affect results of assays used for hormonal evaluations and therapeutic drug monitoring. Plain red tubes can be used for all submissions of hormonal assays, and specific recommendations for certain tests are included in the discussion that follows (Table 5–1).

Disturbances in the secretion of some hormones may be recognized clinically if careful attention is given to the history and physical examination. Particular attention should be paid to the rate of growth and physical development; subsequent changes in body weight and conformation and distribution of body fat; sexual development and reproductive performance; changes in physical activity and stamina; condition of the skin and hair; and the occurrence of polyphagia, polydipsia (PD), or polyuria (PU).

Table 5–1. Handling and Shipping Guidelines—Endocrine Assays*

Assay	Sample
T₃, T₄, cortisol, insulin, progesterone, testosterone, estradiol	Serum
ACTH	Collect whole blood in EDTA; transfer immediately to a plastic container. Centrifuge immediately. Collect *plasma*. Freeze in plastic container. Submit frozen; pack in dry ice.

T₃ triiodothyronine; T₄ thyroxine.
*Never ship whole blood or hemolyzed samples. The reproductive state (i.e., pregnant or stage of estrus) should be noted on samples submitted for T₃, T₄, cortisol, or insulin. Store samples at 4°C or lower if required. Samples should be frozen when storage is expected to exceed 3 days. Avoid administration of medication, especially anesthetics, analgesics, and hormones, prior to testing. Ship early in the week. Avoid shipping on Fridays. Samples should be shipped to arrive at the laboratory early in the week.

............ADRENAL CORTEX

Cortisol, corticosterone, and aldosterone—the principal hormones secreted by the adrenal cortex—regulate carbohydrate and electrolyte metabolism. Cortisol is the main glucocorticosteroid produced by the adrenal cortex, and its rate of secretion is controlled primarily by adrenocorticotropic hormone (ACTH) from the adenohypophysis. Aldosterone is the main mineralocorticoid, and corticosterone has both mineralocorticosteroid and glucocorticosteroid functions. The prime regulator in controlling aldosterone release is the renin-angiotensin system, which is dependent on variations in fluid volume. Aldosterone stimulates sodium and chloride reabsorption, increases the excretion of potassium, and increases the retention of water, thus expanding the vascular compartments.

............Effect of Mineralocorticoids

The mineralocorticoids increase resorption of sodium and chloride, increase the excretion of potassium, and allow an exchange of intracellular potassium with extracellular sodium.

............Effect of Glucocorticosteroids (Cortisol)

Glucocorticosteroids increase protein catabolism, which results in an increased breakdown of muscle protein, interference with the normal production of bone matrix, and increased gluconeogenesis from amino acids. Antibody formation initially increases but later decreases because of the lysis of lymphocytes and lymph nodes. Glucocorticosteroids tend to conserve energy derived from circulating glucose by (1) inhibiting glucose utilization in peripheral tissues, (2) mobilizing fatty acids for energy production, and (3) increasing the flow of amino acids to the liver for new glucose production. Glomerular filtration is increased, and an "anti–antidiuretic hormone" (ADH) effect results in diuresis. Electrolyte effects are evidenced by retention of small amounts of sodium and excretion of potassium. Arteriolar tone and blood pressure are maintained. Inflammatory reactions are reduced because of a decrease in fibroplasia as well as a decrease in the production of histamine and histamine-like substances (serotonin).

Evaluation of Adrenocortical Function
Clinical Syndromes

Signs of *canine hyperadrenocorticism* can result spontaneously from excessive administration of glucocorticoids or from pituitary-dependent or cortisol-producing adrenocortical tumor. The clinical manifestations of hyperadrenocorticism may include PU or PD, polyphagia, panting, weakness, endocrine alopecia, and insulin-resistant diabetes.

Eighty percent to 90% of the dogs with naturally occurring hyperadrenocorticism have pituitary-dependent hyperadrenocorticism (PDH). The balance of the dogs have functional adrenocortical adenomas or carcinomas. Most of the pituitary tumors are microadenomas. Larger (> 4 mm in size) macroadenomas may be present in 10% to 20% of the cases based on computed tomography (CT) scans or magnetic resonance imaging (MRI). Macroadenomas may produce the following clinical signs: dorsal growth of the tumor produces compression or invasion, or both, of the hypothalamic area; animals appear disoriented, develop inappetence and anorexia, are dull and listless, may pace and circle, have difficulty lying down, develop ataxia and head-pressing, or have seizures and visual loss.

Laboratory Tests

The total WBC, differential, hematocrit, and total eosinophil counts should be evaluated. Serum sodium, potassium, chloride, urea, and protein determinations may also be valuable.

The following laboratory tests are helpful in confirming the diagnosis of hyperadrenocorticism: a complete blood count (CBC) that exhibits a stress pattern, including leukocytosis, neutrophilia, lymphopenia, eosinopenia, and monocytosis; slight elevation of serum alanine aminotransferase (ALT; formerly serum glutamate pyruvate transaminase [SGPT]); elevated alkaline phosphatase, associated with induction of the steroid liver isoenzyme of alkaline phosphatase by glucocorticosteroid excess; mild to moderate elevations in serum cholesterol levels; and a slight to moderate elevation in fasting blood glucose levels, associated with increased hepatic gluconeogenesis. Urine specific gravity is low in patients with PU or PD; resting thyroid hormone levels are low; and systolic and diastolic blood pressures are elevated. Urinalysis often reveals proteinuria and evidence of cystitis.

CANINE HYPERADRENOCORTICISM
Dexamethasone Suppression Test

For cortisol determinations collect blood in ethylenediaminetetraacetic acid (EDTA) and separate sample, and refrigerate. Send sample refrigerated.

The dexamethasone test is indicated when there is a need to distinguish among adrenal hyperplasia, pituitary-dependent adrenal hyperplasia, and adrenal neoplasia.

In normal dogs, dexamethasone suppresses the plasma cortisol concentration essentially to zero and maintains the suppression for several hours. Dogs with pituitary-dependent Cushing's disease are less sensitive to the suppression, and a larger dose of dexamethasone is required.

The low-dose dexamethasone suppression (LDDS) test should be done first. The high-dose dexamethasone suppression (HDDS) test can be begun 48 hours later. For the screening test, inject dexamethasone sodium phosphate intravenously (IV) at 0.01 mg/kg and collect samples at 0 (baseline), 2, 4, and 8 hours. Collect blood in heparin. Centrifuge the sample, and remove and freeze the plasma.

In normal dogs, the plasma cortisol level is reduced to less than 1.5 μg/dL within 3 hours and remains suppressed for 8 hours or more. In most dogs with pituitary-dependent Cushing's disease, there is a slight decrease at the 3-hour point, but by 8 hours there is no suppression. No cortisol suppression occurs in the majority of dogs with adrenal tumors and in 25% of those with pituitary-dependent hyperadrenocorticism. The low-dose dexamethasone test can confirm Cushing's disease but cannot reliably differentiate between pituitary-dependent and adrenal tumors. The low-dose dexamethasone suppression test is not used to evaluate mitotane therapy.

A high-dose dexamethasone suppression test can be used in some cases to differentiate between the presence of pituitary-dependent Cushing's disease and autonomous adrenal tumor. Inject dexamethasone phosphate 0.1 mg/kg IV, and collect a baseline sample and later response samples at 2, 6, and 8 hours post injection.

When dexamethasone 0.1 mg/kg is used, complete suppression is defined as plasma cortisol values that are (1) less than 50% of the baseline value or (2) less than 1.5 μg/dL, according to Peterson (using his radioimmunoassay technique). Dogs with pituitary-dependent hyperadrenocorticism (90%) often fulfill this suppression criterion. The high-dose dexamethasone suppression test fails to suppress corticosteroid levels in 20% to 30% of dogs with pituitary-dependent Cushing's disease and 100% of dogs with adrenal tumors.

............Endogenous ACTH

Blood should be collected in tubes containing EDTA and the enzyme inhibitor aprotinin. The tube should be filled to maximum and the blood immediately centrifuged and the plasma removed and placed into plastic tubes and shipped at 4°C. Normal values for dogs, 10 to 80 pg/mL; cats, 5 to 85 pg/mL.

New radioimmunoassay (RIA) tests for endogenous ACTH production can be used to screen dogs for Cushing's disease and to distinguish pituitary-dependent from adrenocortical tumor hyperadrenocorticism. In normal dogs, the resting ACTH levels in early-morning samples have been determined as 46.0 ± 16.85 pg/mL with a range of 20 to 100 pg/mL. In dogs with pituitary-dependent functional hyperplasia, ACTH levels are usually greater than 40 pg/mL; means have been reported as 98 ± 48.6 pg/mL and 132 ± 68 pg/mL, with ranges from 29 to 340 pg/mL. In dogs with adrenocortical tumors, ACTH concentrations were usually less than 20 pg/mL, with a mean of 16 ± 2.0 pg/mL (range = 16 to 36). This form of testing, coupled with dexamethasone suppression testing, is extremely helpful in evaluating the pituitary-adrenal axis in hyperadrenocorticism. The addition of the protease inhibitor aprotinin to whole blood in EDTA tubes prevents degradation of ACTH. Samples are spun in a centrifuge and can be kept up to 4 days at 4°C.

............Plasma Cortisol Determinations—ACTH Stimulation

Plasma cortisol levels can be valuable diagnostic aids in hyperadrenocorticism. Plasma cortisol levels can be determined by competitive protein binding, fluorometric techniques, and radioimmunoassay (RIA). Cortisol values may differ significantly from laboratory to laboratory. RIA is the most sensitive test. In the evaluation of plasma cortisol levels, blood is taken before and 1 hour after administration of 0.5 units/kg aqueous synthetic ACTH IV.* An early morning venous sample, 3 to 5 mL, is obtained in heparin; the blood sample is centrifuged; and the plasma is removed. Plasma should be separated from the blood

....

*Cortrosyn, Organon Pharmaceuticals, West Orange, NJ.

cellular elements within 15 to 30 minutes. The plasma must be kept frozen until the test is run; otherwise, cortisol levels will decrease.

Porcine aqueous gelatin ACTH* can also be used to evaluate adrenocortical function; ACTH gel 2.2 IU/kg (maximum 20 units per dog) can be given intramuscularly (IM) and baseline and plasma collected 2 hours later.

The normal levels of plasma cortisol measured by RIA are variable and depend on which laboratory performs the test. It is recommended that normal levels be established for the laboratory used.

Single plasma cortisol determinations do not provide an adequate assessment of adrenal function because of the normal variation in blood cortisol levels. Testing cortisol levels and response with ACTH is much more effective. In hyperadrenocorticism, there is a hyperresponse of plasma cortisol to ACTH stimulation. In normal dogs, post-ACTH cortisol concentrations are at least two to three times higher than basal levels. In pituitary-dependent Cushing's disease, the post-ACTH cortisol level is higher than the normal level (usually >15 μg/dL). In dogs with adrenocortical tumors, there is a variability in response to ACTH, with some dogs having normal increases (two to three times basal cortisol levels) and other dogs having exaggerated increases. Dogs with carcinoma of the adrenal gland may show an especially elevated cortisol response. Dogs with adrenocortical tumors (approximately 25% of these cases) may show a below-normal response to ACTH stimulation; however, 75% to 80% of dogs with adrenocortical tumors *do not* show at least 50% suppression of baseline cortisol levels when evaluated with dexamethasone 0.1 mg/kg.

The ACTH stimulation test will identify hyperadrenocorticism in more than half of dogs with adrenal tumor hyperadrenocorticism and in 85% of dogs with pituitary-dependent hyperadrenocorticism.

A subnormal response to ACTH and greater than 50% suppression of plasma cortisol by high-dose dexamethasone indicate a diagnosis of iatrogenic hyperadrenocorticism.

The ACTH test is valuable as a screening test for Cushing's disease. However, if the results of the test are normal, Cushing's disease cannot be ruled out because dogs with adrenal tumors can respond normally to ACTH. The test alone cannot reliably distinguish between pituitary-dependent and adrenal tumor–dependent Cushing's disease (Table 5–2).

·········· Cortisol Levels for Cats

Hyperadrenocorticism in cats has also been reported, although the incidence is very low. Typically, cats with hyperadrenocorticism are presented with poorly regulated diabetes mellitus. Cats have polyuria, polydipsia, pendulous abdomen, polyphagia, endocrine alopecia, muscle wasting, hepatomegaly, and thin, easily traumatized skin. Cats are often diabetic and exhibit glycosuria, elevated blood glucose levels, and elevated serum aldosterone levels. Female cats appear to be more susceptible than male cats. Hyperadrenocorticism is a disease of older cats (usually >10 years) and is strongly correlated with the development of insulin-resistant diabetes mellitus.

·········· Pituitary-Adrenal Function Tests in the Cat

Diagnostic tests used to diagnose hyperadrenocorticism in the cat are similar to those used in the dog but there are differences in protocol and interpretations. The ACTH stimulation test is a valuable screening test for hyperadrenocorticism in cats. The ACTH stimulation test can be conducted by:

1. Administering ACTH gel 2.2 units/kg IM and collecting baseline, 60-minute, and 120-minute blood samples or,

*Cortigel-HO, Savage Labs, Melville, NY.

Table 5-2. Diagnostic Tests to Assess the Pituitary-Adrenocortical Axis

Test	Purpose	Protocol	Results		Interpretation
Endogenous ACTH	Differentiate PDH vs. AT	Plasma sample obtained between 8 and 10 AM; special handling required	<20 pg/mL 20-50 pg/mL >50 pg/mL		AT Nondiagnostic PDH
ACTH stimulation	Diagnose Cushing's disease	Dog: 0.25 mg synthetic ACTH/dog IM; plasma pre-ACTH and 1 hr post-ACTH	*Post-ACTH Cortisol:* >24 μg/dL 19-24 μg/dL 8-18 μg/dL <8 μg/dL		Strongly suggestive* Suggestive† Normal Iatrogenic Cushing's disease
		Cat: 0.125 mg synthetic ACTH/cat IM; plasma pre-ACTH, 30 and 60 min post-ACTH	>15 μg/dL 12-15 μg/dL 6-12 μg/dL <6 μg/dL		Strongly suggestive Suggestive Normal Iatrogenic Cushing's disease
Low-dose dexamethasone suppression test	Diagnose Cushing's disease and differentiate PDH vs. AT	0.01 mg dexamethasone/kg IV; plasma pre-dexamethasone, 4 and 8 hr post-dexamethasone	*4 hr Post-Dexamethasone:* — <1.5 μg/dL >1.5 μg/dL	*8 hr Post-Dexamethasone:* <1.5 μg/dL >1.5 μg/dL >1.5 μg/dL	Normal PDH PDH or AT
High-dose dexamethasone suppression test	Differentiate PDH vs. AT	0.1 mg dexamethasone/kg IV, plasma dexamethasone and 4 and 8 hr post-dexamethasone	*Post-Dexamethasone Cortisol:* <50% of pre-value ≥50% of pre-value		PDH PDH or AT

AT, adrenocortical tumor; PDH, pituitary-dependent hyperadrenocorticism.
*Strongly suggestive of hyperadrenocorticism.
†Suggestive of hyperadrenocorticism.

2. Administering synthetic ACTH (cosyntropin) 0.125 mg and collecting baseline, 30-minute, and 60-minute blood samples

The post-ACTH peak plasma level in the cat is 12 μg/dL.

The low-dose dexamethasone suppression test in the cat can be used as in the dog. Most cats with hyperadrenocorticism do not suppress at 3 hours following low-dose dexamethasone testings and have an exaggerated response to ACTH gel. Cats may occasionally not respond to the LDDS test and fall outside of the normal limits after 8-hour measurement. Therefore, it is recommended that the LDDS not be used as the only test for demonstrating hyperadrenocorticism in the cat; rather, the HDDS test along with abdominal radiography and ultrasound should be used in an attempt to differentiate pituitary-dependent hyperadrenocorticism from adrenal tumor hyperadrenocorticism.

Discrimination of pituitary-dependent hyperadrenocorticism from adrenal tumors can be carried out by measuring endogenous plasma ACTH levels (see also p. 632). Elevated plasma ACTH levels are found in cases of PDH. CT and MRI can be used to demonstrate masses in the pituitary fossa.

Megestrol acetate administered to cats causes significant depression of cortisol levels, and the ACTH-stimulated cortisol response is still abnormal for at least 1 or 2 weeks after discontinuation of megestrol.

·········· Canine Primary Hypoadrenocorticism (Addison's Disease)

Hypoadrenocorticism (Addison's disease) is the result of primary adrenocortical failure. The disease is more common in female dogs than in male dogs. Hypoadrenocorticism has been reported in the cat only rarely. Lack of aldosterone leads to inability to conserve sodium and excrete potassium. Loss of sodium leads to a decrease in extracellular fluid volume, weight loss, decreased blood pressure, decreased cardiac output, azotemia, generalized weakness, and depression. Hyperkalemia and mild acidosis also develop. Clinical signs include lethargy, weakness, anorexia, vomiting, weight loss, prerenal azotemia, eosinophilia, microcardia, hypoglycemia, anemia, PU or PD, hypothermia, and bradycardia.

·········· Confirmation of Hypoadrenocorticism

In dogs with hypoadrenocorticism, results of ACTH stimulation testing revealed low to low-normal serum baseline cortisol concentrations that failed to increase after ACTH administration.

The following laboratory test results are helpful in confirming the diagnosis of hypoadrenocorticism: elevated blood urea nitrogen (BUN) associated with prerenal azotemia from reduced renal perfusion and decreased glomerular filtration rate and electrolyte changes consisting of hyponatremia, hypochloremia, and hyperkalemia. The normal sodium-potassium ratio is 27:1 to 32:1. In hypoadrenocorticism, this ratio is 20:1 or less. Hypoadrenocorticism is associated with hyperkalemia, hyponatremia, hypochloremia, and hypercalcemia in 25% to 30% of the cases.

■ CAUSES OF REDUCED SODIUM-TO-POTASSIUM RATIO (<27)

Hypoadrenocorticism
Renal disease
Repeated drainage of effusions (from pleural or peritoneal cavity)
Diarrhea associated with *Trichuris* infection
Diabetic ketoacidosis

A finding of normal serum sodium and potassium levels cannot rule out the possibility of hypoadrenocorticism in all cases. The diagnosis of hypoadrenocorticism should be based on lack of response to ACTH.

In hypoadrenocorticism with hyperkalemia (serum potassium level between 6 and 7 mEq/L), the T waves may become increased in amplitude, spiked, and narrow-based. Serum potassium levels of 7 to 8 mEq/L produce a depression of the P wave. Serum potassium levels above 8 mEq/L produce bradycardia (50 to 70 bpm), absence of P waves, and a widened QRS wave. Concentrations of potassium in the range of 11 to 14 mEq/L lead to ventricular asystole or ventricular fibrillation.

............Hypoadrenocorticism in Cats

Primary hypoadrenocorticism is a rare disease in cats. The most common signs are lethargy, depression, anorexia, and weight loss. Additional signs may include vomiting, PU and PD, and response to nonspecific supportive therapy. Affected cats are depressed, often dehydrated, hypothermic, have slow capillary refill time, and weak femoral pulses. Affected animals have an abnormal sodium-potassium ratio (<24:1). Characteristic T-wave changes associated with the problem in dogs have not been observed in cats.

............Pheochromocytomas

A pheochromocytoma is a tumor of the sympathetic nervous system. The postganglionic fibers are adrenergic and liberate norepinephrine and, in the adrenal medulla of the dog, epinephrine. Feldman and Nelson provide an excellent description of the normal production and metabolism of epinephrine. The endocrine cells of the adrenal medulla are called chromaffin cells. They are capable of secreting norepinephrine and epinephrine. A pheochromocytoma is a catecholamine-producing tumor derived from chromaffin cells. Adrenal pheochromocytomas are diagnosed uncommonly in dogs and rarely in cats and diagnosis is usually made at autopsy. Pheochromocytomas are usually malignant in dogs. There are often signs of many other concurrent problems when a pheochromocytoma is present. The use of abdominal ultrasound as a diagnostic test has been helpful in identifying possible adrenal masses. The most common clinical signs associated with pheochromocytomas are weakness, collapsing episodes, lethargy, vomiting, panting, PU/PD, diarrhea, weight loss, rear limb edema, nasal hemorrhage, acute visual loss, and retinal bleeding. Blood pressure readings are very important in making the diagnosis (see also p. 75).

The use of the clonidine suppression test as an aid to the confirmatory diagnosis of a pheochromocytoma in the dog is described by Feldman and Nelson.

REFERENCES

Barthez PY, Marks SL, Woo J, et al: Pheochromocytoms in dogs: 61 cases (1984–1995), J Vet Intern Med 11:272, 1997.
Feldman EC, Nelson RW: Canine and Feline Endocrinology and Reproduction, ed 2. Philadelphia, WB Saunders, 1996.
Meyer D, Harvey J: Veterinary Laboratory Medicine, ed 2. Philadelphia, WB Saunders, 1998.

............Growth Hormone

Growth hormone (GH, somatotropin) is a polypeptide hormone secreted by the anterior pituitary gland. The hormone stimulates cell growth and mitosis and results in increased cell size and increased numbers of cells. The ability to reach normal body size is dependent on GH. The absence of effective levels of GH results in retarded growth called *dwarfism.* Overproduction of GH can result in acromegaly. The catabolic effect of GH is mediated through interference with the action of insulin on peripheral tissue.

GH is affected by many physiologic factors thought to be mediated by factors produced by the hypothalamus. The release of GH from the anterior pituitary is mediated by a hypothalamic growth hormone–releasing factor (GH-RF). A GH-inhibiting factor, somatostatin, has been located in the median eminence of the hypothalamus and can block GH release.

.... Growth Hormone Excess (Acromegaly)

Acromegaly in dogs has been associated with elevated levels of GH resulting from the treatment of dogs with progestational compounds or, in older dogs, occurring spontaneously during the corpus luteum phase (progestational phase) of the ovarian cycle. All acromegalic dogs are females. Normal GH levels for the dog have been found by RIA to be 10 ng/mL or less. Evidence for excessive GH production includes (1) inspiratory stridor caused by increased soft tissue around the neck and increased soft tissue density around the abdomen, (2) reduced exercise tolerance, (3) PU or PD, and (4) enlargement of the interdental space. The condition is controlled by ovariohysterectomy, which reduces GH levels to the normal range.

Cats may suffer from acromegaly associated with GH-secreting pituitary tumors (macroadenomas). Most acromegalic cats are males. The problem is usually associated with middle-aged and older domestic shorthair (DSH) cats (mean age, 10 years). The most commonly recognized clinical manifestation of feline acromegaly is insulin-resistant diabetes mellitus. Additional signs include PU or PD, cardiomegaly, hepatomegaly, large head, large tongue, and arthritis. Fifty percent of the cats with acromegaly have renal failure.

■ CLINICAL SIGNS OF ACROMEGALY IN THE CAT

Polyuria or polydipsia related to diabetes mellitus
Polyphagia
Organomegaly (kidney, liver, heart)
Prognathia inferior
Weight gain
Large head
Potbelly
Spondylosis
Large tongue
Arthropathy, CNS disease

5

Growth Hormone Response Test In this test, IV xylazine is used to stimulate GH release. Heparinized plasma samples are collected at baseline, 30 minutes, and 60 minutes following IV injection of xylazine 100 μg/kg. Abnormal production of GH may be associated with secretory capacity for GH as well as hyperadrenocorticism with hypothyroidism. Measurement of somatomedin C (insulin-like growth factor) is used as an indirect indicator of GH activity. Reference values are 5 to 70 nmol/L for nondiabetic cats and 150 to 180 nmol/L for acromegalic cats.

.... Growth Hormone Deficiency (Dwarfism)

Endocrine dwarfism occurs most frequently in the German shepherd breed of dogs, in which it is thought to be inherited as an autosomal recessive trait.

The condition in German shepherds is associated with abnormal development of Rathke's pouch and produces partial or total pituitary insufficiency.

Growth hormone–responsive alopecia occurs predominantly in Pomeranians, chow chows, poodles, American water spaniels, keeshonds, and Samoyeds. The onset is usually between 1 and 2 years of age.

............THE POSTERIOR PITUITARY

ADH, or vasopressin, and the oxytocic hormone involved in parturition are both produced in the hypothalamus and released from the pars nervosa of the pituitary.

............Antidiuretic Hormone

Arginine vasopressin is formed in the supraoptic and paraventricular nuclei of the hypothalamus and stored in the posterior lobe of the pituitary. Under normal conditions, the major physiologic controls governing vasopressin release are plasma osmolarity and changes in blood volume. The major physiologic effect of ADH is to increase the permeability of the distal tubules of the kidneys to water.

............Diabetes Insipidus (see also Polyuria and Polydipsia, p. 424)

Diabetes insipidus is a syndrome of excessive excretion of water due to insufficient production or release of ADH. In affected animals, urine volume is 3 to 10 times the normal amount per day; urine specific gravity ranges from 1.001 to 1.005; and urine osmolality ranges from 50 to 200 mOsm/kg.

There are two prerequisites for a diagnosis of diabetes insipidus: (1) persistent diuresis in the presence of stimuli that normally provoke secretion of ADH, and (2) antidiuresis in response to administered ADH.

The release of ADH and its effect on the urine should be measured by urine and plasma osmolality or specific gravity. (Osmolality is a measure of the number of particles in a given weight of fluid and is proportional to the osmotic pressure of that fluid. Osmolality is measured by freezing point depression in an osmometer; see p. 772).

The long-term prognosis for dogs with chronic diabetes insipidus is dependent on the underlying etiology. Dogs with PDI should have a CT or MRI scan to visualize the pituitary gland. Radiation is the treatment of choice for pituitary neoplasia.

............Tests (see also Differential Diagnosis, Polyuria and Polydipsia, p. 424)

............*Vasopressin Response Tests*

............Aqueous ADH Test

1. Place the indwelling catheter in the vein; flush with heparinized saline.
2. Empty the bladder of residual urine.
3. Make a fresh solution of aqueous ADH (Pitressin) in 5% dextrose in water (D5W).
4. Administer ADH 5 mU/lb IV over a 60-minute period. (An addition of 5 units of aqueous vasopressin in 1 L of D5W produces a vasopressin concentration of 5 mU/mL; thus, 1 mL/lb administered over a 60-minute period.)
5. Collect urine at 30, 60, and 90 minutes following vasopressin infusion.
6. The response in dogs with diabetes insipidus may not be as great as that in

normal dogs, and specific gravity may reach only 1.012 or higher, but this is diagnostic for diabetes insipidus.

............Repositol ADH Response Test

1. Inject (after warming and shaking) 5 units of Pitressin tannate in oil subcutaneously (SC). The effects can last 2 to 3 days.
2. Withhold fluids and food during the test period.
3. Empty the bladder immediately, and collect all urine at and 12 hours following ADH administration.

Although precise responses of dogs to this test have not been established, a urine specific gravity value of 1.020 to 1.025 or higher represents a normal response.

Desmopressin acetate (DDAVP) intranasal drops can be used by administering one drop in the nose (20 μg [0.1 mL]) q12h. Urine specific gravity and osmolality can then be checked.

............Infusion of Hypertonic Saline

Infusion of hypertonic saline may also be used to determine whether ADH can be released, but this infusion is rarely required and should be used with caution.

1. Withhold food for 12 hours (however, water may be given for free choice).
2. Administer water 30 mL/kg by stomach tube.
3. One hour later, collect urine and plasma samples and check the osmolality. An indwelling catheter is left in the bladder.
4. Give 10 mL/kg of 5% saline IV over a period of 30 minutes *under close observation*. (This infusion occasionally produces mild to moderately severe seizures and should be discontinued immediately if they occur.)
5. At the 15- and 30-minute marks after the infusion, collect urine and plasma samples and check their osmolality. The hypertonic saline will cause a rise in plasma osmolality, and urine osmolality must be increased above that of the corresponding plasma sample to demonstrate ADH secretion.

............THE THYROID GLAND

Thyroid hormone affects the rate of metabolism, growth, and development. Thyroxine (T_4) and triiodothyronine (T_3) are iodinated amino acids, and their synthesis and secretion are principally under the control of thyroid-stimulating hormone (TSH). In the formation of thyroid hormones, iodine is absorbed from the gastrointestinal tract, is transported to the follicular cells of the thyroid gland, and becomes part of the follicular colloid. When iodine is bound to tyrosine, this monoiodotyrosine is again iodinated to form diiodotyrosine. The oxidative condensation of two diiodotyrosine molecules forms T_4, or one mono-iodo- and one diiodotyrosine form T_3. T_4 is transported in the blood of the dog by at least four serum proteins. Only free T_3 and T_4 are physiologically active and maintain the euthyroid state of the animal. Metabolism of thyroid hormones occurs primarily in the liver by both diiodination and conjugation.

Maintenance of normal thyroid secretion is established through the anterior pituitary via TSH and the free T_3-T_4 feedback system. The control of TSH production is also regulated by the hypothalamus through the production of thyrotropin-releasing hormone (TRH).

The normal blood level of T_4 in the dog is approximately 1 to 4 μg/dL, and the normal level of T_3 is between 60 and 200 ng/dL. Protein-bound iodine (PBI) levels would then be about 2.00 μg/dL for the dog and approximately 1.60 μg/

dL for the cat. In the cat, T_4 levels measured by RIA range from 1 to 4 μg/dL and T_3 levels range from 40 to 110 ng/dL, although these estimates vary with different laboratories.

............Evaluating Thyroid Function

............Hyperthyroidism

Hyperthyroidism is mainly associated with animals that have functional adenomas of the thyroid gland. Thyroid neoplasia accounts for 10% to 15% of head and neck tumors in the dog. Most thyroid neoplasms are carcinomas. Signs seen in the dog are nervousness, weight loss, PU/PD. Hyperthyroidism is the most common endocrinopathy affecting cats older than 8 years of age. Adenocarcinomas are present in 20% of the cats. Seventy percent of cats with hyperthyroidism have bilateral involvement. Normal thyroid glands are not palpable in the cat. Enlarged thyroid glands may be palpable or may be within the thoracic inlet. The major presenting clinical signs are weight loss, polyphagia, hyperactivity, PU or PD, hyperdefecation with marked steatorrhea, heat intolerance, panting, and muscle tremors. Mild to moderate hypertrophic cardiomegaly that is reversible may develop, and tachycardia (> 240 bpm), ventricular hypertrophy, and increased amplitude of the R waves are seen. Eighty percent of the cats with hyperthyroidism are hypertensive.

The differential diagnosis of hyperthyroidism in the cat may include diabetes mellitus, pancreatic exocrine insufficiency, chronic renal disease, primary cardiomyopathy, intestinal malabsorption, hepatic disease, and neoplasia.

RIA for thyroid hormones in hyperthyroid cats gave average values for T_4 of 8 to 24 μg/dL (1.4 to 4.0 μg/dL is normal) and for T_3 of 277 ± 49 ng/dL (40 to 110 ng/dL is normal). Serum T_4 in cats fluctuates from day to day. Many nonthyroidal diseases can lower the T_4 concentration. A single T_4 sample should not rule out hyperthyroidism.

Evaluation of the serum T_4 response to IV administration of 0.1 mg/kg of TRH will differentiate normal from hyperthyroid cats. After IV administration of TRH, normal cats at 4 hours show a twofold increase or greater in T_4 Hyperthyroid cats typically show no increase or a marginal increase in serum T_4 levels. Cats with mild hyperthyroidism have an increase in serum T_4 concentrations less than 50%, whereas normal cats and those with other illnesses have an increase greater than 60%.

Free T_4 by Dialysis (FT$_4$D) as an Aid to Diagnosis of Mild Hyperthyroidism in the Cat FT$_4$D concentrations are useful in the diagnosis of hyperthyroidism in the cat when T_4 levels are normal or only slightly elevated. Cats with mild hyperthyroidism may have T_4 concentrations between 2.5 and 4.0 μg/dL and an elevated FT$_4$D level. FT$_4$D should not be used alone as a screening test for hyperthyroidism in the cat because occasionally elevated FT$_4$D levels have been noted in cats with nonthyroidal illness.

A very reliable procedure for diagnosing hyperthyroidism in cats is a technetium 99m pertechnetate thyroid scan. Clinical pathology demonstrates an increased packed cell volume (PCV) in 45% of the cases, eosinopenia in 40% of the cases, and erythrocytosis in 20% of the cases.

............Occult Hyperthyroidism

Peterson has described cats in which the clinical manifestations of hyperthyroidism are mild with normal to equivocal basal serum thyroid concentrations. In these cases, a T_3 suppression test can be performed utilizing the oral administration of T_3 to detect cats with abnormal elevations of T_4 hormone and clinical hyperthyroidism. In normal cats, administration of T_3 results in inhibition of pituitary TSH secretion and a subsequent fall in T_4 levels. In cats with hyperthyroidism, the autonomous production of T_4 and T_3 by the thyroid has already suppressed the pituitary TSH secretion and therefore exogenous T_3 should have no effect on T_4 levels. To perform a T_3 test, collect serum for T_4 and T_3 and freeze. Liothyronine (T_3; Cytomel, Smith Kline-Beecham, Philadelphia, PA) is started the following morning at a dosage of 5 μg t.i.d. for 2 days. The final dose is given on the morning of the third day, and blood for T_4 and T_3 determination is collected 2 and 4 hours later.

..........Thyroid Gland Neoplasia and Hyperthyroidism in the Dog

Thyroid gland tumors in dogs are usually nonfunctional, large, invasive, metastatic carcinomatous masses. They usually develop in middle-aged dogs. Metastases occur most commonly to the lungs and retropharyngeal lymph nodes.

Clinical features are swelling in the neck, dyspnea, coughing, vomiting or regurgitation, listlessness, depression, dysphagia, weight loss, change in bark, and pain in the cervical area.

..........Hypothyroidism in Dogs

Hypothyroidism is seen most commonly in middle-aged dogs (4 to 10 years of age) of medium-sized to large breeds. Prominent breeds include the golden retriever, Doberman pinscher, Irish setter, miniature schnauzer, dachshund, cocker spaniel, Airedale, Great Dane, and Old English sheepdog. Clinical signs of hypothyroidism may include mental dullness; lethargy; exercise intolerance; weight gain; bilateral symmetrical, nonpruritic alopecia; dull or dry, easily epilated hair coat; hyperpigmentation; poor wound healing; prolonged estrus intervals; lack of libido; seizures; ataxia; facial paralysis; peripheral neuropathy; idiopathic megaesophagus; and ocular, cardiovascular, gastrointestinal, and clotting abnormalities.

Most cases of hypothyroidism in dogs are of primary origin, resulting from idiopathic follicular atrophy or an entity that is being more commonly recognized: immunologically mediated lymphocytic thyroiditis. In lymphocytic thyroiditis, clinical signs of hypothyroidism develop when more than 75% of the gland is destroyed. Lymphocytic thyroiditis is an immune-mediated disease.

Hypothyroidism may also be secondary to a deficiency of pituitary gland TSH or iodine deficiencies.

..........Hypothyroidism in Cats

Hypothyroidism in cats is rare. The most common cause is iatrogenic destruction or removal of the thyroid gland for treatment of hyperthyroidism. Signs include lethargy, obesity, alopecia, thickened skin, edema of the head, failure to have normal reproductive cycles, bradycardia, reduced body size, nonpruritic seborrhea sicca, matting of hair over the back, and loss of hair on the pinnae of the ears. Diagnosis is based on a TSH stimulation test with bovine TSH hormone 1.0 IU/kg IV or 2.5 units per cat IM with a T_4 sample collected 8 to 12 hours following the injection. Normal response to TSH is a T_4 concentration that is 2.0 to 3.0 μg/dL higher than the basal serum T_4 value.

..........Clinical Pathology in Hypothyroidism

1. Hemogram: normocytic, normochromic, nonregenerative anemia
2. Hypercholesterolemia or hypertriglyceridemia in fewer than 30%

...........Laboratory Tests

There are numerous tests for the evaluation of thyroid gland function in dogs; older tests include T_4, T_3, and the TSH stimulation tests. TSH for the TSH stimulation test is no longer available. Several new tests are available for evaluation of thyroid function in dogs and cats: FT_4D, canine thyroid stimulation hormone (cTSH), and thyroglobulin autoantibodies (TgAAs). The Orthopedic Foundation for Animals has established a thyroid registry, and serum concentrations of FT_4D, cTSH, and TgAA will be used as baseline levels. The tests are suggested to be repeated once a year for 5 years.

...........Thyroxine Test

This test determines the total circulating serum T_4 level. The two most commonly used methods for T_4 analysis are competitive protein binding (CPB) assay and RIA. The free T_4 determination by RIA has largely supplanted the CPB assay and is the preferred thyroid test. In the dog, normal values for T_4 determined by RIA are greater than 3 μg/dL. Values below 1.5 μg/dL are abnormal. There is variability in normal canine T_4 levels determined in different laboratories. Also, there is an overlap in values for dogs that may be hypothyroid and those that are euthyroid. The TSH response test may be helpful in these situations. The observation of a low T_4 concentration may be consistent with nonthyroidal disorders, and a single T_4 value outside the normal range does not mean that treatment for hypothyroidism is indicated.

The use of a test dose of TSH is a much more accurate method of measuring thyroid function and is the test of choice. Obtain baseline T_4 levels, and inject 0.1 IU of TSH (Dermathycin) IV. Collect a second blood sample at 6 hours after TSH administration for T_4 determination. Another method involves the IM administration of TSH. Obtain baseline values of T_4 by RIA, and administer aqueous TSH, 0.4 units/kg IM. Obtain a second sample for T_4 RIA 16 hours later. The minimal normal thyroid response is a doubling of the zero-time thyroid response at 16 hours following TSH injection.

...........Canine Thyroid-Stimulating Hormone

When endogenous TSH and FT_4D measurements are run concurrently and concur, the diagnostic accuracy is 100%. With primary hypothyroidism, serum FT_4D levels fall, resulting in increased TSH levels. Dogs with advanced thyroiditis or idiopathic hypothyroidism should have low FT_4D concentrations and elevated cTSH levels. Dogs with compensated hypothyroidism should have normal FT_4D concentrations and normal to elevated cTSH levels.

...........Serum Free T_4 by Dialysis Concentration

Free T_4 is the fraction of T_4 that is not bound to protein. The free fraction of T_4 is not as influenced by extrathyroidal disease, which may lower T_4 levels falsely. FT_4D can be used to monitor thyroid supplementation but offers no direct advantage over T_4 levels.

...........Thyroglobulin Antibodies

Hypothyroidism is associated with antithyroid antibodies and lymphocytic thyroiditis in approximately 80% of cases in the dog. The major action of thyroid hormones is primarily mediated by T_3 at the cellular level. T_4 serves as a prohormone for T_3 (T_4 is converted to T_3). An animal with normal T_4 levels can exhibit clinical hypothyroidism if T_4 is inadequately converted to T_3. Therefore,

T_3 testing with RIA can also be done. In interpreting T_4 values, it is important to realize that certain extrathyroidal factors can influence the levels:

1. Excess endogenous (Cushing's disease) or exogenous corticosteroid can cause lowered T_3 and T_4 test results. Lowered T_4 results from a decrease in thyroid-binding globulin levels and suppression of TSH release.
2. Other diseases resulting in lowered T_4 and T_3 levels are acute infections, diabetes mellitus, malignant disease, and renal disease.
3. Levels can be affected by drug-induced interference with propranolol salicylate therapy, phenylbutazone, phenytoin, phenobarbital, or mitotane.

The efficacy of replacement thyroid hormones can be checked by T_4 and T_3 testing (following replacement with levothyroxine). The animal should be evaluated 4 to 6 weeks after beginning medication. Thyroxine should be measured 4 to 8 hours following administration, and T_3 should be measured 2 to 3 hours following administration. These tests are called postpill tests.

The thyroid gland's ability to trap iodide can be evaluated by its ability to take up iodine 131. This procedure is limited to institutions that are equipped to perform this work. Decreased thyroid uptake indicates hypothyroidism. Serum cholesterol determinations may be coupled with thyroid function tests.

............Thyroid Gland Biopsy

This procedure is very helpful in confirming the diagnosis of hypothyroidism and in distinguishing primary from secondary hypothyroidism. Because most cases of hypothyroidism in dogs are due to primary atrophy of the thyroid gland or destructive thyroiditis, biopsy of the thyroid is almost equal in diagnostic value to measurement of ^{131}I uptake. Furthermore, biopsy often provides confirmatory evidence in cases in which the results of other tests are equivocal or are invalidated by iodine contamination.

The reviews by Feldman and Nelson and by Ferguson on thyroid gland function are excellent references.

............CALCIUM METABOLISM AND DISORDERS OF THE PARATHYROID GLANDS

Calcium is involved in many biologic processes of the body, including neuromuscular excitability, membrane permeability, muscle contraction, enzyme activity, hormone release, and blood coagulation. Total serum calcium consists of three fractions: ionized (free), protein-bound, and complexed fractions. Ionized calcium measurements are superior to total serum calcium measurements. In normal animals and in most animals with hypercalcemia, ionized calcium approximates 55% of total calcium values in dogs and 60% in cats. Determination of ionized calcium should be made from serum.

Primary control of blood calcium is dependent on (1) parathyroid hormone (PTH) secretion, (2) calcitonin hormone secretion, and (3) the presence of cholecalciferol (vitamin D_3). Major control of calcium is dependent on PTH production. Parathyroids are composed of chief cells whose secretory activity is related to levels of ionized calcium circulating in the blood. The biologic effects of PTH are numerous: PTH (1) elevates the blood calcium concentration, (2) decreases the blood phosphate concentration, (3) increases the urinary excretion of phosphate and decreases calcium loss in urine, (4) increases the rate of skeletal modeling and bone resorption, (5) increases the urinary excretion of hydroxyproline-containing peptides, (6) activates adenylate cyclase in target cells, and (7) accelerates the formation of active vitamin D metabolites by the kidney.

Levels of calcium in the body are also controlled by the hormone calcitonin.

Calcitonin is secreted by the parafollicular cell population in the mammalian thyroid gland. Calcitonin-secreting cells are derived embryologically from cells of the neural crest. Calcitonin produces a hypocalcemic effect by decreasing the entry of calcium from the skeleton into plasma through a temporary inhibition of PTH-stimulated bone resorption. In addtion, calcitonin increases the rate of movement of phosphate out of plasma into soft tissue and bone, and PTH and calcitonin are synergistic in decreasing the renal tubular reabsorption of phosphorus. Regulation of calcitonin secretion is governed by the level of ionized calcium.

The final major hormone involved in the regulation of calcium metabolism is 1,25-dihydroxyvitamin D_3 (1,25-DHCC). The target tissue for this metabolite is the small intestine, where it stimulates calcium and phosphate absorption and increases calcium and phosphate utilization from bone. Ultraviolet (UV) irradiation of ergosterol produces vitamin D_2. Vitamin D_2 or vitamin D_3 is transformed by the liver to 25-hydroxyvitamin D and is then actively metabolized in the kidney to 1,25-hydroxyvitamin D. In the skin, UV light converts 7-dehydrocholesterol to vitamin D_3.

...........Disorders of Parathyroid Glands

...........Hypocalcemia

Primary hypoparathyroidism signifies subnormal amounts of PTH or it may indicate that the hormone secreted cannot react normally with the target cells. Decreased secretion of PTH results in hyperphosphatemia, hypocalcemia, and impaired 1,25-dihydroxyvitamin D production. The two most common causes of primary hypoparathyroidism are idiopathic atrophy or destruction of parathyroid tissue, probably immune-mediated, and removal of or injury to parathyroid glands during thyroid surgery. Idiopathic hypoparathyroidism has been found in mature female dogs of small breeds. The clinical manifestations of hypoparathyroidism develop because of reduced bone resorption and progressively diminishing calcium levels (4 to 6 mg/dL). In cats the most common cause of hypocalcemia is following thyroidectomy with damage to the parathyroid glands. Major clinical signs in cats are related to the neuromuscular system, including seizures, nervousness, muscle twitching, tetany, ataxia, and weakness. Patients with primary hyperparathyroidism have high serum ionized calcium and immunoreactive PTH (iPTH) concentrations. In contrast, renal failure patients that subsequently develop hypercalcemia have normal to low ionized calcium in association with a high iPTH concentration.

Sensitive and validated iPTH assays for use in dogs are available. The most popular commercial assay employs a two-site immunoradiometric (IRMA) method that recognizes both the N- and C-terminals of the intact PTH (1–84) molecule. Serum needs to be separated immediately and frozen. It is necessary to interpret PTH concentrations simultaneously with the corresponding calcium concentrations. High PTH at the time of hypercalcemia strongly suggests the diagnosis of primary hyperparathyroidism, although PTH levels in the normal range are occasionally encountered in patients with primary hyperparathyroidism.

Secondary hyperparathyroidism may be nutritional or renal in origin. Both conditions result in altered calcium-phosphorus ratios. In nutritional secondary hyperparathyroidism, secretion of PTH increases to compensate for altered mineral levels associated with dietary abnormalities. Dietary abnormalities that may lead to nutritional secondary hyperparathyroidism are (1) a low level of calcium in the diet, (2) excessive phosphorus with a normal or low calcium level, and (3) inadequate amounts of vitamin D_3. Hypocalcemia results in parathyroid stimulation. Nutritional secondary hyperparathyroidism has been reported in a wide variety of species, including the dog, cat, and primate (Table 5–3).

Secondary hyperparathyroidism of renal origin is a complication of chronic renal failure with progressive loss of glomerular function and retained phosphorus resulting in progressive hyperphosphatemia. Hyperphosphatemia results in lowering of blood calcium levels and secondary stimulation of PTH release. In addition, chronic renal disease is involved in altered vitamin D metabolism, leading to hypocalcemia. Chronic renal disease impairs the production of 1,25-DHCC by the kidney.

............*Hypercalcemia* (see also p. 722)

Consistently elevated blood calcium levels above 11.5 to 12.0 mg/dL can be associated with any of a series of lesions: (1) primary hyperparathyroidism; (2) vitamin D intoxication; (3) malignant neoplasms with osseous metastases; and (4) other malignant neoplasms (pseudohyperparathyroidism), of which lymphosarcoma is the most common. The total calcium level should be corrected:

Corrected Ca (mg/dL) = measured serum total Ca − serum albumin (g/dL) + 3.5.

■ CLINICAL EFFECTS OF HYPERCALCEMIA

Neuromuscular—locomotor weakness, muscle twitching, depression, seizures
Cardiovascular—increased myocardial excitability, potential for cardiac dysrhythmias
Renal—vasoconstriction, renal mineralization

In primary hyperparathyroidism, hormone secretion is autonomous and is usually associated with an adenoma composed of active chief cells. Primary hyperparathyroidism is associated with autonomous secretion of PTH hormone from parathyroid tumors. A palpable parathyroid mass may be felt. In cats, clinical signs are PU or PD, hypercalcemia, increased alanine aminotransferase (ALT), increased alkaline phosphatase, and elevated BUN.

Pseudohyperparathyroidism is a metabolic abnormality in which parathyroid-like hormone is produced by some malignant tumors of nonparathyroid origin. Pseudohyperparathyroidism has been reported in dogs and cats with malignant lymphoma, mammary adenocarcinoma, and apocrine gland adenocarcinoma of the anal sac.

............GLUCOSE METABOLISM—DIABETES MELLITUS

5

The islets of Langerhans secrete two hormones that have important functions in intermediary metabolism: glucagon and insulin.

Glucagon is a polypeptide hormone that elevates the blood glucose level by stimulating hepatic glycogenolysis. Secretion of glucagon is stimulated by lowered blood glucose levels and sympathetic nerve stimulation. Glucagon secretion may help maintain blood glucose levels during starvation. The principal actions of *insulin* are (1) to promote glucose oxidation and triglyceride formation in adipose tissue, (2) to promote protein and glycogen synthesis in muscle, and (3) to promote glycogen and triglyceride synthesis in the liver. Changes in blood glucose levels result in reciprocal changes in the levels of these two hormones.

Many other hormones are important in regulating carbohydrate metabo-

Table 5–3. Differential Diagnosis of Primary Hyperparathyroidism, Renal Secondary Hyperparathyroidism, Pseudohyperparathyroidism, and Hypercalcemia Due to Neoplastic Osteolysis

Factors	Primary Hyperparathyroidism	Renal Secondary Hyperparathyroidism	Pseudohyper-parathyroidism	Neoplastic Osteolysis*
Serum calcium	Elevated	Normal to decreased	Elevated	Elevated
Serum phosphorus	Decreased unless uremic; then normal to increased	Increased	Decreased unless uremic; then normal to increased	Frequently increased
Serum alkaline phosphatase	Normal to increased	Normal to increased	Normal to increased	Normal to increased
Blood urea nitrogen; creatinine	Normal unless uremic; then increased	Increased	Normal unless uremic; then increased	Normal unless uremic; then increased
Bone radiographs	Varying degrees of demineralization	Varying degrees of demineralization	Varying degrees of demineralization	Disseminated osteolytic lesions

*Findings reported in human beings.

From Osborne CA, Stevens JB: Hypercalcemic nephropathy. *In* Kirk RW, ed: Current Veterinary Therapy VI. Philadelphia, WB Saunders, 1977, p 1083.

lism. The catecholamines epinephrine and norepinephrine enhance glucose production by enhancing hepatic glycogenolysis, gluconeogenesis, lipolysis, and proteolysis. Growth hormone (GH) has a catabolic effect on carbohydrate metabolism. Cortisol raises the blood sugar level by increasing gluconeogenesis. Excessive thyroid hormone production can cause increased glucose oxidation.

The major disease associated with an abnormality in glucose metabolism is diabetes mellitus. Persistent hyperglycemia caused by diabetes mellitus may result from subnormal levels of circulating insulin or reduced responsiveness of the organs on which insulin has its effect. Hyperglycemia does not mean lack of insulin in all cases. It is possible to classify spontaneous diabetes mellitus of dogs into types I, II, and III, according to fasting plasma insulinogenic index ($\Delta I/\Delta G$), and total insulin secreted.

Type I, insulin-dependent diabetes mellitus (IDDM) is characterized clinically by sudden onset of symptoms, absence of immunoreactive insulin, a need for insulin to sustain life, and a tendency to develop ketotic diabetes. Most cases of type I are found in mature and older dogs.

Type II, non–insulin-dependent diabetes mellitus (NIDDM) is characterized by glucose intolerance and typical signs of diabetes. Plasma insulin concentrations are usually within acceptable limits in dogs that are not obese but are higher in obese dogs. In both obese and nonobese dogs, there is no insulin response to a glucose load. Breed predilection indicates that dachshunds and poodles are at increased risk.

In *type III diabetes* in dogs, fasting plasma glucose concentrations are nondiagnostic, but glucose intolerance and subnormal insulin response to a glucose load are observed. In obese dogs, glucose intolerance may be improved after weight loss. The most common form of canine diabetes closely resembles type I IDDM or severe type II non–insulin-dependent diabetes. Both cases are characterized by hypoinsulinemia, abnormal response to glucose load, and ketoacidosis.

Because classification of diabetes mellitus on the basis of insulin levels usually does not help with diagnosis, a classification based on other possibly associated diseases is more significant.

In older female dogs that have a higher incidence of diabetes, disease factors may develop that alter their peripheral resistance to insulin. Two such factors are increased levels of GH and excess glucocorticoids, as seen in hyperadrenocorticism. In early hypersomatotropism, hyperinsulinemia and mild to severe hyperglycemia develop. With persistence of hyperglycemia, carbohydrate intolerance and beta cell fatigue produce hypoinsulinemia and diabetes. GH levels greater than 10 ng/mL (measured by RIA) have been observed in female dogs treated with medroxyprogesterone acetate or have been seen naturally during diestrus. These dogs have altered IV glucose tolerance test results associated with insulin insensitivity and glucose intolerance. In this group of dogs, withdrawal of artificial progestational compounds is indicated or an ovariohysterectomy should be performed.

Another factor that can play an important role in diabetes is hyperadrenocorticism. Abnormal glucocorticoid levels lead to insulin resistance and glucose intolerance.

Early-onset diabetes mellitus is uncommon in dogs but has been described in one form as a primary atrophy of beta cells of the pancreas in genetically related keeshonds. Early-onset diabetes in keeshonds develops at 2 to 6 months of age. Affected animals are hypercholesterolemic, ketotic, insulinopenic, and euglycemic. Early-onset diabetes mellitus is inherited as an autosomal recessive trait with incomplete penetrance. The diabetic phenotype has been found to be expressed in 80% of dogs with the diabetes mellitus genotype. Diabetes has also been observed in a variety of breeds and mixed dog populations as a delayed finding related to systemic disease and secondary pancreatic damage.

...........Diabetes Mellitus in the Cat

Cats with diabetes mellitus can be categorized as either type I (IDDM) or type II (NIDDM). In cats, IDDM is characterized by hypoinsulinemia, little or no increase in endogenous serum insulin concentration after the administration of insulin secretagogue, failure to establish glycemic control with diet and oral hypoglycemic drugs, and the need for exogenous insulin to maintain glycemic control. IDDM occurs in the cat but is not commonly observed except secondary to systemic disease such as acute pancreatitis, chronic progestational compound use, hyperthyroidism, GH-producing tumors, and hyperadrenocorticism. The characteristics of NIDDM in cats include mild clinical signs, lack of ketoacidosis, and close association with obesity. Another classification of diabetes that has been used for cats with diabetes is complicated or uncomplicated diabetes. In the uncomplicated cases of diabetes mellitus in the cat, the animals are presented with hyperglycemia but without ketoacidosis or hyperosmolar nonketotic syndrome, and the clinical signs may be transient or permanent. Obesity-induced carbohydrate intolerance in the cat and islet amyloidosis cause NIDDM in cats.

In cats that are not seriously ill with NIDDM or uncomplicated diabetes mellitus, initial therapy may consist of the oral hypoglycemic agent glipizide (Glucotrol*), a high fiber diet, and correction of obesity. Glipizide is administered orally (PO) at 5 mg once a day or b.i.d. Caution must be used because glipizide can also cause hypoglycemia.

For treatment of IDDM in the cat, see p. 143.

Diabetes mellitus occurs predominantly in cats over 5 years of age, and male cats are at increased risk for development of the disease.

...........Glucose Tolerance Test Evaluating Glucose Metabolism

The glucose tolerance test is used to help confirm a diagnosis of diabetes mellitus when results of other tests are equivocal. Either oral or IV tests may be used. The oral glucose tolerance test in the dog is started by obtaining a baseline fasting blood sugar level. Glucose 2 g/kg body weight is then administered in a solution through a stomach tube. The concentration of glucose should not be greater than 25%. Blood samples are taken at 30, 60, 120, 180, and 240 minutes. In nondiabetic animals who have had a high carbohydrate intake for 3 days prior to testing, the fasting blood sugar level is less than 110 mg/dL. The level does not rise above 160 mg/dL at the end of the first hour and returns to normal by the end of the second hour. In diabetic animals, the baseline fasting blood sugar level is usually higher than 150 mg/dL; the level rises markedly during the test and does not return to the pretest value within 2 hours.

The standard IV glucose tolerance test is performed by administering glucose at 0.5 g/kg following a 15-hour fast. A 50% glucose solution is used. A baseline blood sample is obtained prior to testing and again at 5, 15, 30, 45, and 60 minutes.

A high-dose IV glucose tolerance test can be used for the dog. After a baseline fasting blood sugar sample is taken, 50% glucose 1 g/kg, is administered IV and blood samples are taken at 5, 15, 30, 45, and 60 minutes. To shorten the procedure, blood samples can be taken at 5 (T_1) and 60 (T_2) minutes. The glucose disappearance coefficient *(K)* is calculated from the formula:

$$K = 698/T_2 - T_1.$$

*Glucotrol, Pfizer Inc., Roerig Division, New York, N.Y.

Values of K that are 2.0 or less can be considered evidence for latent diabetes mellitus.

...........Provocative Tests for Insulin Release

Insulinomas are found in dogs, in ferrets, and occasionally in cats.

Several diagnostic tests have been used in the diagnosis of hypoglycemia secondary to functional beta cell tumors. Pancreatic adenocarcinomas are functional tumors of the beta cells of the islets of Langerhans. The tumors occur in older dogs, with German shepherds, collies, and setters having the highest incidence. The median age is 9 years, and most of the tumors are malignant. Clinical signs are associated with Whipple's triad (see p. 144). Signs are related to the effect of hypoglycemia on the CNS and may include seizures, including grand mal, focal facial seizures, or status epilepticus; generalized weakness; collapse; poserior paresis; and depression. In ferrets signs are characterized by weakness, lethargy, stupor, collapse, generalized tremors, and ptyalism.

Blood glucose levels in insulinomas are usually below 70 mg/dL and are often in the range of 40 to 50 mg/dL. Some dogs have normal blood glucose levels until they are fasted; then they develop low glucose levels. Fast the suspected insulinoma case after feeding at 8 A.M. Record the blood glucose levels at hourly intervals. When the blood glucose level falls to 60 mg/dL, take a blood sample for simultaneous insulin level. Fasting should not be done for more than 8 hours, which is usually sufficient to see altered blood glucose levels of 60 mg/dL or less. The clinical signs in insulinomas appear to be episodic rather than constant.

Plasma insulin levels can be measured by immunoreactive insulin (IRI) concentrations. The IRI concentrations in normal dogs average 20 µU/mL; values above 54 µU/mL are considered abnormal.

Insulin concentrations closely parallel plasma glucose concentrations. This fact is used in a test involving the amended insulin-glucose ratio (AIGR), which is given by the formula:

Serum insulin (µU/mL $\times$ 100/plasma glucose [mg/dL]) $-$ 30.

Normal ratios are less than 30. Because dogs with functional islet cell adenomas may have normal serum insulin levels, the AIGR may be helpful in making a tentative diagnosis of pancreatic tumor when coupled with clinical signs.

Another evaluation of serum insulin levels is based on the simple glucose-insulin ratio:

Plasma glucose (mg/dL)/serum insulin (µU/mL)

A ratio greater than 5.0 is normal, and less than 2.5 is abnormal.

REFERENCES

Barthez P, Nyland T, Feldman C: Ultrasonography of the adrenal glands in the dog, cat, and ferret. Vet Clin North Am Small Anim Pract 28:869, 1998.

Boothe DM: Effects of drugs on endocrine tests: *In* Bonaguri JD, ed: Kirk's Current Veterinary Therapy XII. Philadelphia, WB Saunders, 1995, p 339.

Campbell KL: Growth hormone–related disorders in dogs. Compend Contin Educ Pract Vet 10:477, 1998.

Chastain CB: Pseudohypothyroidism and covert hypothyroidism. Probl Vet Med 2:693–716, 1990.

Chew D, Nagode LA, Carothers M: Disorders of calcium: Hypercalcemia and hypocalcemia. *In* DiBartola S, ed: Fluid Therapy in Small Animal Practice, Philadelphia, WB Saunders, 1992.

Dunn JJ, Heath MF, Herrtage ME, et al: Diagnosis of insulinoma in the dog: A study of 11 cases. J Small Anim Pract 32:514–520, 1992.

Duesberg CA, Bertoy EH, Feldman EC: Diagnosis and treatment of macrotumors in dogs with pituitary-dependent hyperadrenocorticism. *In* Bonagura JD ed: Kirk's Current Veterinary Therapy XII. Philadelphia, WB Saunders, 1995, p 351.

Duesberg CA, Feldman EC, Nelson RW, et al: Magnetic resonance imaging for diagnosis of pituitary macrotumors in dogs. J Am Vet Med Assoc 206:657–662, 1995.

Elie M, Zerbe C: Insulinoma in dogs, cats, and ferrets; Compend Contin Educ Pract Vet 17:51–60, 1995.

Feldman EC, Nelson RW: Canine and Feline Endocrinology and Reproduction, ed 2; Philadelphia, WB Saunders, 1996.

Feldman EC, Nelson RW, Feldman MS: Use of the low- and high-dose dexamethasone tests for distinguishing pituitary-dependent from adrenal tumor hyperadrenocorticism in dogs. J Am Vet Med Assoc, 209:772–775, 1996.

Ferguson DC: The clinical significance of thyroid autoantibodies. Vet Med Rep 2:32–38, 1991.

Ferguson DC, ed: Thyroid disorders. Vet Clin North Am Small Anim Pract 24:3, 1994.

Ferguson DC, Nachreiner RF: Diagnosis of canine hypothyroidism. Vet Med Rep 3:172–181, 1991.

Ford SL, Feldman EC, Nelson R: Hyperadrenocorticism caused by bilateral adrenocortical neoplasia in dogs. J Am Vet Med Assoc 202:789–792, 1993.

Greco D: Pediatric endocrinology. Curr Vet Ther 12:346, 1995.

Grooters AM, Biller DS, Thiesen SK, et al: Ultrasonographic characteristics of the adrenal glands in dogs with pituitary-dependent hyperadrenocorticism: Comparison with normal dogs, J Vet Intern Med 10:110–115, 1996.

Harb M, Nelson RW, Feldman EC, et al: Central diabetes insipidus in dogs: 20 cases (1986–1995). Am Vet Med Assoc 209:1884, 1996.

Kallett AJ, Richter KP, Feldman EC, et al: Primary hyperparathyroidism in cats: Seven cases (1984–1989). J Am Vet Med Assoc 199:1767–1771, 1991.

Kintzer P: Adrenal disorders. Vet Clin North Am Small Anim Pract 27(2), 1997.

Kintzer P: Advances in testing for canine hyperadrenocorticism. *In* Proceedings of the Annual Forum of the American College of Veterinary Internal Medicine Forum, San Antonio, 1996, p 107.

Kintzer PP, Peterson M: Mitotane (*o,*'-DDD) treatment of 200 dogs with pituitary-dependent hyperadrenocorticism. J Vet Intern Med 5:182–190, 1991.

Kempaineen R, Terrence C: Sample collection and testing protocols in endocrinology. *In* Bonagura JD, ed: Kirk's Current Veterinary Therapy XII. Philadelphia, WB Saunders, 1995, p 335.

Lawrence D, Thompson J, Layton AW: Hyperthyroidism associated with a thyroid adenoma in a dog. J Am Vet Med Assoc 199:81–83, 1991.

Lifton SJ, King LG, Zerbe CA: Glucocorticoid deficient hypoadrenocorticism in dogs: 18 cases (1986–1995). J Am Vet Med Assoc 209:2076–2081, 1996.

Lorenz MD, Cornelius LM: Small Animal Medical Diagnosis, ed 2. Philadelphia, JB Lippincott, 1993.

Lutz TA, Rand J: Pathogenesis of feline diabetes. Vet Clin North Am Small Anim Pract, 25:527–552, 1995.

Mauldin GN, Burk R: The use of diagnostic computerized tomography and radiation therapy in canine and feline hyperadrenocorticism. Probl Vet Med 2:557–564, 1990.

Melian C, Peterson ME: Diagnosis and treatment of naturally occurring hypoadrenocorticism in 42 dogs; J Small Anim Pract 37:268–275, 1996.

Mooney CT, Thoday KL, Doxey DL: Carbimazole therapy of feline hyperthyroidism. J Small Anim Pract 33:228–235, 1992.

Moreau R, Squires RA: Hypercalcemia. Compend Contin Educ Pract Vet 14:1077, 1992.

Myers NC, Bruyette DS: Feline adrenocorical diseases. Semin Veter Med Surg 9:137–143, 1994.

Nelson RW, Feldman EC: Indications and interpretation of endocrine tests used in the dog and cat. Semin Vet Med Surg 7:285–291, 1992.

Nelson RW, Feldman EC: Treatment of feline diabetes mellitus. *In* Kirk RW, ed: Current Veterinary Therapy XI. Philadelphia, WB Saunders, 1992, p 364.

Nelson RW, Feldman EC, Ford S: Topics in the diagnosis and treatment of canine hyperadrenocorticism. Compend Contin Educ Pract Vet 13:1797, 1991.

Nelson RW, Ihle SL, Feldman EC, et al: Serum free thyroxine concentration in healthy dogs, dogs with hypothyroidism and euthyroid dogs with concurrent illness. J Am Vet Med Assoc 198:1401, 1991.

Panciera D: Thyroid-function testing: Is the future here? Vet Med 92:50–57, 1997.

Peterson ME, Gamble DA: Effect of nonthyroidal illness or serum thyroxine concentration in cats: 494 cases. J Am Vet Med Assoc 197:1203, 1990.

Peterson ME, Kintzer PP, Kass PH: Pretreatment clinical and laboratory findings in dogs with hyperadrenocorticism: 225 cases (1979–1993). J Am Vet Med Assoc 208:85–91, 1996.

Peterson ME, Melian C. Nichols R: Measurement of total thyroxine, triiodothyronine, free thyroxine, and thyrotropin concentrations for the diagnosis of hypothyroidism in the dog. J Am Vet Med Assoc, 211:1396–1402, 1997.

Peterson ME, Taylor S, Greco DS: Acromegaly in fourteen cats. J Vet Intern Med 4:192–201, 1990.

Podell M: Canine hyperadrenocorticosm. Probl Vet Med 2:717–737, 1990.

Reimers TJ: Guidelines for collection, storage, and transport of samples for hormone assay. In Kirk RW, ed: Current Veterinary Therapy X. Philadelphia, WB Saunders, 1989.

Richter KP, Kallet AJ, Feldman EC: Primary hyperparathyroidism in seven cats. J Vet Intern Med 4:115, 1990.

Robson M, Taboda J, Wolfsheimer K: Adrenal gland function in cats. Comp Contin Educ Pract Vet 17:1205, 1995.

Rosol T, Capen C: Pathophysiology of calcium, phosphorus, and magnesium metabolism in animals. Vet Clin North Am Small Anim Pract 26:1155, 1996.

Sadek D, Schaer M: Atypical Addison's disease in the dog: A retrospective survey of 14 cases. J Am Animal Hosp Assoc 32:159–163, 1996.

Salisbury KS: Hyperthyroidism in cats. Compend Contin Educ Pract Vet 13:1399, 1991.

Steiner J, Bruyette D: Canine insulinomas. Compend Contin Educ Pract Vet 18:13, 1996.

Waters CB, Moncrieff SC: Hypocalcemia in cats. Compend Contin Educ Pract Vet 14:497, 1992.

Zerbe CA: Islet cell tumors secreting insulin, pancreatic polypeptide, gastrin or glucagon. In Kirk RW, ed: Current Veterinary Therapy XI. Philadelphia, WB Saunders, 1992, p 368.

HEMATOLOGY

Hematology is the branch of medicine that deals with the relationship of changes in the hemogram to underlying primary or secondary disease states and includes the study of morphology of the blood and blood-forming tissues. Hematologic studies in veterinary medicine have five major functions:

1. To confirm the diagnosis of the presence or absence of a blood abnormality
2. To determine the extent of the disease process
3. To find out why there is a blood abnormality
4. To serve as a guide to the prognosis of clinical cases
5. To serve as a guide during therapy to the treatment of clinical disorders

This section covers the interpretation of results obtained from hematologic examination. It includes evaluation of the erythron, the leukogram, leukemias, the sedimentation rate, coagulation disorders, blood parasites, and blood chemistry.

EVALUATION OF THE ERYTHRON

The erythron consists of the circulating erythrocytes in the blood, their precursors, and all the elements of the body concerned with their production. Abnormalities in the erythron include anemia, polycythemia, hemodilution, or hemoconcentration.

.... Tests

.... Hematocrit (Packed Cell Volume)

This test measures the relative red blood cell (RBC) mass. It is an accurate test (error of 1% to 2%). The microhematocrit enables rapid determination using a small amount of blood.

Following high-speed centrifugation, the blood in the hematocrit (Hct) tube will be divided into three layers: the bottom or packed erythrocyte layer; the middle or buffy coat, containing leukocytes and thrombocytes; and the upper plasma layer.

The hemoglobin (Hb) concentration can be predicted from the packed cell volume (PCV) in all conditions except iron deficiency anemia and during the remission phase of acute blood loss and hemolytic anemia. The Hb concentration is approximately equal to one third of the PCV (see MCHC, below). The approximate total erythrocyte count (normocytic, normochromic erythrocytes) can be estimated by dividing the PCV by one sixth. In the dog, the following PCV values are estimated according to the animal's age: 2 to 4 months, 32% to 45%; 4 to 6 months, 35% to 52%; 6 to 8 months, 41% to 55%.

Feline RBCs are smaller than those of many other species. Blood volume and Hct are significantly lower for the cat than for the dog. The blood volume of cats is 50 to 60 mL/kg compared with 80 to 90 mL/kg for the dog. The Hct of normal cats is 30% to 45% compared with 37% to 55% for the dog. Total RBC mass is 20% to 30% lower in cats.

Approximate leukocyte counts can be made by measuring the buffy coat (useful only in the Wintrobe hematocrit tube). The first millimeter of the buffy coat is equal to approximately 10,000 leukocytes, and each additional 0.1 mm equals 2000 leukocytes per cubic millimeter. (This is only a means of obtaining a rough estimate of the total leukocyte count.)

Always examine the color of the plasma layer in the Hct tube: a yellow plasma may indicate icterus, a pale to colorless plasma may indicate bone marrow depression, a cloudy plasma may indicate lipemia, and a red-tinged plasma is indicative of hemolysis. The PCV varies with the age, breed, state of nutrition, environment, degree of activity, and state of hydration of the animal. Care should be taken to avoid excess anticoagulant (EDTA) because this can result in a reduction of the PCV by as much as 25%.

.... Hemoglobin

Hb tests measure the oxygen-carrying ability of the erythrocytes. The Hb value should be approximately one third of the Hct value if the RBCs are of normal size. In the cat there are a greater number of reactive Hb sulfhydryl groups than in other species and there is a greater tendency in cats for their Hb to form Heinz bodies after oxidative injury.

.... Erythrocyte Counts

This determination is the most inaccurate of the tests used to evaluate the erythron (the error may be as high as 20% to 40%). RBC numbers vary with the age of the animal and, in general, the total RBC count is used only in obtaining RBC indices.

.... Red Blood Cell Indices

The conventional method of calculating changes in RBC size involves knowledge of the PCV, total RBC count, and Hb concentration. Because both the total RBC and Hb values are inaccurate, the RBC indices may reflect these inaccuracies. A much more accurate mechanism is used by electrostatic cell counters that compute *mean corpuscular volume (MCV)*, the average volume of RBCs, directly. Basically, these RBC indices determine whether the erythrocyte population is made up of small cells, large cells, or cells with adequate or inadequate amounts of Hb. The average weight of Hb in the average cell is called the *mean corpuscular hemoglobin (MCHb)*. The *mean corpuscular hemoglobin concentration (MCHC)* is the percentage of Hb in the RBC mass. The basic information contained in the RBC indices may also be obtained subjectively by careful examination of the blood smear.

The MCV expresses the average volume of the individual erythrocyte. Normal MCV is seen in normocytic anemias, such as those that may be present with acute hemorrhage and hemolysis, whereas increased MCV (macrocytic cells) is associated with increased activity of the bone marrow, deficiencies in hematopoietic factors, or nonregenerative anemias associated with acute myelogenous leukemia or myelodegenerative syndrome. Decreased MCV (microcytic cells) is associated with iron deficiency or deficiency in hematopoietic factors. Microcytosis has been observed in 75% of dogs with portosystemic shunts.

$$\text{MCV expressed in femtoliters (fL)} = \frac{\text{PCV in mL/10 mL}}{\text{RBC count } (10^6/\mu\text{L})}$$

$$\text{MCH expressed in picograms (pg)} = \frac{\text{Hb in g/dL} \times 10}{\text{RBC count } (10^6/\mu\text{L})}$$

$$\text{MCHC expressed in grams per deciliter (g/dL)} = \frac{\text{Hb in g/dL} \times 100}{\text{PCV}}$$

The normal range for MCHC is 30 to 36 g/dL for all mammals (with few exceptions). Normal MCV for dogs is 60 to 77 fL and for cats is 39 to 55 fL. Normal MCH for dogs is 19.5 to 24.5 pg and for cats is 12.5 to 17.5 pg.

............Blood Smears and Erythrocyte Morphology

The stem cells for mature RBCs in the bone marrow generate a continuous supply of nucleated erythroid precursors. Precursor cells undergo a series of divisions in which nuclear and cytoplasmic maturation take place. As the RBC matures, the numbers of polyribosomes and mitochondria decrease, the cells become smaller, and the cytoplasm loses its basophilic staining properties. During maturation, Hb is synthesized.

Thin blood smears and a good staining technique are needed to evaluate the morphology of RBCs. Examine the smear; evaluate the size, shape, and color of the erythrocytes; and determine the presence of any intracellular or extracellular parasites.

Anisocytosis refers to an abnormal variation in the size of the RBCs due to the presence of both mature and immature RBCs in the circulation. Anisocytosis may be slight, moderate, or marked. Mild anisocytosis is normal in cats.

Macrocytosis refers to an increase in the MCV of the RBC and is most frequently seen in responsive anemias and, rarely, with vitamin B_{12} and folic acid deficiency. Macrocytosis has been seen in miniature poodles and chondroplastic malamutes, in which the cause is unknown.

Poikilocytosis refers to any unusual shape of the RBCs. This condition usually occurs in chronic anemia in which the RBCs are not stable and undergo fragmentation, and it indicates premature destruction or defective formation of the RBCs. Poikilocytosis is seen in disseminated intravascular coagulation (DIC) (see p. 45), and the fragmentation anemia that rapidly develops causes an acute hemolytic anemia. Other disease entities that have been associated with poikilocytosis are massive heartworm disease, hemangiosarcomas, disseminated neoplasia, and chemotherapy with cyclophosphamide (Cytoxan).

Polychromatophilia refers to the bluish tinge of young RBCs.

Howell-Jolly bodies are remnants of nuclear material found in young RBCs.

Normoblasts are immature RBCs, both orthochromophilic and polychromatophilic, that contain Hb, are nucleated, and are capable of carrying oxygen. Their presence indicates that immature RBCs are in demand. Because nucleated RBCs are ordinarily counted as leukocytes in the process of counting white blood cells (WBCs), the WBC count should be corrected for circulating normoblasts.

Nucleated RBCs may be released during periods of accelerated erythropoiesis. (If the response is appropriate for the need, it is called *appropriate*; when nucleated RBCs are released and the numbers are not related to the degree of stimulation, the response is called *inappropriate*). Nucleated RBC release is associated with the following:

  Congestive heart failure
  Chronic pulmonary disease
  Endotoxemia
  Bone marrow neoplasia
  Myelofibrosis
  Myelosclerosis
  Bone marrow necrosis
  Spinal cord disease
  Lead poisoning
  Extramedullary hematopoiesis
  Some healthy schnauzers
  Anemia with increased RBC production
  Anemia with decreased RBC production
  Inflammatory liver disease
  Others

There are three diseases in which nucleated RBCs are frequently seen: canine hemangiosarcoma (HSA), autoimmune hemolytic anemia (AIHA), and lead toxicity.

Leptocytes are thin erythrocytes that have an increased surface area without an increase in cell volume; this gives the cell distinctive morphologic characteristics. The cells are usually seen in chronic disease leading to anemia. Target cells are a form of leptocyte seen most frequently in the dog.

Acanthocytes are RBCs with numerous projections. These cells have been "fractured" or damaged, and this damage is associated with hepatic disease and lipid abnormalities. Acanthocytes are commonly seen in cats with liver disease.

Keratocytes are RBCs with variable numbers of elongated, irregularly spaced projections and are associated with damage from intravascular fibrin such as occurs in DIC.

Hereditary stomatocytosis is a rare hereditary disorder in chondrodysplastic Alaskan malamutes. The abnormality of the RBCs may be associated with abnormalities in the RBC cation pump. The RBCs have a short life span and appear as stomatocytes.

Hypochromasia refers to a decrease in the amount of Hb in erythrocytes. In Wright's- or Giemsa-stained smears, the cells appear abnormally pale.

Punctate basophilia or stippling of the erythrocytes may be due to degenerative changes in the cytoplasm involving ribonucleic acid (RNA) in the young cells. Stippling may also occur in lead poisoning.

Spherocytes are RBCs of decreased diameter in relation to their volume. They appear hyperchromatic and lack central pallor. Spherocytes are readily detected in the dog and are observed in autoimmune and isoimmune hemolytic anemias and following transfusion. These cells are removed from the circulation by the spleen. When fewer than 25% of the cells are spherocytes, the mechanism may be fragmentation or immune-mediated. When 25% to 50% are spherocytes, the mechanism is most likely immune-mediated. When spherocytes constitute more than 50% of the RBCs, the mechanism is immune-mediated. Usually, animals with 50% or 75% spherocytes have good reticulocyte responses and respond readily to treatment. When the spherocytes range from 75% to 100%, the reticulocyte response is lower or nonexistent. Spherocytosis cannot be used as an indicator of immune-mediated hemolytic anemia in cats because normal feline RBCs demonstrate minimal and inconsistent central pallor of RBCs.

Reticulocytes are immature, non-nucleated erythrocytes that retain basophilic staining material (RNA). Although reticulocytes do not contain a nucleus, the cell still has polyribosomes and mitochondria and can therefore synthesize Hb and utilize oxygen. The number of reticulocytes in the peripheral blood is the most commonly used clinical index of erythropoietic activity. The number of reticulocytes can be estimated by counting the RBCs and reticulocytes in a field under oil immersion and expressing reticulocytes as a percentage of RBCs.

Two types of reticulocyte patterns have been identified in the cat and are referred to as punctate and aggregate. Punctate cells have been in the peripheral blood for some time and aggregate cells have been recently produced by erythrogenesis. Cats may normally have up to 10% (500,000/μL) punctate reticulocytes in their peripheral blood. Punctate reticulocytes account for the majority of reticulocytes observed in regenerative anemias in cats.

Reticulocytes can be identified only with supravital stains such as new methylene blue (NMB). An increased reticulocyte count indicates increased erythrogenesis. In the cat, the maturation time for reticulocytes is delayed and peak levels are reached after 11 days (following blood loss of 50%). The normal reticulocyte count in the cat ranges from 1.4% to 10.8%, with a mean of 4.6%. The reticulocyte count should be corrected for PCV:

$$\text{Reticulocyte count} \times \frac{\text{measured Hct}}{\text{normal Hct}} = \text{corrected reticulocyte count.}$$

The reticulocyte index for the dog may be helpful in defining nonregenerative vs. other forms of anemia:

$$\text{Corrected reticulocyte count} \times \frac{1}{\text{maturation factor}} = \text{reticulocyte index.}$$

A reticulocyte index of less than 1.0 is found in nonregenerative anemias, 1.0 to 3.0 is found in hemorrhagic anemia, and greater than 3.0 is found in hemolytic anemia (Table 5–4).

Erythrocyte refractile bodies (ERBs) are round or angular refractile bodies consisting of denatured Hb particles that are best seen with NMB and are commonly called *Heinz bodies*. Healthy cats can have variable numbers of

Table 5–4. Relationship Between Hematocrit Levels and Maturation Factor

Hematocrit	Maturation Factor
45	1.0
35	1.5
25	2.0
15	2.5

erythrocytes with Heinz bodies, and there is no indication of a shortened erythrocyte survival time (normal cat, 69 to 79 days). The refractile bodies are 1 to 3 μm in diameter and are located at the periphery of the cell.

Heinz-Bodies Heinz bodies are formed when Hb is denatured during periods of excessive oxidative stress. There is a greater tendency for feline Hb to form Heinz bodies after oxidative injury. In the cat, RBCs that contain Heinz bodies are not removed efficiently by the spleen. The shortened life span of RBCs that contain Heinz bodies is caused by the binding of the denatured globin molecule of Hb to membrane proteins resulting in loss of membrane integrity, decreased cell deformability, and cell lysis. These anemias are acquired and, in the dog, are often associated with the ingestion of onions (the toxic principle of which is *n*-propyl nitrite). The degree of severity of the hemolytic anemia is variable, and the changes in erythrocytes can best be demonstrated with NMB staining. Heinz body anemia has also been associated with a variety of toxic drugs, including phenothiazines, urinary antiseptics containing methylene blue and phenazopyridine (in the cat), sodium nitrate, and naphthalene. Other causes of Heinz body anemia are zinc toxicity; propylene glycol, which may be found in soft, moist dog foods; and methionine therapy. Acetaminophen in the cat can cause severe Heinz body hemolytic anemia (see p. 662). There is a strong correlation between the development of Heinz bodies in the cat and the development of diabetes mellitus, hyperthyroidism, and lymphoma. Healthy cats may have up to 5% to 10% Heinz bodies. Heinz bodies may cause hemolysis and hemolytic anemia because of splenic removal of these cells or cell membrane damage.

The life span of RBCs in the dog is approximately 110 to 122 days; in the cat, it is approximately 69 to 79 days. The stimulus for increased RBC production is persistent anoxia at the level of the renal cortex, resulting in elaboration of the hormone erythropoietin by the kidney.

..........ANEMIAS

Anemia is a condition in which there is a decrease in the number of erythrocytes or a deficiency in Hb or both. Anemia is a clinical sign of disease, not a diagnosis. The significant clinical signs associated with anemia are pallor, weakness, collapse and shortness of breath, tachycardia, systolic bruits, and malaise. Anemia should not be treated without first trying to understand and eliminate the cause. Anemias may be classified in two basic ways: by morphology or by etiology (Fig. 5–1).

..........Etiologic Classification

Anemias can be subdivided into two categories: those due to excessive loss of erythrocytes through hemorrhage or hemolysis and those due to inadequate production of erythrocytes.

..........Blood Loss Anemias

The anemia of acute blood loss occurs when 25% to 40% of the circulating blood volume is lost over a relatively short period of time. Blood loss anemia may result from overt hemorrhage following trauma or surgery, clotting defects, or rupture of highly vascular malignant tumors such as hemangioendotheliomas. Chronic loss of blood in parasitism may also result in blood loss anemia. In acute uncomplicated blood loss anemia there is a marked regenerative response, and the anemia is characteristically normochromic and normocytic. Chronic blood loss associated with parasitism, gastrointestinal bleeding, or genitourinary tract bleeding may result in a hypochromic, microcytic anemia.

Dogs with hemangiosarcoma may be seen in acute collapse with shock associated with tumor rupture in the peritoneal cavity, thoracic cavity, pericardium, or brain. These dogs may also be seen with a history of weakness, intermittent or progressive lethargy, very pale mucous membranes, panting, and exercise intolerance. Hemangiosarcomas may also produce DIC and thrombocytopenia.

The response of the dog to acute external blood loss is predictable. By the third day following blood loss, reticulocytes in increased numbers are present in the peripheral blood. Peak reticulocyte response occurs between the fifth and sixth days. Normoblasts, Howell-Jolly bodies, and anisocytosis are markedly evident at the time of peak reticulocyte response. The PCV increases from day 4 to day 25, after which it is normal. Cats do not respond as rapidly to blood loss, and the peripheral blood smears do not reflect marked polychromasia and anisocytosis.

Internal blood loss into body cavities results in marked absorption by lymphatics, so that two thirds of the lost blood may be absorbed in 24 hours and the balance completely absorbed after 48 to 72 hours.

...........Hemolysis (Hemolytic Anemias)

A hemolytic state exists when the life span of the RBC is decreased. If destruction is balanced with erythropoiesis, there is no anemia.

Accelerated RBC destruction can be associated with two basic causes: (1) intracorpuscular defects (inherited RBC defects) and (2) extracorpuscular defects (acquired).

Hemolytic anemias are characterized by (1) signs of regenerative anemia (such as reticulocytosis, anisocytosis, macrocytosis, reticulocytosis, polychromasia, and Howell-Jolly bodies); (2) decreased RBC life span; (3) increased osmotic fragility; (4) hyperbilirubinemia and hyperbilirubinuria; (5) elevated fecal urobilinogen; (6) hemoglobinemia and hemoglobinuria; (7) splenomegaly; (8) spherocytes in peripheral smear; and (9) Heinz bodies.

Hemolytic anemias can be peracute, acute, or chronic. In the peracute cases, all signs of regeneration are absent and jaundice and hemoglobinuria may develop rapidly. The spleen may be congested and markedly enlarged.

Most dogs are jaundiced, but dogs with mild extravascular hemolysis may have increased bilirubin without clinical signs of icterus. There are increased bone marrow iron stores.

Acute hemolytic anemia may develop over a period of 1 week. Regenerative signs are usually prominent; jaundice is usually present.

■ HEMOLYTIC DISEASE IN THE DOG

- Immune-mediated hemolytic anemia
- Zinc intoxication—ingestion of pennies
- Onion ingestion—Heinz body anemia
- *Babesia canis* infection
- *Ehrlichia canis* infection
- Phosphofructokinase deficiency—English springer spaniels
- Pyruvate kinase deficiency—Basenjis, beagles, wire-haired fox terriers
- Microangiopathic disease—hemangiosarcoma, DIC, heartworm
- Hypophosphatemia
- Transfusion reactions

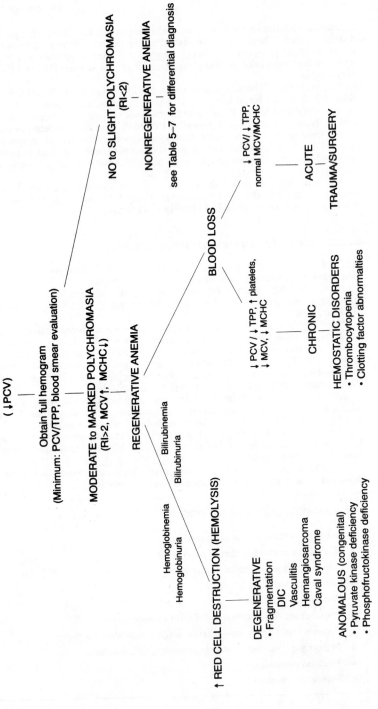

ANEMIA
(↓PCV)

Obtain full hemogram
(Minimum: PCV/TPP, blood smear evaluation)

MODERATE to MARKED POLYCHROMASIA
(RI>2, MCV↑, MCHC↓)

REGENERATIVE ANEMIA

↑ RED CELL DESTRUCTION (HEMOLYSIS)

Hemoglobinemia
Hemoglobinuria

Bilirubinemia
Bilirubinuria

DEGENERATIVE
• Fragmentation
  DIC
  Vasculitis
  Hemangiosarcoma
  Caval syndrome

ANOMALOUS (congenital)
• Pyruvate kinase deficiency
• Phosphofructokinase deficiency

BLOOD LOSS

↓ PCV / ↓ TPP, ↑ platelets,
↓ MCV, ↓ MCHC

CHRONIC

HEMOSTATIC DISORDERS
• Thrombocytopenia
• Clotting factor abnormalties

↓ PCV/ ↓ TPP,
normal MCV/MCHC

ACUTE

TRAUMA/SURGERY

NO to SLIGHT POLYCHROMASIA
(RI<2)

NONREGENERATIVE ANEMIA

see Table 5–7 for differential diagnosis

METABOLIC
- Hypophosphatemia
- Hypo-osmolality

INFECTIOUS
- *Leptospira icterohaemorrhagiae*
- *Haemobartonella canis*
- *Babesia canis, Babesia gibsoni*
- *Ehrlichia canis, Ehrlichia equi*
- *Rickettsia rickettsii*
- *Haemobartonella felis*
- FeLV+
- Fleas
- *Cytauxzoon felis*

IMMUNE-MEDIATED
- 1° or 2° immune-mediated hemolytic anemia
- Neonatal isoerythrolysis (kittens)
- Incompatible red cell transfusion

TOXIC
- Heinz-body anemia (+/- methemoglobinemia)
  methylene blue, acetaminophen,
  benzocaine, phenazopyridine, propyl-
  thiouracil, onions
- Zinc
- Snake venoms

GASTROINTESTINAL
- Ulcers
- Parasitism
- Neoplasia

GENITOURINARY
- Neoplasia

NEOPLASIA
- Hemangioma/sarcoma
  (spleen, liver, heart)
- Nasal (epistaxis)

ECTOPARASITES

HEMOSTATIC DISORDERS
- DIC
- ITP
- Anticoagulant rodenticide toxicity
- von Willebrand's disease

GASTROINTESTINAL
- Ulcers (2° drugs, foreign body, neoplasia)
- Viral infections (parvo, corona)

NEOPLASIA
- Ruptured hemangioma/hemangiosarcoma
  (spleen, liver, heart)

Figure 5–1. Approach to the anemic patient. PCV, packed cell volume; TPP, total plasma protein; MCV, mean corpuscular volume; MCHC, mean corpuscular hemoglobin concentration; RI, reticulocyte index; DIC, disseminated intravascular coagulation; ITP, immune-mediated thrombocytopenia; FeLV, feline leukemia virus.

In determining the cause of a hemolytic anemia, the location of the site of RBC destruction is important.

Intravascular Hemolysis This type of hemolysis usually causes a peracute or acute hemolytic syndrome resulting in hemoglobinemia, hemoglobinuria, increased MCHC, and red discoloration of plasma. If hemolysis is extensive enough and of sufficient duration for bilirubin to be formed in amounts that exceed the liver's ability to conjugate bilirubin, hyperbilirubinemia will be evident. Intravascular hemolysis may be associated with:

1. Bacterial infection (e.g., *Leptospira* sp.)
2. RBC parasites (e.g., *Babesia* sp.)
3. Chemicals that can produce a Heinz body anemia (e.g., phenothiazines, onions, methylene blue, acetaminophen, phenazopyridine, copper, castor beans, severe hypophosphatemia, and the venae cavae syndrome of dirofilariasis)
4. An immune-mediated cause (e.g., neonatal isoerythrolysis and incompatible transfusion)

Extravascular Hemolysis This type of hemolysis usually follows a chronic clinical course. Hb is not evident in plasma or urine. In chronic cases, bone marrow hyperplasia may compensate for RBC destruction and the PCV may be within the normal range. Extravascular hemolysis may be associated with (1) RBC parasites (e.g., *Haemobartonella*); (2) an immune-mediated cause (e.g., AIHA, lupus erythematosus); (3) intrinsic erythrocyte defects (e.g., pyruvate kinase deficiency in Basenjis and beagles); and (4) increased fragmentation of erythrocytes, as seen in DIC.

...........Nonregenerative Anemias

Nonregenerative anemias may be separated into refractory anemias (in which normal or increased numbers of WBCs and platelets are present) and pancytopenia and bicytopenia (anemia with decreased numbers of WBCs or platelets).

In bone marrow depression anemias, erythrocytes are produced at a decreased rate or are improperly formed within the bone marrow (hypoproliferative or hyperproliferative with abnormal maturation). The anemia may be hypoplastic if there is partial or incomplete production of erythrocytes, or aplastic if there is no development of new erythrocytes. Bone marrow depression anemia may be associated with:

1. Adverse physical agents such as excessive irradiation
2. Chemical agents, such as arsenicals, estrogens, and hydrocarbons; and antibiotics, such as chloramphenicol and streptomycin
3. Metabolic inhibition of bone marrow, as occurs with any chronic infection, chronic interstitial nephritis, chronic liver disease, and endocrine diseases (hypothyroidism and hypopituitarism)
4. Myelophthisic tumors such as lymphosarcoma

Anemia may also be associated with various other systemic abnormalities. Anemia is seen in chronic inflammatory disease and is characterized by a shortened erythrocyte life span, disordered iron metabolism, depressed bone marrow response, and disordered iron storage. Abnormalities exist in the release of iron from the reticuloendothelial system. The anemia is usually normocytic, normochromic. Anemia of inflammatory disorders is characterized by hypoferremia, a decreased level of transferrin, reduced saturation of transferrin, and decreased numbers of bone marrow sideroblasts.

The normal serum iron content of the dog is 84 to 233 µg/dL with a mean of 149 µg/dL; the total iron-binding capacity is 284 to 572 µg/dL with a mean of 391 µg/dL; and the total iron-binding capacity saturation is 33% to 37%.

Chronic iron deficiency anemia is found in dogs with chronic blood loss associated with internal parasitism such as hookworm disease, fleas, chronic bleeding from tumors, hemorrhagic colitis, or gastrointestinal bleeding of unknown cause. Characteristically, animals with iron deficiency anemia have an Hct below 37%, an Hb level below 12 g/dL, microcytosis with an MCV of less than 60 fL, and a serum iron level below 84 µg/dL. Total iron-binding capacity is generally normal, and absolute reticulocyte counts may be elevated.

The condition of low serum iron concentration and anemia must be differentiated from the anemia of inflammatory disease (AID). In AID, there is normal to increased storage of iron in the body, but the iron is inadequately released into the plasma to be transported to and metabolized in developing erythroid cells in the bone marrow.

Iron deficiency anemias can be differentiated by examination of bone marrow for stainable iron, which is minimal or absent in iron deficiency and normal or high in the anemia of chronic disease. Stainable iron is not present in the bone marrow of normal cats; therefore a lack of stainable iron does suggest iron deficiency anemia in this species. Low MCHC values may occur in animals with chronic iron deficiency. The MCHC is low in iron deficiency because iron is not adequate for synthesis of normal amounts of Hb.

In iron deficiency anemia, ferrous salts can be administered PO at a dosage of 100 to 300 mg of ferrous sulfate (33 to 100 mg of elemental iron) per day. For systemic administration, iron dextran is the most commonly administered drug. Iron dextran can be administered at an elemental iron level of 10 mg/kg, divided b.i.d., until the total required dose of iron is attained. The total dose of iron needed can be estimated by using the formula:

$$TD \ (mg) = BW \ (kg) + (4.5 \ [15 - Hb]) + 30$$

where TD = total dosage and BW = body weight.

Leukoerythroblastic anemia is characterized by pronounced increases in numbers of nucleated circulating erythrocytes and immature WBCs. This type of anemia is characteristic of myelophthisis, which is caused by metastatic carcinoma or leukemic infiltration of the bone marrow.

Histiocytic medullary reticulosis is characterized by phagocytosis of RBCs by malignant histiocytes, leading to anemia.

Nonmegaloblastic, macrocytic anemias are often associated with feline leukemia virus (FeLV) infection. There may be associated bone marrow hypoplasia. Aplastic anemia may be associated with pancytopenia or may be only RBC aplasia. In some cases, there may be abnormal maturation of RBCs, although bone marrow cellular elements are still adequate.

Pure red cell aplasia (PRCA) exists when the patient's bone marrow fails to produce RBCs, resulting in a normocytic anemia; normal numbers of WBCs and platelets are produced. Reticulocytes are extremely decreased in number or absent from peripheral blood, as are RBC precursors from the bone marrow. Although a distinct cause of this condition is not known, factors to be considered include immune-mediated agents, thymoma, infections, chemicals, and systemic lupus. The majority of PRCA cases in dogs have been consistent with primary PRCA in humans and it is believed to be an immune-mediated disease. Direct Coombs'-positive and direct Coombs'-negative cases have been reported. There may be evidence of peripheral RBC destruction as well as inhibition of RBC precursors. Treatment involves use of agents such as prednisolone at immunosuppressive doses for the first 2 weeks; then, if no response occurs and reticulocyte numbers remain low, cyclophosphamide therapy can be initiated. Repeated blood transfusions are indicated (see also p. 46).

·············Congenital Erythrocyte Enzyme Deficiencies

Mature erythrocytes depend solely on anaerobic glycolysis for adenosine triphosphate (ATP) generation because the physiologic processes, namely the

Krebs cycle and oxidative phosphorylation, reside in the mitichondria. Deficiencies of enzymes involved in glycolysis can significantly influence erythrocyte function.

..........Pyruvate Kinase Deficiency

Congenital hemolytic anemia resulting from erythrocyte pyruvate kinase (PK) deficiency occurs in Basenji, beagle, West Highland white terrier, Cairn terrier, and American Eskimo dogs, and Abyssinian cats. The deficiency is transmitted as an autosommal recessive trait. Affected animals that exhibit clinical signs have decreased exercise tolerance, pale mucous membranes, tachycardia, and splenomagaly. Affected animals have macrocytic hypochromic anemia with uncorrected reticulocyte counts of 15% to 50%.

..........Phosphofructokinase (PFK) Deficiency

Autosomal recessive inherited PFK deficiency occurs in English springer spaniels and American cocker spaniels. Homozygously affected dogs have a compensated hemolytic anemia and episodes of intravascular hemolysis with hemoglobinuria. Affected animals may show clinical signs of lethargy, weakness, and pale mucous membranes.

..........Methemoglobin Reductase Deficiency

Persistent methemoglobinemia associated with methemoglobin reductase deficiency has been observed in the Chihuahua, borzoi, English setter, Welsh corgi, and other mixed breeds of dogs, and in a domestic shorthair cat. There is persistence of cyanotic-appearing tongue and mucous membranes with possible exercise intolerance and lethargy.

■ CAUSES OF FELINE ANEMIA

Chronic disease

Feline immunodeficiency virus infection

Feline leukemia virus infection

Hemobartonellosis

Cytauxzoonosis

Heinz body anemia

Hypophosphatemia

Liver disease

Chronic renal failure

Congenital disorders

Immune-mediated hemolytic disease

..........Diagnosis of Anemias

Several major questions should be answered at the beginning to determine the cause of anemia:

1. *Does a true anemia exist?* This can be determined by evaluating the Hb and PCV together with the presenting clinical signs.
2. *Is the anemia hemolytic or nonhemolytic?* This question can be answered by

testing for excessive bilirubin in the urine or hemoglobinuria, the presence of free Hb in the plasma, the presence of icterus, increased urobilinogen in the urine and feces, and signs of increased bone marrow activity.

3. *Is the anemia responsive (are the bone marrow and other hematopoietic centers responding to the stress) or unresponsive?* A response to anemia is indicated by an increased number of leukocytes and a shift to the left, an increased number of reticulocytes, the presence of nucleated erythrocytes in the peripheral circulation, polychromatophilia, the presence of Howell-Jolly bodies, and an increased platelet count.

The signs of a nonresponsive anemia are a pale or colorless plasma, decreased number of leukocytes, absence of reticulocytes, absence of nucleated erythrocytes, and normal erythrocyte indices. Bone marrow dysfunction may be categorized into bicytopenias in which there is a decrease in at least two circulating blood cell lines resulting in anemia, and leukopenia and pancytopenia in which there is anemia, leukopenia, and thrombocytopenia.

Exceptions to normal erythropoietic indices are iron and vitamin B_6 (microcytic, hypochromic) or folic acid and vitamin B_{12} (macrocytic, hypochromic) deficiencies.

Of primary importance in evaluating nonresponsive anemias is the bone marrow examination. The myeloid-erythroid ratio determines whether erythrocytic precursors are present. Examination for abnormally shaped erythroid precursors or for the presence of leukemic or tumor cells is important in diagnosing refractory anemias.

Examination of the bone marrow can be helpful in determining whether only erythroid precursors are involved in the clinical problem or whether there is also a granulopoietic abnormality.

1. Erythroid hypoplasia and normal granulopoietic abnormality.
   a. Lack of erythropoietin production.
   b. Anemia of chronic inflammatory or neoplastic disease associated with low serum, low iron-binding capacity.
   c. Part of the FeLV complex.
2. Erythroid hypoplasia and granulopoietic hypoplasia. This entity suggests a problem at the stem cell level.
   a. Aplastic anemia that may be associated with radiation.
   b. Myelophthisic anemia—replacement of bone marrow by abnormal accumulation of neoplastic cells.
   c. Infections—feline panleukopenia virus, FeLV complex, ehrlichiosis.
   d. Chemical toxins—chloramphenicol, primidone, phenylbutazone, sulfa drugs, meclofenamic acid.
   e. Chemotherapeutic drugs, including cyclophosphamide, cytosine arabinoside, doxorubicin, vinblastine, hydroxyurea.
   f. Chronic renal failure—impaired erythropoietin.
   g. Endocrine disorders—hypothyroidism, lack of androgens, hypoadrenocorticism.
   h. Impairment of DNA synthesis (macrocytic anemia) can involve vitamin B_{12} and folic acid deficiency with resulting cell arrest in the prorubricyte and rubricyte stages.
3. Defective erythropoiesis with hyperproliferative erythroid bone marrow and defective maturation. Erythropoietic precursors are numerous in the bone marrow, but abnormal maturation of cells leads to defective RBC function and anemia.
   a. Abnormal nucleic acid synthesis associated with vitamin B_{12} and folic acid deficiency.
   b. Impaired hemosynthesis—iron deficiency, pyridoxine deficiency, copper deficiency, lead poisoning.

c. Macrocytosis is a common finding in cats with FeLV-associated anemia and myeloproliferative disorders. It is usually indicative of faulty maturation of erythroid precursors and signals the presence of neoplastic hematopoietic stem cells.

............POLYCYTHEMIA

Polycythemia refers to an increase in the erythrocyte count, Hb concentration, or PCV. *Absolute polycythemia* refers to an excess number of RBCs in the circulation accompanied by an increase in total blood volume. Absolute polycythemia can be further divided into secondary polycythemia and primary polycythemia. *Relative polycythemia* refers to an increase in RBC number associated with a decrease in the volume of plasma and signs such as water deprivation, vomiting, diarrhea, fever, general malnutrition, and acute shock. Shifting of abdominal problems that induce shock and burns can result in polycythemia. The distinction between absolute polycythemia and relative polycythemia can be made by examining the hemogram, or "blood picture."

In absolute secondary polycythemia, there is an increase in the total RBC mass (erythron) in response to hypoxia (Fig. 5–2).

Abnormalities in erythropoietin production may be associated with renal tumors, renal vascular impairment, renal cysts, hydronephrosis, release of erythropoietin-like substance from hepatomas, uterine myoma, or cerebellar hemangiomas. In the dog, secondary polycythemia has been associated with renal carcinomas.

Most cases of secondary polycythemia are associated with generalized hypoxia that can be caused by (1) low ambient oxygen tension, (2) respiratory

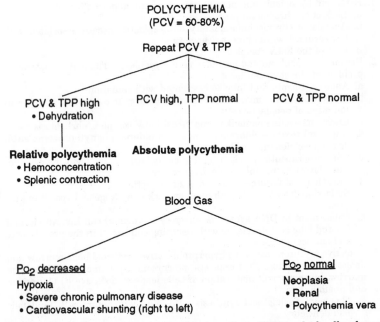

Figure 5–2. Approach to the polycythemic patient. PCV, packed cell volume; TPP, total plasma protein.

hypoventilation, (3) obstructive pulmonary disease, (4) arteriovenous (A-V) shunting, or (5) abnormal Hb. Renal ischemia can result in increased RBC production.

Primary polycythemia (polycythemia vera) is considered to be a myeloproliferative disease, with the development of myeloid metaplasia and acute leukemia as a possible outcome. No excessive erythropoietin is required for this abnormal cloning of erythrocytic precursors. In primary polycythemia, increased RBC mass results in increased RBC viscosity and hypoxia, thromboembolism, and rupture of damaged vessels. This disease is seen in middle-aged dogs and has no sex predilection.

Radioactive chromium (^{51}Cr) labeling of RBCs can be used to document abnormal RBC masses. Serum erythropoietin concentration can be measured.

Various techniques have been used to treat polycythemia vera, including bleeding and immunosuppressive and chemotherapeutic agents, such as hydroxyurea. Hydroxyurea is initially given in a loading dose of 30 mg/kg/day for 7 to 10 days, followed by 15 mg/kg/day in single or divided doses. The PCV is initially reduced to less than 60% with repeated phlebotomies, withdrawing 20 mL/kg of blood, and replacing fluid volume.

···········CROSSMATCHING

A test of the recipient's serum with the donor's RBCs is known as a *major crossmatch*; when the donor's plasma and recipient's RBCs are used, the test is called a *minor crossmatch*. Under most circumstances, a major crossmatch is performed (Table 5–5).

Table 5–5. Crossmatching

	Donor	Recipient
Major crossmatch	Cells	Serum/plasma
Minor crossmatch	Serum/plasma	Cells

*Crossmatching Procedure**

1. Collect 2 mL of EDTA anticoagulated blood from donor and recipient.
2. Centrifuge the blood samples for 1 min (1000 rpm). Remove the plasma to prelabeled tubes.
3. Make a 2% RBC suspension by taking 0.1 mL of the RBCs and add 5 mL of 0.9% saline solution. Mix the suspension.
4. Centrifuge the suspension for 1 min. Discard the supernatant. Resuspend the RBCs in another 5 mL of 0.9% saline, centrifuge, etc. This washing procedure is repeated a total of three times.
5. Place two drops of the recipient's plasma/serum and two drops of the donor cell suspension in a 3-mL test tube (this is the *major crossmatch*). Then place two drops of the recipient's RBCs and two drops of the donor serum/plasma in another test tube (this is the *minor crossmatch*). Mix well and incubate the tubes for 30 min at room temperature.† For *controls,* use the donor and recipient's own cells and plasma (the same procedure as above). Centrifuge for 1 min at 1000 rpm.
6. Reading the tubes: (1) check for agglutination, (2) check for hemolysis, (3) place drop on slide and examine microscopically at ×40 for agglutination.

---

*Modified after the procedure used at the Clinical Hematology Laboratory, University of Minnesota, Minneapolis.

†Optimal is incubation at 4°C, room temperature, and 37°C.

............BONE MARROW
............Interpretation (see Fig. 5-3)

Bone marrow is the site of production of erythrocytes, granulocytes, and thrombocytes. For methods by which bone marrow can be obtained from the dog and cat, see p. 514. When the bone marrow material has been obtained, a differential count of 200 nucleated cells should be made. The myeloid-erythroid (M/E) ratio should be determined by dividing the number of nucleated RBCs into the sum of all cells belonging to the granulocytic series. When the total leukocyte count is within the normal range for the species, the M/E ratio can be used to indicate depression or acceleration of erythrogenesis. Different areas of the bone marrow smear should be included in the cell count. Normal values of the M/E ratio range from 0.75 to 2.5, with a mean of 1.20:1.0. The normal M/E ratio in the cat is 0.60 to 3.90, with a mean of 1.6:1.0. An elevated M/E ratio indicates the opposite situation. The M/E ratio may appear normal in bone marrow hypoplasia if both erythroid and myeloid elements are depressed. Evaluation of the M/E ratio is not as important as the cellularity and the types of cells found in the bone marrow (Table 5-6).

Examples of conditions in which an increased M/E ratio may occur are leukocytosis, leukemoid reaction, granulocytic leukemia, lymphosarcoma, and erythemic hypoplasia. A decreased M/E ratio may be associated with a reduction in the number of myeloid cells, hyperplasia of erythropoietic tissue, metarubricytic (normoblastic) response associated with hemorrhage, hemolysis, iron deficiency, lead poisoning, cirrhosis of the liver, polycythemia vera, and rubriblastic (megaloblastic) response associated with a deficiency of vitamin B_{12}

Table 5-6. Interpretation of Myeloid-Erythroid (M/E) Ratios*

Increased M/E Ratio	Decreased M/E Ratio
Inflammatory leukocytosis	Regenerative anemia
Leukemoid reaction	Polycythemia (absolute)
Myelogenous leukemia	Erythroleukemia
Lymphosarcoma	Myeloid hypoplasia
Erythroid hypoplasia	Drug-induced
Pure RBC aplasia	Immune-mediated
Anemia of chronic disease	Cyclic hematopoiesis
Endocrine hypofunction (thyroid, adrenal, pituitary)	Infectious diseases (FeLV, *Ehrlichia canis*)
Infectious diseases (FeLV, *Ehrlichia canis*)	
Example 1	*Example 2*
Increased M/E ratio (8:1)	Decreased M/E ratio (1:6)
PCV 20%, nonregenerative anemia	PCV 15%, regenerative anemia
WBC 20,000/μL with neutrophilia and left shift	WBC 8000/μL with normal differential
Bone marrow interpretation: myeloid hyperplasia and erythroid hypoplasia	Bone marrow interpretation: erythroid hyperplasia

FeLV, feline leukemia virus, PCV, packed cell volume.
*Complete blood count results facilitate interpretation of the M/E ratio.
From Grindem CB: Bone marrow biopsy and evaluation. Vet Clin North Am Small Anim Pract 19:685, 1989.

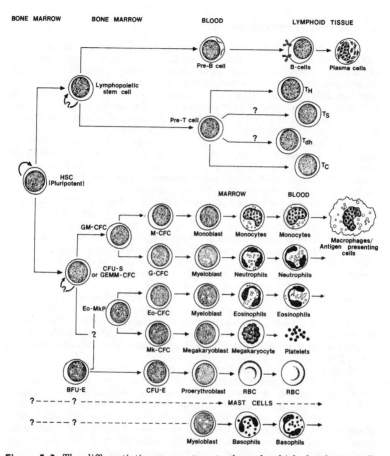

Figure 5–3. The differentiation compartments through which developing cells of the blood pass. The cells arise from the pluripotent hematopoietic stem cell and pass through partially committed precursors and through proliferation and maturation pools to become fully differentiated cells. The anatomical locations of these cells are indicated. HSC, hematopoietic stem cell; T_H, helper T cells; T_S, suppressor T cells; T_C, cytotoxic T cells; T_dh, delayed type hypersensitivity T cells; CFU-S, colony-forming unit, spleen; GEMM-CFC, mixed (granulocytic, erythroid, monocytic, and megakaryocytic) colony-forming cells; GM-CFC, granulocytic-monocytic colony-forming cell; Eo-MkP, eosinophil-megakaryocyte progenitor cell; Eo-CFC, eosinophil colony-forming cell; Mk-CFC, megakaryocyte colony-forming cell; BFU-E, bursa-forming unit, erythroid; CFU-E, colony-forming unit, erythroid; RBC, red blood cells; HSC, self-maintaining stem cell population; ?, inadequate information available. (Modified from Evans RJ, Gorman NT: Myeloproliferative disease in the dog and cat. Part I. Vet Rec 121:437–443, 1987.)

or folic acid. Tumors of RBC-producing tissues (as in erythemic myelosis) can also alter the M/E ratio.

...........THE THROMBON

The thrombon consists of circulating blood platelets and megakaryocytes and megakaryoblasts in the bone marrow. Megakaryocytes do not divide, but platelets are formed when invaginations of the megakaryocyte membrane coalesce; the platelets are released as ribbons that fragment into individual platelets. Approximately 150 to 200 platelets are formed from a single megakaryocyte by fragmentation of a ribbon. Thrombopoietin is a plasma factor that stimulates this fragmentation. Maturation time for the development of a mature platelet is 3 days, and the normal platelet life span is 7 to 10 days.

Blood platelets are involved in both the intrinsic and extrinsic pathways of coagulation and are essential to the formation of the prothrombin-converting enzyme complex in the intrinsic coagulation pathway. The platelet component is called *platelet factor 3* (PF-3). Other platelet factors have been found that are involved in the intrinsic blood-clotting pathway.

The normal number of blood platelets is from 200,000 to 500,000/μL. Platelet number can be estimated by counting platelets under oil immersion (×1000), where each platelet is equivalent to 15,000 platelets per microliter.

Abnormalities of the thrombon can be either quantitative or qualitative.

Effective management of thrombocytopenia involves correction of the underlying problem where possible. Infectious agents such as *Ehrlichia* spp. or *Rickettsia rickettsii* should be eliminated, and DIC should be treated. Avoid the administration of drugs with antiplatelet activity.

When platelet numbers fall to the level at which petechiae and bleeding develop, transfusions of fresh platelets are necessary (see p. 46). Whole fresh blood taken in plastic bags should be used. Enough fresh whole blood should be given to increase the patient's platelet count to 100,000/μL. If platelet-rich plasma can be prepared, it has distinct advantages when administered at a rate of 6 to 10 mL/kg.

Immune-mediated thrombocytopenia is treated with corticosteroids. If corticosteroids are not helpful, vincristine in low doses can be added and has resulted in increased levels of circulating platelets. The dosage of vincristine is 0.01 to 0.025 mg/kg. Corticosteroids reduce the titer of antiplatelet antibody, platelet sequestration, and splenic and hepatic destruction of platelets. Prednisolone may be administered in dosages of 0.5 to 1.5 mg/kg q12h. during the acute phase of thrombocytopenia. Therapy should continue until the platelet count is greater than 100,000/μL; then corticosteroids should be tapered slowly (1 to 2 weeks).

...........EVALUATION OF THE LEUKOCYTE RESPONSE

Leukocytes serve the function of protecting the body against foreign substances. The two basic mechanisms involved are phagocytosis and antibody production.

Granulocytopoiesis involves the progressive development within the bone marrow of the stem cell progranulocyte, myelocyte, metamyelocyte, band cell, and finally mature granulocyte. Within the bone marrow are the (1) stem cell pool of cells, (2) proliferating pool of cells, and (3) maturation storage pool of cells.

Phagocytes consist of the granulocytes (neutrophils, eosinophils, and basophils) and monocytes.

The entire generative process from myeloblast to blood segmenter takes approximately 3½ to 6 days. Neutrophils have a circulating half-life of approximately 5.5 to 7.5 hours in the blood and then marginate and emigrate into the tissues. Neutrophils are viable in the tissues for 1 to 2 days.

The immunocyte system is involved in the production of antibody and in cell-mediated immunity. Cells of the immunocyte system are the thymus-derived lymphocytes (also known as T1, T lymphocytes, and T cells), which are involved in direct cell-mediated immunity, and the "bursa-equivalent" lymphocytes (also known as B1, B lymphocytes, and B cells), involved in antibody production.

Leukocytic changes in the peripheral blood may be associated with (1) diseases that affect the blood-forming organs (such as the bone marrow, lymphoid tissue, spleen, and reticuloendothelial system) and (2) diseases that affect other body tissues in such a way as to mobilize leukocytes to the area of injury or disease. To obtain the maximum information from leukocyte examinations, the total leukocyte count must be correlated with the differential count.

·········· Clinical Interpretation of the Leukogram

The *leukogram* consists of the total and differential leukocyte counts and the morphologic assessment of blood leukocytes. Included in the interpretation of the leukocyte response are the total leukocyte count and differential cell patterns, along with any distinctive morphologic changes.

·········· General Leukocyte Responses

Leukopenia Leukopenia refers to a decrease in the total number of circulating leukocytes. Leukopenia can be associated with infections of viral etiology that destroy young myeloid cells. In the early stages of an infectious disease that is bacterial in origin, there can be a depletion of peripheral blood leukocytes until the bone marrow produces more leukocytes. In cases of shock, leukocytes can become sequestered in capillaries of the lung, liver, and spleen. Bone marrow abnormalities can lead to abnormal production of leukocytes or to an abnormal life span of leukocytes. Bone marrow can be affected by some of the following abnormalities:

1. Hypoplasia associated with metabolic abnormalities, ionizing radiation, or chemical agents
2. Dysplasia, with normal marrow becoming replaced with tumor cells (myelophthisic)
3. Abnormalities of maturation of cells associated with vitamin B_{12} deficiency
4. The action of chemical agents on the bone marrow

Leukocytosis Leukocytosis refers to an increased number of leukocytes beyond the normally accepted range per microliter. In most instances, one predominant cell type is elevated in number; however, simultaneous increases of several types may occur. Neutrophils are usually increased in number over any other cell type; thus, the term *leukocytosis* usually implies neutrophilia unless another specific cell type is designated.

The degree of leukocytosis may be related to numerous factors, including cause, severity of the infection, resistance of the animal, location of the inflammatory response, and species variation. Estimates of the neutrophil-leukocyte ratio can be used to predict an animal's ability to handle the leukocytic response.

·········· Neutrophil Responses

The interpretation of neutrophil responses depends on the total number of neutrophils present per microliter of blood and the presence or absence of morphologic changes in the cells. The following information is pertinent when interpreting neutrophil responses:

1. The primary functions of neutrophils are phagocytosis and bactericidal action.
2. Neutrophil maturation proceeds through morphologic stages in the bone marrow. Differentiation of pluripotential cells in the bone marrow is controlled by colony-stimulating factors.
3. Neutrophil production is regulated by granulopoietin (or a colony-stimulating factor), which is produced by stimulation of bacterial products.
4. Neutrophil release from the bone marrow is promoted by a leukocytosis-inducing factor. The approximate maturation time from myeloblast to metamyelocyte is 48 to 60 hours.
5. *Neutrophilia* is defined as the presence of greater than 11,400 neutrophils per microliter in dogs and greater than 12,500 neutrophils per microliter in cats. Neutropenia is the presence of fewer than 3000 neutrophils per microliter in dogs and fewer than 2500 neutrophils per microliter in cats.

Neutrophilia Without a Left Shift Physiologic events such as increased blood flow associated with muscular activity, increased heart rate, increased blood pressure, and increased production of epinephrine can mobilize neutrophils normally located in the margins of small vessels.

Corticosteroids of endogenous or exogenous origin cause neutrophilia without a left shift, as well as lymphopenia, eosinopenia, and occasional monocytes. Dogs demonstrate these changes most consistently and the cat will occasionally develop a monocytosis.

Neutrophilia can accompany inflammatory disorders in cases in which the tissue reaction does not stimulate large numbers of immature neutrophils to be present.

Neutrophilia With a Left Shift Neutrophilia with a left shift is an increase in the number of immature cells of the granulocytic series in the peripheral blood. This type of neutrophilia indicates the presence of inflammation with a tissue demand for neutrophils. Neutrophil release from the bone marrow is age-related, with the most mature cells being released earliest. The increase in neutrophils is usually orderly, with the number of band neutrophils usually exceeding the number of neutrophilic metamyelocytes. If the production of immature neutrophils is not orderly, granulocytic leukemia may be present.

Normal Neutrophil Count With a Left Shift The presence of a low, normal, or slightly elevated total leukocyte count with an increased number of immature cells in the peripheral blood is called *a degenerative shift to the left.*

If this response exists, it is important to interpret subsequent leukocytic responses to determine whether immature neutrophils are accompanied by an increased WBC count. Continued stress for production of neutrophils by the bone marrow, failure of total neutrophil numbers to increase, and persistence of immature neutrophils may signify severe purulent inflammatory disease and the release of toxic products, as occurs in septicemia or bacterial sepsis.

Neutropenia With or Without a Left Shift Neutropenia indicates a lower-than-normal WBC count and is associated with a deficiency of functional neutrophils in the peripheral blood.

Neutropenia can result from (1) a sudden demand for increased numbers of neutrophilic leukocytes, (2) sequestration of circulating neutrophils, and (3) decreased bone marrow production of neutrophils. Neutropenia may indicate severe bacterial infection and toxemia, as occurs in acute metritis, aspiration pneumonia, acute peritonitis, and bacterial pneumonia. Bone marrow depression can be associated with myelophthisic tumors as a manifestation of systemic disease (such as feline leukemia). Neutropenia can also be associated with a reduction of granulopoiesis in the bone marrow that may be drug-induced or associated with chronic infection or malignancies replacing bone marrow elements. Deficiencies in vitamin B_{12} and folic acid can impair the development of mature neutrophils. Congenital defects of neutrophil development are also known, such as cyclic neutropenia in gray collies.

Immune-Mediated Neutropenia Immune-mediated neutropenia is a disease in which there is persistent neutropenia with monocytosis while other blood cells remain normal. The bone marrow may be hypocellular but has greatly reduced numbers of more mature neutrophils. Progranulocytes and myelocytes predominate, and the M/E ratio is usually high. The absence of more mature, postmitotic granulocytes is described as a "maturation arrest"; however, this term should be used only when there is direct evidence of inhibition of mitosis or intramarrow granulocyte destruction. A definitive diagnosis of immune-mediated neutropenia depends on whether an antineutrophil antibody is evident.

Various causes of immunoneutropenia have been demonstrated, including idiopathic, viral, or bacterial infections; drug therapy; neoplasia; isoimmune neonatal neutropenia; and transfusion-induced isoimmune neutropenia. These causes have most frequently been described in humans.

Antineutrophil antibody in the circulation changes the neutrophil membrane, making the neutrophil more susceptible to damage and resultant phagocytosis by marrow macrophages. These neutrophils have a shortened intravascular survival time. The circulating antineutrophil antibody is predominantly of the immunoglobulin G (IgG) type.

■ NEUTROPENIA IN THE DOG AND CAT

Abnormalities in Bone Marrow Proliferation

Drugs
Infectious agents
  Parvovirus
  Feline leukemia virus
  Feline immunodeficiency virus
  Histoplasmosis
  Ehrlichia canis
Neoplastic
  Myelophthisic
  Testicular Sertoli cell tumor
Additional causes
  Myelofibrosis
  Osteopetrosis
  Cyclic hematopoiesis
  T-lymphocyte suppression of granulopoiesis

Cellular Defects Associated With Abnormal Cell Survival

Increased tissue demand for neutrophils
  Sepsis
  Localized bacterial infections—lungs, uterus, gastrointestinal tract
Accelerated destruction
Drugs
  Chemotherapeutic agents
  Estrogens
  Phenylbutazone
  Chloramphenicol, cephalosporins, trimethoprim-sulfadiazine
  Griseofulvin—cat
  Immune-mediated neutropenia—not proven in dog and cat

5

..........Lymphocyte Responses

Lymphocytes are part of the immune system of the body, which responds to foreign antigens by producing antibody and mounting a direct cellular response. Subpopulations of lymphocytes are functionally different: the thymus-derived T cells are concerned with direct cell-mediated immunity, whereas the gut-derived B cells are concerned with antibody production.

Lymphocytes can be produced in several areas of the body. Lymphocyte production occurs chiefly in the thymus and bone marrow. The circulating small lymphocytes represent two populations of cells: B and T lymphocytes. Lymph nodes are not sites of intense lymphocyte production, but rather are sites of phagocytic activity, with antigen draining into regional lymph nodes and stimulating B lymphocytes. Lymph nodes, spleen, and gut-associated lymphatic tissue are seeded by lymphocytes formed elsewhere; with antigenic stimulation, local lymphopoiesis occurs.

Lymphopenia Lymphopenia is the presence of fewer than 1000 lymphocytes per microliter of blood in dogs and fewer than 1500 lymphocytes per microliter of blood in cats. Lymphopenia denotes decreased numbers of circulating lymphocytes: fewer than 1000 cells per microliter in the dog and fewer than 1500 cells per microliter in the cat. Lymphopenia is associated with (1) lymphocyte destruction or cell redistribution associated with increased endogenous or exogenous corticosteroid levels; (2) loss of lymphatic fluid as in chylothorax or chronic enteric disease; and (3) lysis of lymphocytes, which is associated with systemic infections such as canine distemper, canine hepatitis, radiation injury, and the use of immunosuppressive drugs.

Lymphocytosis Lymphocytosis is the presence of greater than 4800 lymphocytes per microliter of blood in the dog and greater than 7000 lymphocytes per microliter in cats. Lymphocytosis is characterized by a total lymphocyte count above normal and can be associated with (1) a physiologic response to fear, excitement, or handling (especially in the cat; also, young animals have higher lymphocyte counts than older animals); (2) prolonged or abnormal antigenic stimulation; (3) hypoadrenocorticism; and (4) lymphocytic leukemia.

..........Eosinophil Responses

Eosinophils are granulocytes and originate in the bone marrow, where a high percentage of cells (75%) are mature and serve as a reservoir of cell release. Eosinophils are found in various tissues of the gut, respiratory system, and urinary tract that are portals of entry of antigenic agents and sites of potential histamine release. Eosinophils moderate reactions that occur when tissue mast cells and basophils degranulate. The eosinophil chemotactic factor of anaphylaxis (ECF-A) is present in basophils and mast cells. Eosinophilia refers to the presence of more than 750 cells per microliter in the dog and more than 1500 cells per microliter in the cat.

Two characteristics distinguish the eosinophil from the neutrophil and other leukocytes: (1) eosinophils can inactivate mediators released from mast cells and reduce the reaction associated with IgE-mediated degranulation of mast cells, and (2) eosinophils can damage the larval stage of helminth parasites, such as *Schistosoma mansoni*. Eosinophils can also react chemotactically to mediators released in other immunologic reactions, including split products of complement and products of activated lymphocytes (eosinophil stimulation promoter and eosinophil chemotactic factor).

The eosinophil cell contains specific enzymes that reduce IgE-mediated inflammation: (1) 10 to 20 times as much arylsulfatase B as is found in neutrophils, (2) phospholipase D, (3) lysophospholipase activity, and (4) histaminase.

There is evidence that degranulation of the eosinophil releases a major basic protein that may destroy antibody-coated parasites with which it comes in contact.

Diseases and organ function problems that involve the release of histamine, serotonin, and bradykinin can produce elevated levels of eosinophils.

Lower-than-normal levels of eosinophils result in eosinopenia, which can be induced by (1) hyperadrenocorticism; (2) administration of corticosteroids or adrenocorticotropic hormone (ACTH); and (3) prolonged systemic stress associated with inflammation, trauma, or intoxication (Table 5–7).

...........Basophil Responses

Basophils are produced in the bone marrow and may be present in cellular immune reactions. Basophilic granules contain heparin in a bound form with histamine, serotonin, and hyaluronic acid. In addition, basophils contain ECF-A and platelet activating factor (PAF). They appear to be involved in immediate hypersensitivity reactions. At the time of stimulation, basophils will synthesize and release leukotrienes and probably platelet activating substance. The mediators activate platelets, attract eosinophils, cause smooth muscle contraction and edema formation, and may affect coagulation. Tissues that contain mast cells (basophil cells within tissues) are skin and subcutaneous tissue, lung, gastrointestinal tract, uterus, scrotum, and serosal linings.

...........Monocyte Responses

Monocytes are produced in the reticuloendothelial system and are transformed into macrophages when present in tissues. Monocytes are phagocytic cells that

Table 5–7. Etiology of Bicytopenia and Pancytopenia

Decreased Cell Production

Bone marrow hypoplasia/aplasia
  Chemicals
  Hormones (endogenous or exogenous estrogens)
  Drug-related—antibiotics, chemotherapy, nonsteroidal anti-inflammatory
    drugs
  Radiation therapy
  Immune-mediated
  Infectious (parvovirus, FeLV, FIV, *Ehrlichia canis*)
  Idiopathic
Bone marrow necrosis
  Infectious (*E. canis, Histoplasma capsulatum,* sepsis, parvovirus)
  Toxic
  Neoplastic
Bone marrow fibrosis/sclerosis
Myelophthisis—neoplastic infiltration and granulomatous inflammation with
  infiltration
Myelodysplasia

Increased Cell Destruction or Sequestration

Immune-mediated
Sepsis
Microangiopathy—hemangiosarcoma, DIC
Splenomegaly

FeLV, feline leukemia virus; FIV, feline immunodeficiency virus; DIC, disseminated intravascular coagulation.

5

persist for longer periods of time in tissues than do neutrophils and, when present in increased numbers in the leukogram, may indicate chronic suppurative inflammation or acute stress. Macrophages are important in inflammation because they secrete many substances that are biologically active in inflammation, including proteolytic enzymes, prostaglandins, interferon, interleukin-1, and complement.

Monocytosis is the presence of greater than 1350 monocytes per microliter of blood in dogs and 850 monocytes per microliter of blood in cats. Monocytosis usually occurs simultaneously with neutrophilia, although monocytosis may be present alone in bacterial endocarditis and bacteremia. Persistent monocytosis above 15,000 cells per microliter may indicate a diagnosis of leukemia.

REFERENCES

Blue JT, French TW, Kranz TS: Non-lymphoid hematopoietic neoplasms in cats: A retrospective study of 60 cases. Cornell Vet 78:21–42, 1988.

Breitschwerdt B: Infectious thrombocytopenia in dogs. Compend Contin Educ Pract Vet 10:1177–1191, 1988.

Bull RW: Immunohematology. *In* Halliwell EW, Gorman NT, eds: Veterinary Clinical Immunology. Philadelphia, WB Saunders, 1989.

Christopher MM: Relation of endogenous Heinz bodies to disease and anemia in cats: 120 cases (1978–1987). J Am Vet Med Assoc 194:1089, 1989.

Christopher MM, Harvey JW: Specialized hematology tests. Semin Vet Med Surg 7:301–310, 1992.

Eibert M, Lewis D: Evaluation of the feline erythron in health and disease. Compend Contin Educ Pract Vet 19:335, 1997.

Feldman E, Nelson R: Canine and Feline Endocrinology and Reproduction, ed 2. Philadelphia, WB Saunders, 1996.

Giger U: Hereditary disorders of canine erythrocytes. *In* Kirk RW, ed: Current Veterinary Therapy X. Philadelphia, WB Saunders, 1989.

Gilmour M, Lappin M, Thrall MA: Investigating primary acquired pure red cell aplasia in dogs. Vet Med 86:1199, 1991.

Grindem CB: Bone marrow biopsy and evaluation. Vet Clin North Am Small Anim Pract 19:669, 1989.

Halliwell REW, Gorman NT, eds: Autoimmune blood diseases. *In* Halliwell REW: Veterinary Clinical Immunology. Philadelphia, WB Saunders, 1989.

Hansen P, Henotreaux M, Rutten VPMG, et al: Neutrophil phagocyte dysfunction in a Weimaraner with recurrent infections. J Small Anim Pract 36:128–131, 1995.

Harvey JW: Congenital erythrocyte enzyme deficiencies. Vet Clin North Am, Small Anim Pract 26:1003, 1996.

Hosgood G: Canine hemangiosarcoma. Compend Contin Educ Pract Vet 13:1065, 1991.

Jain NC: Essentials of Veterinary Hematology. Philadelphia, Lea & Febiger, 1993.

Klag AR: Hemolytic anemia in dogs. Compend Contin Educ Pract Vet 14:1090, 1992.

Kociba GJ: Feline anemia. *In* Kirk RW, ed: Current Veterinary Therapy X. Philadelphia, WB Saunders, 1989.

Latimer KS, Rakish P: Clinical interpretation of leukocyte responses. Vet Clin North Am Small Anim Pract 19:637, 1989.

Meyer DJ, Coles EH, Rich LJ, eds: Veterinary Laboratory Medicine. Philadelphia, WB Saunders, 1991.

Meyer DJ, Harvey J: Veterinary Laboratory Medicine, ed 2. Philadelphia, WB Saunders, 1998.

Raskin RE: Myelopoiesis and myeloproliferative disorders. Vet Clin North Am Small Anim Pract, 26:1023, 1996.

Raskin RE, Meyer DJ: Update on Clinical Pathology. Vet Clin North Am Small Anim Pract, 26, 1996.

Smith JE: Iron metabolism in dogs and cats. Compend Contin Educ Pract Vet 14:39, 1992.

Weiss DJ, Klausner JS: Drug associated aplastic anemia in dogs. J Am Vet Med Assoc 196:472, 1990.

············HEMATOPOIETIC NEOPLASMS

This group of blood disorders is characterized by malignant neoplasia of the hematopoietic tissues, which may include bone marrow, lymphoid tissue, the reticuloendothelial system (RES), and the plasma cell system. The disease can be classified according to the predominant cell type; however, the parent neoplastic tissues may all be of one stem cell type.

Leukemia is a neoplastic proliferation of hematopoietic cells. Cells may or may not be present in the peripheral blood and may or may not invade organs other than the bone marrow. Leukemia is either acute or chronic. *Lymphoid leukemias* can be divided into acute lymphoblastic, chronic lymphocytic, and large granular lymphoma.

Lymphoma (lymphosarcoma [LSA]) is a lymphoid malignancy originating from solid organs (lymph node, spleen, liver). Seventy percent of cats with lymphoma are positive for FeLV. Canine lymphomas are multifactorial in etiology with a genetic component being present. Four anatomical sites may be involved in lymphomas—multicentric, mediastinal, alimentary, and extranodal.

Reticulum cell sarcoma is a neoplastic proliferation of abnormal lymphocytes or other reticuloendothelial areas, resulting in tumor formation and infiltration of various tissues.

Myeloproliferative disorders are interrelated dysplastic and neoplastic conditions that arise from clonal transformation of nonlymphoid stem cells and their progeny in the bone marrow. Classification of the disorders depends on the morphologic and cytochemical characteristics of the cells. Myelopoiesis is the production of erythroid, granulocytic, monocytic, or megakaryocytic cell lines. The stages of myeloproliferative disorders can be categorized as reticuloendotheliosis, erythemic myelosis, erythroleukemia, granulocytic leukemia, and monocytic leukemia; myelomonocytic disorders can be categorized as myelodysplastic syndrome (MDS) and acute myelogenous leukemia (AML). A patient with more than 30% myeloblasts in the marrow is considered to have AML and can be treated with aggressive chemotherapy. A patient with maturation abnormalities and defects in one or more cell lines with a myeloblast count of less than 30% has MDS.

Myelogenous tumor refers to the presence of primary neoplastic cells in the bone marrow.

Erythemic myelosis, erythroleukemia, and *reticuloendotheliosis* refer to hematopoietic tumors of erythroid precursors. Erythroleukemia is characterized by abnormal proliferation of both erythroid and myeloid cell lines. Myeloproliferative disorders may begin as erythemic myelosis, progress to erythroleukemia, and terminate as granulocytic leukemia. Reticuloendotheliosis refers to a myeloproliferative disorder of the cat with immature, undifferentiated reticuloendothelial cells in the blood and bone marrow.

············RETROVIRUSES

Retroviruses are single-stranded RNA viruses that contain reverse transcriptase, which is an enzyme that is necessary for the synthesis of DNA on an RNA template. The domestic cat is susceptible to infection by five retroviruses, including FeLV, feline sarcoma virus (FeSV), endogenous feline retrovirus (RD-114), and feline immunodeficiency virus (FIV).

............Feline Leukemia Virus (Feline Leukemia Complex)

Leukemia complex is a term used to describe all the neoplastic diseases of hematopoietic or blood-forming cells originating in bone marrow or lymphoid tissue. Approximately one third of all cat tumors are hematopoietic tumors, and 90% are lymphoid tumors. The cause of the feline leukemia complex is an RNA virus termed *C-type virus* classified in the oncornavirus genus and Retroviridae family. The virus contains an enzyme, reverse transcriptase, that allows the virus to produce DNA copy and more viral RNA and thus to form new complete viral units. Cells infected with C-type viruses can begin to proliferate neoplastically. Virus-infected tissue can be identified by (1) demonstration on electron microscopy; (2) demonstration of FeLV structural proteins and glycoproteins in the cytoplasm and on the surface of infected cells as indicated by positive immunofluorescent techniques; and (3) cytotoxicity test.

The FeLV core and envelope are composed of several proteins and glycoproteins, including gp70, p15e, and p27:

1. The gp70 antigen is the major antigen in the viral envelope and is involved in attachment to and penetration of the cell by the virus. The antigen is present on the membrane of the infected cells.
2. The p15e antigen is an envelope protein and a mediator of FeLV-associated immunosuppression. This protein can reduce by 50% to 90% the response of lymphoid cells to stimulation in vitro.
3. The p27 antigen is the viral core protein and is present in the cytoplasm of infected cells and the peripheral blood of infected cats. This antigen is detected in both the enzyme-linked immunosorbent assay (ELISA) and immunofluorescent antibody (IFA) tests for leukemia. Antibodies to p27 do not protect the cat against FeLV infection, FeLV-associated diseases, or neoplastic transformation.

FeLV can cause a variety of hematopoietic neoplasms and anemias, as well as some immundeficiency conditions.

Most tumors caused by FeLV are classified as lymphosarcomas and consist of solid masses of proliferating lymphocytes. Lymphosarcomas are seen in thymic, alimentary, renal, generalized, or miscellaneous forms.

FeLV is widespread in nature. It has been estimated that 1.8% to 3.5% of cats in the general free-roaming cat population are chronic virus carriers. Cats in urban areas and catteries show a much higher incidence of exposure to the virus. The virus is shed in the saliva, urine, and feces of infected cats and is present in the blood cells and platelets. The virus can also be transmitted from mother to offspring, either in utero or following birth through the queen's milk.

Approximately 2% of the cats exposed to FeLV become persistently viremic and develop FeLV-related disorders. Young cats have a much greater incidence of becoming persistently viremic than older cats. Persistently viremic cats with FeLV-related disorders usually die within 3 to 5 years. Most cats exposed to FeLV develop a systemic immune-mediated humoral response and remain free of clinical illness. Approximately one third of transiently infected cats cannot eliminate the virus within 4 to 6 weeks and become latently infected, with the FeLV virus remaining in the bone marrow, and may develop clinically related disease or may extinguish the virus infection.

The period of disease development in healthy cats infected with FeLV is variable; however, studies indicate that 83% of FeLV-infected cats die within 3 years.

Diagnosis of lymphosarcoma in the cat depends on the primary tissues affected. In the gastrointestinal form, vomiting, diarrhea, constipation, and anorexia are the signs most often seen. In the multicentric form, icterus and uremia are often present when there is extensive infiltration of the liver and kidneys. The anterior mediastinal form may be characterized by difficulty in swallowing, dyspnea, coughing, and vomiting after eating. Often, there are nonspecific signs such as lethargy, anemia, loss of weight, anorexia, and dehydration.

Enlargement of peripheral lymph nodes is not commonly found in lymphosarcoma of the cat; nevertheless, all lymph nodes should be carefully examined. In addition, the liver, spleen, mesenteric lymph nodes, and kidneys should be examined for any indication of enlargement.

Aspiration of fluid (thoracentesis or paracentesis) may be helpful in performing cytologic evaluation and confirming the presence of a neoplasm.

Examination of peripheral blood smears in cats with lymphosarcoma reveals that a pronounced normocytic, normochromic anemia is present in 65% to 70% of the cases. A high percentage of these cases involve a nonresponsive anemia. Absolute leukocytosis has been found in 30% of the cases, absolute leukocytopenia in 10% of the cases, and absolute lymphocytopenia in 40% of the cases. Leukemia is present in 10% to 30% of the cases, depending on the stage of the disease at examination.

Most feline lymphosarcomas are of T-cell origin; however, B-cell lymphosarcoma is observed in the alimentary form. Seventy percent of cats with lymphosarcoma are FeLV-positive, and 30% have no detectable FeLV antigens. Both FeLV-positive and FeLV-negative lymphosarcoma cells have tumor-specific feline oncornavirus–associated cell membrane antigen (FOCMA).

Ancillary examinations that may be helpful include radiographs of the thorax and abdomen, thoracentesis and paracentesis coupled with exfoliative cytology, intravenous pyelogram (IVP) examination, pneumoperitoneogram, and biopsy of any suspicious tissue.

FeLV is infectious for cats and is transmitted primarily via the saliva and urine. The prevalence of FeLV among cats depends on their environment. It has been estimated that 33% of cats in a multicat household may be infected, fewer than 1% of cats living alone are infected, and only 1.8% to 3.5% of stray cats with an unknown history of FeLV exposure are infected. In hospital blood donor cats, 12% have been found to be infected with FeLV.

··········· Immunodiagnosis of FeLV Infection

The IFA technique detects group-specific antigen only after it is incorporated into leukocytes and platelets, indicating a persistent viremia.

The extent of disease in FeLV-exposed cats is dependent on the immunologic response to FeLV envelope antigens and to the FeLV- and FeSV-induced tumor-specific antigen. Most cats exposed to FeLV envelope antigen produce high neutralizing antibody titers and become immune to infection; a smaller percentage of FeLV-exposed cats that do not produce an effective immune response will become persistently infected. About 30% of exposed cats develop a latent infection (Fig. 5–4).

Immunity to FeLV antigen can be developed, and two kinds of antibodies have been described: (1) a virus-neutralizing antibody and (2) FOCMA antibodies. The standard tests that are used to demonstrate the presence of FeLV in a host are the IFA test and the ELISA. A positive IFA test is indicative of the presence of infectious FeLV in the cat. About 97% of IFA-positive cats remain infected for life; 3% reject the virus, develop immunity to FeLV, and become IFA-negative. The ELISA detects soluble FeLV p27 antigen in the plasma or serum of FeLV-infected cats. The ELISA has been positive in cases in which the FeLV IFA test is negative, and the virus could be isolated from 68% of the cats with positive ELISAs and from 98.5% of the cats with positive IFA tests. All ELISA-positive cats that do not show signs of FeLV-associated diseases should have the result confirmed by the IFA test or should be retested by the

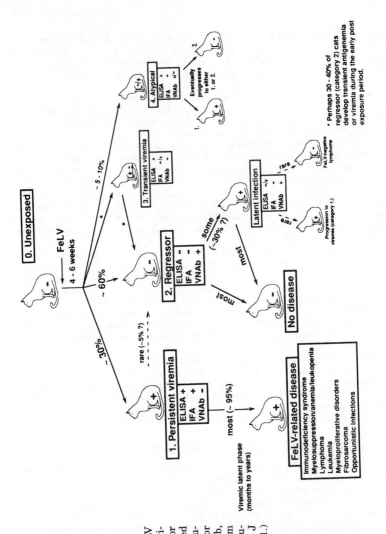

Figure 5–4. The pathways for FeLV p27 antigen of feline leukemia virus (FeLV) infection. See text for description. ELISA, enzyme-linked immunosorbent assay; IFA, immunofluorescent antibody assay (for cell-associated p27 antigen); VNAb, virus-neutralizing antibody. (From Hoover EA, Mullins JI: Feline leukemia virus infection and disease. J Am Vet Med Assoc 199:1287, 1991.)

678

ELISA procedure in 6 to 8 weeks. Approximately 30% of ELISA-positive cats may convert to negative status on a repeat test (Table 5–8).

Cats that have protective titers of FOCMA antibody will not develop lymphosarcoma; however, they can develop the other diseases associated with FeLV. There is currently no commercially available assay for FOCMA antibody.

Most unexposed cats in the general pet cat population and the majority of FeLV-exposed cats do not have protective titers (>1:10) of FeLV-neutralizing antibody. FeLV-infected cats do not have FeLV-neutralizing antibody.

FeLV is capable of growing in canine or human cells in tissue culture. However, FeLV antigen has never been found in any human tumors thus far examined. The cat, a known harborer of an oncogenic virus, is always in very close contact with humans. At this time, there is no evidence to suggest that horizontal transmission of FeLV may occur between the cat and human.

Cats exposed to FeLV can respond in several different ways:

1. Not becoming infected at all.
2. Becoming temporarily infected, developing immunity, and overcoming the infection.
3. Becoming infected and continuing to shed virus indefinitely without becoming ill.
4. Becoming infected, with leukemia or another of the FeLV-related diseases developing. Cats infected with FeLV show a generalized syndrome of immunosuppression and numerous systemic diseases. The veterinarian needs to know whether the cat is infected with FeLV. Basically, FeLV-negative cats (even if they have neutralizing antibody or FOCMA titers) should not be housed with a cat that is infected with FeLV (as proved by at least two positive IFA tests done 3 months apart).

Other forms of diseases associated with infection by FeLV include:

1. Myeloproliferative diseases, in which there is neoplastic proliferation of cells formed in the bone marrow. The four stages of feline myeloproliferative disease are:
   a. Erythemic myelosis.
   b. Erythroleukemia with proliferation of mixed populations of erythemic and granulocytic cells.
   c. Myeloblastic leukemia.
   d. Proliferation of erythroid and myeloid cells in the bone marrow and

Table 5–8. Feline Leukemia Virus (FeLV) Immunofluorescent Antibody Test and Removal Program

1. Remove all FeLV-infected sick cats from the household.
2. If there are no other cats at home, wait 10 days before bringing another cat into the household.
3. Immediately test all remaining cats for FeLV.
4. Remove all FeLV-infected healthy cats from the household.
5. Clean dishes, litter pans, and bedding with detergents.
6. Quarantine all remaining FeLV-uninfected cats in the household.
7. Retest all FeLV-uninfected cats 3 mo after the first test. The incubation period for FeLV infection can be as long as 3 mo.
8. The household can be considered free of FeLV-infected cats only when all cats have tested FeLV-negative in two tests done 3 mo apart.
9. Test all new cats for FeLV before they are introduced into the household.

From Hardy WD: Hematopoietic tumors of cats. J Am Anim Hosp Assoc 17:921, 1981.

spleen and proliferation of fibrous tissue and cancellous bone, producing medullary osteosclerosis or myelofibrosis.

2. Anemias, including nonregenerative anemia unassociated with hematopoietic neoplasia, nonregenerative anemia associated with a panleukopenia-like syndrome, hypoplastic anemia with no bone marrow involvement, myelophthisic-type anemia, and regenerative and nonregenerative anemia associated with *Haemobartonella felis*.

3. Immunosuppression-associated conditions in young cats with thymic involution:
   a. Poor healing of wounds and abscesses.
   b. Chronic general infections.
   c. Glomerulonephritis.
   d. Panleukopenia-like syndrome.
   e. Abortions.
   f. Stomatitis.
   g. Upper respiratory diseases.

■ RECOMMENDATIONS FOR FELINE LEUKEMIA VIRUS TESTING

1. Test new kittens before introduction into the household.
2. Test newly adopted kittens or cats.
3. Test cats whose immune status is not known.
4. Test ill cats.
5. All kittens or adult cats that test negative at the first ELISA screening but with a known or suspected exposure to FeLV should be retested.
6. All FeLV-negative exposed cats in a multiple-cat household (in which an FeLV carrier is found) should be retested at 3-month intervals until all cats within the household or facility test FeLV-negative on at least two consecutive tests.

...........Feline Immunodeficiency Virus

Pedersen and associates in 1987 described a retrovirus of cats, feline immunodeficiency virus (FIV), that suppresses the immune system. FIV is a member of the Retroviridae family (subfamily Lentivirinae). FIV causes lifelong infection. The virus is not highly contagious and is usually transmitted through bite infections. The virus attacks T cells. There are five phases of infection with FIV virus in the cat:

1. An acute stage occurring several weeks after infection and lasting 4 to 16 weeks
2. An asymptomatic carrier stage lasting months to years
3. Persistent generalized lymphadenopathy
4. An acquired immunodeficiency syndrome– or AIDS-related complex (ARC) phase
5. A terminal stage with a variety of opportunistic infections

Clinical signs of infection depend upon the stage of infection with the FIV the cat is in. In the asymptomatic carrier phase, there are no marked clinical signs, but abnormalities in CD4/CD8 lymphocyte cell ratios may develop along with depressed lymphocyte blastogenesis response. The persistent generalized lymphadenopathy phase quickly progresses to the ARC stage. The ARC phase signs may include generalized lymphadenopathy, fever, leukopenia, conjunctivitis, gingivitis, periodontitis, rhinitis, emaciation, diarrhea, and pustular dermatitis. Thirty-five percent to 75% of FIV-infected cats suffer hematologic abnormalities, including anemia, leukopenia, neutropenia, thrombocytopenia, and pancytopenia. Anemias generally are nonregenerative and hemobartonellosis may be associated with the anemia. A Coombs'-positive anemia can also be observed. FIV produces lymphopenia associated with lysis of T lymphocytes, and anemia, neutropenia, and bone marrow abnormalities.

Cats with FIV infections are predisposed to neoplasia development that may include lymphoma, squamous cell carcinoma, and extranodal LSA. FeLV coinfection is increased in cats with FIV infection. The virus has not been transmitted to humans. Cats infected with the virus may remain carriers or may develop a wide variety of diseases that resemble the pathologic changes seen in humans infected with the AIDS virus. A large number of FIV-positive cats are asymptomatic and do not die. In the United States, 1% to 3% of healthy cats and about 13% to 15% of sick cats are infected with FIV. The mean age of FIV-infected cats is 5 to 6 years.

An ELISA for FIV has been developed to detect antibody to FIV. Most of the antibody is directed to the two virus core proteins, p26 and p15. A positive test indicates that the cat has experienced FIV infection and is likely to be infected persistently. A Western blot test can be used to confirm the findings of the ELISA. The Western blot test is more specific than the ELISA or IFA. Adult cats and kittens over 6 months of age that test negative, but with a known or suspected exposure to FIV, should be retested. The determining retest should be at least 120 days post exposure. Periodic annual testing should be performed in cats at risk, that is, outdoor cats, cats that fight, stray cats, cats with bite wounds, recently mated female cats, cats in multicat households, and cats in a household with a known FIV-positive cat. FIV-positive healthy cats may live for months to years. Effective FIV case management involves measures aimed at preserving the health of an infected cat, preventing the spread of FIV infection, and early and aggressive treatment of FIV-related disease.

REFERENCES

American Veterinary Medical Association: Panel report on the colloquium on feline leukemia virus/feline immunodeficiency virus: Tests and vaccination. J Am Vet Med Assoc 199:1271–1485, 1991.

August JR: Husbandry practices for cats infected with feline leukemia virus or feline immunodeficiency virus. J Am Vet Med Assoc 199:1474–1481, 1991.

August RR: Consultations in Feline Internal Medicine, ed 3. Philadelphia, WB Saunders, 1998.

Barr M: FIV, FeLV and FIPV: Interpretation and misinterpretation of serological teat results. Semin Vet Med Surg 11:144–153, 1996.

Blue JT, French TW, Kranz JS: Non-lymphoid hematopoietic neoplasia in cats: A retrospective study of 60 cases. Cornell Vet 78:21–42, 1988.

Cotter S: Feline viral neoplasia. In Greene C: Infectious Diseases of the Dog and Cat, ed 2. Philadelphia, WB Saunders, 1998.

English R: Feline immunodeficiency virus. In Bonagura JD, ed: Kirk's Current Veterinary Therapy XII. 1995, p 280.

Feder BM, Hurvitz AI: Feline immunodeficiency virus infection in 100 cats and association with lymphoma. J Vet Intern Med 4:110, 1990.

Hardy WD Jr: Feline T-lymphotrophic lentivirus: Retrovirus-induced immunosuppression in cats. J Am Anim Hosp Assoc 24:241, 1988.

Jain N, Blue J, Grindem CB, et al: Proposed criteria for classification of acute myeloid leukemia in dogs and cats. Vet Clin Pathol 2:63–82, 1991.

Loar AS: Feline leukemia virus. Vet Clin North Am Small Anim Pract 23:193, 1993.

Meyer DJ, Harvey J: Veterinary Laboratory Medicine, ed 2. Philadelphia, WB Saunders, 1998.

Pedersen NC, Ho EW, Brown ML, et al.: Isolation of a T-lymphotropic virus from domestic cats with an immunodeficiency-like syndrome. Science 235:790–793, 1987.

Raskin RE: Myelopoiesis and myeloproliferative disorders. Vet Clin North Am Small Anim Pract 26:1023, 1966.

Sparger EE: Current thoughts in feline immunodeficiency virus infection. Vet Clin North Am Small Anim Pract 23:173, 1993.

Sparkes AH, Hopper CD, Millard WG, et al: Feline immunodeficiency virus infection. J Vet Intern Med 7:85–90, 1993.

Thomas J, Robinson W: Feline immunodeficiency virus infection. Waltham Focus 5:(2): 1995.

Yamamoto JK, Hensen H, Ho E, et al: Epidemiologic and clinical aspects of feline immunodeficiency virus infection in cats from the continental U.S. and Canada and possible mode of transmission. J Am Vet Med Assoc 194:213, 1989.

............LEUKEMIAS

By definition, leukemia is the neoplastic proliferation of hematopoietic cells in the bone marrow with abnormal cells in the peripheral circulation. Leukemias can be classified as myeloid or lymphoid and placed in four major categories:

1. Acute lymphoblastic leukemia
2. Chronic lymphoid leukemia
3. Acute myelogenous leukemia
4. Chronic myelogenous leukemia

Lymphocytic leukemia is more common than nonlymphocytic leukemia; acute lymphoblastic leukemia is more common than chronic lymphocytic leukemia.

Acute lymphoblastic leukemia (ALL) is primarily a bone marrow disorder that affects lymphoblasts. If untreated, ALL will become a multisystem disorder.

Chronic lymphoid leukemia (CLL) is characterized by small lymphoid cells that are well differentiated. The bone marrow is infiltrated with small lymphocytes (>20%). The clinical signs, which are usually mild and may be nonspecific, include lethargy, anemia, weight loss, partial anorexia, cough, mild lymphadenopathy, hepatomegaly, and splenomegaly.

Acute myelogenous leukemia (AML) involves proliferation of poorly differentiated myeloid cells. Hematologic findings may include leukemic cells (blast cells) in the peripheral circulation, pancytopenia, and macrothrombocytes in the peripheral blood. Ocular signs may be prominent, with immune lymphoblastic cells infiltrating the uveal tract of the eye.

Chronic myelogenous leukemia (CML) is a monoclonal proliferation that affects the pluripotential hematopoietic stem cells and results in overproduction of granulocytes. Bone marrow examination reveals an increased M/E ratio with an abundance of immature cells of the granulocytic series.

A true leukemic blood picture with more than 100,000 cells per microliter rarely develops, although examination of peripheral smears may reveal primitive or atypical cells in more than 60% of the cases. Approximately 50% of affected dogs may have protein values lower than those of normal age-matched dogs. Anemia is present in about one third of the cases.

............Canine Leukemia

Leukemias in the dog represent fewer than 10% of all hematopoietic neoplasms in the dog. Lymphomas outnumber leukemia cases in the dog. Myeloid leukemias are more common than lymphoid leukemias, with three fourths of the acute leukemias being myeloid. Cytochemical staining is required to differentiate myeloid from lymphocytic tumors. Acute leukemias present with a variety of clinical signs, including lethargy, weight loss, lameness, persistent fever, vomiting, diarrhea, splenomegaly, hepatomegaly, and mild LNN enlargement.

Dogs with acute leukemias have a variety of acute hematologic changes that have been reviewed by Couto. These may include:

- Abnormal (leukemic) cells in the peripheral blood count.
- Isolated cytopenias, bicytopenias, and pancytopenias.

- Leukoerythroblastic reactions in 50% of dogs with AML.
- Total WBC count and blast cells are highest in dogs with ALL.
- Severe anemia is present in ALL and AML, as well as thrombocytopenia.

The diagnosis of AML or ALL is based on physical signs, the peripheral blood picture, and biopsy of liver, spleen, LNN, or bone marrow.

.... Canine Lymphoma

Canine lymphomas are multifactorial in origin. The affected animal is usually between 5 and 10 years of age. Dog breeds reported to have epidemiologically confirmed higher incidences of lymphosarcoma are the boxer, basset hound, Saint Bernard, Scottish terrier, Airedale, bulldog, and Labrador retriever. Lymphoma may present as four anatomical forms:

1. Multicentric, with generalized lymphadenopathy, and hepatic, splenic, or bone marrow involvement, individually or severally
2. Mediastinal, with mediastinal lymphadenopathy and possible bone marrow involvement
3. Alimentary, with diffuse focal involvement of the gastrointestinal tract
4. Extranodal, affecting any organ or tissue

The most common type of lymphosarcoma in the dog appears to be lymphoblastic and prolymphocytic lymphosarcoma of the disseminated variety. Most dogs with lymphosarcoma develop bilateral lymphadenopathy and visceral organ involvement (i.e., spleen, liver, kidneys, or intestines).

The signs associated with lymphosarcoma are often related to sites of involvement. In suspected cases of canine lymphosarcoma, examine all peripheral lymph nodes, carefully palpate the spleen and liver, and visually examine the tonsils. The eyes and respiratory and nervous systems may also be involved. More rarely observed sites of lymphosarcoma are the skin and mediastinum.

Most canine lymphosarcomas appear to be of B-cell origin, based on lymphocyte surface markers. The major cell types associated with canine lymphosarcoma are lymphocytic, lymphoblastic, and histiocytic. Lymphoblastic lymphosarcoma is the most poorly differentiated of the cell types. The survival time of dogs treated for lymphoblastic lymphosarcoma ranges from 6 to 18 months and averages 9 months. In histiocytic lymphosarcoma, survival times range from 1 to 6 months.

Hematologic and serum abnormalities associated with lymphoma are involved with bone marrow infiltration with neoplastic cells, splenic abnormalities, paraneoplastic syndromes, and immune-mediated syndromes.

Paraneoplastic syndromes associated with lymphoma in the dog can include hypercalcemia (see p. 169), monoclonal and polyclonal gammopathies (see p. 703) and immune cytopenias, polyneuropathy, and hypoglycemia (see p. 144). Canine lymphosarcoma is the most common cause of hypercalcemia in the dog (see p. 722). Hypercalcemia is observed more frequently in dogs with mediastinal lymphoma. Altered serum calcium levels are frequently associated with bone marrow involvement (see p. 666). Dogs with hypercalcemia associated with lymphosarcoma are very ill, and serum calcium levels may be in the 15- to 20-mg/dL (emergency) range. In vivo findings suggest that in some cases of hypercalcemia associated with canine lymphosarcoma there is a PTH-like humoral factor that can stimulate nephrogenous cyclic adenosine monophosphate (cAMP) excretion and inhibit proximal tubular phosphate reabsorption.

Additional examinations that may be helpful in confirming lymphoma are exfoliative cytology of lymph nodes or fluid aspirates, lymph node biopsy, bone marrow examination, radiology, and exploratory surgery.

After a confirming diagnosis of lymphoma has been made, the disease should be staged in order to better establish a prognosis and treatment regimen.

Unlike feline lymphosarcoma, canine lymphosarcoma is not known to have a viral cause, and there are no reports of clusters of cases. Canine lymphosarcoma and lymphocytic leukemia are transmissible to neonatal pups or to canine fetuses in utero. Dogs with lymphosarcoma have an immunodeficiency in the cellular (T-cell) component, as measured by lymphocyte blastogenesis.

The treatment of lymphosarcoma in the dog should be individualized and depends on the stage of the disease, the location of tumor tissue, and possibly the cell type (see p. 932). For further information about treatment protocols, see the references.

REFERENCES

Couto GC: Clinicopathologic aspects of acute leukemias in the dog. J Am Vet Med Assoc 186:681–685, 1985.

Hahn A, Richardson R: Cancer Chemotherapy. Baltimore, Williams & Wilkins, 1995.

Jain NC, Kociba GJ, Blue J: Proposed criteria for classification of acute myeloid leukemia in dogs and cats. Vet Clin Pathol 20:63–82, 1991.

Nelson RW, Couto C: Essentials of Small Animal Internal Medicine. St Louis, Mosby–Year Book, 1992.

Theilen GH, Madewell BR: Veterinary Cancer Medicine, ed 2. Philadelphia, Lea & Febiger, 1987.

Weir EC, Norrdin RW, Matus KE, et al: Humeral hypercalcemia of malignancy in canine lymphosarcoma. Endocrinology 122:602–608, 1988.

Withrow SJ, MacEwan GE: Clinical Veterinary Oncology. Philadelphia, JB Lippincott, 1989.

..........FELINE INFECTIOUS PERITONITIS

Feline infectious peritonitis (FIP) is a chronic, progressive viral disease of domestic and wild members of the Felidae family. The virus producing FIP and feline enteric coronavirus (FECV) are antigenically very similar. The prevalence of FECV infection in single-cat households in the United States is approximately 25%. There are at least nine different strains of FIP virus. When first characterized, the disease was recognized as a chronic fibrinous peritonitis with abdominal effusion. Both effusive and noneffusive forms of the disease can exist. Effusive FIP may be seen as pleuritis or peritonitis, or both. Noneffusive FIP is characterized by pyogranulomatous inflammation and necrosis of a variety of organs, including kidney, eye, brain, lung, and liver.

FIP is caused by a small RNA virus of the coronavirus variety. The virus is shed by sick, subclinically ill, and asymptomatic carrier cats. The natural route of infection is mainly through oral transmission and contact with infected fecal material. The disease is readily reproduced by parenteral inoculation of infected fluids or tissues, and the virus is present in the blood of infected cats. Maternal transmission, either in utero or neonatal, may also occur.

..........Morbidity (Infection Rate) and Mortality

The FIP virus is widespread in nature. In the United States, the seroprevalence of FECV is 25% in single-cat households and 75% to 100% in multicat households. In problem catteries, the overall morbidity may be 90% or more. In the general population, the morbidity is about 20%. When the virus is introduced into a susceptible population of cats for the first time, the overall mortality during the first 6 months to 1 year may approach 25% or more in some instances.

There is no apparent breed or sex predilection for the clinical disease. The peak incidence of clinical disease is in cats approximately 1 to 2 years of age.

FIP produces a generalized vasculitis associated with phlebitis, thrombophlebitis, and thrombosis in numerous organs. Microscopic disseminated fibrinonecrotic or pyogranulomatous inflammation and necrosis are found in almost every body organ. The form of vasculitis and the generalized inflammation suggest that the inflammatory reaction is immune-mediated.

Cats infected with FIP may also develop DIC characterized by thrombocytopenia, prolonged one-stage prothrombin time (PT), partial thromboplastin time (PTT), and increased levels of fibrin degradation (split) products (FDPs), along with decreased activity of factors VII, VIII, IX, X, XI, and XII.

Among the clinical pathologic abnormalities found in FIP is a mild to moderate normochromic, normocytic nonregenerative anemia. The absolute WBC count is elevated and is associated with an increase in the absolute number of neutrophils. Lymphocyte numbers are reduced. An elevation in the total plasma protein level as determined with a refractometer is a characteristic feature of FIP. An albumin-globulin (A/G) ratio greater than 0.81 of peritoneal or pleural effusions is a factor in ruling out FIP, whereas a γ-globulin content of more than 32% of the effusion is likely to be indicative of FIP. The hyperproteinemia is due to increased concentrations of α_1-, β_2-, and γ-globulins as seen on protein electrophoresis. (Serum fibrinogen levels of 400 mg/dL can be seen.)

FIP is a more significant clinical problem in catteries where concurrent FeLV infections exist.

············Clinical Diagnosis

Despite being in an era of sophisticated in-house diagnostic technology, when certain viral antigens can be detected within minutes of collecting blood, stool, or saliva from the patient, there are no serologic tests that can distinguish FIP virus from FECV. This includes the FIP-specific ELISA for the 7B protein as well as the RT-PCR (reverse transcriptase–polymerase chain reaction) test for coronavirus antigen.

The diagnosis of FIP depends on identifying a series of physical and laboratory abnormalities sufficient to justify a *clinical* diagnosis of FIP. Diagnostic *confirmation*, on the other hand, depends on documenting histologic changes in affected tissues collected at biopsy or, as occurs most often, at necropsy. Yet, it is absolutely critical to note that certain physical and laboratory variables carry much more diagnostic value than others.

············Physical Changes

Abdominal Effusion There is no single physical change that a diagnosis of FIP can be based on. Fever, weight loss, and decreased appetite are reported, but because these findings occur so often in sick cats that do not have FIP, they have minimal diagnostic value. The development of a distended, fluid-filled abdomen is an important clinical finding that must be pursued. Abdominal radiographs will confirm the presence of fluid (vs. tumor or pregnancy). Laboratory evaluation of the fluid is the critical next step in arriving at a diagnosis.

Thoracic Effusion Although about 50% of cats with FIP develop an abdominal effusion, approximately 10% of FIP-infected cats develop an effusion that accumulates in the thoracic (pleural) cavity. Affected cats may present with signs of respiratory distress characterized by tachypnea—rapid respirations and inactivity. A γ-globulin level above 32% in the exudate had a 100% positive predictive value for FIP. An albumin content greater than 48% or an albumin-globulin ratio greater than 0.81 had a 100% negative predictive value for ruling out FIP.

Ocular and Neurologic Signs Other physical changes that support a diagnosis of FIP include sudden-onset uveitis in one or both eyes, development of opaque precipitates in the cornea, or retinal hemorrhage or detachment. The two most common neurologic signs associated with FIP are posterior paresis and seizures. It is important to note that the ocular and neurologic signs typically occur independently of an abdominal effusion.

............Laboratory Findings

Fluid Analysis Among FIP-infected cats having a distended abdomen, abdominal fluid analysis and cytology are the most valuable diagnostic tests. Peritoneal and pleural fluids are light to dark yellow in color and have a sticky, viscous consistency. The fluid is technically classified as an exudate, since its total protein content is typically above 5 g/dL. Cytology reveals a relatively *hypo*cellular fluid containing low numbers of neutrophils and macrophages. A homogeneous, light-blue staining background is evidence of the high protein content in the fluid.

Serum Hematology and Biochemistry Leukocytosis with lymphopenia and anemia are frequently reported in cats with FIP. However, a normal hemogram is quite possible. Elevated serum glucose ("stress" hyperglycemia) and liver enzymes are also reported but cannot be regarded as having diagnostic merit. On the other hand, elevated plasma protein is of particular importance in the diagnosis of FIP, particularly in cats that do *not* have effusions associated with their infection. Approximately 75% of the cats with the noneffusive form of FIP have a plasma protein value greater than 7.8 g/dL. Characteristically, the albumin is less than 3.0 g/dL, while plasma globulin, particularly the γ-globulin fraction, is dramatically elevated. Cats with clinical signs suggestive of FIP along with lymphopenia, an FECV antibody titer over 1:160, and hypergammaglobulinemia have an 88.9% probability of having FIP confirmed at necropsy.

Antibody Titers Antibody titer is incorrectly referred to as the "FIP antibody test" or the "FIP test." A number of commercial laboratories offer coronovirus antibody titers as a diagnostic test for FIP. None of the available antibody tests for FIP are diagnostic. Today, most authorities on FIP agree that (1) an elevated titer does *not* confirm a diagnosis of FIP *nor* does it indicate that a cat is doomed to develop FIP in the future, and (2) a "negative" titer does not rule out a diagnosis of FIP. In fact, determining an antibody titer for coronovirus is among the *least reliable and least effective* means of diagnosing FIP.

Histopathology Today, histopathology is regarded as the only reasonable diagnostic test for FIP. Any diagnosis of FIP made without histologic confirmation must be considered presumptive.

............Prevention

The only FIPV vaccine currently available (Primucell, Pfizer Animal Health, Exton, PA) uses a temperature-sensitive strain of FIPV that replicates well at temperatures below 31°C in the upper respiratory tract but not at higher than 38° to 39°C. The vaccine is not approved for use in pregnant queens or in kittens less than 16 weeks of age.

REFERENCES

Addie D: Interpretation of feline coronavirus serology. Practice 11:232–236, 1989.
Addie D, Jarrett O: Control of feline coronavirus in kittens. Vet Rec 126:164, 1990.
Addie D, Jarrett O: Feline coronavirus infection. *In* Greene C, ed. Infectious Diseases of the Dog and Cat, ed 2. Philadelphia, WB Saunders, 1998, pp 58–69.
Barr M: FIV, FeLV, and FIPV: Interpretation and misinterpretation of serological test results. Semin Vet Med Surg 11:144–153, 1996.

Hoskins JD: Corona virus infection in cats. Vet Clin North Am Small Anim Pract 23:1–16, 1993.

McReynolds C, Macy D: Feline infectious peritonitis: Etiology and diagnosis. Compend Contin Educ Pract Vet 19:1007, 1997.

Wolf AM: Feline infectious peritonitis. *In* Proceedings of the Annual Forum of the American College of Veterinary Internal Medicine. San Diego, 1992, pp 103–106.

⋯⋯⋯⋯BLEEDING AND BLOOD COAGULATION

A thorough medical history can be helpful in evaluating animals with a bleeding problem. Basically, the causes of abnormal bleeding can be divided into five major categories: (1) vascular trauma, (2) defective production of hemostatic factors, (3) dilution of hemostatic factors, (4) use of systemic anticoagulants, and (5) DIC.

Most bleeding is the result of local injuries from a variety of causes. The following types of bleeding should cause the clinican to suspect possible abnormalities in blood coagulation:

1. Bleeding at multiple sites throughout the body involving several body systems
2. Development of spontaneous deep hematomas
3. Unusually prolonged bleeding after injury
4. Delayed onset of extensive hemorrhage after bleeding
5. Inability to find an organic cause of the bleeding

In obtaining a history of the bleeding patient, the following information is important:

1. How old was the animal when the bleeding first occurred? Is this the first episode of bleeding? Hereditary defects usually develop in very young dogs.
2. Do immediate relatives have similar bleeding problems? Are multiple animals in one litter affected? Are both sexes affected?
3. Is the animal allowed to roam freely so that it could be exposed to rodenticides? Has the animal recently received any drugs known to interfere with hemostasis or depress the production of platelets? Is there a history of recent vaccination?

Bleeding and altered mechanisms of blood coagulation may have varied manifestations, including petechial hemorrhages; epistaxis; melena; hematuria; and bleeding into body cavities, joints, and the spinal cord. The clinician must determine whether the bleeding has a local cause or is the manifestation of a disease that produces alteration in bleeding or clotting mechanisms. It is important to establish the site and duration of the bleeding, its history (including any previous episodes of bleeding), and the presence of another disease.

⋯⋯⋯⋯Collection and Handling of Blood Samples to Be Used in Evaluation of Coagulation Abnormalities

1. All blood samples should be taken with plastic-coated or silicone-coated glass syringes by *careful* venipuncture. When collecting blood for coagulation studies a two-syringe technique can minimize the amount of tissue thromboplastin in the final sample. Aspirate 1 mL of blood into the first syringe after making the venipuncture. Change to syringe No. 2 and aspirate sufficient blood for the laboratory test.
2. Trisodium citrate or sodium oxalate is the anticoagulant of choice for coagulation and platelet work (e.g., one part 3.8% trisodium citrate plus nine

parts whole blood). The anticoagulant should be added to the syringe first and the blood drawn directly into the syringe in the required volume.

3. All samples must be kept in plastic-coated or silicone-coated glass test tubes.

4. Plasma samples should be prepared for fresh blood and tested immediately or frozen for testing later. Plasma frozen at −20°C can be stored for a few days, and samples frozen at −40° to −80°C can be stored for several months to a year. Samples to be shipped for specialized coagulation assays should be sent in dry ice. Samples should be assayed in duplicate and kept at refrigerator temperature when tested.

5. Platelet tests must be done on fresh samples within 2 hours of collection. Polycarbonate is an ideal plastic surface for platelet preparation. Samples should be kept at room temperature because platelet shape is altered by heat or cold.

■ SPECIMEN COLLECTION FOR LABORATORY EVALUATION OF HEMOSTASIS

Specimen	Tube Top Color	Test
EDTA blood	Purple	Platelet count
Citrated blood	Blue	OSPT, APTT, fibrinogen
Thrombin	Blue	FDPs

OSPT, one-stage prothrombin time; APTT, activated partial thromboplastin time; FDPs, fibrin degradation products.

..........Practical Screening Diagnostic Tests in Bleeding Disorders (Table 5–9)

..........Initial In-Office Screen

The initial in-office screen for the patient with a bleeding disorder should include: a blood smear (see p. 651), activated coagulation time (ACT) test (see p. 690), fibrin degradation products (FDPs) (see p. 45), total fibrin, and buccal mucosa bleeding time (see p. 690).

■ INTERPRETATION OF THE IN-OFFICE COAGULATION PROFILE

Platelet count in peripheral smear	Low	Thrombocytopenia
ACT	Prolonged	Intrinsic system defect
FDPs	Positive	Enhanced fibrinolysis, DIC
Buccal mucosa bleeding time	Prolonged	Thrombocytopenia, thrombocytopathia

---

Examination of the Blood Smear The average number of platelets per monolayer field should be obtained. In normal dogs there are 11 to 25 platelets per field. Most patients with spontaneous bleeding due to thrombocytopenia have fewer than two platelets per oil immersion field.

..........Activated Coagulation Time of Whole Blood

Measurements of whole-blood clotting time can be performed by using the Lee-White whole-blood clotting time and the capillary tube clotting time. The ACT test is technically more dependable because blood temperature does not vary during the test, some of the variables produced by tissue thromboplastin are eliminated, and the vehicle is more reliable for contact activation of the blood

Table 5-9. Interpretation of Coagulation Screens

Disorder	BT	ACT	OSPT*	APTT*	Platelets	Fibrinogen	FDPs
Thrombocytopenia	↑	N	N	N	↓	N	N
Thrombocytopathia	↑	N	N	N	N	N	N
von Willebrand's disease	↑	N/↑	N	N/↑	N	N	N
Hemophilias	N	↑	N	↑	N	N	N
Warfarin toxicity	N	↑	↑	↑	N/↓	N/↓	N/↑
Disseminated intravascular coagulation	↑	↑	↑	↑	↓	↓	↑

BT, bleeding time; ACT, activated coagulation time; OSPT, one-stage prothrombin time; APTT, activated partial thromboplastin time; FDP, fibrin degradation products; ↑, elevated; N, normal or negative; ↓, decreased.

*OSPT and APTT are considered prolonged if they are 25% or more over the concurrent controls.

From Nelson R, Couto G: Essentials of Small Animal Internal Medicine. St Louis, Mosby–Year Book, 1992.

sample. The ACT test evaluates the integrity of the intrinsic and common clotting pathway (factors XII, XI, IX, VIII, X, V, and II). The ACT test can be used as a reliable screening test for evaluation of secondary hemostasis. Qualitative or quantitative abnormalities of platelet function may result in prolongation of the ACT. Platelet numbers may have to be reduced to below 10,000/mm^3 before an effect of the ACT test is produced (dogs have 12 to 15 platelets per oil immersion microscopic field and cats have 10 to 12 platelets per field). Low fibrinogen levels can also influence the ACT test.

To perform the ACT test, make a cephalic or jugular venipuncture using a disposable 20-gauge, 1-in. needle screwed into a plastic tube holder. Insert a 5-mL Vacutainer tube,* partially evacuated, into the needle holder; withdraw 2 mL of blood, and eliminate any tissue thromboplastin that was present when the needle entered the vein. Remove the first tube, and replace it with a second tube containing 12 mg of diatomite (siliceous earth), partially evacuated to withdraw 2 mL of blood. Prewarm the diatomite tube to 38°C in a calibrated heating block.† When blood first appears in the diatomite tube, begin timing with a stopwatch. When 2 mL of blood is present in the tube, return the tube to the heating block. After 1 minute and at each 5-second interval thereafter, remove the tube from the block, tilt the tube, and observe it for evidence of clotting. Normal values are: median, 75.0 seconds; mean, 77.5 seconds; standard deviation (SD), 14.7 seconds.

..........Buccal Mucosa Bleeding Time (BMBT)

This test evaluates the interaction between platelets and endothelium that produces a primary hemostatic plug. Prolonged BMBT occurs in dogs with thrombocytopenia and platelet dysfunction syndromes.

..........Total Platelet Count

Make a direct platelet count using a hemocytometer. For most animal species, the range is 175,000 to 500,000/mm^3. The tendency for bleeding problems to develop in association with thrombocytopenia will depend on the number and function of the available platelets.

..........Fibrin (Fibrinogen) Degradation Products

FDPs are formed when plasma biodegrades these coagulation proteins. The Thrombo Wellco Test is used as an assay for FDPs in dogs and cats. A positive Thrombo Wellco test is indicative of active fibrinolysis and the most common syndrome associated with this is DIC. Positive FDPs can also be observed in dogs with venous or arterial thrombosis and anticoagulant rodenticide poisoning.

..........Platelet Function

Platelet function can be estimated by clot retraction.

..........Activated Partial Thromboplastin Time

The APTT is a measure of the cumulative effects of clotting factors in the intrinsic or intravascular system (measures intrinsic factors VIII, IX, XI, XII,

....

*Vacutainer tube, No. 3206 or 3865, Becton-Dickinson Co., Franklin Lakes, NJ.
†Dow Diagnostest Heating Block, Model 12/1A, Dow Chemical Co., Midland, MI.

and common factors V, X, II) and fibrinogen pathways. The normal range for the APTT of healthy dogs is 14 to 25 seconds.

.... Prothrombin Time

The PT is a measure of the effects of the extrinsic or tissue fluid system of clotting. Most of the factors involved are synthesized in the liver, and the PT test is one of the screening tests used in liver function. The prothrombin-complex clotting factors are II, VII, and X; these factors interact with factor V and fibrinogen in the presence of tissue thromboplastin and $CaCl_2$.

.... Thrombin Time

The thrombin time is a measure of the amount of functional fibrinogen in plasma. The test is used in DIC when fibrinogen levels may be low. Fibrinogen levels may be normal in DIC, but the thrombin time may still be altered because fibrinogen function is changed by in vivo fibrinolysis.

.... The PIVKA Test

The PIVKA (proteins induced by vitamin K absence or antagonists) test is most useful in vitamin K deficiencies. The test is sensitive to moderate deficiencies of factors II, VII, IX, and X. The test will become prolonged 12 to 24 hours after the PT test is prolonged.

■ CAUSES OF DEFECTIVE PRIMARY HEMOSTASIS

Thrombocytopenia
  Defective thrombopoiesis
  Reduced circulating platelet life spans
Thrombopathia (defective platelet function)
Congenital illness
  von Willebrand's disease
  Other hereditary thrombopathias
Systemic illness
  Uremia
  Hepatic disease
  Pancreatitis
  Ehrlichiosis
  Dysprotinemias
  Myeloproliferative and myelodysplastic disorders
  Disseminated intravascular coagulation
Medications that cause platelet dysfunction
Antibody-mediated platelet dysfunction
Vascular disorders

5

■ CAUSES OF DEFECTIVE SECONDARY HEMOSTASIS
(MEASURED BY ACTIVATED CLOTTING TIME)

Clotting factor deficiency
Decreased production
  Hereditary causes
  Chronic hepatic insufficiency
  Anticoagulant rodenticides

Box continued on following page

■ CAUSES OF DEFECTIVE SECONDARY HEMOSTASIS
(MEASURED BY ACTIVATED CLOTTING TIME) *(Continued)*

Increased consumption
  Disseminated intravascular coagulation
  Hemangiosarcoma
Circulating inhibitors of coagulation
Heparin
Fibrin degradation products

...........IMPORTANT BLEEDING DISORDERS IN SMALL ANIMALS
...........Factor VIII Deficiency (Hemophilia A)

This disease is an X-chromosome–linked recessive trait that is carried by females and manifested in males. Female hemophiliacs can be produced by breeding hemophiliac males to carrier females. The disease has been reported in a wide variety of dog breeds and cats, including the Shetland sheepdog, beagle, English setter, Irish setter, Labrador retriever, German shepherd, collie, Greyhound, Weimaraner, Chihuahua, Samoyed, Vizsla, English bulldog, miniature poodle, miniature schnauzer, and Saint Bernard. The clinical disease can be mild, moderate, or severe and can produce both internal and external bleeding. Signs may be observed shortly after weaning and may include umbilical cord bleeding, gingival bleeding, gastrointestinal hemorrhage, hemarthrosis, and hematoma development. Laboratory tests reveal a prolonged APTT, whereas PT, bleeding time, and thrombin time are normal. Affected animals have very low coagulant activity of factor VIII but normal or elevated levels of factor VIII–related antigen. Carrier female animals can be detected by low factor VIII activity (30% to 60% of normal) and a normal or elevated level of factor VIII antigen.

Von Willebrand's disease (vWD) is a bleeding disorder associated with defects in plasma von Willebrand's protein. Several variants of the disease have been described: vWD type I is associated with a defect in factor VIIIR:protein concentration, and vWD type II is associated with a defect in factor VIIIR:vWF (von Willebrand's factor). Type 1 disease is most common in veterinary medicine. vWD has been recognized in more than 29 breeds of dogs, and the incidence varies from 10% to 60% depending on the breed of origin. There are two forms of genetic expression: (1) an autosomal recessive disease in which homozygous vWD individuals have a bleeding disorder and heterozygous individuals are normal carriers, and (2) an autosomal dominant disease with incomplete expression in which heterozygous individuals are affected carriers and homozygous individuals are severely affected. The disease has a high morbidity and low mortality. Dogs with 30% or less of normal levels of vWF tend to hemorrhage. Dogs with abnormal vWF have increased bleeding times but normal platelet counts. When coagulation factor VIII is less than 50% the APTT can be slightly prolonged. The disease has been found in German shepherds, golden retrievers, miniature schnauzers, Doberman pinschers, standard Manchester terriers, Pembroke Welsh corgis, and Scottish terriers. The recessive disease has been recognized in Scottish terriers and Chesapeake Bay retrievers. The incomplete dominant has been recognized in 25 breeds of dogs.

Routine screening tests for coagulation defects are nondiagnostic in this disease. Diagnosis is based on finding reduced or undetectable levels of factor VIII antigen or platelet-related activities of vWF. Animals with the recessive form of the disease are homozygotes and have zero vWF:Ag; (antigen), a subunit of factor VIII; heterozygotes have reduced levels of the antigen, 15% to 60% of normal. In the incompletely dominant form, reduced levels of vWF antigen are present (<7% to 60%). Signs vary from mild to severe and are usually associated with surgery. Other forms of bleeding that may be associated with vWD are hematuria; diarrhea with melena; penile bleeding; lameness; hematoma formation; excessive bleeding when nails are cut, tails are docked, ears are cropped, and so on; prolonged estrous or postpartum bleeding; nose bleeds; and neonatal deaths. A DNA test to detect carriers of the gene for von Willebrand's disease is available through VetGen in Ann Arbor, MI.

............Factor IX (Christmas Factor) Deficiency (Hemophilia B)

This is an X-linked recessive trait that occurs with less frequency than hemophilia A. The disease has been reported in Scottish terriers, Shetland sheepdogs, Saint Bernards, cocker spaniels, French bulldogs, Old English sheepdogs, Alaskan malamutes, Labrador retrievers, bichon frisés, Airedales, and a family of British shorthair cats. The clinical signs are more severe than those seen with hemophilia A. Carrier females have low (40% to 60% of normal) factor IX activity.

............Factor VII Deficiency

This disease has also occurred in the dog. Congenital deficiencies of factor VII have been reported in beagles, although bleeding tendencies are very mild. The deficiency appears to be inherited as an autosomal, incompletely dominant characteristic; heterozygotes have 50% factor VII deficiency. The PT and the serum prothrombin consumption time are prolonged.

............Factor X Deficiency

This deficiency has been found in cocker spaniels. The disease very closely resembles the fading-puppy syndrome in newborn dogs. Bleeding may be internal or through the umbilicus, and affected dogs frequently die. In adult dogs, bleeding may be mild. In severe cases, factor X levels are reduced to 20% of normal; levels are 20% to 70% of normal in mild cases.

............Factor XII (Hageman Factor) Deficiency

Factor XII deficiency has been found as an inherited autosomal recessive trait in domestic cats. Heterozygotes can be detected because they have a partial deficiency of factor XII, with an average of 50% of normal activity levels. Homozygote cats with factor XII deficiency have less than 2% activity. Deficiency of Hageman factor usually does not result in bleeding or other major disorders.

5

............Factor XI Deficiency

Factor XI deficiency is an autosomal disease in English springer spaniels, Great Pyrenees, and Kerry blue terriers. Protracted bleeding may be observed following surgery. Homozygotes have low factor XI activity (<20% of normal); heterozygotes have 40% to 60% of normal factor XI activity.

............PRIMARY HEMOSTATIC DEFECTS
............Platelet Factors (see also p. 46)

Platelets are essential to normal blood coagulation. When vasoconstriction occurs in an injured vessel, the blood flow is retarded and platelets attach to the injured endothelium. Following adhesion, platelets undergo primary aggregation, release of chemical mediators of the coagulation mechanism, secondary aggregation, and contraction. Certain plasma proteins, including calcium fibrinogen, vWF:Ag, and a part of factor VIII, are required for normal platelet adhesion. The release factors produced by degranulating platelets include vasoactive substances, adenosine diphosphate (ADP), prostaglandins, serotonin, epinephrine, and thromboxane A_2. The secondary aggregation is accompanied by the production of PF-3 (thromboplastin).

■ ABNORMALITIES IN PLATELETS

Decreased platelet production
Decreased platelet function
Increased platelet destruction
Increased platelet consumption
Increased platelet sequestration

..........Qualitative Disorders of Platelets

Alterations in platelet function can affect platelet adhesion, aggregation, or release of vasoactive substances. In vWD there is a deficiency of vWF:Ag, which results in altered platelet adhesion. Vascular purpuras are reported and are seen in collagen abnormalities such as Ehlers-Danlos syndrome, which may be inherited as an autosomal dominant trait with complete penetrance in dogs such as the German shepherd, dachshund, and Saint Bernard.

Thrombasthenic thrombopathia is a hereditary abnormality of platelet aggregation described in otter hounds, foxhounds, and Scottish terriers. This abnormality is inherited as an autosomal dominant trait. Platelets do not aggregate normally in response to ADP and thrombin stimulation.

Evaluation of blood platelets is based on a total thrombocyte count, a clot retraction test, and a bleeding time test.

Platelet function defects (thrombocytopenia, thrombopathia) are autosomally inherited and affect both sexes. This familial disorder has been reported in otter hounds and basset hounds.

The clinical signs may resemble those of vWD. Laboratory tests indicate a prolonged bleeding time but normal platelet count and clotting tests.

..........Causes of Accelerated Platelet Destruction

When accelerated platelet destruction appears to be the cause of thrombocytopenia, the differential diagnosis should include immune destruction associated with autoantibodies, drug antibodies, infection, isoimmune destruction, removal associated with DIC, vasculitis, microangiopathic hemolytic anemia, severe vascular injury, hemolytic uremic syndrome, and gram-negative septicemia.

..........Causes of Thrombocytopenia

A decrease in the number of circulating platelets (thrombocytopenia) can result in increased bleeding time and prolonged clot retraction time. Thrombocytopenia may be due to (1) increased platelet destruction, utilization, or sequestration; or (2) decreased platelet production by the bone marrow. Primary thrombocytopenia of unknown cause has been called *idiopathic thrombocytopenic purpura* (ITP). Recent information indicates that in 80% of the cases, thrombocytopenia is secondary to immune-mediated disorders, including autoimmune hemolytic anemia (AIHA), systemic lupus erythematosus (SLE), rheumatoid arthritis (RA), DIC, and other diseases that can affect the bone marrow. Platelet production in the bone marrow can be reduced primarily or cause the release of PF-3 from fresh homologous platelets. The spleen is the major site of production of this non–complement-fixing antibody. PF-3 can be demonstrated in the blood in up to 70% of cases. Not only peripheral platelets but also megakaryocytes in the bone marrow are affected by PF-3. Bone marrow hypoplasia may involve only platelets or may involve all cell lines. Antibody to an animal's own platelets is usually of the IgG type. A specialized test—the PF-3 release test—can be used to demonstrate antiplatelet antibody. Thrombocytopenia is usually associated with bleeding of the purpuric or capillary type and is characterized by petechiae and ecchymoses of the skin, mucous membranes, and conjunctiva; gingival bleeding; epistaxis; melena; and hematuria.

A summary of the etiology of thrombocytopenia follows:

1. Primary (etiology unknown): ITP, AIHA, amegakaryocytic thrombocytopenia.
2. Secondary:
   a. Aplastic anemia.
   b. Destruction of thrombocytes in peripheral blood caused by incompatible blood transfusions, hypersplenism, sensitivity or allergy to various drugs and chemicals, extensive burns, massive transfusions of citrated stored blood, excessive platelet consumption in pulmonary thrombosis, chronic infection, irradiation, infectious disease, or live virus vaccination.
   c. Platelet sequestration and increased utilization: hypersplenism, hepatomegaly, endotoxemia, DIC, hypothermia, or prolonged hemorrhage.
   d. Myelophthisic—leukemia and bone marrow tumors.
   e. Abnormal platelet function; that is, thrombocytopathic thrombocytopenia resembling vWD in humans. This is a familial disorder in Samoyed dogs.

.... Thrombopathias

Abnormal function of blood platelets is referred to as *thrombopathia*. Abnormal function of platelets does not usually affect the platelet count. Functional abnormalities can be produced by a variety of reactions to drugs and systemic and hematologic disorders.

Drugs: aspirin and other nonsteroidal anti-inflammatory agents, cephalothin, phenothiazines, heparin
Systemic disorders: uremia, liver disease
Hematologic disorders: antiplatelet antibody production, myeloproliferative disorders, dysprotinemias, vWD defects

.... Inherited Thrombopathias

Canine thrombasthenic thrombopathia of the otter hound: autosomal recessive trait
Glanzmann's thrombasthenia in Great Pyrenees
Thrombopathia in the basset hound
Thrombopathia of the spitz
Cyclic hematopoiesis of the grey collie
Platelet storage pool disease of American cocker spaniels

.... Immunologically Mediated Thrombocytopenia in the Dog

Dogs with ITP usually have marked thrombocytopenia with platelets usually less than 50,000/μL. Immune mediated hemolytic anemia is reported in approximately 20% of dogs with ITP. Diagnosis of ITP may be confirmed by:

1. Severity of thrombocytopenia
2. The presence of microthrombocytosis or platelet fragmentation
3. Normal to increased numbers of megakaryocyes in the bone marrow
4. Detection of antiplatelet antibody
5. Increased platelet counts following treatment with glucocorticoid therapy
6. Elimination of other causes of thrombocytopenia

Idiopathic and secondary thrombocytopenias are characterized by petechiae and ecchymoses of the skin and mucous membranes, gingival bleeding, epistaxis, melena, and hematuria. The primary disease entity is associated with an immunologic mechanism, and the secondary disease is due to the effects of certain drugs or toxic agents or to a variety of disease states. Some of the disease states that have been cited are septicemia, lymphoproliferative disorders, incompatible blood transfusions, malignancy, and autoimmune diseases (e.g., AIHA, SLE, and RA). In SLE, 20% to 30% of antinuclear antibody (ANA)–positive dogs may have thrombocytopenia that is immune-mediated. Coombs'-positive anemias are often associated with thrombocytopenia (see p. 705). ITP and AIHA when combined in one patient is called Evan's syndrome. *Ehrlichia canis* infection often produces extensive thrombocytopenia. Other infectious organisms that can cause thrombocytopenia are *Ehrlichia equi* and *Rickettsia rickettsii*, which causes Rocky Mountain spotted fever (see p. 700).

Primary immune-mediated thrombocytopenia has an unknown cause and is most frequently seen in middle-aged female dogs. There is some breed predilection, including German shepherds; cocker spaniels, miniature, toy, and standard poodles; and Old English sheepdogs. Antibody-positive thrombocytopenias are chronic and recurrent. A 7S immunoglobulin has been found to cause the release of PF-3 from fresh homologous platelets. The PF3 test lacks specificity and has variable sensitivity in dogs with ITP. The spleen is the major site of production of this non–complement-fixing antibody.

............Thrombocytopenia in the Cat

Cats can also suffer from thrombocytopenia. Causes have been listed as:
Infectious disease—29%
Neoplasia—20%
Cardiac disease—7%
Primary immune-mediated disease—2%
Multiple diseases—22%
Unknown cause—20%

Feline leukemia and myeloproliferative disease have been found in one study in 44% of cats affected with thrombocytopenia. DIC was diagnosed in 12% of cats with thrombocytopenia.

............Other Causes of Bleeding Disorders

............*Monoclonal Gammopathies*

Bleeding tendencies, including epistaxis, gingival bleeding, and retinal hemorrhages, may be associated with a wide variety of gammopathies. Abnormal proteins may lead to bleeding tendencies by coating platelets, combining with clotting factors, or damaging capillaries.

............*Vitamin K Deficiency*

Significantly lowered levels of vitamin K–dependent clotting factors—factors II, VII, IX, and X—have been associated with ingestion of warfarin and coumarin derivatives, pindone and diphacinone poisoning, administration of the coccidiostat sulfaquinoxaline, and possibly malabsorption syndromes. Coumarin compounds inhibit the epoxidase reaction and deplete active vitamin K, producing coagulopathies. Bleeding associated with vitamin K antagonism is dose dependent and can occur within hours of ingestion or as much as 1 week later. Vitamin K antagonism is best determined by tests that involve factor VII, such as the PIVKA test and the PT test (see p. 687). Abnormalities in these tests are best measured by comparison with results for serum from a normal dog. Patient levels that produce a ratio of greater than 1.3 when compared to normal controls are evidence of significant prolongation of the patient's PT. Proteins induced by vitamin K absence or antagonists are produced in the liver and can be detected in the blood when a relative or absolute vitamin K deficiency develops.

Treatment of vitamin K deficiency should be performed with vitamin K_1 delivered SC with a 25-gauge needle. The initial loading dose is 5 mg/kg followed in 8 hours by 2.5 mg/kg q8h.

REFERENCES

Averis S, Lothrop CD, McDonald TP: Plasma von Willebrand factor concentration and thyroid function in dogs. J Am Vet Med Assoc 196:921–924, 1990.

Badylak SF: Coagulation disorders and liver disease. Vet Clin North Am Small Anim Pract 18:87–92, 1988.

Brooks M, Dodds WJ, Raymond SL: Epidemiologic features of von Willebrand's disease in Doberman pinschers, Scottish terriers, and Shetland sheepdogs: 260 cases (1984–1988). J Am Vet Med Assoc 200:1123, 1992.

Cotter SM: Autoimmune hemolytic anemia in dogs. Compend Contin Educ Pract Vet 14:53–59, 1992.

Crystal MA, Cotter SM: Acute hemorrhage: A hemorrhagic emergency in dogs. Compend Contin Educ Pract Vet 14:60–68, 1992.

Feldman BF: Diagnostic approaches to coagulation and fibrinolytic disorders. Semin Vet Med Surg 7:315–322, 1992.

Greene CE: Prolonged bleeding. In Lorenz M, Cornelius LM, eds: Small Animal Medical Diagnosis. Philadelphia, JB Lippincott, 1989.

Hackner S: Approach to the diagnosis of bleeding disorders. Compend Contin Educ Pract Vet 17:331, 1995.

Halliwell RE, Gorman NT: Autoimmune blood diseases. In Veterinary Clinical Immunology. Philadelphia, WB Saunders, 1989.

Hargis AM, Feldman A: Evaluation of hemostatic defects secondary to vascular tumors in dogs. J Am Vet Med Assoc 198:891–894, 1991.

Honeckman A, Knapp D, Reagan W: Diagnosis of canine immune mediated hematologic disease. Compend Contin Educ Pract Vet 18:113, 1996.

Lewis D, Meyers K: Canine idiopathic thrombocytopenic purpura. J Vet Intern Med 10:207–218, 1996.

Mackin A: Canine immune-mediated thrombocytopenia. Compend Contin Educ Pract Vet 17:353, 515, 1995.

Meric SM: Drugs used for disorders of coagulation. Vet Clin North Am Small Anim Pract 18:1217–1241, 1988.

Meyer DJ, Harvey J: Veterinary Laboratory Medicine, ed 2. Philadelphia, WB Saunders, 1998.

Myers KM, Wardrops JK, Meinkoth J: Canine von Willebrand's disease: Pathobiology, diagnosis and short term treatment. Compend Contin Educ Pract Vet 14:13, 1992.

Peterson J, Couto G, Wellman M: Hemostatic disorders in cats: A retrospective study and review of the literature. J Vet Intern Med 9:298–303, 1995.

Redford RL: Diagnosis of platelet disorders. Semin Vet Med Surg 7:323–329, 1992.

BLOOD PARASITES
Haemobartonella felis (Feline Infectious Anemia)

The rickettsial agent *Haemobartonella felis* causes a disease in cats that may be characterized by fever, anorexia, lethargy, emaciation, splenomegaly, macrocytic normochromic anemia without hemaglobinuria, and occasionally icterus. Cats may carry *H. felis* and be perfectly normal; however, during periods of stress, overt clinical infection may develop. The parasite is seen as coccoid, rodlike, or ringlike bodies on the RBCs in smears stained with Wright's, Giemsa, NMB, or acridine orange. Parasitemic episodes are variable but may last up to a month. Fever is present during parasitemic episodes. Cats become anemic following a parasitemic episode. *Haemobartonella* parasites alter the erythrocyte membrane and produce immune-mediated damage leading to increased RBC fragility and destruction. The anemia produced is characteristically regenerative. Occasionally a nonregenerative anemia characterized by RBC macrocytosis may be observed. The direct Coombs' test can become positive in cats infected with *H. felis*. Parasitized cells become spherical and have a markedly shortened life span. The response to the anemia produced is characteristic of a markedly regenerative anemia.

Transmission can occur by oral, intraperitoneal, and IV inoculation of infective blood. The presence or absence of the spleen has little effect on transmission in cats. *Haemobartonella* organisms can be disseminated by blood-sucking arthropods such as fleas and can be transmitted from female cats to their offspring. Infections can also be transmitted iatrogenically through blood transfusions. The numbers of parasites present in the peripheral blood at any one time can vary greatly; therefore, repeated smears may be needed (3 to 5 consecutive days). In cases of severe infection with *H. felis* and a resultant very low PCV (<20), a whole-blood transfusion can be administered.

Feline infectious anemia *(H. felis)* presents a diagnostic challenge. The absence of the organism from blood smears does not rule out the disease. The true prevalence of the disease is unknown, but estimates are that 4% to 10% of the cat population is infected. A DNA test for feline infectious anemic (FIA) based on polymerase chain reaction (PCR) technology is available. This test allows an immediate, definitive diagnosis or rule-out of FIA.

............*Haemobartonella canis*

The rickettsial agent *Haemobartonella canis* causes a disease in dogs that may be characterized by fever, anorexia, weakness, splenomegaly, macrocytic normochromic anemia, and (rarely) icterus. The infection is usually latent and may be activated by stress or splenectomy. The parasite is seen as coccoid or chainlike forms on the RBCs in smears stained with Wright's, Giemsa, NMB, or acridine orange. The numbers of parasites present in the peripheral blood at any one time can vary greatly; therefore, repeated smears may be needed (3 to 5 consecutive days).

............*Babesia canis*

The hematozoan agent *Babesia canis* causes a disease in dogs that may be characterized by recurrent fever, anorexia, lethargy, splenomegaly, macrocytic normochromic anemia, hemoglobinuria, and variable icterus. Acute babesiosis may produce a shock syndrome. Blood transfusions and other mechanisms of treating hypoxic shock should be instituted (see p. 46). Laboratory findings include hemolytic anemia, thrombocytopenia, bilirubinemia, bilirubinuria, hemoglobinuria, azotemia, and possible development of DIC. An IFA test is available to detect patent or subpatent parasitemia in dogs. The parasite is seen as multiple, basophilic, pear-shaped bodies within the RBCs in smears stained with Wright's, Giemsa, or NMB. The numbers of parasites present in the peripheral blood at any one time can vary greatly; therefore, repeated smears may be needed (3 to 5 consecutive days). Ehrlichiosis and babesiosis may occur simultaneously, and leukocytes should be examined for *Ehrlichia canis* morulas. The brown dog tick, *Rhipicephalus sanguineus*, is the principal vector in the United States. Animals that recover from babesiosis remain carriers.

...........Babesia gibsoni

The protozoan agent *Babesia gibsoni* causes a disease in dogs that may be characterized by recurrent fever, anorexia, lethargy, splenomegaly, macrocytic normochromic anemia, hemoglobinuria, thrombocytopenia, and (very rarely) icterus. The parasite is seen as multiple, basophilic, annular or oval bodies within the RBCs in smears stained with Wright's, Giemsa, or NMB. The parasites are pleomorphic, 1.0 to 2.5 μm in size (one-half the size of *B. canis*). The numbers of parasites present in the peripheral blood at any one time can vary greatly; therefore, repeated smears may be needed (3 to 5 consecutive days). The disease has been reported in California. Affected dogs are thrombocytopenic and have a regenerative anemia with an intermittent fever. The disease can be misdiagnosed as AIHA.

...........Babesia felis (Biliary Fever or Malignant Jaundice)

The protozoan agent *Babesia felis* causes a disease in cats that may be characterized by fever, anorexia, lethargy, macrocytic normochromic anemia, and icterus. The parasite is seen as multiple, basophilic, oval or round bodies within the RBCs in smears stained with Wright's, Giemsa, or NMB. The numbers of parasites present in the peripheral blood at any one time can vary greatly; therefore, repeated smears may be needed (3 to 5 consecutive days).

...........Ehrlichia canis (Canine Ehrlichiosis)

There are three identified *Ehrlichia* species known to cause disease in dogs: *E. canis* (canine ehrlichiosis), which infects mononuclear cells; *E. platys* (canine infectious cyclic thrombocytopenia), which infects platelets; and *E. ewingi* (canine granulocytic ehrlichiosis), which infects neutrophils and rarely eosinophils.

Canine ehrlichiosis appears to be distributed widely throughout the world. The greatest incidence is reported from tropical and subtropical areas, including Vietnam, Thailand, Singapore, and Tunisia. The disease is also prevalent in the southern and southwestern regions of the United States. In dogs, ehrlichia infection is caused by *E. canis*, *E. ewingii*, *E. equi*, *E. platys,* and a species similar to *E. risticii*. Any dog exposed to the infected ticks, *Rhipicephalus sanguineus*, can become infected. Concurrent infection with *Babesia canis* can lead to marked icterus. The *E. canis* organisms are obligate rickettsial parasites and are seen as basophilic, raspberry-shaped bodies. When grouped together in the cytoplasm of WBCs, they are called *morulas*. A strain of *Ehrlichia* that parasitizes neutrophils has also been found and may be similar to *E. equii* in the horse. The *E. canis* organisms persist in infected dogs for at least 29 months and probably for life unless appropriate antibiotic therapy is administered. The vector of *E. canis* is the tick *R. sanguineus*. In the tick, transstadial (larva to nymph to adult) transmission occurs, and the tick transmits the disease only if engorgement develops during the acute phase of the disease. The brown dog tick is the natural reservoir of the organism and can transmit infection and disease to susceptible dogs for at least 155 days after engorgement. Stained blood smears will reveal the morulas of *E. canis* in monocytes. An IFA test is available for serologic diagnosis as well as an ELISA and an immunoblot test.

Serum antibodies to *E. canis* can be detected as early as 7 days after exposure, but some dogs may not become positive for antibodies until 28 days. Paired serum samples are best for confirming the disease. A titer of 1:10 is suspicious and 1:20 or higher is diagnostic. Laboratory results are variable and the cutoff for positive serology may range from 1:10 to 1:80. The presence of antibodies to *E. canis* does not guarantee immunity to the disease. The disease may present in one of three forms:

1. Acute—lymphoid hyperplasia, pyrexia, cytopenias, hemostatic bleeding, splenomegaly, pneumonitis, CNS signs
2. Subclinical—hyperglobulinemia, cytopenia
3. Chronic—lymphoreticular hyperplasia, cytopenias, hyperglobulinemia, hyperplastic splenomegaly, ocular changes

Recently, human infection has been associated with a granulocytic *Ehrlichia* species in the United States. *Ixodes scapularis* ticks are competent vectors for transmission of granulocytic *Ehrlichia*. Ticks are capable of transmitting the organism to a broad range of hosts, including cats, dogs, horses, sheep, goats, rodents, nonhuman primates, and humans.

............*Hepatozoon canis*

The protozoan agent *Hepatozoon canis* causes a disease in cats and dogs. The definitive host for the organism is the brown dog tick *Rhipicephalus sanguineus* and the intermediate host is the dog. Infection with *H. canis* is characterized by cyclic fever, generalized pain and hyperesthesia, muscle atrophy, weakness, depression, emaciation, anemia, mucopurulent ocular discharge, and hepatosplenomegaly. Laboratory findings consist of an increased neutrophil count with a marked left shift. Gametocytes are frequently found in the peripheral blood, especially if the buffy coat is examined. A muscle biopsy may be taken to identify the parasite. The parasites are seen as basophilic, elongate, rectangular bodies with dark, red-purple nuclei and pink cytoplasmic granules within the leukocytes in smears stained with Wright's. Treatment is imidocarb dipropionate (classified as investigational in the United States).

............Infectious Cyclic Thrombocytopenia in the Dog

This disease is caused by a platelet-specific rickettsial organism that is ultrastructurally similar to *Ehrlichia canis* but does not cross-react with *E. canis* serologically. The organism has been tentatively classified as *Ehrlichia platys*. The disease can be transferred from infected to noninfected dogs via blood inoculation and, presumably, is also transmitted by ticks. The geographic distribution of this disease is similar to that of *E. canis*. An IFA test has been developed for detection of serum antibodies to the platelet-specific rickettsial organism that causes this disease.

............*Rickettsia rickettsii* (Rocky Mountain Spotted Fever)

Rocky Mountain spotted fever (RMSF) is a tickborne rickettsial disease; dogs are susceptible hosts. The disease is most prevalent on the East Coast, in the Midwest, and the central Great Plains. Dogs, rabbits, and rodents constitute a mammalian reservoir.

A history of exposure to ticks is present in about 50% to 60% of the cases.

The clinical signs of RMSF are attributible to invasion of endothelial cells of small blood vessels and the vasculitis that results. The vasculopathy may lead to coagulation disorders, edema, and thrombosis. Clinical signs are dependent upon the organ involved. Acute manifestations are characterized by fever, scleral injection, hyperemic mucous membranes, ocular and nasal discharge, coughing, dyspnea, generalized lymphadenopathy, edema, petechial hemorrhages of skin and mucous membranes, hemorrhagic uveitis or retinitis, melena, hematochezia, epistaxis, and hematuria.

Hematologic changes include anemia, thrombocytopenia, and leukopenia proceeding to leukocytosis. Serum chemistries may reveal elevation of ALT and alkaline phosphatase.

Many dogs infected with *Dermacentor andersoni* or *Dermacentor variabilis* develop subclinical rickettsial infections. Epizootiologic studies indicate that titers to RMSF in the dog population range from 4% to 64%, with the highest incidence in working breeds.

Determination of the serum titer of rickettsiae in paired acute and convalescent samples is confirmatory for the diagnosis of RMSF. A fourfold rise in titer is considered diagnostic. IgM titers rise quickly following infection and peak around day 20. IgG titers rise much more slowly and gradually decline over a period of 6 to 9 months.

The latex agglutination test may be a valuable screening test for the diagnosis of RMSF in dogs. Latex agglutination titers greater than 1:16 when used in combination with a test that detects predominantly IgG with either latex agglutination or IgM IFA can identify infected dogs.

Confirmation is by direct immunofluorescence testing for *Rickettsia rickettsii* antigen or serologic and indirect fluorescent antibody tests. Elevations of IgM antibody are seen in acute cases, and elevations of IgG are seen 3 weeks later. Single titers greater than 1:256 in the western United States and greater than 1:1024 in the eastern United States associated with clinical signs is diagnostic for the disease.

REFERENCES

Breitschwerdt EB: Ehrlichiosis: One or many diseases? *In* Proceedings of the 14th Annual Forum of the American College of Veterinary Internal Medicine Forum; San Antonio, 1996, p 608.

Carney HC, England J: Feline hemobartonellosis. Vet Clin North Am Small Anim Pract 23:79–90, 1993.

Comer KM: Rocky Mountain spotted fever. Vet Clin North Am Small Anim Pract 21:27–44, 1991.

Conrad P, Thomford J, Yamane I, et al: Hemolytic anemia caused by *Babesia gibsoni* infection in dogs. J Am Vet Med Assoc 199:601–605, 1991.

Cowell R: Diagnostic Cytology of the Dog and Cat. St Louis, Mosby–Year Book, 1998.

Eng T, Giles R: Ehrlichiosis. J Am Vet Med Assoc 194:497–500, 1989.

Greene CE: Infectious Diseases of the Dog and Cat, ed 2. Philadelphia, WB Saunders, 1998.

Greene CE, Burgdorfer W, Cavagnolo R, et al: Rocky Mountain spotted fever in dogs and its differentiation from canine ehrlichiosis. J Am Vet Med Assoc 186:465–472, 1985.

Greene CE, Marks A, Lappin M, et al: Comparison of latex agglutination, IFA, enzyme immunoassay for the serodiagnosis of RMSF in dogs. Am J Vet Res 54:20, 1993.

Hoskins JD: Tick transmitted diseases. Vet Clin North Am Small Anim Pract 21, 1991.

Johnson NV, Baneth G, Macintire K: Canine hepatozoonosis: Pathophysiology, diagnosis and treatment. Compend Contin Educ Pract Vet, 19:51, 1997.

Kordick D, Lappin M, Breitschwerdt B: Feline rickettsial diseases: *In* Bonagura JD, ed: Kirk's Current Veterinary Therapy XII. Philadelphia, WB Saunders, 1995, p 287.

Meyer D, Harvey J: Veterinary Laboratory Medicine, ed 2. Philadelphia, WB Saunders, 1998.

Sellon R, Breitschwerdt E: Update: Rocky Mountain spotted fever: *In* Bonagura JD, ed: Kirk's Current Veterinary Therapy XII. Philadelphia, WB Saunders, 1995, p 293.

Van Steenhouse JL, Millard J, Taboada J: Feline hemobartonellosis. Compend Contin Educ Pract Vet 15:535, 1993.

Waddle JR, Littmor MP: A retrospective study of 27 cases of naturally occurring canine ehrlichiosis. J Am Anim Hosp Assoc 24:615–620, 1988.

Woody BJ, Hoskins JD: Ehrlichial diseases of dogs. Vet Clin North Am Small Anim Pract 21:75–98, 1991.

...........LYME DISEASE

Lyme disease is caused by a tickborne spirochete, *Borrelia burgdorferi*. The etiologic agent can be transmitted by the nymphal stage of *Ixodes dammini* in the Northeast and Midwest and *Ixodes pacificus* in the West. Whitetail deer *(Odocoileus virginianus)* and the white-footed mouse *(Peromyscus leucopus)* are two of several natural hosts for *I. dammini*. The disease is named after the town in Connecticut where it was first observed. *Ixodes* ticks require three hosts and four different developmental stages to complete their 2-year life cycle. Up to 80% (average of 50%) of the adult ticks in areas endemic for Lyme disease in the northeastern United States may carry *B. burgdorferi*. The proportion of dogs in endemic areas that develop infection is relatively small. Eighty-five percent of reported cases are from northeastern and Mid-Atlantic foci (coastal states from North Carolina to Maine), 10% from midwestern foci, and 4% from western foci (California and Oregon).

The characteristic signs in dogs are fever, inappetence, lethargy, lymphadenopathy, stiffness, pain, intermittent lameness, nonerosive arthritis, and swelling in one or more joints. Antibodies to *B. burgdorferi* have been found in raccoons, whitetail deer, opossums, eastern chipmunks, gray squirrels, white-footed mice, and dogs. An IFA test that can detect titers to *B. burgdorferi* is available, as is an ELISA and a Western blot test. The Diagnostic Laboratory, College of Veterinary Medicine, Cornell University, has developed an ELISA (KELA) that is highly diagnostic in confirming active infection with *Borrelia*. The results of the ELISA have been confirmed with Western blot analysis. Western blot testing has been used to distinguish dogs with titers created by vaccination vs. those with natural infection. More than 50% of dogs in an endemic area may have antibody to *B. burgdorferi*. In serologic samples from endemic areas, IgG samples tested for IFA revealed titers of greater than 1:64 in 53% of dogs. Titers in dogs with clinical illness ranged from 1:256 to 1:16,384. Acute and convalescent titers should be submitted. Synovial specimens from joints infected with *B. burgdorferi* show a microvascular lesion.

REFERENCES

Appel M: Lyme disease in dogs and cats. Compend Contin Educ Pract Vet 12:617–626, 1990.

Greene CE: Infectious Diseases of the Dog and Cat, ed 2. Philadelphia, WB Saunders, 1998.

Greene RT: Canine lyme borreliosis. Vet Clin North Am Small Anim Pract 21:51–64, 1991.

Jacobson R, Chang Yung-Fu, Shin Sang: Lyme disease: Laboratory diagnosis of infected and vaccinated symptomatic dogs. Semin Vet Med Surg 11:172–182, 1996.

Madigan JE: Lyme disease update. Proceedings of the 10th Annual Forum of the American College of Veterinary Internal Medicine, San Diego, 1992, pp 692–695.

Magnarelli LA, Anderson J, Schreier A, et al: Clinical and serologic studies of canine borreliosis. J Am Vet Med Assoc 19:1089–1094, 1987.

IMMUNOLOGIC DISORDERS IN THE DOG AND CAT

Four distinct classes of immunoglobulins have been identified in normal canine serum: IgG, IgA, IgM, and IgE. IgG, IgA, and IgM have also been described in normal feline serum. IgG is the most abundant of the immunoglobulins and is a systemic mediator of numerous systemic infections. IgM is the major immunoglobulin produced in a primary immune response. IgA is the major immunoglobulin found in external secretions of the body and plays an important role in protecting the intestinal, respiratory, and urogenital tracts.

GAMMOPATHIES

Abnormalities in serum immunoglobulins characterized by increased levels are termed *gammopathies*. The basic categories of gammopathies are polyclonal and monoclonal gammopathies.

The monoclonal gammopathies are a group of disorders characterized by proliferation of a single clone of plasma cells, which produce a homogeneous, monoclonal (M) protein. Monoclonal gammopathies are designated by capital letters that correspond to the classes of their heavy chains that are designated by the Greek letters: γ for IgG, α for IgA, μ for IgM, and ϵ for IgE. Subclasses are IgG1, IgG2, IgG3, and IgA1 and IgA2. Myeloma proteins in the dog are usually IgG or IgA. Lymphosarcoma produces proteins of the IgM class.

Initial evaluation of serum for monoclonal gammopathies should be done with electrophoresis on cellulose acetate membrane. Specific identification of an abnormal protein level can be accomplished with immunoelectrophoresis.

Monoclonal gammopathies are characterized by a narrow peak in any of the electrophoretic zones. The abnormal, dense, sharply defined electrophoretic band is composed of a homogeneous monoclonal protein, or M component of paraprotein.

■ DISEASES ASSOCIATED WITH MONOCLONAL GAMMOPATHIES

1. Lymphoproliferative neoplasia: multiple myeloma, macroglobulinemia, lymphoma, leukemia
2. Infectious diseases: canine ehrlichiosis, FIP, FIV
3. Undetermined: myeloma, immune-mediated inflammatory disease

---

Plasma cell dyscrasias are a group of diseases resulting from the uncontrolled proliferation of B lymphocytes, which synthesize abnormal amounts of monoclonal immunoglobulins. Multiple myeloma is the most common form of monoclonal gammopathy seen in veterinary medicine.

Multiple myelomas result in proliferation of monoclonal antibodies other than IgM, plasmacytic cellular infiltration into the bone marrow, Bence Jones proteinuria, and osteolytic lesions seen on radiographic evaluation of the skeletal system (often difficult to locate). Anemia is the most common hematologic abnormality observed. Myelomas with light-chain proteinuria develop in 40% of the cases. Both hyperproteinemia and hypercalcemia can contribute to renal insufficiency. Bence Jones proteins are light-chain proteins (22,000 daltons) that pass through the renal glomerulus and are passed in the urine. These proteins are toxic to renal tubular cells and may be associated with renal failure. These proteins precipitate when heated to 60°C but redissolve as the temperature is raised to 80°C. In cats, plasma cell infiltration of the bone marrow and monoclonal gammopathy may be present in lymphoma and FIP.

Cats reported with monoclonal gammopathy associated with a variety of causes have been FeLV-negative. Monoclonal gammopathy with hyperviscosity syndrome (HVS) may also be associated with *Ehrlichia canis* infection.

Polyclonal gammopathies are characterized by increased production of several immunoglobulin types. This condition usually arises in association with persistent stimulation of the immune system. In the dog, elevation usually occurs in the β region; and in the cat, in the γ region. Abnormalities that can result in polyclonal gammopathies are protracted infections; chronic parasitisms; cirrhosis of the liver; and immunologically mediated diseases such as SLE, RA, thyroiditis, idiopathic hypergammglobulinemia, Aleutian disease of mink, myasthenia gravis, and FIP (Fig. 5–5). In addition to routine evaluation of the serum for abnormal levels of blood proteins, other tests should be performed, including:

1. Evaluation for cryoglobulins. Serum samples should be evaluated at 0°C and incubated at this temperature for 24 hours to detect the presence of a precipitate gel. Dissolution of this precipitate gel at 37°C for 30 minutes indicates the presence of a cryoglobulin.

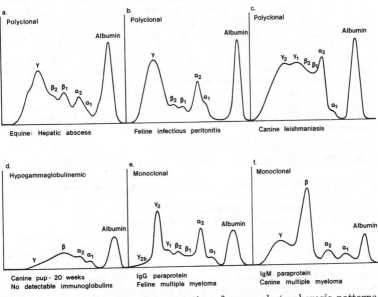

Figure 5–5. Examples of the interpretation of serum electrophoresis patterns on cellulose acetate paper. The proteins are separated by electrophoretic mobility into α, β, and γ regions but cannot be quantitated using this technique. Gross changes in the serum proteins such as polyclonal and monoclonal gammopathies can be identified, as can decreased levels of immunoglobulins. The polyclonal gammopathies are characterized by an elevated level of the proteins in the β and γ region, but no single protein predominates. In monoclonal gammopathy, there is a single sharp peak in either region, which is dependent on the immunoglobulin class involved. In cases in which there is a congenital absence of lowered levels of immunoglobulins, the β region is considerably reduced and the γ region is absent. (From Halliwell REW, Gorman NT: Veterinary Clinical Immunology. Philadelphia, WB Saunders, 1989, p 65.)

2. Evaluation of the urine for abnormal proteins. It is recommended that electrophoresis of the urine be performed. A 24-hour urine sample must be collected for this test.

Major clinical signs associated with monoclonal gammopathies include:

1. Bleeding diathesis, which can often be recognized on retinal examination by hemorrhages and exudative retinal detachments.
2. Hyperviscosity syndrome. Serum viscosity is related to the type, size, shape, and concentration of the abnormal immunoglobulin in the blood. Hyperviscosity is particularly severe in animals suffering from IgM myeloma.
3. Nephrotoxicity caused by proteins in renal tubules.
4. Cryoglobulinemia, which can cause animals to develop gangrenous sloughs of the ear tips, eyelids, digits, and tip of the tail.
5. Hypercalcemia.
6. Skeletal lesions.
7. Infections.
8. Anemia.

Clinical treatment is available for dogs with hyperviscosity syndrome associated with an IgA monoclonal gammopathy resulting from multiple myeloma. The treatment involves continuous plasmapheresis (at least once) to remove abnormal protein constituents, followed by a program of chemotherapy with alkylating agents such as melphalan and cyclophosphamide coupled with systemic prednisolone administration.

·············AUTOIMMUNE HEMOLYTIC ANEMIA

Autoimmune hemolytic anemia is a disease in which the body attempts to destroy its own RBCs. The clinical signs of AIHA are referable to a response anemia that may be acute or chronic. The disease can be seen in dogs of all ages and is more common in females. Antibody may be directed against unaltered RBCs (primary AIHA) or against RBCs that have been antigenically altered by reaction with chemicals or microorganisms (secondary AIHA). Immune-mediated hemolytic anemia is a type II immune reaction. Five immunologic subtypes can produce erythrocyte destruction:

■ CATEGORIES OF IMMUNE-MEDIATED ANEMIA

Subtype	Reaction	Development	Pathophysiology
I	In-saline agglutinins	Peracute	Intravascular hemagglutination
II	Intravenous (IV) hemolysis	Peracute or acute	IgM and IgG with complement and IV agglutination
III	Incomplete agglutination	Acute or chronic	IgG destruction and erythrophagocytosis by mononuclear cells
IV	Cold agglutinins	Chronic	IgM, complete agglutination at low temperature
V	Cold-acting, nonagglutinating	Chronic	IgM erythrophagocytosis; minimal RBC destruction

---

Autoantibodies in AIHA may be of the IgG or IgM class. Most cases of AIHA in dogs and cats are caused by IgG antibodies in combination with complement that react with RBCs at 37°C. IgG does not fix complement efficiently, and acute intravascular hemolysis is not commonly seen. This anemia may coincide with other autoimmune diseases, including SLE, immune-mediated thrombocytopenia, and immune-mediated thyroiditis. Other diseases that have been associated with Coombs'-positive anemia in dogs and cats are lymphosarcoma, hemangiosarcoma, FeLV disease, hemobartonellosis, ehrlichiosis, dirofilariasis, piroplasmosis, leishmaniasis, and glomerulonephritis.

The incidence of immune-mediated hemolytic anemia is highest in Old English sheepdogs, poodles (all varieties), miniature schnauzers, Akitas, beagles, and rottweilers. Increased incidences have been seen in American cocker spaniels, long-haired dachshunds, German shepherds, Irish setters, Shetland sheepdogs, Scottish terriers, and vizslas.

AIHA is seen in cats, and affected animals often have an underlying systemic disease such as FeLV infection, myeloproliferative disease, or *Haemobartonella felis* infection. Cats frequently show autoagglutination of blood, hepatosplenomegaly, and icterus. Cats do not exhibit good spherocytosis, because the RBCs are normally small and dense.

There are several forms of AIHA, with the following characteristics.

In Vivo Hemolysis Animals in this condition are very ill. There is massive destruction of RBCs in the circulation, and both hemoglobinuria and hemoglobinemia can result. In these cases, IgM in combination with complement is the mediating antibody.

Warm Agglutinins Animals in this condition are ill and the prognosis is poor. The blood agglutinates as soon as it is drawn and placed on a slide, regardless of the precautions taken to prevent a drop in temperature.

Incomplete or Nonagglutinating Antibodies This is the most common form of AIHA. The blood cells themselves are not actually destroyed by the allergic reaction, but RBCs coated with antibody tend to be removed by the reticuloendothelial system, particularly the spleen; thus, there is accelerated destruction of RBCs. The onset of the disease is usually gradual.

Cold Agglutinins This form of AIHA is usually mediated by IgM antibodies. In this condition, there is often hemoglobinuria; the blood agglutinates when placed on a slide and allowed to cool. If the slide is heated to 37°C, the agglutination disappears. Skin manifestations involving the extremities arise because of ischemia associated with intravascular agglutination in small blood vessels. Coombs' test results are negative at 37°C but positive at 4°C. The most important mechanism of RBC destruction is removal by the reticuloendothelial system—namely, the spleen.

·············Clinical Signs

Development of clinical signs in AIHA depends on whether the onset is acute or gradual and whether thrombocytopenia is also involved. Acute clinical signs are dependent on sufficient loss of RBC mass with loss of oxygen-carrying ability of blood. Signs include depression, anorexia, pale mucous membranes, splenomegaly, peripheral lymphadenopathy, hemoglobinemia, and icterus. In thrombocytopenia the clinical signs are petechiae of the skin, mucous membranes, and sclera. Thromboembolism and DIC (see p. 45) are complications of AIHA. Dogs with marked reticulocytosis on admission have a significantly lower mortality and dogs with high serum bilirubin levels (>10 mg/dL) have a significantly greater mortality. Absence of reticulocytosis on admission should not be used to rule out AIHA because 20% of cases may exhibit this phenomenon.

·············Laboratory Findings

Laboratory findings include macrocytic, hypochromic, or normochromic anemia; reticulocytosis; spherocytosis; anisocytosis; polychromasia; and leukocytosis with neutrophilia. Spontaneous autoagglutination of RBCs is diagnostic of

AIHA. In the dog, this syndrome may be associated with bone marrow failure and a poor regenerative erythroid response.

.... Coombs' Test (Direct Antiglobulin Test)

Confirmatory diagnosis of AIHA is based on demonstration of a positive reaction in a Coombs' antiglobulin test for the presence of autoantibody on the surface of RBCs or in the serum. Antibodies directed against RBCs can be classified by serologic characteristics into warm autoantibodies, which have maximal activity at 37°C and are usually of the IgG class; and cold autoantibodies, which usually have maximal activity at 2° to 4°C and are of the IgM class. In cats, both IgG and IgM are prevalent.

In immune-mediated hemolytic anemia, the RBCs may be coated with immunoglobulins, immunoglobulins and complement, or complement alone.

In the Coombs' test, a suspension of washed RBCs from the animal (direct test) or of normal homologous RBCs exposed to the animal's serum (indirect test) is allowed to react with species-specific antiglobulin to effect visible agglutination. The direct antiglobulin test demonstrates the presence of autoantibodies on the surface of the RBCs. The indirect test reveals the presence of antibodies in the serum. The indirect Coombs' test is not reliable because of the variability of isoagglutinins present. The direct Coombs' test is usually performed with pooled antisera; however, additional information can be obtained by evaluating agglutination with anti-IgG and anti-C3 (anti-C3 is the most frequent agglutinating agent in dogs). The most common causes of false-negative results in Coombs' test are failure to utilize serial dilutions of the Coombs' antiserum, use of non–species-specific antiserum, and use of antiserum that detects only one class of immunoglobulin. Up to 30% of dogs with presumed AIHA are Coombs'-negative. The most common cause of false-positive results is prior blood transfusion.

For the direct Coombs' test, the blood sample is collected in edetate (EDTA), which prevents in vitro binding of C3 to RBCs.

.... Erythrocyte Osmotic Saline Fragility Test

Spherocytes are less resistant than normal cells, because their spherical shape does not allow for an increase in volume when water enters the cell.

The increased susceptibility of erythrocytes to lysis in hypotonic saline is associated with spherocytosis. The presence of spherocytes associated with AIHA is sufficient to produce gross changes in the saline fragility curve.

.... Clinical Management of Immune-Mediated Hematologic Disease

Dogs with AIHA may also have immune-mediated thyroiditis and hypothyroidism. Evaluation for thyroid function is indicated and treatment with thyroid hormones may be indicated.

Aggressive treatment with corticosteroids is indicated: prednisone or prednisolone 2 mg/kg, q12h for 5 to 7 days, or dexamethasone 0.50 to 0.75 mg/kg, divided q12h for 5 to 7 days. Once response has taken place therapy is reduced by 25% of the original dose each week. Alternate-day steroid therapy may be indicated on a long-term basis.

If more potent and prolonged immunosuppressive immunomodulating therapy is indicated, azathioprine (Imuran) can be used. Azathioprine is administered at 1 mg/lb/day for 7 to 10 days initially, followed by tapering doses.

Immunosuppressive therapy should stabilize the ongoing immune process, and the absolute lymphocyte count should be maintained at one-third the normal range.

In cases where very low PCV is present, blood transfusion will be necessary (see p. 46).

............AUTOIMMUNE THYROIDITIS (LYMPHOCYTIC THYROIDITIS) ((see also p. 639)

Immune-mediated thyroiditis appears to be a common cause of thyroid disease in dogs and results in clinical hypothyroidism. Biopsies of thyroid tissue from dogs with hypothyroidism reveal infiltration of the gland with plasma cells and small lymphocytes.

Experimentally, the disease has been found most frequently in beagles, in which its occurrence may be genetically determined. Antibodies against thyroglobulin, follicular microsomes, and unidentified colloid antigen are usually present. Focal lymphocytic thyroiditis in laboratory beagles is not usually associated with the severe clinical signs and alterations in thyroid function tests observed in pet dogs (see p. 639). Beagles have lower maximal thyroid uptake of ^{131}I and faster loss of ^{131}I than do dogs with mild or no thyroiditis.

............MYASTHENIA GRAVIS

Myasthenia gravis is a disease of neuromuscular transmission associated with a deficiency of acetylcholine receptors (AcHRs) in the neuromuscular postsynaptic membrane. It is an autoimmune disease and autoantibodies to AcHRs are detected in the sera of affected patients.

Myasthenia gravis occurs as both a congenital and an acquired disease in the dog and cat. In congenital myasthenia gravis, there is a deficiency of AcHRs that is not associated with autoantibodies against AcHR sites. Congenital myasthenia gravis is usually recognized at 8 weeks of age and has been described in springer spaniels, Jack Russell terriers, smooth fox terriers, and Siamese cats.

Acquired myasthenia gravis appears to have a bimodal distribution in age of onset, with one group of animals developing problems at 3 years of age and a second group at 10 years of age. Golden retrievers, German shepherds, Labrador retrievers, dachshunds, Akitas, Shetland sheepdogs and cocker spaniels appear to be especially predisposed to the problem. Clinical signs may be focal involving the extraocular muscles, larynx, facial muscles, or esophagus, singly or severally, or the signs may be more generalized, characterized by megaesophagus, facial muscle weakness, pharyngeal muscle weakness, laryngeal muscle weakness, and appendicular muscle weakness. Fulminating myasthenia gravis is characterized by megaesophagus, facial muscle weakness, and pharyngeal muscle weakness. Clinical signs may be characterized by retching, regurgitation, anorexia, megaesophagus, aspiration pneumonia, lack of strength in facial muscles, generalized lack of strength, exercise intolerance, and respiratory difficulty. Routine screening usually shows a normal CBC and blood chemistry results in animals with myasthenia gravis. Ninety percent of dogs with acquired myasthenia gravis have AcHR autoantibodies in their sera.

Myasthenia gravis is also associated with thymomas, which are rare in the dog but reported in middle-aged, mostly female large-breed dogs. Myasthenia has been reported to be present in 18% to 47% of thymoma cases.

Electromyographic findings in patients with myasthenia gravis reveal a decrease in amplitude of action potentials recorded from skeletal muscles during stimulation of motor nerves.

The short-acting anticholinesterase agent edrophonium chloride (Tensilon) is given IV at a dose of 1 to 2 mg to evaluate the response in animals with possible myasthenia. Within 10 to 30 seconds following injection, there should be obvious clinical improvement. If the response test is positive, the dog should respond to anticholinesterase drugs. DO NOT RULE OUT A DIAGNOSIS OF ACQUIRED MYASTHENIA GRAVIS BASED ON A NEGATIVE EDROPHONIUM CHLORIDE TEST because dogs with severe immune-mediated disease may have such low AChR content that acetylcholine will have no effect at neuromuscular junctions. These animals need to be treated with plasmapheresis, intensive immunosuppressive therapy with cortisone, and extensive support therapy, including even positive pressure ventilation.

The prognosis for animals with myasthenia gravis is not grave if megaesophagus is recognized early and severe aspiration pneumonia has not developed; if pharyngeal weakness is not present; and if the dog does not have such a severe form of the disease that marked respiratory and muscle weakness is present.

Feline aquired myasthenia gravis has been observed and may be more commonly seen than reported previously. Cats with focal myasthenia gravis display weakness of esophageal, facial, pharyngeal, and laryngeal muscles. Signs may include difficulty in swallowing, hypersalivation, regurgitation, inability to blink, and dysphonia. Generalized myasthenia gravis includes appendicular muscle weakness, exercise intolerance and weakness, ventroflexion of the neck, dropped jaw, and focal muscle weakness. Diagnosis and treatment are the same as for the dog.

REFERENCES

Bartges JW: Clinical remission following plasmapheresis and corticosteroid treatment in a dog with acquired myasthenia gravis. J Am Vet Med Assoc 196:1276–1278, 1990.

Dewey CW, Bailey CS, Shelton D, et al: Clinical forms of acquired myasthenia gravis in dogs: 25 cases (1988–1995). J Vet Intern Med 11:50–57, 1997.

Ducote JW, Dewey CW, Coates JR: Clinical forms of acquired myasthenia gravis in cats. Compend Contin Educ Pract Vet 21:440, 1999.

Klebanow E: Thymoma and acquired myasthenia gravis in the dog: A case report and review of 13 additional cases. Am Anim Hosp Assoc 28:63, 1992.

Odair HA, Holt E, Pearson GR: Acquired immune mediated myasthenia gravis in a cat with a cystic thymus. J Small Anim Pract 32:198–202, 1991.

Scott-Moncrieff JC, Cook JR Jr, Lantz GC: Acquired myasthenia gravis in a cat with thymoma. J Am Vet Med Assoc 196:1291–1293, 1990.

Shelton D, Schule A, Kass P: Risk factors for acquired myasthenia gravis in dogs: 1,154 cases (1991–1995). J Am Vet Med Assoc 211:1428, 1997.

Shelton DG: Canine myasthenia gravis. In Kirk RW, Bonogura JD, eds: Current Veterinary Therapy XI. Philadelphia, WB Saunders 1992, pp 1039–1042.

Shelton DG: Myasthenia gravis. In Proceedings of the 14th Annual Forum of the American College of Veterinary Internal Medicine, San Antonio, 1996, p 658.

··········· SYSTEMIC LUPUS ERYTHEMATOSUS

5

Systemic lupus erythematosus is a generalized immunologic disorder resulting from a generalized loss of overall control of the specificity of the B cell, possibly associated with abnormal suppressor cell function. Affected dogs (SLE is rarely reported in cats) produce autoantibodies against a wide range of normal organs and tissues, including nucleic acids (DNA).

The disease may be mild or severe in dogs and is associated with the following signs, either individually or in combination:

1. Hemolytic anemia (Coombs'-positive) or thrombocytopenia, or both (PF-3-positive); nonregenerative anemias.
2. Severe polyarthritis characterized by a shifting leg lameness; the arthritis is nonerosive.
3. Glomerulonephritis and proteinuria. Immune complexes with DNA become

deposited in glomeruli and result in a membranous glomerulonephritis. Immune complexes may also be deposited in arterial walls, producing an immune-mediated vasculitis, fibrinoid necrosis, and fibrosis.

4. Skin lesions, usually involving the face and ears (and sometimes mucocutaneous junctions), that are frequently symmetrical. The cutaneous manifestations of SLE are variable and may include discoid lupus erythematosus (LE), macular-papular rashes, vesiculobullous eruptions, mucocutaneous ulceration, alopecia, seborrhea-erythema, panniculitis, vasculitis, secondary pyodermas, lymphedema, and nasal dermatitis.

5. Antimuscle antibodies can lead to myositis; antimyocardial antibodies can lead to myocarditis.

6. Myasthenia gravis.

7. Vasculitis.

8. Leukopenia.

9. Fever of unknown origin, myocarditis, oral ulcers, and polymyositis.

··········· Tests

SLE is a multisystemic autoimmune disease involving blood vessels, kidneys, skin, joints, the hematopoietic system, and the gastrointestinal tract. Immune complexes bind with complement and produce multisystemic inflammatory reactions.

Diagnosis of SLE is based on serologic evidence from the LE test and the ANA test. The LE test is less reliable than the ANA test. Positive results in LE tests have been found in AIHA, RA, lymphosarcoma, leukemia, pulmonary granulomatosis, and warfarin poisoning. In the LE test, nuclear material from fragmenting cells is incubated with leukocytes and serum from patients with SLE. Antinuclear factors, shown to be IgG antibody to native DNA nuclear protein, coat the nuclear material and opsonize it for phagocytosis by polymorphonuclear WBCs. The LE cell is a polymorphonuclear WBC that has ingested nuclear material. Approximately 60% of animals with SLE have a positive LE test on initial examination; therefore, the absence of LE-positive cells does not rule out SLE.

Antinuclear antibody assays are positive in 97% to 100% of dogs with SLE, with titers often higher than 256. Canine SLE is associated with both humoral and cellular immunity disorders. In active SLE there is lymphopenia. Evaluation of lymphocyte subsets indicates an increase in the CD8+ population. The percentage of CD4+ cells increases and the absolute number decreases. The CD4+:CD8+ ratio in dogs with SLE is higher than in control dogs.

■ **IF SYSTEMIC LUPUS ERYTHEMATOSUS IS SUSPECTED THE FOLLOWING ARE INDICATED**

- ■ Radiographs of joints to rule out erosive arthritis
- ■ Joint tap for cytology (see p. 770)
- ■ Direct Coombs' test (see p. 707)
- ■ Antinuclear antibody (ANA) test
- ■ Bone marrow sample if the anemia is nonregenerative (see p. 666)
- ■ Lymph node aspirate (see p. 496)
- ■ Skin biopsy (see p. 492)
- ■ Renal biopsy (see p. 502)

............DISCOID LUPUS ERYTHEMATOSUS (see Dermatologic Examination, p. 364) AND RHEUMATOID ARTHRITIS

Inflammatory joint disease is characterized by inflammation of the synovial membrane and changes in synovial fluid along with signs of systemic illness such as fever, leukocytosis, depression, and increases in fibrinogen and γ-globulins.

Infectious arthritis can be associated with exogenous and endogenous infections. The presence of pus within the joint cavity is characteristic of suppurative arthritis. Nonsuppurative infectious arthritis can be associated with viral organisms, pleuropneumonia-like organisms (PPLOs), and fungal organisms. Infectious arthritis results in thickening of the synovial membrane, distention of the joint capsule, and accumulation of exudate with widening of the joint space. Septic arthritis leads to destruction of the articular cartilage, joint destruction, irregular joint surfaces, periarticular rarefaction, and fibrous bony ankylosis.

In septic or infectious arthritis, the characteristic signs are pain; a warm, tender, swollen joint; and usually associated systemic signs, including fever. Synovial fluid examination is commonly diagnostic. Cellular examination of synovial fluid may indicate a large polymorphonuclear count of 80,000 to 200,000/mm^3.

■ CLASSES OF ARTHROPATHY IN DOGS AND CATS

Erosive Joint Disease	Nonerosive Joint Disease
Rheumatoid arthritis	Systemic lupus erythematosus
Feline progressive polyarthropathy	Immune-mediated inflammation
Greyhound polyarthritis	Infectious arthritis
	Neoplasm
	Drug-induced arthritis

The *noninfectious arthritides* of dogs have been grouped into disease entities that cause erosions on joint surfaces and disease entities that are nonerosive. The erosive arthritides have been seen mainly in the small breeds of dogs, and the changes resemble RA as seen in humans. Dogs with rheumatoid disease have multiple-leg lameness and stiffness of the joints, especially in the morning. There is often generalized joint swelling and pain, intermittent fever, and peripheral lymphadenopathy.

The diagnosis of canine RA (see also p. 346) is based on documentation of at least six of the following nine signs:

1. Morning stiffness
2. Pain and tenderness of one or more joints
3. Soft tissue swelling or effusion in one or more joints
4. Swelling of any other joint
5. Symmetrical onset of joint symptoms and swelling
6. Radiographic evidence of RA
7. Positive test for rheumatoid factor (RF)
8. Poor mucin precipitate of synovial fluid
9. Characteristic changes in the synovium

A canine rheumatoid factor (CRF) test kit is available for in-office use.* The

....

*Canine rheumatoid factor test, Synbiotics.

CRF test kit is of the latex agglutination type. A positive test indicates the presence of RF; however, the presence of RF is not diagnostic, since it is detectable in only about 70% of cases. Another test, the Rose-Waaler test, is performed with rabbit antibody against sheep RBCs.

Newer testing methods for CRF involve ELISAs for IgG, IgM, and IgA, both in the serum and in the joint fluid. Immune complexes, IgG, and IgM have been demonstrated in canine RA. Circulating IgA has been demonstrated in dogs with canine RA and in dogs with arthritis associated with SLE, especially in those having erosive changes in the joints. Only 40% to 75% of canine RA patients have a positive CRF test.

RA in the dog can range, radiographically, from soft tissue changes to marked bone changes involving the joints. Signs may include periarticular rarefaction and the appearance of coarse epiphyseal trabeculae; rarefaction of the subchondral bone plate and cancellous bone of the epiphysis, producing a rough, irregular joint; and, in advanced cases, fibrous ankylosis of joints.

Confirmatory diagnosis is based on immunologic tests, radiography, and cytologic examination of synovial fluid. Cytologic examination of synovial fluid may reveal an increase in nucleated cells, ranging from 3000 to 38,000/mm³, with 20% to 80% mononuclear cells and 20% to 80% neutrophils.

RA is associated with the deposition of immune complexes in the synovia of the joints. Development of autoantibodies to IgG is characteristic of the disease. These autoantibodies are called *rheumatoid factors* and are of the maternal γ-globulin (IgM) class. RFs can also be formed in other conditions in which extensive immune complex formation develops.

Lameness associated with arthritis can be a component in many SLE cases in the dog (see also p. 346). Dogs with SLE exhibit multiple systemic signs, including lethargy, depression, fever, skin lesions, lymphadenopathy, hemolytic anemia, and thrombocytopenia.

A Coombs' test, ANA test, and LE preparation should be carried out as part of the immunologic profile. The ANA test should be strongly positive.

Nonerosive arthritis has been seen with increasing frequency in dogs. The disease appears to be mediated by immunopathologic mechanisms. Joint inflammation usually involves the smaller, distal joints, particularly the carpus and tarsus. Systemic signs of illness may also be present and include cyclic fever, depression, generalized stiffness, and muscle atrophy. During periods of active arthritis, the joints are swollen and hot, fever is present, and leukocytosis is evident. Abnormalities in serum proteins may also be apparent. In most of these cases, no etiologic diagnosis can be established. During acute exacerbations of this disease, swelling and heat in the distal joints, as well as generalized lymphadenopathy, are frequently seen. The results of routinely performed tests for immunologically mediated disease (e.g., LE test, ANA, or RF) are negative.

··········Feline Chronic Progressive Polyarthritis

This proliferative periosteal polyarthritis occurs exclusively in male cats, and the common age of onset is 4.5 years. The disease is characterized by high fever, severe joint pain, stiffness in the carpal and tarsal joints, and regional lymphadenopathy. Radiography shows osteoporosis and periosteal new bone formation, with joint enlargement and ankylosis. Feline syncytia–forming virus (FeSFV) is isolated from all cats with the disease, and FeLV is found in 70% of affected cats. The incidence of FeSFV is two to four times greater in cats with chronic progressive polyarthritis than in the normal feline population, whereas the incidence of FeLV is 6 to 10 times greater than in the normal feline population. The joint disease has been described as being immunologically mediated. Aspiration of joint fluid reveals high numbers of polymorphonuclear neutrophil leukocytes (PMNs) and protein.

·····GLOMERULONEPHRITIS

Immunologic factors contribute to the production of many forms of glomerulonephritis. Two pathogenic mechanisms appear to be operative in the mediation of immunologic glomerular injury. The first is the nephrotoxic or antiglomerular basement membrane type, which produces antibodies capable of reacting with glomerular basement membrane antigens. The second is the immune complex type, which passively traps circulating complexes in the glomerular capillary walls. The antibody involved in this reaction is not directed against glomerular antigens. The antigen may be either endogenous or exogenous in origin. This form of glomerulonephritis has been described in the dog in association with neoplastic, inflammatory, infectious, and autoimmune diseases. Renal lesions associated with dirofilariasis have been described (see p. 754).

In order to detect immune complexes in renal tissue, a needle or wedge biopsy of kidney tissue is required. For the immunofluorescence test, an anti-canine IgG and anti-canine C3 labeled with fluorescein isothiocyanate (FITC) are used to detect immune complexes in the mesangium or on the glomerular basement membrane. Glomerular damage associated with humoral immunologic disease results in a discontinuous granular fluorescent pattern along the glomerular basement membrane when examined with fluorescence microscopy.

·····SKIN DISEASES

Immunologically mediated skin diseases in the dog include the bullous autoimmune abnormalities, including pemphigus vulgaris, pemphigus vegetans, pemphigus foliaceus, pemphigus erythematosus, bullous pemphigoid, discoid LE, and SLE. Antibodies may be directed against intercellular cement substance and the epithelial cell wall or basement membrane zone. Bullous eruption, ulceration, crusting, and scarring characterize these diseases.

Diagnosis is based on skin biopsies that are frozen or stored in Michel's medium and sectioned and examined with immunofluorescence for abnormal location of antibody in the diseased epithelium. However, for all these diseases, a definitive diagnosis must correlate clinical signs, clinical pathology tests, and histopathology with the immunologic tests. Reliance on the latter tests alone may lead to diagnostic errors.

A summary of laboratory diagnosis for immunologic disorders is shown in Table 5–10.

·····PARANEOPLASTIC SYNDROMES (see also p. 169)

Paraneoplastic syndromes refer to the indirect, noninvasive, systemic effect that certain types of tumors can produce in their hosts. The effects are related to the production of abnormal hormones or other protein molecules that affect the metabolism of the host. Paraneoplastic syndromes can be categorized according to the portion of the body that is affected:

1. Hematopoietic syndromes
   a. Leukocytosis—lymphosarcoma
   b. Leukopenia—lymphosarcoma
   c. Thrombocytopenia—lymphosarcoma
   d. Anemias—FeLV; reduced RBC maturation (see p. 662)
   e. Erythrocytosis—renal tumors

Table 5–10. Immunodiagnostic Tests

Test and Sample Requirements	Indications	Method	Disease	Interpretation
Direct Coombs' Test 1 mL whole blood in EDTA; mail on ice; do *not* freeze	Progressive, regenerative, hemolytic anemias; distal extremity dermatoses; anemia with hepatosplenomegaly; *not* a screening test for autoimmune disorders without anemia	Direct hemagglutination for detection of Ig or C3 on patient RBCs incubated with serial dilution of species-specific antisera to IgG, IgM, or C3	Autoimmune hemolytic anemia (AIHA); cold agglutinin disease (distal extremity dermatoses)	Agglutination at one or more serial dilutions of Coombs' antiserum is significant; prior transfusion may cause false-positive results; see text for further details
Indirect Coombs' Test 1 to 2 mL frozen serum; mail on ice	As above	Indirect hemagglutination for detection of circulating autoantibody; dilutions of patient serum are incubated with donor RBC suspension; if no agglutination is observed, a direct Coombs' test is then performed	As above	Titers ≤1:164 are significant; isoantibody to major blood group antigens or prior blood transfusion may give false-positive results; false-negative results can occur if patient RBC autoantigen differs from that represented in donor RBC pool
Antinuclear Antibody (ANA) Test 1 to 2 mL frozen serum; mail on ice	Polysystemic, noninfectious, inflammatory disorders; AIHA; immune-mediated thrombocytopenia; unexplained leukopenia; fever of undetermined origin	Indirect immunofluorescence for detection of circulating ANA, using nuclear substrate and fluorescein-conjugated anti-Ig (species-specific) under fluorescent microscopy	Systemic lupus erythematosus (SLE)	Significant titer levels vary with substrate and laboratory controls: ≥1:20 for mouse liver; ≥1:80 for Vero cell line; ≥1:40 for HeLa cell line

Test / Sample	Indication	Method	Disease	Comments
LE Cell Test 5 to 10 mL whole clotted or heparinized blood; deliver to laboratory within several hours	As above	Sample is processed through wire mesh or agitated with glass beads, stained, and examined for presence of large intracytoplasmic, homogeneous inclusions within PMNs	SLE	Presence of 3 or more LE cells is considered significant; tart cells are sometimes falsely interpreted as LE cells; corticosteroids interfere with the LE cell phenomenon
Platelet Factor 3 (PF-3) Test 3 mL citrated plasma fresh-frozen and mailed (express) on dry ice	Idiopathic thrombocytopenia	Detects antiplatelet antibody in a clotting test system using patient plasma and donor platelets; PF-3 released from antibody-coated platelets results in shortened clotting time compared with controls	Immune-mediated thrombocytopenia (IMT); SLE with thrombocytopenia; Evan's syndrome (AIHA and IMT)	Steroids may interfere; false-positive results can occur owing to platelet activation from improper handling of samples; *use* Vacutainer collection system
Rheumatoid Factor (RF) Test 1 to 2 mL frozen serum; mail on ice	Progressive, erosive, nonseptic polyarthritis	Indirect hemagglutination test; detection of autoantibody (RF) to IgG using rabbit IgG–sensitized sheep RBCs and serial dilutions of patient's serum	Rheumatoid arthritis (RA)	Serum titers $\geq$1:16 are significant; serum RF can be present in other inflammatory disorders; 25%–40% of canine RA cases are RF-negative
Immunoelectrophoresis (IEP) 1 to 3 mL frozen serum; mail on ice	Qualitative screening test for hypoglobulinemia and for monoclonal immunoglobulin class identification	Double immunodiffusion with electrophoresis of patient serum to separate out Ig classes; polyvalent (all classes) or monospecific (single Ig class) antisera can be used (species-specific)	Multiple myeloma; lymphosarcoma (B-cell origin); benign monoclonal gammopathy Waldenström's macroglobulinemia Hypoglobulinemia (all classes) Selective Ig deficiency	Monoclonal precipitin pattern shows restricted electrophoretic band by using dilutions of patient serum compared with control serum Restricted electrophoretic pattern for IgM Decreased or absent precipitin bands for IgG, IgM, and IgA Decreased or absent precipitin band for single Ig class

Table continued on following page

5

Table 5–10. Immunodiagnostic Tests *Continued*

Test and Sample Requirements	Indications	Method	Disease	Interpretation
Immunoglobulin Quantitation 1 to 3 mL frozen serum; mail on ice	Quantitative evaluations for hypoglobulinemia, selective Ig deficiency, and monoclonal hyperglobulinemias	Radial immunodiffusion (RID), rocket immuno-electrophoresis, ELISA, or nephelometry, using species-specific monovalent antiserum	As above	Quantitative excess or deficiency of single or multiple Ig classes
Tissue-Fixed Ig/C3 Skin, kidney, or other organ biopsies fixed in Michel's preservative (2-wk limit for processing) or snap-frozen in liquid nitrogen and mailed express on dry ice	Vesiculobullous skin disorders; protein-losing glomerulonephropathy; detection of immune complex vasculitis	Direct immunofluorescence using fluorescein-labeled antisera (species-specific)	SLE	Ig or C3 deposits at cutaneous dermoepidermal junction; granular Ig or C3 deposits along glomerular basement membrane
			Immune-complex glomerulonephritis	Same as for lupus nephritis
			Pemphigus var.	Intercellular Ig deposits
			Bullous pemphigoid	Linear Ig or C3 deposits along dermoepidermal junction
			Pemphigus erythematosus	Ig or C3 deposits consistent with both lupus and pemphigus
			Immune-complex vasculitis	Ig or C3 deposits in vessel walls

PMNs, polymorphonuclear neutrophils; ELISA, enzyme-linked immunosorbent assay.
From Gorman NT, Werner LL: Diagnosis of immune-mediated diseases and interpretation of immunologic tests. *In* Kirk RW, ed: Current Veterinary Therapy IX. Philadelphia, WB Saunders, 1986, p 432.

2. Excessive production of serum proteins—gammopathies (see also p. 703) and hyperviscosity syndromes
   a. Multiple myeloma tumors (see also p. 704)
   b. Lymphoproliferative diseases
3. Ectopic hormone production
   a. Pituitary adenomas—ACTH
   b. PTH-like hormone-producing hypercalcemia—lymphosarcoma, leukemia, thyroid adenocarcinoma, parathyroid tumors, multiple myeloma, mammary adenocarcinoma, perianal adenocarcinoma
4. Hypoglycemia—associated with lymphosarcoma (see also p. 144)
5. Mast cell tumors—histamine, heparin, serotonin
6. Non–beta cell tumors of pancreas
   a. Production of gastrin leading to Zollinger-Ellison syndrome
7. Metastatic and primary lung tumors, spirocerosis, rhabdomyosarcoma of the bladder, and carcinoma of the liver
   a. Can produce hypertrophic pulmonary osteoarthropathy
8. Hyperestrogenism—Sertoli cell tumors

REFERENCES

Bell SC, Carter SD, May C, et al: IgA and IgM rheumatoid factors in canine rheumatoid arthritis. J Small Anim Pract 34:259–264, 1993.

Bennett D, Taylor DJ: Bacterial infective arthritis in the dog. J Small Anim Pract 20:207–230, 1988.

Chabanne L, Monier JC, Fournel C, et al: Canine systemic lupus erythematosus. Part I. Clinical and biologic aspects. Compend Contin Educ Pract Vet 21:135, 1999.

Chabanne L, Monier JC, Fournel C, et al: Canine systemic lupus erythematosus. Part II. Diagnosis and treatment. Compend Contin Educ Pract Vet 21:402, 1999.

Codner EC: Infectious polyarthritis of the dog and cat. In Kirk RW, Bonagura JD, eds: Current Veterinary Therapy XI. Philadelphia, WB Saunders, 1992.

Cotter SM: Autoimmune hemolytic anemia in dogs. Compend Contin Educ Pract Vet 14:53, 1992.

Dorfman M, Dimski D: Paraproteinemias in small animal medicine. Compend Contin Educ Pract Vet 14:621, 1992.

Gorman NT, Werner LL: Diagnosis of immune-mediated diseases and interpretation of immunologic tests. In Kirk RW, ed: Current Veterinary Therapy IX. Philadelphia, WB Saunders, 1986, p 427.

Halliwell RE, Gorman NT: Autoimmune and other immune-mediated diseases. In Halliwell RE: Veterinary Clinical Immunology. Philadelphia, WB Saunders, 1989.

Hopkins AL: Canine myasthenia gravis. J Small Anim Pract 33:477–484, 1992.

Hopper PE: Immune-mediated nonerosive arthritis in the dog. In Kirk RW, ed: Current Veterinary Therapy X. Philadelphia, WB Saunders, 1989.

Joseph RJ, Carrillo JM, Lennor VA: Myasthenia gravis in the cat. J Vet Intern Med 2:75–79, 1988.

Klag AR, Giger U, Shofer FS: Idiopathic immune mediated hemolytic anemia in dogs: 42 cases. J Am Vet Med Assoc 202:783–788, 1993.

Klein MK, Dow SW, Rosychuk RAW: Pulmonary thromboembolism associated with immune-mediated hemolytic anemia in dogs. J Am Vet Med Assoc 195:2426–250, 1989.

Luttgen PJ: Disorders of the neuromuscular junction and muscle. Semin Vet Med Surg 4:104–146, 1989.

Meric SM: Disorders of the joints. In Nelson RW, Couto GC, eds: Essentials of Small Animal Internal Medicine. St Louis, Mosby–Year Book, 1992, pp 820–830.

Meyer D, Harvey J: Veterinary Laboratory Medicine, ed 2. Philadelphia, WB Saunders, 1998.

Shelton GD, Cardinet GH, Bandman E: Canine masticatory muscle disorders: A study of 29 cases. Muscle Nerve 10:753–766, 1987.

Stewart AF, Feldman B: Immune-mediated hemolytic anemia. Compend Contin Educ Pract Vet 15:372–381, 1993.

Weisser MG: Diagnosis of immunohemolytic disease. Semin Vet Med Surg 17:311–314, 1992.

....

CLINICAL CHEMISTRY

The measurement of various constituents of the blood is an invaluable aid in establishing a diagnosis and in determining the prognosis and course of a clinical disease. Several facts should be remembered when the use of blood chemistry tests is contemplated.

1. Blood chemistry tests are important only when combined with an adequate history and physical examination.
2. Blood chemistry tests should not be used indiscriminately. Selected tests should be used to evaluate a differential diagnosis or confirm a diagnosis.
3. The clinician must realize the limitations of the test being used and must be able to interpret the results of the test.
4. The clinician must be familiar with reference laboratory values used at a particular commercial laboratory. In general, reference values include 95% of all values obtained from normal animals. The other 5% of normal animals will have values that fall outside the reference interval in the third SD above or below the mean. The larger the number of tests run on a serum sample, the greater the chance that a normal animal will have at least one abnormal test result. *Do not base a clinical diagnosis on one abnormal test result!*
5. The reference range of a test is the range of values that includes the central 95% of values from the representative group of disease-free animals. The limits of this range are usually given by 2 SD above and below the arithmetic mean if the data fit a gaussian distribution. Thus, when the test is applied to animals with a disease, the results can fall into four different categories: abnormal, false abnormal, true normal, and false normal.
6. The specificity of a test is the percentage of nondiseased animals whose results are normal. The specificity indicates the ability of the test to detect nondiseased animals. The sensitivity of a test is the percentage of diseased animals whose results are abnormal. The sensitivity indicates the ability of the test to detect diseased animals. There is an inverse relationship between sensitivity and specificity of a test. The predictive value of a test is how well it performs in a given population.

...........SERUM PROTEINS

For total plasma protein measured by refractometer submit an EDTA blood tube greater than half-full and ship in a cold pack. For the protein panel submit 1 ml separated serum or heparinized plasma. Ship in an ice pack. For protein electrophoresis submit 1 to 2 mL serum in a plain plastic or glass tube. Send in an ice pack.

The liver produces all the albumin and most of the globulins; a small amount of γ-globulin is produced by reticuloendothelial tissue (see p. 703 for information about globulins and the albumin-globulin ratio).

Fibrinogen, albumin, and globulins constitute the major proteins of the blood plasma. In determining serum proteins, serum or plasma must be free of hemolysis. Fibrinogen is removed in coagulation; therefore, fibrinogen cannot be determined in serum samples.

In general, plasma protein levels are low in young animals (usually <5 g/dL of plasma). Older animals may have total plasma proteins in the range of 7 to 8 g/dL.

Determination of plasma protein levels may be important when:

1. The nutritive state of the animal is being assessed
2. Kidney and liver functions are being evaluated

3. The role of the reticuloendothelial system in a clinical situation is being assessed
4. Fluid balance in states of shock, dehydration, and hemorrhage is being determined

The albumin fraction exerts the greatest effect on the total volume of plasma protein. Decreases in albumin levels usually result in lowered total plasma volume. A decrease in total serum albumin may be the result of a lowered protein intake resulting from malnutrition, which may be diet-related or associated with malabsorption; deficient synthesis of albumin by the liver associated with chronic hepatic disease (see p. 734); excessive protein breakdown, which may occur with prolonged fever, diabetes mellitus, postsurgical conditions, and trauma; or excessive loss of protein, which may occur with acute nephritis, nephrosis, burns, parasitism, ascites, and hemorrhage associated with damaged vessels and tissue.

The concentration of proteins in the blood determines the colloidal osmotic pressure of the plasma. Lipemic plasma, cloudy plasma, or hemolysis will affect the total serum protein determinations. The concentration of protein in the plasma can be influenced by the nutritional state of the animal, hepatic function (see p. 741), renal function, blood loss, dehydration, various diseases, and metabolic abnormalities. Various individual fractions of the plasma proteins may be helpful in diagnosing certain diseases. These plasma protein fractions may be separated by plasma electrophoresis.

Disorders that cause hypoproteinemia can be associated with diminished production of proteins or increased loss of proteins. Diminished production of proteins (specifically, hypoalbuminemia) can be associated with primary or secondary intestinal malabsorption, exocrine pancreatic insufficiency, malnutrition, parasitism, and liver disease. Increased loss of proteins resulting in hypoalbuminemia could be associated with renal disease (specifically, glomerular disease), protein-losing enteropathies, severe exudative skin diseases, and chronic blood loss. Sequestration of plasma proteins can be associated with ascites or pleural effusion or may be found in vasculopathies, including ehrlichiosis.

Hyperproteinemia can occur in dehydration, shock, administration of quantities of concentrated amino acids, certain neoplasms, and infections. Plasma fibrinogen levels have been used in the interpretation of the response and severity of certain diseases in small animals. The normal range of fibrinogen is 200 to 400 mg/dL of plasma. The total ratio of plasma protein (PP) to fibrinogen (F) is variable, depending on the age of the animal. In general, a PP/F ratio of less than 15:1 indicates an increase in fibrinogen over plasma protein. A ratio below 10:1 indicates a marked increase in fibrinogen. Fibrinogen is a soluble plasma protein produced in the microsomes of hepatic parenchymal cells and stored in the liver. The half-life of canine fibrinogen is 2.3 to 2.7 days. The normal range of fibrinogen levels is 200 to 400 mg/dL in the dog and cat.

Increased fibrinogen levels are associated with inflammation (both acute and chronic) and tissue destruction. Decreased fibrinogen levels can be associated with clotted blood samples, liver disease, DIC, fibrinous exudation into serous cavities, shock, and nutritional disorders.

·············BLOOD AMMONIA

Ammonia is normally absorbed from the lower intestinal tract, removed via the portal circulation, transported to the liver, and converted to urea. Ammonia is normally converted to urea in the liver by the urea cycle. Abnormalities in blood ammonia levels can be seen in hepatoencephalopathic patients. The most common of these conditions is congenital portacaval shunt; however, acquired diseases such as cirrhosis, toxic hepatopathy, and hepatic neoplasia can also lead to this condition. The availability of pre- and postprandial bile acid testing generally precludes the need to perform blood ammonia tests.

In animals with congenital portal vein anomalies, ammonium biurate crystals may be found in the urine in approximately one third of the cases, and fasting venous blood ammonia levels are usually greater than 120 μg/dL. An ammonia tolerance test can be done in the dog. The animal must be fasted for 12 hours. Blood samples should be collected in ammonium-free heparin and placed in ice when held for analysis. Separate the plasma within 30 minutes after sampling by centrifugation of the chilled sample. Administer 0.1 g of NH₄Cl per kilogram of body weight PO following a fast. A maximum of 3 g is administered in 20 to 50 mL of warm water. Samples are collected at 30 minutes, and the results are compared with control values. Values are dependent on the testing procedure being used; thus, paired samples should be run using control samples from a normal dog. (Normal values are usually 19 to 120 μg/dL. Levels above 300 μg/dL are abnormal.) Levels should be compared with those of controls; abnormal levels may be 5- to 10-fold greater than baseline levels.

Blood ammonia levels for the cat following the PO administration of 100 mg/kg ammonium chloride have been reported to be 0.26 to 0.53 mg/dL; normal fasting blood ammonia levels are 0.1 to 0.35 mg/dL.

...........SERUM AMYLASE

In normal animals, a small amount of serum amylase from the pancreas and salivary glands is present in the blood. Inflammation of the pancreas may release abnormal amounts of this enzyme into the blood. Conditions such as renal insufficiency, corticosteroid elevations, and factors that increase the production of pituitary and adrenal glands could also elevate serum amylase levels. Hyperamylasemia associated with renal failure is due in part to the impaired clearance of amylase by glomerular filtration. Primary renal failure is usually associated with an azotemia, impaired ability to concentrate or dilute urine (specific gravity = 1.007 to 1.024), and moderate to severe hyperamylasemia (two to three times normal). In dogs, acute pancreatitis is associated with marked hyperamylasemia, which may be up to seven times normal; occasional prerenal azotemia; and ability of the kidneys to concentrate urine to a specific gravity greater than 1.025.

Normal values for serum amylase levels in dogs are as follows: modified Caraway units (amyloclastic), under 1000; Harding units (amyloclastic), under 3200; Gomori (amyloclastic), 0 to 800; DyAmyl (saccharogenic), under 3200; international units per liter, 185 to 700; and Somogyi units, 100 to 400.

...........PLASMA BICARBONATE (CO_2, TOTAL) (see also p. 591)

Submit 1 mL separated serum or heparinized plasma. Ship in an ice pack.

The bicarbonate–carbonic acid buffer is one of the most important buffer systems in maintaining the normal pH of the body fluid. Normally, these constituents are present in a ratio of 1 part carbonic acid to 20 parts bicarbonate.

Serum bicarbonate is elevated in metabolic alkalosis as occurs with prolonged vomiting or in respiratory acidosis due to hypoventilation. Serum bicarbonate is reduced in metabolic acidosis in conditions such as diabetic ketosis, persistent diarrhea, renal insufficiency, shock, or respiratory alkalosis due to hyperventilation.

............**CARBON DIOXIDE** (see also p. 591)

Serum contains bicarbonate, physically dissolved carbon dioxide, (proportional to the partial pressure of CO_2 [PCO_2]), and carbonic acid. At normal blood pH, the ratio of HCO_3^- to dissolved CO_2 and H_2CO_3 is 20:1. In assessing acid-base status reliably, measurement of arterial blood pH or PCO_2 and total CO_2 is desirable. When the value of any two of these three variables is known, a nomogram can be used to calculate the other.

Practical office evaluation of acid-base abnormalities often depends on the availability of CO_2 determination interpreted along with clinical findings. When one measures the CO_2 content of blood that has been exposed to the air, the total CO_2 that is measured is almost exclusively HCO_3^-. The development of rapid, inexpensive office screening procedures for CO_2 determination makes this a practical test. A low CO_2 level may indicate either metabolic acidosis or respiratory alkalosis, and a high CO_2 level may indicate metabolic alkalosis or respiratory acidosis.

............**SERUM BILIRUBIN** (see p. 734),

BLOOD UREA NITROGEN–SERUM UREA NITROGEN

Submit 1 mL separated serum or heparinized plasma. Send in an ice pack.
Ammonium oxalate or "double oxalate" cannot be used as an anticoagulant if this test is to be performed, because the ammonia will be measured as urea.

Urea, an end product of protein metabolism, is excreted by the kidneys. Forty percent or more of this urea is reabsorbed by the kidney tubules. Thus, blood urea levels are one indication of kidney function and can serve as a rough index of glomerular filtration rate (GFR). The BUN varies directly with protein intake and inversely with the rate of excretion of urea. Nonrenal variables may cause variable increases in urea nitrogen levels:

1. Ingestion and absorption of large quantities of protein
2. Absorption of protein from gastrointestinal hemorrhage
3. Catabolic states in fever, infection, or trauma
4. Administration of catabolic drugs such as glucorticoids or thyroid hormones

The BUN may be elevated in renal insufficiency (acute or chronic); increased nitrogen retention associated with diminished renal blood flow or impaired renal function, as may occur in dehydration and shock; adrenal insufficiency and congestive heart failure; and postrenal obstruction preventing normal urination, as may occur with urethral calculi.

Repeated BUN tests are usually indicated to follow the progress of the animal. An elevation of BUN will not become evident until 70% to 75% or more of the nephrons of both kidneys become nonfunctional.

Azotemia is the presence of abnormally high concentrations of urea, creatinine, and other nonprotein nitrogenous substances in the blood.

............**CREATININE** (see also p. 772)

Creatinine is derived from creatine and phosphocreatine during muscle metabolism and is excreted by way of the glomerulus of the kidney, with a small amount secreted by the proximal tubules. Blood creatinine levels are not affected by dietary protein, protein catabolism, age, sex, or exercise. Excretion is almost entirely dependent on the process of glomerular filtration. Creatinine clearance can be used as a measure of the GFR. Estimation of the degree of reduction of glomerular filtration from the concentration of creatinine in plasma has a basis because there is a steady-state relationship between the GFR and the concentration of creatinine in the plasma. For every 50% reduction in GFR, the creatinine concentration should double. The normal plasma creatinine concentration is 0.5 to 1.0 mg/dL. Assays of 24-hour endogenous urine creatinine are more reliable in evaluating GFR but are more difficult to do. Serial determinations of creatinine should be used when determining the prognosis in renal disease. The significance of an elevated creatinine can be determined only after analyzing other renal function tests. A high creatinine level that persists despite appropriate therapy justifies a guarded prognosis.

............URIC ACID
BLOOD CALCIUM (see also p. 146)

Blood calcium levels should be obtained on fasting serum or heparinized samples. The normal range of blood calcium for the dog is 9 to 11 mg/dL. Calcium is necessary for the normal function of muscle contraction, transmission of nerve impulses, blood coagulation, neuromuscular excitability, and cell membrane permeability. The main store of body calcium is in the bones. Serum calcium exists in two forms: (1) an inactive form that is combined with a serum protein fraction (mainly albumin), and (2) an active form (ionized) that is not combined with a protein. When total serum calcium is measured in the laboratory, the measurement includes ionized calcium, chelated calcium, and protein-bound calcium.

Approximately 50% of the measured total plasma calcium is bound to serum proteins. A number of factors may alter the distribution of calcium in plasma, including hypoalbuminemia, acid-base status, and the presence of abnormal calcium-binding proteins (as may be present in myelomas). Hyperproteinemia can increase the measured calcium, and hypoproteinemia can decrease the measured calcium.

Changes in serum calcium relative to blood albumin levels can be estimated using the following formula (this formula should not be used with dogs 6 to 24 weeks old or with cats):

$$\text{Corrected Ca (mg/dL)} = \text{Ca (mg/dL)} - \text{albumin (g/dL)} + 3.5.$$

The correction formula based on total serum protein is:

$$\text{Corrected Ca (mg/dL)} = \text{Ca (mg/dL)} - (0.4 \times \text{total protein [g/dL]}) + 3.3.$$

There are several clinical situations in which serum calcium levels should be determined, including bone disorders, convulsions, parathyroid abnormalities, renal insufficiency, malabsorption syndromes, pseudohyperparathyroidism, and vitamin D intoxication. Various forms of neoplasia in the dog have been associated with hypercalcemia, including lymphosarcoma, multiple myeloma, mammary gland adenocarcinoma, fibrosarcoma, perianal gland adenoma, apocrine cell adenocarcinoma of the anal sac, perirectal adenocarcinoma, and abdominal adenocarcinoma. Of these, lymphosarcoma is the most common tumor associated with calcium abnormalities (see p. 924). The incidence of hypercalcemia in dogs with lymphosarcoma ranges from 10% to 40%. The anterior mediastinal form of lymphosarcoma is commonly associated with high calcium levels. Cats with lymphosarcoma rarely demonstrate hypercalcemia.

Several factors can alter the ionized (active) serum calcium levels:

1. Alkalosis lowers ionized calcium levels, whereas acidosis may increase ionized calcium levels.
2. Vitamin D levels influence serum calcium levels. Deficiencies of vitamin D may lead to low blood calcium levels. Large excesses of vitamin D cause

high levels of serum calcium and may result in dystrophic calcification. Ingestion of the houseplant day-blooming jasmine *(Cestrum diurnum)* can produce vitamin D intoxication.

3. The parathyroid glands, by producing parathormone, can greatly influence serum calcium levels. Parathormone controls calcium mobilization from the bones and renal excretion of phosphorus, thus controlling the calcium-phosphorus (C/P) ratio.

4. The C/P ratio in the diet can also affect serum calcium levels.

The advent of assays for PTH, ionized calcium, and 1,25-dihydroxyvitamin D_3 have made the diagnostic approach to animals with abnormalities in calcium homeostasis a simpler process. Most of the differentials involved in abnormalities in calcium homeostasis can be ruled out with a good history, physical examination, and routine laboratory workup, including a CBC and blood chemistry.

Increased serum calcium levels are seen in primary hyperparathyroidism. Primary hyperparathyroidism is very rare, is usually caused by a functioning adenoma of the parathyroid gland, and has been reported in dogs (see also p. 639).

Secondary hyperparathyroidism may result from a poor C/P ratio in the diet or from renal insufficiency. The normal C/P ratio in the diet is 1.2:1. Excessively high phosphorus levels, as seen in cats on all-red-meat diets, lead to hyperparathyroidism and mobilization of calcium from the bones. Secondary hyperparathyroidism in renal insufficiency is associated with retention of phosphorus, leading to hyperphosphatemia and hypocalcemia, which stimulate the production of PTH. It is important to remember that in secondary hyperparathyroidism, the serum calcium levels may be normal, decreased, or elevated, depending on the stage of the disease.

Thus, repeated serum calcium, phosphorus, and alkaline phosphatase determinations are needed to assess the condition of an animal with secondary hyperparathyroidism.

Other causes of high serum calcium may be primary hyperparathyroidism (tumor, hyperplasia), pseudohyperparathyroidism, tertiary hyperparathyroidism, overzealous oral or parenteral calcium supplementation, poisonings with vitamin D–containing rodenticides, the recovery phase of acute renal failure, drug-induced (thiazides, spironolactone), adrenocortical insufficiency, hyperthyroidism and hypothyroidism, hypophosphatasia, generalized periostitis, immobilization, use of calcium ion-exchange resins in hemodialysis, and sarcoidosis.

■ CAUSES OF HYPERCALCEMIA IN THE DOG

Laboratory error
Primary hyperparathyroidism
Hypercalcemia of malignancy
  Anal sac adenocarcinoma
  Multiple myeloma
  Bone tumors
  Other nonbone tumors (lymphosarcoma)
Chronic renal failure
Hypoadrenocorticism
Young animals
Hypervitaminosis D
Rodenticide intoxication (see p. 184)
Granulomatous pulmonary disease (blastomycosis)

■ CAUSES OF HYPERCALCEMIA IN THE CAT

Lymphosarcoma
Vitamin D–containing rodenticides
Myeloproliferative diseases
Chronic renal failure
Squamous cell carcinoma
Primary hyperparathyroidism

Signs of hypocalcemia are usually observed once calcium levels fall to below 6.0 to 6.5 mg/dL. Decreased levels of blood calcium can be seen in hypoparathyroidism, azotemia, hypoalbuminemia, starvation, eclampsia, rickets, vitamin D deficiency, and malabsorption syndromes. Excessive dietary calcium produces hypercalcitonism, either by increasing plasma calcium with direct stimulation of the thyroid C cells, or indirectly, via stimulation of gastrin production by the G cells, mainly in the distal pylorus of the stomach. The ultimate results of excessive dietary calcium in balanced proportion to phosphorus are hypocalcemia, hypophosphatemia, and hypophosphatasemia. Hypoalbuminemia is the most common condition associated with hypocalcemia. Hypoalbuminemia involves a reduction in the level of protein-bound calcium, although ionized calcium may remain normal.

Other causes of lowered serum calcium include hypoparathyroidism (surgical, idiopathic), eclampsia, intoxications (ethylene glycol), reduction in serum albumin (malabsorption, short-bowel syndrome, chronic liver disease, nephrotic syndrome, malnutrition), pancreatitis, renal disease (acute and chronic renal tubular dysfunction, renal tubular acidosis), adrenal corticosteroid excess, commercial phosphate-containing enemas (when used in small dogs and cats, these enemas can produce hypocalcemia, because phosphate is absorbed through the colonic wall), increased skeletal avidity due to osteoblastic metastases, infusion of chelating agents, hyperphosphatemia (renal failure, phosphate infusions), rickets and osteomalacia, magnesium deficiency, glucagon administration, mithramycin administration, pseudohypoparathyroidism, medullary carcinoma of the thyroid, and calcitonin-secreting tumors.

■ CAUSES OF HYPOCALCEMIA IN THE DOG

Laboratory error
Primary hypoparathyroidism
Hypoalbuminemia
Chronic renal failure
Acute renal failure (ethylene glycol poisoning)
Puerperal tetany (eclampsia)
Hypomagnesemia
Pseudohypoparathyroidism
Vitamin D deficiency
Intestinal malabsorption diseases
Medications: EDTA, citrate
Phosphate-containing enemas

In the cat, bilateral thyroidectomy for the treatment of feline hyperthyroidism is the most common cause of symptomatic hypocalcemia in the cat.

·········· CREATINE KINASE

The enzyme creatine kinase (CK) splits creatine phosphate in the presence of adenosine diphosphate (ADP) to yield creatine and adenosine triphosphate (ATP). This enzyme is most abundant in mammalian skeletal muscle, heart muscle, and nervous tissue. Variations in CK values can be related to sex, age, and physical activity. Values are elevated in the presence of muscle damage that could result from trauma, infarction, muscular dystrophies, or inflammation. Elevated CK values can also be observed following IM injections of irritating substances, and this factor should be considered in measurement of this enzyme. Elevated CK values do not reveal the underlying muscle disorder. Muscle diseases may be associated with abnormalities of the muscle fiber itself or with neurogenic diseases that result in secondary damage to muscle fibers. Greatly increased CK values are usually associated with myogenic disease.

·········· SERUM PHOSPHORUS (INORGANIC PHOSPHORUS) (see also p. 143)

Phosphorus is the major intracellular anion. Phosphorus is 80% to 85% bound as organic hydroxyapatite in bone and 15% to 20% is found in soft tissue and muscle. Normal phosphorus values may be variable in the dog, depending on age and diet. Young, rapidly growing dogs of large breeds have phosphorus levels of 8.0 to 9.0 mg/dL. Mature dogs have phosphorus values that range from 2.5 to 6.1 mg/dL; cats have values that vary from 3.5 to 7.1 mg/dL.

The level of inorganic phosphorus in the plasma can be influenced by the parathyroid glands, intestinal absorption, renal function, bone metabolism, nutrition, and levels of ionized serum calcium.

Hyperphosphatemia can occur in renal failure with phosphorus retention (when the GFR decreases to <20% of normal, hyperphosphatemia develops), hypoparathyroidism with excessive tubular reabsorption of phosphorus in the absence of adequate levels of PTH, and excessive vitamin D intake associated with phosphate enemas and hemolysis. The most common reason for abnormally elevated phosphate levels is renal failure (see p. 122).

Box continued on following page

■ HYPERPHOSPHATEMIA *(Continued)*

Decreased renal excretion
    Acute or chronic renal failure
    Uroabdomen, urethral obstruction
    Hypoparathyroidism
    Hyperthyroidism
Maldistribution
    Hemolysis
    Tumor cell lysis
    Metabolic acidosis

Hypophosphatemia can occur with inadequate intake of phosphorus, in primary hyperparathyroidism due to the elimination of large amounts of phosphorus in the urine, and after insulin administration. Diabetes mellitus may be associated with hypophosphatemia because of osmotic diuresis and abnormal tubular reabsorption of phosphorus. Deficiency states of phosphorus can be divided into mild (serum phosphorus = 2.5–3.3 mg/dL), moderate (serum phosphorus = 1.0–2.5 mg/dL), and severe (serum phosphorus <1.0 mg/dL). It is estimated that 2% of cats receiving hyperalimentation after being malnourished or dehydrated may develop hypophosphatemia.

Hypophosphatemia can develop when a severely catabolic state is rapidly corrected with movement of phosphorus from blood into cells. Examples are in *diabetic ketoacidosis,* severe burns, and starvation. Phosphate is the major intracellular anion. The clinical features of hypophosphatemia are:

- Detrimental effect on RBCs, granulocytes, and platelets; reduction in RBCs, ATP, and 2,3-diphosphoglycerate (DPG). Severe RBC abnormalities occur when the phosphorus level falls to 1.0 mg/dL.

- Impaired chemotaxis by leukocytes.

- Hemolytic anemia, thrombocytopenia, impaired clot retraction, hemolysis in cats with diabetic ketoacidosis.

- Muscle weakness and pain associated with rhabdomyolysis; anorexia, nausea, vomiting associated with ileus.

■ HYPOPHOSPHATEMIA

Reduced renal reabsorption
    Primary hyperparathyroidism
    Renal tubular disorders
    Proximally acting diuretics (carbonic anhydrase inhibitors)
    Eclampsia
    Hyperadrenocorticism
Maldistribution
    Carbohydrate load, insulin administration
    Treatment of diabetic ketoacidosis
    Respiratory alkalosis, hyperventilation
    Hypothermia
Reduced intestinal absorption
    Vomiting
    Malabsorption
    Phosphate binders administered orally
    Vitamin D deficiency

··········MAGNESIUM METABOLISM

Magnesium is an essential dietary element for animals. Magnesium is an intracellular cation and functions as an activator or catalyst for over 300 enzymes in the body, including phosphates and enzymes that involve ATP. Magnesium balance is primarily controlled by ingestion through the gastrointestinal tract and excretion by the kidney.

Serum magnesium concentrations may range from 1.5 to 5.0 mg/dL, being variable with the species being evaluated. Magnesium is 20% protein-bound and the remaining 80% is free ion or bound to phosphate, citrate, or other compounds. The magnesium status of an animal is difficult to evaluate because plasma magnesium represents less than 1% of total body magnesium.

Critically ill animals may have a higher incidence of hypomagnesemia. The causes of this may include anorexia, receiving long-term fluid therapy, excess gastrointestinal loss, redistribution of magnesium intracellularly (as may occur with insulin or glucose administration or with amino acid administration), and tissue sequestration of magnesium. Some drugs may also increase magnesium loss through the kidneys and may include diuretics such as furosemide, thiazides and mannitol, cardiac glycosides, and aminoglycosides.

Manifestations of hypomagnesemia are nonspecific and often due to concurrent hypokalemia or hypocalcemia or both. Signs may include muscle weakness, dyspnea, muscle twitching, seizures, and alterations in mentation. Hypomagnesemia can lead to refractory hypokalemia. Electrolyte abnormalities, including hypokalemia, hypophosphatemia, hyponatremia, and hypocalcemia, may be accompanied by hypomagnesemia. Mild hypomagnesemia may resolve with treatment of the underlying disease, modified IV fluid therapy, and correction of hypophosphatemia. Supplementation is suggested if magnesium levels are lower than 1 mg/dL (normal range, 1.7 to 2.4 mg/dL).

Both sulfate (8.13 mEq Mg/g) and chloride (9.25 mEq Mg/g) salts are available in 50% solutions. The IV route is preferred. The IV dose is 0.75 to 1.0 mEq/kg/day administered by continuous-rate infusion in D5W. A lower dose (0.3 to 0.5m Eq/kg/day) may be used for an additional 3 to 5 days.

··········SERUM SODIUM AND CHLORIDE (see also p. 585)

Submit 1 mL separated serum or heparinized plasma.

Chloride is the principal inorganic anion of the extracellular fluid and is important in the maintenance of acid-base balance. When chloride in the form of hydrochloric acid or ammonium chloride is lost, alkalosis follows; when chloride is retained or ingested, acidosis follows. Abnormalities in serum chloride levels are uncommon but, when found, may be associated with metabolic acidosis, as seen in diarrhea, chronic draining fistulas, renal tubular acidosis, and administration of ammonium chloride.

Sodium and chloride ions are the greatest part of the osmotically active solute in the plasma and can greatly influence the distribution of water. A shift of sodium ions into cells or a loss of sodium from the body produces a decrease in extracellular fluid that greatly affects circulation, renal function, and the nervous system.

Increases in sodium (hypernatremia) may occur in dehydration or a primary water deficit, hyperadrenocorticism, and CNS trauma or disease. Hyponatremia may be associated with redistribution of body water, overhydration, or factitious changes.

Decreased serum sodium levels can be seen in adrenal insufficiency, inadequate sodium intake, renal insufficiency, physiologic response to burns or trauma, losses from the gastrointestinal tract (as in diarrhea or intestinal obstruction), water intoxication, and uncontrolled diabetes mellitus. The osmolality of the plasma should be determined (see p. 142). In pseudohyponatremia, the plasma sodium is low but the plasma osmolality is normal. This condition may be observed in hyperlipidemia and hyperproteinemia. Hyponatremic patients with volume depletion have lost fluid by renal and nonrenal routes, including the gastrointestinal tract, third space, and skin. Renal loss of sodium can be observed in hypoadrenocorticism, in chronic renal disease, and with diuretic administration. Hypernatremia with hypervolemia can be seen in congestive heart failure, severe liver disease, and nephrotic syndrome.

Metabolic acidosis with evidence of increased anion gap is usually associated with hyperchloremia. Hyperchloremia can be associated with hemoconcentration, hyperchloremic metabolic acidosis, or chronic respiratory alkalosis.

Most cases of hyperchloremic metabolic acidosis are associated with dehydration, loss of sodium bicarbonate or conjugate base from the extracellular space, and increased renal tubular resorption of chloride.

One unusual and interesting disease observed in dogs with hyperchloremia is renal tubular acidosis. Two forms have been described. In proximal renal tubular acidosis (type 2), there is abnormal tubular resorption of HCO_3^- and loss of HCO_3^- in the urine, with retention of chloride. Glycosuria, aminoaciduria, and phosphaturia may also be present. The combination of these syndromes in the dog has been described as a "Fanconi-like" syndrome and is seen in the Basenji breed.

Distal renal tubular acidosis is associated with inability of the distal renal tubules and collecting ducts to secrete hydrogen ions against a pH gradient. Metabolic acidosis develops with retention of chloride and sodium. The urine pH becomes elevated in relationship to blood pH. Confirmation of this problem is based on the ability of the kidneys to excrete an acid load such as ammonium chloride.

Elevated serum chloride levels can be seen in renal insufficiency following administration of ammonium chloride, chronic pyelonephritis, dehydration, overtreatment with saline solution, congestion and edema associated with cirrhosis of the liver, and carbon dioxide deficit (as occurs in hyperventilation). Clinical manifestations are polyuria (PU) or polydipsia (PD), anorexia, weight loss, weakness associated with loss of potassium, acidosis, and progressive renal failure.

Decreased serum chloride levels can be seen in gastrointestinal disease (producing vomiting and diarrhea), renal insufficiency with salt deprivation, overtreatment with certain diuretics, diabetic acidosis, adrenal insufficiency, and hypoventilation (as occurs in pneumonia, emphysema, and pulmonary edema), resulting in respiratory acidosis.

............SERUM POTASSIUM (see also p. 588)

Potassium is the major cation of intracellular fluid. The concentration of potassium in the extracellular fluid normally varies over a narrow range from 3.9 to 5.6 mEq/L in the dog and 4.0 to 4.5 mEq/L in the cat. Cells are highly permeable to K^+ ions, which move passively and freely in and out of the cell. Numerous mechanisms are responsible for regulation of potassium levels: (1) ingestion in the diet, (2) sodium pump (renal), (3) arterial pH, (4) insulin levels, and (5) cell breakdown.

............Hypokalemia

Abnormalities associated with abnormal decreases in potassium can produce metabolic, neuromuscular, cardiovascular, and renal changes:

1. Hypokalemia produces glucose intolerance; release of insulin is impaired.
2. Neuromuscular–skeletal muscle weakness: impaired smooth muscle function.

3. Inability to concentrate urine, resulting in nocturia, PU or PD.
4. Abnormal repolarization of cardiac cell membranes—depression of the S-T segment, prolongation of the Q–T interval, slow heart rate.

Hypokalemia may develop in cats with chronic renal disease where there is metabolic acidosis. Hypokalemia may also develop in cats fed a potassium-deficient diet plus a urinary acidifier, which can lead to significant declines in GFR. When potassium supplementation needs to be administered to cats, oral potassium gluconate 2 to 6 mEq per cat per day and not potassium chloride should be administered.

Hypokalemia (Table 5–11) can result from excessive loss of potassium associated with protracted vomiting or diarrhea. Alkalosis results in the migration of K^+ ions from the extracellular to intracellular fluid and increased urinary loss of potassium. Urinary loss of potassium occurs by secretion in the distal tubules. Excessive potassium loss occurs in hyperadrenocorticism and renal tubular acidosis. Hypokalemia may be evident following the administration of K^+-depleting diuretics. Hypokalemia can also be seen in ketoacidotic diabetes following the administration of insulin, which causes K^+ ions to enter the cell (see p. 118). Administration of fluids low in potassium can result in hypokalemia; lactated Ringer's solution contains only 4 mEq of potassium per liter (see p. 600).

·········· Hyperkalemia

Hyperkalemia (see Table 5–11) is often associated with impaired renal excretion of potassium. Potassium excretion is largely accomplished by tubular secretion, not by glomerular filtration; therefore, hyperkalemia does not occur until late in the course of renal disease, with marked alteration in glomerular filtration and existing uremia. Urethral obstruction, especially in cats, is often associated with elevated serum potassium levels (see p. 122). Clinically significant hyperkalemia occurs when serum potassium exceeds 7.0 to 7.5 mEq/L. Hyperkalemia has also been reported with potassium chloride administration in cats.

The major cardiovascular effects of hyperkalemia are reviewed on p. 61.

Table 5–11. Causes of Hypokalemia and Hyperkalemia

Hypokalemia	Hyperkalemia
Normal Body Potassium Content (Redistribution of Potassium)	*Normal Body Potassium Content (Redistribution of Potassium)*
Insulin excess	Acidosis
Alkalosis, metabolic or respiratory	Insulin deficiency
Aldosterone release	Tissue necrosis
Catecholamine release	Drugs: digitalis, succinylcholine, β-adrenergic blockers
Low Body Potassium Content	
Decreased potassium intake (anorexia and dietary deficiency)	*Increased Body Potassium Content*
Urinary loss: diuretics, primary aldosteronism	Decreased renal excretion
Gastrointestinal loss: vomiting, diarrhea	Toxin-induced acute renal failure
Cutaneous loss: burns	Defects in renin-angiotensin-aldosterone renal axis
Renal potassium wasting in cats	Volume depletion
Intrinsic renal disease	Hypoadrenocorticism

5

Metabolic acidosis contributes to the development of severe hyperkalemia, as does adrenal insufficiency.

············Feline Hypokalemic Polymyopathy–Nephropathy Syndrome

In hypokalemic cats the most common disease is chronic renal disease. Other disease states that may predispose to hypokalemia are diabetes mellitus, systemic infectious disease, feline urologic syndrome (FUS), and hepatic disease. Signs associated with hypokalemia in cats are appendicular muscular weakness, persistent ventroflexion of the neck, a stiff stilted gait and reluctance to walk, and pain on muscle palpation. Serum biochemical abnormalities found in cats with kaliopenic polymyopathy include hypokalemia, metabolic acidosis with or without respiratory compensation, normal anion gap, azotemia, increased serum CK activity, and hyperkaliuria. Chronic dietary acidification in cats can lead to negative imbalance of potassium in adult cats associated with increased urinary and fecal loss of potassium.

············BLOOD GLUCOSE (see also p. 645)

Blood glucose levels are usually determined after a 12-hour fast. Serum is the sample of choice; however, plasma is acceptable. Sodium fluoride is the anticoagulant to use when only the glucose concentration is desired.

The glucose level in the blood is maintained within relatively narrow physiologic limits. Several factors control blood glucose levels, including hepatic gluconeogenesis and glycogenolysis, renal excretion and reabsorption, removal of glucose by the tissues, effects of hormonal processes on tissue metabolism, and intestinal absorption of glucose.

Elevated blood glucose levels (hyperglycemia) can occur in diabetes mellitus, hyperthyroidism, hyperadrenocorticism, hyperpituitarism, anoxia (because of the instability of liver glycogen in oxygen deficiency), production of epinephrine, certain physiologic conditions (digestion, exposure to cold, following general anesthesia), administration of glucose-containing fluids, and acute pancreatic necrosis.

Decreased blood glucose levels (hypoglycemia) may occur in hyperinsulation due to a tumor of the pancreas (islet cell adenoma) or an overdose of exogenous insulin; following severe excretion, starvation, adrenal insufficiency, hypopituitarism, and hepatic insufficiency; as well as in a functional hypoglycemic von Gierke's–like syndrome. Transient hypoglycemia is also reported in working sport breeds and toy breeds.

············Serum Fructosamine

The term *fructosamine* refers to albumin and other plasma proteins that have been linked to sugar by a nonenzymatic chemical reaction via a process known as glycation. Serum fructosamine concentration is proportional to the blood glucose concentration over the life span of the protein being measured (serum albumin in cats has a life span of 1 to 2 weeks). In clinically normal cats, the serum fructosamine concentration ranged from 172 to 410 μmol/L with a median of 252 μmol/L. In cats with transitory stress-induced hyperglycemia, the fructosamine concentration ranged from 154 to 504 μmol/L with a median of 269 μmol/L. No significant difference in fructosamine concentration was noted in normal cats vs. cats with stress-induced hyperglycemia. In cats with untreated diabetes mellitus the median fructosamine concentration was 624 μmol/L which is significantly higher than the value in normal cats or cats with stress hyperglycemia. Serum fructosamine values can be used to differentiate cats with true diabetes mellitus from those with transient stress-induced hyperglycemia.

··········· SERUM TRANSAMINASES (see also p. 735)

Aspartate aminotransferase (AST; formerly SGOT) is found in high levels in the liver, myocardium, and skeletal muscles. Alanine aminotransferase (ALT; formerly SGPT) is found in large concentrations in the liver of the dog and cat. Destruction of liver cells can release these enzymes, resulting in an increase in their concentration in the plasma. Half-lives of ALT in normal dogs average 2.5 hours. Persistently high levels of ALT suggest the presence of a hepatocellular necrosis.

Increased ALT in the dog and cat is usually specific for hepatic necrosis. Values of ALT of 10 to 50 Sigma-Frankel units are considered normal; values of 50 to 400 Sigma-Frankel units indicate moderate liver necrosis; and severe necrosis is indicated by values of more than 400 Sigma-Frankel units.

The simultaneous use of bromsulphalein (BSP) and ALT is of value in differentiating between advanced fibrosis and liver necrosis. In fibrosis, the BSP excretion is decreased and the ALT activity is normal, whereas in necrosis, the reverse situation usually occurs.

The AST activity is not specific for liver necrosis. Pathologic conditions involving the cardiac or skeletal muscles that produce necrosis will also elevate the activity of AST.

Cats with cholestatic liver disease may show signs of lethargy, weakness, vomiting, anorexia, diarrhea, weight loss, jaundice, pyrexia, bleeding disorders, and ascites. Elevation of alkaline phosphatase (ALP) in the cat is not an accurate indication of cholestatic disease (see p. 736). A much better indication is the ALT activity, and elevations in serum bile acids and total cholesterol and a marked elevation in liver copper content are seen in long-present cholestasis.

··········· ALKALINE PHOSPHATASE (see also p. 735)

Serum ALP activity is a summation of the activities of different isoenzymes derived from different body tissues. ALP is present in high concentration in bone, intestinal mucosa, renal cortex, placenta, and bile. The ALP in serum consists of a mixture of isoenzymes that can be separated by electrophoresis. Significant increases in ALP activity can be observed in both intrahepatic cholestasis and extrahepatic bile duct obstruction. High levels of serum ALP are not usually observed in the cat, even with hepatobiliary obstruction. The half-life of hepatic-derived ALP in the cat is 5.8 hours. This enzyme is rapidly cleared from the blood.

Increased ALP activity in clinical cases is associated with liver or bone abnormalities; the serum half-life of these isoenzymes is 3 days.

Serum ALP may be increased in bone diseases, in osteoblastic and osteoclastic changes such as secondary hyperparathyroidism, in obstruction of bile ducts, in certain bone tumors such as osteogenic sarcomas, and in hyperadrenocorticism. Phenobarbital is a potent activator of ALP. In dogs, neoplasms, including adrenocortical adenosarcomas, mixed mammary tumors, and hepatic hemangiosarcomas, may increase serum ALP levels.

Biliary obstruction results in the most dramatic increases in serum ALP levels. The obstruction is not usually a complete extrahepatic obstruction but rather is intrahepatic, associated with swelling of hepatocytes and bile stasis. Alkaline phosphatase is membrane-bound and is produced by epithelial cells forming bile canaliculi. In biliary obstruction these cells proliferate and enzyme activity increases. Serum ALP activity is also increased with steroid-induced hepatopathy, either iatrogenic or associated with Cushing's disease.

..........SERUM LIPIDS (CHOLESTEROL, TRIGLYCERIDES)

Serum lipids in the dog consist of cholesterol, both free and esterified; triglycerides, phospholipids; and unesterified (free) fatty acids.

Triglycerides are the main form in which lipids are stored and are the predominant type of dietary lipid. Variability in triglyceride level depends on the diet of the animal. Animals should be fasted for 12 hours before blood samples are taken for lipid analysis. Normal fasting triglyceride levels range from 30 to 150 mg/dL in the dog and cat, with mean values of about 60 mg/dL.

Cholesterol is a precursor of bile salts and endogenous steroids as a part of cell wall membranes. Total cholesterol levels range from 80 to 280 mg/dL in the dog and 50 to 180 mg/dL in the cat.

Four major classes of endogenous lipoproteins have been characterized in the dog and cat: (1) chylomicrons, (2) very-low-density lipoprotein (VLDL), (3) low-density lipoprotein (LDL), and (4) high-density lipoprotein (HDL).

Hyperlipidemia refers to an abnormally high concentration of triglycerides or cholesterol, or both, in the blood. Lipemic serum (i.e., cloudy or turbid serum) is the result of hypertriglyceridemia. Lipemia becomes grossly detectable as triglyceridemia increases beyond 300 to 400 mg/dL. Elevations of cholesterol cannot be determined by visual inspection of serum or plasma. The hyperlipidemic states can be categorized as primary hyperlipidemias and secondary hyperlipidemias. The primary hyperlipidemias are inherited disorders of lipid metabolism and have not been well characterized in the dog or cat. Primary hyperlipoproteinemia appears to occur in miniature schnauzers and some cats. An unusually large number of miniature schnauzers have lipemia that persists despite a 12-hour or longer fast. Lipid abnormalities may be evident on ocular examination characterized by lipemia retinalis and lipids in the anterior chamber fluid. This idiopathic hyperlipidemia of miniature schnauzers is thought to be hereditary. The major increase is hypertriglyceridemia with chylomicrons predominating. Serum cholesterol is usually normal to moderately elevated. Some miniature schnauzers may exhibit systemic signs with hypertriglyceridemia. The systemic signs resemble pancreatitis and are characterized by recurrent episodes of abdominal pain, vomiting, and pancreatitis. Triglycerides can be elevated to extreme levels even in fasting animals.

Secondary hyperlipidemias are commonly found in dogs and are associated with pancreatitis, diabetes mellitus, hypothyroidism, nephrotic syndrome, glucocorticosteroid administration, and a variety of liver abnormalities. When an animal presents with hyperlipidemia, it is important to evaluate the dietary status. A complete physical examination, including clinical pathologic study, should be performed to evaluate the possible role of systemic diseases.

..........SERUM LIPASE

Submit 1 mL separated serum or heparinized plasma with an ice pack.

Lipase determinations are made on serum samples. Lipase is excreted by the kidneys, and the presence of oliguria or anuria can result in increased levels of serum lipase. Normal values of serum lipase in the dog are Sigma-Tietz units, 0 to 1; Ree-Byler units, 0.8 to 12; and international units, 13 to 200.

Normally, a low concentration of this fat-splitting enzyme is present in the blood. In acute pancreatitis, pancreatic lipase is released into the circulation in elevated amounts. *It has been found that the canine stomach secretes lipase, and elevations of serum lipase can reflect gastroenteritis rather than acute pancreatitis.*

···········SERUM LACTATE DEHYDROGENASE

Lactate dehydrogenase (LDH) catalyzes the reaction:

$$\text{Lactate } + \text{ NAD} \leftrightarrow \text{pyruvate } + \text{ NADH } + \text{ H}^+.$$

This enzyme is found in body tissues that use glucose for energy.

Assay of total serum LDH, because of the ubiquitous origins of the enzyme and consequent difficulties in interpretation of altered levels, has not been widely used as a diagnostic test in veterinary medicine. Analysis of LDH isoenzymes provides more specific diagnostic information. In normal canine serum, five isoenzymes of LDH are demonstrable, with $LDH_1 > LDH_3 > LDH_4 > LDH_2 > LDH_5$. This distribution may be altered following damage to tissues. The nature of the alteration provides a more accurate indication of the organs involved than does assay of total serum LDH. Sources of LDH isoenzyme fractions are LDH_1 and LDH_2—heart, erythrocytes, kidney, and brain; LDH_3—lung, pancreas, adrenals, spleen, thymus, and thyroid; LDH_4 and LDH_5—skeletal muscle and liver.

Analysis of LDH isoenzymes provides a reliable and fairly specific contribution to the diagnosis of active myocardial damage in the dog. There is a rapid rise and fall in the activity of LDH_1 and LDH_2 following experimentally induced myocardial damage in the dog. Increased activity of these isoenzymes in serum provides supportive evidence of recent or continuing myocardial damage. Conversely, the absence of elevated activity of these isoenzymes suggests that myocardial damage is not the cause of the problem, is no longer occurring, or is proceeding at such a low level that it is not reflected in the serum.

Because of the abundance of LDH (LDH_1 and LDH_2) in erythrocytes, samples for analysis should be free of hemolysis; otherwise, pronounced alterations in LDH activity are observed.

Increases in activity of both total LDH and LDH isoenzymes have also been observed in dogs with neoplasia. The isoenzyme patterns observed in these cases vary, but the major increases have been observed in the isoenzymes of intermediate and slow electrophoretic mobility. With liver disease and skeletal damage, assay of LDH isoenzymes does not appear to offer any advantage over the more commonly assayed enzymes.

REFERENCES

Armstrong PJ, Ford RB: Hyperlipidemia. *In* Kirk RW, ed: Current Veterinary Therapy X. Philadelphia, WB Saunders, 1989, pp 1046–1050.

Bruyette D: Disorders of calcium metabolism. *In* Proceedings of the 10th Annual Forum of the American College of Veterinary Internal Medicine Forum. San Diego, 1992, pp 161–164.

Carriere F, Raphel V, Moreau H: Gastric lipase: Stimulation of its secretion in vivo and cytolocalization in mucous pit cells. Gastroenterology 102:1535–1545, 1992.

Crenshaw K, Peterson M, Heeb L, et al: Serum fructosamine concentration as an index of glycemia in cats with diabetes mellitus and stress hyperglycemia. J Vet Intern Med 10:360–364, 1996.

Dhein CR, Wardrop KJ: Hyperkalemia associated with potassium chloride administration in a cat. J Am Vet Med Assoc 206:1565–1566, 1995.

Dhupa N: Magnesium therapy. *In* Bonagura JD, ed: Kirk's Current Veterinary Therapy XII. Philadelphia, WB Saunders, 1995, p 132.

DiBartola, S: Fluid Therapy in Small Animal Practice. Philadelphia, WB Saunders, 1993.

DiBartola SP, Rutgers HC, Zack PM, et al: Clinicopathologic findings associated with chronic renal disease in cats: 74 cases (1973–1984). J Am Vet Med Assoc 190:1196, 1987.

Dow SW, Fettman MJ, Curtis CR, et al: Hypokalemia in cats 136 cases. J Am Vet Med Assoc 194:1604, 1989.

5

Fettman MJ: Feline kaliopenic polymyopathy/nephropathy syndrome. Vet Clin North Am Small Anim Pract 19(3):415, 1989.

Jones BR: Inherited hyperchylomicronemia in the cat. J Small Anim Pract 34:493–499, 1993.

Justin R, Hohenhaus A: Hypophosphatemia associated with enteral alimentation in cats. J Vet Intern Med 9:228–233, 1995.

Lumsden JH, Jacobs RM: Clinical chemistry. Vet Clin North Am Small Anim Pract 19:875–898, 1989.

Martin L, Van Pelt D, Wingfield W: Magnesium and the critically ill patient. *In* Kirk RW, ed: Current Veterinary Therapy I, Philadelphia, WB Saunders, 1995, p 128.

Meyer D, Harvey J: Veterinary Laboratory Medicine, ed 2. Philadelphia, WB Saunders, 1998.

Murtaugh RJ, ed: Clinical pathology. Semin Vet Med Surg 7(4):1992.

Phillips S, Polzin D: Clinical disorders of potassium homeostasis: Hyperkalemia and hypokalemia. Vet Clin North Am Small Anim Pract 28:545, 1998.

Reimers TJ, Lamb SV, Bartells S, et al: Effects of hemolysis and storage in quantification of hormones in blood samples from dogs, cattle and horses. Am J Vet Res 52:1075, 1991.

Rosol T, Capen CT: Pathophysiology of calcium, phosphorus and magnesium metabolism in animals. Vet Clin North Am Small Anim Pract 6:1155, 1996.

Waters CB, Moncrieff S, Catherine R: Hypocalcemia in cats. Compend Contin Educ Pract Vet 14:497, 1992.

Watson TDG, Barrie J: Lipoprotein metabolism and hyperlipidemia in the dog and cat: A review. J Small Anim Pract 34:479–487, 1993.

Whitney MS: Evaluation of hyperlipidemia in dogs and cats. Semin Vet Med Surg 7:292–308, 1992.

Willard MD, Tvedten H, Turnwald GH, eds: Small Animal Clinical Diagnosis by Laboratory Methods. Philadelphia, WB Saunders, 1989.

....

EVALUATION OF LIVER FUNCTION

The liver is of central importance to many different biologic processes. It influences carbohydrate, protein, and fat metabolism; it is important in the homeostasis of the coagulation and fibrinolytic systems; and it influences the balance of and response to many hormones. The liver is an important storage depot for blood, certain vitamins, lipids, glycogen, and iron. The liver is also an important site for protein synthesis, ammonia detoxification, and bilirubin elimination and can undergo extramedullary hematopoiesis when the need arises. In addition, the hepatobiliary system contains a major arm of the reticuloendothelial system (RES) that serves to protect the body from infectious agents and toxic substances. Because of the large size and tremendous regenerative capability of the liver, early detection of functional impairment may be difficult.

CLINICAL SIGNS IN HEPATOBILIARY DISEASE

General, Nonspecific	Specific
Anorexia	Abdominal enlargement
Depression	Jaundice, hyperbilirubinuria
Lethargy	Acholic feces
Weight loss	Coagulopathy
Nausea, vomiting	Polyuria, polydipsia
Diarrhea	Metabolic encephalopathy
Dehydration	

■ CHANGES IN LIVER SIZE

Generalized Hepatomegaly

Infiltration associated with neoplasia, chronic hepatitis complex, cholangiohepatitis, extramedullary hematopoiesis, amyloidosis
Passive congestion associated with right heart failure, pericardial disease, caudal vena cava obstruction
Hepatocellular hypertrophy associated with idiopathic or secondary lipidosis, hyper-adrenocorticism, anticonvulsant drug therapy

Focal or Symmetrical Enlargement

Primary or metastatic neoplasia
Nodular hyperplasia
Chronic hepatic disease with fibrosis

Generalized Microhepatica

Congenital portosystemic shunts
Chronic liver disease with liver atrophy
Hypovolemia, Addison's disease

■ FOUR GROUPS OF TESTS USED TO EVALUATE THE LIVER:

Tests indicative of hepatocellular leakage: serum alanine transaminase, aspartate transaminase, dehydrogenase, alkaline phosphatase, γ-glutamyltransferase
Tests related to hepatic uptake, conjugation, and secretion: bilirubin and bile acids
Tests related to portal clearance (bile acids, ammonia)
Tests related to hepatic synthesis (albumin, glucose, BUN, coagulation factors)

···········LIVER ENZYME ACTIVITY

Although liver enzymes are sensitive indicators of hepatobiliary disorders, they lack specificity and provide no evidence of the sufficiency of hepatic function. The extent to which enzyme leakage occurs depends on the severity and number of cells damaged. Elevated enzyme levels do not indicate the reversibility of liver disease or the functional state of the liver. Enzymes should be used as screening tests in association with concentrations of total bilirubin, albumin, glucose, urea, and cholesterol, and consideration of the hemogram and urinalysis. Severe chronic hepatic failure may be associated with normal serum enzyme activity as a result of a paucity of surviving hepatocytes. Minor liver disorders and drug-induced enzyme activity can be associated with marked increases in certain enzymes.

Increased serum activity of alkaline phosphatase (ALP), γ-glutamyltransferase (GGT), alanine aminotransferase (ALT), and aspartate aminotransferase (AST) may result from reversible or irreversible changes in hepatocellular membranes associated with necrosis, cholestasis, hypoxia, hypoperfusion, inflammation, infectious agents, and toxins or from excessive stores of hepatocyte lipid, copper, or glycogen. In the dog, enzyme induction is common and can result in profound increases in serum enzyme activities. In the cat, hyperthyroidism is commonly associated with increased liver enzymes, especially ALP. Careful palpation of the thyroid should therefore be done and the baseline thyroxine (T_4) level should be evaluated in middle-aged to old cats with increased liver enzyme activity.

In some cases, the pattern of abnormal enzyme activity suggests a specific abnormality. The ALT is considered a liver-specific enzyme in the dog and cat, although it is present in limited concentrations in other tissues. AST is also present in substantial concentrations in muscle, so increases in AST without concurrent increases in ALT should be carefully scrutinized. Because ALT and AST are located in the hepatocellular cytosol, they can be elaborated rapidly when membrane permeability changes. AST is largely associated with mitochondria. When AST activity is markedly increased, a more serious cellular injury should be suspected rather than a transient change in membrane permeability. Both ALP and GGT are membrane-associated enzymes. Enzyme induction occurs before marked increases in the serum are realized. These enzymes are associated with pericanalicular areas, biliary structures, and the endoplasmic reticulum. Smaller increases in serum ALP activity develop in the cat than in the dog. Nevertheless, this enzyme is an important indicator of liver disease in the cat. The use of ALP in the cat is improved by concurrent consideration of GGT. In the cat, GGT seems to be a more sensitive indicator of liver disease than ALP, although ALP appears to be more specific. Arginase can be used in the recognition of acute hepatic necrosis and as a prognostic indicator. Used in conjunction with the transaminases, arginase activity can reflect the likelihood of continued hepatocellular injury. Large quantities of arginase are immediately released at the time of acute injury, along with the transaminases. If the injurious situation is rectified, arginase activity will decline over several days, whereas the transaminase activity will persist for several weeks.

Extrahepatic bile duct occlusion is typically associated with huge increases in ALP and GGT activities, severe hyperbilirubinemia, and moderate increases in transaminase activity. Acute parenchymal inflammation or necrosis is associated with huge increases in AST and ALT activities. Following necrosis or inflammation, it takes several days for marked changes in the ALP and GGT activities in serum to be realized. Drug-associated enzyme induction (anticonvulsants, glucocorticoids) in the dog is usually characterized by remarkable increases in ALP with lesser changes in GGT, ALT, and AST. Most hepatic disorders in the cat are associated with greater increases in GGT than in ALP. The exception is hepatic lipidosis in cats, in which ALP activity is markedly increased in comparison with GGT. Animals with congenital portosystemic shunts may have normal, mildly increased, or moderately increased liver enzyme activities. Since this disorder is often recognized before 9 months of age, increased ALP activity is presumably due to bone growth. Dogs with portosystemic shunts that have been treated with anticonvulsants to control neurologic signs develop drug-induced enzyme activity.

···········SERUM BILIRUBIN

The major bilirubin pigment is derived from hemoprotein (hemoglobin) released from senescent RBCs. Other sources include hepatic hemoproteins (cytochrome P-450, peroxidase, and catalase) and overproduction of heme in bone marrow. Released hemoglobin is transported bound to haptoglobin, which restricts it to the vascular compartment. In the RES, hemoglobin is enzymatically degraded to yield biliverdin under the influence of heme oxygenase, and then biliverdin is degraded to unconjugated bilirubin under the influence of biliverdin reductase. Unconjugated bilirubin (UB) is insoluble in water and is circulated avidly bound to albumin, which restricts it from urinary excretion. At the hepatocyte surface, albumin facilitates the hepatic uptake of UB, and the UB binds to a cytosolic storage protein, ligandin, prior to the conjugation reactions. Conjugated bilirubin (CB) is soluble in water and is excreted in bile. The CB is transported into canaliculi and excreted into bile ducts, stored in the gallblad-

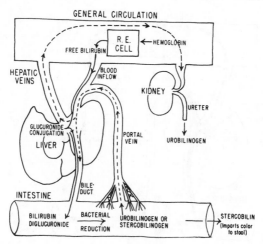

Figure 5–6. Normal enterohepatic circulation of bile pigments. R.E., reticuloendothelium. (From Cornelius CE: Liver function. *In* Kaneko JJ, ed: Clinical Biochemistry of Domestic Animals, ed 4. San Diego, Academic Press, 1989, p 368.)

der, and eventually expelled into the small intestines. In the small intestine, the bacterial flora reduces bilirubin to urobilinogen and stercobilinogen (Fig. 5–6).

Cholestasis refers to the stagnation of bile flow and may be caused by intrahepatic or extrahepatic factors. Cholestasis is associated with altered permeability of hepatic membranes and injury to the microfilaments in the canalicular areas. Various noxious influences may induce intrahepatic cholestasis, including hypoxia; exposure to various toxins, infectious agents, or drugs; and excessive concentrations of toxic bile acids that may accumulate secondary to impaired bile excretion.

■ CAUSES OF FELINE CHOLESTASIS

Feline cholangiohepatitis
Primary neoplasms of the liver
Feline hepatic lipidosis
Feline infectious peritonitis
Liver cirrhosis

5

Increases in serum bilirubin cause jaundice when the serum concentration exceeds 1.5 mg/dL. Jaundice can develop from (1) increased bilirubin pigment liberation and hemolysis causing an increased influx of hemoglobin (prehepatic or hemolytic jaundice [Fig. 5–7]); (2) decreased bilirubin excretion due to impaired hepatocellular uptake, storage, conjugation, or transport into the biliary tree (hepatic jaundice); or (3) blockage of the biliary excretory pathways (posthepatic jaundice [Fig. 5–8]).

⋯⋯⋯⋯ICTERUS INDEX

The icterus index is an approximate measure of the severity of hyperbilirubinemia. This index is based on gross visual inspection of the color of plasma or

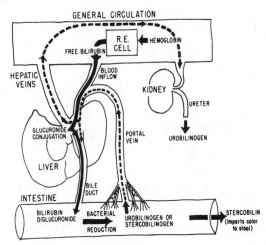

Figure 5–7. Hemolytic crisis. Note the increase in the quantities of unconjugated bilirubin (indirect-reacting) in the serum (unable to pass the renal filter), stercobilin in the stool (imparting a darker color to the stool), and urinary urobilinogen. Increased urinary urobilinogen may be partly due to secondary liver damage (less reexcreted into the bile and hence lost to the serum and urine) in addition to the increased quantity of bile pigments metabolized owing to erythrocyte hemolysis. If secondary liver damage is extensive from hemosiderosis or bile pigment overload, some bilirubin glucuronide may be regurgitated and lost to the urine (not in diagram). R.E., reticuloendothelium. (From Cornelius CE: Liver function. *In* Kaneko JJ, ed: Clinical Biochemistry of Domestic Animals, ed 4. San Diego, Academic Press, 1989, p 368.)

serum and comparison with the color of standards prepared from a potassium dichromate solution.

⋯⋯⋯⋯SERUM BILIRUBIN FRACTIONATION

Differentiation of the total bilirubin into the UB and CB components is possible. Nearly all diseases associated with hyperbilirubinemia in cats and dogs are characterized by a mixture of conjugated and unconjugated bilirubinemia. This means that the van den Bergh test is not that clinically significant. CB reacts directly or rapidly with the diazo reagent and is therefore termed *direct* (-reacting) bilirubin. Unconjugated bilirubin reacts slowly with the diazo reagent and requires a facilitator. Therefore, UB is termed *indirect* (-reacting) bilirubin. In theory, increased concentrations of UB or indirect bilirubin indicate increased hemoprotein release by hemolysis. Unfortunately, veterinary patients with hemolytic disorders are presented long after initial pigment release and after the liver has conjugated a large component of the UB. In clinical practice, there are few circumstances in which the fractionation of bilirubin serves an important diagnostic function. Measurement of total bilirubin provides the most essential information.

⋯⋯⋯⋯URINE BILIRUBIN

Most urine bilirubin is CB because of its water solubility, less avid protein binding, and potential for glomerular filtration. The renal tubules in the dog

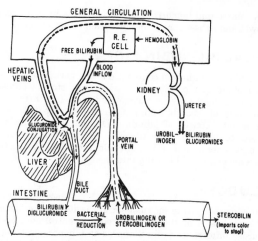

GENERAL CIRCULATION

Figure 5–8. Hepatocellular pathology. Increased levels of bilirubin conjugates (direct-reacting) can be present in the serum; lesser amounts of unconjugated bilirubin may also be elevated in the serum owing to a decreased uptake of the pigment. During recovery from cholestasis, increased serum levels of direct-reacting covalently bound bilirubin conjugates (biliprotein) may persist without bilirubinuria. Observe the presence of bilirubin glucuronide and increased amounts of urobilinogen in the urine. Increased urinary urobilinogen is due to the inability of the altered hepatic cells to reexcrete this pigment into the bile. R.E., reticuloendothelium. (From Cornelius CE: Liver function. *In* Keneko JJ, ed: Clinical Biochemistry of Domestic Animals, ed 4. San Diego, Academic Press, 1989, p 369.)

are capable of metabolizing hemoglobin to bilirubin, of conjugating bilirubin, and of secreting bilirubin. The renal threshold for bilirubin in the dog is thus said to be low. Male dogs have more bilirubin in urine than do females. The detection of trace to 1+ bilirubin on urine tests is considered normal in a concentrated sample (specific gravity, ≥ 1.030) in the dog. Consistent detection of 2+ or 3+ bilirubin in the urine of the dog at any urine specific gravity indicates hyperbilirubinuria and probable hyperbilirubinemia.

Bilirubinuria is abnormal in cat urine at any specific gravity. Bilirubinuria in cat urine indicates hyperbilirubinemia and thus may be used to detect a hepatic or hemolytic process before tissue jaundice becomes clinically evident.

·············URINE UROBILINOGEN

Urobilinogen is formed in the bowel by bacterial reduction of bilirubin. Most urobilinogen is excreted in the feces, but up to 20% is reabsorbed into the portal vein and circulated to the liver for reexcretion in bile or to the kidneys for elimination by glomerular filtration. The absence of urine urobilinogen in the presence of jaundice suggests the possibility of extrahepatic bile duct occlusion (see Fig. 5–8). Unfortunately, the test has many shortcomings. False-negative results may be obtained because of urine dilution, antibiotic alteration of normal enteric flora, a low urine pH, storage of urine for too long, storage of urine in light, or accelerated intestinal transit. False-positive reactions in the presence of extrahepatic bile duct occlusion may develop because of the tendency for gastrointestinal hemorrhage, which results in "jaundiced" blood entering the bowel and subsequently the formation of urobilinogen.

............FECAL BILIRUBIN PIGMENTS

Urobilinogen and stercobilinogen contribute to the normal brown color of feces. Increased stercobilinogen produces a dark-orange stool, whereas decreased amounts produce a light-gray or clay-colored stool (see Figs. 5–8 and 5–9). Increased amounts of fecal bilirubin pigments develop in association with hemolytic or hepatic causes of jaundice. Decreased amounts or absence of stercobilinogen occurs in extrahepatic bile duct obstruction. Stercobilinogen can develop in patients with complete bile duct occlusion, again associated with hemorrhagic tendencies and bleeding into the bowel.

............GLUCOSE

Many aspects of carbohydrate metabolism are influenced by hepatic function. The effect of liver disease on the blood glucose concentration is highly variable. Apparent glucose intolerance (mild inappropriate hyperglycemia), euglycemia, and hypoglycemia have each been observed. The liver provides a large glycogen reservoir for gluconeogenesis, and this is the principal source of glucose during acute starvation. During chronic starvation, the liver is the principal site of gluconeogenesis from branched-chain amino acids and glycerol. The liver is also involved in regulation of blood insulin, glucagon, and glucocorticoids, hormones that have a major influence on the blood glucose concentration.

Severe hepatic insufficiency, as seen in endstage cirrhosis and in animals with portosystemic shunts, may be associated with profound hypoglycemia. Neuroglycopenia may cause neurologic signs that are mistakenly interpreted

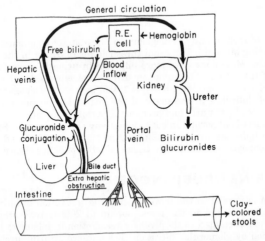

Figure 5–9. Extrahepatic obstruction. Note regurgitation to the serum and subsequently the urine of all bilirubin diglucuronides conjugated in the liver. Biliprotein may also be present in the serum during cholestasis. Urinary urobilinogen and fecal stercobilin are absent. R.E., reticuloendothelium. (From Cornelius CE: Liver function. *In* Kaneko JJ, ed: Clinical Biochemistry of Domestic Animals, ed 4. San Diego, Academic Press, 1989, p 369.)

as evidence of encephalopathic toxins. Abnormal responsivity to glucagon and reduced glycogen stores are thought to be etiologic. The hepatic reserve for gluconeogenesis is immense. Reduction in hepatic function to less than 25% to 30% is necessary before hypoglycemia becomes a critical problem. Other causes of hypoglycemia should be considered, as outlined on p. 144, before hepatic failure is accepted as the cause.

············CHOLESTEROL

The liver is of central importance to lipoprotein metabolism and to the regulation of the serum cholesterol concentration. Cholesterol is esterified in the liver and is used in the synthesis of bile acids and steroid hormones. A primary route of cholesterol excretion is in bile. Both hypercholesterolemia and hypocholesterolemia can be associated with serious hepatic disease.

Hypercholesterolemia develops in patients with major bile duct occlusion and is thought to be caused by an increase in cholesterol synthesis, as well as reflux from bile into blood. Increased synthesis appears to be related to a lack of normal feedback inhibition due to abnormal lipoprotein metabolism. Other causes of hypercholesterolemia should be considered, including diabetes mellitus, hypothyroidism, hyperadrenocorticism, pancreatitis, nephrotic syndrome, idiopathic hyperlipidemia of schnauzers (and other breeds), and postprandial hyperlipidemia.

Hypocholesterolemia develops in some animals with severe hepatic insufficiency due to endstage cirrhosis, anticonvulsant-associated liver disease, and congenital portosystemic shunts. Intestinal lymphangiectasia should be ruled out when severe hypocholesterolemia is identified.

The ratio of esterified to total cholesterol has been reported to be abnormal in 90% of patients with liver disease. Normal ratios range between 0.64 and 0.80. In dogs with acute severe hepatic necrosis, cholesterol esterification may be reduced, but this defect normalizes within a week or two.

············PROTEIN METABOLISM

Regulation and synthesis of many essential proteins has been a well-documented liver function. Proteins dependent on normal hepatic function include, but are not restricted to, albumin; many globulins, including important hormone and drug-transport proteins; fibrinogen and most other coagulation proteins; and important inhibitors of coagulation, including antithrombin III, plasminogen, antiproteases, and the protein components of lipoproteins.

Albumin constitutes 25% of the major hepatic export proteins. Albumin is essential as a plasma transport protein and as the major determinant of the plasma oncotic pressure. Fortunately, there is a tremendous hepatic reserve for albumin synthesis. The normal liver works at only 30% of its maximum albumin-synthesizing potential. The half-life of albumin in the dog is approximately 7.5 days but can be extended if synthetic capabilities are reduced. In health, albumin degradation occurs in the liver as well as in other tissues. The rates of synthesis and degradation are balanced to maintain the plasma oncotic pressure. A feedback mechanism operating at the surface of the hepatocyte adjusts the rate of albumin synthesis.

The concentration of albumin depends on nutritional status, the adequacy of liver function, and the presence or absence of disorders causing pathologic losses from the body or into body cavities. Mild to moderate hypoalbuminemia can develop during starvation in animals with normal liver function. Moderate to marked hypoalbuminemia can develop in patients with hepatic insufficiency. Although synthetic failure is often causal, third-space sequestration of albumin in ascitic fluid may be a major contributing factor. Whenever serious hypoalbuminemia is identified, other causes must be carefully considered, including protein-losing nephropathies, protein-losing enteropathies, albumin sequestration into body cavities, and albumin loss through extensive cutaneous lesions. Hypoalbuminemia is an important cause of adverse drug reactions in patients with hepatic disease. Drugs that are highly protein-bound will have a large unbound component free to bind to cellular receptors.

Although many globulins are synthesized by the liver, serious hepatic disease is frequently associated with hyperglobulinemia. This hyperglobulinemia consists primarily of immunoglobulins derived from immunocompetent cells in other areas of the body. Reduced hepatic RES function results in the systemic circulation of antigens of gut origin that are normally entrapped and detoxified in the liver. As a result of hyperglobulinemia, measurement of total protein does not accurately reflect the serum albumin concentration. Fractionation into the albumin and globulin fractions is essential to reliable detection of hypoalbuminemia.

···········BLOOD COAGULATION

Most of the coagulation proteins, their activators and inhibitors, and the proteins responsible for fibrinolysis are synthesized or regulated by the liver. Bleeding tendencies can develop in patients with serious hepatic insufficiency or major bile duct occlusion. The underlying mechanisms include deficient coagulation factor synthesis or activation; deficient synthesis of antithrombin III; insufficient synthesis, activation, or inhibition of plasminogen resulting in insufficient or unrestricted fibrinolysis; an increase in anticoagulant factors such as fibrin degradation products (FDPs), increased surface contact activation of the coagulation cascade by hepatic endothelial lesions, or increased release of tissue thromboplastin; and platelet defects such as thrombocytopenia and acquired platelet dysfunction (increased or decreased platelet aggregation).

Spontaneous hemorrhage is uncommon in patients with liver disease. Bleeding is usually provoked by invasive diagnostic procedures, trauma, or disease processes that create localized lesions. Abnormalities are not reliably detected by the routinely used coagulation tests—prothrombin time (PT), activated partial thromboplastin time (APTT), or activated clotting time (ACT)—because factor activity must be reduced to 30% of normal before test abnormalities are evident. Assays to detect the activity of specific factors or tests completed on diluted plasma are more sensitive, although they are not practical for routine use. The measurement of fibrinogen is complicated by the fact that, although it is synthesized in the liver, there is a huge synthetic reserve and it is an acute-phase protein. Any type of systemic inflammation can cause hyperfibrinogenemia, and acute or chronic low-grade DIC can cause hypofibrinogenemia.

Jaundiced animals should be carefully examined for bleeding tendencies attributable to vitamin K depletion. Interruption of the enterohepatic bile acid circulation in extrahepatic bile duct occlusion leads to malabsorption of the fat-soluble vitamins. Vitamin K deficiency results in insufficient activation of coagulation factors II, VII, IX, and X. The earliest abnormality may be an increased PT or APTT. Treatment with vitamin K_1 will correct abnormal coagulation times by 80% to 90% within 12 to 24 hours. Animals with major parenchymal lesions causing jaundice will not substantially improve. Because of its high degree of efficacy in correcting vitamin depletion, vitamin K_1 5 to 10 mg IM once daily or b.i.d. should be given to any jaundiced animal 24 to 48 hours before hepatic biopsy.

The coagulation system is tenuously balanced in many animals with liver disease. Invasive procedures may disrupt this balance and provoke a hemorrhagic crisis. Therefore, a fresh, compatible blood transfusion should be arranged before any surgical procedures. In patients with normal results in coagulation tests, transfusion is not given unless hemorrhagic tendencies develop during or after surgery. In patients with abnormal test results or with clinical signs of a bleeding tendency, a transfusion is initiated prior to surgery. In these patients, it is prudent to demonstrate test normalization before biopsy is undertaken. If routine coagulation tests are normal, evaluation of a bleeding time will help predict the presence of platelet dysfunction or von Willebrand's disease that might cause hemorrhage. If the bleeding time is abnormal, a transfusion is indicated.

In animals with severe parenchymal disease, especially those with acute necrosis, DIC seems to be common. Unrestricted clotting seems to be associated with excessive factor activation due to sinusoidal endothelial lesions, excessive release of tissue thromboplastin, insufficient antithrombin III, decreased hepatic removal of FDPs, and thrombocytopenia. These patients may require treatment with whole blood, heparin, or low-dose aspirin, or any combination of these, depending on the features and severity of their coagulopathy (see the section on DIC, p. 45). If heparin therapy is deemed necessary, measurement of antithrombin III activity is useful. Antithrombin III is the most important natural inhibitor of thrombin generation and is necessary for the anticoagulant effect of heparin. It is the most dependable indicator of DIC among the routinely used coagulation tests. Antithrombin III is synthesized in the liver and is a useful prognostic indicator of the severity of liver disease. Normal values in the dog and cat seem to range between 80% and 120% of normal activity. Antithrombin III activity of less than 70% is associated with a moderate risk of unrestricted clotting and thromboembolism. Values less than or equal to 50% are associated with a marked risk of thromboembolism, severe liver disease, and a poor prognosis. Other causes of subnormal antithrombin III activity include protein-losing nephropathies, protein-losing enteropathies, and excessive consumption, as occurs in DIC. If antithrombin III is subnormal, a fresh whole-blood transfusion can be used to correct the deficit.

If a blood transfusion is necessary for a patient with hepatic insufficiency, only fresh, whole compatible blood should be used. Stored blood may generate a substantial quantity of ammonia, which might induce encephalopathic effects. In addition, stored blood has reduced erythrocyte viability, which can result in the release of a substantial quantity of protein requiring hepatic detoxification. Fresh blood also supplies viable platelets for recipient use.

···········AMMONIA

The liver is the major site of ammonia detoxification by metabolism to urea in the Krebs-Henseleit urea cycle (see p. 719 for a more complete discussion of ammonia metabolism). Quantification of the blood ammonia concentration and assessment of ammonia tolerance can be used to detect hepatic insufficiency. To conduct this test under optimal conditions, proper sample management is imperative. Samples should be transported in an ice bath; plasma should be separated immediately in a refrigerated centrifuge and analyzed within several hours. Assessment of ammonia tolerance following the oral administration of ammonium chloride (NH_4Cl) is superior to measurement of baseline ammonia concentrations. NH_4Cl may be administered in a dilute solution or in a gelatin capsule. The recommended dose is 0.1 g/kg or 100 mg/kg, up to a maximum of 3 g. Blood samples are collected into an ammonia-free heparin Vacutainer before and 30 minutes following dose administration. Although ammonia is regarded as a major toxin responsible for hepatic encephalopathy, it is not the only toxin that can produce the neurologic signs. Therefore, baseline hyperammonemia is inconsistently associated with hepatic encephalopathy. The ATT (ammonia tolerance test) will be abnormal in these patients.

Hyperammonemia was reported once in two dogs with what was thought to be a congenital urea cycle enzyme defect. Hyperammonemia has also been recognized in patients with uropathies associated with urine retention and infection with urease-producing organisms capable of metabolizing urea to ammonia.

In patients that have urate urinary calculi, hyperammonemia as a result of hepatic insufficiency should be ruled out by demonstrating normal hepatic function with either the serum bile acid test or the ATT. Some animals with congenital portosystemic shunts have been primarily presented for obstructive uropathies due to urate calculi. The young age of these animals, their stunted body size, and other typical historical abnormalities should alert the clinician to evaluate hepatic function. In approximately one third of the animals with congenital portosystemic shunts, ammonium biurate crystals can be visualized in urine sediment.

............UREA

Since urea is synthesized from ammonia in the liver, a subnormal BUN can develop in patients with severe hepatic insufficiency. A low BUN can also be seen in animals undergoing fluid diuresis, in animals on restricted protein diets, or as a normal variation. The concurrent development of dehydration or any other cause of reduced GFR complicates the use of BUN as an indicator of hepatic function. Likewise, the BUN cannot be used as a reliable indicator of renal function in patients with reduced hepatic function. Serum creatinine should be used in this circumstance.

............URIC ACID

Uric acid is converted to allantoin in the liver by uricase. Dalmatian dogs have a genetic defect limiting the transmembrane transport of uric acid, although they have adequate uricase activity. These dogs may have recurrent formation of urate urinary calculi due to their increased urinary excretion of uric acid. Affected animals may be successfully managed by chronic administration of allopurinol, which inhibits the formation of uric acid and promotes the formation of water-soluble products. In addition, affected males may benefit from a permanent prescrotal urethrostomy.

In liver disease, the amount of uric acid in the blood may increase. Test results have been highly variable, so uric acid determinations are not routinely used.

............ORGANIC ANION TESTS OF LIVER FUNCTION

............Bile Acids

Measurement of serum bile acids to estimate hepatic function is now used more commonly than are the organic anion dyes or the ATT. Bile acids are synthesized in the liver from cholesterol and are then transported in the biliary tree to the gallbladder, where they are stored and concentrated. At mealtime, neurohumoral stimuli invoke the release of cholecystokinin, which stimulates gallbladder contraction and expulsion of bile into the intestines. Bile acids are essential to optimal digestion and absorption of dietary fats. The bile acids are resorbed throughout the intestines but most prominently in the ileum, where an active transport process provides more than 90% absorption efficiency. The resorbed bile acids are transported into the portal circulation, which presents them to the liver for extraction. The hepatocyte has an efficient uptake capability for bile acids and achieves 90% extraction during first pass. The overall efficiency of the enterohepatic circulation of bile acids is so great that very low serum concentrations are maintained. The enterohepatic circulation of bile acids is illustrated in Figure 5–10. The efficiency of the uptake systems and

BILE ACID ENTEROHEPATIC CIRCULATION

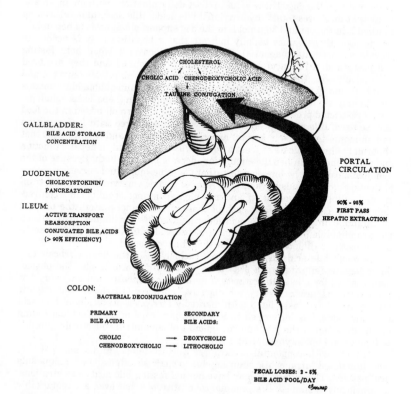

CHOLESTEROL

CHOLIC ACID CHENODEOXYCHOLIC ACID

TAURINE CONJUGATION

GALLBLADDER:
**BILE ACID STORAGE
CONCENTRATION**

DUODENUM:
**CHOLECYSTOKININ/
PANCREAZYMIN**

ILEUM:
**ACTIVE TRANSPORT
REABSORPTION
CONJUGATED BILE ACIDS
(> 90% EFFICIENCY)**

PORTAL
CIRCULATION

90% - 95%
FIRST PASS
HEPATIC EXTRACTION

COLON:
BACTERIAL DECONJUGATION

PRIMARY
BILE ACIDS:

SECONDARY
BILE ACIDS:

CHOLIC   ⟶ DEOXYCHOLIC
CHENODEOXYCHOLIC ⟶ LITHOCHOLIC

FECAL LOSSES: 2 - 5%
BILE ACID POOL/DAY

Figure 5-10. Patterns of total serum bile acid concentrations (12-hour fasting and 2-hour postprandial) commonly observed in certain hepatic disorders. These patterns are often, but not always, observed in these specified disorders. Abbreviations: PSS = portosystemic shunt, CIRR = cirrhosis, CHOLE = intrahepatic cholestasis, EHBDO = extrahepatic bile duct occlusion. (From Center SA: Serum bile acid concentrations for hepatobiliary function testing in cats. *In* Kirk RW, ed: Current Veterinary Therapy X. Philadelphia, WB Saunders, 1989.)

portal circulation can be appraised by measurement of bile acids at a specified interval after feeding during which maximal ileal presentation, portal vein transportation, and hepatocellular presentation of the bile acids are thought to occur. The optimal interval following a diet with a composition similar to that of p/d and c/d Hill's pet diets for the healthy dog and cat, respectively, has been demonstrated to be 2 hours. To conduct the fasting and postprandial bile acid test, a blood sample is collected before feeding and again 2 hours after confirmed meal ingestion. The meal size should approximate a normal meal to ensure adequate stimulus.

The following test performance statistics are relevant to the direct enzymatic method for determination of total serum bile acid values. Normal baseline bile acid concentrations in the dog and cat are less than or equal to 5 μmol/L.

Two hours following a meal, normal values are up to 10 μmol/L in the cat and 15.5 μmol/L in the dog. These values reflect determinations with an enzymatic assay that measures total 3-hydroxylated bile acids. Bile acid values exceeding 20 μmol/L in the cat and 30 μmol/L in the dog support a diagnosis of hepatobiliary disease (these values usually indicate that a hepatic biopsy is needed to provide an accurate diagnosis). The test functions best when both fasting and postprandial bile acid concentrations are determined and they are used adjunctively with the routine biochemical profile screening tests (enzyme and total bilirubin) for gastric emptying, intestinal transit, and gallbladder contraction. In animals with adverse reactions to dietary protein (hepatic encephalopathy), a restricted protein diet with a few milliliters of corn oil mixed in the food may be used. Bile acid concentrations have been compared with ICG excretion and ammonia tolerance in several experimental models, and it is thought that abnormal values indicate at least a 60% to 70% impairment in hepatic function due to a reduction in hepatic circulation, hepatic mass, or both. Because of the dynamic nature of the bile acid test, there is some individual variation among patients. Some animals have altered rates of gastric emptying, intestinal transit, and gallbladder evacuation, and may have spontaneous gallbladder contraction during a prolonged fast; each of these circumstances alters the optimal postprandial interval for bile acid determination. When higher fasting than postprandial bile acid concentrations are observed, alterations in gastrointestinal transit or gallbladder evacuation should be suspected.

Although bile acids are synthesized exclusively in the liver, cirrhosis and acute hepatic failure are not associated with low bile acid levels. The physiologic reserve for bile acid synthesis is seemingly immense, and only very low concentrations are necessary for digestive purposes. Cirrhosis and hepatic failure are always associated with markedly increased postprandial bile acid concentrations. Fasting concentrations may be normal or increased, depending on the duration of the fast and the amount of circulation collectively afforded to functional hepatocytes during the fast.

Patients with congenital or acquired portosystemic shunts and patients with functional intrahepatic shunting due to cirrhosis often show a unique bile acid pattern. These animals may have normal fasting bile acid concentrations, as previously explained. Postprandial concentrations, however, are remarkably increased. Other predictive, but inconsistent, patterns have also been noted. The highest bile acid values are seen in patients with severe cholestasis, usually associated with extrahepatic bile duct occlusion.

The bile acid test for liver function has strengthened the ability of the veterinarian in practice to diagnose occult liver disease and congenital portosystemic shunts and to decide when a liver biopsy is appropriate. Current recommendations state that hepatic biopsy is needed when fasting serum bile acid concentration using enzymatic method exceeds 20 μmol/L in cats and 30 μmol/L in dogs. The test is completed on serum samples that can be routinely mailed to a laboratory for analysis. Hemolysis greatly interferes with the enzymatic assay, so serum must be separated carefully before mailing. Measurement of total serum bile acids or the taurine-conjugated bile acids is recommended. Procedures in which the glycine-conjugated bile acids are determined cannot be recommended, since dogs and cats primarily conjugate their bile acids to taurine.

■ DIAGNOSTIC EFFICACY OF 12-HOUR FASTING AND 2-HOUR POSTPRANDIAL SERUM BILE ACIDS IN CATS

A fasting serum bile acid (FSBA) greater than 15 mmol/L and a postprandial serum bile acid (PSBA) greater than 20 mmol/L in the cat give the highest specificities of any single test to determine liver disease. The overall test efficacy for all cats with

Box continued on following page

■ DIAGNOSTIC EFFICACY OF 12-HOUR FASTING AND 2-HOUR
POSTPRANDIAL SERUM BILE ACIDS IN CATS *(Continued)*

liver disease (excluding cats with portosystemic vascular anomaly) was 66% for FSBA
greater than 15 mmol/L, 81% for PSBA greater than 20 mmol/L, and 83% for FSBA
and PSBA interpreted in parallel. The efficacy of PSBA in cats with portosystemic
vascular anomaly is 100%.

Center S: Diagnostic procedures for evaluation of hepatic disease. *In* Guilford WG,
Center SA, Strombeck DR, et al, eds: Strombeck's Small Animal Gastroenterology, ed 3.
Philadelphia, WB Saunders, 1996, p 130.

REFERENCES

Anderson M, Sevelius E: Circulating autoantibodies in dogs with chronic liver disease. J
  Small Anim Pract 33:389–394, 1992.
Barr F: Ultrasonographic assessment of liver size in the dog. J Small Anim Pract 33:359–
  364, 1992.
Blaxter AC, Holt PE, Pearson GR: Congenital portosystemic shunts in the cat: A report of
  nine cases. J Small Anim Pract 29:631–645, 1989.
Bunch SE: Hepatobiliary and exocrine pancreatic disorders. *In* Nelson RW, Couto C, eds:
  Essentials of Small Animal Internal Medicine. St Louis, Mosby–Year Book, 1992.
Center S: Diagnostic procedures for evaluation of hepatic disease. *In* Guilford WG, Center
  SA, Strombeck DR, et al, eds: Strombeck's Small Animal Gastroenterology, ed 3. Phila-
  delphia, WB Saunders, 1996, p 130.
Center SA: Chronic liver disease: Current concepts of disease mechanisms. J Small Anim
  Pract 40:101–114, 1999.
Cornelius CE: Liver function. *In* Kaneko JJ, ed: Clinical Biochemistry of Domestic Ani-
  mals, ed 4. San Diego, Academic Press, 1989, pp 364–397.
Day D: Feline cholangiohepatitis complex. Vet Clin North Am Small Anim Pract 25:375,
  1995.
Dial S: Clinicopathologic evaluation of the liver. Vet Clin North Am Small Anim Pract
  25:257, 1995.
Dill-Macky E: Chronic hepatitis in dogs. Vet Clin North Am SmallAnim Pract, 25:387, 1995.
Dimski D, Taboada J: Feline idiopathic hepatic lipidosis. Vet Clin North Am Small Anim
  Pract 25:357, 1995.
Guilford WG, Center SA, Strombeck DR, et al: Strombeck's Small Animal Gastroenterol-
  ogy, ed 3. Philadelphia, WB Saunders 1996.
Meyer DJ, Harvey J: Veterinary Laboratory Medicine ed 2. Philadelphia, WB Saunders,
  1998.
Meyer DJ, Williams DA: Diagnosis of hepatic and exocrine pancreatic disorders. Semin
  Vet Med Surg 7:275–284, 1992.
Paugh BP, Biller D: Hepatic imaging with radiology and ultrasound. Vet Clin North Am
  Small Anim Pract 25:305, 1995.
Saunders M: Ultrasonography of abdominal cavitary parenchymal lesions. Vet Clin North
  Am Small Anim Pract 28:755, 1998.
Sutherland RJ: Biochemical evaluation of the hepatobiliary system in dogs and cats. Vet
  Clin North Am Small Anim Pract 19:899–927, 1989.
Zawie DA, Shaker E: Diseases of the liver. *In* Sherding RG, ed: The Cat: Diseases and
  Clinical Management. New York, Churchill Livingstone, 1989.

ANTIMICROBIAL SENSITIVITY TESTING

Susceptibility of microorganisms to antibiotics can be measured in commercial
laboratories by dilution techniques, with results reported as minimal inhibitory
concentrations (MICs). Smaller laboratories use the agar diffusion technique,
in which the zone of inhibition of microbial growth around a disk containing a

fixed amount of antibiotic is directly related to the MIC of the organism being tested.

These in vitro tests are classically performed with a pure culture growth of the infecting agent obtained by culture isolation from the primary specimen (see p. 466). The test indicates the susceptibility or resistance of the organism to specific antimicrobial agents. A response showing resistance should eliminate that agent from therapeutic consideration; however, a test showing susceptibility may not always guarantee similar results in vivo. In general, the following hold true: If the test shows resistence, the organism is not likely to respond to therapy with the antibiotic. If the test response is intermediate, the organism is susceptible if the dosage is high or if the antibiotic is concentrated, as in the urine. If the test shows susceptibility, the organism is susceptible to an ordinary dosage. The tests, properly performed, do serve as a useful guide.

The tests *are not* indicated in the following circumstances:

1. When organisms are of unvarying susceptibility. Beta-hemolytic streptococci, *Pasteurella, Actinobacillus, Actinomyces,* and anaerobes (except for *Bacteroides fragilis*) are susceptible to penicillin or ampicillin.
2. When the number of organisms as determined by culture is deemed to be insignificant for infection.
3. When the primary specimen yields a mixture of infecting organisms and it is uncertain which, if any, is the etiologic agent. Interpretation of tests run on such samples is difficult and unreliable.

The tests *are* indicated in the following circumstances:

1. When body defenses may be defective and the utmost antimicrobial efficacy is necessary.
2. When the antibiotic allows the organisms to develop resistance easily.
3. When infections are caused by bacterial species that commonly have many strains of differing antibiotic susceptibility. Among bacteria that commonly show variable strains are *Staphylococcus aureus, Staphylococcus intermedius,* and members of the Enterobacteriaceae (such as *Escherichia coli, Proteus, Enterobacter, Klebsiella,* and *Salmonella*).

REFERENCES

Hirsh DC: Antimicrobial sensitivity testing. *In* Kirk RW, ed: Current Veterinary Therapy X. Philadelphia, WB Saunders, 1989.

Kilgore RW: Clavulanate-potentiated antibiotics. *In* Kirk RW, ed: Current Veterinary Therapy X. Philadelphia, WB Saunders, 1989.

MYCOLOGY

DERMATOPHYTES

Wood's light fluorescence of affected hair and skin may be observed in many infections due to *Microsporum canis*, a common dermatophyte of small animals. A similar response is often observed with *Microsporum audouini* and *Microsporum distortum*, rare animal dermatophytes. Not all specimens of these fungi fluoresce. When they do, the typical fluorescence is a yellow-green color. Other colors of fluorescence (purple, blue) may be due to medications, mineral oil, scales, or mineral particles. Fluorescing hair and skin make excellent samples for culture, and the distribution of these areas may indicate foci of infection not otherwise apparent.

Table 5–12. Features of Direct Smears Helpful in Identification of Soft Tissue Mycoses

Agent	Important Features
Systemic Mycoses	
Blastomycosis	Direct smear with Parker ink and KOH: large, thick-walled budding yeast
Coccidioidomycosis	Direct smear with Parker ink and KOH: thick-walled spherules with endospores and smaller spherules devoid of spores
Cryptococcosis	Direct smear in India ink and water: small, round budding yeast surrounded by a capsule (halo); culture at both 20° and 37°C without cyclohexamide, which inhibits growth
Histoplasmosis	Usually need culture; direct smear with blood stain may show small oval bodies, yeast cells within macrophages
Subcutaneous Mycoses	
Aspergillosis	Nasal washings, biopsies, and scrapings in KOH for hyphae and aspergillus heads: culture on Sabouraud dextrose agar
Mycetoma	*Actinomycotic*—crush granules and use Gram stain to observe gram-positive filaments; culture granules after washing in sterile saline, and place on Sabouraud dextrose agar without antibiotics and on blood agar; incubate one set at 37°C and one at 25°C
	Eumycotic—crush granules, mix with KOH, and examine for hyphae and chlamydospores
Phaeohyphomycosis	Exudate or tissue mixed with KOH to see black septate hyphae with unusual dilations; culture on Sabouraud dextrose agar at 25°C
Phycomycosis	Exudates and tissue mixed with KOH and examined for wide, nonseptate hyphae; culture on Sabouraud dextrose agar at 25°C
Prototuecosis	Exudates mixed with KOH and examined for oval to globoid structures containing two or more autospores; easily cultured on blood or Sabouraud dextrose agar; yeast colonies in 24 hr
Rhinosporidiosis	Crush a polyp, mix with KOH, and examine for sporangia with endospores; culture not needed
Sporotrichosis	Direct smears of little value; dimorphic; culture on Sabouraud dextrose agar; use special fungal stains on tissues

5

Potassium hydroxide 20% for digestion of hair and scale preparations may clear the sample of debris so that fungal mycelia can be observed more easily. Unless the fungal growth is abundant, the test may be negative, and even if mycelia are observed, one cannot make valid conclusions about the pathogenicity of the organism. A positive test does help confirm suspicions and is a mandate for cultures and further identification.

Fungal cultures (see p. 476) afford the only accurate way to identify pathogenic organisms, and positive laboratory reports provide a definitive diagnosis.

1. The great majority of dermatomycoses of small animals are caused by *M. canis, Microsporum gypseum,* or *Trichophyton mentagrophytes*.
2. *Candida albicans*, a yeast, causes a mycosis of intermediate depth (moniliasis) that may affect skin and mucous membranes. *C. albicans* is often an opportunist associated with moist or macerated skin or mucous membranes, and the clinician should search carefully for another etiologic agent. *C. albicans* and *Malassezia pachydermatis* are yeasts commonly found in otitis externa, but they may be present as secondary invaders.

Wet-mount or acetate tape preparations can be made from fungal cultures for precise identification of fungal species. To visualize the morphologic aspects, collect small masses of cultured growth with a sterile loop, suspend in saline, and place them under a coverslip. Another method is to press clear acetate (Scotch) tape onto the surface growth of a fungal culture. Place a drop of lacto cotton phenol blue stain onto a microscope slide. Then place the tape, sticky side down, on top of the stain, cover with a coverslip, and examine for morphologic identification.

............DEEP MYCOSES

Subcutaneous mycoses develop in the host at the site of inoculation and are usually soil saprophytes that do not spread to other animals. Debilitating diseases, immunodeficiencies, and long-term antibiotic or corticosteroid therapy are common findings in affected animals.

Systemic mycoses are usually chronic, low-grade, debilitating, nonpainful infections that are not usually transmitted naturally between animal hosts. Young animals that may have a depressed immune system show enlarged nodes, abscesses, draining fistulas, or granulomatous lesions. The rare acute infections are usually diagnosed at necropsy.

Direct smears from exudates or node aspirates and scrapings from granulomas or affected skin usually provide suitable specimens for identification of soft tissue mycoses (Table 5–12). Centrifuge transtracheal washing, cerebrospinal fluid (CSF), or urine, and collect the sediment. Suspend the material in 10% to 20% potassium hydroxide (KOH) and ink (one part ink, two parts KOH) to help outline the fungi. India ink and water can also be used to help outline budding yeast forms in cryptococcosis. The ink outlines the clear capsule so that it appears as a halo. Cultures require up to 6 weeks of growth and an extensive isolation procedure.

Histopathology is often helpful in diagnosis. Soft tissue specimens of affected organs should be fixed in 10% buffered formalin. Stains of special value for preparation of these specimens are hematoxylin-eosin (H&E), Gridley, Gomori's methenamine silver, and periodic acid–Schiff (PAS).

REFERENCES

Greene CE, ed: Infectious Diseases of the Dog and Cat, ed 2. Philadelphia, WB Saunders, 1998.

Jackson JA: Immunodiagnosis of systemic mycoses in animals: A review. J Am Vet Med Assoc 7:702, 1986.

Scott, Miller, Griffin: Muller and Kirk's Small Animal Dermatology, ed 5. Philadelphia, WB Saunders, 1997.

Sharp N: Nasal aspergillosis. *In* Kirk RW, ed: Current Veterinary Therapy X. Philadelphia, WB Saunders, 1989.

Wolf AM, Troy GC: Deep mycotic diseases. *In* Ettinger SJ, ed: Textbook of Veterinary Internal Medicine. Philadelphia, WB Saunders, 1989, pp 341–372.

INTERNAL PARASITES OF DOGS AND CATS

............ANCYLOSTOMIASIS (ANCYLOSTOMA CANINUM, ANCYLOSTOMA BRAZILIENSE, UNCINARIA STENOCEPHALA)

The life cycles of all three species of hookworm are similar. Infection with hookworms can occur in the following ways:

1. Skin penetration—third-stage larvae can infect by active skin penetration followed by somatic migration. The minimum prepatent period is 14 to 17 days in puppies.
2. Oral infection—the minimum prepatent period is 14 to 17 days.
3. Transmammary or intrauterine infection—for *A. caninum*.

Adult worms live in the small intestine. Growth and maturation after the ingestion of infective ova require between 18 and 21 days. Females lay large quantities of eggs that are passed in the feces and, under the proper conditions, hatch in 48 to 72 hours. The larvae develop to the infective third stage within 5 to 7 days.

............Transmission to Humans

Infective larvae can penetrate the skin of humans, causing cutaneous larval migrans (creeping eruption).

............Diagnosis

A diagnosis can be made by demonstrating eggs or larvae in the feces. In puppies prenatally or neonatally infected with hookworms, severe clinical disease may occur during the prepatent period, and diagnosis must be based on signs of the disease.

............ASCARIASIS (TOXOCARA CANIS, TOXOCARA CATI, TOXASCARIS LEONINA)

The pattern of migration of these three helminths is variable. *T. canis* in the dog and *T. cati* in the cat follow a tracheal migration route. Second-stage larvae hatch in the stomach after ingestion, penetrate the bowel wall, enter the portal bloodstream, wander in the hepatic parenchyma, enter the postcava, and arrive in the lungs—breaking out of the capillaries to the alveoli and migrating up the bronchial tree and trachea to the pharynx, where they are swallowed. Following a molt in the stomach wall, the parasite matures in the small intestine. The prepatent period for direct infection in young puppies is 4 to 5 weeks.

If the *Toxocara* larvae hatch in numerous foreign hosts, the pattern of migration is altered and somatic migration results.

T. canis infections in puppies less than 1 month of age are produced by migration of second-stage larvae from the bitch to the pups in utero. Infected puppies can have third-stage larvae in their lungs when born, and a molt from third-stage to fourth-stage larvae occurs during the first week of life; fourth-stage larvae may be present in the intestinal tract at 3 days after birth. The prepatent period for intrauterine infection of puppies is 19 to 23 days.

T. canis has a life span averaging 4 months. Females can produce up to 200,000 eggs per day within a temperature range of 15° to 35°C and humidity of 85%. *Toxocara* eggs can become infective within 2 to 5 weeks, whereas *Toxascaris* eggs may require only 1 week. Infective larvae are third stage.

T. leonina follows a mucosal migration in both dogs and cats. The second and third molts occur in the intestinal wall, and the fourth-stage larvae enter the lumen of the gut to mature. The prepatent period is normally 10 to 11 weeks.

The life cycle of *T. cati* is similar to that of *T. canis*; however, there is no placental transfer of larvae. Neonatal infection of kittens can develop via transmammary passage of larvae in the queen's milk.

When the eggs of *T. canis* hatch, they can be ingested by several noncanid species, including humans. The invading larvae do not invade the intestinal tract but may reach other tissues, including the skin, liver, and eye. Other species such as earthworms, mice, rats, chickens, pigeons, lambs, and pigs may be infested by *T. canis* larvae, and if dogs eat infected tissues, the encysted larvae may mature within the dog. This is called a *paratenic cycle*.

............Diagnosis

The diagnosis is based on finding parasitic eggs on fecal examination or parasites in the stool or vomitus.

............Transmission to Humans

Toxocara larvae have been implicated in an increasing number of cases of visceral larva migrans infestations in the liver and eyes of young children. It is the responsibility of the veterinarian to keep pets as free as possible of *Toxocara* and to inform pet owners that children should avoid contact with parasite-laden feces. An ELISA has been developed for detecting human exposure to ascarids.

............TRICHURIASIS (*TRICHURIS* SPECIES)

Three species of *Trichuris* are important in small animals: *T. vulpis* in the dog and *T. campanula* and *T. terrata* in the cat. The infective eggs are ingested by the host, hatch in the small intestine, where the larvae develop in the jejunal glands, and then migrate posteriorly, where they mature. The prepatent period is 70 to 197 days. Adult *T. vulpis* may live in the cecum and colon for 16 months, and eggs may remain viable under proper conditions for 5 years.

............Diagnosis

The diagnosis is based on finding eggs in the feces. Repeated fecal examinations may have to be performed with a flotation fluid with a specific gravity of 1.4 in order to find eggs.

............STRONGYLOIDIASIS (*STRONGYLOIDES*)

Species of *Strongyloides* important in small animals are *S. stercoralis* in the dog and *S. tumefaciens* in the cat. This parasite lives in the mucosae of the anterior half of the small intestine in dogs, cats, foxes, and humans. The parasitic worms are all females, and the eggs develop parthenogenetically. The eggs develop rapidly and hatch before evacuation in the feces. Some of the larvae develop into infective larvae, whereas other develop into free-living males and females. Infective larvae may enter by the oral route or may penetrate the skin. Percutaneous infections may cause focal dermatitis. First-stage larvae are usually found in fresh feces. After a fecal culture has been made for at least 18 hours, the diagnosis may be confirmed by finding free-living adult worms and infective third-stage larvae. Larvae migrate by way of the circulation and lungs, going to the intestine as fourth-stage larvae. Progeny may be shed in the feces 7 to 20 days after infection.

...........Diagnosis

The diagnosis is based on recovery of the characteristic infective larvae in the feces after incubation in sterile sand for 48 hours. Direct smears of fresh feces should be examined for the presence of rhabditiform larvae or eggs. Larvae may be diagnosed by fecal flotation or by using a Baermann apparatus and incubating fresh feces for 36 to 72 hours.

...........Transmission in Humans

Strongyloidiasis in humans is a chronic debilitating disease. Humans and dogs can readily infect each other; therefore, caution should be used in handling infected dogs. Infected dogs should be isolated, and extreme care should be taken to avoid human contamination.

...........TAPEWORMS

In the United States, most dogs and cats are domesticated and eat prepared, cooked foods; therefore, cestode parasitism in both humans and animals is not a major problem. Exceptions to this general statement can be found with infections in dogs of *Dipylidium caninum*, in which the intermediate host is the flea, and *Taenia pisiformis*, in which the natural reservoir is the rabbit. Cats frequently harbor *Taenia taeniaeformis*, the larval stage of which is found in rats and mice.

...........LUNGWORMS

The metastrongyloid nematodes *Aelurostrongylus abstrusus*, *Paragonimus kellicotti*, and *Capillaria aerophilia* are parasites that reproduce in the air passages and pulmonary vessels or parenchyma of the lungs.

Adult *Aelurostrongylus* worms live in the terminal respiratory bronchioles, alveolar ducts, and small branches of the pulmonary arteries. Eggs are forced into the alveolar ducts and alveoli. The first-stage larvae escape into the airways, are coughed up and swallowed, and thus pass into the feces. The first-stage larvae can survive in moist soil for up to 5½ months, in live mollusks for 5 months, and in dead mollusks for 3 weeks. Various transport hosts (amphibians, birds, reptiles, and rodents) may eat infected mollusks and serve as a source of infection when eaten by cats and dogs. When ingested, the infective third-stage larvae penetrate the mucosa of the esophagus, stomach, and small intestine and travel to the bloodstream and lymphatics and finally to the lungs. The prepatent period is 34 to 42 days.

The life cycle of *C. aerophilia* may be direct or may involve earthworms as facultative intermediate hosts. *C. aerophilia* lives in the mucosa of the nasal passages or the trachea and larger bronchi. *Paragonimus* lung flukes have a natural host, the mink, but also occur in the dog, cat, pig, and other animals. Eggs that are coughed up or swallowed by the adult host are passed in the feces or sputum, and the miracidia hatch. The miracidia then enter a snail. Crayfish become infected by eating snails or cercariae. The definitive host becomes infected by eating the crayfish. Geographic distribution of this parasite is in the Great Lakes region and midwestern and southern United States.

Adults live in the trachea and produce eggs, which are coughed up and passed in the feces. The eggs are ingested, and the prepatent period is about 6 weeks.

............Diagnosis

Fecal examination is the most practical diagnostic technique. First-stage larvae of *Aelurostrongylus* have a characteristic notched or S-shaped tail and appear in the feces. The most accurate way to find larvae in the feces is by use of a Baermann apparatus. Fecal examination will not reveal early infections (<5 to 6 weeks) of *Aelurostrongylus* when adult parasites are not yet mature, or late infections when eggs are no longer produced. In addition to fecal examination, transtracheal washes and needle biopsies of the lung can be very helpful.

There has been recent experimental and clinical evidence of low-grade infection of the lungs of dogs with *Filaroides hirthi*. These very small nematodes, 0.5 to 2.0 mm long, are found in the alveolar spaces and terminal bronchioles of dogs. The infections are most prevalent in beagle colonies. The first-stage larvae of *F. hirthi* are infectious directly from the feces. Zinc sulfate flotation is much more efficient than a Baermann technique in concentrating larvae and demonstrating them in the feces; however, eggs may be difficult to find. Transtracheal washes may be helpful in finding parasites.

............SPIROCERCOSIS

The nematode *Spirocerca lupi* is a parasite of carnivores. It is found primarily in dogs but has also been reported in other animals, including cats, foxes, and jackals. The infection is seen most frequently in the southeastern United States. Adult spirurids are large worms (males are 3 to 4 cm long and females 6 to 7 cm long) that reside in nodules in the wall of the thoracic esophagus with a tract open into the lumen of the esophagus through which the eggs pass. The eggs enter the gastrointestinal tract of the host and hatch after they are ingested by a coprophagous beetle. The eggs become infective within the beetle after 2 months. Transport hosts for this parasite include domestic and wild birds, amphibians, reptiles, and certain small animals. Infective larvae are consumed with the beetle by the definitive host. The larvae hatch in the stomach, migrate through the mucosa of the stomach, burrow into the gastric artery and into the wall of the aorta, and move cranially into the thoracic aorta after 3 weeks. Worms leave the aorta 102 to 124 days after infection and enter the esophagus.

............Diagnosis

Diagnosis of spirocercosis is based on finding the embryonated eggs in the feces on a direct fecal smear or by fecal flotation. Thoracic radiographs and barium swallows can be helpful. Esophagoscopy and gastroscopy may enable visualization of the encysted parasites.

............DIROFILARIASIS (HEARTWORMS)

............Diagnosis

............History

A suggestive history of exposure to an endemic heartworm region of the country should prompt a laboratory examination.

............Clinical Pathology

Heartworms must reach maturity before tests for either antigens or microfilariae become positive. This normally occurs about 6½ months after infection, and detectable antigenemia may precede or follow by a few weeks the presence of microfilariae. There is no validity in testing dogs or cats younger than 6 months for heartworms.

The diagnosis of heartworm disease is made by finding microfilariae of *Dirofilaria immitis* in the bloodstream or the use of occult screening tests to detect microfilarial antigens. The microfilariae must be differentiated from the microfilariae of *Dipetalonema* spp. Several different tests have been advocated for the detection of microfilariae, including the direct wet smear, membrane filtration test, capillary sedimentation test, saponin lysis test, and modified Knott test. New data show that monthly preventives for heartworm disease eventually cause sterility in the heartworms leading to a lack of circulating microfilariae and false-negative Knott testing. Dogs being administered diethylcarbamazine citrate as a daily preventive can be tested by a concentration test (Knott). Dogs that have been on monthly preventives (ivermectin and milbemycin) should have the occult heartworm test run. When using the occult test to detect heartworm disease, about 4% of normal dogs will show a false-positive result. In the asymptomatic dog that has been on monthly preventives for less than 2 years with a positive occult test for heartworm, consider running a Knott test for possible remaining microfilariae and use physical and radiographic findings to confirm the diagnosis.

The presence of eosinophilia may be associated with heartworm disease, but this finding is nonspecific. Any animal with an unexplained eosinophilia should have a blood check, a chest radiographic examination, and an electrocardiogram (ECG).

Occult dirofilariasis is *D. immitis* infestation without circulating microfilariae in peripheral blood. The percentage of cases of adult heartworm disease without microfilaremia is variable, from 20% to 67%. Occult *Dirofilaria* infection can be clinically important in (1) determining that a dog is free of heartworm disease before beginning a preventive program with diethylcarbamazine, (2) demonstrating the presence of adults and microfilariae in heartworm-infected dogs, and (3) determining heartworm infection as a cause of cardiopulmonary disease in dogs.

There are several demonstrated causes of occult dirofilariasis: (1) prepatent infections in which clinical, pulmonary arterial signs may develop but microfilariae are not produced and the IFA test for antimicrofilarial antibody is negative; (2) unisexual infections with nongravid female worms; (3) drug-induced sterility of adult *D. immitis*; and (4) immune-mediated sterile infection, which appears negative in a routine check for microfiliariae but positive in an IFA test.

Clinical signs include weight loss, extreme fatigue, chronic cough, and dyspnea. Radiographic findings are dilated and tortuous caudal lobar pulmonary arteries in the dorsoventral view. The caudal lobar arteries should not be larger than the ninth rib. Additionally, radiographs may reveal enlargement of the right ventricle, enlargement of the pulmonary outflow tract, and pulmonary infiltrative disease, which is most demonstrable radiographically in the peripheral areas of the diaphragmatic lobes. The ECG shows changes of right ventricular hypertrophy in advanced heartworm disease. Tests used to detect antifilarial host antibody are the ELISA and IFA assay. These tests are not satisfactory for screening purposes because they are usually negative when microfilariae are numerous. The IFA assay is for host antibody to microfilarial cuticular antigen.

In the ELISA, a semipurified antigen derived from adult parasites is used to bind antifilarial antibody. A significant rise in antibody titer occurs about 3 months after infection and reaches a peak at patency in 6 to 7 months. The ELISA is very sensitive and can detect antibody against *D. immitis* even in lightly infected dogs. The test can be useful in identifying dogs with occult heartworm disease and has a strong negative predictive value; that is, occult dirofilariasis can be almost positively excluded when antibody is not detected by the ELISA.

The development of monoclonal antibodies to *D. immitis* antigen coupled with ELISA testing has made *D. immitis* antigen screening clinically feasible. Antigen detection is the preferred method of serodiagnostic testing for *D. immitis* infection.

Both host antibody and parasite antigen can be used to evaluate the efficiency of treatment of adult *D. immitis* infection. After successful treatment, antigen to *D. immitis* disappears from the serum within 12 weeks and positive antibody titers may remain for up to 8 months.

■ CLASSIFICATION OF CANINE HEARTWORM DISEASE

Class 1—Asymptomatic to mild. Patients with mild disease may have such vague or nonspecific signs as general loss of body condition, fatigue during exercise, or occasional cough; however, no definitive radiographic signs, anemia, or other abnormal laboratory findings are present.

Class 2—Moderate heartworm disease. Radiographic signs, mild anemia (packed cell volume between 20% and 30%), or other hematologic abnormalities are evident. Mild proteinuria (2+) may be present. Radiographic signs may include enlargement of the right ventricle, slight enlargement of the pulmonary artery, or circumscribed perivascular densities plus mixed alveolar or interstitial lesions. History and physical examination findings may be normal or may include general loss of condition, fatigue during exercise, or occasional cough. The patient may need to be stabilized before treatment.

Class 3—Severe heartworm disease. Prognosis is guarded. Patients may exhibit cardiac cachexia (wasting), constant fatigue, persistent cough, dyspnea, or other signs associated with enlargement of the right side of the heart. On radiographs, the pulmonary artery may be severely enlarged and there may be circumscribed to chronic mixed patterns and diffuse patterns of pulmonary density or signs of thromboembolism. Significant anemia (packed cell volume <20%) or other hematologic abnormalities may be present. Proteinuria (>2+) may be present. A case is categorized as class 3 if clinical signs are moderate and laboratory or radiographic alterations are significant if clinical signs are significant but laboratory or radiographic alterations are moderate. Patients with class 3 disease should be stabilized before treatment and then given the alternate dose regimen.

Class 4—Caval syndrome in dogs with severe pulmonary hypertension when the worm burden exceeds 60 worms. Because of retrograde migration, 55% to 84% of these worms reside in the cranial and caudal venae cavae and the right atrium. The worm mass interferes with the tricuspid valve and causes tricuspid insufficiency with resultant systolic murmur, jugular pulsations, elevated central venous pressure, and dramatically decreased cardiac output. Hemolytic anemia, disseminated intravascular coagulation, hemoglobinemia, hemoglobinuria, and hepatic and renal dysfunction are common sequelae. Prognosis is poor unless the worms are removed from the right atrium and venae cavae.

Cats are also susceptible to heartworm disease. The frequency of the disease is correlated with the dog population in an area. In cats, only 1% to 25% of the infective larvae develop into adults. Heartworm infection in cats may be by singular sex infections (approximately one third of infections). The occult nature of the disease in cats makes diagnosis difficult.

Most cats with heartworm disease are presented in the late summer or early fall. Clinical signs in cats may be acute, characterized by collapse, dyspnea, convulsions, vomiting, diarrhea, tachycardia, and syncope. More chronic signs of heartworm disease may include coughing, dyspnea, lethargy, and increased bronchovesicular sounds with systolic murmur. Respiratory signs are reported in 50% of the cases. A dorsoventral view on radiographs for cats is best to evaluate caudal lobar arteries. Radiographic signs are characterized by alveolar infiltration of the middle and caudal lung lobes, generalized interstitial pattern in the lungs, right ventricular cardiac enlargement, and enlargement of the right caudal pulmonary arteries. The most consistent laboratory signs are hyperglobulinemia and eosinophilia (one third of affected cats have eosinophilia). The presence of glomerulonephropathy in cats with heartworms is high. Occult dirofilariasis appears to be common. Only 20% of cats with *D. immitis* may have circulating microfilariae. Both the serologic IFA-microfilaria slide test and the ELISA are useful in detecting prepatent or nonpatent infection.

A feline heartworm ELISA antibody test for circulating IgG antibodies to a specific heartworm antigen has been developed. A positive result indicates the animal was infected with *D. immitis* at least 50 to 60 days ago. Cats have the ability to spontaneously clear heartworms, and infection with heartworms in cats should be confirmed with the aid of additional tests such as clinical evaluation and radiographs.

Adult antigen (ELISA) screening in cats is often positive; however, a negative test does not rule out heartworm disease. A differential diagnosis in cats should include infestation with *Aelurostrongylus abstrusus, Paragonimus kellicotti,* asthma, and cardiomyopathy.

The American Heartworm Society is recommending the use of heartworm prophylaxis in cats in endemic heartworm areas. Milbemycin can be used monthly at the same dosage used for dogs, whereas ivermectin is used at four times the regular dog dosage. A new medication, melarsomine dihyrochloride (Immidicide, Merial, Ltd, Iselin, NJ), has been developed for treating heartworms. Indications for use are the same as for sodium thiacetarsemide. Melarsomine is administered by two deep IM injections 24 hours apart in the two paralumbar muscles. It must be administered with small-gauge needle deep into the muscle. Injections may cause pain on injection. The dose is 2.5 mg/kg (1 mL/10 kg).

Microfilaricide therapy is begun 3 weeks after the administration of melarsomine. A single oral dose of ivermectin 0.05 mg/kg is administered in the hospital with the animal observed for side effects in the hospital for 1 day. If adverse reactions develop they will usually develop 5 to 10 hours after administration.

Dogs should be rechecked for microfilaria 1 week after treatment. If negative, a regimen of heartworm prevention is begun. If results of the test are positive, then ivermectin is repeated and the dog is returned in another week for microfilaria testing.

············ *OLLULANUS TRICUSPIS* (GASTRIC NEMATODE IN CATS)

Persistent vomiting in cats may be associated with parasitism by *Ollulanus.* This is a minute nematode whose life cycle is viviparous, with the third- and fourth-stage larvae and adults existing in the host's stomach and expelled in vomitus. The parasites cause chronic gastritis. The parasites are 0.8 to 1.0 mm long and can be recognized when vomitus is examined with a dissecting microscope. *Aelurostrongylus* parasite infection may cause similar clinical signs, but the larvae migrate or are coughed up in the trachea, are swallowed, and are then passed in the feces. *Aelurostrongylus* adults are much larger than *Ollulanus* adults.

············ *PLATYNOSUM CONCINNUM* (LIVER FLUKE)

In the southern United States, and especially in southern Florida and in Hawaii, the digenetic trematode *Platynosum* may infect the liver of cats. In stray cats and "ranging" feral cats that have access to the intermediate hosts—land snails, lizards, and toads—the incidence may be as high as 50%. The adult flukes are 1.1 mm wide and 2.7 mm long, and their eggs are 30 to 40 μm in size. Infected cats develop fibrotic livers, portal fibrosis, and biliary epithelial hyperplasia and become chronically debilitated and icteric, signs associated with chronic liver disease.

The drug of choice for treatment at this time appears to be albendazole.

■ FORMALIN-ETHER SEDIMENTATION TECHNIQUE FOR DETECTING PLATYNOSUM

1. Mix 1 g of feces in 25 mL saline; filter through a fine-mesh screen.
2. Centrifuge solution for 5 minutes at 155 rpm; discard supernate.
3. Resuspend the pellet in the bottom of the tube with 7 mL of 10% neutral formalin; let stand 10 minutes.
4. Shake vigorously for 1 minute; centrifuge for 3 minutes at 1500 rpm.
5. Discard supernate, resuspend pellet in several drops of saline, and prepare slide.

Adapted from Bielsa LM, Greiner EC: Liver flukes *(Platynosum concinnum)* in cats. J Anim Hosp Assoc 21:269–274, 1985.

REFERENCES

Atkins CE: Feline cardiovascular disease: Therapeutic considerations. *In* Proceedings of the 14th Annual Forum of the American College of Veterinary Internal Medicine, San Antonio, 1996, p 175.
Bielsa LM, Greiner EC: Liver flukes *(Platynosum concinnum)* in cats. J Am Anim Hosp Assoc 21:269–274, 1985.
Bowman DD: Georgis' Parasitology for Veterinarians, ed 7. Philadelphia, WB Saunders, 1999.
Brunner CJ, Hendrix C, Blagburn B, et al: Comparison of serologic tests for detection of antigen in canine heartworm infections. J Am Vet Med Assoc 192:1423–1427, 1988.
Calvert CA: Heartworm disease. *In* Miller MS, Tilley LP, eds: Manual of Canine and Feline Cardiology, ed 2. Philadelphia, WB Saunders, 1995, pp 225–259.
Egerton JR, Eary CH, Suhayda D: Use of ivermectin against *Ancylostoma caninum* and *Uncinaria stenocephala* infections. Am J Vet Res 46:1057, 1985.
Fox S, Burns J, Hawkins J: Spirocercosis in the dog. Compend Contin Educ Pract Vet 10:807–822, 1988.
Grieve R (ed): Parasitic infections. Vet Clin North Am Small Anim Pract 17(6):1987.
Holmes RA: Feline dirofilariasis. Vet Clin North Am Small Anim Pract 23:125, 1993.
Hoskins J: Canine heartworm disease. Compend Contin Educt Pract Vet 18:348, 1996.
Jenkins CC, Lewis DD, Brock K: Extrahepatic biliary obstruction associated with *Platynosum concinnum* in a cat. Compend Contin Educ Pract Vet 10:628, 1988.
Kilpatrick CE, Edward A: Paragonimiasis in a dog: Treatment with praziquantel. J Am Vet Med Assoc 187:75, 1985.
Knight DH: Guidelines for diagnosis and management of heartworm infection. *In* Kirk RW, Bonagura JD, eds: Current Veterinary Therapy XII. Philadelphia, WB Saunders, 1995, pp 879–887.
Rawlings C, McCall J: Melarsomine: A new heartworm adulticide. Compend Contin Educ Pract Vet 18:373, 1996.
Ware W: Heartworm disease. *In* Nelson RW, Couto GC, eds: Essentials of Small Animal Internal Medicine. St Louis, Mosby–Year Book, 1992.
Zanotti S, Kaplan P: Feline dirofilariasis. Compend Contin Educ Pract Vet 11:1005–1015, 1989.

·········· COCCIDIOSIS

Included in the subclass Coccidia are the genera *Isospora, Eimeria, Sarcocystis, Cryptosporidium, Besnoitia, Hammondia,* and *Toxoplasma. Isospora bigemina,*

Isospora rivolta, and *Isospora felis* are the three common types of organisms causing coccidiosis in the United States.

Coccidiosis usually affects young dogs and cats, especially those from kennels, pet shops, catteries, or other places where large numbers of animals are kept together.

Infection of the host results from ingestion of infective oocysts. The coccidia undergo repeated cycles of asexual multiplication (schizogony) that finally terminate in the formation of sexually differentiated gametes that combine to form zygotes. At this stage, a protective covering is formed (oocyst). Sporulation (sporogony) may occur in the intestinal tract or after the oocyst is eliminated in the feces. In the genus *Isospora*, there are two sporocysts, each containing four sporozoites.

⋯⋯⋯⋯ Diagnosis

Diagnosis is based on finding oocysts in the feces coupled with the clinical history. The diarrhea may precede a heavy outpouring of oocysts by a few days and may continue even after oocyst levels become low. It is, therefore, not always possible to confirm a clinical diagnosis of coccidiosis by finding oocysts in the feces. Other intestinal parasites and systemic diseases such as distemper may also complicate the picture.

⋯⋯⋯⋯ TOXOPLASMOSIS

Cats and other Felidae family members are the only definitive hosts for *Toxoplasma gondii*. *Toxoplasma* is an intestinal coccidian of cats, with a wide range of intermediate hosts. Cats, especially kittens younger than 6 months of age, can become infected and shed *Toxoplasma* oocysts after eating mice, rats, birds, or meat containing *Toxoplasma* cysts. Cats can acquire infection by ingesting any of three infectious stages of *Toxoplasma*: tachyzoites, bradyzoites in the encysted form in muscle tissue, and oocysts or zygotes found within the feces of definitive hosts. Fewer than 50% of cats shed oocysts after ingesting cysts. The prepatent period to the shedding of oocysts is 3 to 5 days after the ingestion of mice or meat containing *Toxoplasma* cysts and 20 to 34 days after the ingestion of oocysts. Oocysts are shed by infected cats for 1 to 5 weeks during primary infection and in reduced numbers or not at all following reinfection. The oocysts are not infectious until sporulation, which requires 1 to 5 days (or longer, depending on environmental temperature and oxygenation). Under favorable circumstances, oocysts remain infectious for several months to a year or longer.

The oocysts of *Toxoplasma* develop two sporocysts and four sporozoites. *Isospora felis* and *Isospora rivolta* are the two common coccidian parasites found in young cats. The oocysts of *I. felis* measure 40 by 30 μm and those of *I. rivolta*, 25 by 20 μm. Oocysts of *Toxoplasma* are much smaller, 10 by 12 μm, or about twice the size of an RBC.

Standard techniques of fecal flotation at specific gravity of 1.15 will concentrate the oocysts in the supernatent. Cats infected with *Toxoplasma* shed oocysts for only a 2-week period; finding oocysts in cat feces during this limited time period is unlikely.

From serologic evidence, it appears that humans and animals can suffer from asymptomatic infections with *Toxoplasma* organisms. *Toxoplasma* antibodies have been found in varying percentages of cats, depending on the types of populations tested. Forty percent to 60% of cats in the Kansas-Iowa area had *Toxoplasma* antibodies, and reports indicate that 24% to 57% of dogs in the United States have *Toxoplasma* antibodies.

Clinical signs in cats depend on the cat's age at the time of infection, the cat's immune status, and the route of infection. In utero infection may result in pneumonitis, myocarditis, retinitis, and chronic encephalitis.

Confirmation of *Toxoplasma* infection can be based on serologic evidence or isolation of *Toxoplasma* organisms by inoculating tissues into mice. Serologic examination should be done with paired serum samples taken 1 or 2 weeks apart.

The most specific of the tests is the IgM ELISA. IgM is detectable in serum by ELISA in approximately 80% of subclinically ill cats within 4 weeks following experimental induction by toxoplasmosis. These titers are generally negative after 16 weeks of infection. Toxoplasmosis titers greater than 1:256 have been detected within the first 12 weeks of infection. Persistent IgM titers greater than 12 weeks have been documented in cats coinfected with FIV virus. IgG can be detected in serum of *Toxoplasma*-infected cats 3 weeks following infection. Titers generally last for years following infection. A single sample for IgG only indicates previous exposure, not recent or active disease.

Based on currently available serologic procedures (ELISA, Diagnostic Laboratory, Colorado State University), the following results are consistent with, but not diagnostic of, recent or active infection with *T. gondii* in cats:

1. Fourfold or greater increase in IgG antibody titer over 2 to 3 weeks
2. IgM antibody titer greater than 1:256
3. Positive serum antigen test with negative serum antibody tests
4. Positive serum immune complex tests with negative serum antibody tests

The presence of IgG antibody against *Toxoplasma* does not mean that a cat is currently infected or in need of treatment. Immune cats are safer pets than nonimmune cats because, on reinfection, they shed few or no oocysts. Clinical diagnosis of toxoplasmosis can be detected by the following four diagnostic criteria:

1. Demonstration of serologic evidence of infection
2. Clinical signs of disease referable to toxoplasmosis
3. Exclusion of other common causes
4. Positive response to appropriate treatment

REFERENCES

Dubey JP: Toxoplasmosis. Vet Clin North Am Small Anim Pract 17:1389–1404, 1987.

Frenkel JK: Transmission of toxoplasmosis and the role of immunity in limiting transmission and illness. J Am Vet Med Assoc 196:233–240, 1990.

Greene CE: Infectious Diseases of the Dog and Cat, ed 2. Philadelphia, WB Saunders, 1998.

Greene CE, Lappin MA: Feline toxoplasmosis: New diagnostic and therapeutic implications. Feline Med 5:22–24, 1988.

Lappin M: CVT update: Feline toxoplasmosis. *In* Bonagura JD, ed: Kirk's Current Veterinary Therapy XII. Philadelphia, WB Saunders, 1995, p 309.

Lappin M, Greene C, Winston S, et al: Clinical feline toxoplasmosis. J Vet Intern Med 3:139–143, 1989.

Lappin MR: Feline toxoplasmosis: Interpretation of diagnostic test results. Semin Vet Med Surg 11:154–160, 1996.

Wilson M, Ware D, Juranek D: Serologic aspects of toxoplasmosis. J Am Vet Med Assoc 196:277–280, 1990.

············ GIARDIASIS

Giardia species are flagellate protozoan parasites. The trophozoite is the active feeding stage of the parasite, and the cyst is the dormant resistant stage. The trophozoites are teardrop-shaped, are bilaterally symmetrical, and measure 15 mm long, 10 mm wide, and 3 mm thick. Organelles consist of four pairs of flagella, two nuclei, axonemes, and microtubules.

The life cycle of *Giardia* is direct, with the prepatent period being 5 to 16 days. Infection with *Giardia* occurs when the host ingests the cyst stage of the parasite (direct life cycle, no intermediate host needed). Excystation occurs in the duodenum, and maturation of the trophozoite occurs in the upper small intestine of the dog and lower small intestine of the cat. Trophozoites attach to the brush borders of the villous epithelium, and reproduction is by binary fission. Cyst formation can occur 5 to 10 days following onset of infection. Clinical signs are acute small bowel diarrhea, occasional chronic large bowel diarrhea, and intermittent vomiting.

............Diagnosis

Diagnosis is based on finding cysts or trophozoites in the feces. Two techniques advocated for diagnosis are the direct smear and the modified zinc sulfate concentration technique. On initial examination of direct fecal smears, positive results are obtained in only 20% of cases; repeated examinations at 3-day intervals increase the known positives to 43%. In the zinc sulfate technique, 15 to 20 g of feces are mixed with tap water in a small paper cup to achieve a suspension. The suspension is placed through a wire-mesh screen and centrifuged in a 15-mL tube for 10 minutes at 400 *g*. The sediment is resuspended with zinc sulfate solution of specific gravity 1.18. The tube is centrifuged in a swing-head centrifuge or placed in a fixed-head centrifuge at 1500 rpm for 5 minutes. A hanging drop on a coverslip with either technique is examined by phase microscopy for evidence of cysts or trophozoites.

Treatment involves the systemic (PO) administration of metronidazole (Flagyl, G.D. Searle, Chicago) or albendazole at 25 mg/kg PO q12h for four doses.

REFERENCES

Barr SC, Bowman DD, Erb H: Evaluation of two test procedures for the diagnosis of giardiasis in dogs. Am J Vet Res 53:2028, 1992.
Barr SC, Bowman DD, Erb HN, et al: Albendazole efficacy against *Giardia* infections in dogs (abstract). Am Coll Vet Intern Med 7:131, 1993.
Bowman DD: Georgis' Parasitology for Veterinarians, ed 7. Philadelphia, WB Saunders, 1999.
Dubey JP: Intestinal protozoa infections. Vet Clin North Am Small Anim Pract 23:37–55, 1993.
Kirkpatrick CE: Giardiasis. Vet Clin North Am Small Anim Pract 17:1377–1387, 1987.
Leib M: Giardiasis. *In* Proceedings of the 10th Annual Forum of the American College of Veterinary Internal Medicine, San Diego, 1992, pp 78–79.
Zimmer JF, Burrington DG: Comparison of four protocols for the treatment of canine giardiasis. J Am Anim Hosp Assoc, 22:161–167, 1986.

5

FECAL SAMPLE COLLECTION AND EXAMINATION

............COLLECTION

Fresh fecal samples should always be used. Closed 2- to 4-oz containers are best suited for fecal collections. Fecal samples can be picked up with disposable wooden tongue blades after the animal defecates, or they can be taken directly from the rectum. An enema may be administered; however, soapy or oily enemas should not be used because they interfere with examination of the stool. Material left on thermometers is not usually adequate for fecal examinations except in a few heavy parasitic infestations. If samples must be kept for a few hours to several days, refrigeration or chemical fixation should be used. Refrigeration at 4°C preserves eggs and larvae for up to 72 hours. Formalin may be added to fecal specimens, one part 10% formalin to four parts fecal specimen, to preserve parasitic material.

...........GROSS EXAMINATION

Examine the stool for adult worms or tapeworm segments. Note the presence of blood, mucus, fat, or other undigested material. Characterize the odor of the stool. Note the amount of stool passed, and observe whether it is formed on unformed. Fecal volume is determined by the content of water and fiber. Normal feces contain 60% to 70% water. The volume of formed feces in a 15-kg dog should be about 40 mL/day (Guilford et al.). The longer the total gastrointestinal passage time, the firmer the feces. If the stool is formed, note its shape and diameter.

...........COLOR

Feces are usually brown in color due to the pigments urobilin and stercobilin derived from the bacterial action of bilirubin. A dark-brown to black tarry stool can indicate that the animal is on a high-meat diet or that there are blood pigments in the stool from upper gastrointestinal bleeding. Excessive amounts of bilirubin may produce a darker orange-brown stool. Charcoal and bismuth can produce black feces, whereas sulfobromophthalein causes the feces to be purple. A grayish-white, clay-colored stool is associated with biliary obstruction and pancreatic acinar insufficiency. A light-brown or tan-colored stool is frequently seen in nursing puppies or dogs on a diet high in milk. A very white or acholic stool can be associated with an absence of bile pigments, overt bacterial infections of the gastrointestinal tract, or diarrhea with rapid passage of material through the intestinal tract. A green stool may be seen in dogs with unchanged bilirubin in the stool. Fresh red blood in the stool indicates recent bleeding into the colon or rectum.

...........MUCUS

Normal stools contain only a small amount of mucus, which may not be easily observed. Excess mucus in the stool is a sign of lower bowel disease and is associated with acute and chronic inflammatory disease of the terminal ileum, cecum, and colon.

...........ODOR

Odor is produced by indole and skatole, which are products of bacterial action on tryptophan. Byproducts of the breakdown of sulfur-containing amino acids and hydrogen sulfide also contribute to the odor. Alterations in the diet or bacterial flora can markedly change fecal odor.

...........MICROSCOPIC EXAMINATION OF THE FECES

...........Smear Technique

The smear technique is used when small quantities of material are available or when the fecal examination must be completed in a short period of time.

The procedure involves mixing a small amount of fecal material in a drop or two of saline on a slide and examining the material microscopically. This method is qualitative and is useful only if positive; a negative result is inconclusive.

............Qualitative Concentration Method

This is the routine method for examination for parasites. The concentration of parasite ova or oocysts may be determined in a number of ways. All the methods depend on mixing the fecal sample with a material whose specific gravity is higher than that of most of the parasitic ova or oocysts and lower than that of the fecal debris. Solutions of sodium chloride, sucrose, glycerine, zinc sulfate, or magnesium sulfate may be used to float the parasitic ova. Sugar flotation, although satisfactory for most parasitic ova, will not float the ova of tapeworms and flukes. Saturated sodium nitrate is routinely used for flotation with canine feces. Tapeworms are most easily diagnosed by gross examination of the feces for the typical segments.

............METHODS FOR PROTOZOAL EXAMINATIONS

The protozoan parasites *Trichomonas, Giardia,* and *Balantidium* disappear rapidly from fecal samples. For these parasites to be identified, the stool must be either examined or placed in a fecal fixative immediately after removal from the rectum. Polyvinyl alcohol is a good fecal fixative. Wet smears are satisfactory in some cases of protozoan infections if the feces can be examined immediately and the infection is heavy. The wet smears can be stained with Lugol's iodine to better visualize *Giardia* cysts. Routine fecal examination with sugar and salt solutions destroys *Giardia* cysts, and they are microscopically unrecognizable. The zinc sulfate centrifugation technique allows *Giardia* cysts to be recognized. The $ZnSO_4$ solution is prepared by mixing 331 g of $ZnSO_4$ in 1 L of warm tap water to a specific gravity of 1.18. Fecal smears stained with iron hematoxylin trichrome, or Giemsa are best for visualizing *Giardia* organisms. Better results are obtained in isolating *Giardia* from dogs when duodenal aspirations are used rather than fecal examinations (88% recovery in duodenal aspirates vs. 39% recovery in a single fecal flotation).

A second technique involving fixed feces provides the advantages of concentration and delayed examination. Prepare PAF fixative: phenol crystals (white), 20 g; normal saline (0.85%), 825.0 mL; ethanol (95%), 125 mL; and formaldehyde solution, 50 mL (23 mL of liquefied phenol may be substituted for the crystals). Cover the fresh feces with the PAF fixative, and allow them to stand at room temperature for 1 hour or longer. Strain the fixed sample through gauze, and then centrifuge the collected fluid at 1000 rpm for 2 or 3 minutes. Decant the excess fluid, and wash and centrifuge the sediment twice with normal saline. Stain several drops of the sediment with thionin or azure A to permit easy identification. If concentration is not desired, examine the sediment directly from the fixed feces.

............Methods for *Strongyloides* Examination

The rhabditiform larvae of *Strongyloides stercoralis* can be found in smears prepared from fresh feces. These larvae can easily be confused with other larval parasites and can be definitively identified by incubating the fecal specimen for 24 hours at room temperature or by culturing the feces on sterile sand for 48 hours. The infective filariform larvae will develop and can be identified by the esophageal length (one-third the total body length). A Baermann apparatus may also be used for examination of the larvae.

The feces should also be examined for the presence of undigested muscle (creatorrhea), fat (steatorrhea), or starch (amylorrhea) and for the presence or absence of pancreatic proteolytic enzymes. Fat droplets are demonstrated with a Sudan III stain. Muscle fibers are seen microscopically in direct fecal smears. One drop of Lugol's solution will turn undigested starch blue. Fecal trypsin can be identified by using the film strip digestion test or the more accurate gelatin tube test.

REFERENCES

Bowman DD: Georgis' Parasitology for Veterinarians, ed 7. Philadelphia, WB Saunders, 1999.
Guilford WG, Center SA, Strombeck DR, et al: Strombeck's Small Animal Gastroenterology, ed 3. Philadelphia, WB Saunders, 1996.
Kirkpatrick C, Farrell JP: Giardiasis. Compend Contin Educ Pract Vet 4:367, 1982.

...........SPECIFIC TESTS FOR EVALUATION OF GASTROINTESTINAL FUNCTION

...........Fecal Weight

Twenty-four-hour fecal weight depends on the nature of the diet and the fluid content of the feces. Dogs fed dry dog food have bulkier, softer feces that weigh roughly twice as much as the feces from dogs fed canned dog food that contains 70% water, most of which is absorbed in the gastrointestinal tract. To attempt to standardize fecal weight against a norm, feed the dog a canned meat-based dog food, 50 g/kg of body weight, once daily for 2 or 3 days; then make a 24-hour collection, weigh the feces, and divide by the weight of dog in kilograms.

...........Exocrine Pancreatic Function and Insufficiency
(see also p. 645)

Exocrine pancreatic insufficiency (EPI) in the dog is typically due to pancreatic acinar atrophy. It occurs in many purebred and mixed-breed dogs but is most common in German shepherds, in which there is a genetic predisposition to the disease. Clinical signs of EPI depend on the duration, nature, and severity of the condition but usually include degrees of polyphagia, weight loss, and voluminous, semiformed feces. Affected dogs usually are not depressed or lethargic and do not show signs of systemic disease.

In the gelatin tube test, two tubes containing 2 mL of 7.5% gelatin are warmed to 37°C to liquefy the gelatin. To one tube, 2 mL of a feces mixture is added, and to both tubes, 2 mL of 5% sodium bicarbonate is added. Incubate both tubes at 37°C for 1 hour, and refrigerate for 20 minutes. Failure to gel indicates the presence of trypsin, which has digested the gelatin.

Feces can be evaluated for proteolytic enzyme activity by using the "film test" to detect digestion of the gelatin in the film emulsion and the gelatin tube test to detect digestion of the gelatin.

These tests usually identify animals with complete loss of pancreatic exocrine function. False-positive results (identifying animals as having no proteolytic enzymes) may occur because pancreatic enzymes can be destroyed by intestinal bacteria and autodigestion. These tests are not very accurate, and the canine serum trypsin-like immunoreactivity (TLI) test is the recommended test for the diagnosis of EPI.

...........*Serum Trypsin-like Immunoreactivity Test*

The TLI test gives the concentration of proteins recognized by antibodies against the pancreatic digestive enzyme trypsin. The cationic isoenzyme levels of trypsinogen in normal dogs range from 5 to 35 µg/L. Pancreatic acinar atrophy can result in TLI levels less than 2.5 µg/L. The enzyme is stable in serum, and samples can be shipped to diagnostic laboratories without any special preservatives.

············Serum Trypsin-like Immunoreactivity Test in the Cat

Pancreatitis is the most common condition of the feline exocrine pancreas. RIA for feline serum trypsin-like immunoreactivity shows the control value of 17 to 49 µg/L. Serum TLI concentration in cats showing evidence of acute pancreatitis ranged from 14.8 to 540 µg/L, with a mean of 100 µg/L.

············Fecal Fat

The presence of excessive amounts of fat in the feces (steatorrhea) can be a prominent sign of a severe gastrointestinal disturbance, such as malabsorption. The normal dog excretes 3 to 5 g of fat in the stool per day, and the amount excreted is not greatly affected by normal dietary intake of fat.

Steatorrhea can be demonstrated by staining a fresh stool with a lipophilic stain such as Sudan II and examining the material under the microscope. Levels of split and unsplit fats in fecal samples can be detected with Sudan III. Mix a 3-mm-diameter pellet of fecal material with a drop of 36% acetic acid on a glass slide. Add one drop of Sudan III stain, apply a coverslip, and pass the slide over a Bunsen burner or alcohol lamp, bringing the mixture to a boil three times. Under the microscope, split fats will appear as orange globules when cooled. When 10 or more globules of fat 20 µm or larger are seen per high-power field, the test is positive for split fats.

CAUSES OF STEATORRHEA

Maldigestion
Exocrine pancreatic insufficiency
   Pancreatic atrophy
   Chronic pancreatitis
   Pancreatic duct obstruction
Hepatobiliary disease
   Liver failure
   Intrahepatic cholestasis
   Extrahepatic cholestasis

Malabsorption
   Inflammatory bowel disease
   Neoplasia of the small intestine
   Lymphangiectasia

············Fat Absorption and Excretion Tests

To perform a gross fat absorption test (plasma turbidity test), draw a heparinized blood sample from a fasted animal and separate the plasma. Feed the animal a meal enriched with corn oil (2 mL/kg) or peanut oil (0.5 to 2.0 mL/kg). An alternative product is Lipomul (Pharmacia & Upjohn, Inc., Kalamazoo, MI.) 2 to 3 mL/kg. Take a second blood sample 2 hours after the ingestion of the fat meal, and compare plasma turbidity between pre- and postfat ingestion samples. If the blood sample is not lipemic after 2 hours, wait 4 hours and take a second blood sample. In the normal situation, the second plasma sample shows increased turbidity because of neutral fat droplets or chylomicrons. If both plasma samples are clear, either pancreatic exocrine function is inadequate or the intestine is not absorbing nutrients properly. Pancreatic exocrine insufficiency can be eliminated by repeating the test but predigesting the fat meal with pancreatic extracts. If the second sample of plasma still remains clear, a diagnosis of malabsorption should be considered.

............D-Xylose Absorption Test

The D-xylose absorption test measures the ability of the proximal jejunum to absorb five-carbon sugar. The rate at which xylose is absorbed is determined by the amount administered, the rate of gastric emptying, the size of the area of absorption in the small intestine, and the intestinal circulation. For adequate evaluation of the test, the gastric emptying time should be normal. The major defects leading to abnormal xylose absorption are abnormalities in mucosal absorption area and circulation. Lymphangiectasia has no effect on xylose absorption. Fast the patient for 24 hours, and empty the patient's bladder prior to the administration of D-xylose. Administer a 10% to 25% solution of D-xylose at 500 mg/kg in 200 mL of warm water by stomach tube. Collect all urine for the next 5 hours; the bladder must be rinsed on final collection. Collection of 8 to 12 g of D-xylose can indicate a malabsorption problem. Kidney function must be normal for accurate interpretation of this test. Serum xylose levels can also be measured. Measurement in serum may be preferable to measurement in urine. Blood samples are taken every 30 minutes for 3 hours. Peak D-xylose concentrations at 60 to 90 minutes are 60 to 70 mg/dL. In the normal dog, serum xylose levels peak between 1 and 2 hours after administration (mean concentration, 142 mg/dL). Values at 30 minutes range from 25 to 160 mg/dL. At 1 hour, serum levels of D-xylose are 63 ± 12 mg/mL. Values less than 45 mg/dL after 1 hour are considered abnormal. A control dog (normal) should be evaluated with the animal being tested.

The D-xylose absorption test's sensitivity and specificity may be as high as 98% and 95% respectively. However, the test is influenced by nonintestinal disorders, and the absorption curves can be underestimated if there is pancreatic insufficiency or bacterial overgrowth. D-Xylose is decreased in its clearance if there is renal failure.

The oral glucose tolerance test measures the ability of the proximal jejunum to absorb a six-carbon sugar (see p. 645).

............Serum Cobalamin (Vitamin B$_{12}$)

Serum cobalamin is a water-soluble vitamin found in large amounts in canine diets. Small intestinal disease involving the ileum may lead to a functional loss of cobalamin–intrinsic factor receptors on enterocytes leading to malabsorption. Small intestinal bacterial overgrowth (SIBO) may lead to low serum cobalamin concentrations. Pancreatic deficiency may lead to low levels of cobalamin absorption. Absorption of cobalamin in dogs occurs via specific receptors located exclusively in the distal small intestine. Cobalamin malabsorption can produce subnormal serum levels when malabsorption is severe and body stores of vitamin B$_{12}$ are depleted. Pancreatic function must be normal for cobalamin to be absorbed; therefore, both pancreatic acinar atrophy and small intestinal disease can produce low levels of vitamin B$_{12}$. There are various assay procedures for cobalamin. Normal levels should be established for individual laboratories. Normal levels established by competitive binding assay are in the range of 300 to 800 ng/L.

............Serum Folate

Folate is a water-soluble vitamin. It is dependent upon intestinal mucosa deconjugase to increase availability for receptor-mediated absorption. These enzymes and receptors are found primarily in the proximal small intestine with little folate absorption taking place in the small intestine. Decreases are seen with proximal small intestinal disease. SIBO leads to increased production of folate by bacterial folate synthesis. Folate is absorbed in the proximal (jejunal) small intestine. Serum folate concentrations can increase in dogs with bacterial overgrowth as a result of folate synthesis by abnormal microflora. Serum folate levels can be assayed by a number of techniques, and normal levels for individual laboratories should be obtained. Normal levels obtained by competitive binding assay range from 7.5 to 17.5 µg/L.

⋯⋯⋯Vitamin A Absorption Test

The oral vitamin A absorption test measures the ability of the intestine to digest and absorb lipids. Administer 300,000 units of vitamin A (White's cod liver oil concentrate drops) to the fasting dog. Collect heparinized blood samples prior to administration and after 2, 4, 6, 8, and 24 hours. Mean fasting vitamin A concentrations in serum range from 112 to 278 µg/dL. Normal dogs show a two- or threefold increase in vitamin A levels. A flat curve may indicate lack of bile or pancreatic enzymes, malabsorption, or disease of the ileum.

⋯⋯⋯Iodine 131–Labeled-Triolein Test

Another test for lipid absorption involves PO administration of ^{131}I-labeled triolein. On the day before the test, administer 0.3 mL of Lugol's iodine in a capsule PO to block thyroidal uptake of the ^{131}I label. On the day of the test administer 30 µCi of ^{131}I-labeled triolein. Collect blood samples at 2, 4, 6, 8, and 10 hours. Normal dogs show 8% to 15% absorption after a 10-hour period.

The same test can be performed with oral administration of ^{131}I-labeled oleic acid instead of triolein. Normal values are 10% to 15% absorption in 10 hours.

Performing the ^{131}I triolein and oleic acid tests in sequence aids in differentiating steatorrhea. In steatorrhea associated with lack of pancreatic lipase, absorption of oleic acid will be normal; however, absorption of triolein, which requires lipolysis, will be reduced. The absorption of both compounds is reduced in malabsorption syndrome. Absorption of oleic acid may also be reduced in cases of longstanding pancreatic insufficiency.

REFERENCES

Batt RM: Exocrine pancreatic insufficiency. Vet Clin North Am Small Anim Pract 23:595, 1993.
Guilford WG, Center SA, Strombeck DR, et al: Strombeck's Small Animal Gastroenterology, ed 3. Philadelphia, WB Saunders, 1996.
Jacobs RM, Norris AM, Lumsden JH, et al: Laboratory diagnosis of malassimilation. Vet Clin North Am Small Anim Pract 19:951, 1989.
Ludlow C: Methods for testing small intestinal function. Veterinary Medicine, October 1995, pp 934–948.
Steiner J: Feline trypsinlike immunoreactivity in feline exocrine pancreatic disease. Compend Contin Educ Pract Vet 18:543, 1996.
Steiner J, Williams DA: Feline exocrine pancreatic disorders: Insufficiency, neoplasia and uncommon conditions. Compend Contin Educ Pract Vet 19:836, 1997.
Tams T: Handbook of Small Animal Gastroenterology. Chronic Diseases of the Small Intestine. Small Intestinal Bacterial Overgrowth. Philadelphia, WB Saunders, 1996.
Willard M: Disorders of the intestinal tract. In Nelson RW, Cuoto CG, eds: Essentials of Small Animal Internal Medicine. St Louis, Mosby–Year Book, 1992, pp 334–359.
Williams D: Feline TLI—An update. In Proceedings of 14th Forum of the American College of Veterinary Internal Medicine, 1996, p 141.

5

••

EXAMINATION OF FLUIDS

All serous cavities and tissue spaces of the body contain a small amount of fluid. Under normal circumstances, this fluid consists of a low protein blood filtrate. Abnormal amounts of fluid in body cavities are termed *effusions*. Aspirates of these fluids are studied in an attempt to classify the origin of the fluids as transudative (a noninflammatory accumulation of fluid associated with physiochemical disturbance) or exudative (an accumulation of fluid associated with an inflammatory response). Not all body fluids can be strictly classified as transudates or exudates. Transudates that are longstanding can be transformed into modified transudates by the accumulation of inflammatory cells, chemotactic substances, and increased protein levels.

••••••••••••PHYSICAL EXAMINATION

1. Measure the volume of fluid removed.
2. Evaluate the fluid for color and transparency.
   a. A pinkish to reddish color usually indicates the presence of erythrocytes.
   b. A yellowish color is imparted by excessive bilirubin, a high protein content, or degenerated erythrocytes.
   c. A milky-white color may indicate chyle (see also p. 248). If the cloudiness of the fluid is caused by the presence of chylomicrons, the fluid will clear upon adding ether and shaking.
   d. A thick, creamy fluid usually indicates the presence of a large number of leukocytes.
3. Note whether the fluid coagulates. The ability to clot is dependent on the amount of fibrin present. Exudates may show rapid coagulation, whereas transudates usually do not coagulate. Lysis of the clot may occur in exudates and may not be demonstrated.
4. Determine the specific gravity of the fluid. In general, the specific gravity is closely correlated with the protein content of the fluid. If a refractometer is used to measure specific gravity, a specific gravity of 1.020 is approximately equivalent to 3 g/dL of protein, with an additional 1 g/dL of protein increasing specific gravity 0.0004 unit. Attempt to characterize the fluid as representing a transudate, modified transudate, septic exudate, nonseptic exudate, chylous effusion, neoplastic effusion, or hemorrhage.
5. Smell the fluid. Puncture fluids are usually odorless unless contaminated by putrefying bacterial organisms such as *Escherichia coli* from the intestinal tract or urine from a ruptured bladder.

••••••••••••CHEMICAL EXAMINATION
••••••••••••Seromucin Test

This test can be used to help distinguish a transudate from an exudate. Exudates are usually seromucin-positive, and transudates are usually seromucin-negative.

••••••••••••Total Proteins

Exudates usually have a high protein content (>3 g/dL); transudates usually have a lower total protein content. Animals with diseases that cause low plasma proteins, especially albumin, may develop abdominal effusion, subcutaneous edema, or a combination of these signs. This low protein may develop because the liver fails to synthesize protein or because protein is lost through the skin, intestinal tract, or kidneys. If hypoalbuminemia is the only cause of abdominal effusions, total protein levels are usually less than 1.5 g/dL before fluid accumulates in the abdomen.

............Urea Nitrogen

Urea nitrogen determinations can be used to determine the presence of nitrogenous material within the abdominal cavity in such conditions as rupture of the bladder or to evaluate the efficiency of fluid that has been used in peritoneal dialysis.

A transudate is clear and has a specific gravity of less than 1.017, a protein concentration of less than 2.5 g/dL, and fewer than 500 cells per unit.

A modified transudate has been altered by protein and cells and often appears serosanguineous. The protein concentration is 2.5 g/dL, with 1000 to 5000 cells of mixed population. Effusions associated with right heart failure or neoplasia are usually modified transudates.

Exudates may be nonseptic or septic. Septic exudates are usually more cellular and contain degenerating neutrophils, high protein levels, degenerating RBCs, and infectious organisms. Septic exudates in the abdomen indicate that an exploratory laparotomy is indicated. Prior to an exploratory laparotomy the following additional tests may be helpful in discovering the source of the sepsis:

1. Bilirubin levels of abdominal fluid vs. levels of serum bilirubin
2. Abdominal fluid creatinine vs. serum creatinine
3. Serum triglycerides vs. abdominal fluid triglycerides to evaluate possible chyloperitoneum

............MICROSCOPIC EXAMINATION
............Total Cell Counts

The numbers and types of cells in a fluid will depend on how the fluid accumulated within the body cavity. Pure transudates are usually acellular with small numbers of macrophages and lymphocytes coming from the blood. The accumulation of fluids in body cavities is usually associated with changes in mesothelial lining cells. Mesothelial cells exfoliate, become cuboidal, and increase in size, and their cytoplasm shows strong basophilic staining.

The presence of large numbers of inflammatory cells and an elevated protein content generally characterize an exudate. The presence of polymorphonuclear leukocytes and elevated protein levels in exudative fluid is not always indicative of a septic inflammation. If neutrophils exhibit degenerative morphologic changes (karyolysis, karyorrhexis, and pyknosis), the presence of microorganisms should be suspected.

The following cell types may also be found in pleural and peritoneal effusions:

1. Macrophages can be found in both acute and chronic effusions.
2. Neutrophils are nondegenerative in transudates, nonseptic exudates, and septic exudates in which the etiologic agent is of low toxicity. Neutrophils are degenerative in most severe septic infections.
3. Plasma cells indicate chronicity.
4. Giant cells indicate granulomatous inflammation.
5. Neoplastic cells.
6. Eosinophils, basophils, mast cells, and other cells that have exfoliated from body cavities may be present in exudates or modified exudates.
7. Traumatic or neoplastic rupture of major lymphatic ducts can result in the accumulation of chyle in the pleural or peritoneal cavity. Chyle usually has a milky appearance when removed. Microscopically, chyle contains large numbers of lymphocytes, chylomicrons, and RBCs.

8. Diagnosis in chronic pleuritis, pleural effusion, and pneumonias can be aided by thoracentesis (see p. 620) and fine-needle aspiration biopsy of the lung. The presence of a bloody exudative fluid with yellow flecks or granules may be indicative of nocardial or actinomycotic infection. The granules should be crushed on a microscope slide and examined, and a culture should be obtained of the fluid. In actinomycotic infections, the granules contain gram-positive branching filamentous rods, and *Actinomyces viscosus* is the most common organism isolated from the thoracic cavity of dogs. If a modified acid-fast staining technique is used, *Nocardia* will stain acid-fast and *Actinomyces* will not stain.

·········· Differential Smear

Large numbers of neutrophils indicate a purulent exudate, and one should look for a causative organism. Lymphocytes indicate a chronic exudative or viral reaction. Very young, bizarrely shaped lymphocytes may indicate tumor formation. If an allergy or parasitic problem is causing the formation of an exudate, eosinophils may be found. If a tumor is suspected, examination of cells by a cytologist may prove very helpful in making a diagnosis. Smears should be fixed while still wet with a commercial fixative. These smears can be stained by the method of Papanicolaou or Sano and then examined.

··········BACTERIOLOGIC EXAMINATION

Bacteriologic examination involves the following procedures:

1. Prepare new methylene blue or Gram stains of aspirated material.
2. Culture (see p. 466).
3. Animal inoculations may be indicated.

REFERENCES

Clinkenbeard K, Walker D, Cowell R, et al: Diagnostic cytology: Bacterial infections. *In* Compend Contin Educ Pract Vet 17:71, 1995.
Cowell R: Diagnostic Cytology of the Dog and Cat. St Louis, Mosby–Year Book, 1998.
Cowell RL, Tyler RD, Meinkoth JH: Abdominal and thoracic fluid. *In* Cowell RL, Tyler RD, eds: Diagnostic Cytology of the Dog and Cat. Goleta, Calif, American Veterinary Publications, 1989, pp 151–166.
Meyer DJ, Harvey J: Veterinary Laboratory Medicine, ed 2. Philadelphia, WB Saunders, 1998.

SYNOVIAL FLUID

Synovial fluid is a protein dialysate of plasma that contains mucin produced by the synovial cells. Synovial fluid can be obtained by arthrocentesis (aseptic aspiration of a joint cavity).

··········EXAMINATION OF SYNOVIAL FLUID (see also p. 346)

1. The physical characteristics should be noted, including color, turbidity, viscosity, clot formation, and quantity. Normal synovial fluid does not clot but forms a gel that returns to a liquid following shaking. Clotting of synovial

Table 5–13. Characteristics of Canine Joint Fluid Analysis

Condition	Total Cells (per mm³)*	Cells in Direct Smear	Neutrophils (%)	Color	Mucin Clot	Culture	Rheumatoid Factor
Normal	750 (250–3000)	1/2–5 per HPF	10	Clear	Good	–	–
Degenerative joint disease	1000 (250–3000)	1/2–5 per HPF	10 (0–20)	Clear	Good	–	–
Septic arthritis	200,000 (100,000–300,000)	3–15/HPF	80 (70–95) Many toxic	Turbid	Poor	+	–
Lyme arthritis	50,000 (10,000–100,000)	2–8/HPF	75 (50–90) Toxic forms rare	Clear to turbid	Fair to poor	±	–
Lupus arthritis	20,000 (5000–30,000)	1–4/HPF	70 (50–90) Occasional LE cells	Clear to turbid	Fair	–	±|
Nonerosive arthritis	50,000 (6000–200,000)	2–8/HPF	70 (50–90)	Clear to turbid	Fair	–	±|
Rheumatoid arthritis	10,000 (5000–50,000)	2–5/HPF	70 (10–90)	Clear to turbid	Poor	–	± to +

HPF, high-power field; –, negative; +, positive; ±, positive or negative.
*Approximate mean (and range).
From Halliwell REW, Gorman NT: Veterinary Clinical Immunology. Philadelphia, WB Saunders, 1989, p 349.

771

fluid is abnormal and is associated with abnormal vascular permeability or degeneration of synovial membrane.

2. The total cell count and a differential cell count should be obtained. Collect synovial fluid in an EDTA-containing vial to prevent clotting.

3. A total protein estimation should be made.

4. A mucin clot test can be performed. A poor mucin clot may indicate a septic arthritis producing bacterial enzymes or excessive effusions into the joint (Table 5–13).

5. Bacteriologic examination, including culture, should be performed. Cell counts in aspirates from the carpal, elbow, shoulder, hip, stifle, and hock joints of dogs showed 0 to 2900/mm^3 with a mean of 430/mm^3. The anticoagulant to be used with synovial fluid is EDTA.

The cell count of normal synovial fluid should contain fewer than 10% polymorphonuclear leukocytes. The following mean percentages have been reported for the dog: monocytes, 39.72; lymphocytes, 44.16; clasmatocytes, 4.20; and polymorphonuclear leukocytes, 1.38.

In traumatic osteoarthritis, clasmatocytes increase in number.

In traumatic or degenerated joint lesions, there may be an increase in the nonmucin protein content of the joint fluid because of the degeneration or change in the permeability of blood vessels. Mucin concentration is usually decreased in infectious arthritis but stays normal in traumatic or degenerative joint lesions.

Polyarthritis associated with systemic lupus erythematosus (SLE) has been described in the dog, and LE cells have been located in the synovial fluid.

When joint effusions of unknown cause are present, it can be advantageous to obtain a synovial membrane biopsy.

Normal joint fluid should be sterile when cultured (see p. 466).

REFERENCES

Bennett D: Immune-based erosive inflammatory joint disease of the dog: Canine rheumatoid arthritis. 1. Clinical radiological and laboratory investigations. J Small Anim Pract 28:779–797, 1987.

Bennett D: Immune-based non-erosive inflammatory joint disease of the dog: Canine rheumatoid arthritis. 3. Canine idiopathic polyarthritis. J Small Anim Pract 28:909–928, 1987.

Bennett D, Kelly DF: Immune-based non-erosive inflammatory joint disease of the dog: Canine systemic lupus erythematosus. J Small Anim Pract 28:871–889, 1987.

Cowell R: Diagnostic Cytology of the Dog and Cat. St Louis, Mosby–Year Book, 1998.

Halliwell RE, Gorman NT: Immune-mediated joint disease. In Halliwell RE, Gorman NT, eds: Veterinary Clinical Immunology. Philadelphia, WB Saunders, 1989.

Meric SM: Disorders of the joints. In Nelson RW, Couto GC, eds: Essentials of Small Animal Internal Medicine. St Louis, Mosby–Year Book, 1992, pp 820–830.

Meyer D, Harvey J: Veterinary Laboratory Medicine, ed 2. Philadelphia, WB Saunders, 1998.

URINALYSIS

Evaluation of urine often provides information that is essential to safe and effective management of patients requiring urgent medical attention. Results of the urinalysis are particularly helpful in verifying or eliminating diagnostic possibilities formulated on the basis of observations obtained from the history and physical examination. Urinalyses provide information about the adequacy of renal perfusion with blood and the integrity of the excretory pathway, as well as many other body systems. The speed and economy with which information can be obtained with simple laboratory equipment adds to the usefulness of the urinalysis in the emergency setting. For these reasons, we include urinalyses as a part of the initial evaluation of all patients with illnesses of unknown cause that require hospitalization.

............URINE COLLECTION

Several methods are used to collect urine. However, under most conditions, cystocentesis is the preferred method because it is a safe, simple, and rapid method of obtaining urine for diagnostic and therapeutic evaluation. In addition, cystocentesis (see also p. 486) provides samples free of vaginal and preputial contaminants. When proper technique is used in a relaxed patient, cystocentesis has virtually no adverse effects. If the urinary bladder is difficult to palpate, ultrasound can be used to guide the cystocentesis needle into the bladder lumen. We routinely use a 1.5 in., 22-gauge needle attached to a dry sterile syringe. When anticipating removal of large volumes of urine (e.g., additional urine for further testing or urinary bladder decompression to minimize the consequences of urethral obstruction), IV tubing and a three-way stopcock are attached between the needle and syringe. This configuration of equipment allows the syringe to be filled and emptied repeatedly without movement of the needle within the bladder lumen.

Voided urine samples can be collected from patients if the urinary bladder cannot be localized or stabilized sufficiently for cystocentesis. Collection of midstream samples minimizes contamination with unwanted material located in the distal urethra, prepuce, vagina, or vulva. Collection of samples by voiding is recommended for collecting urine from patients with ascites in which sampling of ascitic fluid can be mistaken for urine. In addition, analysis of voided urine is recommended as an aid in evaluation of urethral disease.

If urine cannot be obtained by cystocentesis or voluntary voiding, manual bladder expression or transurethral catheterization of the urinary bladder can be performed. If possible, manual expression of the bladder should not be attempted in patients with suspected urethral obstruction, a devitalized bladder wall, urinary tract infection (UTI), or generalized coagulopathies for fear of rupturing the bladder wall, inducing reflux of bacteria into the ureters and kidneys, or exacerbating urinary hemorrhage.

Urinary catheterization is associated with risk of iatrogenic trauma and nosocomial infection. Bacteria appear to be frequently introduced into the bladder as a result of contact of the catheter tip with genital and urethral mucosa. In one study, 20% of normal female dogs developed UTI following catheterization for urine sampling. This percentage is likely to be higher in patients that are systemically ill, are immunosuppressed, or have an abnormal lower urogenital tract.

............PERFORMING THE URINALYSIS

When performing the urinalysis examine fresh urine whenever possible. If samples cannot be analyzed within 30 minutes, the urine should be refrigerated and warmed prior to analysis. It is important to recognize that although refrigeration will minimize bacterial multiplication and reduce enzyme activation, the propensity for in vitro crystalluria is intensified.

Because detection of abnormal findings by urinalysis may dictate the need for further evaluation of urine, banking an additional 1 to 5 mL in a separate sterile dry tube at the time of collection is advised. The additional urine can be used to culture for bacteria, screen for toxins, or quantitate protein and electrolyte concentrations.

The following procedure is helpful in standardizing urine analysis

1. Warm urine to room temperature if refrigerated.
2. Thoroughly mix the sample.
3. Evaluate color and turbidity.
4. Determine the urine specific gravity.
5. Immerse test portions of reagent strips into urine sample and rapidly remove. Gently tap the edge of the strip on the edge of the collection container to remove excess urine. At the proper time intervals, compare the color of various reagent pads with the color scale provided by the manufacturer.
6. Transfer a standard volume (5 mL) to a conical-tip centrifuge tube. The remainder of the urine sample should be saved in the event that additional testing is needed.
7. Centrifuge 5 mL of urine in a conical-tip centrifuge tube at 300 rpm for 3 to 5 minutes. Remove the supernatant, and save it for potential chemical analysis. Allow a standard volume (usually 0.5 mL) of supernate to remain in the test tube.
8. Thoroughly resuspend the urine sediment in the 0.5 mL of urine remaining in the tube.
9. Transfer a drop of resuspended sediment to a microscope slide and place a coverslip over it.
10. Subdue the intensity of the microscope light by lowering the condenser.
11. Systematically examine the entire specimen under the coverslip with the low-power objective, assessing the quality and type of sediment (casts, cells, crystals). Examine the sediment with the high-power objective to identify the structure of elements and to detect microbes. The number of casts is recorded per low-power field (LPF), and the numbers of RBCs, WBCs, and epithelial cells are recorded per high-power field (HPF).
12. If the uncentrifuged urine specimen was visibly bloody or very turbid, repeat the dipstick analysis on the urine supernate.

...........INTERPRETING RESULTS

Before attempting to interpret the significance of results, determine whether any medications have been given, the type of diet the patient is receiving, the method of urine collection, the method of urine preservation, and the specific gravity. A common cause of abnormal urinalysis results and potential misdiagnosis is associated with therapy prior to sample collection. Consider the following example. How would you treat a vomiting, dehydrated dog with increased serum concentrations of amylase and urea nitrogen? What disease are you managing? Fluid administration to correct dehydration results in a variable reduction of urine concentration. In animals with pancreatitis urine is adequately concentrated; urine is inappropriately concentrated in those with renal failure. Therefore, differentiation of acute pancreatitis from acute renal failure requires collection of a urine sample prior to administration of fluids. Likewise, attempting to culture bacteria from urine following antimicrobial administration to treat a suspected UTI is likely to produce unreliable results. Because most critically ill patients require rapid therapeutic intervention to sustain life, we recommend that urine samples be collected prior to therapy when possible. If diagnostic or therapeutic agents have been given prior to sample collection, the time and sequence of therapy with sampling should be recorded to facilitate meaningful interpretation of results. For example, administration of diuretics for heart disease can result in an inappropriately concentrated urine in a clinically dehydrated patient. Without knowledge that diuretics have been used to treat the patient, the clinician may erroneously conclude that a disorder of urine concentration is present when in fact the diuretics reduce urine concentration. Consumption of diets containing low quantities of protein also promote formation of increased quantities of marginally concentrated or even dilute urine.

Collection of urine by cystocentesis, catheterization, or manual expression of the bladder often causes varying degrees of iatrogenic transient hematuria. Likewise, the degree of crystalluria is likely to increase in urine samples stored by refrigeration.

The specific gravity is important because interpretation of other results of the urinalysis is dependent on this value. Tests of the routine urinalysis are typically performed on a relatively small volume of urine without regard to the rate of urine formation or to total urine volume. Semiquantitative interpretation of results is more reliable if compared to the specific gravity. The dipstick determination of protein can be used as an example. A 2+ proteinuria at a specific gravity of 1.008 reflects a much greater loss of protein than a 2+ proteinuria at a 1.035 specific gravity. The same concept is applicable to interpretation of the significance of glucose, bilirubin, and constituents in urine sediment.

............Solute Concentration of Urine (Specific Gravity)

Urine specific gravity is a measurement of the density of urine compared to the density of pure water. Urine is more dense than water because it contains several solutes. However, the relationship between specific gravity and total solute concentration is only approximate. In addition to the number of molecules of solute, specific gravity is influenced by other factors, including the molecular size and molecular weight of solutes, and the temperature of urine. Determination of urine osmolality by freezing point depression or vapor pressure osmometry is considered the gold standard for determining urine solute concentration. However, this procedure requires special equipment and additional time. Urine specific gravity determined by refractometers is a simple and rapid procedure and has become the standard clinical method for assessing urine solute concentration. Reagent strip determination of specific gravity is unsatisfactory because dipsticks only detect urine to approximately 1.025 to 1.030. These values are too low to detect adequate renal concentrating ability in dogs and cats.

Urine specific gravity is used to assess the ability of the renal tubules to concentrate (remove water in excess of solute) or dilute (remove solute in excess of water) glomerular filtrate. Isosthenuria refers to urine of the same concentration as altered glomerular filtrate (specific gravity approximately 1.007 to 1.012 or 300 mOsm/kg).

Hyposthenuria refers to urine less concentrated than glomerular filtrate (specific gravity <1.007; <300 mOsm/kg). Hypersthenuria refers to urine more concentrated than glomerular filtrate (specific gravity >1.012; >300 mOsm/kg). The normal range for the total solute concentration in urine from dogs and cats is wide (dogs, approximately 1.001 to 1.065; cats, approximately 1.001 to 1.080). Despite this wide range, dogs and cats usually excrete urine that is moderately concentrated. Dogs and cats less than approximately 3 months of age do not have the same degree of urine concentrating ability as adult animals.

Complete inability of the nephrons to modify glomerular filtrate typically results in a urine with a specific gravity that is similar to that of glomerular filtrate (1.008 to 1.012). However, urine specific gravity values between approximately 1.007 and 1.029 for dogs and 1.007 and 1.035 for cats with clinical dehydration and azotemia are physiologically inappropriate and suggest disease. Interpretation of urine specific gravity values depends on knowledge of the patient's hydration status and serum concentrations of urea nitrogen or creatinine.

............Color, Appearance, and Odor

Normal urine is yellow because of the presence of urochrome pigment. Very concentrated urine may be deep amber in color, and very dilute urine may be almost colorless. A red or reddish-brown color is usually due to RBCs, hemoglobin, or myoglobin. A yellow-brown to yellow-green color may be due to bilirubin.

Normal urine is usually clear. Cloudy urine often contains increased levels of cellular elements, crystals, or mucus. The most common abnormal odor is ammoniacal and is due to the release of ammonia from urea by urease-producing bacteria.

............pH

Urine pH varies with diet and acid-base status. Normal urine pH for dogs and cats is approximately 5.0 to 7.5. Causes of acidic urine include meat diets, administration of acidifying agents, metabolic acidosis, respiratory acidosis, paradoxical aciduria in metabolic alkalosis, and protein catabolic states. Causes of alkaline urine pH include cereal diets, urine allowed to stand open to air at room temperature, postprandial alkaline tide, UTI by urease-positive organisms, administration of alkalinizing agents, metabolic alkalosis, respiratory alkalosis, and distal renal tubular acidosis.

............Protein

Random urine samples from normal dogs contain small amounts of protein. Commonly used dipstick methods for protein determination are much more sensitive to albumin than to globulin. Results must be interpreted in consideration of urine specific gravity. Very alkaline urine may result in a false-positive dipstick determination of protein. If the urine sediment examination is normal and urine protein tests are positive, urine protein excretion should be quantitated. Calculation of urine protein-creatinine ratios from randomly collected spot urine samples can be used to estimate the quantity of protein excreted in a 24-hour period.

In interpreting the significance of proteinuria, it is critical to localize the origin of protein loss. This can often be done by history, physical examination, evaluation of blood, and examination of urine sediment. Persistent, moderate-to-heavy proteinuria in the absence of urine sediment abnormalities (i.e., RBCs, WBCs, bacteria) in a properly collected urine sample is highly suggestive of glomerular disease. With evidence of intravascular hemolysis, muscle damage, or hyperproteinemia, consider preglomerular causes. The hallmark of postglomerular proteinuria (urinary tract trauma, infection, or neoplasia) is proteinuria associated with urinary sediment abnormalities consistent with extravasation of blood cells and protein, and tissue proteins.

............Glucose

Glucose filtered by glomeruli is almost completely reabsorbed in the proximal tubules and therefore is not normally present in the urine of dogs or cats. If the plasma glucose concentration exceeds the renal threshold (approximately 180 mg/dL in the dog and 300 mg/dL in the cat), glucose will appear in the urine (glycosuria). Most dipstick tests for glucose involve a colorimetric test based on an enzymatic reaction (glucose oxidase) specific for glucose. Causes of hyperglycemic glucosuria include diabetes mellitus (most common), stress of excitement (especially cats), and administration of glucose-containing fluids. Normal glycemic glucosuria occurs with renal tubular diseases such as acute tubular necrosis, Fanconi's syndrome, and primary renal glucosuria.

.... Ketones

β-Hydroxybutyrate, acetoacetate, and acetone are collectively referred to as ketones, the products of exaggerated and incomplete oxidation of fatty acids. They are not normally detected by standard tests in the urine of dogs and cats. The nitroprusside reagent present in dipstick tests reacts with acetone and acetoacetate, although it is much more reactive with acetoacetate. It does not react with β-hydroxybutyrate. Causes of ketonuria include diabetic ketoacidosis (most common), starvation or prolonged fasting, glycogen storage disease, low carbohydrate diet, persistent fever, and persistent hypoglycemia. Ketonuria occurs more readily in young animals and, of the causes listed above, diabetic ketoacidosis is the most important cause in adult dogs and cats requiring urgent medical attention.

.... Occult Blood

Dipstick tests for occult blood are very sensitive but do not differentiate between RBCs, hemoglobin, and myoglobin. The test is more sensitive to hemoglobin than to intact RBCs. A positive test must be interpreted in light of urine sediment findings (i.e., the presence or absence of RBCs). Free hemoglobin secondary to intravascular hemolysis or lysis of RBCs in urine is most common. Causes of intravascular hemolysis include immune-mediated hemolytic anemia, transfusion reaction, DIC, postcaval syndrome of dirofilariasis, splenic torsion, and heat stroke. Myoglobinuria is less common but may occur following severe rhabdomyolysis.

.... Bilirubin

Bilirubin is derived from the breakdown of heme by the reticuloendothelial system. Bilirubin is transported to the liver, where after being conjugated with glucuronic and sulfuric acids it is excreted in bile. Conjugated bilirubin is not bound to plasma carrier proteins and therefore passes through glomerular capillary walls. Because the renal threshold for bilirubin is low in dogs, small quantities of bilirubin are commonly observed in concentrated urine samples of normal dogs, especially males. Detection of bilirubin in less concentrated urine samples or persistent bilirubinuria should prompt consideration of disorders characterized by prehepatic, hepatic, or posthepatic disorders of bile metabolism. Unlike in dogs, mild bilirubinuria is not a finding in normal feline urine. Common causes of bilirubinuria are RBC hemolysis, liver disease, extrahepatic biliary obstruction, diabetes mellitus, feline infectious peritonitis, and feline leukemia.

.... Leukocyte Esterase Reaction for White Blood Cells

Indoxyl released by esterases from intact or lysed leukocytes reacts with diazonium salt and is detected as a blue color reaction after oxidation by atmospheric oxygen. This test is specific for pyuria in canine urine samples but has low sensitivity (many false-negative results). Thus, a positive leukocyte esterase reaction indicates pyuria, but a negative result is not reliable. This test is not specific for pyuria in feline urine. Urine from most cats is positive, even though leukocyte numbers in urine are absent or insignificant.

.... Red Blood Cells Evaluated in Urine Sediment

Occasional RBCs are considered normal in the urine sediment (0 to 5/HPF utilizing a standard technique of sediment preparation). Hematuria may be microscopic or macroscopic. Hematuria can result from a generalized coagulopathy or localized bleeding (i.e., the urogenital tract). Causes of hematuria include urinary tract trauma (urolithiasis, contusion or rupture, vigorous exercise, hypertension, catheterization, cystocentesis, renal biopsy), neoplasia, inflammation (idiopathic feline lower urinary tract disease, bacterial infection, fungal infection, cyclophosphamide-induced cystitis), parasites *(Cappillaria* spp., *Dioctophyma renale)*; genital tract contamination (prostate, prepuce, vagina); and systemic hemorrhage (e.g., warfarin intoxication, DIC, thrombocytopenia, von Willebrand's disease).

............White Blood Cells Evaluated in Urine Sediment

Utilizing a standard technique of sediment preparation, occasional leukocytes are considered normal. In properly collected samples or concentrated urine, WBCs rarely exceed 3 to 5/HPF. Detection of abnormal increased numbers of WBCs does not localize their origin. Bacterial infection of the urinary tract is the most common cause of pyuria, but genital tract contamination may also cause pyuria, especially from voided or catheterized samples.

............Epithelial Cells

Both squamous and transitional epithelial cells may be found in the urine sediment, but often they are of little diagnostic value. Squamous cells are large, polygonal cells with small round nuclei. Squamous cells are common in voided or catheterized samples because they originate in the urethra and vagina. Increased numbers of squamous cells may be present during estrus.

Transitional epithelial cells of variable size are derived from the urothelium lining the renal pelvis to the urethra. Caudate cells are transitional cells with tapered ends and are thought to originate from the renal pelvis. Occasional transitional cells are normal. Increased numbers occur in association with infection and noninfectious inflammation, and neoplasia. Renal cells are small epithelial cells from the renal tubules; their renal origin can be determined only if they are observed in cellular casts.

............Casts

Casts are cylindrical molds of the renal tubules composed of aggregated proteins that may contain cells. Casts are formed in the distal nephron, possibly because of maximal urine acidity, high solute concentration, and low flow rate in this area. Detection of significant numbers of casts in the urinary sediment indicates renal involvement and thus is of localizing value. Occasional transient hyaline and granular casts per LPF are considered insignificant. Cellular casts are not normal findings in urine sediment. The types of casts observed in the urine sediment include hyaline, granular, cellular, and waxy. Hyaline casts are protein precipitates (primarily Tamm-Horsfall mucoprotein). These casts may be difficult to detect because their refractive index is similar to urine and because they may dissolve in dilute or alkaline urine. Small numbers of hyaline casts may be observed in association with fever or exercise. Hyaline casts are commonly seen in renal diseases associated with proteinuria (e.g., amyloidosis and glomerulonephritis). Granular casts represent the degeneration of tubular epithelial cells or WBCs trapped in Tamm-Horsfall mucoprotein matrix, or precipitation of large plasma proteins that have passed through glomeruli. Fatty casts are a type of cast containing lipid granules and may be seen in nephrotic syndrome or diabetes mellitus. Cellular casts include WBC casts (suggestive of pyelonephritis), RBC casts (fragile and rarely observed in dogs and cats), and renal epithelial cell casts (suggestive of acute tubular necrosis). Waxy casts, representing the final stage of degeneration of granular casts, are relatively stable and suggest chronic intrarenal stasis. They often are very convoluted, with cracks and blunt ends.

·············Microbes

Urine from the bladder of clinically healthy patients is sterile. However, voided or catheterized urine samples may be contaminated with bacteria normally present in the distal urethra, genital tract, or skin. Contaminants from the urethra in voided or catheterized specimens usually do not result in sufficient numbers of bacteria to be visualized in urine sediment. However, if allowed to incubate at room temperature, these contaminants may proliferate. For bacteria to be seen microscopically, there must be more than 10^4 rods per milliliter of urine or more than 10^5 cocci per milliliter of urine. Large numbers of bacteria in urine collected by cystocentesis is highly suggestive of UTI. Usually, there is accompanying pyuria. Particulate debris in the sediment may be confused with bacteria, resulting in false-positive reports. Failure to detect bacteria in the sediment does not rule out urinary tract infection. Yeast and fungal hyphae in sediment may represent contaminants or pathogens.

·············CRYSTALS

Precipitation of crystals in urine is dependent on urine pH, temperature, specific gravity, and concentration of lithogenic substances. Detection of crystals indicates that urine is supersaturated with lithogenic precursors and therefore a risk factor for urolith formation. For most animals, however, crystals pass out of the urinary tract before attaining sufficient size to initiate disease.

Care must be used so as not to overinterpret or underinterpret the significance of crystalluria. Factors helpful in assessing the significance of crystalluria include their type, number, and persistence, as well as the clinical condition of the patient. Small numbers of struvite crystals in the urine of normal animals are often of little diagnostic or therapeutic significance. However, crystalluria in patients with urinary tract signs or persistent crystalluria should be evaluated further for underlying disease processes. For example, calcium oxalate crystals can be associated with calcium oxalate uroliths, hypercalcemia, or ethylene glycol intoxication. Struvite crystals may provide clues to an underlying UTI by bacteria that produce urease. Animals with urate crystals may have an inherited defect in purine metabolism (e.g., Dalmatians and English bulldogs) or a hepatic portosystemic vascular shunt. The presence of cystine crystals in urine of dogs and cats is abnormal and suggestive of inherited cystinuria.

·············Other Findings in Sediment

Sperm commonly are found in urine samples from normal intact male dogs. Parasite ova of *Dioctophyma renale* or *Capillaria plica* or microfilaria of *Dirofilaria immitis* may be observed in the urine sediment. Retractile lipid droplets may occur in diabetes mellitus or nephrotic syndrome and may also be observed in normal cats due to degeneration of lipid-laden tubular cells.

·············URINALYSIS ABNORMALITIES THAT WARRANT URGENT CONSIDERATION OF FURTHER DIAGNOSTIC OR THERAPEUTIC INTERVENTION

The rapidity with which accurate information can be obtained from analysis of urine makes urinalysis an ideal test for assessment of patients requiring urgent medical attention (Table 5–14).

Table 5–14. Urinalysis

Urine Abnormality	Disorders That May Require Urgent Diagnostic and Therapeutic Intervention
Glucosuria	Diabetes mellitus
	Acute renal failure
	Acute pancreatitis
Ketonuria	Uncontrolled diabetes mellitus
Bilirubinuria	Liver disease
Hemoglobinuria	Intravascular hemolysis
WBC casts	Bacterial pyelonephritis
Bacteriuria	Bacteremia
	Pyelonephritis
	Prostatitis
	Pyometra
Calcium oxalate crystalluria	Ethylene glycol toxicity
	Hypercalcemia
	Urinary obstruction with uroliths
Urate crystalluria	Hepatic encephalopathy
	Urinary obstruction with uroliths that are radiolucent by survey radiography
Hyposthenuria	Central or renal diabetes insipidus
Neoplastic epithelial cells	Urinary tract neoplasia

...........ADDITIONAL URINE TESTS

Urine represents the end product of many metabolic processes. Substances that are rapidly metabolized in the body and filtered by the kidney may be more easily detected in urine. Therefore, additional tests using urine may be helpful in the diagnosis and management of hospitalized patients (Table 5–15).

RENAL FUNCTION TESTS

Creatinine clearance can be used to estimate glomerular filtration rate (GFR) in the dog and cat because creatinine excretion by the kidney is accomplished almost entirely by glomerular filtration. There is minimal tubular reabsorption and secretion of creatinine by the kidney. Creatinine clearance determinations are useful in detecting reductions in GFR prior to increases in BUN and serum creatinine concentrations. Measurement of *endogenous* creatinine clearance requires collection of a timed urine sample. Measurement of *exogenous* creatinine clearance requires administration of a creatinine-containing solution but is more accurate than measurement of endogenous clearance because the effect of noncreatinine chromagens on the laboratory measurement of serum creatinine is minimized.

...........ENDOGENOUS CREATININE CLEARANCE
...........Method

1. Weigh the dog and empty its bladder.
2. Collect all urine produced over a specified time (e.g., 24 hours).

3. At the end of the collection period, empty the bladder and add the urine obtained to that already collected. Measure the total volume of urine collected, and submit an aliquot for measurement of urine creatinine concentration and urine protein concentration.
4. Submit a blood sample for measurement of serum creatinine concentration.
5. Calculate the endogenous creatinine clearance:

$$\text{Creatinine clearance (mL/min/kg)} = U_{Cr}V/S_{Cr}BW$$

where U_{Cr} = urine creatinine (mg/dL), V = urine volume/time of collection (mL/min), S_{Cr} = serum creatinine (mg/dL), and BW = body weight (kg). Reported normal values for endogenous creatinine clearance in the dog and cat are approximately 2.8 to 3.7 mL/min/kg for the dog and 2 to 3 mL/min/ kg for the cat.

···········EXOGENOUS CREATININE CLEARANCE

A simplified technique for measurement of exogenous creatinine clearance in the dog using a single subcutaneous (SC) injection of creatinine has been described.

···········Method

1. Weigh the dog.
2. Administer water per stomach tube at a dose equal to 3% of body weight.
3. Inject creatinine solution (50 mg/mL) at 100 mg/kg SC with a maximum of 10 mL per site.
4. Wait 60 minutes.
5. Empty the dog's bladder, and rinse the bladder twice with sterile saline (50 mL). Discard the rinses.
6. Submit a blood sample for measurement of serum creatinine concentration.
7. Wait 20 minutes.
8. Empty the bladder, and save all urine obtained. Rinse the bladder once with sterile saline (50 mL), and add this rinse to the urine previously collected.
9. Submit another blood sample for measurement of serum creatinine concentration.
10. Calculate the creatinine clearance (as described above) using the mean serum creatinine concentration.

···········URINE PROTEIN–URINE CREATININE RATIO

The severity of proteinuria can be estimated by calculating the ratio of the urine protein concentration as measured by a quantitative technique (e.g., Coomassie Brilliant Blue) to the urine creatinine concentration. The urine protein–urine creatinine ratio has been shown to be highly correlated with 24-hour protein excretion in urine in dogs and cats. The urine protein–creatinine ratio is obtained by dividing the protein concentration (mg/dL) by the creatinine concentration (mg/dL). Less than 0.5 is normal; between 0.5 and 1.0 is questionable; greater than 1.0 is abnormal. Dogs with glomerular amyloidosis have very high urine protein–creatinine ratios (>10), whereas dogs with glomerulonephritis demonstrate a wide range of values (1 to >40).

···········ABRUPT WATER DEPRIVATION TEST

The water deprivation test may be used to evaluate renal function in patients with suspected renal disease but without azotemia. If overt azotemia exists

Table 5–15. Additional Urine Tests

Test	Indication	Methodology	Interpretation
Protein-creatinine ratio	Diagnose, monitor, and evaluate therapy for protein-losing glomerulonephropaties	Urine is submitted for determination of protein (mg/dL) and creatinine (mg/dL) concentrations; complete urinalysis including sediment should be evaluated from the same sample	Values >1 to 2 are consistent with glomerular disease; higher ratios can exceed 40; higher values are consistent with more severe disease *Caution:* Increased ratio can occur in association with preglomerular proteinuria (e.g., intravascular hemolysis) and lower urinary tract diseases (e.g. infection, uroliths, neoplasia)
Creatinine concentration	To differentiate ascites from uroabdomen	Obtain urine by voiding or catheterization; simultaneously determine serum and ascitic fluid creatinine concentrations	Similar creatinine concentrations between ascitic fluid and urine are consistent with uroperitoneum
Basic fibroblast growth factor	To identify transitional cell carcinoma as a cause of urinary tract signs	Basic fibroblast growth factor can be assayed by a commercially available ELISA kit (Quantikine HS, R & D systems, Minneapolis); simultaneously determine urine creatinine concentration	Values >7.37 ng/g of creatinine indicate the need for intensive diagnostic evaluation and close monitoring for bladder neoplasia

Test	Indication	Comments	Interpretation
Quantitative aerobic bacterial culture	Patients at risk of urinary tract infection	Collection by cystocentesis is preferred; evaluation should include antimicrobial susceptibility	From urine obtained by cystocentesis; numbers ≥1000 are consistent with infection and numbers ≤100 are considered contaminants; identification of multiple species may indicate contamination
γ-Glutamyl transpeptidase–creatinine ratio (Rivers et al.)	A sensitive marker of renal tubular damage associated with gentamicin toxicity	Simultaneously determine urine creatinine concentration	In one study normal dogs did not exceed 0.42; increasing values are consistent with worsening disease
Arsenic (Neiger)	Arsenic is commonly found in roach and ant baits; cats are more commonly affected than dogs		Evaluation of urine is more reliable than blood; values >2 ppm are consistent with toxicity, values rapidly decline within days of eliminating exposure
Ethylene glycol (Thrall A, et al.)	Patients suspected of ethylene glycol intoxication		Mean urine concentration was 3975 mg/dL 6 hr after dogs ingested 10.5 g/kg and 1500 mg/dL after cats ingested 1.6 g/kg

5

and the urine is not concentrated, renal dysfunction is obvious and further dehydration by water deprivation testing may further aggravate renal function. If dehydration is clinically evident and the animal has not concentrated its urine, the animal has already failed the test and further water deprivation could be dangerous.

.... Method

1. Empty the bladder and weigh the animal.
2. Withhold water during the test. Dry food may be given if the test lasts more than 24 hours.
3. Monitor the animal for evidence of dehydration every 2 to 4 hours by measuring body weight (using the same scale each time), total plasma proteins, hematocrit, skin turgor, and serum osmolality.
4. Monitor for urinary concentrating ability every 2 to 4 hours by measuring urine specific gravity (SG), urine osmolality, and the urine-plasma osmolality ratio. The bladder should be emptied after each collection.
5. Continue the test until the patient demonstrates adequate concentrating capacity or becomes dehydrated, based on loss of 5% or more of its body weight.
6. If there has been less than a 5% increase in urine osmolality or less than a 10% change in urine SG for three consecutive determinations or if the animal has lost more than 5% of its body weight, 0.25 to 0.5 units/kg aqueous vasopressin (Pitressin) (up to a total dose of 5 units) or 1 µg/kg desmopressin (DDAVP) may be given SC and parameters of urinary concentrating ability monitored at 1 and 2 hours after antidiuretic hormone (ADH) injection.

Normal dogs achieve urine SG values of 1.050 to 1.076 after water deprivation, sufficient to cause dehydration. Their urine osmolality values are expected to be 1787 to 2791 mOsm/kg and their urine-plasma osmolality ratios, 5.7 to 8.9. Normal cats achieve urine SG values of 1.047 to 1.087 and urine osmolality values of 1581 to 2984 mOsm/kg after water deprivation, sufficient to induce 5% loss of body weight.

.... GRADUAL WATER DEPRIVATION

Gradual water deprivation can be performed before abrupt water deprivation to eliminate diagnostic confusion caused by medullary solute washout.

1. Instruct the owner to reduce water consumption by approximately 20% per day over a 3- to 5-day period (but not to <60 mL/kg/day). In dogs with psychogenic polydipsia, this will promote release of endogenous vasopressin, increase permeability of the inner medullary collecting ducts to urea, and restore the normal gradient of medullary hypertonicity. This approach should only be used in animals that are otherwise healthy on initial clinical evaluation, and the owner should provide dry food ad libitum and weigh the dog daily to monitor for loss of body weight.
2. At the end of the 3- to 5-day period, proceed with the abrupt water deprivation test as described above.

.... EXOGENOUS VASOPRESSIN (ANTIDIURETIC HORMONE) TEST

This test is indicated for patients that are unable to concentrate their urine after water deprivation testing or for debilitated patients in which water deprivation is deemed hazardous.

Table 5–16. Normal Values for Fractional Clearance of Electrolytes in Dogs and Cats

	Value (%)	
	Dogs	Cats
Sodium	<1	<1
Chloride	<1	<1.3
Potassium	<20	<20
Phosphate	<40	<73

............Method for Repositol ADH Test

1. Administer 3 to 5 units of vasopressin tannate in oil IM.
2. Provide water ad libitum.
3. Empty bladder 3 to 6 hours after injection.
4. Measure urine SG at 0, 6, 12, 18, and 24 hours, and empty the bladder at each measurement.

The expected response in normal dogs is a maximal urine SG value of 1.024 to 1.060 at approximately 8 hours and a maximal urine osmolality of 1033 to 2001 mOsm/kg. The maximal urine-plasma osmolality ratio obtained should be 3.8 to 7.4.

............FRACTIONAL ELECTROLYTE CLEARANCE

The extent to which specific electrolytes appear in the urine is the net result of glomerular filtration, tubular reabsorption, and tubular secretion. The fractional clearance (FC) of electrolytes can be used to evaluate tubular function and is defined as the ratio of the clearance of the electrolyte, x, to that of creatinine:

$$FC_x = \frac{U_xV/P_x}{U_{Cr}V/P_{Cr}} = \frac{U_xP_{Cr}}{U_{Cr}P_x}$$

where U = urine, V = volume, P = plasma, x = electrolyte, and Cr = creatinine. The number obtained is multiplied by 100 to express the fractional clearance as a percentage. Fractional clearances can be determined by using random urine samples; a timed urine collection is not necessary. The fractional clearance of sodium may be useful in the differentiation of prerenal and primary renal azotemia. The FC_{Na} should be low (1%) in prerenal azotemia because of avid conservation of sodium. The FC_{Na} should be high (>1%) in primary renal azotemia. Values for fractional clearances of electrolytes in dogs and cats are listed in Table 5–16.

REFERENCES

Adams LG, et al: Correlation of urine protein/creatinine ratio and twenty four hour protein excretion in normal cats and cats with surgically induced chronic renal failure. J Vet Intern Med 6:36, 1992.

Bagley RS, Center S, et al: The effect of experimental cystitis and iatrogenic blood contamination on urine protein/creatinine ratios in the dog. J Vet Intern Med 5:66–70, 1991.

Chew DJ, DiBartola SP: Manual of Small Animal Nephrology and Urology. New York, Churchill Livingstone, 1986.

Dorfman M, Barsanti J: Diseases of the canine prostate gland. Compend Contin Educ Pract Vet 17:791, 1995.

Finco D, Barsanti JA, Brown SA: Solute fractional excretion rates. *In* Kirk RW, ed: Current Veterinary Therapy XI. Philadelphia, WB Saunders, 1992 p 818.

Kruger JM, Osborne C, Nachreiner R, Refsal K: Hypercalcemia and renal failure: Etiology, pathophysiology, diagnosis, and treatment. Vet Clin North Am Small Anim Pract 26:1417–1446, 1996.

Lulich JP, Osborne C: Interpretation of urine protein-creatinine ratios in dogs with glomerular and nonglomerular disorders. Compend Contin Educ Pract Vet 12:59–72, 1990.

Meyer DJ, Harvey J: Veterinary Laboratory Medicine, ed 2. Philadelphia, WB Saunders, 1998.

Monroe WE, Davenport DJ, Saunders GK: Twenty-four hour urinary protein loss in healthy cat and the urinary protein-creatinine ratio as an estimate. Am J Vet Res 50:1906, 1989.

Osborne C, Finco D: Canine and Feline Nephrology and Urology. Baltimore, Williams & Wilkins, 1995.

Polzin DJ, ed: Renal dysfunction. Vet Clin North Am Small Anim Pract 26(6):1996.

Section 6

CHARTS AND TABLES

OPTIMAL BODY WEIGHTS—BY BREED

See Table 6–1.

Table 6–1. Optimal Body Weight of Mature Dogs [kg (lb)]*

Giant Breeds [Ht 66–79 cm (26–31 in.)]		
Bloodhound	36–50	(80–110)
Borzoi	34–48	(75–105)
Bullmastiff	45–59	(100–130)
Great Dane	52–55	(115–145)
Great Pyrenees	41–57	(90–125)
Irish wolfhound	48–61	(105–135)
Komondor	34–48	(75–105)
Kuvaszok	34–55	(75–120)
Mastiff	77–89	(170–195)
Newfoundland	50–68	(110–150)
Rottweiler	32–45	(70–100)
Saint Bernard	68–82	(150–180)
Scottish deerhound	34–50	(75–110)
Large Breeds [Ht 58–64 cm (23–25 in.)]		
Afghan hound	23–27	(50–60)
Alaskan malamute	34–39	(75–85)
American foxhound	27	(60)
Belgian sheepdog	27	(60)
Bernese mountain dog	30	(66)
Black-and-tan coonhound	27	(60)
Blue tick hound	27–32	(60–70)
Bouvier des Flandres	32	(70)
Boxer	32	(70)
Briard	32	(70)
Chesapeake Bay retriever	25–34	(55–75)
Collie	23–34	(50–75)
Curly-coated retriever	32	(70)
Doberman pinscher	32	(70)
English foxhound	32	(70)
English setter	30	(66)
Eskimo	34	(75)
Flat-coated retriever	27–32	(60–70)
German shepherd	27–39	(60–85)
German short-haired pointer	21–32	(45–70)
Golden retriever	27–34	(60–75)
Gordon setter	21–36	(45–80)
Greyhound	27–32	(60–70)
Irish setter	27–32	(60–70)
Irish water spaniel	21–29	(45–65)
Kuvosz	32	(70)
Labrador retriever	25–34	(55–75)
Old English sheepdog	30	(66)
Otterhound	27–32	(60–70)
Pointer	27	(60)
Redbone hound	30–32	(65–70)
Rhodesian ridgeback	18–27	(40–60)
Saluki	27	(60)

Table 6–1. Optimal Body Weight of Mature Dogs [kg (lb)]* *Continued*

Schnauzer—giant	34	(75)
Standard poodle	25	(55)
Vizsla	21–30	(45–65)
Weimaraner	25–38	(55–85)

Medium Breeds [Ht 43–56 cm (17–22 in.)]

Airedale	23	(50)
American water spaniel	11–20	(25–45)
Border collie	18–23	(40–50)
Brittany spaniel	14–18	(30–40)
Bulldog	18–23	(40–50)
Bull terrier	23	(50)
Chow chow	27	(60)
Clumber spaniel	16–29	(35–65)
Dalmatian	21	(45)
English springer spaniel	20–25	(45–55)
Field spaniel	16–23	(35–50)
Harrier	21	(45)
Keeshond	18	(40)
Kerry blue terrier	15–18	(33–40)
Norwegian elkhound	23	(50)
Puli	16	(35)
Samoyed	25	(55)
Schnauzer—standard	16	(35)
Siberian husky	16–27	(35–60)
Staffordshire terrier	21	(45)
Sussex spaniel	16–21	(35–45)
Welsh springer spaniel	17	(37)
Wire-haired pointing griffon	25	(55)
Whippet	5–12	(10–28)

Toy Breeds [Ht 13–28 cm (5–11 in.)]

Affenpinscher	3.6	(8)
Australian terrier	5.5–6.5	(12–14)
Brussels griffon	3.5–5.5	(8–12)
Chihuahua	1–3	(2–6)
Dachshund—miniature	3.6	(8)
English toy spaniel	4–5.5	(9–12)
Fox terrier–toy	1.8–3.4	(4–7)
Italian greyhound	4.1	(9)
Japanese spaniel	3.6	(8)
Maltese	2–3	(4–6)
Manchester terrier	2.5–5.5	(5–12)
Mexican hairless	5.5	(12)
Miniature pinscher	3.6	(8)
Norwich terrier	5–5.5	(11–12)
Papillon	5	(11)
Pekingese	4.1	(9)
Pomeranian	2–3	(4–6)
Poodle—toy	3.2	(7)
Silky terrier	3.5–4.5	(8–10)
Yorkshire terrier	3.2	(7)

Small Breeds [Ht 30–41 cm (12–16 in.)]

Basenji	10–11	(22–24)
Basset hound	11–25	(25–55)

Table continued on following page

Table 6-1. Optimal Body Weight of Mature Dogs [kg (lb)]* *Continued*

Small Breeds [Ht 30–41 cm (12–16 in.)]

Breed	kg	(lb)
Beagle	8–14	(18–39)
Bedlington terrier	10–11	(22–24)
Border terrier	5.5–7	(12–15)
Boston terrier	6–11	(13–25)
Cairn terrier	6–6.5	(13–14)
Cocker spaniel	11.5	(25)
Dachshund	9	(20)
Dandie Dinmont	8–11	(18–24)
English cocker spaniel	12–15	(25–34)
French bulldog	8–13	(18–28)
Fox terrier	7–8	(16–18)
Irish terrier	11–12	(25–27)
Lakeland terrier	7.7	(17)
Lhasa apso	6.8	(15)
Manchester terrier	5.5–10	(12–22)
Poodle—miniature	7.3	(16)
Pug	6–8	(14–18)
Schipperke	6.8	(15)
Schnauzer—miniature	6.8	(15)
Scottish terrier	8–10	(18–22)
Sealyham	9–10	(20–22)
Shetland sheepdog	7.3	(16)
Shih Tzu	5.5–7	(12–15)
Skye terrier	11.4	(25)
Smooth fox terrier	7.7	(25)
Spitz	7.3	(16)
Welsh corgi	8–11	(18–24)
Welsh terrier	8–10	(18–22)
West Highland white terrier	7.3	(16)
Whippet	9.1	(20)
Wire-haired fox terrier	7.7	(17)

*Weight varies depending on body size and build. Males are larger than females. For dogs of mixed of unknown breed, use weight of dog of similar height at shoulder of a breed similar in appearance.

From Lewis LD, Morris ML, Hand MS: Small Animal Clinical Nutrition III. Topeka, Kan, Mark Morris Associates, 1987.

FRENCH SCALE CONVERSION TABLE

See Table 6–2.

Table 6–2. Conversion Table for Standard French (Charrière) Scale

The standard French, or Charrière, scale (abbreviated F or Fr) is generally used in the size calibration of catheters and other tubular instruments. It is based on the metric system, with each unit being approximately 0.33 mm, with a difference of 0.33 mm in diameter between consecutive sizes. Example: 27F indicates a diameter of 9 mm; 30F, a diameter of 10 mm.

A convenient conversion table from the French scale to the English and American scales that is sometimes used for certain instruments is given below.

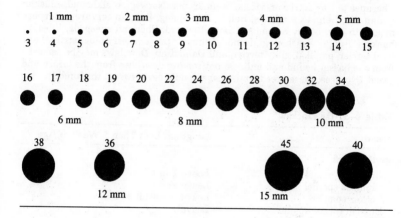

....

TAIL DOCKING AND DEWCLAW REMOVAL

The data on tail docking and dewclaw removal were based on official standards published by the American Kennel Club or on information obtained directly from judges, veterinarians, dog breeders, and professional handlers (Table 6–3).

> *Note:* Because of the ambiguous descriptions used in many standards and because of changes in breed fashions, veterinarians are cautioned *to use these figures as suggestions only!* Always obtain *specific instructions* from the owner as to length of dock or whether to remove dewclaws.

Because dewclaws may become torn during field exercise, they are often removed from all four feet of many hunting and working breeds. Removing dewclaws makes the legs of a dog appear smooth and clean.

Breeds from which dewclaws should be removed include the following: Chesapeake Bay retriever, vizsla, Weimaraner, Norwegian elkhound, Alaskan malamute, Belgian malinois, Belgian sheepdog, Belgian tervuren, Bernese mountain dog, boxer, Komondor, Saint Bernard, Shetland sheepdog, Siberian husky, Cardigan Welsh corgi, Dandie Dinmont terrier, Kerry blue terrier, Lakeland terrier, papillon, silky terrier, and Dalmatian. Dewclaws may be removed from the basset hound and puli. Do not remove dewclaws from the briard and Great Pyrenees; these breeds must have double dewclaws on the hindleg.

Table 6–3. Tail Docking*

Breed	Length at Less Than 1 Week of Age
Sporting Breeds	
Brittany spaniel	Leave 1 in.†
Clumber spaniel	Leave ¼–⅓
Cocker spaniel	Leave ⅓ (about ¾ in.)
English cocker spaniel	Leave ⅓
English springer spaniel	Leave ⅓
Field spaniel	Leave ⅓
German short-haired pointer	Leave ⅖‡
German wire-haired pointer	Leave ⅖‡
Sussex spaniel	Leave ⅓
Vizsla	Leave ⅔†
Weimaraner	Leave ⅗ (about 1½ in.)
Welsh springer spaniel	Leave ⅓–½
Wire-haired pointing griffon	Leave ⅓
Working Breeds	
Bouvier des Flandres	Leave ½–¾ in.
Boxer	Leave ½–¾ in.
Doberman pinscher	Leave ¾ in. (two vertebrae)
Giant schnauzer	Leave 1¼ in. (three vertebrae)
Old English sheepdog	If necessary—close to body (leave one vertebra)‡
Rottweiler	If necessary—close to body (leave one vertebra)‡
Standard schnauzer	Leave 1 in. (two vertebrae)
Welsh corgi (Pembroke)	Close to body (leave one vertebra)†

Table 6–3. Tail Docking* Continued

Breed	Length at Less Than 1 Week of
Terrier Breeds	
Airedale terrier	Leave ⅔–¾§
Australian terrier	Leave ⅖‡
Fox terrier (smooth and wire-haired)	Leave ⅔–¾§
Irish terrier	Leave ¾‡
Kerry blue terrier	Leave ½–⅔
Lakeland terrier	Leave ⅔§
Miniature schnauzer	Leave about ¾ in.—no more than 1 in.
Norwich terrier	Leave ¼–⅓
Sealyham terrier	Leave ⅓–½
Soft-coated wheaten terrier	Leave ½–¾
Welsh terrier	Leave ⅔§
Toy Breeds	
Affenpinscher	Close to body (leave ⅓ in.)
Brussels griffon	Leave ¼–⅓
English toy spaniel	Leave ⅓
Miniature pinscher	Leave ½ in. (two vertebrae)
Silky terrier	Leave about ⅓ (about ½ in.)
Toy poodle	Leave ½–⅔ (about 1 in.)
Yorkshire terrier	Leave about ⅓ (about ½ in.)
Nonsporting Breeds	
Miniature poodle	Leave ½–⅔ (about 1⅛ in.)
Schipperke	Close to body†
Standard poodle	Leave ½–⅔ (about 1½ in.)
Miscellaneous Breeds (not registered by American Kennel Club)	
Cavalier King Charles spaniel	Optional; leave at least ⅔; always leave white tip in broken-colored dogs
Spinoni Italiani	Leave ⅗

* This list gives *approximate* guides for docking when done before the puppy is 1 week old. If definite information was not given in the official breed standard, *opinions* were obtained from judges, breeders, veterinarians, and professional handlers. Breeds not listed are those not usually docked. Docking disqualifies the Boston terrier, Cardigan Welsh corgi, and West Highland white terrier for showing. An improperly docked tail may ruin a puppy for show purposes. If one is in doubt, consultation with an established breeder is suggested. There may be variations among puppies, and a knowledge of breed characteristics is important in determining the correct length to dock. M. Josephine Deublner, V.M.D., compiled most of these data.

† May be naturally tailless.

‡ Taken from official breed standard.

§ The tip of the docked tail should be approximately level with the top of the skull with the puppy in show position.

LINICAL NUTRITION FOR
ƷS AND CATS

L PRINCIPLES

a animal nutrition is to maximize health and longevity.
hed by feeding prepared diets to dogs and cats. A diet is
...es all the essential nutrients for a given animal, including
specific requirements for species, breed, age, and physiologic status. A diet is
balanced if it provides all the required nutrients in (optimal) proportion to the
animal's needs.

............MAINTENANCE ENERGY REQUIREMENTS

The *maintenance energy requirement (MER)* is loosely defined as the amount
of energy necessary to "maintain" an adult healthy dog or cat in a comfortable
environment with moderate activity. It is estimated as a multiple of the animal's resting energy requirement (RER). Any estimate of MER needs to account
for individual variation in activity, as well as variation in environmental demands on metabolism (e.g., what is the energy cost of spending a day out in
the cold?). What is not clear is just which figure or multiple to use. For both
dogs and cats the values have declined each time they have been critically
evaluated. Until more data are acquired, the current "best estimate" for dogs
is 1.6×110 kcal/kg$^{.75}$, and for cats it is 1.4×110 kcal/kg$^{.75}$. Nutrition textbooks
will list values for MER in cats which range from 60 to 80 kcal/kg/day, and a
value of 70 kcal/kg/day is suggested for "inactive" cats.

These calculations provide an estimate of maintenance requirements. Table
6–4 demonstrates individual variation with respect to an animal's energy needs
since maintenance depends on activity or work level, environment, and physiologic state. The formulas in Table 6–4 do not apply to growing animals. Growth
in puppies and kittens is dynamic and nutrient (energy) needs change almost
daily depending on breed and stage of growth (Table 6–5).

............LIFE STAGE NUTRITION

The theory behind life stage nutrition is that the use of a complete and balanced
diet specific for a particular life stage allows animals in different physiologic
states to be fed, or to eat, their energy requirements and simultaneously obtain
all of their nutrient needs. In practical terms this is the best way to approach
feeding normal dogs, cats, kittens, and puppies since the nutrient requirements
for each life stage are indeed different. Body condition scoring criteria for adult
dogs and cats are listed in Table 6–6.

Table 6–4. Canine Energy Requirements in Different Physiologic States

Activity	Estimate of Energy Needs
Light work (1 hr/day)	$1.1 \times$ MER
Light work (all day)	$1.5 \times$ MER
Heavy work	2–$4 \times$ MER
Gestation (1st 6 wks)	$1 \times$ MER
Gestation (last 3 wks)	$1.3 \times$ MER
Peak lactation	2–$4 \times$ MER

MER, maintenance energy requirement.

Table 6–5. Energy Requirements for Puppies and Kittens

Age	Energy Needs*
Puppies	
Birth–3 mo	2.0 × MER
3–6 mo	1.6 × MER
6–12 mo	1.2 × MER
3–9 mo (giant)	1.6 × MER
9–24 mo (giant)	1.2 × MER
Kittens	
5 wk	~250 kcal ME/kg
30 wk	~100 kcal ME/kg
50 wk	~85 kcal ME/kg

MER, maintenance energy requirement; ME, metabolizable energy.
* Multiples of MER for an adult dog of the same body weight.

............Canine Nutrition

............Gestation, Lactation, Pregnancy

From a nutritional view pregnancy in the dog is a nonevent until the last trimester when most of fetal growth and development occur. Therefore no changes in diet composition or food intake need to be made until the last trimester (starting at weeks 5 to 6). In fact, increased food intake or a switch to a more energy-dense or palatable diet earlier in pregnancy simply encourages excess fat deposition which could complicate delivery of puppies.

Starting at weeks 5 to 6, things begin to change. Rapid fetal development places increased nutritional demands on the bitch. Thus, nutrient intake needs to increase. One recommendation is to increase food intake by 15% each week, starting at week 5, until delivery. That presents practical problems because most owners will not be able to (or may not be that interested in) accurately increasing food intake by 15% per week. Also, depending on litter size there may be limited room in the abdomen for more digesta, and in addition appetite and activity are often decreased during the last trimester, meaning that voluntary increases in food intake are unlikely. Feeding frequent small meals is one way to overcome the problem (four to five times per day). *A more practical solution is to change the diet beginning the last trimester (weeks 5 to 6) to an energy-dense diet.* Most commonly, growth diets are used to support gestation and lactation. Changing to such a diet during the last trimester, before birth, provides the increased nutrients necessary to support fetal development and allows the bitch to adapt to the new diet before undergoing the stress of lactation (rather than adding to the stress by changing the diet around parturition).

Depending on litter size the energy cost of lactation can be as much as two to four times more than maintenance. The easiest way to accommodate the increased metabolic demands is to feed the lactating bitch ad libitum. This would not be appropriate for small litters which do not place a significant burden on the bitch.

............Feeding Puppies

6

A useful rule of thumb is that pups should gain approximately 1 to 2 g/lb of adult body weight per day. Gruel is typically introduced at about 3 weeks, and fed until 5 weeks, when solid food is introduced. Weaning is usually at 6 to 7

Table 6–6. Body Condition Scoring Criteria

Score		Criteria
Dogs		
1	Ribs:	Easily palpable with no fat cover
Very thin	Tailbase:	Prominent raised bony structures with no subcutaneous tissue
	Abdomen:	Severe abdominal tuck, accentuated hourglass shape
2	Ribs:	Easily palpable with minimal fat cover
Underweight	Tailbase:	Raised bony structure with little subcutaneous tissue
	Abdomen:	Abdominal tuck, marked hourglass shape
3	Ribs:	Palpable with slight fat cover
Ideal	Tailbase:	Smooth contour or some thickening; bony structures palpable under thin layer of subcutaneous fat
	Abdomen:	Abdominal tuck, well-proportioned lumbar "waist"
4	Ribs:	Difficult to palpate, moderate fat cover
Overweight	Tailbase:	Smooth contour or some thickening; bony structures remain palpable
	Abdomen:	Little or no abdominal tuck or waist; back slightly broadened
5	Ribs:	Very difficult to palpate; thick fat cover
Obese	Tailbase:	Appears thickened, difficult to palpate bony structures
	Abdomen:	Pendulous ventral bulge, no waist, back markedly broadened
		Trough may form when epaxial areas bulge dorsally
Cats		
1	Ribs:	Easily palpable with no fat cover
Very thin	Bony prominences:	Easily palpable
	Abdomen:	Severe abdominal tuck
2	Ribs:	Easily palpable with minimal fat cover
Underweight	Bony prominences:	Easily palpable
	Abdomen:	Obvious waist, minimal abdominal fat palpable
3	Ribs:	Palpable with slight fat cover
Ideal	Abdomen:	Well-proportioned waist, minimal abdominal fat pad
4	Ribs:	Difficult to palpate, moderate fat cover
Overweight	Abdomen:	Little or no waist, abdominal rounding, moderate abdominal fat pad
5	Ribs:	Very difficult to palpate, thick fat cover
Obese	Abdomen:	Distended with extensive fat deposit, no waist
		Fat deposits over lumbar area, ± limbs

From Armstrong J, Lund E: Changes in body composition and energy balance with aging. Vet Clin Nutrition 3:83–87, 1996.

weeks. Once puppies are weaned many nutritional mistakes can and have been made which affect the entire life of the dog. There are numerous approaches to feeding puppies and normal dogs. Historically, the recommendations have varied from feeding puppies ad libitum to feeding all they can eat two or three times per day. Intuitively this makes sense since they are growing rapidly. Unfortunately, this is the worst thing to do! *Overnutrition is the most common form of malnutrition in companion animals! In adults the result is obesity. During growth excessive energy intake can be particularly devastating, especially in puppies of large breeds. Overnutrition during growth exacerbates developmental skeletal diseases, including hip dysplasia, osteochondritis dissicans, and wobbler's syndrome.* In contrast, caloric restriction leads to an increase in both life span and overall health in every species studied. Therefore, except for the toy and miniature breeds, some form of controlled feeding should be instituted for puppies. Subsequently, recommendations were to feed on a time-restricted basis (all the puppy could eat in 15 to 20 minutes). Current recommendations are even more severe, and puppies should generally be fed all they can eat for 5 to 10 minutes three to four times daily until they are 50% of adult body weight. Feeding frequency is then reduced to twice daily. The exception to this is feeding miniature breeds ad libitum, or at least four to five times per day because they have a large metabolic body size and limited fuel stores.

............Feeding Adult Dogs

Puppies should be switched from growth diets to maintenance or adult diets when they have reached about 90% of their adult body weight. Generally, adult dogs can be fed once daily, although twice daily is more appropriate. Maintenance energy requirements need to be met, beyond the fact that the type and amount of food will depend on the individual dog (whether it is a lap dog or working dog, etc.). Obesity is the most common nutritional disorder of adult dogs, is more common in neutered dogs, and is more easily prevented than treated. It is important to inform owners that despite the fact that neutering reduces the risk of certain other diseases and prevents pet overpopulation, after neutering their pet is at increased risk for obesity, and food intake needs to be regulated!

............Feeding Senior Dogs

Life expectancy for dogs and cats has increased as a result of better veterinary health care, improved nutrition, and humans manipulation of what used to be "natural selection." Although specific recommendations are given to the special requirements of senior animals, there is little in the way of factual information available. The gaps can be filled superficially using knowledge available from human geriatric studies. In humans the aging process is accompanied by a decrease in food and energy needs due to changes in hormonal balance (drifting towards sexual neutrality with aging) and a decrease in metabolic rate due to decreases in bone mineral mass, lean tissue mass, and an increase in body fat. Some, if not all, of these changes can be slowed or reversed by enhanced physical conditioning. There is some evidence that in dogs a similar decrease in voluntary food intake occurs with aging and that digestive "efficiency" decreases. In general it can be argued that nutrient digestibility should be increased in senior diets to account for any possible loss of digestive or absorptive capacity. This is fine so long as diets are reduced in energy while being enriched in other nutrients to prevent obesity.

............Feeding Working and Athletic Dogs

Nutritional requirements have only recently been investigated. Working (field) dogs generally can be fed standard maintenance diets at increased amounts on days when exercise is increased substantially. This is in contrast to canine "athletes" such as endurance dogs that run across the Arctic for weeks or search-and-rescue dogs used to find survivors of natural or manmade disasters. These dogs are under incredible metabolic demands. In fact recent work with sled dogs in Alaska has shown that the metabolic rate of these dogs exceeds what was previously thought to be the theoretical maximum for dogs (food requirements during racing are six to seven times maintenance!). Generally, for these types of canine athletes, performance is a function of the degree of conditioning and the digestibility and fat content of the diet. It is the fat that is important as a concentrated source of energy to meet the increased metabolic demands. *Performance is not dependent on dietary protein level and protein needs do not increase with exercise!* Also, there is some evidence that vitamin and mineral requirements may be increased, although not enough data are available to make specific recommendations. Potential candidates include vitamins C and E and selenium, in part to counter increased oxidative stress in muscle. Practical feeding recommendations are obvious; under such circumstances athletic dogs need to be fed a very energy-dense (or high fat) diet which has been formulated so that the other nutrients are more concentrated (in keeping with the complete and balanced concept). They should be fed well before the day's events to avoid working on a full gastrointestinal tract.

............Feline Nutrition

The unique metabolism and subsequent nutrient needs of cats warrants a thorough discussion, since the domestic cat is growing in popularity and it is the only common obligate carnivore seen in veterinary practice. Domestic-cats are strict carnivores, having descended from the African wild cat (*Felis lybica*), a small desert cat native to North Africa. *As obligate carnivores of desert origin they have adapted to a high protein, high fat, low carbohydrate, and low fiber diet.* Subsequently, they have lost certain metabolic abilities, and have modified others. From a teleological view these adaptations have an evolutionary advantage, but can be problematic with respect to feline nutrition and clinical medicine. The desert origin provides for *differences in renal physiology* not found in other domestic species. For example, similar to some marine mammals, cats have the ability to concentrate urine to a much greater degree than other domestic species, and are able to maintain adequate hydration by drinking hypertonic solutions such as seawater, because of their ability to extract and excrete salt loads. While this seems merely a physiologic curiosity it begs important questions: What other aspects of renal physiology are different and do these influence nutrient needs? For example, data regarding acid-base balance and renal gluconeogenesis are not readily available, and in a clinical setting we are left to assume that these aspects of nutrition and physiology are similar to what is known in other species. These differences have practical implications in a clinical setting. When using commercially available nutrition support products we often end up diuresing cats in the process of providing adequate calories. Furthermore, the relationship between potassium balance, acid-base balance, and renal function is only now being addressed after the realization that cats develop a *hypokalemic polymyopathy* associated with renal failure. This may be precipitated by the chronic use of acidifying diets for the prevention of lower urinary tract disorders and is in stark contrast to the hyperkalemia observed in other mammals with renal failure.

Other aspects of feline nutrition and metabolism, perhaps better characterized than those above, include increased requirements for protein, arginine, and taurine. In addition and in contrast to most other mammals, cats have an obligate dietary requirement for arachidonic acid, vitamin A, and niacin. The most common nutritional diseases in cats are *obesity, hypervitaminosis A* (producing painful skeletal disease due to bony exostoses and fusion of joints, usually the result of overfeeding liver or kidney) and *thiamine deficiency* (neurologic symptoms including fits, ataxia, and weakness from diets high in thiaminases, e.g., raw fish or overcooked cereal diets). Pansteatitis (painful necrosis of fat stores) used to be seen in cats fed high fat diets with insufficient antioxidants, especially vitamin E. The main differential was feline infections peritonitis (FIP) because of the resulting neutrophilic exudate. This is a very rare disease but underscores the importance of a good dietary history!!!

Cats have high protein requirements compared to other species. *Adult maintenance requirements are four to six times higher than for dogs, and six to eight times higher than for humans.* This is a reflection of the need for protein as an energy source. As a result, cats, unlike omnivores or herbivores, do not downregulate protein degradative enzymes or urinary nitrogen excretion in response to changes in dietary protein intake. The clinical implications of obligate protein oxidation have not been investigated in obese cats undergoing weight loss or in the hospital setting in anorectic cats, but are of obvious practical importance.

In addition to a generalized increase in protein requirements, cats have an obligate need for dietary *arginine.* This appears to be due primarily to an inability to synthesize ornithine, meaning that the carbon skeleton for the urea cycle must be provided by dietary arginine. Cats fed a single meal of an arginine-deficient diet will quickly show signs of ammonia toxicity and hepatic encephalopathy, which is fatal within hours. This results from an inability to dispose of the ammonia generated by the obligate oxidation of protein coupled with an inability to maintain urea cycle function in the face of an arginine-deficient state. The importance of dietary arginine for the cat is further demonstrated by the results of a series of comparative studies which evaluated the ratio of intestinal transport capacity to physiologic load for a number of nutrients across a variety of species. The ratio of transport capacity to physiologic load for arginine is higher in the cat than for any other nutrient in any other species evaluated. Although naturally occurring arginine-deficient diets do not exist, a state of relative arginine deficiency accompanying anorexia or diminished food intake may play an important role in the clinical signs associated with certain disease conditions, especially the hepatic encephalopathy that is seen in feline liver diseases such as hepatic lipidosis.

Cats also have an obligate requirement for dietary *taurine,* a sulfur-containing β-amino acid. Taurine is the most abundant free intracellular amino acid in mammalian tissues and concentrations are highest in the brain, retina, heart, and platelets. The exact biologic function of taurine has not been elucidated, but it does play a role in development and maintenance of neural, myocardial, and reproductive tissue. As a result, several clinical syndromes associated with taurine deficiency occur in cats: *the earliest reported was feline central retinal degeneration.*

Additionally, taurine deficiency is associated with reproductive failure, poor neonatal survival, and abnormal development of embryonic neural tissues. Perhaps the most common and most significant clinical syndrome seen with taurine deficiency is a form of dilated cardiomyopathy. Dilated cardiomyopathy in the cat is proved to be associated with taurine deficiency. The dietary requirement for several other nutrients reflects the adaptation of the cat to a high protein, high fat diet. Not surprisingly cats are unable to utilize β-carotene, since they lack the dioxygense necessary to cleave this plant-derived precursor of vitamin A and instead rely on a preformed source of vitamin A, as found in animal tissue. Cats also require a preformed source of niacin, because they do not convert significant amounts of dietary tryptophan to niacin. Although they have a full complement of enzymes necessary to do so, the majority of dietary tryptophan is diverted to other pathways and subsequently metabolized. This is an adaptation which allows ingestion of a tryptophan-rich diet while maintaining normal circulating levels of tryptophan (and subsequently serotonin). Cats also require a preformed source of arachidonic acid that can only be found in animal tissue.

............*Pregnancy and Lactation*

From a nutritional view, pregnancy and gestation in cats are quite different than in other mammals in that nutrient needs, and thus food intake, begin to increase soon after mating, and gradually increase throughout gestation. Fortunately, meeting nutrient needs is rather easy since during gestation and lactation, queens can be fed ad libitum with little risk of obesity. As for the dog, energy requirements during lactation are three to four times MER.

............*Growth*

Generally, the previous comments made for dogs apply to kittens; however, kittens grow faster than puppies and reach mature body weight sooner. Therefore, kittens generally start on solid food sooner. Generally, by 3 to 4 weeks they will eat substantial amounts of food when offered. There are some interesting changes which occur in nutrient absorption, digestion, and transport in kittens early in life. One of the most important changes is the loss of intestinal lactase activity after about 8 to 12 weeks. As a result, older kittens and adult cats should not be fed substantial amounts of milk, as it can result in diarrhea and certainly can lead to exuberant production of flatulence.

Similar to the nutritional differences between dogs and puppies, kittens have increased needs for a number of nutrients, relative to the needs of an adult cat. Kittens have especially increased needs for protein, taurine, sulfur-containing amino acids, arginine, and calcium and phosphorus. In contrast to most puppies (except the miniature breeds), most kittens have reached 75% of their adult body size by 6 months and can be safely switched to adult cat food by then. Some growth and development still occurs between 6 and 12 months, but the rate and, subsequently, the nutritional needs are substantially lower.

............*Feeding Adult Cats*

MER for adult cats is approximately $1.4 \times$ RER, lower than that for other domestic species. This is probably due to the degree of metabolic efficiency related to the fact that "catnaps" lower the metabolic rate. In a "natural environment," cats tend to eat multiple small meals a day. In a domestic environment, most cats are nibblers and will eat dry food in small quantities until they have met their needs. Cat owners may elect to feed a combination of wet and canned food in conjunction with dry kibble.

............*Obesity and Neutering*

Obesity is the number one form of malnutrition in dogs and cats. Predisposing factors involved in obesity are living indoors and neutering. Prevention of obesity is much easier than treatment, especially since treatment is not terribly successful and tends to be a lot of work for veterinarians and owners. Along the lines of prevention, owners need to be aware of the fact that after neutering, because of changes in (hormonal) physiology, their pets' nutritional needs have been altered forever. In other species in which the effects of neutering have been studied (mainly rats, mice, and humans), there is a loss of lean body mass and bone mineral content and a gain in fat mass, often without significant change in body weight. It is important to inform owners that body weight and food intake need to be monitored closely in neutered animals.

...........Feeding Senior Cats

What is a senior cat? The definition is perhaps more vague than "senior dog!" The genetic maximum life span for cats is about 28 years. Some texts suggest that by the age of 7 or 8 years, cats are geriatric. Again, as with dogs, it would be good in theory to feed senior cats a highly digestible diet. Equally important is to maintaining oral hygiene through the use of abrasive foods. This is easier in dogs since they can be given "chew toys" and biscuits. Minimizing the buildup of tartar and subsequent gingival disease will prevent the decrease in food intake and the burden placed on the immune system and kidneys as a result of food particles and bacteria that enter the bloodstream. This is especially important since renal failure is one of the most common causes of serious disease in older cats. The debate over whether dietary protein should be decreased in otherwise healthy old cats to prevent kidney damage is still present. What is clear is that in cats with overt renal failure, protein and the associated phosphorus should be decreased.

...........When and How to Feed

There are three types of feeding regimens that may be used when feeding dogs and cats. These regimens are called free-choice (also called ad libitum or self-feeding), time-controlled feeding, and portion-controlled feeding. One method of feeding may be preferred over another, depending on the owner's daily schedule, the number of animals that are being fed, and acceptability of the method by the pet.

Free-choice feeding involves having a surplus amount of food available at all times. The pet is able to consume as much food as desired at any time of the day. This type of feeding relies on the animal's ability to self-regulate food intake so that energy and nutrient needs are met. Dry pet food is most suitable for this type of feeding because it will not spoil as quickly as canned food or dry out as easily as semimoist products. However, even if dry food is used, the food bowl or dispenser should be cleaned and refilled with fresh food daily. Disadvantages to free-choice feeding are food wastage, overeating, and increased risk of developmental bone disease because of overconsumption in the large and giant breeds of dogs. Free-choice feeding is contraindicated in these type of "at risk" dogs until they have reached skeletal maturity at 12 months of age or 80% to 90% of mature body weight.

Time-controlled feeding involves contolling the amount of time that the pet has access to food. Similar to a free-choice regimen, time-controlled feeding relies somewhat on the pet's ability to regulate its daily energy intake. At mealtime, a surplus of food is provided, and the pet is allowed to eat for a predetermined period of time. Most adult dogs and cats that are not physiologically stressed are able to consume enough food within 15 to 20 minutes to meet their daily needs. Although one meal per day can be sufficient for feeding adult pets during maintenance, providing two meals per day is healthier and more satisfying. There is some evidence that feeding once daily can lead to gastric changes that are associated with gastric dilatation in large breeds of dogs. Moreover, feeding two times per day reduces hunger between meals and minimizes food-associated behavior problems such as begging and stealing food.

Portion-contolled feeding is the feeding method of choice in most situations. This procedure allows the owner the greatest amount of control over the pet's diet. One or several meals are provided per day, and they are premeasured to meet the pet's daily caloric and nutrient needs. Many adult pets can be maintained on one meal, but providing two or more daily meals is preferable. Portion-controlled feeding enables the owner to carefully monitor the pet's food consumption and immediately observe any changes in food intake or eating behavior. The pet's growth and weight can be strictly controlled with this

6

method by adjusting either the amount of food or the type of food that is fed. As a result, conditions of underweight, overweight, or inappropriate growth rate can be corrected at an early stage.

............Determining How Much to Feed

In all animals, food intake is governed principally by energy requirements. When companion animals are fed free-choice, the underlying control over the amount of food that is consumed is primarily the pet's need for energy. Although highly palatable or energy-dense foods can override the natural tendency to eat to meet energy needs, energy is still the dietary component that most strongly governs the amount of food consumed. When companion animals are fed on a portion-controlled basis, owners will select a quantity of food based primarily on the pet's weight response and energy needs. If the pet gains too much weight (energy surplus), the owner will decrease the amount that is fed. Conversely, if weight is lost, an increased amount of food is provided. Energy requirements are described in Tables 6–4 and 6–5. Once the daily caloric requirement has been calculated in kilocalories per day, divide this number by the energy density of the food to determine the amount of food to feed per day.

Another way to determine the amount to feed a dog or cat is to use the guidelines that are included on the commercial pet food label. All pet foods that carry the complete and balanced claim are required to include feeding instructions on the product label. These guidelines usually provide estimates of the quantity to feed for several different ranges in body size. Such instructions provide only a rough estimate which can be used as a starting point when first feeding a particular brand of food. Adjustments to in these estimates should be made based on the owner's knowledge of the individual animal and on the animal's response to feeding.

............NUTRITIONAL SUPPORT OF THE SURGICAL PATIENT

Nutritional requirements of the surgical patient are dependent on the patient's metabolic rate and nutritional status. In hypermetabolic surgical patients that are unable or unwilling to eat voluntarily, nutritional supplementation is indicated. Common causes of hypermetabolism in the surgical patient include trauma; sepsis; surgery; disease states, especially cancer; and drug therapy.

■ PHYSICAL EXAMINATION AND HISTORY INDICATING NUTRITIONAL ABNORMALITY.

Recent loss of body weight > 10%
Recent major surgery or extensive trauma
Altered food intake with restriction over a 10-day period
Increased metabolic loss associated with diarrhea, vomiting, malabsorption, draining abscesses, wounds, and burns
Increased nutritional needs associated with burns, infection, trauma, cancer, fever, pregnancy, or lactation
Use of drugs that alter appetite
Disease that produces chronic organ dysfunction

The nutritional status of the surgical patient can have a major impact on wound healing and immunity characterized by reduced immunoglobulin synthesis and altered cell-mediated immunity, hypoproteinemia, intestinal mucosal atrophy, and reduced cell synthesis.

■ ENERGY REQUIREMENTS FOR THE SURGICAL PATIENT

Body Condition	Factor × Maintenance
Hypermetabolism	
Mild stress	1.0–1.2
Moderate stress	1.2–1.5
Severe stress	1.5–2.0

Protein requirements for the surgical patient may be 25% to 48% of the metabolizable energy. High fat diets are recommended for the surgical patient, utilizing triglycerides as the principle energy source. Cancer patients require increased levels of proteins of high-quality biologic value and high in carbohydrates. Food for cancer patients should avoid simple sugars.

REFERENCES

Case L, Carey D, Hirakawa D: Canine and Feline Nutrition. St Louis, Mosby–Year Book 1995.

Richardson D, Toll P: Relationship of nutrition to developmental skeletal disease in young dogs. Vet Clin Nutrition 4:6–13, 1997.

Prymak C, Gorman N: Nutritional support of the surgical canine patient. Waltham Focus 4(4):1997.

··········· VETERINARY DIETS

Several special diets developed for dogs and cats with acute, as well as chronic, illness are available through veterinary practices exclusively. Nutrient reference charts are listed for several of these diets in Tables 6–7 and 6–8.

Table 6–7. Canine Nutrient Reference Charts

	As Fed, Caloric Basis (g/100 kcal)	
	Canned	Dry
Eukanuba Veterinary Diets The Iams Company Dayton, OH 45414 800-525-4267		
Product Name: Response Formula KO/Canine		
Protein		4.9
Fat		3.6
Carbohydrate		12.0
Fiber		0.69
Calcium		0.16
Phosphorus		0.13
Sodium		0.12
Potassium		0.15
Magnesium		0.04
Chloride		—
ME (kcal/can)		
ME (kcal/cup)		381

6

Table continued on following page

Table 6–7. Canine Nutrient Reference Charts *Continued*

	As Fed, Caloric Basis (g/100 kcal)	
	Canned	Dry
Product Name: Restricted Calorie Formula/Canine		
Protein		4.7
Fat		1.6
Carbohydrate		17.2
Fiber		0.47
Calcium		0.20
Phosphorus		0.18
Sodium		0.10
Potassium		0.18
Magnesium		0.016
Chloride		0.15
ME (kcal/can)		
ME (kcal/cup)		238
Product Name: Nutritional Kidney Formula Early Stage		
Protein		4.72
Fat		3.3
Carbohydrate		13.6
Fiber		0.56
Calcium		0.17
Phosphorus		0.099
Sodium		0.12
Potassium		0.16
Magnesium		0.019
Chloride		0.27
ME (kcal/can)		
ME (kcal/cup)		285
Product Name: Response Formula FP/Canine		
Protein	8.0	5.5
Fat	6.7	3.1
Carbohydrate	5.9	11.6
Fiber	0.3	0.5
Calcium	0.29	0.24
Phosphorus	0.21	0.22
Sodium	0.16	0.13
Potassium	0.49	0.37
Magnesium	0.024	0.034
Chloride	0.25	0.26
ME (kcal/can, 14 oz)	518	
ME (kcal/cup)		301
Product Name: Low Residue Canine		
Protein	7.5	5.9
Fat	4.5	2.5
Carbohydrate	7.5	12.9
Fiber	0.54	0.48
Calcium	0.19	0.23
Phosphorus	0.18	0.18
Sodium		0.1

Table 6–7. Canine Nutrient Reference Charts *Continued*

| | As Fed, Caloric Basis (g/100 kcal) | |
	Canned	Dry
Potassium		0.2
Magnesium		0.017
Chloride		—
ME (kcal/can, 14 oz)	447	
ME (kcal/cup)		328

Product Name: Nutritional Kidney Formula Advanced Stage

Protein		3.27
Fat		3.31
Carbohydrate		13.6
Fiber		0.41
Calcium		0.13
Phosphorus		0.06
Sodium		0.1
Potassium		0.1
Magnesium		0.01
Chloride		0.3
ME (kcal/can)		
ME (kcal/cup)		310

Product Name: Low Residue Formula for Puppies

Protein		6.7
Fat		4.5
Carbohydrate		7.2
Fiber		0.39
Calcium		0.24
Phosphorus		0.19
Sodium		0.08
Potassium		0.16
Magnesium		0.018
Chloride		0.17
ME (kcal/can)		
ME (kcal/cup)		435

Product Name: Maximum Calorie/Canine

Protein	7.5	7.8
Fat	7.1	5.6
Carbohydrate	1.3	4.4
Fiber	0.28	0.45
Calcium	0.19	0.26
Phosphorus	0.15	0.20
Sodium	0.05	0.08
Potassium	0.18	0.29
Magnesium	0.013	0.018
Chloride	0.14	0.24
ME (kcal/kg, 6 oz)	2,000	4,870

Table continued on following page **6**

Table 6–7. Canine Nutrient Reference Charts *Continued*

	As Fed, Caloric Basis (g/100 kcal)	
	Canned	Dry

Product Name: Glucose Control

Protein		8.1
Fat		2.2
Carbohydrate		14.7
Fiber		0.81
Calcium		0.31
Phosphorus		0.25
Sodium		0.18
Potassium		0.3
Magnesium		0.045
Chloride		0.37
ME (kcal/can)		
ME (kcal/cup)		253

WALTHAM Veterinary Diets
Vernon, CA 90058-0853
800-925-8426

Product Name: Canine Low Phosphorus/Low Protein

Protein	3.50	3.91
Fat	5.55	3.57
Carbohydrate	11.90	17.45
Fiber	0.31	0.54
Calcium	0.22	0.17
Phosphorus	0.06	0.08
Sodium	0.04	0.04
Potassium	0.15	0.16
Magnesium	0.012	0.022
Chloride	0.14	0.15
ME (kcal/can)	607.2	N/A
ME (kcal/cup)	N/A	287.3

Product Name: Canine Low Phosphorus/Medium Protein

Protein	4.81	4.70
Fat	7.20	3.63
Carbohydrate	6.52	15.06
Fiber	0.25	0.53
Calcium	0.17	0.19
Phosphorus	0.08	0.11
Sodium	0.06	0.04
Potassium	0.18	0.16
Magnesium	0.014	0.022
Chloride	0.36	0.02
ME (kcal/can)	625.3	N/A
ME (kcal/cup)	N/A	307.2

Product Name: Canine Low Fat

Protein	9.07	6.87
Fat	1.72	1.87
Carbohydrate	15.77	17.15
Fiber	0.44	0.62

Table 6–7. Canine Nutrient Reference Charts *Continued*

	As Fed, Caloric Basis (g/100 kcal)	
	Canned	Dry
Calcium	0.47	0.34
Phosphorus	0.35	0.32
Sodium	0.20	0.13
Potassium	0.27	0.20
Magnesium	0.025	0.029
Chloride	0.30	0.29
ME (kcal/can)	375.1	N/A
ME (kcal/cup)	N/A	264.1

Product Name: Canine High Fiber

Protein		6.21
Fat		2.50
Carbohydrate		16.42
Fiber		1.45
Calcium		0.38
Phosphorus		0.42
Sodium		0.08
Potassium		0.28
Magnesium		0.046
Chloride		0.29
ME (kcal/can)		N/A
ME (kcal/cup)		226.8

Product Name: Canine Selected Protein with Lamb and Rice

Protein	7.80	
Fat	4.76	
Carbohydrate	9.84	
Fiber	0.64	
Calcium	0.31	
Phosphorus	0.20	
Sodium	0.15	
Potassium	0.16	
Magnesium	0.021	
Chloride	0.16	
ME (kcal/can)	387.3	
ME (kcal/cup)	N/A	

Product Name: Canine Selected Protein with Rice and Catfish

Protein		7.21
Fat		2.65
Carbohydrate		14.98
Fiber		1.29
Calcium		0.64
Phosphorus		0.42
Sodium		0.12
Potassium		0.19
Magnesium		0.031
Chloride		0.27
ME (kcal/can)		N/A
ME (kcal/cup)		258.2

Table continued on following page

Table 6–7. Canine Nutrient Reference Charts *Continued*

| | As Fed, Caloric Basis (g/100 kcal) | |
	Canned	Dry
Product Name: Canine Calorie Control		
Protein	12.05	8.76
Fat	5.80	2.78
Carbohydrate	3.35	13.06
Fiber	0.90	0.99
Calcium	0.50	0.61
Phosphorus	0.33	0.55
Sodium	0.17	0.12
Potassium	0.59	0.38
Magnesium	0.055	0.048
Chloride	0.39	0.40
ME (kcal/can)	195.6	N/A
ME (kcal/cup)	N/A	212.1

ME, metabolizable energy; NA, not applicable.

Table 6–8. Feline Nutrient Reference Charts

| | As Fed, Caloric Basis (g/100 kcal) | |
	Canned	Dry
Eukanuba Veterinary Diets		
The Iams Company		
Dayton, OH 45414		
800-525-4267		
Product Name: Maximum Calorie/Feline		
Protein	7.5	8.2
Fat	7.1	5.5
Carbohydrate	1.3	3.5
Fiber	0.28	0.27
Calcium	0.19	0.25
Phosphorus	0.15	0.20
Sodium	0.05	0.10
Potassium	0.18	0.17
Magnesium	0.013	0.017
Chloride	0.14	0.19
Taurine		
ME (kcal/kg)	2,000	4,870
Product Name: Response Formula LB/Feline		
Protein	7.9	
Fat	4.9	
Carbohydrate	4.7	
Fiber	0.3	
Calcium	0.24	
Phosphorus	0.21	

Table 6–8. Feline Nutrient Reference Charts *Continued*

	As Fed, Caloric Basis (g/100 kcal)	
	Canned	Dry
Sodium	0.08	
Potassium	0.13	
Magnesium	0.012	
Chloride	0.07	
Taurine	0.07	
ME (kcal/can, 6 oz)	222	
ME (kcal/cup)		

Product Name: Restricted Calorie Formula/Feline

Protein		8.4
Fat		2.4
Carbohydrate		10.7
Fiber		0.49
Calcium		0.26
Phosphorus		0.20
Sodium		0.08
Potassium		0.20
Magnesium		0.02
Chloride		0.16
Taurine		0.07
ME (kcal/can)		
ME (kcal/cup)		298

Product Name: Nutritional Urinary Formula Low pH/S

Protein	9.5	7.8
Fat	6.2	3.9
Carbohydrate	3.5	8.0
Fiber	0.21	0.40
Calcium	0.24	0.24
Phosphorus	0.19	0.20
Sodium	0.09	0.11
Potassium	0.18	0.20
Magnesium	0.02	0.018
Chloride	0.14	0.19
Taurine	0.13	0.05
ME (kcal/can, 6 oz)	197	
ME (kcal/cup)		441

Product Name: Nutritional Urinary Formula Moderate pH/O

Protein	9.2	7.7
Fat	5.9	3.9
Carbohydrate	3.2	8.0
Fiber	0.20	0.4
Calcium	0.23	0.24
Phosphorus	0.17	0.21
Sodium	0.099	0.10
Potassium	0.27	0.31
Magnesium	0.023	0.019
Chloride	0.15	0.15
Taurine	0.12	0.045

6

Table continued on following page

Table 6–8. Feline Nutrient Reference Charts *Continued*

	As Fed, Caloric Basis (g/100 kcal)	
	Canned	Dry
ME (kcal/can, 6 oz)	197	
ME (kcal/cup)		451

Product Name: Low Residue Formula/Feline

	Canned	Dry
Protein	10.4	8.5
Fat	4.2	3.3
Carbohydrate	7.9	9.7
Fiber	0.5	0.43
Calcium	0.30	0.24
Phosphorus	0.24	0.23
Sodium	0.13	0.08
Potassium	0.28	0.24
Magnesium	0.021	0.025
Chloride	0.27	0.21
Taurine	0.12	0.05
ME (kcal/can, 6 oz)	165	
ME (kcal/cup)		369

WALTHAM Veterinary Diets
Vernon, CA 90058-0853
800-925-8426

Product Name: Feline Low Phosphorus/Low Protein

	Canned	Dry
Protein	5.72	5.83
Fat	8.55	5.19
Carbohydrate	2.83	10.14
Fiber	0.28	1.11
Calcium	0.19	0.18
Phosphorus	0.08	0.10
Sodium	0.12	0.04
Potassium	0.21	0.17
Magnesium	0.031	0.017
Chloride	0.50	0.09
Taurine		
ME (kcal/can)	286.6	N/A
ME (kcal/cup)	N/A	380.6

Product Name: Feline Calorie Control

	Canned	Dry
Protein	12.44	12.89
Fat	5.70	2.40
Carbohydrate	2.98	9.85
Fiber	0.66	1.20
Calcium	0.41	0.67
Phosphorus	0.34	0.40
Sodium	0.40	0.20
Potassium	0.37	0.28
Magnesium	0.023	0.024
Chloride	0.41	0.51
Taurine	0.140	0.355
ME (kcal/can)	110.7	N/A
ME (kcal/cup)	N/A	211.2

Table 6–8. Feline Nutrient Reference Charts *Continued*

	As Fed, Caloric Basis (g/100 kcal)	
	Canned	Dry
Product Name: Feline Selected Protein with Rice and Duck		
Protein		9.34
Fat		3.45
Carbohydrate		10.83
Fiber		1.32
Calcium		0.52
Phosphorus		0.37
Sodium		0.19
Potassium		0.21
Magnesium		0.023
Chloride		0.41
Taurine		
ME (kcal/can)		N/A
ME (kcal/cup)		264.3
Product Name: Feline Selected Protein with Venison and Rice		
Protein	11.14	
Fat	4.31	
Carbohydrate	7.68	
Fiber	0.72	
Calcium	0.34	
Phosphorus	0.27	
Sodium	0.26	
Potassium	0.33	
Magnesium	0.02	
Chloride	0.21	
Taurine	0.97	
ME (kcal/can)	151.5	
ME (kcal/cup)	N/A	
Product Name: S/O Feline Control pHormula Diet		
Protein	7.50	8.77
Fat	8.00	4.73
Carbohydrate	1.90	8.27
Fiber	0.24	0.51
Calcium	0.17	0.17
Phosphorus	0.21	0.21
Sodium	0.21	0.22
Potassium	0.21	0.23
Magnesium	0.015	0.015
Chloride	0.18	0.51
Taurine	0.186	0.097
ME (kcal/can)	177.5	N/A
ME (kcal/cup)	N/A	385.1

ME, metabolizable energy; N/A, not applicable.

6

Maternal milk and milk substitutes for puppies and kittens, along with dosing information, are provided in Tables 6–9, 6–10, and 6–11.

Table 6–9. Range of Intakes During First 4 Weeks of Life (kcal/g Body Weight)

Week 1	0.13–0.2
Week 2	0.15–0.22
Week 3	0.18–0.28
Week 4	0.2–0.3

* To estimate milk (Esbilac liquid) intake in milliliters, multiply intake (kcal/g body weight) by neonate body weight in grams, and divide product by energy content of milk (kcal/mL). For example, a 200-g pup at 7 days of age would need about 0.15 kcal/g × 200 g = 30 kcal ÷ 0.9 kcal/mL = 33 mL/day. This amount should be divided into four feedings. The animal should be fed until it is satiated, or, if feeding by gavage, until the abdomen is slightly distended. It should be fed again when it wakes up and vocalizes again. The ranges are broad to reflect large variation in reported recommendations. Younger animals in the ranges should be started at lower volumes. Orphans should be weighed daily and food intake adjusted to assure regular increase in body weight.

Table 6–10. Composition of Maternal Milk and Substitutes

	kcal/mL	% Solids	% Fat	% Protein	% Carbohydrate
Bitch milk	1.5	24.0	44.1	33.2	15.8
Esbilac powder*†	1.0	98.4	44.1	33.2	15.8
Esbilac liquid*	0.9	15.3	44.1	33.2	15.8
Cow milk	0.7	12.0	30.0	25.6	38.5
Evaporated milk‡	1.2	14.0	15.8	13.9	19.5
Cat milk	0.9	18.2	25.0	42.2	26.1
KMR*	0.9	18.2	25.0	42.2	26.1

* Manufactured by Pet-Ag, Inc., Elgin, IL.
† 1 volume to 3 volumes water.
‡ 4 volumes to 1 volume water.

Table 6–11. Ambient Temperature Guide for Raising Orphans*

Age of Orphan	Environmental Temperature
Birth–7 days	85°–90°F
7–28 days	80°–85°F
28–35 days	70°–80°F

* Younger animals should be maintained at the higher values of the range.

RECIPES FOR HOMEMADE DIETS

See Table 6–12.

Table 6–12. Recipes for Homemade Diets

Recipe I
Highly Digestible Diet for Dogs

½	cup farina (113 mL) (Cream of Wheat) cooked to make 2 cups (490 g)
1½	cups (340 g) creamed cottage cheese
1	large egg (50 g), hard-cooked
2	T (25 g) brewer's yeast
3	T (45 g) sugar
1	T (15 g) vegetable oil
1	t (5 g) potassium chloride
1	t (4.5 g) dicalcium phosphate
1	t (5 g) calcium carbonate

Balanced supplement which fulfills the canine MDR for all vitamins and trace minerals.
Cook farina according to package directions, including salt. Cool. Add remaining ingredients to farina and mix well. Yield: 2.2 lb (980 g).

	Nutrient Contents	
	As Fed	Dry Matter
Moisture (%)	75.8	0
Protein (%)	7.1	29.3
Fat (%)	3.7	15.3
Carbohydrate (%)	11.2	46.3
Fiber (%)	0.1	0.4
Ash (%)	2.1	8.7
Calcium (%)	0.33	1.4
Phosphorus (%)	0.19	0.8
Sodium (%)	0.16	0.7
Potassium (%)	0.36	1.5
ME (kcal/lb)	485	2008

Recipe 2
Restricted Protein-Phosphorus Diet for Dogs

¼	lb (115 g) ground beef (regular)*
1	large egg (50 g), hard-cooked
2	cups (350 g) cooked rice without salt
3	slices (75 g) white bread, crumbled
1	t (5 g) calcium carbonate

Balanced supplement which fulfills the canine MDR for all vitamins and trace minerals.
Braise the meat, retaining fat. Combine all ingredients and mix well. This mixture is somewhat dry. The palatability can be improved by adding some water (not milk). Yield: ¼ lb (595 g).

Table continued on following page

6

Table 6–12. Recipes for Homemade Diets *Continued*

	Nutrient Contents	
	As Fed	Dry Matter
Moisture (%)	65.5	0
Protein (%)	6.9	29.0
Fat (%)	5.5	15.9
Carbohydrate (%)	21.1	61.1
Fiber (%)	0.01	0.04
Ash (%)	1.0	2.9
Calcium (%)	0.36	1.03
Phosphorus (%)	0.1	0.29
Sodium (%)	0.1	0.26
Potassium (%)	0.1	0.27
Magnesium (%)	0.01	0.04
ME (kcal/lb)†	750	2175

* Do not use lean ground round or chuck.

† This diet supplies 17% protein calories, 30% fat calories, and 53% carbohydrate calories.

Recipe 3
Restricted Protein-Phosphorus Ultralow Protein Diet for Dogs

2½	cups (440 g) cooked rice
2	T (1 oz/28 g) vegetable oil
1	large egg (50 g), hard-cooked
¼	t (1.25 g) calcium carbonate
¼	t (1.25 g) potassium chloride

Balanced supplement which fulfills the canine MDR for all vitamins and trace minerals.

Cook rice as per package instructions, except use only ¼ salt. Add other ingredients and mix well. Yield: 1.1 lb (520 g).

	Nutrient Contents	
	As Fed	Dry Matter
Moisture (%)	69.2	0
Protein (%)	3.0	9.7
Fat (%)	6.7	21.7
Carbohydrate (%)	20.5	66.6
Fiber (%)	0.01	0.03
Ash (%)	0.6	2.1
Calcium (%)	0.12	0.39
Phosphorus (%)	0.07	0.22
Sodium (%)	0.10	0.32
Potassium (%)	0.17	0.55
Magnesium (%)	0.01	0.03
§ME (kcal/lb)*	690	2240

* This diet supplies 8% protein calories, 39% fat calories, and 53% carbohydrate calories.

Table 6–12. Recipes for Homemade Diets *Continued*

Recipe 4
Low Fat Reducing Diet for Dogs

¼	lb (115 g) lean ground beef
½	cup (75 g) cottage cheese, *uncreamed*
2	cups (310 g) carrots, canned solids
2	cups (270 g) green beans, canned solids
1½	t (7 g) dicalcium phosphate

Balanced supplement which fulfills the canine MDR for all vitamins and trace minerals.
Cook beef, drain fat, and cool. Add the remaining ingredients and mix.
  Yield: 1¾ lb (775 g).

	Nutrient Contents	
	As Fed	Dry Matter
Moisture (%)	86.4	0
Protein (%)	5.5	40.4
Fat (%)	1.7	12.5
Carbohydrate (%)	4.1	30.1
Fiber (%)	0.7	5.1
Ash (%)	1.6	11.8
Calcium (%)	0.17	1.3
Phosphorus (%)	0.17	1.3
Sodium (%)	0.23	1.7
Potassium (%)	0.14	1.0
ME (kcal/lb)	220	1614

Recipe 5
Low Sodium Diet for Dogs

¼	lb (115 g) lean ground beef
2	cups (350 g) cooked rice without salt
1	T (15 g) vegetable oil
2	t (9 g) dicalcium phosphate

Balanced supplement which fulfills the canine MDR for all vitamins and trace minerals.
Braise meat, retaining fat. Add the remaining ingredients and mix.
  Yield: 1.1 lb (490 g).

	Nutrient Contents	
	As Fed	Dry Matter
Moisture (%)	68.5	0
Protein (%)	6.3	20.0
Fat (%)	5.5	17.4
Carbohydrate (%)	17.6	55.8
Fiber (%)	0.07	0.22
Ash (%)	2.0	6.3
Calcium (%)	0.44	1.4

Table continued on following page

6

Table 6–12. Recipes for Homemade Diets *Continued*

Phosphorus (%)	0.44	1.4
Sodium (%).	0.016	0.052
Sodium (mg/100 kcal ME).	11	11
Potassium (%)	0.44	1.4
ME (kcal/lb)	660	2100

Recipe 6
Hypoallergenic Diet for Dogs or Cats

 ¼ lb (115 g) lamb
 1 cup (175 g) cooked rice
 1 t (5 g) vegetable oil
 1½ t (7 g) dicalcium phosphate
 ⅛ t (0.6 g) potassium chloride (salt substitute or no-sodium salt)

Balanced supplement which fulfills the canine or feline MDR for all vitamins
 and trace minerals.
Combine all ingredients and mix well. Yield: ⅔ lb (300 g).

	Nutrient Contents	
	As Fed	Dry Matter
Moisture (%)	66.0	0
Protein (%)	7.0	20.6
Fat (%)	10.0	29.4
Carbohydrate (%)	14.0	41.2
Fiber (%)	0.06	0.2
Ash (%)	2.9	8.5
Calcium (%)	0.53	1.6
Phosphorus (%)	0.51	1.5
Sodium (%).	0.24	0.7
Potassium (%)	0.24	0.7
ME (kcal/lb)	795	2340

Recipe 7
Liquid Diet for Dogs and Cats

 ½ can (224 g) Prescription Diet Feline p/d canned
 ¾ cup (170 mL) water

Blend to smooth consistency in a blender. Strain through a kitchen strainer
(1-mm mesh). Yield: 390 mL.

	Nutrient Contents	
	As Fed	Dry Matter
Moisture (%)	83.0	0
Protein (%)	7.4	44.2
Fat (%)	5.0	29.6
Carbohydrate (%)	2.8	17.0
Calcium (%)	0.19	1.1

Table 6–12. Recipes for Homemade Diets *Continued*

Phosphorus (%)	0.13	0.8
Sodium (%)	0.10	0.6
ME (kcal/lb)*	0.8/mL	4.75/g

Daily dose (dog or cat)—1 oz/lb (60 mL/kg) body weight. Fulfills all normal fluid and nutrient needs. Excessive fluid losses must be replaced by additional water or parenteral fluids.

---

* This diet supplies 33% protein calories, 55% fat calories, and 12% carbohydrate calories.

Recipe 8
Restricted Mineral and Sodium Diet for Cats

1	lb (450 g) regular ground beef, cooked
¼	lb (115 g) liver
1	cup (175 g) cooked rice without added salt
1	t (5 g) vegetable oil
1	t (5 g) calcium carbonate

Balanced supplement which fulfills the feline MDR for all vitamins and trace minerals.
Combine all ingredients. Yield: 1¾ lb (750 g).

	Nutrient Contents	
	As Fed	Dry Matter
Moisture (%)	64.0	0
Protein (%)	14.3	39.7
Fat (%)	13.9	38.6
Carbohydrate (%)	6.3	17.5
Fiber (%)	0.02	0.06
Ash (%)	1.4	3.9
Calcium (%)	0.27	0.75
Phosphorus (%)	0.16	0.44
Sodium (%)	0.06	0.16
Potassium (%)	0.20	0.56
Magnesium (%)	0.014	0.04
Magnesium (mg/100 kcal ME)	7	7
ME (kcal/lb)	940	2610
Taurine (%)	—	0.20

Recipe 9
Restricted Protein/Phosphorus Diet for Cats

¼	lb (115 g) liver
2	large eggs (100 g), hard-cooked
2	cups (350 g) cooked rice without added salt
1	T (15 g) vegetable oil
1	t (5 g) calcium carbonate
¼	t (1 g) potassium chloride (salt substitute or no-sodium salt)

Table continued on following page

6

Table 6–12. Recipes for Homemade Diets *Continued*

Balanced supplement which fulfills the feline MDR for all vitamins and trace minerals.

Dice and braise the liver, retaining fat. Combine all ingredients and mix well. This mixture is somewhat dry and the palatability may be improved by adding some water (not milk). Yield: 1¼ lb (585 g).

	Nutrient Contents	
	As Fed	Dry Matter
Moisture (%)	70.0	0
Protein (%)	7.3	24.3
Fat (%)	5.3	17.7
Carbohydrate (%)	15.8	52.7
Fiber (%)	0.06	0.2
Ash (%)	1.5	5.0
Calcium (%)	0.36	1.20
Phosphorus (%)	0.14	0.47
Phosphorus (mg/100 kcal ME)	100	100
Sodium (%)	0.05	0.17
Potassium (%)	0.21	0.70
Magnesium (%)	0.01	0.04
Magnesium (mg/100 kcal ME)	7	7
ME (kcal/lb)*	635	2140
Taurine (%).	—	0.09

*This diet supplies 21% protein calories, 35% fat calories, and 44% carbohydrate calories.

Recipe 10
Low Fat Reducing Diet for Cats

1¼	lb (565 g) liver, cooked and ground
1	cup (175 g) cooked rice
1	t (5 g) vegetable oil
1	t (5 g) calcium carbonate

Balanced supplement which fulfills the feline MDR for all vitamins and trace minerals.

Combine all ingredients. Yield: 1¾ lb (750 g).

	Nutrient Contents	
	As Fed	Dry Matter
Moisture (%)	70.0	0
Protein (%)	15.5	51.7
Fat (%)	3.4	11.3
Carbohydrate (%)	9.2	30.7
Fiber (%)	0.02	0.07
Ash (%)	1.9	6.3
Calcium (%)	0.28	0.9
Phosphorus (%)	0.28	0.9
Sodium (%)	0.19	0.6
Potassium (%)	0.22	0.7

Table 6–12. Recipes for Homemade Diets *Continued*

Magnesium (%)	0.012	0.04
Magnesium (mg/100 kcal ME)	9	9
ME (kcal/lb)	585	1950
Taurine (%).	—	0.10

ME, metabolizable energy; MDR, minimum daily requirement; T, tablespoon; t, teaspoon.

From Lewis LD, Morris ML, Hand MS: Small Animal Clinical Nutrition III. Topeka, Kan, Mark Morris Associates, 1987.

....

SHIPPING REGULATIONS FOR SMALL ANIMALS

..........INTERSTATE REGULATIONS

For the exact requirements regarding the entry of dogs and cats into the various states of the United States and Puerto Rico, inquiry should be made to the state veterinarian in the state of destination.

Under most circumstances, no animal that is affected with or has recently been exposed to any infectious, contagious, or communicable disease or that originates from a rabies-quarantine area shall be shipped or in any manner transported or moved into any state until written permission for such entry is first obtained from the state veterinarian or chief animal health official of the state to which the animal is to be transported.

Common carriers will usually not accept dogs or cats for interstate movement without health certificates; thus, it would seem advisable, even if not specifically required, that such certificates be issued by the accredited practicing veterinarian in the state of origin.

..........INTERNATIONAL REGULATIONS

Travelers from the United States to foreign countries on vacations and duty assignments frequently want to take their pets with them. Similarly, persons returning from abroad need to make arrangements for the reentry of their pets and for animals acquired in other countries. For both importations and exportations, there are usually health requirements with which one must comply.

..........MOVEMENT INTO FOREIGN COUNTRIES

There are no United States regulations governing the movement of dogs and cats to any foreign country. The regulations that must be complied with are those of the receiving country. These regulations are many, varied, and subject to change. If pets are to be moved to any foreign country except Canada, the owner should obtain from the nearest consulate of the country of destination that country's regulations and procedural instructions governing the importation of pets, such as the number of copies of the health certificate to be furnished, an indication of whether it must be validated by the consulate, and whether certified copies of the pedigree or photograph of the pet must accompany the health certificate.

Dogs from the United States may be imported into Canada through any Canadian customs port of entry when accompanied by a certificate signed by a veterinarian licensed in Canada or the United States. The certificate must show that the dog has been vaccinated against rabies during the preceding 12 months.

6

............IMPORTATION OR REENTRY OF DOGS INTO THE UNITED STATES

The entry of dogs into the United States from all foreign countries is under the jurisdiction of the Public Health Service of the United States Department of Health, Education, and Welfare, Centers for Disease Control and Prevention, Division of Quarantine, E-03, Atlanta, GA 30333. An excerpt from the United States Public Health Service regulations regarding importation of dogs is quoted:

Vaccination for rabies shall be accomplished with nerve tissue vaccine more than one month but not more than 12 months before the dog's arrival, or with chicken embryo vaccine more than one month but no more than 36 months before arrival.

............MOVEMENT INTERSTATE

Veterinarians should contact the individual state animal health control agency for confirmation of guidelines (see Table 6–13).

Table 6–13. State Travel Requirements

State	Telephone	Dogs	Cats	Rabies Vaccination Requirements	Exempt Under
AL	334-240-7255	Yes	Yes	Within 12 months	3 mo
AK	907-745-3236	Yes	Yes	Per Compendium	3 mo
AZ	602-542-4293	Yes		Per Compendium; permit number if from rabies quarantined area	4 mo
AR	501-225-5138	Yes	Yes	Within 12 months	3 mo
CA	916-654-0881	Yes		Per Compendium	4 mo
Canada	613-995-5433	Yes	Yes	Within 3 yr; rabies certificate tag with animal	3 mo
CO	303-239-4161	Yes	Yes	Within 12 months	3 mo
CT	203-566-4616	Yes	Yes	Over 21 days and within 6 mo or not exposed to rabies within 100 days	3 mo
DE	302-739-4811	Yes	Yes	Per Compendium	Dog, 4 mo; Cat, 6 mo
FL*	904-488-8280	No		Permit number required if from a rabies quarantined area	4 mo
GA	404-656-3671		Yes	Per Compendium; H.C. with commercial carrier shipment	3 mo
Guam	617-734-3940	No		120-day quarantine at facility; H.C. within 10 days	None
HI	808-483-7100		Yes	120-day quarantine at quarantine facility; inactivated vaccine only; other vaccination required; H.C. within 14 days	3 mo
ID	208-332-8560	Yes	Yes	Per Compendium	3 mo
IL	217-782-4944	Yes	Yes	Per Compendium	4 mo
IN	317-232-1344	Yes	Yes	Within 12 mo	3 mo
IA	515-281-5305	Yes		Per Compendium	4 mo
KS	913-296-2326	Yes	Yes	Per Compendium	3 mo
KY	502-564-3956	Yes	Yes	KV, 12 mo; MLV, 24 mo (dogs only)	4 mo
LA	504-925-3980	Yes	Yes	Within 12 mo	3 mo
ME	207-287-3701	Yes	Yes	No H.C. required unless for resale. Vaccination within 24 mo; approval by CDC	Dog, 6 mo; Cat, 3 mo
MD	410-841-5810	Yes	Yes	Within 12 mo; not exposed to rabies within 120 days	4 mo
MA	617-727-3018	Yes	Yes	Within 12 mo	4 mo
MI	517-373-1077	Yes		Per Compendium	6 mo
MN	612-296-2942	Yes	Yes	Per Compendium	3 mo

Table continued on following page

6

821

Table 6–13. State Travel Requirements *Continued*

State	Phone	Dogs	Cats	Rabies Vaccination Requirements	Exempt Under
MS	601-354-6089	Yes	Yes	Within 12 mo	3 mo
MO	573-751-3377	Yes	Yes	Per Compendium	4 mo
MT	406-444-2043	Yes	Yes	Per Compendium	3 mo
NE	402-471-2351	Yes	Yes	Per Compendium	3 mo
NV	702-688-1180	Yes	Yes	Per Compendium	3 mo
NH	603-271-2404	Yes	Yes	Per Compendium; ferrets require rabies vaccination	3 mo
NJ	609-292-3965	No		H.C.; if vaccination, per compendium	None
NM	505-841-4000	Yes	Yes	Within 12 mo	3 mo
NY	518-457-3502	Yes	Yes	Rabies vaccination within 12 mo	3 mo
NC	919-733-7601	Yes	Yes	Within 12 mo	4 mo
ND**	701-328-2655	Yes	Yes	Per Compendium; not exposed within 100 days	3 mo
OH	614-728-6220	Yes		Within 12 mo	6 mo
OK	405-521-3864	Yes		Within 12 mo; not exposed within 6 mo	4 mo
OR	503-986-4680	Yes	Yes	Per Compendium (permit number required if commercial carrier)	4 mo
PA	717-783-5301	Yes	Yes	Per Compendium; not exposed to rabies within 100 days	3 mo
Puerto Rico	809-725-1685	Yes	Yes	Within 6 mo; rabies certificate attached to H.C.	4 mo
RI	401-222-2781	Yes	Yes	KV, over 30 days and within 6 mo	3 mo
SC	803-788-2260	Yes	Yes	Within 12 mo	3 mo
SD	605-773-3321	Yes	Yes	Within 12 mo	Dog, 3 mo Cat, 6 mo
TN	615-360-0120	Yes	Yes	Within 12 mo	3 mo
TX	512-719-0700	Yes	Yes	Within 12 mo, do not require H.C. on dogs or cats	4 mo
UT	801-538-7160	Yes	Yes	KV, 12 mo; MLV, 24 mo	4 mo
VT	802-828-2421	Yes	Yes	3-year vaccine	4 mo
VA	804-786-2481	Yes	Yes	Within 12 mo; inactivated virus	

State	Phone			Requirement	
Virgin Islands	809-772-4781	Yes	Yes	Within 6 mo; rabies certificate attached to H.C.	2 mo
WA	360-902-1878	Yes	Yes	Per Compendium	3 mo
WV	304-558-2214	Yes	Yes	Within 12 mo	6 mo
WI	608-224-4872	Yes	Yes	Per Compendium	4 mo***
WY	307-777-7515	Yes	Yes	Per Compendium; within 24 mo; H.C. within 10 days of shipment	3 mo

Inspection should be made and health certificate (H.C.) issued within 30 days of shipment; if shipment is subject to the USDA Animal Welfare Act (wholesalers, researchers), H.C. must be issued within 10 days of shipment. If in doubt, call state of destination.

NOTE: Health Certificates for animals in commerce must be issued within 10 days of shipment to conform with the Animal Welfare Act, and cats and dogs must be over 8 weeks of age. Cats and dogs for resale must be inoculated against distemper not more than 30 nor less than 7 days before entry.

*H.C. must state no infectious disease, not from a rabies quarantine area, and no exposure to rabies. If animal is to remain in state less than 6 months, no H.C. required.

**Rabies vaccination required 30 days or more before entry for hunting dogs.

***Grace period of one month allowed.

SMALL ANIMAL EXPORT REQUIREMENTS: The following countries require Health Certificates for pets be endorsed by USDA:

Argentina	Dominican Republic	Hong Kong	Romania
Belgium	Egypt	Hungary	Trinidad/Tobago
Bulgaria	France	India	Uruguay
Chile	French Guiana	Italy	Venezuela
	French West Indies	Ivory Coast	
	Germany	Japan	Madagascar
	Guatemala	Lebanon	Mauritius
		Luxembourg	Netherlands
			Reunion

The Interstate Health Certificate for small animals, issued by the Arizona State Veterinarian's Office, is acceptable for endorsement by USDA. Please print your name under your signature.

CANADA: Dogs and cats from the United States need interstate health certificates, including statement of rabies inoculation administered within preceding 3 years, and endorsement by a licensed veterinarian. Non-psittacine birds from the United States must have an interstate health certificate from the USDA. A maximum of two non-psittacine birds from the United States may be brought into Canada in any 90-day period, if accompanied by owner, who must certify in writing that birds have not been in contact with any other birds and have been in owner's possession for preceding 90 days. Import permits must be obtained for birds not accompanied by owner, more than two birds, psittacine birds, and birds from countries other than the United States. Apply in advance to Canada for permit.

MEXICO: Veterinary certificates (in duplicate) are necessary listing inoculations (rabies and distemper) and including dates and types of vaccines. Certificates showing full description of the animal, including tag number, must be signed by a licensed veterinarian. Health certificates need *not* be endorsed.

Certificate in dual language required by Austria, Germany, and Italy. Bi-lingual health certificates (English/German) can be obtained from the State Veterinarian's or the USDA, APHIS, VS Office. These requirements are subject to change. If in doubt, contact the USDA, APHIS, VS Office. Table courtesy of State of Minnesota Board of Animal Health, St. Paul, Minnesota.

6

823

··

INHERITED DISEASES

This area of disease recognition and evaluation is undergoing very rapid change, especially as related to dogs. New genetic tests are being developed with rapid frequency as the dog genome is mapped. Table 6–14 serves as an introduction to this area of medicine.

The James A. Baker Laboratories at the New York State College of Veterinary Medicine has been actively involved in developing genetic screening tests for inherited diseases in purebred dogs. The emphasis has been on ocular disorders, including congenital stationary night blindness in the briard, PRA (progressive retinal atrophy) in the the Irish setter, and PRCD (progressive rod-cone degeneration), a form of PRA, in numerous breeds of dogs.

The dog genome project, conducted as a collaborative study at the University of California, Berkeley, the University of Oregon, and the Fred Hutchinson Cancer Research Center, is trying to map all of the chromosomes of the dog.

OptiGen LLC is a commercial genetic service licensing its technology from the James A. Baker Research Institute. They are offering genetic testing for PRCD in a variety of purebred dogs and congenital stationary night blindness (CSNB) in the briard.

VetGen is a commercial genetic service started as a collaboration between Michigan State University and the University of Michigan. They are offering numbers of genetic-based tests for von Willebrand's disease (vWD), phosphofructokinase deficiency (PFK), and PRCD.

All of the above-menbioned centers have websites, and information regarding inherited disorders in the dog can be obtained. New genetic tests are being developed at a rapid pace.

Table 6–14. Breed Predilection for Diseases and Congenital and Hereditary Disorders

Breed	Disorder
Aberdeen terrier	Primary uterine inertia
Abyssinian cat	Psychogenic alopecia/dermatitis
Affenpinscher (monkey terrier)	Anasarca (puppies) Cleft palate Elongated soft palate Oligodontia Patellar luxation Patent ductus arteriosus
Afghan hound	Cataract (bilateral) Elbow joint malformation Hypothyroidism Necrotizing myelopathy Persistent pupillary membranes Progressive retinal atrophy
Airedale terrier	Cerebellar hypoplasia Corneal dystrophy Distichiasis Progressive retinal atrophy Hyposomatotropism Trembling of the hindquarters Umbilical hernia

Table 6–14. Breed Predilection for Diseases and Congenital and Hereditary Disorders *Continued*

Breed	Disorder
Akita (Japanese deerhound)	Corneal dystrophy
	Deafness
	Entropion
	Pemphigus foliaceus
	Progressive retinal atrophy
	Umbilical hernia
	Vogt-Koyanagi-Harada–like syndrome
Alaskan malamute	Anemia with chondrodysplasia
	Cataracts
	Corneal dystrophy
	Dwarfism
	Factor VII deficiency, factor VIII deficiency, hemophilia A
	Hemeralopia
	Progressive retinal atrophy
	Renal cortical hypoplasia
	Zinc-responsive dermatosis
American foxhound	Deafness
	Microphthalmia
	Spinal osteochondrosis
	Thrombocytopathy
American Staffordshire terrier (pit bull)	Cataract
	Cleft palate
	Deafness
	Entropion
American water spaniel	Hermaphroditism
Antarctic husky	Entropion
	Hemophilia A
Australian cattle dog (Australian heeler)	Deafness
Australian kelpie (kelpie, Australian sheepdog)	Microphthalmia
	Multiple colobomas
Australian shepherd	Cataracts
	Cleft palate
	Colobomas
	Deafness
	Dwarfism
	Hip dysplasia
	Microphthalmia
	Progressive retinal atrophy
	Retinal detachment/atrophy
	Spina bifida
	Umbilical hernia
Australian terrier	Cataract
	Diabetes mellitus
	Legg-Perthes disease
	Progressive retinal atrophy

Table continued on following page

6

Table 6–14. Breed Predilection for Diseases and Congenital and Hereditary Disorders *Continued*

Breed	Disorder
Basenji	Cataract
	Coliform enteritis
	Corneal leukomas
	Hemolytic anemia
	Inguinal hernia
	Intestinal malabsorption
	Persistent pupillary membrane
	Progressive retinal atrophy
	Pyruvate kinase deficiency
	Renal tubular dysfunction
	Umbilical hernia
Basset hound	Achondroplasia
	Anomaly of third cervical vertebra
	Ectropion
	Entropion
	Glaucoma
	Inguinal hernia
	Osteochondritis dissecans
	Osteodystrophy
	Patellar luxation
	Platelet disorder
	Progressive retinal atrophy
	Retinal dysplasia
	Torsion of stomach, spleen, lung
Beagle	Atopic dermatitis
	Bladder cancer
	Bundle-branch block
	Cataract (unilateral)
	Cataract with microphthalmia
	Cleft lip and palate
	Deafness
	Demodicosis
	Ectasia syndrome
	Epilepsy
	Factor VII deficiency
	Hemophilia A
	Hypercholesterolemia
	Intervertebral disk disease
	Lymphocytic thyroiditis
	Microphthalmia
	Mononephrosis
	Multiple epiphyseal dysplasia
	Necrotizing panotitis
	Otocephalic syndrome
	Perianal gland tumor
	Primary glaucoma
	Progressive retinal atrophy
	Pulmonic stenosis
	Renal hypoplasia
	Retinal dysplasia
	Sebaceous gland tumors

Table 6–14. Breed Predilection for Diseases and Congenital and Hereditary Disorders *Continued*

Breed	Disorder
Beagle *(Continued)*	Short tail Thyroiditis Unilateral kidney aplasia
Bearded collie (Highland collie)	Cataracts Persistent pupillary membrane Progressive retinal atrophy Retinal dysplasia Subvalvular aortic stenosis
Bedlington terrier	Abnormal copper metabolism Cataract Distichiasis Lacrimal duct atresia Microphthalmia Osteogenesis imperfecta Recessive retinal dysplasia Renal cortical hypoplasia
Belgian malinois	Epilepsy Hip dysplasia Progressive retinal atrophy
Belgian sheepdog	Cataracts Chronic superficial keratitis Epilepsy Hip dysplasia
Belgian tervuren	Cataracts Epilepsy Hypothyroidism
Bernese mountain dog (Bernese sennehund)	Cataracts Cerebellar degeneration Cleft lip and palate Entropion Hip dysplasia Osteochondritis dissecans Umbilical hernia
Bichon frisé	Cataract Deafness Entropion Epilepsy Medial patellar luxation
Black-and-tan coonhound	Ectropion Factor IX deficiency, hemophilia B Hip dysplasia Polyradiculoneuritis Progressive retinal atrophy
Bloodhound (slot hound)	Bloat Ectropion Entropion Malocclusion Uterine inertia

Table continued on following page

6

Table 6–14. Breed Predilection for Diseases and Congenital and Hereditary Disorders *Continued*

Breed	Disorder
Blue tick hound	Globoid cell leukodystrophy
Border collie	Central progressive retinal atrophy Corneal dystrophy Deafness Lens luxation
Border terrier	Aortic and carotid body tumors Cataract (bilateral) Craniomandibular osteopathy Cryptorchidism Hemivertebra Mastocytoma Oligodendroglioma Patellar luxation Pituitary tumor Primary uterine inertia Ventricular septal defects
Borzoi (Russian wolfhound)	Bloat Calcinosis circumscripta Deafness Hygroma Microphthalmia Missing teeth Retinal dysplasia
Boston terrier	Anasarca Atopy Aortic and carotid body tumors Cataracts Cleft lip and palate Craniomandibular osteopathy Cushing's syndrome (hyperadrenocorticism) Deafness Demodicosis Distichiasis Dystocia Endothelial (corneal) dystrophy Esophageal achalasia Hemivertebra Heterochromia, iris Hydrocephalus Hypertrophy of nictitans gland Inguinal hernia Intussusception Mastocytoma Patellar luxation Patent ductus arteriosus Pituitary tumor Pseudocyesis (pyometra) Sebaceous gland tumor Stenotic nares

Table 6–14. Breed Predilection for Diseases and Congenital and
Hereditary Disorders *Continued*

Breed	Disorder
Boston terrier *(Continued)*	Strabismus Swimmer puppies Tail fold dermatitis
Bouvier des Flandres (Belgian cattle dog)	Cataracts Cleft palate Cystic ovaries Dystocia Ectropion Endometritis Entropion Gastric torsion Glaucoma Umbilical hernia
Boxer	Abnormal dentition Acne Atopy Atrial septal defects Cystinuria Deafness Demodicosis Dermoid cysts Distichiasis Esophageal dilation Endocardial fibroelastosis Factor II hypoprothrombinemia Gastric torsion Granulomatous colitis Gingival hyperplasia Histiocytoma Hyperadrenocorticism Hypothyroidism Mastocytoma Pododermatitis Progressive retinal atrophy Sertoli cell tumor Spondylosis Squamous cell carcinoma Sternal callus Subaortic stenosis Superficial corneal ulcer Ulcerative keratitis Vaginal hyperplasia
Briard (French sheepdog)	Cataracts Hypothyroidism Progressive retinal atrophy
Brittany spaniel	Cataracts Cleft palate Hemophilia A, factor VIII deficiency Lens luxation Retinal dysplasia

Table continued on following page

6

Table 6–14. Breed Predilection for Diseases and Congenital and Hereditary Disorders *Continued*

Breed	Disorder
Brussels griffon	Cataracts
	Distichiasis
	Short skull
	Shoulder abnormalities
Bulldog	Abnormal dentition
	Acne
	Arteriovenous fistula
	Cleft lip and palate
	Deafness
	Demodicosis
	Distichiasis
	Dystocia
	Ectropion
	Elongated soft palate
	Entropion
	Facial fold dermatitis
	Folliculitis and furunculosis
	Hemivertebra
	Hip dysplasia
	Hydrocephalus
	Hypoplasia of trachea
	Hypothyroidism
	Keratitis sicca
	Mitral valve defects
	Muzzle pyoderma
	Oligodendroglioma
	Perianal gland tumors
	Pulmonary stenosis
	Pyloric stenosis
	Short tail
	Short skull
	Spina bifida
	Tail fold dermatitis
	Vaginal hyperplasia
Bullmastiff	Abnormal dentition
	Bloat
	Cleft palate
	Cervical vertebra malformation
	Distichiasis
	Entropion
	Glaucoma
	Hip dysplasia
	Progressive retinal atrophy
	Screw tail
	Short tail
	Vaginal hyperplasia
Bull terrier	Deafness
	Ectropion
	Entropion
	Furunculosis
	Hernias (inguinal, umbilical)

Table 6–14. Breed Predilection for Diseases and Congenital and Hereditary Disorders *Continued*

Breed	Disorder
Bull terrier *(Continued)*	Mastocytoma
	Squamous cell carcinoma
	Zinc deficiency
Cairn terrier	Aberrant cilia
	Cataracts
	Cerebellar hypoplasia
	Craniomandibular osteopathy
	Cystinuria
	Glaucoma
	Globoid cell leukodystrophy
	Hemophilia A
	Hemophilia B
	Inguinal hernia
	von Willebrand's disease
Cardigan Welsh terrier	Cystinuria
	Dystocia
	Glaucoma (lens luxation)
	Intervertebral disk disease
	Progressive retinal atrophy
Cats (general)	Abscess
	Acne
	Dermatophytosis
	Eosinophilia, plaque, granuloma
	Flea bite hypersensitivity
	Plasma cell pododermatitis
	Psychogenic alopecia/dermatitis
	Stud tail
Cavalier King Charles spaniel	Cataracts
	Deafness
	Diabetes mellitus
	Patellar luxation
Chesapeake Bay retriever	Distichiasis
	Entropion
	Progressive retinal atrophy
Chihuahua	Cleft palate
	Collapsed trachea
	Deafness
	Dislocation of shoulder
	Glaucoma (lens luxation)
	Hemophilia A
	Hydrocephalus
	Hypoglycemia
	Hypoplasia of dens
	Iris atrophy
	Mitral valve defects
	Patellar luxation
	Progressive retinal atrophy
	Pulmonary stenosis

Table continued on following page

6

Table 6–14. Breed Predilection for Diseases and Congenital and Hereditary Disorders *Continued*

Breed	Disorder
Chow chow	Bloat
	Cerebellar hypoplasia
	Cleft palate
	Color mutant alopecia
	Deafness
	Disposition abnormalities
	Distichiasis
	Elbow dysplasia
	Elongated soft palate
	Entropion
	Hip dysplasia
	Hyposomatotropism
	Hypothyroidism
	Pemphigus foliaceus
	Short tail
Clumber spaniel	Abnormal teeth
	Ectropion
	Entropion
	Hip dysplasia
	Undershot jaw
	Uterine inertia
Cocker spaniel	Allergies
	Apocrine gland tumor
	Anasarca
	Basal cell tumor
	Behavioral abnormalities
	Cataract (bilateral)
	Cataract with microphthalmia
	Cleft lip and palate
	Corneal dystrophy
	Cranioschisis
	Cutaneous asthenia
	Deafness
	Distichiasis
	Ectropion
	Elbow dysplasia
	Entropion
	Epidermoid cyst
	Epilepsy
	Factor X deficiency
	Glaucoma
	Hemophilia B
	Hip dysplasia
	Hydrocephalus
	Hypothyroidism
	Inguinal hernia
	Intervertebral disk disease
	Lip fold dermatitis
	Melanoma
	Otitis externa
	Over- and undershot jaw

Table 6–14. Breed Predilection for Diseases and Congenital and Hereditary Disorders *Continued*

Breed	Disorder
Cocker spaniel *(Continued)*	Patellar luxation
	Patent ductus arteriosus
	Perianal gland tumor
	Progressive retinal atrophy
	Renal cortical hypoplasia
	Retinal dysplasia
	Sebaceous gland tumor
	Seborrhea
	Skin neoplasms
	Tail abnormalities
	Umbilical hernia
	Ununited anconeal process
Collie	Bladder cancer
	Bullous pemphigoid
	Collie eye syndrome
	Corneal dystrophy
	Cyclic neutropenia
	Deafness
	Demodicosis
	Dermatomyositis
	Discoid lupus
	Distichiasis
	Dwarfism
	Epilepsy
	Fibrous histiocytoma
	Hemophilia A
	Inguinal hernia
	Iris heterochromia
	Microphthalmia
	Nasal pyoderma
	Nasal solar dermatitis
	Optic nerve hypoplasia
	Patent ductus arteriosus
	Pemphigus erythematosus
	Progressive retinal atrophy
	Umbilical hernia
Curly-coated retriever	Cataracts
	Ectropion
	Entropion
Dachshund	Acanthosis nigricans
	Achondroplasia
	Cataracts
	Cleft lip and palate
	Color mutant alopecia
	Cystinuria
	Deafness
	Demodicosis
	Diabetes mellitus
	Ectasia syndrome
	Folliculitis and pododermatitis

Table continued on following page

6

Table 6–14. Breed Predilection for Diseases and Congenital and Hereditary Disorders *Continued*

Breed	Disorder
Dachshund *(Continued)*	Hyperadrenocorticism
	Hypothyroidism
	Intervertebral disk disease
	Iris heterochromia
	Juvenile cellulitis
	Linear IgA dermatosis
	Microphthalmia
	Nodular panniculitis
	Osteopetrosis
	Over- and undershot jaw
	Pattern alopecia
	Pemphigus foliaceus
	Renal hypoplasia
	Sebaceous gland tumor
	Sterile pyogranuloma syndrome
	Sternal callus
	Vasculitis
Dalmatian	Atopy
	Blue eyes
	Deafness
	Demodicosis
	Entropion
	Folliculitis and furunculosis
	Glaucoma
	Globoid cell leukodystrophy
	Squamous cell carcinoma
	Uric acid calculi and uric acid excretion abnormalities
Dandie Dinmont terrier	Abnormal dentition
	Cataracts
	Elbow subluxation
	Hip dysplasia
	Intervertebral disk disease
	Patellar luxation
	Shoulder luxation
Doberman pinscher	Abnormal dentition
	Acne
	Acral lick dermatitis
	Bundle of His degeneration
	Cataracts
	Color mutant alopecia
	Craniomandibular osteopathy
	Deafness
	Demodicosis
	Entropion
	Flank sucking
	Folliculitis and pododermatitis
	Hypopigmentation, lips and nose
	Hypothyroidism
	Microphthalmia
	Polyostotic fibrous dysplasia

Table 6–14. Breed Predilection for Diseases and Congenital and Hereditary Disorders *Continued*

Breed	Disorder
Doberman pinscher *(Continued)*	Renal cortical hypoplasia Spondylolisthesis (wobbler's syndrome) Storage abnormality in liver for copper von Willebrand's disease
English cocker spaniel	Cataracts Cryptorchidism Deafness Ectropion Entropion Glaucoma Hemophilia A Juvenile amaurotic idiocy Neuronal ceroid lipofuscinosis Progressive retinal atrophy Pseudohermaphrodism Swimmer puppies
English foxhound	Deafness Spinal osteochondrosis
English setter	Color mutant alopecia Craniomandibular osteopathy Deafness Eclampsia Hip dysplasia Hemophilia A, factor VIII deficiency Hypoglycemia Juvenile amaurotic idiocy Progressive retinal atrophy Uterine eclampsia
English springer spaniel	See Cocker spaniel
English toy spaniel (King Charles and Ruby Blenheim spaniels)	Cataracts Cleft palate Diabetes mellitus Entropion Hanging tongue Patellar luxation Umbilical hernia
Field spaniel	Cataracts Anesthetic idiosyncrasy Hypothyroidism
Fox terriers (wire-haired and smooth-haired)	Abnormal dentition Atopy Cataract Deafness Dislocation of shoulder Distichiasis Esophageal achalasia Glaucoma Goiter

Table continued on following page

6

Table 6–14. Breed Predilection for Diseases and Congenital and Hereditary Disorders *Continued*

Breed	Disorder
Fox terriers (wire-haired and smooth-haired) *(Continued)*	Legg-Perthes disease Lens luxation Persistent aortic arch Pulmonic stenosis Spinal cord demyelination (ataxia)
French bulldog	Cataract Cleft palate and lip Deafness Distichiasis Elongated soft palate Entropion Hemivertebra Hemophilia A, factor VIII deficiency Hemophilia B, factor IX deficiency
German shepherd	Atopic dermatitis Behavioral abnormalities Calcinosis circumscripta Cataract (bilateral) Cellulitis (folliculitis and furunculosis) Celft lip and palate Cystinuria Deafness Dermoid cyst Discoid lupus erythematosus Ectasia syndrome Enostosis Entropion Epilepsy Esophageal achalasia Eversion of nictitating membrane Hemophilia A Hip dysplasia Keratoacanthoma Malabsorption syndrome Nasal pyoderma Osteochondritis dissecans Osteosarcoma Otitis externa Pancreatic insufficiency Pannus Pemphigus erythematosus Perianal fistulas Persistent right aortic arch Pituitary dwarfism Progressive retinal atrophy Renal cortical hypoplasia Seborrhea Silica uroliths Subaortic stenosis Systemic lupus erythematosus Ulcerative colitis

Table 6–14. Breed Predilection for Diseases and Congenital and Hereditary Disorders *Continued*

Breed	Disorder
German shepherd *(Continued)*	Ununited anconeal process von Willebrand's disease
German short-haired pointer	Amaurotic idiocy Cataracts Entropion Eversion of nictitating membrane Fibrosarcoma Lymphedema Melanoma Pannus Subaortic stenosis Thrombocytopathy von Willebrand's disease
German wire-haired pointer	Entropion Subcutaneous cysts
Giant schnauzer	Cataracts Hip dysplasia Osteochondritis dissecans Seborrhea
Golden retriever	Acral lick dermatitis Acute moist dermatitis Atopy Cataract Central progressive retinal atrophy Distichiasis Entropion Folliculitis and furunculosis Hemophilia A, factor VIII deficiency Hypothyroidism Juvenile cellulitis Lymphosarcoma von Willebrand's disease
Gordon setter	Cataracts Cerebellar cortical abiotrophy Generalized progressive retinal atrophy Hip dysplasia Tail deformities
Great Dane	Acne Acral lick dermatitis Bloat Calcinosis circumscripta Cerebellar hypoplasia Color mutant alopecia Cystinuria Deafness Demodicosis Dermoid cyst Distichiasis

Table continued on following page

6

Table 6–14. Breed Predilection for Diseases and Congenital and Hereditary Disorders *Continued*

Breed	Disorder
Great Dane	Ectropion
	Entropion
	Eversion nictitating membrane
	Histiocytoma
	Hygroma
	Hypothyroidism
	Iris heterochromia
	Metabolic bone disease
	Microphthalmia
	Mitral valve defects
	Necrotizing myelopathy
	Osteochondritis dissecans
	Osteosarcoma
	Pododermatitis
	Progressive ataxia
	Spondylolisthesis (wobbler's syndrome)
	Stockard's paralysis
Great Pyrenees	Achondroplasia
	Acute moist dermatitis
	Anophthalmia
	Cataracts
	Deafness
	Demodicosis
	Ectropion
	Entropion
	Factor XI deficiency
	Hip dysplasia
	Malocclusion
	Patellar luxation
	Persistent hyaloid artery
	Swimmer puppies
Greyhound	Anesthesia idiosyncrasy
	Dystocia
	Esophageal achalasia
	Hemophilia A, factor VIII deficiency
	Short spine
Harrier	None recognized
Ibizan hound	Allergies
	Anesthetic idiosyncracy
	Cataract
	Cryptorchidism
	Deafness
Irish setter	Atopy
	Acral lick dermatitis
	Carpal subluxation
	Cataract
	Color mutant alopecia
	Deformed tail
	Entropion
	Epilepsy

Table 6–14. Breed Predilection for Diseases and Congenital and Hereditary Disorders *Continued*

Breed	Disorder
Irish setter *(Continued)*	Folliculitis and furunculosis
	Generalized myopathy
	Generalized progressive retinal atrophy
	Hemophilia A
	Hypothyroidism
	Metabolic bone disease
	Osteochondritis dissecans
	Persistent right aortic arch
	Quadriplegia with amblyopia
	Seborrhea
	Uterine inertia
Irish terrier	Cystinuria
	Progressive retinal atrophy
Irish water spaniel	Hip dysplasia
	Hypotrichosis
	Malocclusion
Irish wolfhound	Entropion
	Hygroma
	Hypothyroidism
Italian greyhound	Anesthetic idiosyncrasy
	Cataracts
	Color mutant alopecia
	Cryptorchidism
	Deafness
	Epilepsy
	Persistent right aortic arch
Jack Russell terrier	Ataxia
	Deafness
	Lens luxation
Japanese chin	Cataracts
	Cryptorchidism
	Distichiasis
Keeshond	Aberrant cilia
	Castration-responsive dermatosis
	Conus septal defects
	Epilepsy
	Hyposomatotropism
	Hypothyroidism
	Keratoacanthoma
	Melanoma
	Mitral valve defects
	Renal cortical hypoplasia
	Sebaceous cyst
	Tetralogy of Fallot
Kerry blue terrier	Cerebellar and extrapyramidal abiotrophy
	Distichiasis
	Entropion

Table continued on following page

6

Table 6–14. Breed Predilection for Diseases and Congenital and Hereditary Disorders *Continued*

Breed	Disorder
Kerry blue terrier	Hair follicle tumors Keratoconjunctivitis sicca Narrow palpebral fissures Ununited anconeal process
Komondor (Hungarian sheepdog)	Cataracts Entropion Hip dysplasia Miscellaneous skin disorders
Kuvasz	Deafness Hip dysplasia
Labrador retriever	Abnormal dentition Acral lick dermatitis Acute moist dermatitis Atopy Carpal subluxation Cataract Central progressive retinal atrophy Coloboma Craniomandibular osteopathy Cystinuria Deafness Dacrocystitis Diabetes mellitus Distichiasis Dwarfism Entropion Hip dysplasia Hypertrophic osteodystrophy Hypoglycemia Hypothyroidism Melanoma Persistent hyaloid artery Persistent pupillary membrane Prolapsed rectum Prolapsed uterus Seborrhea Shoulder dysplasia Type II muscle fiber deficiency
Lakeland terrier	Cataracts Cryptorchidism Distichiasis Entropion Lens luxation Undershot jaw Ununited anconeal process
Lhasa apso	Aberrant cilia Atopy Cataracts Distichiasis Entropion

Table 6–14. Breed Predilection for Diseases and Congenital and Hereditary Disorders *Continued*

Breed	Disorder
Lhasa apso *(Continued)*	Inguinal hernia
	Lissencephaly
	Patellar luxation
	Progressive retinal atrophy
	Renal cortical hypoplasia
Maltese	Aberrant cilia
	Blindness
	Cryptorchidism
	Deafness
	Distichiasis
	Hydrocephalus
	Hypoglycemia
	Patellar luxation
Manchester terrier	Cataracts
	Cutaneous asthenia
	Epilepsy
	Glaucoma
	Legg-Perthes disease
Mastiff	Bloat
	Ectropion
	Entropion
	Persistent pupillary membrane
	Vaginal hyperplasia
Mexican, Turkish, and Chinese breeds	Hairlessness
Miniature bull terrier	None recognized
Miniature pinscher	Cataracts
	Deafness
	Dislocation of shoulder
	Entropion
	Inguinal hernia
	Legg-Perthes disease
	Progressive retinal atrophy
Miniature poodle	See Poodle
Miniature schnauzer	Atopy
	Cataract
	Cryptorchidism
	Cystitis and cystic calculi
	Esophageal achalasia
	Hyperlipidemia
	Hypothyroidism
	Legg-Perthes disease
	Pseudohermaphroditism
	Pulmonary stenosis
	Schnauzer comedo syndrome
	Sinoatrial syncope
	Subcorneal pustular dermatosis
	von Willebrand's disease

Table continued on following page

6

Table 6–14. Breed Predilection for Diseases and Congenital and Hereditary Disorders *Continued*

Breed	Disorder
Newfoundland	Avulsion fractures Cardiomyopathy Dermoid cyst Ectropion Entropion Eversion of nictitating membrane Hypothyroidism Kinked tail Patent ductus arteriosus Subaortic stenosis Ununited anconeal process Ventricular septal defect
Norwegian dunkerhound	Deafness Microphthalmia
Norwegian elkhound	Generalized progressive retinal atrophy Keratoacanthoma Renal cortical hypoplasia Sebaceous gland tumors Seborrhea Subcutaneous cysts
Norwich terrier	None recognized
Old English sheepdog	Cataract Deafness Demodicosis Distichiasis Entropion Folliculitis—pododermatitis Hip dysplasia Microphthalmia Retinal detachment Spondylolisthesis (wobbler's syndrome)
Otter hound	Hip dysplasia Platelet disorder Sebaceous cysts
Papillon	Anasarca Cataract Deafness Entropion Patellar luxation
Pekingese	Cataract Distichiasis Entropion Facial fold dermatitis Hypoplasia of dens Inguinal hernia Intervertebral disk disease Lacrimal duct atresia Microphthalmia Pannus

Table 6–14. Breed Predilection for Diseases and Congenital and Hereditary Disorders *Continued*

Breed	Disorder
Pekingese *(Continued)*	Progressive retinal atrophy
	Sertoli cell tumor
	Short skull
	Swimmer puppies
	Umbilical hernia
Pembroke Welsh corgi	Cervical disk disease
	Cutaneous asthenia
	Cystinuria
	Dystocia
	Epilepsy
	Generalized progressive retinal atrophy
	Glaucoma (lens luxation)
Persian cat	Facial fold dermatitis
	Dermatophytosis
	Hair mats
Pointer	Acral mutilation
	Bithoracic ectomelia
	Calcinosis circumscripta
	Cataract
	Deafness
	Demodicosis
	Entropion
	Juvenile cellulitis
	Neuromuscular atrophy
	Neurotropic osteopathy
	Panosteitis
	Progressive retinal atrophy
	Umbilical hernia
Pomeranian	Cryptorchidism
	Dislocation of shoulder
	Distichiasis
	Entropion
	Epiphora
	Glycogen storage disease
	Hypoplasia of dens
	Hyposomatotropism
	Nasolacrimal puncta atresia
	Cranial fontanel
	Patellar luxation
	Patent ductus arteriosus
	Progressive retinal atrophy
	Tracheal collapse
Poodle (miniature and toy)	Achondroplasia
	Atopy
	Basal cell tumors
	Behavioral defects
	Cerebrospinal demyelination
	Deafness
	Distichiasis

Table continued on following page

Table 6–14. Breed Predilection for Diseases and Congenital and Hereditary Disorders *Continued*

Breed	Disorder
Poodle (miniature and toy) *(Continued)*	Ectodermal defects Ectopic ureters Entropion Epiphora Epiphyseal dysplasia Epilepsy Granulomatous sebaceous adenitis Hemeralopia Hemophilia A, factor VIII deficiency Hyperadrenocorticism Hyposomatotropism Hypothyroidism Intervertebral disk syndrome Iris atrophy Lacrimal duct atresia Microphthalmia Osteogenesis imperfecta Otitis externa Pannus Patellar luxation Patent ductus arteriosus Progressive retinal atrophy Renal detachment Sebaceous gland tumor Squamous cell carcinoma von Willebrand's disease
Poodle (standard)	Atopy Behavioral abnormalities Bloat Cataract Distichiasis Epilepsy Epiphora Hemophilia A, factor VIII deficiency Iris atrophy Lacrimal duct atresia Microphthalmia Osteogenesis imperfecta Pannus Progressive retinal atrophy von Willebrand's disease
Pug	Cleft palate and lip Distichiasis Elongated soft palate Entropion Fold dermatitis (face and tail) Legg-Perthes disease Pannus Pigmentary keratitis Pug encephalitis Pseudohermaphroditism (male)

Table 6–14. Breed Predilection for Diseases and Congenital and Hereditary Disorders *Continued*

Breed	Disorder
Puli	Behavioral abnormalities Cataract Deafness Hip dysplasia
Rhodesian ridgeback	Cervical vertebral abnormality Deafness Dermoid sinus (midline) Entropion Hip dysplasia
Rottweiler	Behavioral abnormalities Cataracts Deafness Diabetes mellitus Distichiasis Ectropion Entropion Folliculitis Hip dysplasia Vasculitis Vitiligo
Saint Bernard	Bloat Colobomas with aphakia Deafness Dermoid cysts (cornea) Distichiasis Ectropion Entropion Epilepsy Eversion of nictitating membrane Factor I deficiency Genu valgum Hemophilia A, factor VIII deficiency Hemophilia B, factor IX deficiency Hepatic arteriovenous fistula Hip dysplasia Lip fold dermatitis Metabolic bone disease Osteosarcoma Stockard's paralysis Vaginal hyperplasia
Saluki	Anesthesia idiosyncrasy Behavioral abnormalities Cataracts Progressive retinal atrophy Retinal detachment
Samoyed	Atrial septal defects Diabetes mellitus Distichiasis Hemophilia A, factor VIII deficiency

Table continued on following page

6

Table 6–14. Breed Predilection for Diseases and Congenital and Hereditary Disorders *Continued*

Breed	Disorder
Samoyed *(Continued)*	Hip dysplasia
	Perianal gland tumor
	Progressive retinal atrophy
	Pulmonary stenosis
	Sebaceous cysts
Schipperke	Cataracts
	Distichiasis
	Ectropion
	Entropion
	Legg-Perthes disease
	Narrow palpebral fissure
	Pemphigus foliaceous
Scottish deerhound	Bloat
	Deafness
	Gastric torsion
Scottish terrier	Achondroplasia
	Atopy
	Cataracts
	Craniomandibular osteopathy
	Cystinuria
	Deafness
	Folliculitis
	Lymphosarcoma
	Melanoma
	Scotty cramp
	Squamous cell carcinoma
	Uterine inertia
Sealyham terrier	Atopy
	Cataracts
	Deafness
	Lens luxation
	Retinal dysplasia and detachment
Shar Pei	Atopy
	Blepharospasm
	Demodicosis
	Ectropion
	Entropion
	Fold dermatitis
	Folliculitis
	Hip dysplasia
	Hypothyroidism
	Lens luxation
	Lipfold dermatitis
	Otitis externa
	Patellar luxation
	Seborrhea
	Stenotic nares
	Undershot jaw
Shetland sheepdog	Achondroplasia
	Cataract
	Central progressive retinal atrophy

Table 6–14. Breed Predilection for Diseases and Congenital and Hereditary Disorders *Continued*

Breed	Disorder
Shetland sheepdog	Choroidal hypoplasia
	Coloboma
	Deafness
	Dermatomyositis
	Discoid lupus erythematosus
	Distichiasis
	Ectasia syndrome
	Epidermolysis bullosa
	Folliculitis
	Hemophilia A, factor VIII deficiency
	Heterochromia iridis
	Hip dysplasia
	Patent ductus arteriosus
	Systemic lupus erythematosus
Shih Tzu	Cataracts
	Cleft lip and palate
	Entropion
	Renal cortical hypoplasia
	von Willebrand's disease
Siamese cat	Hypotrichosis
	Periocular leukotrichia
	Psychogenic dermatitis/alopecia
Siberian husky	Castration-responsive dermatosis
	Cataracts
	Corneal dystrophy
	Deafness
	Discoid lupus erythematosus
	Entropion
	Eosinophilic granuloma
	Progressive retinal atrophy
	von Willebrand's disease
	Zinc-responsive dermatosis
Silky terrier	Cataracts
	Cryptorchidism
	Diabetes mellitus
	Hydrocephalus
	Legg-Perthes disease
	Patellar luxation
	Tracheal collapse
Skye terrier	Behavioral abnormalities
	Enlarged foramen magnum
	Hypoplasia of larynx
	Kinked tail
	Ulcerative colitis
Soft-coated wheaten terrier	Atopy
	Cataracts
	Deafness
	Glomerulonephritis
	Posterior retinal atrophy

Table continued on following page

Table 6–14. Breed Predilection for Diseases and Congenital and Hereditary Disorders *Continued*

Breed	Disorder
Standard schnauzer	Atresia of nasolacrimal puncta
	Cataract
	Conjunctivitis
	Hemophilia A, factor VIII deficiency
	Perianal adenoma
	Pulmonary stenosis
Sussex spaniel	Cardiomyopathy
	Deafness
Tibetan terrier	Anesthetic idiosyncrasy
	Cataracts
	Deafness
	Lens luxation
Toy Manchester	None recognized
Vizsla	Cataracts
	Craniomandibular osteopathy
	Entropion
	Facial nerve paralysis
	Granulomatous sebaceous adenitis
	Hemophilia A, factor VIII deficiency
Weimaraner	Bloat
	Color mutant alopecia
	Distichiasis
	Entropion
	Eversion of nictitating membrane
	Hemophilia A
	Hip dysplasia
	Mastocytoma
	Myasthenia gravis
	Spinal dysraphism
	Sterile pyogranuloma syndrome
	Syringomyelia
	Umbilical hernia
	Undershot jaw
Welsh springer spaniel	Cataracts
	Hip dysplasia
West Highland white terrier	Atopy
	Cataracts
	Craniomandibular osteopathy
	Deafness
	Epidermal dysplasia
	Globoid cell leukodystrophy (Krabbe's disease)
	Inguinal hernia
	Keratoconjunctivitis sicca
	Legg-Perthes disease
	Seborrhea
	Westie armadillo syndrome

Table 6–14. Breed Predilection for Diseases and Congenital and Hereditary Disorders *Continued*

Breed	Disorder
Whippet	Cataracts Color mutant alopecia Cryptorchidism Deafness Demodicosis Lens luxation Partial alopecia
Wire-haired pointing griffon	Hip dysplasia Otitis externa
Yorkshire terrier	Cataracts Deafness Distichiasis Entropion Hydrocephalus Hypoplasia of dens Keratoconjunctivitis sicca Legg-Perthes disease Patellar luxation Portosystemic shunt

Types of Animals Sharing Some Common Defects

All-white animals	Commonly deaf
Brachycephalic breeds	Pituitary cysts Stenotic nares and elongated palates
Giant breeds	Elbow dysplasia Hip dysplasia Metabolic bone disorders Osteogenic sarcoma
Miniature breeds	Tracheal collapse Glycogen storage disease Legg-Perthes disease Patellar luxation Predisposition to dystocia

Material in this table was derived from experienced clinicians' *strong* clinical impressions, but primarily from the following references: Clark RD, Stainer JR: Medical and Genetic Aspects of Purebred Dogs. Edwardsville, Kan, Veterinary Medical Publications, 1983; Kirk RW, (ed): Current Veterinary Therapy IX. Philadelphia, WB Saunders, 1986; and Muller GH, Kirk RW, Scott DW: Small Animal Dermatology. Philadelphia, WB Saunders, 1989.

PHYSIOLOGIC DATA: LABORATORY AND EXOTIC ANIMALS
See Tables 6–15 through 6–24.

6

Table 6–15. Useful Laboratory Animal Information

	Hamster	Rabbit	Mouse	Rat	Gerbil	Guinea Pig
Weight at birth	2 g	100 g	1.5 g	5.5 g	3 g	100 g
Puberty	(F) 28–31 days (M) 45 days (best to breed 70 days)	4–9 mo	35 days	50–60 days	(F) 3–5 mo (M) 10–12 wk	(F) 20–30 days (M) 70 days
Duration of estrous cycle*	4 days	Ovulation not spontaneous; stimulated by copulation; doe ovulates 10–13 hr after	4 days	4 days	4 days	16 days
Gestation (days)	16	28–36	19–21	21–23	24	62–72
Separation of adults during parturition and weaning	Yes	Yes	No	No	No (mates for life)	No
Number per litter	4–10	7	10	8–10	1–12	1–4
Eyes open	15 days	10 days	11–14 days	14–17 days	16–20 days	Prior to birth
Wean at	25 days	42–56 days	21 days	21 days	21 days	14–21 days or 160 g
Postpartum estrus	Within 24 hr	14 days	Within 24–48 hr	Within 24–48 hr	Within 24–72 hr	Within 24 hr
Breeding life	11–18 mo	1–3 years (max. 6 yr)	12–18 mo	14 mo	15–20 mo	3–4 yr

Adult weight	(F) 120 g (M) 108 g	(F) 4.0 kg (M) 4.3 kg	(F) 30 g (M) 39 g	(F) 300 g (M) 500 g	(F) 75 g (M) 85 g	(F) 850 g (M) 1000 g
Life span (yr)	2–3	5–7	3.0–3.5	3	4	4–5
Body temperature	97°–101°F (36.1°–38.3°C)	101°–103.2°F (38.3°–39.5°C)	96.4°–100°F (35.8°–37.7°C)	99.5°–100.6°F (37.5°–38.1°C)	100.8°F (32.8°C)	100.4°–102.5°F (38°–39.2°C)
Daily adult water consumption	8–12 mL/day	80 mL/kg body weight	3–3.5 mL/day	20–30 mL/day	4 mL/day	10 mL/100 g body weight
Daily adult food consumption (varies with age and condition)	7–12 g/day	100–150 g/day	2.5–4.0 g/day	20–40 g/day	10–15 g/day	30–35 g/day
Diet	Commercial rat, mouse, or hamster chow supplemented with kale,† cabbage,† apples, milk	Commercial rabbit pellets, greens in moderation	Commercial mouse chow	Commercial rat or mouse chow	Commercial mouse or rat chow (lowest fat possible); sunflower seeds	Commercial guinea pig chow, good-quality hay, kale, cabbage, fruits (cannot rely on vitamin C levels of commercial ration)
Room temperature	65°–75°F (18.3°–24°C)	62°–68°F (17°–20°C)	70°–80°F (21°–27°C)	76°–78°F (24.5°–25.5°C)	65°–80°F (18.3°–26.6°C)	65°–75°F (18.3°–24°C)
Humidity (%)	50	50	50	50	<50	50

* All species listed except rabbits are seasonally polyestrous.
† Better source of vitamin C than lettuce.

From Schuchman SM: Individual care and treatment of rabbits, mice, rats, guinea pigs, hamsters, and gerbils. *In* Kirk RW, ed: Current Veterinary Therapy X. Philadelphia, WB Saunders, 1989, p 739.

6

Table 6–16. Determination of the Sex of Mature and Immature Laboratory Rodents and Lagomorphs

Mature Hamsters, Mice, Rats, Guinea Pigs, and Gerbils

Male	Female
1. Anogenital distance longer in the male.	1. Anogenital distance shorter in the female.
2. Manipulate "genital papilla" (prepuce) to protrude penis.	2. Look for three external openings in the inguinal area:
3. Palpate for testicles either in a scrotal sac (if present) or subcutaneous in inguinal region.	a. Anus (most caudal opening).
4. Males have only two external openings in the inguinal region.	b. Vaginal orifice (middle opening)—look carefully.
a. Anus.	c. Urethral orifice at tip of urethral papilla (most anterior opening).
b. Urethral orifice at tip of penis.	In these animals the urethral papilla is located outside the vagina
In very fat males there may be a depression between the penis and the anus. This depression can be obliterated by manipulating the skin in that area.	(unlike dogs and cats). In very fat females or young females, the vaginal orifice may be either hidden by folds of skin (the former) or sealed (latter). Gentle manipulation of the skin in this area will divulge the orifice.

Mature Rabbits

Male	Female
1. Protrude penis by manipulating skin of prepuce.	1. There is a common orifice for both the vagina and urethra (like dogs and cats).
2. Palpate for testicles.	2. No structure like a "penis" can be protruded from the urogenital orifice.
3. Anogenital distance is longer.	3. Anogenital distance is shorter.

From Schuchman SM: Individual care and treatment of rabbits, mice, rats, guinea pigs, hamsters, and gerbils. *In* Kirk RW, ed: Current Veterinary Therapy X. Philadelphia, WB Saunders, 1989, p 740.

Table 6–17. Blood Values and Some Values of Chemical Constituents of Serum*

Laboratory Test	Rats	Mice	Hamsters	Guinea Pigs	Rabbits	Mongolian Gerbils
AST (Sigma-Frankel units)	25–42	32–41	22–36	10–25	14–27	—
Alkaline phosphatase (Bodansky units)	4.1–8.6	2.4–4.0	2.0–3.5	1.5–8.1	2.1–3.2	18–24
BUN (mg/dL)	10–20	8–30	10–40	8–20	5–30	18–24
Sodium (mEq/L)	144	114–154	106–185	120–155	100–145	144–158
Potassium (mEq/L)	5.9	3.0–9.6	2.3–9.8	6.5–8.2	3.0–7.0	3.8–5.2
Bilirubin, total (mg/dL)	0.42	0.18–0.54	0.3–0.4	0.24–0.30	0.15–0.20	—
Blood glucose (mg/dL)	50–115	108–192	32.6–118.4	60–125	50–140	69–119
RBCs (10^6 cells/mm³)	7.2–9.6	9.3–10.5	4.0–9.3	4.5–7.0	3.2–7.5	8.3–9.3
Hemoglobin (g/dL)	14.8	12–14.9	9.7–16.8	11–15	10–15	10–16
Hematocrit (%)	40–50	35–50	40–52	35–50	35–45	35–45
WBCs (10^3 cells/mm³)	8–14	8–14	7–15	5–12	8–10	9–14
Segmented (%)	30	26	8	42	30–50	10–20
Nonsegmented (%)	0	0		0	0	0
Lymphocytes (%)	65–77	55–80	64–78	45–81	30–50	70–89
Eosinophils (%)	1	3	1	5	1	1
Monocytes (%)	4	5	2	8	9	0
Basophils (%)	0	0	0	2	0	0

AST, aspartate aminotransferase; BUN, blood urea nitrogen; RBCs, red blood cells; WBCs, white blood cells.
*These are values found in healthy-appearing animals and can be used as guides but should not be interpreted as physiologic norms for the species listed.
Modified from Schuchman SM: Individual care and treatment of rabbits, mice, rats, guinea pigs, hamsters, and gerbils. *In* Kirk RW, ed: Current Veterinary Therapy X. Philadelphia, WB Saunders, Co, 1989, p 746.

6

Table 6–18. Ketamine and Ketamine in Combination Anesthetic Dosages (mg/kg IM)

1. Recommended dose of ketamine:

Rabbit	Guinea pig	Rat	Hamster	Mouse
25–55	22–55	22–24	—	22–44

2. Addition of acetylpromazine to ketamine (ketamine dose is maintained at full strength as shown above):

Rabbit	Guinea pig	Rat	Hamster	Mouse
0.75	0.75	0.75	—	0.75

3. Xylazine dosage used in conjunction with steps 1 and 2:

Rabbit	Guinea pig	Rat	Hamster	Mouse
2–5	2–5	2–5	2–5	2–5

(Xylazine is best administered 10–15 min prior to giving ketamine-acetylpromazine):

Example

Combination surgical anesthetic for a 4-kg rabbit:
   220 mg ketamine
   3 mg acetylpromazine
   20 mg xylazine

The anesthetic described in this example is usually suitable for a surgical procedure that has the potential to elicit deep pain. Duration of anesthesia is 20 min and blood pressure is severely reduced. However, the prospect for recovery is good.

From Sedwick C: Anesthesia for rabbits and rodents. *In* Kirk RW, ed: Current Veterinary Therapy VII. Philadelphia, WB Saunders, 1980, p 708.

Table 6–19. Ferret Species Information

Data	Range or Value
Physiologic Data	
Life span	5–9 yr (average 5–7)
Commercial breeding life	2–5 yr
Body temperature	101°–104°F (38°–40°C)
Respiratory rate	32–36 breaths/min
Heart rate	220–250 bpm (average 240)
Water consumption	75–100 mL/day
Chromosome number	2n = 40
Anatomical Data	
Dental formula	2 (I3/3, C1/1, P3/4, M1/2)
Vertebral formula	C-7, T-14, L-6, S-3, Cd-14–Cd-18
Reproductive Data	
Gestation	39–46 days (average 42)
Litter size	2–17 kits (average 8)
False pregnancy	40–42 days
Placentation	Zonal
Implantation time	12–31 days
Weaning	5–6 wk
Ovulation	30–40 hr post coitus

From Randolph RW: Medical and surgical care of the pet ferret. *In* Kirk RW, ed: Current Veterinary Therapy X. Philadelphia, WB Saunders, 1989, p 766.

Table 6–20. Hematologic Values for Normal Ferrets*

Laboratory Test	Mean	Range
Hematocrit (%)	52.3	42–61
Hemoglobin (g/dL)	17.0	15–18
RBCs (10^6 cells/mm^3)	9.17	6.8–12.2
WBCs (10^3 cells/mm^3)	10.1	4.0–19
WBCs		
Lymphocytes (%)	34.5	12–54
Neutrophils (%)	58.3	11–84
Monocytes (%)	4.4	0–9.0
Eosinophils (%)	2.5	0–7.0
Basophils (%)	0.1	0–2.0
Reticulocytes (%)	4.6	1–14
Platelets (10^3 cells/mm^3)	499	297–910
Total protein (g/dL)	6.0	5.1–7.4

* Values are for both sexes.
From Ryland L, Bernard S, Gorham J: A clinical guide to the pet ferret. Compend Contin Educ Pract Vet 5:25, 1983, which was adapted from Thornton, et al: Lab Anim 13:119, 1979.

Table 6–21. Serum Chemistry Values for Normal Ferrets*

Analyte	Unit	Mean	Range
Glucose	mg/dL	136	94–207
BUN	mg/dL	22	10–45
Albumin	mg/dL	3.2	2.3–3.8
Alkaline phosphatase	IU/L	23	9–84
AST	IU/L	65	28–120
Total bilirubin	mg/dL	<1.0	
Cholesterol	mg/dL	165	64–296
Creatinine	mg/dL	0.6	0.4–0.9
Sodium	mEq/L	148	137–162
Potassium	mEq/L	5.9	4.5–7.7
Chloride	mEq/L	116	106–125
Calcium	mg/dL	9.2	8.0–11.8
Phosphorus	mg/dL	5.9	4.0–9.1

BUN, blood urea nitrogen; AST, aspartate aminotransferase.
* Values for both sexes.
From Ryland L, Bernard S, Gorham J: A clinical guide to the pet ferret. Compend Contin Educ Pract Vet 5:25, 1983, which was adapted from Thornton, et al: Lab Anim 13:119, 1979.

6

Table 6–22. Electrocardiographic Data for Normal Ferrets*

Parameter	Mean	Range
Rate Rhythm	224 ± 51	150–340
Normal sinus rhythm		
Sinus arrhythmia		
Measurements		
P wave		
Width	0.03 ± 0.009	0.015–0.04 s
Height	0.106 ± 0.03	0.05–0.20 mV
P–R interval		
Width	0.05 ± 0.01	0.04–0.08 s
QRS complex		
Q wave	Usually none	
R wave		
Width	0.049 ± 0.008	0.04–0.06 s
Height	1.59 ± 0.63	0.6–3.15 mV
S wave		
Height	0.166 ± 0.101	0.1–0.25 mV
S–T segment		
Width	0.030 ± 0.016	0.01–0.06 s
Q–T interval		
Width	0.13 ± 0.027	0.10–0.18 s
T wave		
Width	0.06 ± 0.01	0.03–0.1 s
Height	0.24 ± 0.12	0.10–0.45 mV
Mean Electrical Axis (Frontal Plane)		*+65–100 degrees*

* Ferrets in right lateral recumbency; sedation with ketamine and xylazine.

Table 6–23. Ferret Anesthetic Regimen

Drug	Dosage	Route of Administration
Acepromazine	0.1–0.25 mg/kg	Subcutaneous, intramuscular
Ketamine*	20–35 mg/kg	Intramuscular
Halothane or isoflurane	Low flow, low concentration, to effect	Face mask
Nitrous oxide†	Low flow, 50:50 with oxygen	Face mask

* Administered 5 to 30 minutes after the acepromazine.
† Optional.
From Randolph RW: Medical and surgical care of the pet ferret. *In* Kirk RW, ed: Current Veterinary Therapy X. Philadelphia, WB Saunders, 1989, p 771.

Table 6–24. Maximum Intramuscular Doses of Ketamine (100 mg/mL) for Use With Xylazine (20 mg/mL)*

Species	Intramuscular (mL of each)	Intravenous (mL of each)
Budgerigars	0.01	0.005
Cockatiels	0.02	0.01
Conures	0.05	0.025
Lorikeets, rosellas	0.07	0.035
Amazons, miniature macaws	0.05–0.10	0.025–0.05
African greys	0.08–0.10	0.04–0.05
Cockatoos	0.12–0.15	0.06–0.07
Macaws	0.15–0.20	0.075–0.10

* Amount given in volume (mL) of ketamine to be mixed with an equal *volume* of xylazine before administering.

From Harrison GJ: Anesthesiology. *In* Harrison GJ, Harrison LH, eds: Clinical Avian Medicine and Surgery. Philadelphia, WB Saunders, 1986, p 555.

....

EPIPHYSEAL FUSION
See Table 6–25.

Table 6–25. Time of Epiphyseal Fusion of Bones as Shown by Radiographs

Tuber scapulae	4½–6 mo
Humeral head and tubercles	10–12 mo
Condyles and medial epicondyle of humerus	8 mo
Radius	
Proximal epiphysis	9–11 mo
Distal epiphysis	10–12 mo
Ulna	
Olecranon	8–10 mo
Distal epiphysis	10–12 mo
Epiphysis of accessory carpal bone	4½ mo
Distal epiphysis of the metacarpal bones and proximal epiphysis of first and second phalanges	6–7 mo
Fusion of the ilium, ischium, pubis, and os acetabuli	5–6 mo
Proximal end of femur	9–11 mo
Distal epiphysis of femur	9–12 mo
Epiphysis of tibial tuberosity	
Fuses with proximal epiphysis	6–9 mo
Fuses with shaft of tibia	10–14 mo
Proximal articular epiphysis of tibia	10–14 mo
Proximal articular epiphysis of fibula	9–11 mo
Distal epiphysis of tibia	9–11 mo
Distal epiphysis of fibula	8–13 mo
Epiphysis of tuber calcanei with calceneus	6 mo

Data from Habel RE: Applied Veterinary Anatomy, ed 2. Ithaca, NY, 1981.

6

....

LABORATORY SAMPLE REQUIREMENTS
See Table 6–26.

Table 6–26. Sample Requirements for Laboratory Tests

These recommendations are only guidelines. Sample requirements may vary depending on each laboratory's protocol. Consult your own laboratory for specific instructions.

Test Description	Specimen
Acid-base balance	3 mL heparinized whole blood (arterial sample preferred)
ACTH (adrenocorticotropic hormone)	12 mL plasma; frozen—separate into two 6-mL vials
A/G (albumin-globulin) ratio	2 mL serum
ALA (aminolevulinic acid)	20-mL aliquot of 24-hr urine; add 6N HCl to pH 1–2; note 24-hr volume
Albumin	2 mL serum
Alkaline phosphatase	1 mL serum
Alkaline phosphatase isoenzymes	2 mL serum, frozen
Ammonia, blood	3 mL heparinized plasma; freeze immediately
Amylase, fluid	1 mL fluid
Amylase serum	1 mL serum
Amylase, urine	10 mL random urine
ANA (antinuclear antibody)	2 mL serum
ALT (alanine aminotransferase)	1 mL serum
AST (aspartate aminotransferase)	1 mL serum
Bence Jones protein	30 mL fresh random urine
Bile, urine, qualitative	2 mL random urine
Bile acids	1 mL serum (fasting); and 1 mL serum (postprandial)
Bilirubin, direct	1 mL serum (do not expose to light)
Bilirubin, total	1 mL serum (do not expose to light)
Bilirubin, urine, qualitative	5 mL random urine
Brucella titer, canine	1 mL serum
Buffy coat preparation	EDTA tube
BUN (blood urea nitrogen)	1 mL serum
Calcium, serum	2 mL serum
Calcium, serum, ionized	3 mL serum
Calcium, urine	25-mL aliquot of 24-hr urine; add 6N HCl to pH 1–2; note 24-hr volume

Table continued on following page

859

6

Table 6–26. Sample Requirements for Laboratory Tests *Continued*

Test Description	Specimen
Carbon dioxide content	2 mL serum
Carbon monoxide (carboxyhemoglobin)	1 gray top
Chloride, CSF	1 mL CSF
Chloride, fluid	1 mL fluid
Chloride, serum	1 mL serum
Chloride, urine	24-mL aliquot of 24-hr urine; note 24-hr volume
Cholesterol	1 mL serum
Cholinesterase, RBC	2 mL heparinized blood
Cholinesterase, serum	1 mL serum
CK (creatine kinase) isoenzymes	1 mL serum
Coagulation factors	
Activated partial thromboplastin time (APTT)	Plasma, frozen: two 1-mL aliquots—blue top
Factor VIII	Plasma, frozen: two 1-mL aliquots—blue top
Factor IX	Plasma, frozen: two 1-mL aliquots—blue top
Factor XI	Plasma, frozen: two 1-mL aliquots—blue top
Factor XII	Plasma, frozen: two 1-mL aliquots—blue top
Factor XIII	Plasma, frozen: two 1-mL aliquots—blue top
Fibrin split products	Plasma, 2 ml: collect in special blue-top vial containing thrombin and special enzyme inhibitor
Fibrin stabilizing factor (factor XIII)	Plasma, frozen: two 1-mL aliquots—blue top
Fibrinogen titer	Plasma, frozen: two 1-mL aliquots—blue top
Partial thromboplastin time (see APTT)	Plasma, frozen: two 1-mL aliquots—blue top
Plasma clot lysis	Plasma, frozen: two 1-mL aliquots—blue top
Platelet count	EDTA tube
Prothrombin consumption time	1-mL serum, frozen; two 1-mL aliquots
Prothrombin time	Plasma, frozen; two 1-mL aliquots—blue top
Russell's viper venom time	Plasma, frozen; two 1-mL aliquots—blue top
Coccidioidomycosis antibody, screening	2 mL serum
Cold agglutinins	2 mL serum

Coombs', direct, canine or feline	1 mL whole blood in EDTA
Coombs', indirect, canine or feline	1 red top
Copper, serum	2 mL serum
Copper, urine	100-mL aliquot 24-hr urine; note 24-hr volume
Cortisol, serum or plasma	3 mL serum or heparinized plasma
Cortisol, urine	10-ml aliquot of 24-hr urine, frozen; note 24-hr volume
Creatine kinase (CK)	2 mL serum
Creatinine, serum	2 mL serum, frozen
Creatinine, urine	10-ml aliquot of 24-hr urine, frozen; note 24-hr volume
Creatinine clearance	2 mL serum–10-mL aliquot of specifically timed (12 or 24 hr) urine; note total volume and time
Cryoglobulins, qualitative	1 red top
11-Deoxycortisol (compound S)	3 mL heparinized plasma; separate immediately
11-Deoxy-11-oxy ratio of 17-ketogenic steroids	100-mL aliquot of 24-hr urine; note 24-hr volume
Digitoxin, RIA (radioimmunoassay)	2 mL serum
Digoxin, RIA	2 mL serum
Dirofilariasis	EDTA tube
Electrolytes (includes Na^+, K^+, Cl^-, CO_2)	2 mL serum
Electrophoresis, CSF	1 mL CSF
Electrophoresis, hemoglobin	EDTA tube
Electrophoresis, protein, serum	1 mL serum
Electrophoresis, protein, urine	20-mL aliquot of 24-hr urine; note 24-hr volume
Eosinophil count, direct	EDTA tube
Erythropoietin, quantitative	2 mL serum
ESR (erythrocyte sedimentation rate)	EDTA tube
Estradiol, serum, RIA	5 mL heparinized plasma or serum, frozen
Fatty acids, free	4 mL serum
Feline infectious peritonitis, fluid examination	3 mL fluid in EDTA tube, fixed smear of sediment
Feline leukemia virus antigen (ELISA)	0.25 mL serum or whole blood
Feline leukemia virus antigen (immunofluorescent antibody)	3 thin blood smears
Fibrinogen, quantitative	1 blue top

Table continued on following page

6

Table 6–26. Sample Requirements for Laboratory Tests *Continued*

Test Description	Specimen
GGTP (γ-glutamyltranspeptidase)	1 mL serum
γ-Globulins, quantitative (immunoglobulins) (includes IgG, IgA, and IgM)	1 mL serum
Glucose, blood, fasting	1 gray top
Glucose, CSF	1 mL CSF
Glucose, fluid	1 gray top
Glucose, urine, quantitative	25-mL aliquot of 24-hr urine; add 250 mg NaF to aliquot and mix; note 24-hr volume
Glucose tolerance (3 tests) each additional glucose	3 gray tops (indicate time) 1 gray top (indicate time)
Heavy metal screen (includes antimony, arsenic, mercury, and bismuth)	50 mL random urine
Hemoglobin, free, urine	10 mL random urine
Hemoglobin electrophoresis	EDTA tube
Hemogram (includes WBC, RBC, Hb, Hct, MCV, MCH, and MCHC)	EDTA tube
Histoplasmosis, serologic screen only	1 red top
Immunoelectrophoresis	1 mL serum; avoid hemolysis
Immunoglobulins, quantitative (includes IgG, IgA, and IgM in most species)	1 mL serum
Insulin, plasma	2 mL serum or plasma, frozen
Iron, total, and iron-binding capacity	4 mL serum
Lactic acid	Mix 4 mL blood from gray top with 4 mL 7% perchloric acid (remove tourniquet before blood withdrawal)
LDH (lactic acid dehydrogenase), serum	1 mL serum (do not freeze)
LDH isoenzyme pattern	1 mL serum (do not freeze)
LE preparation	1 red top (do not mail)
Lead, blood	1 green top
Lead, urine	100-mL aliquot of 24-hr urine; note 24-hr volume

Leptospira agglutinins	2 mL serum
Lipase	2 mL serum
Lipase, total, serum	2 mL serum
Magnesium, serum	1 mL serum
Methemalbumin (Schumm's test)	2 mL serum
Methemoglobin	1 gray top; deliver immediately
Microfilaria	1 mL, EDTA tube
Mucopolysaccharides, qualitative	30 mL random urine
Ornithine carbamyltransferase (OCT)	3 mL serum
Osmolality, serum	2 mL serum
Osmolality, urine	2 mL urine
Oxalate	50-mL aliquot of 24-hr urine; note 24-hr volume
Parathyroid hormone (PTH)	8 mL serum, frozen
Phosphatase, alkaline	1 mL serum
Phospholipids	2 mL serum
Phosphorus, serum	1 mL serum
Phosphorus, urine	25-mL aliquot of 24-hr urine; note 24-hr volume
Plasma clot lysis	Plasma, frozen; two 1-mL aliquots
Platelet factor 3	1 lavender or blue; sample must be free of any clot formation
Potassium, fluid	1 mL fluid
Potassium, serum	1 mL serum
Potassium, urine	10-mL aliquot of 24-hr urine; note 24-hr volume
Protein, total, CSF	2 mL CSF
Protein, total, urine	100-mL aliquot of 24-hr urine; note 24-hr volume
Protein, total, serum	1 mL serum
Protein electrophoresis, serum	1 mL serum
Protein electrophoresis, urine	20 mL random urine
Reticulocyte count	EDTA tube
Rheumatoid factor, canine	1 mL serum
Salicylates	1 mL serum
Sodium, fluid	1 mL fluid
Sodium, serum	1 mL serum

Table continued on following page

863

6

Table 6-26. Sample Requirements for Laboratory Tests *Continued*

Test Description	Specimen
Sodium, urine	10-mL aliquot of 24-hr urine; note 24-hr volume
Specific gravity, fluid	1 mL fluid
T₃ (triiodothyronine) uptake (resin)	1 mL serum
T₄ (thyroxine) by RIA	2 mL serum
Free T₄ by equilibrium dialysis	3 mL serum
Testosterone, serum (RIA)	2 mL serum
Testosterone, urine (RIA)	25-mL aliquot of 24-hr urine; refrigerate sample; note 24-hr volume
Thrombin time	Plasma, frozen: two 1-mL aliquots
Total protein, serum	1 mL serum
Toxoplasma, fluorescent antibody	1 mL serum
Triglycerides	3 mL serum
Trypsin-like immunoreactivity (TLI)	1 mL serum
Urea nitrogen, urine	10-mL aliquot of 24-hr urine; note 24-hr volume
Uric acid, serum	1 mL serum
Uric acid, urine	25-mL aliquot of 24-hr urine; note 24-hr volume
Viscosity, serum	6 mL serum
Xylose tolerance	100-mL aliquot of 5-hr urine plus 250 mg NaF; note 5-hr volume
Zinc, serum	5 mL serum

EDTA, ethylenediaminetetraacetic acid; CSF, cerebrospinal fluid; RBC, red blood cell; WBC, white blood cell; Hb, hemoglobin; Hct, hematocrit; MCV, mean corpuscular volume; MCH, mean corpuscular hemoglobin; MCHC, mean corpuscular hemoglobin concentration.

NORMAL LABORATORY VALUES FOR DOGS AND CATS

See Tables 6–27 through 6–48.

6

Table 6–27. Normal Blood Values

	Adult Dog	Average	Adult Cat	Average
Erythrocytes				
Erythrocytes ($10^6/\mu L$)	5.5–8.5	6.8	5.5–10.0	7.5
Hemoglobin (g/dL)	12.0–18.0	14.9	8.0–14.0	12.0
Packed cell volume (PCV) (%)	37.0–55.0	45.5	24.0–45.0	37.0
Mean corpuscular volume (fL)	66.0–77.0	69.8	40.0–55.0	45.0
Mean corpuscular hemoglobin (pg)	19.9–24.5	22.8	13.0–17.0	15.0
Mean corpuscular hemoglobin concentration (g/dL)				
Wintrobe	31.0–34.0	33.0	31.0–35.0	33.0
Microhematocrit	32.0–36.0	34.0	30.0–36.0	33.2
Reticulocytes (%) (excludes punctate reticulocytes)	0.0–1.5	0.8	0.2–1.6	0.6
Resistance to hypotonic saline (% saline solution producing)	0.40–0.50	0.46	0.66–0.72	0.69
Minimum				
Initial and complete hemolysis				
Maximum	0.32–0.42	0.33	0.46–0.54	0.50
Erythrocyte sedimentation rate	PCV 37	13%	PCV 35–40	7–27
(mm at 60 min)	PCV 50	0%		

RBC life span (days)	100–120		66–78	
RBC diameter (μm)	6.7–7.2	7.0	5.5–6.3	5.8
Leukocytes				
Leukocytes (cells/μL)	6000–17,000	11,500	5500–19,500	12,500
Neutrophils—bands (%)	0–3	0.8	0–3	0.5
Neutrophils—mature (%)	60–77	70.0	35–75	59.0
Lymphocytes (%)	12–30	20.0	20–55	32.0
Monocytes (%)	3–10	5.2	1–4	3.0
Eosinophils (%)	2–10	4.0	2–12	5.5
Basophils (%)	Rare	0.0	Rare	0.0
Neutrophils—bands (cells/μL)	0–300	70	0–300	100
Neutrophils—mature (cells/μL)	3000–11,500	7000	2500–12,500	7500
Lymphocytes (cells/μL)	1000–4800	2800	1500–7000	4000
Monocytes (cells/μL)	150–1350	750	0–850	350
Eosinophils (cells/μL)	100–1250	550	0–1500	650
Basophils	Rare	0	Rare	0

From Schalm OW, Tain NC, Carroll EJ: Veterinary Hematology, ed 3. Philadelphia, Lea & Febiger, 1975.

6

Table 6–28. Canine Blood Values at Different Ages—Average Values

Age	RBC (10⁶/μL)	Retic (%)*	NRBC/ 100 WBC*	Hb (g/dL)	PCV (%)	WBC/μL	Neut/μL	Bands/μL	Lymph/μL	Eos/μL
Birth	5.75	7.1	1.8	16.70	50	16,500	1300	400	2500	600
2 wk	3.92	7.1	1.8	9.76	32	11,000	6500	100	3000	300
4 wk	4.20	7.1	1.8	9.60	33	13,000	8600	0	4000	40
6 wk	4.91	3.6	1.8	9.59	34	15,000	10,000	0	4500	100
8 wk	5.13	3.9	0.3	11.00	37	18,000	11,000	234	6000	270
12 wk	5.27	3.9	Rare	11.60	36	15,300	9400	115	4600	322

RBC, red blood cells; Retic, reticulocytes; NRBC, nucleated RBCs; Hb, hemoglobin; PCV, packed cell volume; WBC, white blood cells; Neut, neutrophils; Lymph, lymphocytes; Eos, eosinophils.
*See Ewing GO, Schalm OW, Smith RS: J Am Vet Med Assoc, 161:1669, 1972.
From Andersen AC, Gee W: Vet Med 53:135, 1958.

Table 6–29. Canine Blood Values

Blood Test	Weanling Puppies (6 wk)			Rapid Growth Phase (12–24 wk)			Young Adults (6–12 mo)			Adult Males (1–11 yr)		
Male	5th Percentile	Median	95th Percentile	5th Percentile	Median	95th Percentile	5th Percentile	Median	95th Percentile	5th Percentile	Median	95th Percentile
RBCs ($\times 10^6/\mu L$)	3.33	3.88	4.49	4.71	5.32	6.03	5.74	6.44	7.14	5.87	6.66	7.59
PCV (%)	22.2	26.9	32.6	30.9	36.4	42.0	39.0	44.5	50.3	41.1	48.2	55.0
Hemoglobin (g/dL)	7.4	8.6	10.2	11.1	12.8	14.9	14.0	16.0	18.0	14.5	17.1	19.2
MCV (fL)	60	69	76	63	68	74	65	69	74	66	71	79
WBCs (cells/μL)	7222	12,100	17,605	7770	12,150	16,340	8314	12,075	18,623	6869	9509	13,985
Bands (cells/μL)	0	67	466	0	0	291	0	0	234	0	0	212
Neutrophils (cells/μL)	4766	7656	12,582	4533	7590	11,286	5043	7245	13,416	4121	6745	10,350
Lymphocytes (cells/μL)	1617	3615	6588	2009	3618	5754	1923	2943	5254	1108	2038	3303
Monocytes (cells/μL)	0	0	366	0	0	440	0	0	333	0	0	118
Eosinophils (cells/μL)	0	140	640	0	333	978	38	663	2251	95	528	1749
Basophils (cells/μL)	0	0	107	0	0	0	0	0	110	0	0	93
Female												
RBCs ($\times 10^6/\mu L$)	3.40	3.98	4.56	4.72	5.51	6.32	5.67	6.61	7.23	5.61	6.60	7.46
PCV (%)	23.2	27.7	33.9	31.1	38.1	42.7	39.5	45.9	52.0	40.4	46.5	55.3
Hemoglobin (g/dL)	7.7	8.8	10.3	11.0	13.1	15.0	14.8	16.6	18.3	14.2	16.6	18.9
MCV (fL)	61	70	76	63	68	74	65	70	76	65	70	80
WBCs (cells/μL)	7908	12,331	17,360	7374	12,200	18,700	7503	10,825	15,063	5939	10,350	16,650
Bands (cells/μL)	0	0	433	0	95	390	0	0	223	0	0	421
Neutrophils (cells/μL)	4769	7726	13,505	4370	7349	12,469	4119	6882	10,446	4424	7209	11,706
Lymphocytes (cells/μL)	1706	3433	6462	2036	3839	5913	1638	2866	5308	1034	2193	4406
Monocytes (cells/μL)	0	0	334	0	105	445	0	0	298	0	0	402
Eosinophils (cells/μL)	0	128	630	0	335	932	0	445	1859	0	582	1853
Basophils (cells/μL)	0	0	166	0	0	0	0	0	105	0	0	50
Breeds												
	English setter			German shepherd			Siberian husky			Beagle		
	English pointer			Labrador retriever			Saint Bernard			Doberman pinscher		
	Poodle									Black and tan coonhound		
	Miniature schnauzer											

From Lawler DF: Reference Intervals for Canine Blood Values. St. Louis, Ralston Purina, 1986.

6

Table 6–30. Feline Blood Values at Different Ages

Age	RBCs ($10^6/\mu L$)	Hb (g/dL)	PCV (%)	WBCs/μL	Neutrophils/μL	Lymphocytes/μL
Birth	4.95	12.2	44.7	7500		
2 wk	4.76	9.7	31.1	8080		
5 wk	5.84	8.4	29.9	8550		
Average	4.80	7.5	26.2	11,770	4600	6970
Range	3.90–5.70	6.6–8.4	21.0–33.5	7500–14,500		4500–9400
6 wk	6.75	9.0	35.4	8420		
8 wk	7.10	9.4	35.6			4900
Average	5.90	7.5	26.2	12,400	7500	
Range	3.30–7.30	7.6–15.0	22–38	6900–23,100		1925–10,100

RBCs, red blood cells; Hb, hemoglobin; PCV, packed cell volume; WBCs, white blood cells.
From Jain Nemi C: Essentials of Veterinary Hematology. Philadelphia, Lea & Febiger, 1993.

Table 6–31. Feline Blood Values

Blood Test*	Rapid Growth Phase (12–20 wk)			Young Adult (6–12 mo)			Adult Male (1–13 yr)		
Male	5th Percentile	Median	95th Percentile	5th Percentile	Median	95th Percentile	5th Percentile	Median	95th Percentile
RBCs ($\times 10^6$/µL)	5.64	6.99	8.11	6.00	7.24	8.90	5.71	7.36	9.67
PCV (%)	26.9	35.5	40.2	28.5	34.3	42.8	26.2	35.2	46.3
Hemoglobin (g/dL)	8.4	10.4	12.8	9.2	10.9	13.2	8.7	11.2	14.4
MCV (fL)	42	48	54	43	47	51	43	48	53
	10th† Percentile	Median	90th† Percentile	10th† Percentile	Median	90th† Percentile	10th† Percentile	Median	90th† Percentile
WBCs (cells/µL)	9985	16,400	24,430	8689	16,950	29,020	6450	9985	19,070
Bands (cells/µL)	0	0	156	0	0	198	0	0	97
Neutrophils (cells/µL)	6339	11,570	19,879	5521	10,725	22,595	3651	6947	13,412
Lymphocytes (cells/µL)	989	2925	6064	1855	3480	6938	1486	2785	4938
Monocytes (cells/µL)	0	0	292	0	107	448	0	0	208
Eosinophils (cells/µL)	352	851	1663	223	847	1816	211	533	1260
Basophils (cells/µL)	0	0	0	0	0	0	0	0	0

Table continued on following page

6

Table 6-31. Feline Blood Values *Continued*

Blood Test* Female	Rapid Growth Phase (12–20 wk)			Young Adult (6–12 mo)			Adult Male (1–13 yr)		
	5th Percentile	Median	95th Percentile	5th Percentile	Median	95th Percentile	5th Percentile	Median	95th Percentile
RBCs (× 10⁶/μL)	5.71	6.85	8.27	6.28	7.42	8.97	5.54	7.24	8.75
PCV (%)	27.4	32.8	39.3	30.2	36.1	45.0	26.9	34.4	42.5
Hemoglobin (g/dL)	8.6	10.5	12.9	9.2	11.1	13.8	9.0	11.4	13.5
MCV (fL)	42	47	54	42	48	52	42	47	52
	10th† Percentile	Median	90th† Percentile	10th† Percentile	Median	90th† Percentile	10th† Percentile	Median	90th† Percentile
WBCs (cells/μL)	8680	16,050	28,250	8232	14,600	25,920	6728	10,500	16,905
Bands (cells/μL)	0	0	0	0	0	199	0	0	114
Neutrophils (cells/μL)	5939	11,199	22,502	5116	9997	19,988	3842	6897	12,201
Lymphocytes (cells/μL)	921	2942	6193	1604	3048	5622	1055	2465	4647
Monocytes (cells/μL)	0	0	286	0	33	313	0	68	329
Eosinophils (cells/μL)	276	1007	1715	229	850	1955	210	552	1454
Basophils (cells/μL)	0	0	0	0	0	0	0	0	5

RBCs, red blood cells; PCV, packed cell volume; MCV, mean corpuscular volume; WBCs, white blood cells.
* Data collected with domestic short-hair (American short-hair) cats.
† Narrower interval reported as a result of wide range below 10th and above 90th percentiles.

Table 6–32. Effect of Pregnancy and Lactation on Blood Values of the Dog

| | Gestation | | | Term | Lactation | | |
	2 Weeks	4 Weeks	6 Weeks	8 Weeks	0 Weeks	2 Weeks	4 Weeks	6 Weeks
RBCs ($10^6/\mu L$)	8.85	7.48	6.73	6.26	4.53	5.13	5.65	6.15
PCV (%)	53	47	44	37	32	34	38	42
Hemoglobin (g/dL)	19.6	16.4	14.7	13.8	11.0	11.7	12.8	13.4
Sedimentation rate (mm at 60 min)	0.6	11.0	31.0	14.0	12.0	14.0	14.0	13.0
WBCs ($10^3/\mu L$)	12.0	12.2	15.7	19.0	18.9	16.9	17.1	15.9

From Jain Nemi C: Essentials of Veterinary Hematology. Philadelphia, Lea & Febiger, 1993.

Table 6–33. Effect of Pregnancy and Lactation on Blood Values of the Cat

	Gestation					Term	Lactation	
	1 Day Past Conception	2 Weeks	4 Weeks	6 Weeks	8 Weeks	0 Weeks	2 Weeks	4 Weeks
RBCs ($10^6/\mu L$)	8.0	7.9	7.1	6.7	6.2	6.2	7.4	7.4
PCV (%)	36.1	37.0	33.0	32.0	28.0	29.0	33.0	33.0
Hemoglobin (g/dL)	12.5	12.0	11.0	10.8	9.5	10.0	11.5	11.2
Reticulocytes (%) (includes punctate reticulocytes)	9%	11%	9%	10%	20.1%	15%	9%	6%

	Adult Dog	Average	Adult Cat	Average
Thrombocytes $\times 10^5/\mu L$	2–5	3–4	3–8	4.5
Icterus index	2–5 units		2–5 units	
Plasma fibrinogen (g/L)	2.0–4.0		0.50–3.00	

From Jain Nemi C: Essentials of Veterinary Hematology. Philadelphia, Lea & Febiger, 1993.

Table 6–34. Normal Bone Marrow

	Dog	Cat
Erythrocytic Cells		
Rubriblasts	0.2	1.71
Prorubricytes	0.9	12.50
Rubricytes	27.0	
Metarubricytes	15.3	11.68
Total	46.4	25.89
Granulocytic Cells		
Myeloblasts	0.0	1.74
Progranulocytes	1.3	0.88
Neutrophilic myelocytes	9.0	9.76
Eosinophilic myelocytes	0.0	1.47
Neutrophilic metamyelocytes	7.5	7.32
Eosinophilic metamyelocytes	2.4	1.52
Band neutrophils	13.6	25.80
Band eosinophils	0.9	—
Neutrophils	18.4	9.24
Eosinophils	0.3	0.81
Basophils	0.0	0.002
Total	53.4	52.542
M/E ratio—average	1.15:1.0	2.47:1.0
M/E ratio—range	0.75–2.50:1.0	0.60–3.90:1.0
Other Cells		
Lymphocytes	0.2	7.63
Plasma cells	0	1.61
Reticulum cells	0	0.13
Mitotic cells	0	0.61
Unclassified	0	1.62
Disintegrated cells	0	4.60

M/E, myeloid-erythroid.
From Bentinck-Smith J, French TW: A roster of normal values for dogs and cats. *In* Kirk RW, ed: Current Veterinary Therapy X. Philadelphia, WB Saunders, 1989, p 1338, as seen in Jain Nemi C: Essentials of Veterinary Hematology. Philadelphia, Lea & Febiger, 1993.

Table 6–35. Hematology Reference Ranges and Units*

	Adult Dog	Adult Cat
RBCs ($10^6/\mu L$)	5.6–8.5	5.5–10.3
Hemoglobin (g/dL)	13.7–19.6	8.4–15.0
Hematocrit (%)	39–56	25–45
Mean cell volume (fL)	65–72	41–51
Mean cell hemoglobin conc. (g/dL)	32–37	32–36
Mean cell hemoglobin (pg)	21–26	14–17
RBC distribution width	12–15	15–20
WBCs ($10^3/\mu L$)	7.5–19.9	6.1–21.1
Platelets ($10^3/\mu L$)	179–510	215–760
Mean platelet volume (fL)	8–12	11–15

* Based on results from 50 clinically normal individuals of each species as determined at the New York State College of Veterinary Medicine, Ithaca, N.Y. The results obtained from this model may vary with the exact instrument settings employed.

6

Table 6-36. Système International (SI) Conversion Factors for Common Hematology and Clinical Chemistry Tests*

	Example Values Expressed in		Conversion Factors (×)	
Analyte	**Traditional Units**	**SI Units**	**Traditional Units to SI Units**	**SI Units to Traditional Units**
Hematology				
RBCs	$6.0 \times 10^6/mm^3$	$6.0 \times 10^{12}/L$	10^6	10^{-6}
PCV	45%	0.45 L/L	0.01	100
Hemoglobin	15.0 g/dL (%)	150 g/L	10	0.1
MCV	75 μm^3	75 fl	No change	No change
MCHC	33 g/dL (%)	330 g/L	10	0.1
MCH	25 pg	25 pg	No change	No change
WBCs	$15.0 \times 10^3/mm^3$	$15.0 \times 10^9/L$	10^6	10^{-6}
Platelets	$250 \times 10^3/mm^3$	$250 \times 10^9/L$	10^6	10^{-6}
Clinical Chemistry				
Albumin	3.0 g/dL	30 g/L	10.0	0.10
Ammonia (NH_3)	20.0 $\mu g/dL$	12 $\mu mol/L$	0.5871	1.7
Bicarbonate	25 mEq/L	25 mmol/L	No change	No change
Bile acids (total)	1.0 mg/L	2.5 $\mu mol/L$	2.547	0.3926
Bilirubin (total)	0.2 mg/dL	3 $\mu mol/L$	17.1	0.0585
Bilirubin (direct)	0.1 mg/dL	2 $\mu mol/L$	17.1	0.0585
Calcium	10.0 mg/dL	2.5 mmol/L	0.250	4.008

	Traditional Units	SI Units	Conversion Factor	Reverse Factor
Chloride	100 mEq/L	100 mmol/L	No change	No change
Cholesterol	200 mg/dL	5.17 mmol/L	0.02586	38.7
Creatinine	1.0 mg/dL	90 μmol/L	88.40	0.0113
Globulins (total)	3.0 g/dL	30 g/L	10.0	0.10
Glucose	100 mg/dL	5.6 mmol/L	0.05551	18.02
Iron	100 μg/dL	18 μmol/L	0.1791	5.59
Iron-binding capacity	300 μg/dL	54 μmol/L	0.1791	5.59
Lead	25 μg/dL	1.21 μmol/L	0.04826	20.7
Magnesium	2.0 mg/dL	0.82 mmol/L	0.4114	2.43
Phosphate (P_i)	4.0 mg/dL	1.29 mmol/L	0.3229	3.10
Potassium	4.0 mEq/L	4.0 mmol/L	No change	No change
Protein (total)	7.0 g/dL	70 g/L	10.0	0.1
Sodium	145 mEq/L	145 mmol/L	No change	No change
Triglycerides	50 mg/dL	0.56 mmol/L	0.01129	88.5
Urea nitrogen	15 mg/dL	5.4 mmol/L	0.3570	2.8

RBCs, red blood cells; PCV, packed cell volume; MCV, mean corpuscular volume; MCHC, mean corpuscular hemoglobin concentration; MCH, mean corpuscular hemoglobin.

* Système International is the system for reporting clinical laboratory data currently used in most countries worldwide. This table gives arbitrary examples of common hematology and clinical chemistry test results, expressed in both traditional and SI units, and supplies the multiplication factors for converting results between the two systems.

From Bentinck-Smith J, French TW: A roster of normal values for dogs and cats. *In* Kirk RW, ed: Current Veterinary Therapy X. Philadelphia, WB Saunders, 1989, p 1339.

Table 6-37. Chemistry Reference Values

Test	Units	Canine	Feline
Arterial blood gas			
pH		7.36–7.44	7.36–7.44
P_{CO_2}	mm Hg	36–44	28–32
P_{O_2}	mm Hg	90–100	90–100
T_{CO_2}	mEq/L	25–27	21–23
HCO_3	mEq/L	24–26	20–22
Venous blood gas			
pH		7.34–7.46	7.33–7.41
P_{CO_2}	mm Hg	32–49	34–38
P_{O_2}	mm Hg	24–48	35–45
T_{CO_2}	mEq/L	21–31	37–31
HCO_3	mEq/L	20–29	22–24
A/G ratio (calculated)		0.89–2.68	0.80–1.68
Albumin	g/dL	3.2–4.7	3.0–4.6
ALP (alkaline phosphatase)	IU/L	0–90	4–81
ALT (SGPT)	IU/L	10–94	23–109
Ammonia (resting)	μg/dL	25–92	30–100
Amylase	IU/L	371–1503	531–1660
AST (SGOT)	IU/L	10–62	14–41
Bile acid (fasting)	μmol/L	0.0–15.3	0.0–7.6
Bile acid (2 hour)	μmol/L	0.0–20.3	0.0–10.9
Bilirubin—total and direct	mg/dL	0.1–0.6	0.1–0.7
BSP		0–5%	0–5%
BUN	mg/dL	7–32	18–41
Calcium	mg/dL	9.0–11.9	8.4–11.5
Cholesterol	mg/dL	116–317	64–229
CK	IU/L	51–529	91–326
Creatinine	mg/dL	0.5–1.4	0.7–2.2

Electrolyte profile			
Sodium (Na)	mEq/L	146–156	153–162
Potassium (K)	mEq/L	3.9–5.5	3.6–5.8
Chloride (Cl)	mEq/L	113–123	119–132
TCO_2	mEq/L	16.9–26.9	12.5–24.5
Anion gap		9–22	10–27
GGT	IU/L	1–6	1–3
Globulin	g/dL	1.5–3.5	2.1–4.0
Glucose	mg/dL	53–117	57–131
LDH	IU/L	42–130	63–193
Lipase	U/L	90–527	
Lipase	Sigma-Tietz units	0.1–1.3	0.1–0.4
Magnesium	mg/dL	1.36–2.09	1.38–2.36
Osmolality–serum			
Calculated	mOsm/kg	302–325	319–371
Determined	mOsm/kg	293–321	290–320
Osmolality–urine	mOsm	200–2000	200–2000
Phosphorus	mg/dL	1.9–7.9	2.9–8.3
SDH	IU/L	5.4–33.3	0.4–10
Total protein	g/dL	5.3–7.6	5.5–7.7
Triglyceride	mg/dL	10–500	10–500
Uric acid	mg/dL	0–1	0–1
Serum iron (Abbott)	µg/dL	61–255	34 122
Iron profile*			
Total iron	µg/dL	84–233*	68–215
UIBC	µg/dL	142–393	105–205
TIBC	µg/dL	284–572	†
Saturation	%	20–59	†

Table continued on following page

6

Table 6–37. Chemistry Reference Values *Continued*

		Dogs and Cats					
	Sex	Birth to 12 Mo	Average	1–5 Yr	Average	6 Yr and Older	Average
Total protein (S) (g/dL) (dogs)	Male	3.90–5.90	5.15	4.90–9.60	6.33	5.5–7.3	6.4
	Female	4.00–6.40	5.58	5.50–7.80	6.34	4.7–7.5	6.2
Total protein (S) (g/dL) (cats)	Male	4.3–10.0	6.4	6.8–10.0	8.1	6.2–8.5	7.2
	Female	4.8–9.1	6.4	6.6–8.9	7.4	6.0–9.0	7.3

Electrophoresis	Dog	Cat
Albumin (S) (g/dL)	2.3–3.4	2.3–3.5
Globulin (S) (g/dL)	3.0–4.7	2.6–5.0
α_1 (S) (g/dL)	0.3–0.8	0.3–0.5
α_2 (S) (g/dL)	0.5–1.3	0.4–1.0
β (S) (g/dL)	0.7–1.8	0.6–1.9
γ (S) (g/dL)	0.4–1.0	0.5–1.5
Albumin-globulin (A/G) ratio	0.7–1.1	0.5–1.0

S, serum; LDH, lactate dehydrogenase; AST, aspartate aminotransferase; ALT, alanine aminotransferase; CK, creatine kinase; GGT, γ-glutamyltransferase.
* Harvey JW, French TW, Meyer DJ: Chronic iron deficiency anemia in dogs. JAAHA 18:946–960, 1982.
† Values not directly determined.
From Willard M, Tvedten H, Turnwald G: Small Animal Clinical Diagnosis by Laboratory Methods, ed 3. Philadelphia, WB Saunders, 1999.

Table 6-38. Chemistry Reference Values: Part II

Other Analytes	Adult Dog	Adult Cat
Lactic acid (S) (mg/dL)	3–15	
Pyruvate (B) (mEq/L)	0.1–0.2	
Cholesterol esters (S) (mg/dL)	84–168	45–120
Free cholesterol (S) (mg/dL)	28–84	15–60
Total lipid (P) (mg/dL)	47–725	145–607
Free glycerol (S) 24-hr fast (mg/dL)	14.2–23.2	145–607
Iron (S) (μg/dL)	94–122	68–215
Total iron-binding capacity (S) (μg/dL)	280–340	170–400
Lead (B) (μg/dL)	0–35	0–35

Blood Gases	Adult Dog	Adult Cat
Po_2 (B) mm Hg (arterial)	85–95	—
Po_2 (B) mm Hg (venous)	40–60	—
Pco_2 (B) mm Hg (arterial)	29–36	—
Pco_2 (B) mm Hg (venous)	29–42	—
Base excess (B) (mEq/L)	±2.5	±2.5
Bicarbonate (P) (mEq/L)	17–24	17–24

S, serum; B, blood; P, plasma.

From Bentinck-Smith J, French TW: A roster of normal values for dogs and cats. *In* Kirk RW, ed: Current Veterinary Therapy X. Philadelphia, WB Saunders, 1989, p 1341.

6

Table 6–39. Tests of the Endocrine System*

Hormone	Unit	Dogs	Cats
Adrenocorticotrophic hormone, basal (ACTH, plasma)	pmol/L	2–15	1–20
Aldosterone† (plasma)			
Basal	pmol/L	14–957	194–388
Post-ACTH	pmol/L	197–2103	277–721
Cortisol (serum or plasma, urine)			
Basal	nmol/L	25–125	15–150
Post-ACTH	nmol/L	200–550	130–450
Post-low-dose dexamethasone (0.01 or 0.015 mg/kg)	nmol/L	≤40	≤40
Post-high-dose dexamethasone (0.1 or 1.0 mg/kg)†	nmol/L	≤40	≤40
Urinary cortisol-creatinine ratio	$\times 10^{-6}$	8–24,† 10‡	—
Insulin, basal (serum)	pmol/L	35–200	35–200
Intact parahormone§ (serum)	pmol/L	2–13	0–4
Progesterone (serum or plasma, female)	mmol/L	≤3.0 in anestrus, proestrus	≤3.0 in anestrus, proestrus
		50–220 in diestrus, pregnancy	50–220 in diestrus, pregnancy
Testosterone (serum or plasma, male)	nmol/L	1–20	1–20

Thyroxine (T$_4$, serum)			
Basal	nmol/L	12–50	10–50
Post-thyroxine-stimulating hormone (TSH)	nmol/L	>45	>45
Triiodothyronine (T$_3$) suppression‖	nmol/L	—	≤20
Triiodothyronine, basal (T$_3$, serum)	nmol/L	0.7–2.3	0.5–2.0

* Prepared with the assistance of M.E. Peterson, The Animal Medical Center, New York, N.Y. Unless indicated otherwise, values in this table are adapted from Kemppainen RJ, Zerbe CA: Common endocrine diagnostic tests: Normal values and interpretations. *In* Kirk RW, ed: Current Veterinary Therapy X. Philadelphia, WB Saunders, 1989, pp 961–968. Hormone determinations are variable between laboratories. The laboratory performing the analysis should provide reference values. Before submitting samples for hormone determinations, consult the laboratory for sample specifications, use of anticoagulants, and sample preservation. General sampling conditions are discussed in Reimers TJ: Guidelines for collection, storage, and transport of samples for hormone assay. *In* Kirk RW, ed: Current Veterinary Therapy X. Philadelphia, WB Saunders, 1989, pp 968–973. Factors that affect serum thyroid and adrenocortical hormone concentrations in dogs are discussed in Reimers TJ, Lawler DF, Sutaria PM, et al: Effects of age, sex, and body size on serum concentrations of thyroid and adrenocortical hormones in dogs. Am J Vet Res 51:454, 1990.

† This test is used after adrenocortical hyperfunction has been confirmed. It is used to differentiate adrenal tumor (where no suppression is seen) from pituitary-dependent cases (where suppression occurs but is variable).

‡ From Stolp R, Rijnberk A, Meiher JC, et al: Urinary corticoids in the diagnosis of canine hyperadrenocorticism. Res Vet Sci 34:141, 1983; Rijnberk A, van Wees A, Mol JA: Assessment of two tests for the diagnosis of canine hyperadrenocorticism. Vet Rec 122:178–180, 1988.

§ Provided by R.F. Nachreiner, Animal Health Diagnostic Laboratory, Endocrine Diagnostic Section, Michigan State University, East Lansing.

‖ From Peterson ME, Ferguson DC: Thyroid diseases. *In* Ettinger SJ, ed: Textbook of Veterinary Internal Medicine. Diseases of the Dog and Cat, ed 3. Philadelphia, WB Saunders, 1989, pp 1632–1675.

From Bonagura JD, ed: Current Veterinary Therapy XII. Philadelphia: WB Saunders, 1995, p 1410.

Table 6-40. Conversion Table for Hormone Assay Units

Hormone	Unit		Conversion Factors	
	Traditional	SI	Traditional to SI	SI to Traditional
Aldosterone	ng/dL	pmol/L	27.7	0.036
Corticotropin (ACTH)	pg/mL	pmol/L	0.22	4.51
Cortisol	μg/dL	nmol/L	27.59	0.36
β-Endorphin	pg/mL	pmol/L	0.289	3.43
Epinephrine	pg/mL	pmol/L	5.46	0.183
Estrogen (estradiol)	pg/mL	pmol/L	3.67	0.273
Gastrin	pg/mL	ng/L	1.00	1.00
Glucagon	pg/mL	ng/L	1.00	1.00
Growth hormone (GH)	ng/mL	μg/L	1.00	1.00
Insulin	μU/mL	pmol/L	7.18	0.139
α-Melanocyte-stimulating hormone (α-MSH)	pg/mL	pmol/L	0.601	1.66
Norepinephrine	pg/mL	nmol/L	0.006	169
Pancreatic polypeptide (PP)	mg/dL	mmol/L	0.239	4.18
Progesterone	ng/mL	nmol/L	3.18	0.315
Prolactin	ng/mL	μg/L	1.00	1.00
Renin	ng/mL/hr	ng/L/s	0.278	3.60
Somatostatin	pg/mL	pmol/L	0.611	1.64
Testosterone	ng/mL	nmol/L	3.47	0.288
Thyroxine (T$_4$)	μg/dL	nmol/L	12.87	0.078
Triiodothyronine (T$_3$)	ng/dL	nmol/L	0.0154	64.9
Vasoactive intestinal polypeptide (VIP)	pg/mL	pmol/L	0.301	3.33

Contributed by M.E. Peterson, The Animal Medical Center, New York, N.Y.
From Bonagura JD, ed: Kirk's Current Veterinary Therapy XII. Philadelphia: WB Saunders, 1995, p 1411.

Table 6–41. Approximate Normal Ranges for Common Measurements in Dogs and Cats

Measurement	Dog	Cat
Heart rate (bpm)	60–180	140–220
Capillary refill time	<2 s	<2 s
Body temperature	99.5°–102.5°F	100.5°–102.5°F
	37.5°–39.2°C	38.1°–39.2°C
Mean arterial pressure (mm Hg)	90–120	100–150
Blood volume (ml/kg)	75–90	47–66
Cardiac output		
(mL/kg/min)	100–200	167 ± 39
(L/m²/min)	4.72 ± 1.09	
Systemic resistance		
(mm Hg/mL/kg/min)	0.64 ± 0.16	
(dynes/s/cm)	2162 ± 458	
Mean pulmonary arterial pressure	14 ± 3	
(mm Hg)		
Central venous pressure (cm H_2O)	3 ± 4	
Pulmonary artery occlusion pressure	5 ± 2	
(mm Hg)		
Urine output	1–2 mL/kg/hr	1–2 mL/kg/hr
Breathing rate (breaths/min)	10–30	24–42
Minute ventilation (mL/kg/min)	170–350	200–350
Oxygen delivery		
(mL/kg/min)	29 ± 8	
(mL/m²/min)	815 ± 234	
Oxygen consumption		
(mL/kg/min)	4–11	3–8
(mL/m²/min)	198 ± 53	
Arterial P_{O_2} (mm Hg)	85–105	100–115
Arterial S_{O_2}	>95	>95
Arterial P_{CO_2} (mm Hg)	30–44	28–35
Arterial pH	7.36–7.46	7.34–7.43
Bicarbonate (mEq/L)	20–25	17–21
Base deficit (mEq/L)	0 to −4	−1 to −8
Total plasma proteins (g/dL)	6.0–8.0	6.8–8.3
Albumin (g/dL)	2.5–3.5	1.9–3.9
Packed cell volume (%)	37–55	29–48
Hemoglobin (g/dL)	12–18	9–15.1
Sodium (mEq/L)	145–154	151–158
Potassium (mEq/L)	4.1–5.3	3.6–4.9
Chloride (mEq/L)	105–116	113–121
Total CO_2 (mEq/L)	16–26	15–21

S_{O_2}, oxygen saturation; P_{O_2}, partial pressure of oxygen; P_{CO_2}, partial pressure of carbon dioxide; s, seconds.

Modified from Aldrich J, Haskins SC: Monitoring the critically ill patient. *In* Bonagura JD, ed: Kirk's Current Veterinary Therapy XII. Philadelphia: WB Saunders, 1995, pp 98–105.

6

Table 6-42. Chemistry Reference Values: Part III[a]

Hormones	Adult Dog		Adult Cat	
	Resting Level	Post-ACTH[b]	Resting Level	Post-ACTH[b]
Cortisol (S) (RIA) (mg/dL)[c]	1.8–4.0	3–4 × Pretreatment	1–3	3–4 × Pretreatment
Cortisol (S) (CPB) (mg/dL)[c]	2–6	3–4 × Pretreatment	2–5	3–4 × Pretreatment
Cortisol (S) (fluorometric) (µg/dL)[c]	5–10	10–20		
	Resting Level	Post-TSH[d]	Resting Level	Post-TSH
T_4 (P) (RIA) (µg/dL)[e]	1.52–3.60	At least 3- to 4-fold	1.2–3.8	
T_3 (P) (RIA) (ng/dL)[e]	48–154	More than 10-ng increase		
Protein-bound iodine (µg/dL)[f]	1.6–3.0	Increase of 3 µg/dL (mean)		

T_4 Changes With Age	Dog	Cat
T_4 (S) (RIA)	Decrease of 0.07 µg/dL per year of age	No values for cat
T_4 (S) (CPB) (µg/dL)[g]		
10–12 wk	3.24 ± 0.51	2.82 ± 0.73
1 hr	2.25 ± 0.33	2.43 ± 0.55

	Adult Dog	Adult Cat
Thyroid uptake of ^{131}I (%)	17–30	—
Insulin (S) (RIA) (µU/mL)[h]	0–30	0–50

886

Plasma Proteins

	Basenji Dogs		Cats	
Age	Plasma Proteins (gm/dL)[j]	Age	Plasma Proteins (g/dL)[j]	
6–8 wk	5.33 ± 0.29	Adults (younger animals have lower values)	6–8	
9–12 wk	5.87 ± 0.46			
4–6 mo	6.6 ± 0.24			
1–2 yr	7.03 ± 0.33			

S, serum; P, plasma; RIA, radioimmunoassay; CPB, competitive protein binding; TSH, thyroid-stimulating hormone; T_4, thyroxine; T_3, triiodothyronine; ACTH, adrenocorticotropic hormone.

a Chemical analytes are liable to show markedly different values depending on the method employed.

b Two μg ACTH gel IM 2 hours after injection.

c Cortisol (S) (RIA) data from Thomas J. Reimers, Assistant Professor and Director of the Endocrinology Laboratory, New York State College of Veterinary Medicine, Cornell University, Ithaca, N.Y. Cortisol (S) (CPB) data from R. Wallace, Research Support Specialist, New York State College of Veterinary Medicine, Cornell University, Ithaca, N.Y. Cortisol (S) (CPB) pretreatment data from D.W. Scott, Assistant Professor of Clinical Sciences, New York State College of Veterinary Medicine, Cornell University, Ithaca, N.Y.

d Five μg TSH IV 4–6 hours after injection.

e T_4 and T_3 (P) (RIA) values from Belshaw BE, Rijnberk, 1979: J Am Anim Hosp Assoc 15:17, 1979.

f Protein-bound iodine values from Benjamin M: An Outline of Veterinary Clinical Pathology, ed 3. Ames, Iowa State University Press, 1978.

g T_4S (CPB) and thyroid uptake values from R.A. Kallfelz FA, Erali RP: Am J Vet Res 34:1449, 1973; personal communication from R.A. Kallfelz, Associate Professor of Clinical Nutrition, Department of Large Animal Medicine, Obstetrics, and Surgery, New York State College of Veterinary Medicine, Cornell University, Ithaca, N.Y.

h Insulin (S) (RIA) data from R.J. Wilkins: Animal Medical Center, New York, N.Y.

i Basenji dogs plasma protein values from Ewing GO, Schalm OW, Smith RS: J Am Vet Med Assoc 161:1661, 1972.

j Cat plasma protein values from Schalm OW, Jain NC, Cornell EJ: Veterinary Hematology, ed 3. Philadelphia, Lea & Febiger, 1975.

From Bentinck-Smith J, French TW: A roster of normal values for dogs and cats. In Kirk RW, ed: Current Veterinary Therapy X. Philadelphia, WB Saunders, 1989, p 1342.

6

Table 6–43. Coagulation Profiles*

	Adult Dog	**Adult Cat**
Bleeding time		
Dorsum of nose (min)	2–4	1–5
Lip (s)	85–110	
Ear (min)	2.5–3	
Abdomen (min)	1–2	
Whole-blood coagulation time		
Glass (Lee and White) (min)	6–7.5	8
Silicone (Lee and White) (min)	12–15	
Capillary tube (min)	3–4	5.2 ±0.2
Activated coagulation time of whole blood		
Room temp (s)	60–125	A limited number of cats have shown a range similar to that of the dog
37°C (s)	64–95	
Prothrombin time (s)	6–10	8.6 ±0.5
Puppies		
1–4 hr old	42.2	
6–12 hr old	49.1	
16–48 hr old	36.8	
Russell's viper venom time	11	9
Partial thromboplastin time	15–25	
Prothrombin consumption	20.5	20
Fibrin degradation products (μg/mL)	<10	

* *Note:* Test should be interpreted with an accompanying normal control.

From Willard M, Tvedten H, Turnwald G: Small Animal Clinical Diagnosis by Laboratory Methods, ed 3. Philadelphia, WB Saunders, 1999.

Table 6–44. Conversion to Systéme International (SI) Units for Hormone Assays

Measurement	SI Unit	Traditional Unit	Traditional to SI Unit*	SI to Traditional Unit*
Aldosterone	pmol/L	ng/dL	27.7	0.036
Corticotropin (ACTH)	pmol/L	pg/mL	0.220	4.51
Cortisol	nmol/L	μg/dL	27.59	0.036
C peptide	nmol/L	ng/mL	0.331	3.02
β-Endorphin	pmol/L	pg/mL	0.292	3.43
Epinephrine	pmol/L	pg/mL	5.46	0.183
Estrogen (estadiol)	pmol/L	pg/mL	3.67	0.273
Gastrin	ng/L	pg/mL	1.00	1.00
Gastrointestinal polypeptide	pmol/L	pg/mL	0.201	4.98
Glucagon	ng/L	pg/mL	1.00	1.00
Growth hormone	μg/L	ng/mL	1.00	1.00
Insulin	pmol/L	μU/mL	7.18	0.139
α-Melanocyte-stimulating hormone	pmol/L	pg/mL	0.601	1.66
Norepinephrine	nmol/L	pg/mL	0.006	169
Pancreatic polypeptide	mmol/L	mg/dL	0.239	4.18
Progesterone	nmol/L	ng/mL	3.18	0.315
Prolactin	μg/L	ng/mL	1.00	1.00
Renin	ng/L/s	ng/mL/hr	0.278	3.60
Somatostatin	pmol/L	pg/mL	0.611	1.64
Testosterone	nmol/L	ng/mL	3.47	0.288
Thyroxine	nmol/L	μg/dL	12.87	0.078
Triiodothyronine	nmol/L	μg/dL	0.0154	64.9
Vasoactive intestinal polypeptide	pmol/L	pg/mL	0.301	3.33

* Factor to multiply to convert from one unit to the other.
From Feldman EC, Nelson RW: Canine and Feline Endocrinology and Reproduction, ed 2. Philadelphia, WB Saunders, 1996.

Table 6–45. Conversion to Systéme International (SI) Units for Common Serum Chemistry Data

Measurement	SI Unit	Traditional Unit	Traditional to SI Unit*	SI to Traditional Unit*
Albumin	g/L	g/dL	10.0	0.100
Bile acids	μmol/L	mg/L	2.55	0.392
Bilirubin	μmol/L	mg/dL	17.10	0.058
Calcium	mmol/L	mg/dL	0.250	4.00
Carbon dioxide content	mmol/L	mEq/L	1.00	1.00
Cholesterol	mmol/L	mg/dL	0.026	38.7
Chloride	mmol/L	mEq/L	1.00	1.00
Creatinine	μmol/L	mg/dL	88.40	0.011
Creatinine clearance	mL/s	mL/min	0.017	60.0
Glucose	mmol/L	mg/dL	0.056	18.0
Inorganic phosphorus	nmol/L	mg/dL	0.323	3.10
Osmolality	nmol/kg	mOsm/kg	1.00	1.00
Potassium	mmol/L	mEq/L	1.00	1.00
Protein, total	g/L	g/dL	10.0	0.100
Sodium	mmol/L	mEq/L	1.00	1.00
Urea nitrogen	mmol/L	mg/dL	0.357	2.8

* Factor to multiply to convert from one unit to the other.
From Feldman EC, Nelson RW: Canine and Feline Endocrinology and Reproduction, ed 2. Philadelphia, WB Saunders, 1996.

6

Table 6–46. Normal Renal Function and Urine Values*

	Adult Dog	Adult Cat
Urine		
Specific gravity		
Minimum	1.001	1.001
Maximum	1.060	1.080
Usual limits (normal water and food intake)	1.018–1.050	1.018–1.050
Volume (mL/kg body weight/day)	24–41	22–30
Osmolality urine (mOsm/kg)		
Usual range	500–1200	
Maximal limits	2000–2400	
Osmolality plasma (mOsm/kg)	300	
Urine Constituents		
Creatinine (mg/dL)	100–300	110–280
Urea nitrogen (g/dL)	1.0–2.5	1.0–3.0
Protein (mg/dL)	0–30	0–20
Amylase (Somogyi units)	50–150	30–120
Sodium (mEq/L)	20–165	
Potassium (mEq/L)	20–120	
Calcium (mEq/L)	2–10	
Inorganic phosphorus (mEq/L)	50–180	
Urinalysis—Semiquantitative Values		
Protein sulfosalicylic acid	0–trace	0–trace
Protein Multistix	0–1+	0–1+
Glucose	0	0
Ketones	0	0
Bilirubin	0	0
10%–20% Dogs—high specific gravity	1+	
5% Cats—high specific gravity		1+
Urobilinogen (Ehrlich unit)	0–1	0–1
(Wallace-Diamond)	<1:32	<1:32

Daily Urine Protein Excretion in Normal Cats and Dogs*

Protein (mg/kg/d)				
Range	Mean	Method of Analysis	Species	Number Evaluated
0.6–5.1	2.3	Coomassie brilliant blue	Canine	16
1.8–22.4	7.66	Coomassie brilliant blue	Canine	14
0.2–7.7	2.45	Trichloroacetic acid ponceau-S	Canine	19
1.9–11.7	4.76	Trichloroacetic acid ponceau-S	Canine	8
2.7–23.2	6.6	Trichloroacetic acid ponceau-S	Canine	29
4.55–28.3	13.9	Trichloroacetic acid ponceau-S	Canine	17
2.99–8.88	4.93	Coomassie brilliant blue	Feline	30

* Urine values, renal function values (dog), and values for creatinine (endogenous clearance) from Osborne C, Finco D: Canine and Feline Nephrology and Urology. Baltimore, Williams & Wilkins, 1995.

Table 6–47. Cerebrospinal Fluid and Synovial Fluid

Cerebrospinal Fluid*	Adult Dog	Adult Cat
Color	Clear, colorless	Clear, colorless
Pressure (mm H_2O)	<170	<100
Cells/µL	<5 lymphocytes	<5 lymphocytes
Protein (mg/dL)	<25	<20
Glucose (mg/dL)	61–116	85

Normal Synovial Fluid—Carpal, Elbow, Shoulder, Hip, Stifle, and Hock Joints	Adult Dog	
	Range	Mean
Amount (mL)	0.01–1.00	0.24
pH	7–7.8	7.33
Leukocytes ($\times 10^3$/µL)	0–2.9	0.43
Erythrocytes ($\times 10^3$/µL)	0–320.0	12.15
Neutrophils/µL	0–32	3.63
Neutrophils (%)	10	
Monocytes/µL	0–838	230.77
Lymphocytes/µL	0–2436	245.6
Clasmatocytes/µL	0–166	14.69
Mononuclear cells (%)	90	
Mucin clot	Tight, ropy clump; clear supernatent	

* Data from A. deLahunta, Professor of Anatomy, Department of Clinical Sciences, New York State College of Veterinary Medicine, Cornell University, Ithaca, N.Y.

From Bentinck-Smith J, French TW: A roster of normal values for dogs and cats. *In* Kirk RW, ed: Current Veterinary Therapy X. Philadelphia, WB Saunders, 1989, p 1344.

6

Table 6–48. Canine Semen*

Regular Collection by Hand Manipulation With a Teaser (125 Ejaculates From Small Dogs, Mostly Beagles)	Mean	Standard Deviation	Range
Volume (mL)	5	4.3	0.5–20.4
% Motile sperm	75	7.5	30–90
% Normal sperm	86	14.7	34–97
pH	6.72	0.19	6.49–7.10
Concentration/mm^3 ($\times 10^3$)	148	84.6	27.2–388.8
Total sperm per ejaculate ($\times 10^6$)	528	321.0	94–1428

Fractionated Ejaculates (Based on 65 Ejaculates)	Mean	Range	pH
First fraction	0.8 mL	0.25–2.00	6.37
Section fraction	0.6 mL	0.40–2.00	6.10
Third fraction	0.4 mL	1.0–16.3	7.20

Ejaculates From Purebred Labrador Retrievers, 18–48 Months Old	Mean	Range
Volume (mL)	2.2	0.5–6.5
% Motile sperm	93	75–99
% Unstained sperm (eosin-nigrosin)	84	61–99
Concentration/mm^3 ($\times 10^3$)	564	103–708

*Revisions and corrections courtesy of R.H. Foote, Professor of Animal Physiology, Department of Animal Science, New York State College of Life Sciences, Cornell University, Ithaca, N.Y.

From Bentinck-Smith J, French TW: A roster of normal values for dogs and cats. *In* Kirk RW, ed: Current Veterinary Therapy X. Philadelphia, WB Saunders, 1989, p 1345.

●●

ANTIMICROBIAL THERAPY
See Tables 6–49 through 6–56.

Table 6–49. Antibacterial Therapy Against Specific Pathogens

Organism	Agent	First Choice	Second Choice	Alternatives
Acinetobacter	Gram-negative bacilli	Enrofloxacin	Gentamicin	Other aminoglycosides
Actinomyces	Gram-positive (variable) anaerobic, filamentous rods	Penicillin G (high dose)	Clindamycin	Chloramphenicol
Aspergillus	Saprophytic fungi	Itraconazole; information on the use of this drug in cats is not available	Ketoconazole (oral)	Thiabendazole (oral and topical via surgically implanted nasal tubes)
Babesia	Hematozoan parasite	Diminazene aceturate (dog only) Primaquine phosphate (cat only)	Pentamidine isethionate (dog only)	Imidocarb dipropionate (dog only)
Bacillus piliformis	Gram-negative bacilli (Tyzzer's disease)	Unknown	Unknown	Unknown
Bacteroides	Gram-negative anaerobic coccobacilli	Clindamycin	Metronidazole	Chloramphenicol
Blastomyces dermatitidis	Systemic fungi	Itraconazole	Amphotericin B followed by ketoconazole	Amphotericin B alone
Bordetella bronchiseptica	Gram-negative bacilli	Tetracycline	Chloramphenicol	Erythromycin
Borrelia burgdorferi	Tick-borne spirochete	Tetracycline	Ampicillin	Erythromycin
Brucella canis	Gram-negative coccobacilli	Minocycline + gentamicin	Tetracycline + dihydrostreptomycin	Repositol tetracycline + dihydrostreptomycin
Chlamydia psittaci	Obligate intracellular bacteria	Chlortetracycline ophthalmic ointment	Oxytetracycline ophthalmic ointment	Chloramphenicol ophthalmic ointment

Table continued on following page

6

893

Table 6–49. Antibacterial Therapy Against Specific Pathogens *Continued*

Organism	Agent	First Choice	Second Choice	Alternatives
Citrobacter	Gram-negative facultative anaerobe			
Clostridium spp. *Corynebacterium* *Ehrlichia*	Gram-positive large rods Gram-positive bacilli Obligate intracellular parasite in the family Rickettsiaceae	Penicillin G Erythromycin Doxycycline	Chloramphenicol Penicillin Tetracycline	Clindamycin Clindamycin Chloramphenicol
Enteric protozoa: *Giardia* *Entamoeba* *Balantidium* *Pentatrichomonas*	Protozoan parasites	Metronidazole	Tinidazole (dog only)	Furazolidone (cat only)
Enterobacter *Escherichia coli*	Gram-negative bacilli Gram-negative bacilli	Enrofloxacin Ampicillin (parenteral)	Aminoglycosides Enrofloxacin	Carbenicillin Trimethoprim-sulfonamide
Haemobartonella	Gram-negative non-acid-fast rickettsia	Tetracycline	Chloramphenicol	Thiacetarsamide (dog only)
Klebsiella	Gram-negative bacilli	Enrofloxacin	Aminoglycoside	Trimethoprim-sulfonamide Other aminoglycosides
Listeria monocytogenes	Gram-negative facultative anaerobe	Gentamicin + ampicillin	Trimethoprim-sulfonamide	Tetracycline
Leptospira spp.	Spirochete	Penicillin G + dihydrostreptomycin	Ampicillin (parenteral) + doxycycline	

894

Organism	Description			
Mycobacterium	Aerobic, non–spore-forming, nonmotile bacteria	Combination therapy for active infection: isoniazid-ethambutol-rifampin for 6–9 mo	Dihydrostreptomycin	Pyrazinamide
Mycoplasma spp.	Prokaryotes	Erythromycin (long-term therapy required)	Tetracycline (long-term therapy required)	Enrofloxacin
Nocardia	Gram-positive filamentous rods	Amikacin	Imipenem-cilastin	Sulfonamides*
Pasteurella	Gram-negative bacilli	Penicillin G	Ampicillin (parenteral)	Tetracycline
Proteus	Gram-negative bacilli	Ampicillin (parenteral)	Enrofloxacin	Gentamicin
Pseudomonas aeruginosa	Gram-negative bacilli	Enrofloxacin	Carbenicillin	Aminoglycoside
Rickettsia	Obligate intracellular parasite in the family Rickettsiaceae	Doxycycline	Tetracycline	Chloramphenicol
Salmonella spp.	Gram-negative bacilli	Enrofloxacin	Chloramphenicol	Trimethoprim-sulfonamide
Shigella spp.	Gram-negative bacilli	Ampicillin (parenteral)	Enrofloxacin	Chloramphenicol
Staphylococcus aureus	Gram-positive cocci	Oxacillin	Lincomycin	Trimethoprim-sulfonamide
Staphylococcus epidermidis	Gram-positive cocci	Oxacillin	Lincomycin	Trimethoprim-sulfonamide
Streptococcus spp.	Gram-positive cocci	Penicillin G or V	Cephalexin	Chloramphenicol
Streptomyces	Gram-positive filamentous rods	Penicillin G	Amoxicillin	Chloramphenicol
Yersinia pestis	Gram-negative facultative anaerobe, non–spore-forming, nonmotile coccobacillus	Gentamicin	Streptomycin	Chloramphenicol

*Sulfonamides have demonstrated good in vivo efficacy in the treatment of nocardiosis, despite the fact that they do *not* demonstrate in vitro activity.

6

Table 6–50. Antibiotic Sensitivity to Major Canine Urinary Bacteria

Agent	Escherichia coli	Staphylococci	Proteus mirabilis	Klebsiella pneumoniae	Pseudomonas aeruginosa	Streptococcus viridans	Streptococcus canis
Trimethoprim-sulfonamide	+*	+	+			+	+
Amoxicillin-clavulanate	+	+	+			+	+
Amoxicillin		+	+			+	+
Cephalexin	+	+	+	+			+
Enrofloxacin	+	+	+	+	+		+
Gentamicin	+	+	+	+	+†	+	+
Ampicillin		+				+	+
Chloramphenicol		+				+	+
Kanamycin		+					+

*More than 90% of strains susceptible (based on minimum inhibitory concentration [MIC] tests).
†Only 89% of strains susceptible (based on MIC tests).
Courtesy of Dr. G.V. Ling, University of California, Davis; from Urinary tract infections. *In* Managing Microbes. Smith Kline Beecham Animal Health and Veterinary Learning Systems, 1995, p 36.

Table 6–51. Dosage and Mean Urinary Concentration of Drugs Commonly Used to Treat Urinary Tract Infections

Agent	Dosage	Route	Concentration ($\pm$ SD) (μg/mL)	Minimum Inhibitory Concentration (μg/mL)
Penicillin G	16,665 units/lb, t.i.d.	PO	295 ($\pm$ 211)*	74*
Penicillin V	12 mg/lb, t.i.d.	PO	148 ($\pm$ 99)	37
Ampicillin	12 mg/lb, t.i.d.	PO	309 ($\pm$ 55)	77
Hetacillin	12 mg/lb, t.i.d.	PO	300 ($\pm$ 156)	75
Amoxicillin	5 mg/lb, t.i.d.	PO	202 ($\pm$ 93)	50
Tetracycline	8 mg/lb, t.i.d.	PO	138 ($\pm$ 65)	35
Chloramphenicol	15 mg/lb, t.i.d.	PO	124 ($\pm$ 40)	31
Cephalexin	15 mg/lb, t.i.d.	PO	500 (–)	125
Sulfisoxazole	10 mg/lb, t.i.d.	PO	1466 ($\pm$ 832)	366
Trimethoprim-sulfonamide	5 mg/lb, t.i.d.	PO	246 ($\pm$ 150)	62
	1 mg/lb, t.i.d.		55 ($\pm$ 19)	14
Kanamycin	2.5 mg/lb, t.i.d.	SC	530 ($\pm$ 151)	132
Gentamicin	1 mg/lb, t.i.d.	SC	107 ($\pm$ 33)	27
Amikacin	2.3 mg/lb, t.i.d.	SC	342 ($\pm$ 143)	85
	(10 mg/kg, b.i.d.)	(SC or IM)		
Tobramycin	1 mg/lb, t.i.d.	SC	145 ($\pm$ 86)*	36

*Units per milliliter.
Courtesy of Dr. G.V. Ling, University of California, Davis; from Urinary tract infections. *In* Managing Microbes, Smith Kline Beecham Animal Health and Veterinary Learning Systems, 1995, p 36.

6

Table 6–52. Systemic Antibiotics for Dogs with Staphylococcal Pyoderma

Antibiotic	Recommended Dosage*
Amoxicillin trihydrate–clavulanate potassium (Clavamox, Pfizer Animal Health)	14–22 mg/kg q12h
Cefadroxil (Cefa-Tabs, Cefa-Drops, Fort Dodge)	22 mg/kg q12h
Cephalexin (Generics [various])	22 mg/kg q12h
Cephradine (Generics [various])	22 mg/kg q12h
Clindamycin hydrochloride (Antirobe, Pharmacia & Upjohn)	5.5–11 mg/kg q12h
Enrofloxacin (Baytril, Bayer)	2.5–5.0 mg/kg q12h
Erythromycin (Stearate and estolate generics [various])	10–15 mg/kg q8h
Lincomycin hydrochloride (Lincocin, Pharmacia & Upjohn)	22 mg/kg q12h
Ormetoprim-sulfadimethoxine (Primor, Pfizer Animal Health)	55 mg/kg q24h, day 1 *then* 27.5 mg/kg q24h
Oxacillin	22 mg/kg q8h
Rifampin (Rifadin, Marion Merrell Dow; Rimactane, Novartis)	5–10 mg/kg q24h
Trimethoprim-sulfadiazine	20–30 mg/kg q12h
Trimethoprim-sulfamethoxazole	20–30 mg/kg q12h

*All antibiotics listed are given orally. Dosages from Kwochka KW: Recurrent pyoderma. *In* Griffin CE, Kwochka KW, MacDonald JM, eds: Current Veterinary Dermatology: The Science and Art of Therapy. St Louis, Mosby–Year Book, 1993, pp 3–21.

From Dermatologic infections. *In* Managing Microbes. Smith Kline Beecham Animal Health and Veterinary Learning Systems, 1995, p 25.

Table 6–53. Treatment Regimens for Bacterial Infections

Indications	Drug
Anaerobic infections (*Clostridium, Bacteroides, Fusobacterium*)	Amoxicillin-clavulanate (Clavamox, Pfizer Animal Health) Cefoxitin (Mefoxin, Merck) Chloramphenicol Clindamycin (Antirobe, Pharmacia & Upjohn) Metronidazole Penicillin
Actinomyces, Pasteurella, Streptococcus, or anaerobic bacteria	Penicillin Ampicillin Amoxicillin (Amoxi-Inject or Amoxi-Tabs, Pfizer Animal Health) Amoxicillin-clavulanate (Clavamox, Pfizer Animal Health)
Skin infections (*Staphylococcus intermedius*)	Amoxicillin + β-lactamase inhibitor (Clavamox, Pfizer Animal Health or Unasyn, Roerig) Cefadroxil (Cefa-Tabs, Fort Dodge) Cephalexin (Keflex, Dista) Cloxacillin Oxacillin
Bacterial prostatitis in dogs (*Proteus, Escherichia coli*)	Ormetoprim or trimethoprim *plus* Sulfonamides
Infections of the central nervous system	Cefotaxime (Claforan, Hoechst-Roussel) Ceftazidime (Ceptaz, Glaxo-Wellcome Pharmaceuticals) Trimethoprim-sulfonamides Penicillin antibiotics (e.g., sodium penicillin)
Intracellular infections	Tetracyclines Chloramphenicol Fluoroquinolones Azithromycin (Zithromax, Pfizer)
Urinary tract infections (*Escherichia coli, Staphylococcus* spp., *Proteus mirabilis, Enterococcus, Pseudomonas aeruginosa*)	Ampicillin Amoxicillin Amoxicillin-clavulanate (Clavamox, Pfizer Animal Health) Cephalexin (Keflex, Dista) Enrofloxacin (Baytril, Bayer) Tetracyclines (not doxycycline) Trimethoprim (various) combinations Ormetoprim-sulfonamide (Primor, Pfizer Animal Health) combinations

From Antiinfective therapy. *In* Managing Microbes. SmithKline Beecham Animal Health and Veterinary Learning Systems, 1995, p 10.

6

Table 6–54. Empirical Antibiotic Choices for Infections in Dogs and Cats*

Site of Infection	First Choice	Alternate Choice
Skin		
Superficial pyoderma	Amoxicillin-clavulanate	Trimethoprim/ormetoprim-sulfonamide
Soft tissue infection	Cephalexin/cefadroxil	Enrofloxacin
	Oxacillin/cloxacillin	Chloramphenicol
		Clindamycin/lincomycin
Urinary tract	Amoxicillin/ampicillin	Enrofloxacin
	Amoxicillin-clavulanate	Oxytetracycline
	Trimethoprim/ormetoprim-sulfonamide	
	Cephalexin/cefadroxil	
	Amoxicillin-clavulanate	
Respiratory tract	Doxycycline	Enrofloxacin
Pneumonia	Cephalexin/cefadroxil	Chloramphenicol
Bronchitis	Amoxicillin-clavulanate	Aminoglycosides
	Cephalexin/cefadroxil	Enrofloxacin
Bones	Cefazolin + amikacin/gentamicin	Clindamycin
Osteomyelitis		Enrofloxacin + clindamycin
Septicemia	Ampicillin sodium + amikacin/gentamicin	Enrofloxacin + ampicillin
		Third-generation cephalosporin

* The "first choice" is ordinarily the dose that has a high likelihood of success. If the first choice cannot be tolerated, or if there is resistance, the alternative choice should be considered.

From Antiinfective therapy. *In* Managing Microbes, SmithKline Beecham Animal Health and Veterinary Learning Systems, 1995, p 7.

Table 6–55. Antibiotic Dosage Reference Guide for Psittacines Based on Pharmacokinetic Studies

Drug	Form and Route	Avian Species in Which Pharmacokinetic Study Has Been Performed	Recommended Dose
Penicillins			
Procaine penicillin G +	IM	Turkey	100 mg/kg once daily
Benzathine penicillin G	IM		100 mg/kg once daily
Amoxicillin	IM	Pigeon	150 mg/kg q.i.d.
Ticarcillin	IM	Budgerigar	200 mg/kg t.i.d.
Piperacillin	IM	Blue-fronted Amazon	200 mg/kg t.i.d.
			100 mg/kg q.i.d.
Cephalosporins			
Cephalexin	PO		100 mg/kg t.i.d.
Cefotaxime	IM	Blue-fronted Amazon	100 mg/kg 3 to 6 times daily
Aminoglycosides			
Gentamicin	IM	Rose-breasted cockatoo	2.5 mg/kg b.i.d.
		Scarlet macaw	
Amikacin	IM	Blue-fronted Amazon	10–15 mg/kg b.i.d.
		Cockatiel	
		Goffin's cockatoo	
		Orange-winged Amazon	
		African grey parrot	
Macrolides and Lincosamides			
Clindamycin	PO	Pigeon	100 mg/kg once daily

Table continued on following page

6

901

Table 6–55. Antibiotic Dosage Reference Guide for Psittacines Based on Pharmacokinetic Studies *Continued*

Drug	Form and Route	Avian Species in Which Pharmacokinetic Study Has Been Performed	Recommended Dose
Tetracyclines			
Chlortetracycline	Medicated diets	Psittacines	0.25%–1.0% during 45 days
Doxycycline	IM (Vibramycin IV, Pfizer, Rotterdam, Netherlands)*	Psittacines	100 mg/kg once a week during 45 days
	Medicated diet	Amazons, cockatoos, African grey parrot	0.1% in diet (see text)
	Vibramycin hyclate IV (Roerig)	Psittacines	25 mg/kg
	PO	Psittacines	25 mg/kg b.i.d.
Quinolones			
Enrofloxacin	PO, IM	Amazons, African grey parrot, cockatoos	7.5–15 mg/kg b.i.d.
Chloramphenicol			
Chloramphenicol	IM	Budgerigar	50 mg/kg b.i.d.
		Macaw	50 mg/kg q.i.d.
		Sun conure	
		Nanday conure	
Potentiated Sulfonamides			
Trimethoprim + sulfamethoxazole	PO	Pigeon	50 mg/kg once daily
			25 mg/kg b.i.d.

* Not available in the United States.
Modified from Antimicrobial Therapy in Caged Birds and Exotic pets. International Symposium Hay Miles Inc. Animal Health Products and Veterinary Learning Systems, 1995, p 41.

Table 6–56. Recommended Dosages of Antimicrobial Drugs for Small Mammals

Drug	Species	Dosage, Frequency, Route	Comments
Ampicillin	Mouse	20–100 mg/kg in divided doses t.i.d., PO/SC	Do not use in hamsters, guinea pigs, rabbits, or chinchillas.
	Gerbil	20–100 mg/kg in divided doses t.i.d., PO/SC	
Cephalothin	Rabbit	12.5 mg/kg q.i.d. for 6 days	
Chloramphenicol palmitate	Mouse	50–200 mg/kg t.i.d. PO	Remember to warn clients to avoid contamination of skin, eyes, and gastrointestinal tract. Potential human toxicity.
	Gerbil	50–200 mg/kg t.i.d. PO	
	Hamster	50–200 mg/kg t.i.d. PO	
	Rat	50–200 mg/kg t.i.d. PO	
	Guinea pig	50 mg/kg b.i.d. PO	
	Chinchilla	50 mg/kg/b.i.d. PO	
	Rabbit	50 mg/kg b.i.d. PO	
	Ferret	50 mg/kg b.i.d. PO	
Chloramphenicol succinate	Mouse	30–50 mg/kg b.i.d. IM/SC	Remember to warn clients to avoid contamination of skin, eyes, and gastrointestinal tract. Potential human toxicity.
	Gerbil	30–50 mg/kg b.i.d. IM/SC	
	Hamster	30–50 mg/kg b.i.d. IM/SC	
	Rat	30–50 mg/kg b.i.d. IM/SC	
	Guinea pig	30–50 mg/kg b.i.d. IM/SC	
	Chinchilla	30–50 mg/kg b.i.d. IM/SC	
	Rabbit	30–50 mg/kg b.i.d. IM/SC	
	Ferret	30–50 mg/kg b.i.d. IM/SC	
Enrofloxacin	Mouse	2.5–5.0 mg/kg b.i.d. IM/SC/PO	Not to be used in rapidly growing young animals due to potential erosion of joint cartilage.
	Gerbil	2.5–5.0 mg/kg b.i.d. IM/SC/PO	
	Hamster	2.5–5.0 mg/kg b.i.d. IM/SC/PO	
	Rat	2.5–5.0 mg/kg b.i.d. IM/SC/PO	
	Guinea pig	2.5–5.0 mg/kg b.i.d. IM/SC/PO	
	Chinchilla	2.5–5.0 mg/kg b.i.d. IM/SC/PO	
	Rabbit	5 mg/kg b.i.d. IM/SC/PO	
	Ferret	3–5 mg/kg b.i.d. IM/SC/PO	

Table continued on following page

6

Table 6–56. Recommended Dosages of Antimicrobial Drugs for Small Mammals *Continued*

Drug	Species	Dosage, Frequency, Route	Comments
Gentamicin	Mouse	5 mg/kg once daily IM/SC	Potentially nephrotoxic and ototoxic. Keep animals hydrated.
	Gerbil	5 mg/kg once daily IM/SC	
	Hamster	5 mg/kg once daily IM/SC	
	Rat	5 mg/kg once daily IM/SC	
	Guinea pig	5 mg/kg once daily IM/SC	
	Chinchilla	5 mg/kg once daily IM/SC	
	Rabbit	4 mg/kg once daily IM/SC	
	Ferret	5 mg/kg once daily IM/SC	
Metronidazole	Mouse	2.5 mg/mL of water for 5 days	The addition of sucrose helps reduce the aftertaste.
	Gerbil	7.5 mg/70–90 g of body weight t.i.d. PO	
	Hamster	7.5 mg/70–90 g of body weight t.i.d. PO	
	Rat	10–40 mg/rat once daily PO	
	Guinea pig	10–40 mg/kg once daily PO	
	Chinchilla	10–40 mg/kg once daily PO	
	Rabbit	40 mg/kg once daily PO for 3 days	
	Ferret	50 mg/kg once daily PO	
Neomycin	Mouse	50 mg/kg once daily SC	Nephrotoxicity and ototoxicity may occur. Neuromuscular blockade possible.
	Gerbil	100 mg/kg once daily SC	
	Hamster	100 mg/kg once daily PO	
	Rat	50 mg/kg once daily PO	
	Guinea pig	8 mg/kg once daily PO	
	Chinchilla	15 mg/kg once daily PO	
	Rabbit	30 mg/kg b.i.d. PO	
	Ferret	10 mg/kg q.i.d. PO	
Oxytetracycline	Mouse	10–20 mg/kg b.i.d. PO; 0.4 mg/mL water	Tooth discoloration in neonatal animals. Renal disease is common in geriatric animals.
	Gerbil	10 mg/kg t.i.d. PO; 0.8 mg/mL water	
	Hamster	16 mg/kg once daily SC; 0.25–1.0 mg/mL water	
	Rat		
	Guinea pig	10–20 mg/kg t.i.d. PO; 0.4 mg/mL water	

Drug	Animal	Dosage	Comments
Sulfadimethoxine	Chinchilla	50 mg/kg b.i.d. PO; 1 mg/mL water	
	Rabbit	50 mg/kg b.i.d. PO; 1 mg/mL water	
	Ferret	50 mg/kg b.i.d. PO; 1 mg/mL water; 20 mg/kg t.i.d. PO	
	Ferret	30–50 mg/kg once or twice daily PO	Animals must remain hydrated to prevent nephrotoxicosis. Renal disease is common in geriatric animals.
Sulfamerazine	Mouse	1 mg/kg of feed or 0.02% water	Animals must remain hydrated to prevent nephrotoxicosis. Renal disease is common in geriatric animals.
	Rat	1 mg/4 g of feed or 0.02% water	
Sulfamethazine	Mouse	1 mg/mL water	Animals must remain hydrated to prevent nephrotoxicosis. Renal disease is common in geriatric animals.
	Gerbil	1 mg/mL water	
	Hamster	1 mg/mL water	
	Rat	1 mg/mL water	
	Guinea pig	1 mg/mL water	
	Chinchilla	1 mg/mL water	
	Rabbit	1 mg/mL water or 5–10 g/kg of feed	
	Ferret	1 mg/mL water	
Sulfaquinoxaline	Mouse	1 mg/mL water	Animals must remain hydrated to prevent nephrotoxicosis. Renal disease is common in geriatric animals.
	Gerbil	1 mg/mL water	
	Hamster	1 mg/mL water	
	Rat	0.025%–0.1% water or 0.05% of diet	
	Guinea pig	1 mg/mL water	
	Chinchilla	1 mg/mL water	
	Rabbit	1 mg/mL water or 0.6 g/kg of feed	
Tetracycline	Mouse	10–20 mg/kg b.i.d./t.i.d. PO; 2–5 mg/mL water	Tooth discoloration in neonatal animals. Renal disease is common in geriatric animals.
	Gerbil	10–20 mg/kg b.i.d./t.i.d. PO; 2–5 mg/mL water	
	Rat	10–20 mg/kg b.i.d./t.i.d. PO; 2–5 mg/mL water	
	Guinea pig	10–20 mg/kg b.i.d./t.i.d. PO; 0.7 mg/mL water	
	Chinchilla	50 mg/kg b.i.d./t.i.d. PO; 0.3–2.0 mg/mL water	
	Rabbit	50 mg/kg b.i.d./t.i.d. PO; 0.7 mg/mL water	
	Ferret	20 mg/kg t.i.d. PO	

Table continued on following page

6

Table 6-56. Recommended Dosages of Antimicrobial Drugs for Small Mammals *Continued*

Drug	Species	Dosage, Frequency, Route	Comments
Trimethoprim-sulfadiazine, Trimethoprim-sulfamethoxazole	Mouse	30 mg/kg b.i.d. SC/PO	Animals must remain hydrated to prevent nephrotoxicosis. Renal disease is common in geriatric animals.
	Gerbil	30 mg/kg b.i.d. SC/PO	
	Hamster	30 mg/kg b.i.d. SC/PO	
	Rat	30 mg/kg b.i.d. SC/PO	
	Guinea pig	30 mg/kg b.i.d. SC/PO	
	Chinchilla	30 mg/kg b.i.d. SC/PO	
	Rabbit	30 mg/kg b.i.d. SC/PO	
	Ferret	30 mg/kg b.i.d. SC/PO	
Tylosin	Mouse	10 mg/kg once daily IM/SC/PO; 500 mg/L water	
	Gerbil	10 mg/kg once daily IM/SC/PO; 500 mg/L water	
	Hamster	2–8 mg/kg b.i.d. IM/SC/PO; 500 mg/L water	
	Rat	10 mg/kg once daily IM/SC/PO; 500 mg/L water	
	Guinea pig	10 mg/kg once daily IM/SC/PO	
	Chinchilla	10 mg/kg once daily IM/SC/PO	
	Rabbit	10 mg/kg once daily IM/SC/PO	
	Ferret	10 mg/kg t.i.d. PO; 5–10 mg/kg b.i.d., IV/IM	

Modified from Antimicrobial Therapy in Caged Birds and Exotic Pets. International Symposium. Miles Inc. Animal Health Products and Veterinary Learning Systems, 1995, pp 5–6.

....

IMMUNIZATION PROCEDURES
See Tables 6–57 through 6–60.

Table 6–57. Rabies Control Guidelines—1999 Compendium of
Animal Rabies Control

A. Principles of rabies control
  1. Rabies exposure. Rabies is transmitted only when the virus is introduced into bite wounds, open cuts in skin, or onto mucous membranes.
  2. Human rabies prevention. Rabies in humans can be prevented either by eliminating exposures to rabid animals or by providing exposed persons with prompt local treatment of wounds combined with appropriate passive and active immunization. The rationale for recommending preexposure and postexposure rabies prophylaxis and details of their administration can be found in the current recommendations of the Immunization Practices Advisory Committee (ACIP), of the Public Health Service (PHS). These recommendations, along with information concerning the current local and regional status of animals rabies and the availability of human rabies biologics, are available from state health departments.
  3. Domestic animals. Local governments should initiate and maintain effective programs to ensure vaccination of all dogs, cats, and ferrets and to remove strays and unwanted animals. Such procedures in the United States have reduced laboratory-confirmed cases in dogs from 6949 in 1947 to 126 in 1997. Since more rabies cases are reported annually involving cats (300 in 1997) than dogs, vaccination of cats should be required. The recommended vaccination procedures and the licensed animal vaccines are specified in Parts I and II of the Compendium.
  4. Rabies in wildlife. The control of rabies among wildlife reservoirs is difficult. Vaccination of free-ranging wildlife or selective population reduction may be useful in some situations, but the success of such procedures depends on the circumstances surrounding each rabies outbreak.
B. Control methods in domestic and confined animals
  1. Preexposure vaccination and management. Parenteral animal rabies vaccines should be administered only by, or under the direct supervision of, a veterinarian. This is the only way to ensure that a responsible person can be held accountable to assure the public that the animal has been properly vaccinated. Within 1 month after primary vaccination, a peak rabies antibody titer is reached and the animal can be considered immunized. An animal is currently vaccinated and is considered immunized if it was vaccinated at least 30 days previously, and all vaccinations have been administered in accordance with this Compendium. Regardless of the age at initial vaccination, a second vaccination should be given 1 year later. (See Parts I and II for recommended vaccines and procedures.)
    a. Dogs, cats, and ferrets. All dogs, cats and ferrets should be vaccinated against rabies at 3 months of age and revaccinated in accordance with Part II of this Compendium. If a previously vaccinated animal is overdue for a booster, it should be revaccinated with a single dose of vaccine and placed on an annual or triennial schedule depending on the type of vaccine used.

Table continued on following page

6

Table 6–57. Rabies Control Guidelines—1999 Compendium of
Animal Rabies Control *Continued*

    b. Livestock. It is neither economically feasible nor justified from a
       public health standpoint to vaccinate all livestock against rabies.
       However, consideration should be given to vaccination of livestock
       that are particularly valuable or may have frequent contact with
       humans.

    c. Other animals
      i. Wild. No parenteral rabies vaccine is licensed for use in wild
        animals. Because of the risk of rabies in wild animals (especially
        raccoons, skunks, coyotes, foxes, and bats), the AVMA, the
        NASPHV, and the CSTE strongly recommend the enactment of
        state laws prohibiting the importation, distribution, relocation,
        or keeping of wild animals or hybrids as pets.
      ii. Maintained in exhibits and in zoological parks. Captive animals
        not completely excluded from all contact with rabies vectors can
        become infected. Moreover, wild animals may be incubating
        rabies when initially captured; therefore, wild-caught animals
        susceptible to rabies should be quarantined for a minimum of
        180 days before exhibition. Employees who work with animals at
        such facilities should receive preexposure rabies immunization.
        The use of pre- or postexposure rabies immunizations of
        employees who work with animals at such facilities may reduce
        the need for euthanasia of captive animals.

2. Stray animals. Stray dogs, cats, or ferrets should be removed from the
  community. Local health departments and animal control officials can
  enforce the removal of strays more effectively if owned animals are
  confined or kept on leash. Strays should be impounded for at least 3
  days to give owners sufficient time to reclaim animals and to determine
  if human exposure has occurred.

3. Importation and interstate movement of animals
    a. International. The Centers for Disease Control and Prevention
       (CDC) regulates the importation of dogs and cats into the United
       States, but present PHS regulations (42 CFR No. 71.51) governing
       the importation of such animals are insufficient to prevent the
       introduction of rabid animals into the country. All dogs and cats
       imported from countries with endemic rabies should be currently
       vaccinated against rabies as recommended in this Compendium. The
       appropriate public health official of the state of destination should
       be notified within 72 hours of any unvaccinated dog or cat imported
       into his or her jurisdiction. The conditional admission of such
       animals into the United State is subject to state and local laws
       governing rabies. Failure to comply with these requirements should
       be promptly reported to the Division of Quarantine, CDC, 404-639-
       8107.
    b. Interstate. Prior to interstate movement, dogs, cats, and ferrets
       should be currently vaccinated against rabies in accordance with the
       Compendium's recommendations (Part III, B.1. Preexposure
       Vaccination and Management). Animals in transit should be
       accompanied by a currently valid NASPHV Form #51, Rabies
       Vaccination Certificate.

4. Adjunct procedures. Methods or procedures that enhance rabies control
  include:
    a. Licensure. Registration or licensure of all dogs, cats, and ferrets may
       be used to aid in rabies control. A fee is frequently charged for such
       licensure, and revenues collected are used to maintain rabies or animal
       control programs. Vaccination is an essential prerequisite to licensure.

Table 6–57. Rabies Control Guidelines—1999 Compendium of
Animal Rabies Control *Continued*

  b. Canvassing of area. House-to-house canvassing by animal control
    personnel facilitates enforcement of vaccination and licensure
    requirements.
  c. Citations. Citations are legal summonses issued to owners for
    violations, including the failure to vaccinate or license their animals.
    The authority for officers to issue citations should be an integral
    part of each animal control program.
  d. Animal control. All communities should incorporate stray animal
    control, leash laws, and training of personnel in their programs.
 5. Postexposure management. Any animal potentially exposed to rabies
  virus (Part III, A.1. Rabies Exposure) by a wild, carnivorous mammal
  or a bat that is not available for testing should be regarded as having
  been exposed to rabies.
  a. Dogs, cats, and ferrets. Unvaccinated dogs, cats, and ferrets exposed
    to a rabid animal should be euthanized immediately. If the owner is
    unwilling to have this done, the animal should be placed in strict
    isolation for 6 months and vaccinated 1 month before being released.
    Animals with expired vaccinations need to be evaluated on a case-
    by-case basis. Dogs, cats, and ferrets that are currently vaccinated
    should be revaccinated immediately kept under the owner's control,
    and observed for 45 days.
  b. Livestock. All species of livestock are susceptible to rabies; cattle
    and horses are among the most frequently infected. Livestock
    exposed to a rabid animal and currently vaccinated with a vaccine
    approved by the U.S. Department of Agriculture (USDA) for that
    species should be revaccinated immediately and observed for 45
    days. Unvaccinated livestock should be slaughtered immediately. If
    the owner is unwilling to have this done, the animal should be kept
    under very close observation for 6 months.
    The following are recommendations for owners of unvaccinated
    livestock exposed to rabid animals.
   i. If the animal is slaughtered within 7 days of being bitten, its
     tissues may be eaten without risk of infection, provided liberal
     portions of the exposed area are discarded.Federal meat
     inspectors must reject for slaughter any animal known to have
     been exposed to rabies within 8 months.
   ii. Neither tissues nor milk from a rabid animal should be used for
     human or animal consumption. However, since pasteurization
     temperatures will inactivate rabies virus, drinking pasteurized
     milk or eating cooked meat does not constitute a rabies
     exposure.
   iii. It is rare to have more than one rabid animal in a herd, or
     herbivore-to-herbivore transmission; therefore, it may not be
     necessary to restrict the rest of the herd if a single animal has
     been exposed to or infected by rabies.
  c. Other animals. Other animals bitten by a rabid animal should be
    euthanized immediately. Animals maintained in USDA-licensed
    research facilities or accredited zoological parks should be evaluated
    on a case-by-case basis.

Table continued on following page

6

Table 6–57. Rabies Control Guidelines—1999 Compendium of Animal Rabies Control *Continued*

6. Management of animals that bite humans. A healthy dog, cat, or ferret that bites a person should be confined and observed for 10 days; it is recommended that rabies vaccine not be administered during the observation period. Such animals should be evaluated by a veterinarian at the first sign of illness during confinement. Any illness in the animal should be reported immediately to the local health department. If signs suggestive of rabies develop, the animal should be euthanized, its head removed, and the head shipped under refrigeration (not frozen) for examination of the brain by a qualified laboratory designated by the local or state health department. Any stray or unwanted dog, cat, or ferret that bites a person may be euthanized immediately and the head submitted as described above for rabies examination. Other biting animals that might have exposed a person to rabies should be reported immediately to the local health department. Prior vaccination of an animal may not preclude the necessity for euthanasia and testing if the period of virus shedding is unknown for that species. Management of animals other than dogs, cats, and ferrets depends on the species, the circumstances of the bite, the epidemiology of rabies in the area, and the biting animal's history, current health status, and potential for exposure to rabies.

C. Control methods in wildlife. The public should be warned not to handle wildlife. Wild mammals and hybrids that bite or otherwise expose people, pets, or livestock should be considered for euthanasia and rabies examination. A person bitten by any wild mammal should immediately report the incident to a physician who can evaluate the need for antirabies treatment. (See current rabies prophylaxis recommendations of the ACIP.)

1. Terrestrial mammals. The use of licensed oral vaccines for the mass immunization of free-ranging wildlife should be considered in selected situations, with the approval of the state agency responsible for animal rabies control. Continuous and persistent government-funded programs for trapping or poisoning wildlife are not cost effective in reducing wildlife rabies reservoirs on a statewide basis. However limited control in high-contact areas (picnic grounds, camps, suburban areas) may be indicated for the removal of selected high-risk species of wildlife. The state wildlife agency and state health department should be consulted for coordination of any proposed vaccination or population reduction programs.

2. Bats
   a. Indigenous rabid bats have been reported from every state except Hawaii, and have caused rabies in at least 32 humans in the United States. It is neither feasible not desirable, however, to control rabies in bats by programs to reduce bat populations.
   b. Bats should be excluded from houses and adjacent structures to prevent direct association with humans. Such structures should then be made bat-proof by sealing entrances used by bats.

Modified from Compendium of Animal Rabies Control, 1999. J Am Vet Med Assoc 214:202–202, 1999.

Table 6–58. 1999 Canine Vaccination Guidelines*

Antigen	Primary Vaccination (Puppy)	Primary Vaccination (Adult)	Booster	Recommendation
Canine distemper virus (MLV)	2–3–4 mo of age	1 dose	Annually	*Highly recommended.* Duration of immunity (DOI) for rCDV has not been established beyond 1 yr; adult dogs challenged 30 mo following MLV vaccination were protected.
Canine distemper virus (rCDV) (recombinant)	2–3–4 mo of age	2 doses, 3–4 wk apart	Annually	*Highly recommended.* May be used interchangeably with MLV-CDV vaccine. Level of protection conferred by the recombinant CDV vaccine is comparable to that provided by MLV vaccines. DOI is at least 12 mo.
Distemper-measles (D-M; MLV) Administer *IM* only	One dose between 6 and 12 wk of age only (one MLV-CDV or rCDV vaccine follows D-M at 14 to 16 wk of age)	Not indicated for use in dogs over 12 wk of age	Not recommended	*Optional – not recommended for routine use.* Intended to provide *temporary* protection in young dogs only. Indicated for use in households/kennels where distemper is a recognized problem. *Do not administer to female dogs >12 wk of age.*
Canine adenovirus-1 (CAV-1) (MLV)	2 doses every 3–4 wk until 12 wk of age	2 doses, 3–4 wk apart	Annually	*Not recommended.* Infectious canine hepatitis is uncommon in the United States. Considering the low (to absent) prevalence, the risk of "hepatitis blue-eye" reactions, and the fact that CAV-2 will cross-protect against CAV-1, vaccines containing this antigen are *not* recommended for use in routine vaccination protocols.

Table continued on following page

6

911

Table 6–58. 1999 Canine Vaccination Guidelines* *Continued*

Antigen	Primary Vaccination (Puppy)	Primary Vaccination (Adult)	Booster	Recommendation
Canine adenovirus-2 (CAV-2) (MLV or killed)	2–3–4 mo of age	1 dose (if using MLV) 2 doses, 3–4 wk apart (if using killed vaccine)	Annually	*Recommended.* Demonstrated cross-protection against canine hepatitis (CAV-1) and CAV-2, one of the agents known to be associated with infectious tracheobronchitis (ITB). Usually combined with CDV and CAV vaccine. Currently this product is not available as a monovalent vaccine.
Parainfluenza virus (CPiV) (MLV)	2–3–4 mo of age	1 dose	Annually	*Recommended.* Usually combined with CDV and CAV vaccine. Currently this product is not available as a monovalent vaccine.
Bordetella bronchiseptica (killed bacterin)	6–8 wk of age, then 10–12 wk of age	2 doses, 2–4 wk apart	Annually	*Optional.* The parenteral vaccine may be less efficacious than the topical *B. bronchiseptica* plus parainfluenza virus vaccines in their ability to stimulate a local immune response (upper respiratory tract).
B. bronchiseptica (live avirulent bacterin) + parainfluenza virus (MLV) TOPICAL (intranasal) USE ONLY	Administer a single dose as early as 2 WEEKS OF AGE. (See product literature for specific age recommendations)	Not stipulated, although a single dose is recommended	Annually and/or 1 wk prior to possible exposure	*Recommended* for dogs housed in kennels, shelters, pounds; prior to boarding in kennels. Transient (3–10 days) coughing, sneezing, or nasal discharge occurs in a small percentage of vaccinates. Antimicrobial therapy may be indicated (doxycycline, 5–7 days) to manage postvaccination upper respiratory signs (persistent cough and nasal discharge).

Vaccine	Initial vaccination	Booster	Revaccination	Comments
B. bronchiseptica (live avirulent bacterin) + parainfluenza virus (MLV) + canine adenovirus-2 (MLV) *TOPICAL (intranasal) USE ONLY*	Administer a single dose at NOT LESS THAN 8 WEEKS OF AGE	A single dose is recommended	Annually	*Note:* Topically administered vaccines for canine infectious tracheobronchitis may provide a superior local immune response compared to parenterally administered vaccines. *Recommended* for dogs considered to be at risk of exposure to any of the pathogens listed. *Note:* Topically administered vaccines for canine ITB may provide a superior local immune response compared to parenterally administered vaccines.
Canine parvovirus (MLV)	2–3–4 mo of age	1 dose	Annually	*Highly recommended.* Although annual boosters are recommended by vaccine manufacturers, studies have shown protection against challenge 2 yr post vaccination with MLV vaccine. It has been suggested that adult dogs vaccinated against parvovirus with MLV vaccine will remain immune for at least 3 yr post vaccination. *Recommended.* A suitable alternative to the MLV canine parvovirus vaccine; advantages of the killed virus product, as claimed by the manufacturer, include: (1) no postvaccination shedding; (2) no vaccination reactions; (3) may be given to pregnant bitches.
Canine parvovirus (killed)	2–3–4 mo of age	2 doses, 3–4 wk apart	Annually	

Table continued on following page

6

Table 6–58. 1999 Canine Vaccination Guidelines* Continued

Antigen	Primary Vaccination (Puppy)	Primary Vaccination (Adult)	Booster	Recommendation
Canine parvovirus (killed)				HOWEVER, killed parvovirus products are susceptible to maternal antibody interference in puppies as old as 16 wk (or older?).
				Although annual boosters are recommended by vaccine manufacturers, studies have shown protection against challenge 16 mo post vaccination with killed vaccine.
Borrelia burgdorferi or Lyme disease (killed bacterin)	Initial dose may be given at 12 wk of age and a required second dose 3–4 wk later	2 doses, 3–4 wk apart	Annually	*Optional.* Lyme disease has limited regional prevalence. Recommendation for use is limited to dogs with a known high risk of exposure, particularly dogs living in the northeastern United States and the upper Midwest (Wisconsin, Michigan) or perhaps those traveling to endemic areas when the risk of tick exposure is considered to be high.
B. burgdorferi; also, rLyme disease (recombinant)	Initial dose may be given at 9 wk of age and a required second dose 2–3 wk later	2 doses, 2–3 wk apart	Annually	*Optional.* Lyme disease has limited regional prevalence. Recommendation for use is strictly limited to dogs with a known high risk of exposure, particularly dogs living in the northeastern United States and the upper Midwest (Wisconsin, Michigan) or perhaps those traveling to endemic areas when the risk of tick exposure is considered to be high.

Vaccine	Initial vaccination	Number of doses	Revaccination	Comments
Canine coronavirus (killed and MLV)	Every 2–4 wk of age until 12 wk of age (MLV) Begin as early as 6 wk of age: every 2–3 wk with the final dose at 12 wk of age (killed vaccine)	1 dose (if using MLV) 2 doses, 2–3 wk apart (if using killed vaccine)	Annually	*Optional.* Prevalence of clinical cases of confirmed canine coronavirus infection does not justify routine inoculation of all dogs. Clinical infections are most likely to occur in puppies <6 wk of age. Clinical signs are mild and typically resolve spontaneously.
Leptospira (*L. canicola* combined with *L. icterohaemorrhagiae*) (killed bacterin)	12 and 16 wk; do not administer to dogs <12 wk of age	2 doses, 2–4 wk apart	Annually; some authors recommend a booster every 6 mo. in dogs considered to be at *significant* risk of exposure	*Optional.* Anecdotal reports from veterinarians and breeders suggest that the incidence of postvaccination reactions (acute anaphylaxis) in puppies (<12 wk of age) and small-breed dogs is high.
Giardia (killed)	Initial dose may be given at 8 wk of age; a second dose should be given 2–3 wk later	2 doses, 2–3 wk apart	Annually	*Optional.* The value of using this vaccine on a routine basis has not been established. Although giardiasis is the most common intestinal parasite among people in the United States, the source of human infection is contaminated water. Infections in dogs and cats are not likely to be zoonotic.

Table continued on following page

6

915

Table 6–58. 1999 Canine Vaccination Guidelines* *Continued*

Antigen	Primary Vaccination (Puppy)	Primary Vaccination (Adult)	Booster	Recommendation
Rabies *1-year* (killed) or ROUTE OF ADMINISTRA-TION MAY *NOT* BE OPTIONAL—see product literature for details	Administer 1 dose as early as 3 mo of age	Administer a single dose	The *1-year* rabies vaccine may be used as a booster vaccine when dogs are required to be vaccinated annually against rabies; local statues apply	*Required.* MLV vaccines are not available; state and local statutes govern the frequency of administration of products labeled as "1-year rabies." *Note:* The rabies (1-yr) vaccine is generally administered as the initial dose followed, 1 yr later, by administration of the rabies (3-yr) vaccine. State and local statutes may dictate otherwise.
rRabies *1-year* (recombinant)	Administer 1 dose as early as 3 mo of age	Administer a single dose	The *1-year* rabies vaccine may be used as a booster vaccine when dogs are required to be vaccinated annually against rabies; local statues apply	*Required.* State and local statutes govern the frequency of administration of products labeled as "1-year rabies." The *recombinant* rabies approved for dogs can be used an alternative vaccine to the 1-yr killed virus vaccine (above). The recombinant product does not contain an adjuvant. *Note:* The rabies (1-yr) vaccine is generally administered as the initial dose followed, 1 yr later, by administration of the rabies (3-yr) vaccine. State and local statutes may dictate otherwise.

Rabies 3-year (killed) ROUTE OF ADMINISTRATION MAY *NOT* BE OPTIONAL—see product literature for details				
Note: In selected situations, the 3-yr rabies vaccine may be used as an alternative to the 1-yr rabies vaccine for initial and subsequent doses; local statutes apply Administer 1 dose as early as 3 mo of age	*Note: In selected situations, the 3-yr rabies vaccine may be used as an alternative to the 1-yr rabies vaccine for initial and subsequent doses; local statutes apply* Administer a single dose	The *second* rabies vaccination is recommended 1-yr following administration of the initial dose regardless of the animal's age at the time the first dose is administered Depending on local statutes, booster vaccines should be administered annually or every 3 yr	*Required.* State and local statutes govern the frequency of administration for products labeled as rabies (3 yr). These statutes vary throughout the United States. *Note:* The rabies (1-yr) vaccine is generally administered as the initial dose followed, 1 yr later, by administration of the rabies (3-yr) vaccine. State and local statutes may dictate otherwise.	

6

* Route of administration is SC or IM unless otherwise noted by the manufacturer.
Note: Letter designation "r" preceding the name of the antigen indicates a recombinant vaccine.

Table 6–59. 1999 Feline Vaccination Guidelines*

Antigen	Primary Vaccination (Kitten)	Primary Vaccination (Adult—Over 6 Months of Age)	Booster	Comment
Panleukopenia (parenteral MLV, killed, OR topical [intranasal/intraocular] MLV) Note: The topical panleukopenia vaccine is combined with FHV-1 and FCV (see below)	9 and 12 wk of age; repeat a single dose in 12 mo	1 dose (if using MLV) 2 doses, 3–4 wk apart (if using killed)	Every 3 yr	*Highly recommended.* In most cats, protection derived following administration of panleukopenia vaccines at 12 wk of age is considered to persist for at least 3 yr and has been shown to persist for up to 6 yr based on titer.
Feline herpesvirus-1 (FHV-1) and feline calicivirus (FCV) (combined parenteral product: MLV or killed)	9 and 12 wk of age; repeat a single dose 12 mo later	1 dose (if using MLV) 2 doses, 3–4 wk apart (if using killed)	Annually to every 3 yr depending on risk of exposure	*Highly recommended* (see also the topical vaccine below). The degree of local immunity derived from parenterally administered vaccines is minimal to absent, although a sustained serologic response is obtained. Recent challenge data support booster intervals of up to 3 yr in cats considered to be at low risk of exposure.

Vaccine	Initial dose schedule		Revaccination	Comments
FHV-1 with FCV (combined product: MLV only) *TOPICAL (intranasal/intraocular) USE ONLY*	9 and 12 wk of age when risk of exposure is low; or in high-risk environments, beginning as early as 3 wk of age, then every 3 wk until 12 wk old; repeat a single dose 12 mo later	1 dose	Annually to every 3 yr depending on risk of exposure	*Highly recommended.* Recommended over the parenteral products in households with a definable risk of exposure to cats with viral respiratory infection, especially cats living in multiple cat households. *Note:* Maternal antibody does NOT appear to interfere with local immune responses occurring within the upper respiratory tract.
Chlamydia psittaci (bacterin) (*Note:* both avirulent live and killed products are available)	9 and 12 wk of age	2 doses, 3–4 wk apart	Annually	*Not recommended for routine use.* Use of this vaccine should be limited to those households/catteries in which *C. psittaci* infection has been confirmed or in which the risk of exposure is deemed to be high (e.g., multiple cat households with high rates of kitten/cat turnover).

Table continued on following page

6

Table 6–59. 1999 Feline Vaccination Guidelines* *Continued*

Antigen	Primary Vaccination (Kitten)	Primary Vaccination (Adult—Over 6 Months of Age)	Booster	Comment
Feline leukemia virus (killed)	9 and 12 wk of age	2 doses, 3–4 wk apart	Annually	*Recommended* for any cat, especially kittens, NOT restricted to a closed, indoor environment. *Optional* for adult cats that only occasionally go outside and adult cats that are strict indoor pets and have no exposure to other cats. *Note:* FeLV (and FIV in cats >6 mo of age) testing by enzyme-linked immunosorbent assay (ELISA), is appropriate prior to initial vaccination. FIV antibody tests (ELISA) are NOT reliable in cats <6 mo of age because of potential false-positive test results associated with maternally derived FIV antibody.
Feline infectious peritonitis (FIP) (MLV) *FOR TOPICAL (intranasal) USE ONLY*	2 doses, 3–4 wk apart *beginning* at 16 wk of age	2 doses, 3–4 wk apart	Annually	*Optional–not recommended for routine use.* There is no consensus among veterinarians on a routine FIP vaccination protocol.

Vaccine	Age/approval	Primary dose	Revaccination	Comments
Microsporum canis (inactivated whole dermatophyte) *Administer SC*	Not approved for use in cats <4 mo of age	1st dose is administered SC to cats that are at least 4 mo of age; 2nd dose is administered SC 12–16 days following the 1st dose; 3rd dose is administered SC 26–30 days following the 2nd dose	Not stipulated	*Optional – not recommended for routine use.* At this time, only one *M. canis* vaccine is available; the product is approved for both "prevention and treatment of clinical signs of disease caused by *Microsporum canis*." *Note:* Although skin lesions in cats with active *M. canis* infection do resolve subsequent to vaccination, spores affixed to the hair of infected cats may not be eliminated. The manufacturer emphasizes the fact that *M. canis* vaccination is only one part of a comprehensive program to control ringworm.
Feline *Bordetella bronchiseptica* (avirulent live bactrin) *FOR TOPICAL (intranasal) USE ONLY*	Administer 1 dose as early as 8 wk of age.	1 dose	Annually; in endemic environments, the manufacturer recommends vaccinating twice yearly or at least 72 hr prior to a "stressful situation in which the risk of exposure exists"	*Optional – not recommended for routine use.* Recommended for use in households with a definable risk of exposure to cats with viral respiratory infection, especially cats living in multiple cat households. This vaccine is NOT the same as the *canine B. bronchiseptica* vaccine; therefore the feline and canine products should NOT be interchanged. Total dose is 0.2 mL. Demonstrated onset of immunity is 72 hr post vaccination. The duration of immunity (DOI) has not been established for this product, but is under study at this writing.

Table continued on following page

6

Table 6–59. 1999 Feline Vaccination Guidelines* Continued

Antigen	Primary Vaccination (Kitten)	Primary Vaccination (Adult—Over 6 Months of Age)	Booster	Comment
Rabies (*1-year vaccine*) ROUTE OF ADMINISTRATION MAY NOT BE OPTIONAL—see product literature for details.	Administer 1st dose as early as 3 mo of age	Administer a single dose	The *1-year* rabies vaccine may be used as a booster vaccine when cats are required to be vaccinated annually against rabies; local statutes apply	*Highly recommended for all cats—required by law in some states and municipalities.* MLV vaccines are not available. State and local statutes govern the frequency of administration for products labeled as rabies (1-yr).
Note: Vaccination of cats against Rabies is NOT required by all states; local statutes apply				*Note:* The rabies (1-year) vaccine is generally administered as the initial dose followed, 1 yr later, by administration of the rabies (3-year) vaccine. State and local statutes may dictate otherwise.
rRabies (*1-year recombinant vaccine*)	Administer 1st dose as early as 3 mo of age	Administer a single dose	The *1-year* rabies vaccine may be used as a booster vaccine when cats are required to be vaccinated annually against rabies; local statutes apply	*Highly recommended for all cats—required by law in some states and municipalities.* MLV vaccines are not available. State and local statutes govern the frequency of administration for products labeled as rabies (1-yr).
Note: Vaccination of cats against rabies is NOT required by all states; local statutes apply				The *recombinant* rabies vaccine approved for cats can be used as an alternative vaccine to the 1-yr killed virus vaccine (above). The recombinant product does not contain an adjuvant.

Rabies (3-year vaccine) ROUTE OF ADMINISTRATION MAY NOT BE OPTIONAL—see product literature for details. *Note:* Vaccination of cats against rabies is NOT required by all states; local statutes apply	*Note: In selected situations, the 3-yr rabies vaccine may be substituted for the 1-yr rabies vaccine for initial and subsequent doses; local statutes apply* Administer 1 dose as early as 3 mo of age	*Note: In selected situations, the 3-yr rabies vaccine may be substituted for the 1-yr rabies vaccine for initial and subsequent doses; local statutes apply* Administer a single dose	The *second* rabies vaccination is recommended 1-yr following administration of the initial dose regardless of the animal's age at the time the first dose is administered Depending on local statutes, booster vaccines should be administered annually or every 3 yr	*Highly recommended—required by law in some states and municipalities.* State and local statutes govern the frequency of administration for products labeled as rabies (3-yr). These statutes vary considerably throughout the United States. *Note:* The rabies (1-yr) vaccine is generally administered as the initial dose followed, 1 yr later, by administration of the rabies (3-yr) vaccine. State and local statutes may dictate otherwise.

* Route of administration is SC or IM unless otherwise noted by the manufacturer.
Note: Letter designation "r" preceding the name of the antigen indicates a recombinant vaccine.

6

Table 6–60. Species Susceptibilities of Nondomestic Carnivores*

Species	Feline Panleukopenia	Canine Distemper	Canine Infectious Hepatitis	Feline Rhinotracheitis	Feline Calicivirus	Canine Parvovirus	Rabies
Canidae (coyote, fox, jackal, wolf, dingo)	−	+	+	−	−	+	+
Felidae (tiger, leopard, lion, cheetah, lynx, ocelot, margay, golden cat, mountain lion)	+	±	−	+	+	−	+
Procyonidae (raccoon, coatimundi, kinkajou, lesser panda)	+	+	±	−	−	−	+
Mustelidae (ferret, mink, otter, skunk, weasel, marten, sable, fisher)	+	+	±	−	−	−	+
Viverridae (mongoose, civet)	+	+	±	−	−	−	+
Ursidae (bear)	−	−	+	−	−	−	+
Hyaenidae (hyena)	±	+	−	−	−	−	+

+, susceptible; −, not susceptible; ±, susceptibility controversial.

* Private ownership of wild animal species as pets is strongly discouraged. State and local statutes determine which nondomestic species, if any, can be kept as pets or vaccinated. Contact your local zoo or American Association of Zoo Veterinarians diplomate before vaccinating any nondomestic species.

Modified from Phillips LG: Preventive medicine in nondomestic carnivores. *In* Kirk RW, ed: Current Veterinary Therapy X. Philadelphia, WB Saunders, 1989, p 729.

ONCOLOGY

BASIC PRINCIPLES

1. Once a definitive diagnosis has been established, early therapeutic intervention is best. As a general rule, the first treatment is the most effective one.
2. A sound therapeutic plan based on knowledge of the tumor type and including whatever treatment modalities are appropriate is imperative. This plan should be presented to the owner *before* any of it is undertaken. The piecemeal addition of therapies of no benefit to either the patient or owner.
3. *Consultation with or referral to an oncologist is warranted in the management of oncology cases and especially infrequently encountered and complex cases.*

EVALUATION OF THE CANCER PATIENT

1. Cancer diagnosis rests on an evaluation of cells. Fine-needle aspiration cytology and incisional or excisional biopsy of various types should provide material appropriate for diagnosis. (See also p. 496.)
   a. The primary utility of fine-needle aspiration cytology is to differentiate inflammatory from neoplastic conditions. Nonetheless, neoplasms may at least be identified as carcinomas or sarcomas; definitive diagnosis of discrete cell tumors is usually possible (although in most cases, there is still additional valuable information to be gained from histopathology).
   b. Histopathologic evaluation of biopsy material definitively diagnoses malignancy. On the basis of pathologic description and knowledge of the biologic behavior of the tumor, the clinician is best able to advise owners about options for therapy and prognosis.
2. The owner's role in the process of evaluation and subsequent decision making cannot be overestimated.
   a. Cancer is a disease seen most often, but not exclusively, in middle-aged and old animals. These animals have usually been in the home a long time, and there are often very strong emotional bonds between owner and pet. In addition, a diagnosis of cancer carries with it a great emotional burden for many owners. These factors cannot be ignored at any step in the process of providing the proper workup and care for a cancer patient.
   b. These animals may have concurrent diseases that have an impact on both the diagnosis and management of the case.
3. A minimum database should be established for each problem defined. Not only may the information gained help define the extent of the disease or disclose concurrent problems, it will also help the clinician assess potential areas of concern in light of proposed therapies.
   a. Minimum databases are problem-specific. Depending on the particular organ system involved or the tumor type, special tests may be indicated, but in every cancer patient for whom therapy is contemplated a complete blood count, including platelet evaluation; a profile biochemical screen, including electrolytes; and urinalysis are warranted.
      i. For some patients, bone marrow aspiration cytology or biopsy is indicated to assess both the impact of the disease and the ability to withstand therapy.
      ii. Other patients may require additional hematologic or cytologic tests.
   b. Radiographs of the affected part are beneficial in assessing the presence of neoplastic disease but do not themselves confirm a diagnosis of cancer.
      i. To evaluate the presence of pulmonary metastases, thoracic radiographs (two lateral views, a ventrodorsal view) should be made for all

patients with solid tumors and are also helpful in evaluating those with hematopoietic neoplasia.

ii. Abdominal radiographs, ultrasonographic imaging, and computed tomography (CT) may contribute meaningful information.

4. Clinical staging is the process of information gathering that leads to an assessment of the extent of the disease. The World Health Organization has defined a system based on evaluation of the primary site, lymph nodes, and distant metastases: the TNM system. This system, unfortunately, has not been extremely successful in providing prognostic guidelines, but it does provide a useful shorthand for descriptive purposes.

a. In general, the greater the tumor burden and the more clinically affected the patient, the poorer the prognosis for response and prolonged survival.

·········· TREATMENT

1. Psychological and emotional issues of treatment are often very tricky. Almost everyone has some experience with cancer patients, either human or animal. Unfortunately, much of this experience is bad. Protocols for animal patient are usually less aggressive than those for people and, therefore, better tolerated.

a. Owners are usually unsure of what course to take and the clinician's input—optimistic or pessimistic—can strongly influence the course. If the clinician is uncertain about the impact of therapy on either the disease or the quality of life of the patient, owners are less likely to undertake treatment.

b. Pessimistic clinician attitudes may deny a patient useful therapy and an extend happy comfortable life. Consultation with an oncologist will ensure an informed opinion.

2. The three widely accepted modalities of cancer therapy are surgery, radiotherapy, and chemotherapy. Biologic response modification (immuno-therapy), hyperthermia, and photodynamic therapy have been useful in some situations, but they must by and large still be considered investigational. Also of growing interest in the management of cancer patients is the use of alternative or nonconventional therapies. These remedies are unproven but probably innocuous. Their use in lieu of approaches more scientifically evaluated in terms of outcome could, however, prevent patients from receiving known effective therapy.

a. Surgery is the oldest means of treating cancer and the one most likely to rid the patient of the largest part of its tumor quickly. However, surgery is a local therapy and does not address the problem of disseminated disease.

b. Radiotherapy is a useful method of treatment for some cancers. Again, treatment is effective against localized disease but does not deal with widespread disease.

i. Radiotherapy is effective in the adjuvant setting for many soft tissue sarcomas and selected mast cell tumors. Radiotherapy is also useful in the primary setting for brain tumors and nasal malignancies.

ii. Palliative treatment is useful for pain management in osteosarcoma and selected spinal malignancies.

c. Chemotherapy is most effective against very small tumor burdens in most cases and is therefore useful as an adjunct to surgery or radiotherapy. Chemotherapy is intended to have systemic effect against small residual deposits and micrometastatic disease.

i. Chemotherapy is limited by the ability of the patient to tolerate the effects of cytotoxic drugs, not by the ability of these drugs to kill neoplastic cells.

ii. Chemotherapeutic drugs are not tumor cell–specific and will affect normal cells as well as cancer cells. Although protocols for animal patients are designed to be minimally toxic, *the clinician must be prepared to assess and manage chemotoxicity of various organ systems.* Table 6–61 provides a summary of pertinent clinical information for selected chemotherapeutic agents. It is not intended as the sole guide to the use of these drugs.

   iii. Anticancer drugs are powerful cytotoxic chemicals, and all aspects of their storage, preparation, administration, and disposal warrant prudent and informed care (see Tables 6–62, 6–63, and 6–64).

3. Multimodality approaches bring to bear the best aspects of surgery, radiotherapy, and chemotherapy. This philosophy allows each modality to attack the disease in its most effective manner.

Table 6–61. Pertinent Clinical Information for Selected Chemotherapeutic Agents

	Brand Name/ (Manufacturer/ Formulation)	Possible Indications	Suggested Dosages	Potential Toxicity
Alkylating Agents				
Cyclophosphamide	Cytoxan (Mead Johnson/ 25- and 50-mg tablets, 100- and 200-mg vials for injection)	Lymphoreticular neoplasms, mammary and lung carcinomas, miscellaneous sarcomas	50 mg/m² PO or IV 4 days/wk, or 200 mg/m² IV weekly	Leukopenia, anemia, thrombocytopenia (less common), nausea, vomiting, sterile hemorrhagic cystitis
Chlorambucil	Leukeran (Burroughs Wellcome/2-mg tablets)	Lymphoreticular neoplasms, chronic lymphocytic leukemia	2 mg/m² PO 2–4 days/wk	Mild leukopenia, thrombocytopenia, anemia, nausea, vomiting (not common)
Nitrogen mustard	Mustargen (Merck Sharp & Dohme/10-mg vial for injection)	Lymphoreticular neoplasms	5 mg/m² IV; cautious topical application (10 mg/50 mL water)	Leukopenia, thrombocytopenia, nausea, vomiting, anrexia, contact dermatitis
Melphalan	Alkeran (Burroughs Wellcome/2-mg tablets)	Multiple myeloma, monoclonal gammopathies, neoplams	1.5 mg/m² PO for 7–10 days; repeat cycle	Leukopenia, thrombocytopenia, anemia, anorexia, vomiting
Dacarbazine	DTIC (Miles/Dome Laboratories/100- and 200-mg vials for injection)	Malignant melanoma, various sarcomas	850–1000 mg/m² IV every 3–4 wk	Leukopenia, thrombocytopenia, anemia, nausea, vomiting, diarrhea
Busulfan	Myleran (Burroughs Wellcome/2 mg tablets)	Chronic myelogenous leukemia, polycythermia vera	2 mg/m² PO q24h	Leukopenia, thrombocytopenia

Antimetabolites

Methotrexate	Methotrexate (Lederle and others/2.5-mg tablets, 50-mg vials for injection)	Lymphoreticular neoplasms, myeloproliferative disorders, various carcinomas and sarcomas	Many possible schedules—2.5 mg/m² PO, 15–25 mg/m² IV (10–15 mg/m² for cats)	Leukopenia, thrombocytopenia, anemia, stomatitis, diarrhea, hepatopathy, renal tubular necrosis
6-Mercaptopurine	Purinethol (Burroughs Wellcome/50-mg tablets)	Lymphoreticular neoplasms, acute lymphocytic and granulocytic leukemia	50 mg/m² PO daily until response or toxicity noted, then as needed	Leukopenia, nausea, vomiting, hepatopathy
6-Thioguanine	Thioguanine (Burroughs Wellcome/40-mg tablets)	Acute lymphocytic and granulocytic leukemia	40 mg/m² PO daily × 4–5 days; 20 mg/m² PO daily × 1–5 days for cats	Leukopenia, thrombocytopenia (potentially severe in cats), anemia, nausea, hepatopathy
5-Fluorouracil	Fluorouracil (Roche Laboratories and others/500-mg vial for injection), Efudex Ceram (Roche)	Various carcinomas and sarcomas	150 mg/m² IV weekly; DO NOT USE IN CATS	Leukopenia (usually mild), thrombocytopenia, neurologic signs, anemia, gastrointestinal upset
Cytosine arabinoside	Cytosar-U (Upjohn and others/100- and 500-mg vials for injection)	Lymphoreticular neoplasms and myeloproliferative disorders	100 mg/m² SC or IV drip × 4 days (2 days for cats)	Leukopenia, thrombocytopenia, anemia, anorexia, nausea, vomiting
Antibiotics				
Doxorubicin	Adriamycin (Adria Laboratories and others/10- and 50-mg vials)	Lymphoreticular neoplasms, osteosaroma, various carcinomas and sarcomas	30 mg/m² IV every 3 wk (20–25 mg/m² IV in cats); *caution—highly vesicant if administered perivascularly!*	Leukopenia, thrombocytopenia, nausea, anorexia, vomiting, cardiomyopathy, allergic reactions during administration

Table continued on following page

929

Table 6-61. Pertinent Clinical Information for Selected Chemotherapeutic Agents *Continued*

	Brand Name/ (Manufacturer/ Formulation)	Possible Indications	Suggested Dosages	Potential Toxicity
Actinomycin D	Cosmegen (Merck Sharp & Dohme/0.5-mg vial)	Lymphoreticular neoplasms, various carcinomas and sarcomas	0.75–1.0 mg/m² IV every 2–3 wk; *caution—highly vesicant if administered perivascularly!*	Leukopenia, gastrointestinal upset
Mitoxantrone	Novantrone (Lederle/ 20-, 25-, and 30-mg vials for injection)	Lymphoreticular neoplasms, squamous cell carcinoma, various carcinomas and sarcomas	5 mg/m² IV every 3 wk	Leukopenia, anorexia, gastrointestinal upset
Bleomycin	Blenoxane (Bristol Myers/15-unit vials for injection)	Squamous cell carcinoma, lymphoreticular neoplams, various carcinomas	10 units/m² IV or SC daily × 3–9 days, then weekly; maximum cumulative dose 200 units/m²	Allergic reactions after administration, pulmonary fibrosis
Alkylating Agents Vincristine	Oncovin (Lilly and others/1- and 2-mg vials for injection)	Lymphoreticular neoplasms, various carcinomas and sarcomas, transmissible venereal tumor	0.5–0.75 mg/m² IV weekly; *caution—highly vesicant if administered perivascularly!*	Peripheral neuropathy, constipation, leukopenia (at higher doses)
Vinblastine	Velban (Lilly and others/ 10-mg vials for injection)	Lymphoreticular neoplasms, some carcinomas	2 mg/m² IV weekly; *caution—highly vesicant if administered perivascularly!*	Leukopenia, nausea, vomiting

Hormones				
Prednisolone Prednisone	Many suppliers and strengths available	Lymphoreticular neoplasms, mast cell tumors, central nervous system neoplasms	Vary widely depending on indications: 20–60 mg/m² q24–48h	Signs of corticosteroid excess, secondary adrenal insufficiency
Diethylstilbestrol	Diethylstilbestrol (Lilly/ 1-mg tablets)	Perianal gland adenoma, prostatic neoplasms (adjunctively)	1 mg PO q72h	Feminization, irreversible bone marrow toxicity; NOT ROUTINELY RECOMMENDED
Miscellaneous				
L-Asparaginase	Elspar (Merck Sharp & Dohme/10,000-IU vial)	Lymphoreticular neoplasms	10,000–20,000 IU/m² IM weekly	Anaphylaxis, pancreatitis, coagulopathies, hepatopathy
o,p′-DDD	Lysodren (Bristol Myers/ 500-mg tablets)	Adrenocortical tumors	25 mg/kg PO q12h to effect, then 25 mg/kg PO every 7–14 days as needed	Adrenocortical insufficiency
Hydroxyurea	Hydrea (Immunex/500-mg capsules)	Chronic granulocytic leukemia, polycythemia vera	50 mg/kg PO until effective or toxic, then as needed to maintain effect	Leukopenia, anemia, thrombocytopenia, altered nail growth
Cisplatin	Platinol (Bristol Myers/ 10- and 50-mg vials for injection)	Osteosarcoma, various carcinomas	60–70 mg/m² IV every 3–5 wk; brisk saline diuresis required before treatment; DO NOT USE IN CATS	Nausea, vomiting, renal insufficiency, myelosuppression
Carboplatin	Paraplatin (Bristol Myers/50-mg, 150-mg, and 450-mg vials for injection)	Osteosarcoma, various carcinomas	Dogs: 300 mg/m² IV every 3 wk; cats: 200 mg/m² every 3–4 wk as WBC count allows	Leukopenia (many cats are still leukopenic at 3 wk)
Piroxicam	Feldene (Pfizer and others/1- and 20-mg capsules)	Transitional cell carcinoma, possibly nasal and oral neoplasms	0.3 mg/kg PO q24h	Nephrotoxicity, gastrointestinal irritation or ulceration

6

Table 6–62. Guidelines to Treatment Modalities for Selected
Neoplastic Diseases

Carcinomas

1. Mammary carcinoma, canine (wide variety of histopathologies)
   S: Very beneficial, may be curative
   R: N/A
   C: Not fully evaluated; not proven beneficial but reasonable in theory for
      some
   O: N/A
2. Mammary carcinoma, feline
   S: Radical mastectomy increases disease-free interval but not survival
   R: N/A
   C: Not fully evaluated; reasonable in theory and may be beneficial
   O: N/A
3. Squamous cell carcinoma, oral
   S: Wide excision beneficial, not as feasible with tonsillar involvement
   R: Potentially useful adjunct to surgery
   C: Potentially useful but yet unproven adjunct to surgery
   O: N/A
4. Squamous cell carcinoma, nail bed
   S: Amputation
   R: Potentially beneficial
   C: N/A, limited likelihood of measurable impact
   O: N/A
5. Perianal adenocarcinoma
   S: Reduces tumor burden, palliates signs
   R: Potentially useful adjunct
   C: Useful adjunct in theory, true benefit unproven
   O: N/A
6. Anal sac adenocarcinoma
   S: Reduces tumor burden, palliates signs
   R: Potentially useful adjunct
   C: Useful adjunct in theory; true benefit unproven
   O: N/A
7. Nasal carcinoma (including squamous cell)
   S: May diminish survival due to postoperative complications
   R: Beneficial and prolongs median survival time
   C: N/A
   O: Photodynamic therapy may be helpful
8. Thyroid carcinoma
   S: Beneficial but often very difficult (invasive and vascular tumor)
   R: ^{131}I potentially helpful; requires long isolation; limited availability
   C: Adjuvant or neoadjuvant potentially beneficial; not fully proven
   O: N/A
9. Prostatic carcinoma
   S: Beneficial with early diagnosis (not usually the case)
   R: Not proven beneficial
   C: Potentially useful adjunct in theory; precise protocols not defined
   O: N/A
10. Renal carcinoma
    S: Beneficial in unilateral disease
    R: N/A
    C: Adjunctive role not evaluated
    O: N/A

Table 6–62. Guidelines to Treatment Modalities for Selected Neoplastic Diseases *Continued*

11. Pulmonary carcinoma
    S: Beneficial for limited disease
    R: N/A
    C: Potentially useful adjunct in theory; precise protocols not evaluated
    O: N/A
12. Gastric and intestinal carcinoma
    S: Beneficial in early, limited disease
    R: N/A
    C: N/A
    O: N/A

Sarcomas

1. Fibrosarcoma, canine
   S: Beneficial but local recurrence likely
   R: May be a useful adjunct but response difficult to predict
   C: N/A
   O: Biologic response modification has not been shown to be helpful
2. Fibrosarcoma, feline vaccine–associated
   S: Wide surgical excision
   R: Useful adjunct to surgery
   C: Doxorubicin (best with surgery and radiotherapy)
   O: Biologic response modification has not been shown to be helpful
3. Hemangiosarcoma, spleen
   S: May be palliative but postoperative survival time is usually short
   R: N/A
   C: Doxorubicin-cyclophosphamide useful adjunct to surgery
   O: N/A
4. Hemangiosarcoma, cutaneous
   S: Wide excision may be beneficial; survival times usually considered better than splenic
   R: N/A
   C: May be beneficial surgical adjunct with aggressive disease
   O: N/A
5. Osteosarcoma, extremity
   S: Palliative but does not increase survival as single modality
   R: May be palliative without impact on survival
   C: Cisplatin useful adjunct to amputation (median survival 12 + mo)
   O: Liposome-encapsulated muramyl tripeptide effective (not generally available)
6. Osteosarcoma, skull
   S: Often difficult due to location
   R: N/A
   C: Not fully evaluated as primary therpay
   O: N/A
7. Hemangiopericytoma
   S: Beneficial; local recurrence likely, may require amputation
   R: May be beneficial as adjunct to surgery; best after first surgery
   C: N/A
   O: N/A

Table continued on following page

6

Table 6–62. Guidelines to Treatment Modalities for Selected Neoplastic Diseases *Continued*

8. Melanoma, oral
   S: Wide excision beneficial, especially with small lesions
   R: Response unpredictable
   C: N/A, generally not very beneficial to date; still under evaluation
   O: *Corynebacterium parvum* shown effective with surgery; other biologic response modification?
9. Melanoma, cutaneous
   S: Wide surgical excision beneficial
   R: N/A
   C: N/A
   O: N/A
10. Liposarcoma
    S: May be difficult to excise completely; expect local recurrence
    R: N/A
    C: N/A
    O: N/A
11. Leiomyosarcoma
    S: Beneficial, depending on ability to excise completely
    R: N/A
    C: N/A
    O: N/A

Discrete Cell Tumors

1. Lymphoma, dogs
   S: N/A
   R: Half-body radiotherapy not effective; may be useful with chemotherapy
   C: Very responsive to combinations of drugs; median survival approaches 12 mo
   O: N/A
2. Lymphoma, cats
   S: N/A
   R: Thoracic radiotherapy may palliate signs of effusion, decrease mediastinal mass
   C: Effective for some; does not affect feline leukemia virus status
   O: N/A
3. Mast cell tumors, dogs
   S: Appropriate alone for solitary lesions, well-differentiated disease
   R: Useful adjunct, prolongs disease-free interval and survival times
   C: Low response rates for prednisone or vincristine as single agents; combined vinblastine-cyclophosamide-prednisone may be beneficial as an adjunct to surgery in the absence of radiotherapy
   O: N/A
4. Mast cell tumors, cats
   S: Useful for splenic disease, not needed for most cutaneous presentations
   R: N/A
   C: Corticosteroid benefit questionable
   O: N/A

Table 6–62. Guidelines to Treatment Modalities for Selected
Neoplastic Diseases *Continued*

5. Transmissible venereal tumor
   S: May be palliative depending on site and clinical indication; usually
   not necessary
   R: Responsive to radiation; usually not necessary
   C: Beneficial effects of vincristine are well recognized, usually curative
   O: N/A
6. Histiocytoma
   S: Can be curative but often not necessary
   R: N/A
   C: N/A
   O: N/A

S, surgery; R, radiotherapy; C, chemotherapy; O, other treatment modalities; N/A,
not applicable.

Table 6–63. Conversion of Body Weight in Kilograms to Body Surface Area
in Meters Squared for Dogs

kg	m²	kg	m²
0.50	0.06	26.00	0.88
1.00	0.10	27.00	0.90
2.00	0.15	28.00	0.92
3.00	0.20	29.00	0.94
4.00	0.25	30.00	0.96
5.00	0.29	31.00	0.99
6.00	0.33	32.00	1.01
7.00	0.36	33.00	1.03
8.00	0.40	34.00	1.05
9.00	0.43	35.00	1.07
10.00	0.46	36.00	1.09
11.00	0.49	37.00	1.11
12.00	0.52	38.00	1.13
13.00	0.55	39.00	1.15
14.00	0.58	40.00	1.17
15.00	0.60	41.00	1.19
16.00	0.63	42.00	1.21
17.00	0.66	43.00	1.23
18.00	0.69	44.00	1.25
19.00	0.71	45.00	1.26
20.00	0.74	46.00	1.28
21.00	0.76	47.00	1.30
22.00	0.78	48.00	1.32
23.00	0.81	49.00	1.34
24.00	0.83	50.00	1.36
25.00	0.85		

Table 6–64. Conversion of Body Weight in Kilograms to Body Surface Area in Meters Squared for Cats

kg	m²
0.50	0.06
1.00	0.10
1.50	0.12
2.00	0.15
2.50	0.17
3.00	0.20
3.50	0.22
4.00	0.24
4.50	0.26
5.00	0.28
5.50	0.29
6.00	0.31
6.50	0.33
7.00	0.34
7.50	0.36
8.00	0.38
8.50	0.39
9.00	0.41
9.50	0.42
10.00	0.44

ANESTHETIC DRUGS AND DOSAGES
See Tables 6–65 through 6–67.

Table 6–65. Recommended Dosages of Anesthetic Drugs*

	Dosage (mg/kg)	
Agent	Dog	Cat
Premedication		
Anticholinergics		
Atropine sulfate	0.02–0.04	Same
Glycopyrrolate	0.01–0.02	Same
Ataractics		
Major		
Acepromazine	0.1–0.2	Same
Promazine	0.6–1.0	1.0–3.0
Chlorpromazine	0.2–0.4	Same
Droperidol	0.2–1.0	0.2–1.0
Minor		
Diazepam	0.1 IV	0.1 IV
Midazolam	0.06–0.1 IV, IM	0.06–0.1 IV, IM
Sedative		
Xylazine	0.4–1.0	0.4–1.0
Medetomidine	10 μg/kg IV	40 μg/kg IV
	40 μg/kg IM	80 μg/kg IM
Pentobarbital	1–3	—

Table 6–65. Recommended Dosages of Anesthetic Drugs* *Continued*

Agent	Dosage (mg/kg)	
	Dog	Cat
Narcotic agonists		
Morphine	0.4–1.5	0.1
Oxymorphone	0.11–0.22	0.04–0.22
Meperidine	2–6	2–4
Pentazocine	1–2	Same
Fentanyl	0.02–0.04	—
Butorphanol	0.4	0.4
Dissociative		
Ketamine	6–10 (use with ataractic)	4–20
Neuroleptanalgesics		
Fentanyl-droperidol		
(Innovar-Vet)	1 mL/10–30 kg IM	—
Acepromazine	0.1	0.05–0.1
Oxymorphone	0.1–0.2	0.02–0.2
Acepromazine	0.1	0.1
Meperidine	2–6	2–6
Diazepam	0.1 IV	0.1 IV
Oxymorphone	0.1–0.2	0.02–0.2
Combination		
Ketamine	5–10	Same
Acepromazine	0.1–0.2	Same
Ketamine	5–10	Same
Diazepam	0.1–0.25 IV	Same
Ketamine†	5–10	Same
Xylazine†	0.4–1.0	Same
Fentanyl-droperidol	1 mL/20 kg	—
Narcotic neuromuscular blocking agent	See individual dose schedules	
Induction		
Sedative-hypnotics		
Thiamylal	12–18	Same
Thiopental	12–18	Same
Methohexital	10–12	—
Pentobarbital	20–25	Same
Propofol (Dog)	4.8 mg/kg IV	Same
Neuroleptanalgesics		
Fentanyl/droperidol	1 mL/10–30 kg	Same
Oxymorphone	0.2	0.2
Acepromazine	0.1	0.1
Oxymorphone	0.2	0.1–0.2
Diazepam	0.2–0.5	0.1–0.2
Meperidine	4–6	4–6
Acepromazine	0.1	0.1
Dissociative		
Ketamine¶	10 IV	10–20 IM
		10 IV

Table continued on following page

Table 6–65. Recommended Dosages of Anesthetic Drugs* *Continued*

Agent	Dosage (mg/kg)	
	Dog	Cat
Maintenance		
Inhalation Agents‡	MAC‡§ value (vol/%)	
Methoxyflurane	0.23	Same
Halothane	0.87	1.19
Enflurane	2.2	2.37
Isoflurane	1.5	1.61
Sevoflurane	2.4	2.6
Desflurane	7.2	9.8
Nitrous oxide	188	150

* All by intramuscular (IM) route unless noted.

† *This combination may cause a high incidence of serious heart block.*

‡ Induction "dose" of 2.5–3.0 × MAC is used for all agents except N_2O. The maintenance level of 1.5–2.0 × MAC is usually satisfactory. Nitrous oxide is mixed with oxygen in a 1:1 to 2:1 ratio and may decrease levels required of other inhalation agents.

¶ Must administer with diazepam, midazolam, or acepromazine.

§ MAC is the minimum alveolar concentration of anesthetic at 1 atm that produces immobility in 50% of the animals exposed to a noxious stimulus.

Table courtesy of Dr. Mark Raffe, Professor of Anesthesiology, University of Minnesota, Minneapolis.

Table 6-66. Important Characteristics of Common Neuromuscular Blocking Agents

Generic Name	Trade Name	Manufacturer	Mode of Action	Dose, Initial (mg/kg)/ Repeat	Metabolism and Excretion		Cardiovascular Effects	Time of Onset	Duration of Effect
					Major	Minor			
Succinylcholine chloride	Anectine	Glaxo Wellcome, Research Triangle Pk., N.C.	Depolarizing	0.1–0.4/100 mg in 500 D5W*	Plasma	—	Some blood pressure ↑ due to ganglionic stimulation	0.75 min	20–30 min—dog 3–5 min—cat
Gallamine triethiodide	Flaxedil	Davis & Geck American Cyanamid, Pearl River, N.Y.	Nondepolarizing	1.0–2.0/0.1	Renal	—	Marked increase in heart rate; mild increase in blood pressure	1.5–2.0 min	30 min
Pancuronium bromide	Pavulon	Organon, West Orange, N.J.	Nondepolarizing	0.06–0.10/0.01	Renal	Liver	Slight ↑ heart rate due to vagal block	0.75–1.0 min	45–60 min
Tubocurarine chloride	Tubocurarine	Abbott Labs, North Chicago	Nondepolarizing	0.2–0.4/0.05	Renal	Liver	Slight heart rate ↑; hypotension from histamine release	2.0–4.0 min	60–90 min

Table continued on following page

6

939

Table 6-66. Important Characteristics of Common Neuromuscular Blocking Agents *Continued*

Generic Name	Trade Name	Manufacturer	Mode of Action	Dose, Initial (mg/kg)/ Repeat	Metabolism and Excretion		Cardiovascular Effects	Time of Onset	Duration of Effect
					Major	Minor			
Dimethyltubocurarine	Metubine iodide	Eli Lilly, Indianapolis	Nondepolarizing	0.2–0.4/ 0.1–0.1	Renal	Liver	Some blood pressure changes due to ganglionic blocking ↓; slight increase in heart rate	1.5–2.0 min	30–45 min
Atracurium besylate	Tracrium	Burroughs Wellcome, Research Triangle Pk, N.C.	Nondepolarizing	0.2–0.4/0.2	Plasma cholinesterase	Metabolism	Slight decrease in blood pressure	1.5–3.0 min	30–45 min
Vecuronium bromide (ORG NC 45)	Norcuron	Organon	Nondepolarizing	0.05/0.05	Liver	Kidney	—	1.5–4.0 min	30–45 min

* Start with minidrip set (60 drops = 1 mL), and begin rate at 0.003 to 0.01 mg/kg/min = 1–3 drops/kg/min.

Table 6–67. Anesthetic Reversal

Agent	Dosage (mg/kg)
Narcotic antagonists	
Naloxone	0.1–0.2 IV
Levallorphan	0.2–1.0 IV
Nalbuphine	0.1–0.2 IM or IV
Arousal agents	
Doxapram	0.5–1.0 IV
Yohimbine	0.1–0.2

ADVERSE DRUG REACTIONS
See Tables 6–68 and 6–69.

6

Table 6–68. Adverse Drug Reactions Reported in Dogs

Drug	Clinical Signs and Lesions
Analgesics	
Aspirin	Bleeding disorders
Meclofenamic acid–corticosteroids	Diarrhea, gastrointestinal bleeding, death
Phenylbutazone	Anemia, leukopenia, thrombocytopenia, emesis, hemorrhagic enteritis, epistaxis, elevated liver enzymes, death
CNS Depressants	
Acetylpromazine	Atypical behavior, aggression, apprehension, lameness of injected leg, prolonged effect, respiratory distress, bradycardia, pallor, seizures, syncope, weak irregular pulse, urination, defecation
Butorphanol	Sedation, ataxia, salivation, gasping, crying, emesis, depression, anorexia, respiratory and cardiac arrest, anaphylaxis, cyanosis, death
Fentanyl-droperidol	Behavior change, lameness, ataxia, hyperthermia, aggression, seizures, bradycardia, tachycardia, hyperpnea, apnea, tremors, hyperventilation, hyperexcitability, hyperkinesia, nystagmus, cardiac arrest, prolonged recovery, death
Ethylisobutrazine	Hyperexcitability
Halothane	Cardiac arrhythmia, malignant hyperthermia, nystagmus, torticollis, emesis
Ketamine	Convulsions, cyanosis
Lidocaine	Laryngeal and facial edema, respiratory arrest, seizures, ataxia, tremors
Methoxyflurane	Cardiac arrest, hepatitis after 2 wk, death
Oxymorphone	Bradycardia
Prochlorperazine-isopropamide	Tachycardia
Promazine	Depression, hypotension, hyperthermia, death
Thiamylal	Cardiac arrest, respiratory arrest, prolonged anesthesia, cyanosis, apnea, cardiac arrhythmias, bradycardia, temporary hearing loss, prolonged recovery, death
Thiopental	Cardiac arrest, prolonged recovery, pulmonary edema, slough at injection site, death
Xylazine	Viciousness, bradycardia, cardiac arrest, death

Anticonvulsants	
Phenytoin	Ataxia, hepatotoxicity, leukopenia, emesis, coma, death
Primidone	Liver failure, icterus, emesis, alopecia, polydipsia, polyuria, death
Antiparasitics	
Arecoline-tetrachlorethylene	Mydriasis, ataxia, emesis, diarrhea, severe colic, inability to walk, depression, hypothermia
Bunamidine	Dyspnea, ataxia, emesis, weakness, bloat, gastroenteritis, lung hemorrhage, seizures, sudden death
Butamisole	Dyspnea, ataxia, muscle tremors, collapse, coma, depression, icterus, swelling at injection site, abscess formation, death
n-Butyl chloride	Stupor, ataxia, death
Dichlorophene-toluene	Incoordination, convulsions, emesis, disorientation, mydriasis, lethargy, anorexia, fever, death
Dichlorvos	Diarrhea, emesis, ataxia, tremors, weakness, death
Diethylcarbamazine	Pruritus, weakness, emesis, diarrhea, icterus, anaphylactoid reaction, death
Diethylcarbamazine-styrylpyridinium	Diarrhea, emesis, sterilization, teratogenesis, death
Disophenol	Hyperthermia, hyperventilation, ataxia, collapse, dyspnea, respiratory distress, swelling at injection site, death
Dithiazazine iodide	Emesis, diarrhea, depression, apprehension, hyperpyrexia, anorexia, lethargy, death
Glycobiarsol	Emesis
Levamisole	Dyspnea, pulmonary edema, emesis
Mebendazole	Icterus, emesis, anorexia, diarrhea, lethargy, abnormal liver function tests, hepatotoxicity, death
Piperazine	Paralysis, death
Metronidazole	Lethargy, rearlimb weakness
Phthalofyne	Hepatitis, splenitis, ataxia, death
Praziquantel	Irritation at injection site, weakness, bradycardia, seizures, emesis, ataxia
Pyrantel pamoate	Emesis
Ronnel	Emesis, twitching, depression
Thenium closylate	Emesis, diarrhea, enteritis, anaphylaxis, hemorrhagic enteritis and liver, seizures, dyspnea, cyanosis, death

Table continued on following page

6

943

Table 6-68. Adverse Drug Reactions Reported in Dogs *Continued*

Drug	Clinical Signs and Lesions
Thiacetarsamide	Emesis, icterus, bilirubinuria, elevated liver enzymes, depression, anorexia, cough, renal failure, swelling at injection site, alopecia, dermatitis, bleeding disorders, death
Toluene	Collapse
Trichlorfon	Anorexia, weakness, lethargy
Uredofos	Emesis, diarrhea, death
Hormones	
Betamethasone	Shock, polydipsia, polyuria
Dexamethasone	Polydipsia, polyuria, emesis, diarrhea, bloody diarrhea, melena, panting
Prednisolone	Anorexia, polyphagia, pica, anemia, lethargy, diarrhea, polyuria, elevated liver enzymes
Methylprednisolone	Disorientation, panting
Triamcinolone	Cushing's syndrome, emesis, depression, urticaria, dyspnea, seizures, shock
Estradiol cypionate	Pain at injection site, pyometra, bone marrow suppression
Megestrol acetate	Polyphagia, hydrometra, uterine inertia, uterine rupture, anorexia, depression, death
Mibolerone	Elevated liver function tests, icterus, vaginal discharge, behavioral changes, urinary incontinence
Antimicrobials	
Amoxicillin	Skin rash, emesis
Ampicillin	Wheals, injection site inflammation, emesis, diarrhea
Bacitracin-polymyxin B-neomycin (ophthalmic)	Eye irritation
Cephalexin	Panting, salivation, hyperexcitability
Chloramphenicol	Emesis, depression, ataxia, diarrhea, death
Gentamicin	Injection site inflammation, edema of lips, eyelids, and vulva; elevated BUN, acute renal failure
Hetacillin	Emesis
Lincomycin	Emesis, soft stools, diarrhea, shock after IM injection, death
Nitrofurantoin	Emesis
Potassium penicillin G	Increased respiration and heart rate

Procaine penicillin G	Ataxia, edema, dyspnea
Procaine and benzathine penicillin G	Sterile abscess, anaphylaxis
Sulfachlorpyridazine	Ataxia, hyperirritability
Sulfaguanidine	Keratoconjunctivitis
Sulfamerazine-sulfapyridine	Emesis, dyspnea
Tetracycline	Emesis
Trimethoprim-sulfadiazine	Emesis, diarrhea, anorexia, elevated liver function tests, icterus, hepatitis, bilateral keratoconjunctivitis, swelling and pain at injection site, urticaria, hives, exfoliative dermatitis, fascial swelling, hemolytic anemia, aplastic anemia, polydipsia, polyarthritis, seizures

Miscellaneous

Aminopropazine	Injection site necrosis
Aminophylline	Emesis, anorexia, polyphagia, polydipsia, polyuria, hyperexcitability
Asparaginase	Ataxia, muscle weakness, lethargy
Atropine	Paradoxical bradycardia, heart block
Calcium edetate	Emesis, diarrhea, anorexia, depression
Copper naphthenate (topical)	Skin burns
Dichlorphenamide	Disorientation
Dinoprost tromethamine	Panting, hypersalivation, discomfort, emesis
Digoxin	Emesis, anorexia
Epinephrine-pilocarpine (ophthalmic)	Conjunctivitis
Ibuprofen	Depression, emesis, gastric ulcers, death
Metrizamide	Seizures after myelogram
Neostigmine-physostigmine (ophthalmic)	Emesis, diarrhea, bradycardia, pannus
Neostigmine methylsulfate	Apnea, cardiac arrest, death
Pyridostigmine	Diarrhea, emesis
Sulfurated lime (topical)	Skin burns, edema, dehydration
Theophylline	Diarrhea

BUN, blood urea nitrogen.
From Aronson AL, Riviere JE: *In* Kirk RW, ed: Current Veterinary Therapy IX. Philadelphia, WB Saunders, 1986, pp 171–172.

Table 6-69. Adverse Drug Reactions Reported in Cats

Drug	Clinical Signs and Lesions
Analgesics	
Acetaminophen	Depression, death
Acetaminophen-codeine	Restlessness, excitement, fear, mydriasis, death
Aspirin	Depression or excitability, ataxia, nystagmus, anorexia, emesis, weight loss, hyperpnea, hepatitis, bone marrow depression, anemia, gastric lesions, death
Phenylbutazone	Inappetence, weight loss, alopecia, dehydration, emesis, severe depression, death
CNS Depressants	
Acetylpromazine	Prolonged effect, cardiac arrest, hyperactivity, convulsions, death
Ketamine, ketamine-acetylpromazine	Anoxia, apnea, hypopnea, ineffective and prolonged recovery, tremors, convulsions, excitement, hyperpyrexia, dyspnea, cardiac arrest, bladder and renal hemorrhage, nephrosis, fatty liver, lung edema, deafness, death
Halothane	Cardiac arrest, apnea, shock
Methoxyflurane	Ataxia, death
Thiamylal	Cardiac arrest, respiratory arrest, apnea, prolonged anesthesia, ataxia, shock, death
Xylazine	Prolonged anesthesia, apnea, convulsions
Proparacaine	Mydriasis
Antiparasitics	
Bunamidine	Seizures, coughing, dyspnea, pulmonary congestion, choking, lethargy, pallor, coma, hypersalivation, anorexia, fever, hypothermia, oral lesion, tongue edema, sudden death
n-Butyl chloride	Emesis
Dichlorophene-toluene	Ataxia, twitching, seizures, mydriasis, disorientation, posterior weakness, incoordination, hypersalivation, emesis, hyperpnea, tachycardia, death
Dichlorvos	Death
Glycobiarsol	Emesis, icterus, death
Levamisole	Salivation, excitement, diarrhea, mydriasis

Niclosamide	Depression, ataxia, hypothermia
Piperazine	Emesis, dementia, ataxia, hypermetria, hypersalivation
Praziquantel	Irritation at injection site, lameness, emesis, ataxia, hypothermia
Hormones	
Megestrol acetate	Polyphagia, hydrometra, uterine rupture
Triamcinolone	Nervousness, hypersalivation, disorientation, syncope
Antimicrobials	
Ampicillin	Diarrhea
Amoxicillin	Emesis
Amphotericin B	Marked elevation of BUN and serum creatinine following single dose
Cephalexin	Emesis, fever
Chloramphenicol	Anaphylactoid-type reaction, anorecia, ataxia, emesis, depression, diarrhea, neutropenia, death
Gentamicin	Pruritus, alopecia, erythema
Lincomycin	Diarrhea, emesis, collapse and coma following IM injection
Tetracycline	Malignant hyperthermia, emesis, dehydration
Tylosin	Irritation at injection site
Hexachlorophene	Anorexia, ataxia
Miconazole	Erythema, alopecia
Sulfasoxazole	Emesis
Procaine penicillin–dihydrostreptomycin	Ataxia
Trimethoprim-sulfadiazine	Emesis, hypersalivation, mydriasis, ataxia seizures
Miscellaneous	
Bethanechol	Emesis

BUN, blood urea nitrogen.
From Aronson AL, Riviere JE: Adverse drug reactions. *In* Kirk RW, ed: Current Veterinary Therapy IX. Philadelphia, WB Saunders, 1986, p 170.

6

••

EMERGENCY INFORMATION, EQUIPMENT, AND DRUGS

See Tables 6–70 and 6–71.

Table 6–70. Emergency Information, Equipment, and Drugs

General Equipment

Anesthesia machine with isoflurane
Argyle double-seal chest drainage unit
Aspirator bulbs or 50-mL syringes*
Bachus towel clamps, 4
Blankets and towels*
Blender
Blood banking equipment
  Blood bags and administration sets
  Anticoagulant
  Plasma separation press
  Refrigerator for blood products
Blood pressure monitors
  Direct pressure
  Doppler
  Oscillometric
  Neonatal blood pressure cuffs sizes 1 to 5 and manometer
Buckets
Cage padding and grates
Central venous pressure manometer, tubing, and stopcocks
Circulating water blanket
Closed-ended stomach tubes—small, medium, and large
Colon tubes—1/4-, 3/8-, and 1/2-in. OD, 5-ft rubber
Crash cart
Defibrillator
Dose syringes—30, 50, and 100 mL
ECG monitor/printer
Electronic thermometer
Endotracheal tube stylet
Endotracheal tubes (cuffed) and Cole tubes for cats; sizes from 3.0 to 15.0 mm
  ID (see Table 1–4)*
Enema can and tubing*
Esophageal stethoscope and earpiece
Face masks—small, medium, and large
Flashlight
Fleece pads—small, medium, and large; long and square
Fluid warmer—cabinet and in-line device
Foley catheters—5-, 8-, 12-, 16-, 24-, and 30F sizes
Funnels
Graduated cylinder for water measurement
Hair clippers
Heat lamp
Heimlich chest drain valve
Hot-water heating pads or blankets and controls
Instrument packs (see below)
Instrument table
Intravenous fluid stand/pole
Large-animal stomach pump

Table 6–70. Emergency Information, Equipment, and Drugs *Continued*

Laryngoscope with small, medium, and large blades
Mechanical respirator
Mouth speculum
Nasogastric tubes—12-, 16-, and 18F sizes (see also p. 537)
Nebulizer, disposable
Neonatal incubator
Ophthalmoscope/otoscope set
Oxygen enclosure–induction chamber
Oxygen tank, reducing valves, flowmeters, Ambu bag*
Peritoneal dialysis catheter (see p. 614)
Pleur-evac water trap aspiration and collection sets
Pliers—side-cutting, for removal of foreign objects
Pressure sleeve—rapid fluid administration
Pulse oximeter
Refrigerator
Scale, electronic or mechanical, including pediatric capability
Schiøtz tonometer
Stethoscope
Stomach pump—large-animal
Stomach tubes—1/4-, 3/8-, and 1/2-in. OD, clear polyethylene*
Stretcher/gurney
Suction unit—portable, Yankauer suction tip
Thermometers—clinical and electronic*
Tie-down ropes
Tracheostomy sets—small, medium, and large; metal and plastic
Vacuum cleaner
Vaginal speculum
Waste containers—plastic
Wood's lamp

General Supplies

Adhesive tape
Aero-flo tip suction catheters—5-, 8-, 12-, 14-, and 18F sizes
Alcohol
Argyle trocar catheters—8-, 10-, 16-, and 28F sizes
Bandage material
Bandage scissors
Catheter caps
Catheters, urinary—canine male and female
Catheters, urinary—feline male and female
Chest tubes—12-, 16-, 20-, 26-, 30-, and 36F sizes
Cotton-tipped applicators
Disposable gloves
Elizabethan collars
Extension tubing
Finger cots
Fluorescein stain
Gauze sponges—sizes 2×2 in. and 4×4 in.
Gauze, 1-in. roll*
Graduated burettes for small-volume infusions
Heimlich one-way valves
Hydrogen peroxide
Hypodermic needles
Intravenous catheters—various gauges*
　Over-the-needle design

Table continued on following page

Table 6–70. Emergency Information, Equipment, and Drugs *Continued*

Through-the-needle design
Wing-tip catheters
Intravenous fluids
  Lactated Ringer's solution
  0.9% NaCI
  0.45% NaCI
  Hypertonic (7%) NaCI
  2.5%, 5.0%, and 50% dextrose
  2.5% dextrose in 0.45% NaCI
Intravenous fluid administration sets
Irrigation solution
Kimwipe disposable wipes
Latex gloves (sterile)
Lubricating jelly (sterile)
Nasogastric feeding tubes
Nasal oxygen catheters
Newspaper
Nonsterile fecal cups and caps
Paper drapes (sterile)
Penrose drains
Peritoneal dialysis catheter
Plastic bags
Plastic garbage bags—small, medium, and large
Schirmer tear test strips
Specimen collecting bottles—plastic, wide-mouth, 4 oz to 1 pt*
Syringes—assorted sizes*
Thoracostomy tubes
Three-way stopcocks
Tongue depressor blades
Tracheal suction catheters
Tracheostomy tubes
Urinary catheters (Foley, Tom-Cat, male)
Urinary collection bags
Urine specimen containers
Venostomy set—regular IV*
Venostomy set—scalp vein infusion

Clinical Laboratory Equipment and Supplies

Activated clotting tubes and heating block
Blood collection tubes
Centrifuge (microhematocrit and blood tube)
Culture broth
Culture plates
Culture tubes
Fecal containers
Glucose reagent strip analyzer
Gram stain solution
Hemocytometer
Incubator
Microhematocrit tubes and clay base
Microscope
Microscope slides and covers
Quick-staining solutions
Reagent strips
  BUN
  Glucose

Table 6–70. Emergency Information, Equipment, and Drugs *Continued*

Ketones
Urine
Refractometer
Emergency Surgical Packs

Individual Packaged

Forceps
  Adson
  DeBakey cardiovascular forceps
  Large and small Forrester sponge forceps or alligator forceps
  Obstetric, clamshell
  Splinter, small 1
  Sponge, rongeur
Hemostat
  Carmalt, curved
  Kelly, curved
Needle holder, 1
Scalpel blades—assorted sizes
Scalpel handle, 1
Scissors
  Bandage
  Iris or strabismus
  Mayo
  Metzenbaum, curved
Suture material
  Maxon 00 to 6-0
  Monofilament nylon 0 to 6-0
  Polyglycolic acid (Vicryl) 0 to 4-0
  Silk on cutting needle 0 to 4-0

Tracheostomy/Thoracostomy Pack

4 drape towels
4 towel forceps
1 scalpel handle
4 mosquito forceps
2 Allis tissue forceps
1 Mayo scissors
1 Metzenbaum scissors
1 Adson forceps
1 Mayo needle holder
1 Weitlander or Gelpi self-retaining retractor
1 Finochetto rib retractor
1 Satinsky vascular forcep
  Gauze sponges
  Saline basin

Laceration Pack

4 drape towels
4 towel forceps
1 scalpel handle
4 mosquito forceps
2 Allis tissue forceps
1 Mayo scissors
1 Metzenbaum scissors
1 Adson or rat tooth forceps
1 Mayo needle holder

6

Table continued on following page

Table 6–70. Emergency Information, Equipment, and Drugs *Continued*

Ophthalmic Pack

1 Adson tissue forceps
4 Mosquito forceps
Stevens' tenotomy scissors
Stevens' tenotomy scissors—blunt tips
1 Metzenbaum scissors
Castroviejo needle holder
1 scalpel handle
Barraquer wire eyelid speculum
1 eye drape
    Gauze sponges
    Saline basin
    Sterile cotton applicators

Bandage Materials

Sterile
    4 × 4-in. sponges
    Paper drapes
    Conforming gauze—1-, 2-, 3-, and 4-in. (Kling)
    Nonadherent dressing pads (Telfa)
    Adaptic nonadherent dressing
Nonsterile
    Adhesive tape—various sizes
    Elastic tape (Elasticon)—various sizes
    Vetrap bandage 2- and 4-in.
    Gauze sponges
    Cast padding
    Conforming gauze 1-, 2-, 3-, and 4-in. (Kling)
    Cotton roll
    Stockinette
    Fiberglass or plaster case material (2- to 4-in.)
    Cast cutter and spreader
    Aluminum splint rod
    Mason Meta splints

Drugs and Solutions†

Acetic acid, 0.5%
Aminophylline, 25 mg/mL
Ammonia water, 0.2%
Antibiotics—gentamicin, ampicillin Na, cephalosporins
Apomorphine*
Atropine sulfate—-parenteral, 0.4 mg/mL*
Bretylium (Bretylol)
Calcium borogluconate*
Calcium gluconate—parenteral, 10%
Charcoal, activated*
Chlorpromazine hydrochloride, 25 mg/mL
Cimetidine or ranitidine
Copper sulfate, 0.2 to 0.4% solution*
Desoxycorticosterone
Dexamethasone sodium phosphate, 2 and 4 mg/mL
Dextran solution (regular and low-molecular-weight)
Dextrose in water, 5% and 50% solution
Diazepam (Valium), 5 mg/mL*
Digoxin

Table 6–70. Emergency Information, Equipment, and Drugs *Continued*

Dimercaprol (BAL)*
Diphenhydramine hydrochloride (Benadryl)—parenteral, 10 mg/mL
Dipyrone (Novin), 500 mg/mL
Doxapram hydrochloride, 20 mg/mL
Edetic acid (EDTA)
Calcium disodium EDTA in 5% dextrose*
Epinephrine hydrochloride—1:10,000, 0.1 mg/mL; 1:1000, 1.0 mg/mL
Ethanol, 50%*
Furosemide (Lasix)
Heparin, parenteral
Hetastarch (Hespan), colloidal replacement solution
Hydrocortisone sodium succinate, ampules
Hydrogen peroxide, 3%
Hypertonic saline—7% solution or 23% ampules
Isoproterenol
Ketamine hydrochloride
Levallorphan
Lidocaine hydrochloride, 2% (20 mg/mL) without epinephrine
Lidocaine hydrochloride, 10% topical spray
Magnesium sulfate, 20 solution*
Mannitol ampules, 30%
Meperidine hydrochloride (Demerol)
Metaraminol bitartrate (Aramine), parenteral
Methcarbamol (Robaxin)*
Methylprednisolone
Milk of magnesia*
Mineral oil*
Morphine hydrochloride
Naloxone (Narcan), 0.4 mg/mL*
Nicotinamide (nicotinic acid, niacin)*
Norepinephrine
Olive oil emollient
Ouabain
Oxymorphone
Oxytocin (Pitocin)
D-Penicillamine*
Pentobarbital sodium, parenteral*
Phenobarbital sodium, parenteral, 130 mg/mL
Phenylephrine hydrochloride, parenteral
Potassium chloride, 2 mEq/mL*
Pralidoxime chloride (2-PAM)*
Prednisolone—prednisolone sodium succinate, 100 mg/10-mL vial
Procainamide hydrochloride (Pronestyl)
Propranolol (Inderal)*
Prussian blue*
Quinidine gluconate, 80 mg/mL
Ringer's lactate and 1/2 strength Ringer's lactate with 2.5% dextrose
    solution*
Sodium bicarbonate*
Sodium chloride, 0.9%
Sodium ferrocyanide*
Sodium nitroprusside dihydrate, 10 mg/mL
Sodium sulfate, 20% solution and salt*
Syrup of ipecac*
Tannic acid*

6

Table continued on following page

Table 6–70. Emergency Information, Equipment, and Drugs *Continued*

Thiamylal (Biotal, Surital) or thiopental (Pentothal) sodium, 2.5% solution
Vitamin K₁ (AquaMEPHYTON injection)*
Yohimbine

OD, outside diameter; ECG, electrocardiogram; ID, internal diameter; IV, intravenous;
BUN, blood urea nitrogen.
*Drugs and equipment useful in poisonings.
†See also Cardiovascular Emergency Drugs and Equipment, p. 61.

Table 6–71. Tube Sizes for Toxicologic Procedures

Weight of Animal	Endotracheal Tubes*	Stomach Tubes†	Colon Tubes‡
2 kg	3.0–4.5 mm	1/8–1/4-in. OD	1/8-in. OD
2–5 kg	3.5–6.0 mm	1/4-in. OD	1/4-in. OD
5–10 kg	5.0–7.5 mm	3/8-in. OD	3/8-in. OD
10–20 kg	7.5–11.0 mm	1/2-in. OD	3/8-in. OD
20–30 kg	8.5–15.0 mm	5/8-in. OD	1/2-in. OD

OD, outside diameter.
* Cuffed endotracheal tubes are recommended. The size is based on internal diameter.
† Clear polyethylene tubing or rubber is satisfactory.
‡ Soft rubber tubes are recommended.
From Aronson AL: Emergency and general treatment of poisonings. *In* Kirk RW, ed:
Current Veterinary Therapy V. Philadelphia, WB Saunders, 1974.

COMMON DRUGS: APPROXIMATE DOSAGES
See Table 6–72.

Table 6-72. Common Drugs: Approximate Doses

Drug Name	Dog	Cat
Acepromazine	0.55–2.2 mg/kg PO 0.025–0.200 mg/kg IV 0.10–0.25 mg/kg IM, PO	1.1–2.2 mg/kg PO 0.05–0.10 mg/kg IV, IM, SC (max 1 mg)
Acetazolamide	10 mg/kg q.i.d. PO	50 mg/kg once IV 7 mg/kg t.i.d. PO
Aluminum hydroxide	30–90 mg/kg once to three times daily PO	30–90 mg/kg/day PO
Amikacin	2–10 mL q2–4h PO 5 mg/kg t.i.d. IM, IV, SC	Same
Amitraz	10.6 mL in 2 gal water; dip every 2 wk for 3–6 wk	0.0125% applied topically weekly
Amitriptyline	2.2–4.4 mg/kg once daily PO 1–6 mg/kg once or twice daily PO	5–10 mg once daily PO 0.5–1.0 mg/kg/day PO 5–10 mg/cat PO once daily
Ammonium chloride	200 mg/kg divided t.i.d. PO	1.1 mg/kg PO b.i.d.
Amoxicillin-Clavulanate	13.75 mg/kg b.i.d. PO	20 mg/kg b.i.d. PO
Carprofen	1 mg/lb b.i.d., dogs only	62.5 mg b.i.d. PO
Cephadrine	20–40 mg/kg PO, IV, IM	Same
Cephalothin	20–35 mg/kg PO, IV, IM	Same
Chlorpropramide	10–40 mg/kg PO once daily	Unknown
Cisapride	0.1–0.5 mg/kg b.i.d.–t.i.d. PO	Same
Clemastine	0.05–0.1 mg/kg b.i.d. PO	0.68 mg b.i.d. PO
Clonazepam	1–10 mg once to four times daily PO	0.016 mg/kg once to four times daily PO
Clorazepate	1.5 mg/kg divided t.i.d. PO 2 mg/kg b.i.d. PO; 0.55–2.2 mg/kg once or twice daily PO	Same
Cyclosporine	20 mg/kg once daily PO	10 mg/kg b.i.d. PO or 8–10 mg/kg/day PO
Cythioate	3.3 mg/kg PO every 3rd day or twice weekly	Same
Dantrolene	3–15 mg b.i.d.–t.i.d. PO 1–5 mg/kg b.i.d. PO	Same 0.5–2.0 mg/kg t.i.d. PO

Table continued on following page

6

955

Table 6–72. Common Drugs: Approximate Doses *Continued*

Drug Name	Dog	Cat
Dextran 40 and 70	10–20 mL/kg/day IV, then 10 mL/kg/day	Same
Dextromethorphan	2–5 mL/kg/hr IV infusion	
Dimethyl sulfoxide	2 mg/kg t.i.d.–q.i.d. PO	2 mg/kg q.i.d. PO, SC, IV
	Apply topically t.i.d.–q.i.d.; 1 g/kg IV slowly over 45 min for CNS edema	None
Diphenoxylate	2.5–10 mg q.i.d. PO	0.6–1.2 mg b.i.d.–t.i.d. PO
Docusate calcium	50–100 mg once or twice daily PO	50 mg once or twice daily PO
Enalapril	0.5 mg/kg once to twice daily PO	0.25–0.5 mg/kg once or twice daily PO
Espirantel	5.5 mg/kg once daily PO	2.75 mg/kg once daily PO
Erythropoietin	100 µg 3 times weekly SC until PCV in normal range, then decrease dose to twice weekly	Same
Ethacrynic acid	0.2–0.4 mg/kg q4–12h IM, IV	Same
Etodolac	10–15 mg/kg PO once daily for dogs	Unknown
Etretinate	1 mg/kg PO once daily	None
Fentanyl-droperidol (Innovar-Vet)	0.3–0.5 mL/55 kg IV (tranquilization); 1 mL/20 kg IM (preanesthetic)	
Fluconazole	2.5–5 mg/kg divided b.i.d. with food	50 mg/kg b.i.d. PO (cryptococcosis)
Flunixin meglumine		0.25 mg/kg once daily SC; can be repeated in 12–24 hr
Fluoxetine		1 mg/kg/day
Fomepizole	20 mg/kg IV loading dose; then 15 mg/kg at 12 hr, 15 mg/kg at 24 hr, 5 mg/kg at 36 hr; then 5 mg/kg b.i.d. prm	
Glipizide	0.25–0.5 mg/kg b.i.d. PO	Same or 2.5–5.0 mg b.i.d.–t.i.d. PO
Glycopyrrolate	0.005–0.010 mg/kg IV or 0.01–0.02 mg/kg SC, IM	Same
Gonadorelin	50–100 µg SC, IV	25 µg; IM after mating (stimulate ovulation)
Granulocyte colony-stimulating factor	5 µg/kg once daily SC	Same

Drug	Dog	Cat
Guaifenesin	44–88 mg/kg IV or 33–88 mg/kg IV with 1.1 mg/kg ketamine (restraint)	None
Hetatarch	20 mL/kg/day IV, then 10 ml/kg/day IV or	
Hydrocodone	0.22 mg/kg b.i.d.–t.i.d. PO	2.5–5.0 mg b.i.d.–t.i.d. PO (with caution)
Imipenem-cilastatin	2–5 mg/kg t.i.d. IV	Same
Imipramine	0.5–1.0 mg/kg t.i.d. PO	2.5–5.0 mg b.i.d. PO
Ipecac (syrup)	5–15 mL PO or 3–6 mL PO	Same
Isoproterenol	15–30 mg q4h PO	Same
	0.1–0.2 mg q.i.d. IM, SC	Same
	1 mg in 250 mL D5W at 0.01 µg/kg/min IV	0.5 mg in 250 mL D5W IV to effect
Isotretinoin	1–3 mg/kg/day PO	Same
Itraconazole	2–5 mg/kg b.i.d.; 5 mg/kg once daily PO	10 mg/kg/day PO or 50 mg/day cats <3.2 kg
	5 mg/kg b.i.d. PO for 60 days (blastomycosis)	≥2 mo beyond clinical remission (cryptococcosis)
Ketamine HCl	5.5–22 mg/kg IV, IM	11 mg/kg IM (restraint)
		2–25 mg/kg IM: 2.0–4.4 mg/kg IV (anesthesia)
Ketoprofen	2 mg/kg IM, IV, SC on day 1, then continue 1 mg/kg once daily PO for 4 days	Same
	2 mg/kg initially PO, then 1 mg/kg/day (chronic pain)	
Ketorolac	0.5 mg/kg t.i.d. up to 48 hr IM or slowly IV, dose can be increased to 0.75 mg/kg if pain persists	Same
	0.3–0.5 mg/kg b.i.d.–t.i.d. IV, IM for 1–2 treatments (surgical pain)	
Levothyroxine (T$_4$)	22 µg/kg b.i.d. PO or 0.02 mg/kg b.i.d.	20 to 30 µg/kg/day PO, or 0.1–0.3 mg/day PO
Loperamide	0.08 mg/kg t.i.d. PO	0.1–0.3 mg/kg once to twice daily (caution)
Meclofenamic acid	1.1 mg/kg/day PO for 5–7 days	No indication

Table continued on following apge

Table 6–72. Common Drugs: Approximate Doses *Continued*

Drug Name	Dog	Cat
Medroxyprogesterone acetate	20 mg/kg once IM; repeat in 3–6 mo if needed; 10 mg/kg prn, IM, SC (behavioral problems)	50–100 mg once IM repeat in 3–6 mo if needed; 10–20 mg/kg prn, SC (behavioral problems)
Melarsomine HCl	2.5 mg/kg IM twice; 24 hr apart via deep lumbar injection	None
Metamucil	2–10 g once or twice daily	2–4 g once or twice daily
Methylphenidate HCl	5–10 mg b.i.d.–t.i.d. PO (narcolepsy)	None
Medetomidine HCl	2–4 mg/kg prn, PO (narcolepsy) 750 µg IV or 1000 µg IM/m² (dogs only)	Same
Methylene blue	8.8 mg/kg (1% solution) slowly IV; repeat prn 100–300 mg/day PO (methemoglobinemia)	Same
Methytestosterone	1–2 mg/kg once daily PO	Same
Midazolam	0.066–0.22 mg/kg IM, IV	Same
Milbemycin oxine	Up to 4.5 kg, 2.3 mg q30d 5–11 kg, 5.75 mg q30d 12–22 kg, 11.5 mg q30d 23–45 kg, 23 mg q30d	None
Minocycline	5–15 mg/kg b.i.d. PO	Same
Misoprostol	2–5 µg/kg b.i.d.–t.i.d. PO	Non indication
Nandrolone decanoate	1–5 mg/kg/wk IM	10–20 mg/wk IM
Nitroglycerin	0.25–1.0 in. t.i.d.–q.i.d. topically 0.125–0.25 in. t.i.d.–q.i.d.	
Nitroprusside	1–10 µg/kg/min IV	Same
Nitroscante	50 mg/kg; PO	Same
Omeprazole	0.7 mg/kg once daily PO >20 kg, 1 cap daily PO	Same
Orbifloxacin	2.5 mg/kg once daily PO; dose may be increased to 7.5 mg/kg if needed	Same
Oxitriptyline	14 mg/kg t.i.d.–q.i.d. PO	6 mg/kg b.i.d.–t.i.d. PO

Drug	Dog	Cat
Oxymorphone	0.05–0.1 mg/kg IV or 0.1–0.2 mg/kg IM SC	0.02 mg/kg IV (caution)
Paregoric	0.05–0.06 mg/kg b.i.d.–t.i.d. PO	Same (caution)
Pentastarch (10%)	10–20 mL/kg/day over 1–24 hr as indicated for up to 3 days	5–10 mL/kg/day over 1–24 hr as indicated for up to 3 days
Pentosan polysulfate	3 mg/kg (1 mL/33 kg) SC every 5 to 7 days for 4 treatments	None
Phenobarbital	2–8 mg/kg PO q12h	1–2 mg/kg PO IM, IV
	10–30 mg/kg IV	25 mg/kg IV
Phenytoin	15–40 mg/kg t.i.d. PO; 2–4 mg/kg up to 10 mgkg total dose IV for arrhythmias	No indication
Plicamycin	25 µg/kg IV (hypercalcemia)	Unknown
Piroxicam	0.3 mg/kg q.48h. PO	No indication
Potassium citrate	100–150 mg/kg/day PO	No indication
Potassium gluconate	2.2 mEq/100 kcal of energy/day PO	5–8 mEq PO 1 to 2 times daily
Potassium iodide	40 mg/kg t.i.d. PO	20 mg/kg b.i.d. PO (with food); 30–100 mg/cat daily for 10–14 days
Potassium phosphate	0.01–0.03 mM/kg/hr	Same
Prednisolone and prednisone	0.2–0.4 mg/kg once to four times daily PO (hypoadrenocortical maintenance); 0.5 mg/kg b.i.d. PO, IM (allergy); 2–4 mg/kg/day PO, IM (immunosuppression)	Same
Primidone	11–22 mg/kg t.i.d. PO	Same
Prochlorperazine	0.13 mg/kg IM or 0.1–0.5 mg/kg t.i.d.–q.i.d. IM, SC	Same
Propofol	4 mg/kg IV with premedication; 6.5 mg/kg without premedication	6 mg/kg IV with premedication; 8 mg/kg IV without premedication
Prostaglandin $F_{2\alpha}$	0.25 mg/kg once daily SC for 5 days (pyometra)	0.1–0.25 mg/kg SC once to twice daily for 3–5 days (pyometra)
Protamine sulfate	1 mg for every 100 IU heparin used over 60 min	Same

Table continued on following page

6

Table 6–72. Common Drugs: Approximate Doses *Continued*

Drug Name	Dog	Cat
Pseudoephedrine	15–30 mg b.i.d.–t.i.d. PO (urinary incontinence)	Unknown
Rifampin	10–20 mg/kg b.i.d. PO	Same
Selegiline	1–2 mg/kg day PO (pituitary-dependent hyperadrenocorticism)	Unknown
Sodium iodide	20–40 mg/kg b.i.d.–t.i.d. PO for 4–6 wk	20 mg/kg/day for PO 4–6 wk
Sodium polystyrene sulfonate	8–15 g t.i.d. PO	No indication
Spironolactone	1–2 mg/kg b.i.d. PO	Same
Sucralfate	0.5–1.0 g b.i.d.–t.i.d. PO	0.25 g b.i.d.–t.i.d. PO
Sulfadimethoxine ormetoprim	55 mg/kg/day, then 27.5 mg/kg once daily for max of 21 days	None
Sulfasalazine	10–30 mg/kg b.i.d.–t.i.d. PO	20 mg/kg b.i.d. PO
Terbutaline	2.5 mg/dog t.i.d. PO, SC	1.25 mg b.i.d. PO; 0.625 mg b.i.d. PO, SC
Thiamine (vitamin B_1)	1–2 mg/kg IM	Same
	2 mg/kg once daily PO	4 mg/kg once daily PO
Thiopental sodium	25–30 mg/kg IV to effect; 11 mg/kg after narcotic sedation	Same
Ticarcillin	40–75 mg/kg t.i.d.–q.i.d. IM, IV	Same
Ticarcillin-clavulanate	30–50 mg/kg t.i.d.–q.i.d. IV	Same
Tiletamine-zolazepam	9.9–13.2 mg/kg IM	9.7–11.9 mg/kg IM
	6.6–9.9 mg/kg IM	10.6–12.5 mg/kg IM
	6–13 mg/kg IM	Same
Tobramycin	1 mg/kg t.i.d. IM, IV, SC	2 mg/kg t.i.d. SC
Tocainide	10–20 mg/kg t.i.d. PO	No indication
Triamcinolone	0.05 mg/kg b.i.d.–t.i.d. PO	0.25–0.5 mg/kg once daily
Trimeprazine	1.1–4.4 mg/kg q.i.d. PO	Same
Valproic acid	75–200 mg/kg t.i.d. PO	No indication
Warfarin	0.1 mg/kg once daily PO	0.1–0.2 mg/kg once daily PO
Zinc acetate	5–10 mg/kg b.i.d. PO	No indication
Zinc sulfate	220 mg once or twice daily PO	No indication

PCV, packed cell volume.

HOTLINES
See Table 6–73.

Table 6–73. Hotlines Every Veterinarian Should Know

USP Veterinary Practitioners' Reporting Program	800-487-7776	Veterinary product failure and adverse reaction reporting; to report to the USP or request reporting forms for product quality problems, medication mishaps, and adverse reactions regarding drugs, biologics, chemicals, pesticides, medical devices, and other products used for companion, food, zoo, and exotic animals
FDA/CVM drugs, devices, animal feeds	888-FDA-VETS (888-322-8387)	For health professionals to report adverse events, particularly with drugs
FDA Medical Advertising Line	800-AD-US-FDA (800-238-7332)	Assists health professionals seeking interpretive information on FDA policy
USDA veterinary biologics and diagnostics	800-752-6255	A 24-hour hotline to report adverse reactions involving veterinary diagnostic and biologic products; weekdays 7:30 A.M. to 4 P.M. CT; message service available other hours
USDA meat and poultry	800-535-4555	
USDA Voice Response Service	800-545-8732	Up-to-date interstate shipping regulations, emergency notices, and animal care regulations for shipping pets on airlines; available 24 hours a day, including weekends and holidays
EPA National Pesticide Telecommunications Network	800-858-7378	Toll-free telephone service by pesticide information
DEA Office of Diversion Control, Registration Section	800-882-9539	A registration assistant is available from 8:30 A.M. to 5 P.M. ET, or leave a voice-mail message to request registration and order forms
National Animal Poison Control Center	800-548-2423	Fee $30 per case unless covered by a sponsoring company; credit cards only; with the 800 access only, follow-up calls are included
	900-680-0000	Fee $20 for first 5 minutes, $2.95 for each additional minute ($20 minimum); if product is covered by a sponsoring company, call will be switched to the 800 line and no fee charged
Impaired Veterinarians Information	800-321-1473	Information on chemical impairment with referrals by assistance; sponsored by the AVMA
Pet Loss Support (grief counseling)	916-752-4200	Staffed by University of California, Davis veterinary students; weekdays, 6:30 P.M. to 9:30 P.M., PT
	904-392-4700, then dial 1 and 4080	Staffed by University of Florida veterinary students; weekdays, 7 P.M. to 9 P.M., ET
	517-432-2696	Staffed by Michigan State University veterinary students; Tuesday through Thursday, 6:30 P.M. to 9:30 P.M., ET

Organization	Phone	Description
	708-603-3994	Staffed by Chicago VMA veterinarians and trained volunteers; leave voice-mail message; calls will be returned 7 P.M. to 9 P.M. CT (long-distance calls will be returned collect)
	540-231-8038	Staffed by Virginia-Maryland Regional College of Veterinary Medicine; Tuesday, Thursday, 6 P.M. to 9 P.M., ET
	614-292-1823	Staffed by the Ohio State University veterinary students; Monday, Wednesday, Friday, 6:30 P.M. to 9:30 P.M., ET (voice-mail messages will be returned, collect, during operating hours)
	508-839-7966	Staffed by Tufts University veterinary students; Tuesday, Thursday, 6 P.M. to 9 P.M., ET (voice-mail messages will be returned daily, collect outside Massachusetts)
Food Animal Residue Avoidance Data Bank	888-USFARAD (888-873-2723)	Sponsored by the USDA Extension Service; information on animal drugs and chemicals with the potential to cause foodborne residues; regional access centers reached by this new toll-free number are located at the University of California, Davis and North Carolina State University
Dr. Louis J. Camuti Memorial Feline Consultation and Diagnostic Service	800-KITTY-DR (800-548-8937)	Sponsored by the Cornell Feline Health Center, a source of information on feline diseases and management; Monday, Wednesday, Friday, 9 A.M. to noon and 2 P.M. to 4 P.M., ET; fee $25 per call, $20 for members of the center
Healthline	606-224-2849	A referral service limited to veterinarians; will direct practitioners to other veterinarians with experience in equine health areas for free phone consultation; co-sponsored by the AAEP and Grayson-Jockey Club Foundation
HEMOPET	714-252-8455	A national, full-service, nonprofit blood bank and educational network for animals, in Irvine, Calif.; accessible 24 hr
Animal Blood Bank	800-243-5759	A 24-hr hotline that focuses on transfusion medicine (particularly blood component therapy), recommending dosages and infusion rates, at no cost to caller
Eastern Veterinary Blood Bank	800-949-EVBB (800-949-3822)	A 24-hr commercial blood bank that focuses on transfusion medicine; gives recommendations and referrals to distribution centers when it cannot ship the requested product; for complicated cases, offers a paid consultation service; available to callers nationwide except California and Oregon

USP, United States Pharmacopeia; FDA/CVM, Food and Drug Administration/Center for Veterinary Medicine; USDA, U.S. Department of Agriculture; CT, Central Time; EPA, Environmental Protection Agency; DEA, Drug Enforcement Administration; ET, Eastern Time; PT, Pacific Time; AAEP, American Association of Equine Practitioners. Adapted from the J AM Vet Med Assoc © 1996. Provided as a service of the USP Veterinary Practitioners' Reporting Program.

6

INDEX

Note: Page numbers in *italics* refer to figures; page numbers followed by t refer to tables; page numbers followed by b refer to text in boxes.

A

A CRASH PLAN, as examination mnemonic, 3–6
Abdomen, acute, 15–22
  auscultation of, 281
  enlargement of, associated signs in, 384
    differential diagnosis of, 386t
  insufflation of, 525
  palpation of, 280
    in cardiovascular examination, 285–286
    in urinary tract evaluation, 381
  percussion of, 281
  skin lesions on, 378t
Abdominal cavity, hemorrhage in, from neoplasms, 171
Abdominal effusion, in feline infectious peritonitis, 685
Abdominal paracentesis, 452–453, *453*
Abdominal radiography, in acute abdomen, 18
Abdominal trauma, blunt, 16
  penetrating, 15–16
    and bowel perforation, 115
Abdominal ultrasonography, in acute abdomen, 18
Abdominocentesis, 18–19
Abducens nerve, evaluation of, 343t
Aberdeen terrier, inherited disorders in, 824t
Abortion, 137–138
Abrasion, corneal, 91
Abrupt water deprivation test, 781, 784
Abscess, of teeth, 277
  retrobulbar, 315
Abyssinian cat, inherited disorders in, 824t
Acanthocyte(s), 654
ACE inhibitor(s). See *Angiotensin-converting enzyme (ACE) inhibitor(s).*
Acepromazine, dosage of, 955t
  for hypertension, 77t, 78
Acetaminophen, adverse reactions to, in cat, 946t

Acetaminophen *(Continued)*
  toxicity of, 207t
Acetate tape test, for skin disease, 493
Acetazolamide, dosage of, 955t
Acetylpromazine, adverse reactions to, in cat, 946t
  in dog, 942t
Acid(s), toxicity of, 194t
Acid-base balance, 591–595, 593t, *595*
  compensatory responses in, 593, 593t
  interpretation of, 592–593
  laboratory values in, 593t
  studies of, laboratory sample requirement for, 859t
Acidosis, from blood component therapy, 576t
  in thermal burns, 27
  metabolic. See *Metabolic acidosis.*
  respiratory. See *Respiratory acidosis.*
Acidurin. See *Ammonium chloride.*
Acinetobacter, antibiotic sensitivity of, 893t
Acromegaly, 637
ACT (activated coagulation time), 688, 689t, 690
ACTH. See *Adrenocorticotropic hormone (ACTH).*
Actinomyces infection(s), antibiotics for, 899t
Actinomycin D, 930t
Activated charcoal, dosage of, 212t
  for poisoning, 226–227
Activated clotting time, 47–48, 48t
Activated coagulation time (ACT), 688, 689t, 690
Activated partial thromboplastin time (APTT), 689t, 690–691
Acute abdomen, 15–22
  with known trauma, 16–22
    diagnosis of, 18
    differential diagnosis of, 17–18
    history in, 16
    physical examination in, 16–17
Acute intrinsic renal failure (AIRF), 124–125, 126t

965

Bird, antibiotic dosage for, 901t–902t

Bisacodyl, toxicity of, 207t

Bismuth subsalicylate (Pepto-Bismol), toxicity of, 207t

Bitch, breeding in, 327–328
  infections and, 326
  insemination of, 463, 465

Bite(s), snake, 230–234. See also *Snake bite(s)*.

Biventricular enlargement, diagnosis of, electrocardiography in, 302
  radiography in, 308

Black widow spider(s), bites from, 235

Bladder, calculi in, radiopacity of, 532t
  chemotherapy and, 183
  manual expression of, 773

Bladder function, evaluation of, in neurologic examination, 340–341

Blastomyces dermatitidis, antibiotic sensitivity of, 893t

Blastomycosis, diagnosis of, 749t

Bleach, toxicity of, 195t–196t

Bleeding, anemia from, 656–657
  continuing, 19
  external, control of, 3
  in neoplastic syndromes, 170–173
  intraocular, and visual loss, 445b
  minor, bandaging of wounds with, 555–557
  retinal, from trauma to globe, 93
  spontaneous, 437–441, 440t
    associated signs in, 439
    definition of, 437, 439
    diagnosis of, 439–441
    differential diagnosis of, 440t
  subconjunctival, 89–90

Bleeding disorder(s), 46–54. See also specific disorder(s).
  classification of, 687
  clinical features of, 47t
  diagnosis of, 46–49, 47t–48t
    history in, 46
    laboratory studies in, 47–48, 48t
    physical examination in, 46–47
  differential diagnosis of, 48t
  etiology of, 691b–692b
  evaluation of, activated coagulation time in, 688, 689t, 690
    handling of blood samples in, 687–688, 688b
    initial in-office, 688

Bleeding disorder(s) *(Continued)*
  from monoclonal gammopathy, 696
  from vitamin K deficiency, 696–697
  in liver disease, 742
  primary, 693–697, 694b
    etiology of, 691b
  secondary, etiology of, 691b–692b
  treatment of, 49–50

Bleeding time, 689t, 888t

Bleomycin (Blenoxane), 930t

Blindness. See *Visual loss.*

Blood, ammonia levels in, 719–720
  in urine, 777
  parasitic infections of, 697–701
  pH of, maintenance of, 591–592
  whole, activated coagulation time of, 688, 689t, 690
    transfusion of, 596–597

Blood banks, 580

Blood chemistries, 718–733. See also specific study.

Blood collection, 453–460, 454t, *458–460*
  arterial, 460
  for clinical chemistry procedures, 456–457
  for hematology studies, 456
  in bleeding disorders, 687–688, 688b
  prevention of hemolysis after, 455
  restraint for, 454
  skin preparation for, 454
  tubes for, 454t
  Vacutainer for, 455

Blood component therapy, 571–582
  complications of, 576t
  crossmatching before, 572
  in cat, 578–579
  in dog, 579–581
  preparation of component for, 572
  principles of, 571b–572b
  prior transfusion history and, 572
  storage of component for, 575t, 580
  with fresh frozen plasma, 574–575
  with red cells, 572–574, 573t–577t
  with simultaneous fluid therapy, 572

Blood culture(s), 467, 469t, 470
  recommendations for, 469t

Blood donor, selection of, 579–580

Blood film(s), 456

Blood gas(es), arterial. See *Arterial blood gas(es).*

ISBN 0-7216-7166-7

90071